Plant Natural Products for Human Health

Plant Natural Products for Human Health

Special Issue Editors

Chun-Tao Che

Hongjie Zhang

MDPI • Basel • Beijing • Wuhan • Barcelona • Belgrade

Special Issue Editors

Chun-Tao Che	Hongjie Zhang
University of Illinois at Chicago	Hong Kong Baptist University
USA	China

Editorial Office
MDPI
St. Alban-Anlage 66
4052 Basel, Switzerland

This is a reprint of articles from the Special Issue published online in the open access journal *International Journal of Molecular Sciences* (ISSN 1422-0067) from 2018 to 2019 (available at: https://www.mdpi.com/journal/ijms/special_issues/plant_natural_products_human_health)

For citation purposes, cite each article independently as indicated on the article page online and as indicated below:

LastName, A.A.; LastName, B.B.; LastName, C.C. Article Title. *Journal Name* **Year**, *Article Number*, Page Range.

ISBN 978-3-03897-712-4 (Pbk)
ISBN 978-3-03897-713-1 (PDF)

Contents

About the Special Issue Editors

Chun-Tao Che is the Harry H.S. Fong Professor of Pharmacognosy at the Department of Medicinal Chemistry and Pharmacognosy, College of Pharmacy, University of Illinois at Chicago (UIC). He is also the Director of the World Health Organization Collaborating Centre for Traditional Medicine at UIC. In 2000–2010, he served as a professor and Director of the School of Chinese Medicine at the Chinese University of Hong Kong. His main research interest is in natural products chemistry, including the discovery of biologically active substances from medicinal herbs, as well as establishing quality standards for herbal drugs and botanical products. He has published over 300 scientific research papers in the areas of pharmacognosy, natural products, and Chinese medicines, and he holds editorial positions in over ten journals.

Hongjie Zhang graduated from Yunnan University with a Bachelor's degree of Chemistry, and obtained his Master and Ph.D. degrees in Phytochemistry at the Kunming Institute of Botany (KIB), the Chinese Academy of Sciences. He was a faculty member (Assistant/Associate/Full Professor) at KIB from 1991 to 2002, and a research faculty member (Research Assistant/Research Associate Professor) in the College of Pharmacy, the University of Illinois at Chicago (UIC) in 2003–2011. He is currently a professor at the School of Chinese Medicine, the Hong Kong Baptist University. Dr. Zhang has more than 30 years of research experience in the isolation, identification, structure elucidation, analysis, synthesis, and biological evaluation of natural products and other small molecules, leading to publication of more than 140 peer reviewed papers and a number of granted patents. His current research interest is in natural products drug discovery from natural resources. Specifically, Dr. Zhang is interested in finding natural lead compounds from plants against different disease targets, such as cancer, HIV, bird flu, Ebola/Marburg, and cancer chemoprevention.

International Journal of *Molecular Sciences*

MDPI

Editorial

Plant Natural Products for Human Health

Chun-Tao Che [1,*] and Hongjie Zhang [2]

1 Department of Medicinal Chemistry and Pharmacognosy, and the World Health Organization Collaborating Center for Traditional Medicine, College of Pharmacy, University of Illinois at Chicago, Chicago, IL 60612, USA

2 School of Chinese Medicine, Hong Kong Baptist University, Kowloon, Hong Kong, China; zhanghj@hkbu.edu.hk

* Correspondence: chect@uic.edu; Tel.: +1 (312) 996-5234; Fax: +1 (312) 996-7107

Received: 6 February 2019; Accepted: 8 February 2019; Published: 15 February 2019

Abstract: The aim of this Special Issue on "Plant Natural Products for Human Health" is to compile a series of scientific reports to demonstrate the medicinal potential of plant natural products, such as in vitro and in vivo activities, clinical effects, mechanisms of action, structure-activity relationships, and pharmacokinetic properties. With the global trend growing in popularity for botanical dietary supplements and phytopharmaceuticals, it is hoped that this Special Issue would serve as a timely reference for researchers and scholars who are interested in the discovery of potentially useful molecules from plant sources for health-related applications.

Keywords: plant natural product; drug discovery; human health

---

Plants have served mankind as an important source of foods and medicines. While we all consume plants and their products for nutritional support, a majority of the world population also rely on botanical remedies to meet their health needs, either as their own "traditional medicine" or as "complementary and alternative medicine" [1,2]. Today we are witnessing a global resurgence in interest and use of plant-based therapies and botanical healthcare products. For example, herbal supplement sales in the U.S. increased 8.5% (compared to the previous year), reaching an estimated total of 8 billion USD in 2017 [3]. The increased interest in herbal medicine and products by the general public has stimulated a greater scientific awareness in exploring and understanding the pharmacologically active constituents of medicinal plants.

From the pharmaceutical point of view, many compounds obtained from plant sources have long been known to possess bio/pharmacological activities, and historically plants have yielded many important drugs for human use, from morphine discovered in the early nineteenth century to the more recent paclitaxel and artemisinin. Although most mega pharmaceutical companies are not focusing on developing natural drugs at this time, natural products remain an important and viable source of lead compounds in many drug discovery programs. After all, development of natural products for the prevention and treatment of diseases continue to attract worldwide attention.

This Special Issue on "Plant Natural Products for Human Health" is intended to be a compilation of scientific reports to cover different aspects of biologically active plant natural products, such as chemical characterization, in vitro and in vivo activities, clinical effects, mechanism of action, structure-activity relationship, and pharmacokinetic/pharmacodynamic properties. With the global trend growing in popularity for botanical dietary supplements and plant-based drugs, it is our hope that this Special Issue would serve as a reference for researchers and scholars who are interested in the discovery of potentially useful molecules from plant sources for health-related applications.

We were overwhelmed to receive many high-quality manuscripts from all over the world. A total of 26 articles have been published in this Special Issue in 2018, covering a wide range of disease targets such as diabetes, inflammation, cancer, neurological disease, cardiovascular disease, liver damage, bacterial and fungus infection and malarial. They provide important insights into the current state of research on drug discovery and new techniques in the following areas of plant natural products.

In the diabetes area, Kang et al. reported that the Amadori rearrangement compounds obtained from heat-processed onion extract were able to suppress carbohydrate absorption through inhibition of intestinal sucrose, thereby reducing the postprandial increase of blood glucose [4]. On the other hand, Nagappan et al. reported the in vitro protective activity of gomisin N (obtained from *Schisandra chinensis*) against cannabinoid type-1 receptor-induced impairment of insulin signaling, as well as the in vivo effect of the compound on gluconeogenesis in high-fat-diet-induced-obese mice [5].

The neurological effects of natural products are demonstrated in three reports. Thus, Li et al. described the neuroprotective activity of phenylethanoid glycosides such as salidroside, acteoside, isoacteoside, and echinacoside, which were found to interfere with the Nrf2 binding site in Keap1 protein in the adrenal phaeochromocytoma PC12 cells [6]. Gugliandolo et al. reported the anti-inflammatory and anti-oxidant effects of cannabigerol (obtained from *Cannabis sativa*) on NSC-34 motor neurons, as demonstrated by a reduction in the IL-1β, TNF-α, IFN-γ and PPARγ protein levels [7]. Furthermore, Tang et al. demonstrated that catechin and procyanidin A2 (obtained from lychee seed) were able to suppress neuroinflammation in amyloid-β-treated microglial BV-2 cells [8].

Asperuloside and asperulosidic acid were reported by He et al. to possess anti-inflammatory activity in lipopolysaccharide-treated RAW 264.7 macrophages through suppression of the NF-κB and MAPK signaling pathways [9]. A glucan fraction prepared from the stalk of *Pleurotus eryngii* mushroom was also shown by Vetvicka et al. to suppress inflammation in a dextran sulfate sodium-induced mouse model of inflammatory bowel disease. The glucan fraction displayed downregulation effects on IFN-γ and MIP-2 levels [10].

In cancer studies, the potential of hinokitiol in lung cancer chemoprevention was described by Jayakumar et al. The compound was shown to inhibit the migration of lung adenocarcinoma A549 cells through several pathways, such as activation of capases-3 and -9, induction of p53/Bax and the antioxidant enzymes CAT and SOD, as well as reduction of MMP-2 and -9 activities [11]. In another study, Zheng et al. demonstrated that the flavonoids isolated from *Glycyrrhiza uralensis* (Chinese liquorice) could induce differentiation of melanoma B16-F10 cells or promote apoptosis [12].

Four papers have focused on cardioprotection. In a study by Czompa et al., the effects of raw and aged black garlic were compared using a rat model of post-ischemic cardiac recovery. Both types of garlic were found to display cardioprotective activity as demonstrated by an enhancement of post-ischemic cardiac function and a reduction in cardiac infarct size [13]. In another study, Hsia et al. reported that morin hydrate could inhibit platelet activation through an inhibition of the PLCγ2-PCK cascade and subsequent suppression of Akt and MAPK activation [14]. On the other hand, Guo et al. reported dihyromyricetin being able to ameliorate myocardial hypertrophy in a transverse aortic constriction mouse model, and the authors suggested that the activity of the compound was related to the suppression of oxidative stress and an upregulation of the SIRT3 pathway [15]. Moreover, Hung et al. reported that the polar extract and chemical ingredients (such as astragaloside IV) of *Astragalus membranaceus* root, which is often used as a tonic herbal drug, exhibited a protective effect on cardiomyocytes exposed to oxidative stress through an increase in the respiratory capacity and mitochondrial ATP production [16].

Liver protection formed the theme of three papers. Using a hepatic steatosis model of HepG2 cells treated with free fatty acids, Guo et al. described the preventive activity of pinocembrin and its glucosides against hepatic steatosis, possibly through the regulation of the SIRT1/AMPK pathway [15]. In another study, fucoidan, a sulphated polysaccharides found in seaweeds, was reported by Wang et al. to be able to protect against hepatotoxicity induced by acetaminophen in a mouse model, with a plausible mechanism related to Nrf2-mediated oxidative stress [17]. Furthermore, the pharmacokinetics of the hepatoprotective triterpenic acids obtained from *Ziziphus jujube* fruits was reported by Li et al. using an UHPLC-MS method to analyze the plasma samples in normal and CCl_4-treated rats [18].

In a screen of phytochemicals isolated from Himalayan medicinal plants, Wangchuk et al. reported scoulerine and bergapten as immunomodulators [19]. A series of cinnamamide derivatives were reported by Pospisilova et al. to possess significant antibacterial, antitubercular, and antifungal activities [20].

The herb-drug interaction between *Panax notoginseng* saponins and aspirin was investigated by Subramanya et al. The saponins were found to inhibit aspirin hydrolysis in HepaRG cells, the effect being ascribed to a suppression of the carboxylesterase-2 enzyme [21].

There are a total of seven review articles included in this Special Issue. They cover various biomedical areas including antimalarial (Pan et al., [22]), anti-arthritic (Dudics et al., [23]), hair growth stimulating (Choi, [24]), and anti-hepatotoxic (Subramanya et al., [21]) properties. Two other reviews have focused on the medicinal plants of *Copaifera* (da Trindade et al., [25]) and *Citrus* species (Dosoky and Setzer, [26]), respectively. Lastly, a review by Thomford et al. discussed the potential of applying innovative technologies such as automation technology, analytical and computational techniques to the next generation of plant-based drug discovery [27].

In conclusion, it is clear from these studies that many plant natural products display interesting bio/pharmacological activities. To better understand their medicinal properties and to establish stronger evidence of potentials for further development, preclinical and clinical investigations regarding their mechanisms of action, safety and efficacy are warranted.

Conflicts of Interest: The authors declare no conflict of interest.

References

1. World Health Organization. *WHO Traditional Medicine Strategy: 2014–2023*; WHO Press: Geneva, Switzerland, 2013.
2. Jonas, W.B.; Eisenberg, D.; Hufford, D.; Crawford, C. The Evolution of Complementary and Alternative Medicine (CAM) in the USA over the Last 20 Years. *Forsch Komplementmed.* **2013**, *20*, 65. [CrossRef] [PubMed]
3. Smith, T.; Kawa, K.; Eckl, V.; Morton, C.; Stredney, R. Herbal Supplements Sales in US Increases 8.5% in 2017, Topping $8 Billion. *HerbalGram* **2018**, *119*, 62.
4. Kang, Y.; Choi, H.; Lee, J.; Jang, S.; Kang, H.; Oh, J.; Jang, H.; Kwon, Y. Calorie Restriction Effect of Heat-Processed Onion Extract (ONI) Using In Vitro and In Vivo Animal Models. *Int. J. Mol. Sci.* **2018**, *19*, 874. [CrossRef] [PubMed]
5. Nagappan, A.; Jung, D.; Kim, J.; Jung, M. Protective Effects of Gomisin N against Hepatic Cannabinoid Type 1 Receptor-Induced Insulin Resistance and Gluconeogenesis. *Int. J. Mol. Sci.* **2018**, *19*, 968. [CrossRef] [PubMed]
6. Li, M.; Xu, T.; Zhou, F.; Wang, M.; Song, H.; Xiao, X.; Lu, B. Neuroprotective Effects of Four Phenylethanoid Glycosides on H2O2-Induced Apoptosis on PC12 Cells via the Nrf2/ARE Pathway. *Int. J. Mol. Sci.* **2018**, *19*, 1135. [CrossRef] [PubMed]
7. Gugliandolo, A.; Pollastro, F.; Grassi, G.; Bramanti, P.; Mazzon, E. In Vitro Model of Neuroinflammation: Efficacy of Cannabigerol, a Non-Psychoactive Cannabinoid. *Int. J. Mol. Sci.* **2018**, *19*, 1992. [CrossRef] [PubMed]
8. Tang, Y.; Xiong, R.; Wu, A.; Yu, C.; Zhao, Y.; Qiu, W.; Wang, X.; Teng, J.; Liu, J.; Chen, H.; Wu, J.; Qin, D. Polyphenols Derived from Lychee Seed Suppress Aβ (1-42)-Induced Neuroinflammation. *Int. J. Mol. Sci.* **2018**, *19*, 2109. [CrossRef]
9. He, J.; Lu, X.; Wei, T.; Dong, Y.; Cai, Z.; Tang, L.; Liu, M. Asperuloside and Asperulosidic Acid Exert an Anti-Inflammatory Effect via Suppression of the NF-κB and MAPK Signaling Pathways in LPS-Induced RAW 264.7 Macrophages. *Int. J. Mol. Sci.* **2018**, *19*, 2027. [CrossRef]
10. Vetvicka, V.; Gover, O.; Hayby, H.; Danay, O.; Ezov, N.; Hadar, Y.; Schwartz, B. Spatial Distribution of Glucan Type and Content between Caps and Stalks in Pleurotus eryngii: Impact on the Anti-inflammatory Functionality. *Int. J. Mol. Sci.* **2018**, *19*, 3371. [CrossRef]
11. Jayakumar, T.; Liu, C.; Wu, G.; Lee, T.; Manubolu, M.; Hsieh, C.; Yang, C.; Sheu, J. Hinokitiol Inhibits Migration of A549 Lung Cancer Cells via Suppression of MMPs and Induction of Antioxidant Enzymes and Apoptosis. *Int. J. Mol. Sci.* **2018**, *19*, 939. [CrossRef]

12. Zheng, Y.; Wang, H.; Yang, M.; Peng, G.; Dong, T.; Xu, M.; Tsim, K. Prenylated Flavonoids from Roots of Glycyrrhiza uralensis Induce Differentiation of B16-F10 Melanoma Cells. *Int. J. Mol. Sci.* **2018**, *19*, 2422. [CrossRef] [PubMed]
13. Czompa, A.; Szoke, K.; Prokisch, J.; Gyongyosi, A.; Bak, I.; Balla, G.; Tosaki, A.; Lekli, I. Aged (Black) versus Raw Garlic against Ischemia/Reperfusion-Induced Cardiac Complications. *Int. J. Mol. Sci.* **2018**, *19*, 1017. [CrossRef] [PubMed]
14. Hsia, C.; Wu, M.; Velusamy, M.; Hsia, C.; Chou, D.; Tsai, C.; Hsu, C.; Jayakumar, T.; Chung, C.; Sheu, J. Novel Therapeutic Agent against Platelet Activation In Vitro and Arterial Thrombosis In Vivo by Morin Hydrate. *Int. J. Mol. Sci.* **2018**, *19*, 2386. [CrossRef] [PubMed]
15. Guo, W.; Wang, X.; Chen, X.; Ba, Y.; Zhang, N.; Xu, R.; Zhao, W.; Wu, X. Flavonones from Penthorum chinense Ameliorate Hepatic Steatosis by Activating the SIRT1/AMPK Pathway in HepG2 Cells. *Int. J. Mol. Sci.* **2018**, *19*, 2555. [CrossRef] [PubMed]
16. Huang, Y.; Kwan, K.; Leung, K.; Wang, H.; Kong, X.; Dong, T.; Tsim, K. The Extracts and Major Compounds Derived from Astragali Radix Alter Mitochondrial Bioenergetics in Cultured Cardiomyocytes: Comparison of Various Polar Solvents and Compounds. *Int. J. Mol. Sci.* **2018**, *19*, 1574. [CrossRef] [PubMed]
17. Wang, Y.; Wei, J.; Tu, M.; Gu, J.; Zhang, W. Fucoidan alleviates acetaminophen-induced hepatotoxicity via oxidative stress inhibition and Nrf2 translocation. *Int. J. Mol. Sci.* **2018**, *19*, 4050. [CrossRef] [PubMed]
18. Li, Y.; Guo, S.; Ren, Q.; Wei, D.; Zhao, M.; Su, S.; Tang, Z.; Duan, J. Pharmacokinetic Comparisons of Multiple Triterpenic Acids from Jujubae Fructus Extract Following Oral Delivery in Normal and Acute Liver Injury Rats. *Int. J. Mol. Sci.* **2018**, *19*, 2047. [CrossRef] [PubMed]
19. Wangchuk, P.; Apte, S.; Smout, M.; Groves, P.; Loukas, A.; Doolan, D. Defined Small Molecules Produced by Himalayan Medicinal Plants Display Immunomodulatory Properties. *Int. J. Mol. Sci.* **2018**, *19*, 3490. [CrossRef] [PubMed]
20. Pospisilova, S.; Kos, J.; Michnova, H.; Kapustikova, I.; Strharsky, T.; Oravec, M.; Moricz, A.; Bakonyi, J.; Kauerova, T.; Kollar, P.; Cizek, A.; Jampilek, J. Synthesis and Spectrum of Biological Activities of Novel N-arylcinnamamides. *Int. J. Mol. Sci.* **2018**, *19*, 2318. [CrossRef] [PubMed]
21. Subramanya, S.; Venkataraman, B.; Meeran, M.; Goyal, S.; Patil, C.; Ojha, S. Therapeutic Potential of Plants and Plant Derived Phytochemicals against Acetaminophen-Induced Liver Injury. *Int. J. Mol. Sci.* **2018**, *19*, 3776. [CrossRef] [PubMed]
22. Pan, W.; Xu, X.; Shi, N.; Tsang, S.; Zhang, H. Antimalarial Activity of Plant Metabolites. *Int. J. Mol. Sci.* **2018**, *19*, 1382. [CrossRef] [PubMed]
23. Dudics, S.; Langan, D.; Meka, R.; Venkatesha, S.; Berman, B.; Che, C.; Moudgil, K. Natural Products for the Treatment of Autoimmune Arthritis: Their Mechanisms of Action, Targeted Delivery, and Interplay with the Host Microbiome. *Int. J. Mol. Sci.* **2018**, *19*, 2508. [CrossRef] [PubMed]
24. Choi, B. Hair-Growth Potential of Ginseng and Its Major Metabolites: A Review on Its Molecular Mechanisms. *Int. J. Mol. Sci.* **2018**, *19*, 2703. [CrossRef] [PubMed]
25. da Trindade, R.; da Silva, J.; Setzer, W. Copaifera of the Neotropics: A Review of the Phytochemistry and Pharmacology. *Int. J. Mol. Sci.* **2018**, *19*, 1511. [CrossRef] [PubMed]
26. Dosoky, N.; Setzer, W. Biological Activities and Safety of Citrus spp. Essential Oils. *Int. J. Mol. Sci.* **2018**, *19*, 1966. [CrossRef] [PubMed]
27. Thomford, N.; Senthebane, D.; Rowe, A.; Munro, D.; Seele, P.; Maroyi, A.; Dzobo, K. Natural Products for Drug Discovery in the 21st Century: Innovations for Novel Drug Discovery. *Int. J. Mol. Sci.* **2018**, *19*, 1578. [CrossRef] [PubMed]

International Journal of
Molecular Sciences

MDPI

Article

Fucoidan Alleviates Acetaminophen-Induced Hepatotoxicity via Oxidative Stress Inhibition and Nrf2 Translocation

Yu-qin Wang [1,†,*], Jin-ge Wei [1,†], Meng-jue Tu [1], Jian-guo Gu [1,2] and Wei Zhang [1,*]

1 Department of Pharmacology, School of Pharmacy and Key Laboratory of Inflammation and Molecular Drug Target of Jiangsu Province, Nantong University, Nantong 226001, China; weijinge1@sina.com (J.W.); dreamjojojo@sina.com(M.T.); jgu@tohoku-mpu.ac.jp (J.G.)

2 Division of Regulatory Glycobiology, Institute of Molecular Biomembrane and Glycobiology, Tohoku Medical and Pharmaceutical University, Sendai, Miyagi 981-8558, Japan

* Correspondence: wangyuqin@ntu.edu.cn (Y.W.); weizhangntu611@aliyun.com (W.Z.); Tel.: +86-513-8505-1726 (Y.W.); +86-513-8505-1727 (W.Z.)

† These authors equally contributed to this work.

Received: 25 November 2018; Accepted: 12 December 2018; Published: 14 December 2018

Abstract: Acetaminophen (APAP) is a widely used analgesic and antipyretic drug that leads to severe hepatotoxicity at excessive doses. Fucoidan, a sulfated polysaccharide derived from brown seaweeds, possesses a wide range of pharmacological properties. However, the impacts of fucoidan on APAP-induced liver injury have not been sufficiently addressed. In the present study, male Institute of Cancer Research (ICR) mice aged 6 weeks were subjected to a single APAP (500 mg/kg) intraperitoneal injection after 7 days of fucoidan (100 or 200 mg/kg/day) or bicyclol intragastric administration. The mice continued to be administered fucoidan or bicyclol once per day, and were sacrificed at an indicated time. The indexes evaluated included liver pathological changes, levels of alanine aminotransferase (ALT) and aspartate aminotransferase (AST) in the serum, levels of reactive oxygen species (ROS), malondialdehyde (MDA), superoxide dismutase (SOD), glutathione (GSH) and catalase (CAT) in the liver, and related proteins levels (CYP2E1, pJNK and Bax). Furthermore, human hepatocyte HL-7702 cell line was used to elucidate the potential molecular mechanism of fucoidan. The mitochondrial membrane potential (MMP) and nuclear factor-erythroid 2-related factor (Nrf2) translocation in HL-7702 cells were determined. The results showed that fucoidan pretreatment reduced the levels of ALT, AST, ROS, and MDA, while it enhanced the levels of GSH, SOD, and CAT activities. Additionally, oxidative stress-induced phosphorylated c-Jun N-terminal protein kinase (JNK) and decreased MMP were attenuated by fucoidan. Although the nuclear Nrf2 was induced after APAP incubation, fucoidan further enhanced Nrf2 in cell nuclei and total expression of Nrf2. These results indicated that fucoidan ameliorated APAP hepatotoxicity, and the mechanism might be related to Nrf2-mediated oxidative stress.

Keywords: fucoidan; acetaminophen; Nrf2; oxidative stress; hepatotoxicity

1. Introduction

Drug-related hepatotoxicity is a common adverse event in clinic, since a large number of drugs are metabolized in the liver [1,2]. Acetaminophen (APAP) is a widely used analgesic and antipyretic drug, which is safe at therapeutic doses. However, severe hepatotoxicity resulting from excessive doses is the leading cause of acute liver failure in the western world [3]. At therapeutic doses, APAP is mainly metabolized to nontoxic water-soluble metabolites by glucuronidation and sulfation in the liver, and only a small fraction of APAP is metabolized by various cytochrome P450s (CYPs) such as

CYP2E1, CYP3A4, CYP1A2, and CYP1A1 to a toxic active product, *N*-acetyl-p-benzoquinoneimine (NAPQI) [4,5]. NAPQI forms APAP-glutathione, APAP-cysteine, and APAP-*N*-acetylcysteine by conjugating with glutathione (GSH) [6]. However, an APAP overdose exhausts glucuronidation and sulfation pathways and produces excess NAPQI, subsequently consuming GSH excessively. Excessive NAPQI forms cysteine adducts by binding to hepatocyte proteins, triggering oxidative stress, mitochondrial dysfunction, cellular necrosis, apoptosis, and even hepatic injury [7].

Nuclear factor-erythroid 2-related factor 2 (Nrf2), a crucial transcription factor, is required for the progress of various diseases, particularly those arising from oxidative stress [8]. Upon exposure to stressors or inducers, Nrf2 enters the nucleus from the cytoplasm and binds to antioxidant response elements (ARE), then activates downstream target genes, including nicotinamide adenine dinucleotide phosphate (NAD(P)H)-quinone oxidoreductase 1 (NQO1) and heme oxygenase-1 (HO-1). It has been reported that Nrf2-deficient mice have a greater severity than wild-type mice in APAP-induced liver injury [9]. In addition, activation of Nrf2/ARE signaling alleviates cerebral ischemia and reperfusion injury by inhibiting reactive oxygen species (ROS) generation and neuronal apoptosis [10]. Thus, targeting Nrf2 activation might be effective for the prevention of hepatotoxicity. Furthermore, oxidative stress also contributes to the phosphorylation of c-Jun N-terminal protein kinases (JNKs) [11]. The translocation of phosphorylated JNK to the mitochondria further aggravates the mitochondrial oxidant stress and evokes mitochondrial dysfunction and DNA fragmentation, thus ultimately causing hepatocyte necrosis [12].

Currently, in addition to *N*-acetylcysteine (NAC), there is no other effective drug for the treatment of liver damage caused by excess APAP. However, it is most beneficial only at an early phase of APAP intoxication, and the efficacy decreases at later times [13]. Therefore, it is urgent to explore novel candidates in preventing and treating APAP-induced hepatotoxicity. Fucoidan, which is mainly found in various species of brown seaweed, is a sulfated polysaccharide containing L-fucose and sulfate groups. Numerous studies have indicated that fucoidan exhibited several therapeutic properties both in vivo and in vitro, such as anticoagulant, antitumor, antiviral, antidiabetic, and anti-inflammatory activities [14]. It has been reported that cotreatment of fucoidan ameliorated APAP-induced liver damage and cell death in rats [15]: However, the impacts of fucoidan on APAP-induced liver injury have not been sufficiently addressed yet. Bicyclol, a synthetic antihepatitis drug in China, possesses protective effects against experimental liver injury induced by several chemical toxins and alcohol [16]. Since the hepatoprotective mechanism of bicyclol is partly related to the clearance of ROS [17], it was used as the positive control in this study. The aim of the present study was to investigate the effect of fucoidan on APAP-induced liver injury and to explore potential molecular mechanisms.

2. Results

2.1. Fucoidan Attenuated APAP-Induced Acute Liver Injury in Mice

The serum levels of alanine aminotransferase (ALT) and aspartate aminotransferase (AST) are usually used as biomarkers for evaluating hepatic function [18,19]. To explore the role of fucoidan against APAP hepatotoxicity, first we detected serum ALT and AST levels in different groups. Starting from 4 h after APAP injection, a massive hepatic toxicity was induced, as revealed by increased serum levels of ALT and AST (Figure 1A,B), and these elevations continued until 48 h after APAP administration (Figure 1E,F). These results indicated that the APAP-induced acute liver injury model was successful, whereas the increased serum levels of ALT and AST were significantly inhibited in the mice treated with fucoidan and bicyclol. Furthermore, the histological examination corroborated the serum ALT and AST results. As shown in Figure 1C, APAP-induced accumulation of erythrocytes in the central vein and sinusoids, infiltration of inflammatory cells, and disordered arrangement in hepatocytes were effectively attenuated by fucoidan or bicyclol treatment. However, the liver ratio in different groups had no significant difference after APAP administration (Figure 1D). These results indicated that treatment with fucoidan or bicyclol prevented APAP-induced acute liver injury.

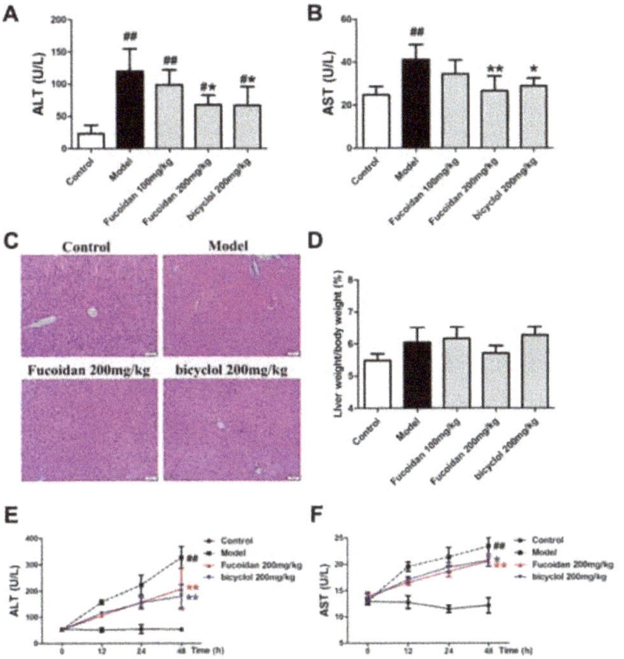

Figure 1. Fucoidan attenuated acetaminophen (APAP)-induced acute liver injury in mice. Male Institute of Cancer Research (ICR) mice were randomly divided into control, model, fucoidan 100 mg/kg, fucoidan 200 mg/kg, and bicyclol 200 mg/kg groups. After pretreating with fucoidan or bicyclol for 7 days, the acute hepatic injury model was induced by intraperitoneal injection of 500 mg/kg APAP, and the normal group was injected with an equal amount of saline. The mice continued to be administered fucoidan or bicyclol once per day, and were sacrificed at an indicated time. (**A**) Serum level of aminotransferase (ALT) in different groups 4 h after intraperitoneal injection of APAP ($n = 8$). (**B**) Serum level of aspartate aminotransferase (AST) in different groups 4 h after intraperitoneal injection of APAP ($n = 8$). (**C**) Representative images of hematoxylin and eosin (H&E) stained liver sections from different groups after APAP treatment (bar = 50 μm). (**D**) Liver ratio in different groups after APAP treatment ($n = 8$). (**E**) Serum levels of ALT at different time points after APAP injection ($n = 6$). (**F**) Serum levels of AST at different time points after APAP injection ($n = 6$). Data are expressed as mean ± SD, $^{\#}$ $p < 0.05$, $^{\#\#}$ $p < 0.01$ versus control group; * $p < 0.05$, ** $p < 0.01$ versus model group.

2.2. Fucoidan Enhanced Antioxidant Capacity and Reduced the Levels of Malondialdehyde (MDA) and ROS in the Liver of APAP-Treated Mice

Overdose of APAP produces excessive NAPQI, which binds to hepatocyte proteins to form cysteine adducts, leading to cellular processes such as oxidative stress, mitochondrial damage, and ultimately hepatocytes necrosis. Oxidative stress is critical in the pathophysiological mechanism of hepatic injury [12,20], and ROS may be the common pathogenesis of hepatic disease [21,22]. ROS fluorescence probe–dihydroethidium (DHE) staining was performed on frozen sections of mice liver. As shown in Figure 2A, fluorescence intensity in the model group significantly increased at 4 h after APAP exposure, and meanwhile, pretreatment with fucoidan and bicyclol attenuated the increase of fluorescence intensity. The level of MDA suggested tissue lipid peroxidation, and the response was consistent with the ROS staining (Figure 2B,F). APAP-induced oxidative stress is normally detoxified by the enzymatic antioxidant defense system. At 4 h after APAP exposure, GSH level, superoxide dismutase (SOD), and catalase (CAT) activities remarkably decreased compared to those of the control group, whereas treatment with fucoidan or bicyclol attenuated the above changes (Figure 2C–E).

With the aggravation of liver damage, fucoidan continued its protective effects against hepatotoxicity by enhancing SOD activity at 48 h after APAP injection (Figure 2G). However, no significant change in CAT activity and GSH content was observed at other time points after APAP administration (Figure 2H–I). Thus, we speculated that fucoidan postponed the consumption of GSH in the early phase of liver injury, and this effect was significantly diminished in the later stage. These data suggested that fucoidan treatment might reduce oxidative stress and restore endogenous antioxidant systems to prevent APAP-induced hepatotoxicity.

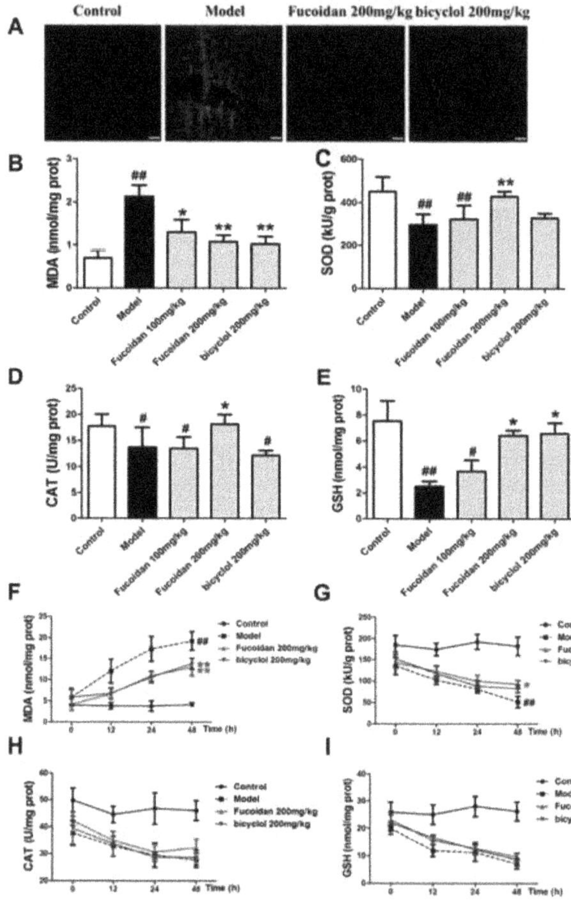

Figure 2. Fucoidan inhibited APAP-induced oxidative stress in mice. Male ICR mice were randomly divided into control, model, fucoidan 100 mg/kg, fucoidan 200 mg/kg, and bicyclol 200 mg/kg groups. After pretreating with fucoidan or bicyclol for 7 days, the acute hepatic injury model was induced by intraperitoneal injection of 500 mg/kg APAP, and the normal group was injected with an equal amount of saline. The mice continued to be administered fucoidan or bicyclol once a day, and were sacrificed at an indicated time. Hepatic tissues were taken for frozen sections and other detections. (**A**) Hepatic sections (4 h) were stained with dihydroethidium (DHE) fluorescent dye, and the levels of superoxide anion were observed with a confocal microscope (bar = 100 μm). (**B**,**F**) Malondialdehyde (MDA) and (**E**,**I**) glutathione (GSH) levels, (**C**,**G**) superoxide dismutase (SOD) and (**D**,**H**) catalase (CAT) activities in the liver were measured for evaluating the level of hepatic oxidative stress. Data are expressed as mean ± SD, $n = 8$, # $p < 0.05$, ## $p < 0.01$ versus control group; * $p < 0.05$, ** $p < 0.01$ versus model group.

2.3. Fucoidan Decreased Phosphorylation of JNK and Expression of Bax in the Liver of APAP-Treated Mice

It is well known that excessive ROS induced by APAP results in phosphorylation of JNK, which further amplifies mitochondria oxidative stress [23]. Moreover, the pro-apoptotic protein Bax, which belongs to the Bcl-2 family of proteins, is highly expressed exposed to an APAP overdose [24–26]. The pathophysiological importance of Bax in APAP hepatotoxicity has been shown by the temporary inhibition of nuclear DNA fragmentation and delayed cell death in Bax-deficient mice [27]. In the present study, the APAP-induced upregulation of phosphorylated JNK was abrogated by pretreatment with fucoidan and bicyclol (Figure 3A,B). Additionally, fucoidan and bicyclol also attenuated the increased protein expression of Bax after APAP injection (Figure 3C,D). Our results indicated that fucoidan, like bicyclol, significantly suppressed JNK phosphorylation and Bax protein expression, and then protected hepatocytes from APAP-induced damage.

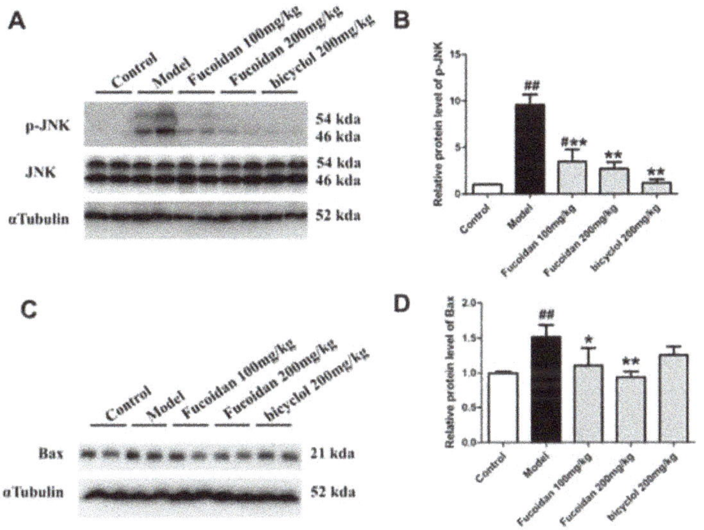

Figure 3. Fucoidan inhibited APAP-induced c-Jun N-terminal protein kinase (JNK) phosphorylation and Bax protein expression in mice. Male ICR mice were randomly divided into control, model, fucoidan 100 mg/kg, fucoidan 200 mg/kg, and bicyclol 200 mg/kg groups. After pretreating with fucoidan or bicyclol for 7 days, the acute hepatic injury model was induced by intraperitoneal injection of 500 mg/kg APAP, and the normal group was injected with an equal amount of saline. Four hours after injection, the hepatic tissue was taken for further detections. The (**A**,**B**) phosphorylation level of JNK and (**C**,**D**) protein expression of Bax were determined by Western blotting analysis. The quantification of relative protein expression was performed by densitometric analysis, and α Tubulin was used as an internal control. All results were expressed as mean ± SD, $n = 6$, # $p < 0.05$, ## $p < 0.01$ versus control group; * $p < 0.05$, ** $p < 0.01$ versus model group.

2.4. Fucoidan Attenuated APAP-Induced Acute Injury in HL-7702 Cells

Previous results have indicated that pretreatment with fucoidan attenuated APAP-induced acute liver injury in vivo. In addition, many studies have reported that fucoidan exhibited several biological activities in vitro [14]. In order to elucidate the protective mechanism of fucoidan on APAP-induced liver injury, an acute APAP injury model was established in human normal hepatocyte HL-7702 cell line. 3-[4,5-dimethylthiazol-2-yl]-2,5- diphenyl tetrazolium bromide (MTT) assay was used to observe the effect of fucoidan pretreatment on the survival rate of HL-7702 cells injured by APAP. As shown in Figure 4A, the survival rate of cells was significantly inhibited by incubation with 20 mM APAP for 24 hours, while pretreatment with 50 or 100 μg/mL fucoidan significantly rescued the decreased cell survival rate. The result was further confirmed by detection of lactate dehydrogenase (LDH) in the culture medium (Figure 4B). In addition, levels of ALT and AST were markedly increased due to incubation with APAP, while fucoidan pretreatment ameliorated the damage of APAP to HL-7702 cells (Figure 4C,D).

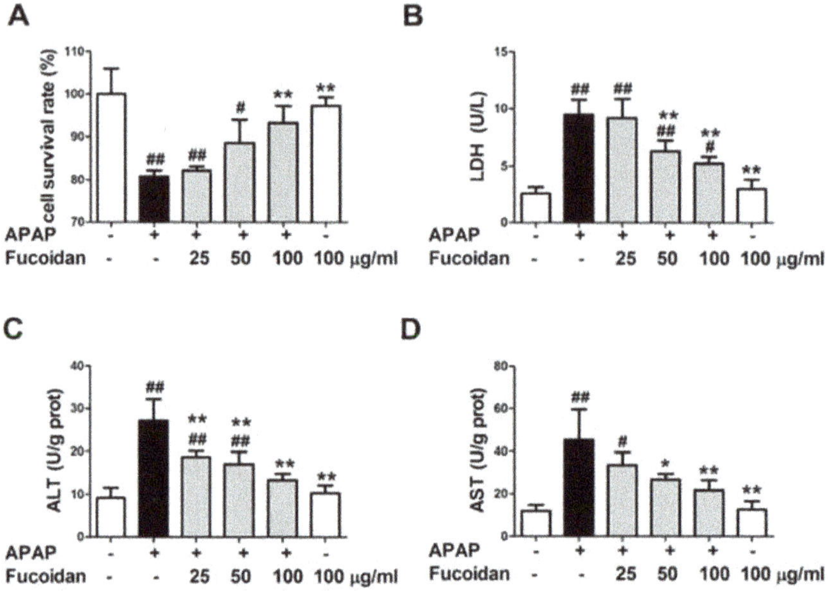

Figure 4. Effect of fucoidan on APAP-induced acute injury in HL-7702 cells. Cells were treated with various concentrations of fucoidan (25, 50, or 100 μg/mL) for 4 h and subsequently stimulated with APAP (20 mM) for 24 h. (**A**) MTT assay was used to observe the survival rate of HL-7702 cells. (**B**) The levels of lactate dehydrogenase (LDH), (**C**) ALT, and (**D**) AST were determined to evaluate the damage of cells. Similar results were obtained from three independent experiments. All results were expressed as mean ± SD, $n = 3$, $^{\#}\ p < 0.05$, $^{\#\#}\ p < 0.01$ versus control group; $^{*}\ p < 0.05$, $^{**}\ p < 0.01$ versus APAP-treated group.

2.5. Fucoidan Enhanced Antioxidant Capacity and Reduced the Levels of MDA and ROS in APAP-Damaged HL-7702 Cells

As shown in Figure 5A, DHE staining showed that the fluorescence intensity was remarkably enhanced in APAP-treated cells. Comparing to the model group, fucoidan attenuated the fluorescence intensity of DHE staining after APAP incubation. Moreover, the variation trend of MDA was similar to that of ROS (Figure 5B). Furthermore, compared to the control group, an overdose of APAP resulted in a significant decrease in GSH, CAT, and SOD activities after 24 h of APAP administration. However, as expected, pretreatment with fucoidan (100 μg/mL) induced a significant increase in GSH content, CAT, and SOD activities (Figure 5C–E). These data suggested that fucoidan attenuated APAP-induced oxidative stress by upregulating the activities of antioxidant enzymes in HL-7702 cells.

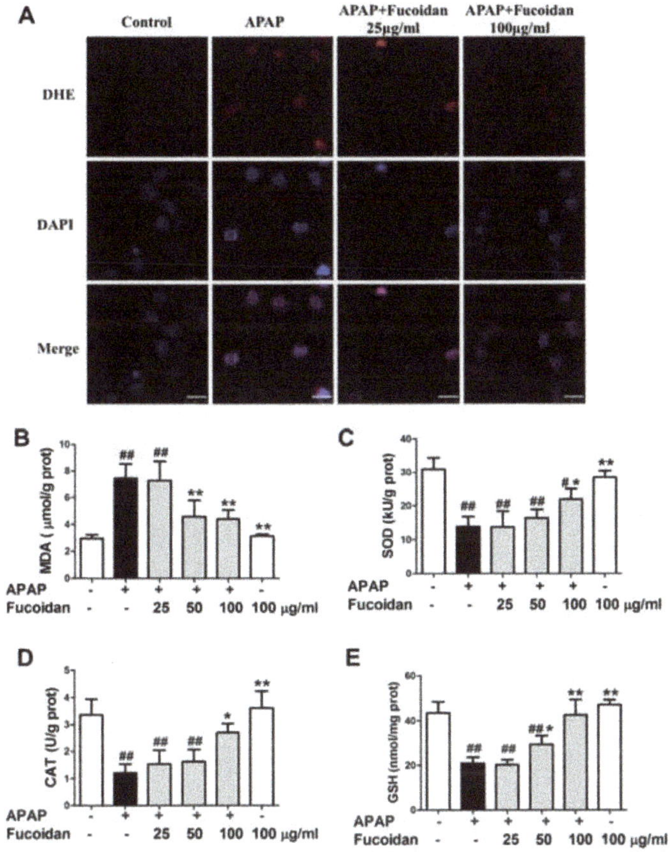

Figure 5. Effect of fucoidan on APAP-induced oxidative stress in HL-7702 cells. Cells were treated with various concentrations of fucoidan (25, 50, or 100 μg/mL) for 4 h and subsequently stimulated with APAP (20 mM) for 24 h. (**A**) HL-7702 cells were stained with DHE fluorescent dye (red), and the levels of reactive oxygen species (ROS) were observed with a confocal microscope (Bar = 25 μm). The nuclei were stained with DAPI (blue). The levels of (**B**) MDA, (**C**) SOD, (**D**) CAT, and (**E**) GSH were measured to evaluate the level of oxidative stress in cells. Similar results were obtained from three independent experiments. All results were expressed as mean ± SD, $n = 3$, $^{\#}$ $p < 0.05$, $^{\#\#}$ $p < 0.01$ versus control group; * $p < 0.05$, ** $p < 0.01$ versus APAP-treated group.

2.6. Fucoidan Suppressed the Protein Expression of CYP2E1 Both In Vivo and In Vitro

It is widely accepted that the highly reactive intermediate of NAPQI is metabolized by the CYP pathway (primarily by CYP2E1) [4]. According to the data of protein expression levels of CYP2E1 using Western blot, we observed that APAP alone enhanced the protein levels of CYP2E1 both in liver tissues and in HL-7702 cells. Meanwhile, with fucoidan or bicyclol, the expression of CYP2E1 was significantly suppressed (Figure 6). These findings suggested that the hepatoprotective effect of fucoidan might be partially associated with the suppression of CYP enzymes.

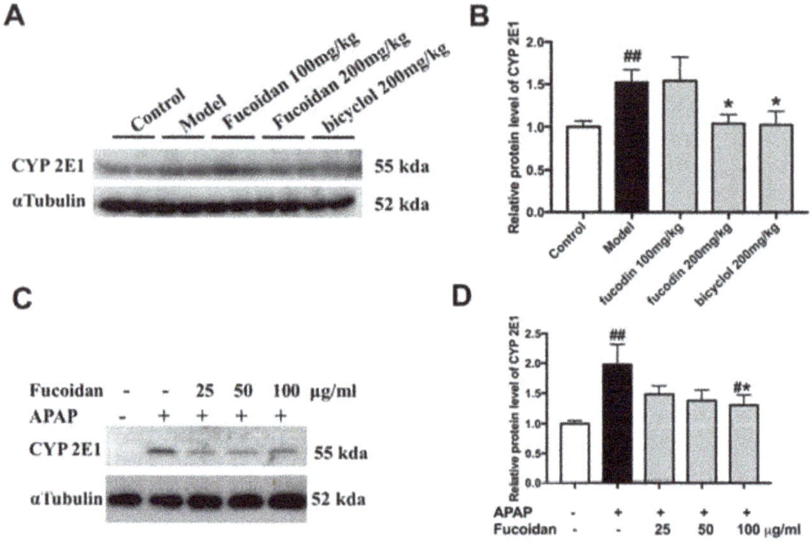

Figure 6. Effect of fucoidan on protein expression of CYP2E1 following an APAP overdose. (**A**) Representative blots of CYP2E1 and α Tubulin expression in hepatic tissues. (**B**) Quantification of CYP2E1 protein levels in liver tissues (n = 6). (**C**) Representative blots of CYP2E1 and α Tubulin expression in HL-7702 cells. (**D**) Quantification of CYP2E1 protein levels in HL-7702 cells (n = 3). Similar results were obtained from three independent experiments. All results were expressed as mean ± SD, $^{##}$ $p < 0.01$ versus control group; * $p < 0.05$ versus APAP-treated group.

2.7. Fucoidan Attenuated APAP-Induced Alteration of Mitochondrial Membrane Potential and Phosphorylation of JNK in HL-7702 Cells

In the case of an APAP overdose, high level of NAPQI depletes cellular glutathione and forms protein adducts, especially on mitochondria, which then inhibits the electron transport chain, resulting in leakage of electrons and oxidative stress [28]. The decline of mitochondrial membrane potential (MMP) is a landmark event in the early stages of mitochondria dysfunction. Compared to the control group, red fluorescence intensity produced by J-aggregates was markedly attenuated after APAP treatment, while incubation with fucoidan alleviated this situation (Figure 7A). As a pro-apoptotic protein, Bax was induced by APAP, and the increased protein expression was inhibited in fucoidan-treated HL-7702 cells (Figure 7B,C). Apoptosis signal-regulating kinase 1 (ASK1) has been identified in a JNK cascade during APAP-induced hepatotoxicity [29]. After APAP incubation, the levels of phosphorylated ASK1 and JNK were also enhanced, and meanwhile being pretreated with fucoidan suppressed phosphorylation of ASK1 and JNK (Figure 7D–G). Taken together, these results indicated that the protective effect of fucoidan against APAP-induced injury might be associated with alleviating mitochondria dysfunction.

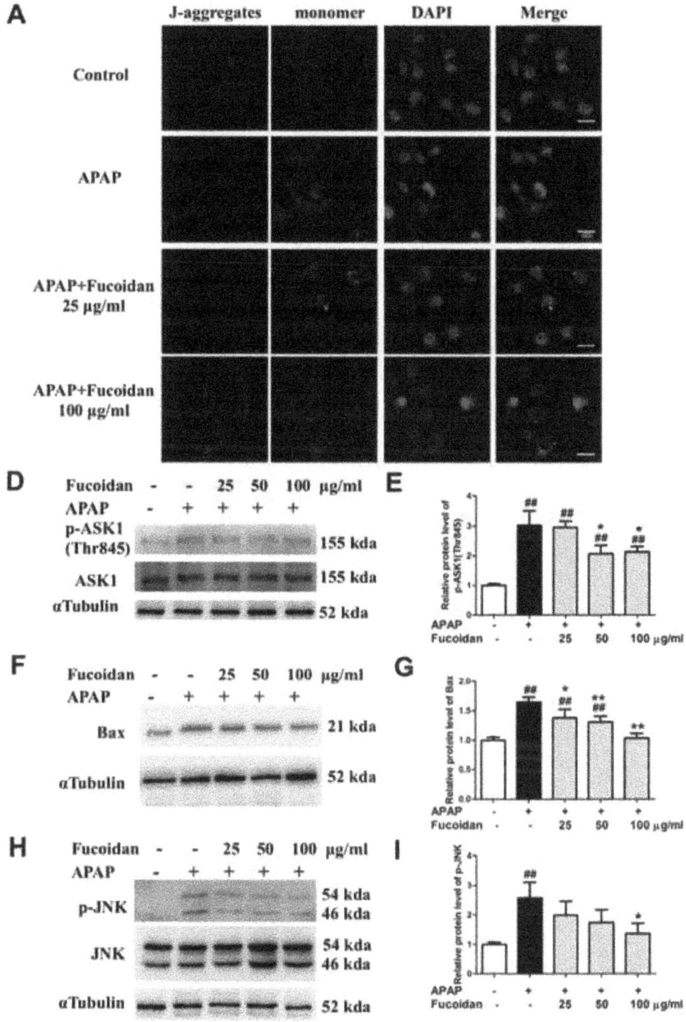

Figure 7. Effect of fucoidan treatment on APAP-induced mitochondrial membrane potential (MMP) and the JNK pathway in HL-7702 cells. Cells were treated with various concentrations of fucoidan (25, 50, or 100 µg/mL) for 4 h, and were subsequently exposed to APAP (20 mM) for 24 h. (**A**) The effect of fucoidan on mitochondrial membrane potential was tested using the JC-1 method and determined by a confocal microscope. The J-aggregates produced red fluorescence, and the monomer emitted green fluorescence (Bar = 25 µm). The nuclei were stained with DAPI (blue). (**B**,**C**) Expression of Bax, (**D**–**G**) phosphorylated ASK1, and phosphorylated JNK were determined by Western blotting analysis. Quantification of relative protein expression was performed by densitometric analysis, and α Tubulin was used as an internal control. Similar results were obtained from three independent experiments. All results were expressed as mean ± SD, $n = 3$, ## $p < 0.01$ versus control group; * $p < 0.05$, ** $p < 0.01$ versus APAP-treated group.

2.8. Fucoidan Enhanced Nrf2 Expression in the Nucleus of HL-7702 Cells

Oxidation damage is one major factor in APAP-induced liver injury. Since the Nrf2-mediated signaling pathway is essential for the inhibition of oxidative stress, Nrf2 plays an important role in the amelioration of APAP-induced hepatotoxicity. Therefore, we examined the expression of Nrf2 in the cytoplasm and nucleus of HL-7702 cells from different groups by immunofluorescence staining and Western blot assay. Exposed to APAP, the expression of Nrf2 in the nuclei remarkably increased, while that in the cytoplasm significantly decreased. In addition, pretreatment with fucoidan further enhanced the expression of Nrf2 in the nucleus, but had no significant effect on Nrf2 in the cytoplasm (Figure 8). In brief, protein expression of total Nrf2 and nuclear Nrf2 were enhanced by fucoidan pretreatment, which might provide a possible mechanism for fucoidan to alleviate APAP-induced oxidative stress and thus protect against APAP hepatotoxicity.

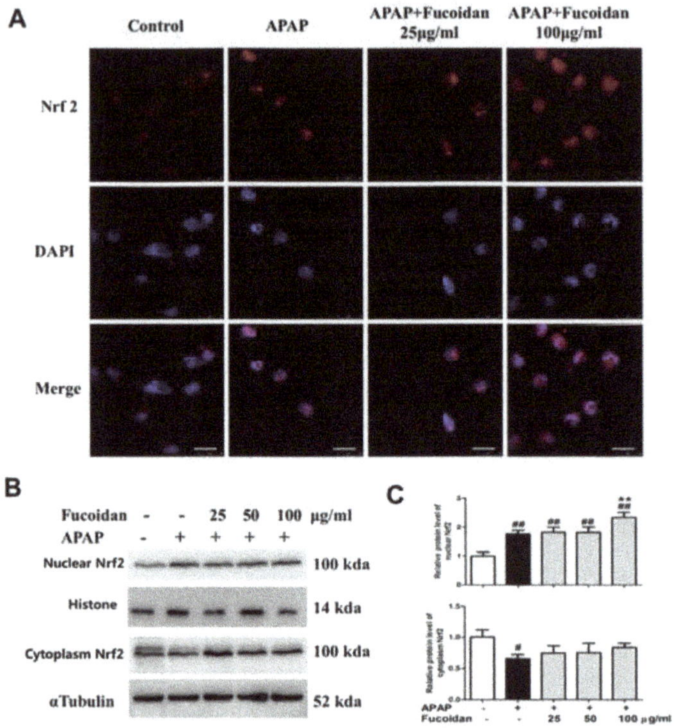

Figure 8. Effect of fucoidan on APAP-induced nuclear factor-erythroid 2-related factor 2 (Nrf2) expression and translocation in HL-7702 cells. Cells were treated with various concentrations of fucoidan (25, 50, or 100 μg/ml) for 4 h, and were subsequently exposed to APAP (20 mM) for 24 h. (**A**) The effect of fucoidan on Nrf2 (red) translocation was tested by immunofluorescence staining and determined by a confocal microscope. The nuclei were stained with DAPI (blue) (Bar = 25 μm). (**B**,**C**) Expression levels of nuclear Nrf2 and cytoplasm Nrf2 were determined by Western blotting analysis. Quantification of relative protein expression was performed by densitometric analysis, with histone and α Tubulin acting as controls. Similar results were obtained from three independent experiments. All results were expressed as mean ± SD, $n = 3$, $^{##}$ $p < 0.01$ versus control group; ** $p < 0.01$ versus APAP-treated group.

3. Discussion

Currently, APAP overdose-induced hepatotoxicity has become one of the most common causes of acute liver failure in many countries. NAC, the only Food and Drug Administration (FDA)-approved antidote, is used for treatment of APAP hepatotoxicity when administered within 8 to 10 h after APAP overdose [30]. Since the therapeutic options for this disease are rather limited, it is urgent to seek safe and effective agents for the treatment. Fucoidan, which is available for use in cosmetics, functional foods, and dietary supplements, is nontoxic and can be easily extracted from brown seaweeds [31]. A large number of studies have demonstrated that oral or intraperitoneal injection of fucoidan inhibits metastases in various cancers [32]. It has also been reported that fucoidan ameliorated steatohepatitis and insulin resistance by suppressing oxidative stress in experimental non-alcoholic fatty liver disease [33]. In addition, fucoidan also possesses protective effects against CCl_4-induced liver injury by inhibiting oxidative stress [34]. Due to its broad spectrum of desirable biological functionalities, fucoidan has become one of the extensively studied macromolecules in the last few decades.

The liver is an important metabolic organ that is able to be impaired or even to be pathologically damaged by various chemical reagents and drugs [35]. Oxidative stress is generally seen in several liver diseases, and ROS plays important roles in the pathogenesis of APAP-induced hepatotoxicity. The prevention of ROS generation and lipid peroxidation is the most common mechanism of hepatoprotective natural compounds [36]. In the current study, mice subjected to fucoidan pretreatment showed significantly decreased lipid peroxidation by scavenging ROS generation. On the other hand, there is an antioxidant system existing to protect the body against oxidative stress. GSH conjugation is the major detoxification pathway for the reactive metabolites generated from APAP. SOD, an important antioxidant enzyme, converts superoxide anion radical induced by NAPQI into hydrogen peroxide (H_2O_2) and oxygen. CAT catalyzes the reaction that removes excess H_2O_2 in mitochondria. In the present study, GSH level, SOD, and CAT activities in liver tissues were significantly reduced after APAP administration, and meanwhile, treatment with fucoidan significantly alleviated the reduction at 4 h APAP exposure. However, the effect of fucoidan on the enhancement of GSH content was not obvious after 24 h of APAP treatment in vivo (Figure 2). Meanwhile, APAP-induced elevations of serum ALT and AST levels continued until 48 h after APAP administration, whereas the increased serum levels of ALT and AST were significantly inhibited in the mice treated with fucoidan or bicyclol (Figure 1). In addition, pretreatment with fucoidan also significantly alleviated the reduction in GSH level, SOD, and CAT activities at 24 h after APAP exposure in vitro (Figure 5). Thus, the protective effects of fucoidan associated with its antioxidant properties might play a role in the early phase of liver injury, although the effects of fucoidan on APAP-induced hepatotoxicity could last for 48 h or longer (Figure 1). Since NAPQI is mainly metabolized by the CYP pathway, especially CYP2E1, the antioxidant properties of fucoidan in APAP hepatotoxicity might be partially associated with the suppression of CYP enzymes (Figure 6).

JNK, which is expressed in a variety of tissues, is activated in response to a variety of stress stimuli, including DNA damage, growth factors, oxidative, and genotoxic stresses [29]. Additional NAPQI leads to increased ROS accumulation (triggering JNK phosphorylation), further amplifies the mitochondria oxidative stress, and triggers mitochondrial dysfunction [23]. Bax is a pro-apoptotic Bcl-2 family member located predominantly in the cytosol. Exposed to an APAP overdose, it is highly expressed [24–26]. It has been reported that APAP-induced mitochondrial Bax expression was attenuated by the inhibition of JNK activation [11]. Moreover, the upstream kinases of JNK activation have been reported to be activated by ASK1 in APAP-induced liver injury [37]. The hepatotoxicity induced by an overdose of APAP was suppressed in ASK knockout mice [38]. Actually, the release of apoptosis inducing factor (AIF) and endonuclease G into the cytosol and the induction of mitochondrial permeability transition were caused by amplified oxidative stress combined with translocation of Bax from the cytosol to the mitochondria [28]. Our data demonstrated that ASK1 and JNK phosphorylation and Bax protein expression were markedly inhibited in fucoidan-pretreated groups after APAP administration (Figures 3 and 7), which suggests that fucoidan reducing APAP-induced toxicity might be associated with alleviating mitochondria dysfunction.

Besides SOD, GSH, and CAT, Nrf2 also belongs to the antioxidant system, which maintains the balance of ROS in hepatocytes. As a key nuclear transcription factor, Nrf2 enters the nucleus from the cytoplasm when exposed to stressors or inducers. Subsequently, Nrf2 binds to ARE and regulates the expression of a battery of cytoprotective genes encoding intracellular detoxifying enzymes, including

SOD, GSH, and CAT, which are responsible for APAP elimination and detoxification [39,40]. In the current study, APAP treatment increased the translocation of Nrf2. However, pretreatment with fucoidan further upregulated nuclear Nrf2 in HL-7702 cells (Figure 8). These observations revealed that fucoidan pretreatment efficiently stimulated Nrf2 translocation from the cytoplasm into the nucleus, then enhanced the ability of antioxidant stress and suppressed APAP-induced ROS accumulation (Figure 9).

In summary, the present study provided an investigation into the protective activities of fucoidan against APAP-induced liver injury, and the potential mechanism was upregulating the Nrf2 antioxidant pathway. Thus, our study suggested a possible therapeutic application of fucoidan in APAP hepatotoxicity.

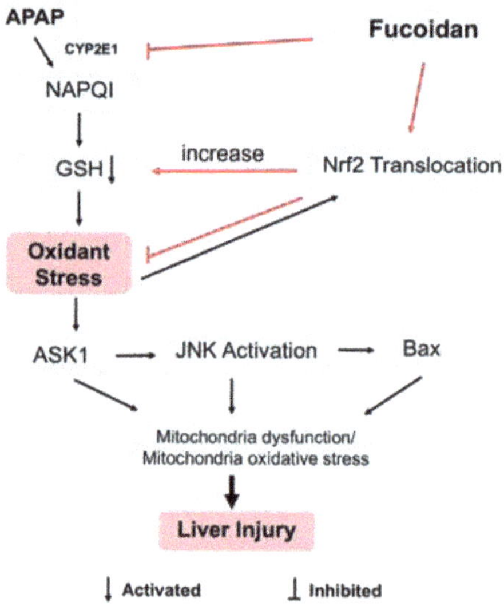

Figure 9. Nrf2 was involved in the protective effect of fucoidan against acetaminophen-induced hepatotoxicity. Fucoidan could regulate Nrf2 translocation, which contributes to the inhibition of APAP-induced oxidant stress. In addition, the inhibition of CYP2E1 by fucoidan might be related to the enhancement of GSH levels. Moreover, fucoidan attenuated the phosphorylation of ASK1 and JNK and further decreased the protein expression of Bax. Subsequently, fucoidan alleviated mitochondria dysfunction and protected hepatocytes against APAP toxicity.

4. Materials and Methods

4.1. Chemicals and Reagents

Fucoidan (purity >98%) was obtained from Cool Chemistry CO., Ltd (Beijing, China). APAP was provided by Santa Cruz Biotechnology (Santa Cruz, CA, USA). Bicyclol was obtained from Beijing Union Pharmaceutical Plant (Beijing, China). ALT, AST, MDA, GSH, CAT, and SOD activity test kits were from Nanjing Jiancheng Bioengineering Institute (Nanjing, China). ROS Fluorescent Probe-Dihydroethidium (DHE) was from Vigorousbio. CO., Ltd. (Beijing, China). The mitochondrial membrane potential assay kit (JC-1 Kit) and the LDH kit were obtained from Beyotime Biotechnology (Haimen, China). Antibodies against Nrf2, CYP 2E1, and ASK1 were obtained from Abcam (Cambridge, United Kingdom). Antibodies against histone, pASK1, pJNK, JNK, and Bax were obtained from Cell Signaling Technology (Beverly, MA, USA). Antibody against α tubulin was from Proteintech (Wuhan, China).

4.2. Animals and Treatment

ICR mice were obtained from Nantong University Experimental Animal Center. Animal experiments were performed in accordance with the National Institutes of Health (NIH) guidelines for Care and Use of Laboratory Animals. The study was approved by the University Animal Ethics Committee of Nantong University (approval no. NTU-20170316, 16 March 2017) and was conducted in accordance with the Declaration of Helsinki.

After 1 week of adaptive rearing, 6-week-old male ICR mice were divided into control, model, fucoidan (100 and 200 mg/kg), and bicyclol 200 mg/kg groups. The drugs were dissolved in saline and orally administered for 7 consecutive days. The mice in the control and model groups were intragastrically administered with an equivalent volume of saline. Two hours after final administration of medication, the mice were intraperitoneally injected with 500 mg/kg APAP [41], and the normal group was injected with an equal amount of saline. The mice continued to be administered fucoidan or bicyclol once per day, and were sacrificed at an indicated time.

4.3. Cell Culture and Treatment

A human normal hepatocyte HL-7702 cell line was obtained from the China Cell Line Bank (Beijing, China). The HL-7702 cells were cultured in Dulbecco modified Eagle medium (DMEM) medium containing 10% fetal bovine serum (FBS), 100 U/mL of streptomycin, 100 U/mL of penicillin, and 3 mM glutamine. The cells were grown in a humidified atmosphere containing 5% CO_2 at 37 °C. Besides the control and APAP group, all the cells were treated with fucoidan (25, 50, and 100 μg/mL) for 4 h and were exposed to APAP (20 mM) for 24 h.

4.4. Biochemical Indexes Assay

All mice were killed 4 h after APAP injection, and the serum and liver were collected for detection of biochemical indexes. For HL-7702 cells, medium and cells were collected at 24 h after APAP administration. The levels of ALT and AST were determined according to the manufacturer's protocol available with the respective kits. In addition, live tissues and cells were homogenized to analyze the MDA, SOD, CAT, and GSH levels in accordance with the manufacturer's instructions. All the results were normalized by the total protein concentration in each sample.

4.5. MTT and LDH Analysis

Cell viability was determined by MTT assay according to the manufacturer's instructions. Briefly, the HL-7702 cells were plated into 96-well plates and treated with APAP for 24 h. After the incubated period, MTT (5 mg/mL) was added to each well and incubated for another 4 h. Then the supernatant was removed, and dimethyl sulphoxide (DMSO) was used to lyse the cells. The absorbance values of each group were measured at 570 nm. LDH levels were detected with an LDH Cytotoxicity Assay Kit, following the manufacturer's protocol. The absorbance was measured at 490 nm.

4.6. Histology and Immunofluorescence

The livers were harvested, fixed in 4% paraformaldehyde, and embedded in paraffin. Hematoxylin and eosin (H&E) staining was used to detect the degree of liver injury. For immunofluorescence staining, cells were fixed with 4% paraformaldehyde and washed with 0.01 M PBS three times, then treated with PBS containing 0.3% Triton-X-100 for 30 min. After blocking with 4% bovine serum albumin (BSA) for 1 h, an antibody against Nrf2 (1:100) was added and incubated overnight at 4 °C. The next day, cells were washed three times with 0.01 M PBS and incubated with Alexa Fluor 488-conjugated immunoglobulin G (IgG) (1:1000) for 2 h at room temperature. The nuclei were stained with DAPI. The images were finally captured with a laser confocal fluorescence microscope.

4.7. DHE Staining

Liver tissue was embedded in an optimal cutting temperature compound, performed on a frozen section. Approximately 6 μm thick sections were washed with 0.01 M PBS twice. DHE (2 μM/L) in hydroxyethyl piperazine ethanesulfonic acid (HEPES) buffer was added on the tissue and mixed well, and placed in the dark at 37 °C for 30 min, then washed with PBS three times. For HL-7702 cells, DHE was directly added into the medium, and the final concentration was 2 μM/L. After incubation in the dark for 30 min, the cells were washed with PBS. Laser confocal fluorescence microscopy was used to photograph the fluorescence intensity.

4.8. JC-1 Assay for Mitochondrial Membrane Potential (MMP)

MMP was measured by JC-1 staining. HL-7702 cells were seeded into 12-well plates at a density of 2×10^5 cells/well for 12 h. Subsequently, the cells were subjected to different dosages of fucoidan (25 or 100 μg/mL) for 4 h, followed by exposure to 20 mM APAP for 24 h. Next, the cells were washed with PBS and incubated with JC-1 (10 μg/mL) at 37 °C in the dark for 20 min. Photos were taken by a laser confocal fluorescence microscope.

4.9. Western Blot Analysis

Hepatic tissues and cells were homogenized and lysed in Radio Immunoprecipitation Assay (RIPA) Lysis buffer supplemented with phenylmethanesulfonyl fluoride (1:100) for 30 min on ice, and the protein concentration was determined using a bicinchoninic acid (BCA) kit (Haimen, China). Cytosolic and nuclear extracts were prepared with a commercially available kit (Beyotime Biotechnology, Haimen, China) in accordance with the manufacturer's instructions. Equal amounts of extracted protein (10–40 μg) were separated on 10% or 12% sodium dodecyl sulfate polyacrylamide gel electrophoresis (SDS-PAGE), and proteins were transferred to a polyvinylidene fluoride (PVDF) membrane and blocked with tris-buffered saline and Tween 20 (TBST) containing 5% nonfat milk for 2 h at room temperature. Subsequently, the membranes were incubated overnight at 4 °C with primary antibodies and incubated with secondary antibodies for 2 h at room temperature. The relative protein levels were calculated by quantification of band intensity with a Bio-red imaging system (Bio-red, Berkeley, CA, USA).

4.10. Statistical Analysis

Data are represented as mean ± SD. Statistical differences were assessed by one-way ANOVA analysis of Tukey's multiple comparison test using GraphPad Prism 7.0 software (San Giego, CA, USA), and $p < 0.05$ was considered statistically significant.

Author Contributions: Y.W., J.G., and W.Z. conceived and designed the experiments; Y.W. and J.W. performed the experiments; M.T. contributed analysis tools; Y.W. and W.Z. wrote the paper; J.G. contributed to the improvement of the writing. All authors reviewed and approved the contents of the manuscript.

Funding: This work was supported by grants from the National Natural Science Foundation of China (31500649, 31670807), grants from the Natural Science Foundation of Nantong City (MS12015101), and the Nantong University Cooperative Innovation Program of Small Molecular Compound R&D-NTU2016-1.

Conflicts of Interest: The authors declare no conflicts of interest.

Abbreviations

APAP	acetaminophen
ALT	alanine aminotransferase
AST	aspartate aminotransferase
ROS	reactive oxygen species
MDA	malondialdehyde
SOD	superoxide dismutase

GSH	glutathione
CAT	catalase
MMP	mitochondrial membrane potential
NAQPI	*N*-acetyl-q-benzoquinoneimine
JNK	c-Jun N-terminal protein kinases
Nrf2	nuclear factor-erythroid 2-related factor 2
NAC	*N*-acetylcysteine
ASK1	apoptosis signal-regulating kinase 1
DHE	dihydroethidium

References

1. Chen, X.; Zhang, J.; Yi, R.; Mu, J.; Zhao, X.; Yang, Z. Hepatoprotective Effects of Lactobacillus on Carbon Tetrachloride-Induced Acute Liver Injury in Mice. *Int. J. Mol. Sci.* **2018**, *19*, 2212. [CrossRef] [PubMed]
2. Wang, F.; Liu, J.C.; Zhou, R.J.; Zhao, X.; Liu, M.; Ye, H.; Xie, M.L. Apigenin protects against alcohol-induced liver injury in mice by regulating hepatic CYP2E1-mediated oxidative stress and PPARalpha-mediated lipogenic gene expression. *Chem. Biol. Interact.* **2017**, *275*, 171–177. [CrossRef] [PubMed]
3. Gong, S.; Lan, T.; Zeng, L.; Luo, H.; Yang, X.; Li, N.; Chen, X.; Liu, Z.; Li, R.; Win, S. Gut microbiota mediates diurnal variation of acetaminophen induced acute liver injury in mice. *J. Hepatol.* **2018**, *69*, 51–59. [CrossRef]
4. McGill, M.R.; Sharpe, M.R.; Williams, C.D.; Taha, M.; Curry, S.C.; Jaeschke, H. The mechanism underlying acetaminophen-induced hepatotoxicity in humans and mice involves mitochondrial damage and nuclear DNA fragmentation. *J. Clin. Investig.* **2012**, *122*, 1574–1583. [CrossRef] [PubMed]
5. Reid, A.B.; Kurten, R.C.; McCullough, S.S.; Brock, R.W.; Hinson, J.A. Mechanisms of acetaminophen-induced hepatotoxicity: Role of oxidative stress and mitochondrial permeability transition in freshly isolated mouse hepatocytes. *J. Pharmacol. Exp. Ther.* **2005**, *312*, 509–516. [CrossRef] [PubMed]
6. Lv, H.; Xiao, Q.; Zhou, J.; Feng, H.; Liu, G.; Ci, X. Licochalcone A Upregulates Nrf2 Antioxidant Pathway and Thereby Alleviates Acetaminophen-Induced Hepatotoxicity. *Front. Pharmacol.* **2018**, *9*, 147. [CrossRef] [PubMed]
7. Huo, Y.; Yin, S.; Yan, M.; Win, S.; Aung-Than, T.; Aghajan, M.; Hu, H.; Kaplowitz, N. Protective role of p53 in acetaminophen hepatotoxicity. *Free Radic. Biol. Med.* **2017**, *106*, 111–117. [CrossRef]
8. Kumar, H.; Kim, I.S.; More, S.V.; Kim, B.W.; Choi, D.K. Natural product-derived pharmacological modulators of Nrf2/ARE pathway for chronic diseases. *Nat. Prod. Rep.* **2014**, *31*, 109–139. [CrossRef]
9. Enomoto, A.; Itoh, K.; Nagayoshi, E.; Haruta, J.; Kimura, T.; O'Connor, T.; Harada, T.; Yamamoto, M. High sensitivity of Nrf2 knockout mice to acetaminophen hepatotoxicity associated with decreased expression of ARE-regulated drug metabolizing enzymes and antioxidant genes. *Toxicol. Sci.* **2001**, *59*, 169–177. [CrossRef]
10. Sandberg, M.; Patil, J.; D'Angelo, B.; Weber, S.G.; Mallard, C. NRF2-regulation in brain health and disease: Implication of cerebral inflammation. *Neuropharmacology* **2014**, *79*, 298–306. [CrossRef]
11. Gunawan, B.K.; Liu, Z.X.; Han, D.; Hanawa, N.; Gaarde, W.A.; Kaplowitz, N. c-Jun N-terminal kinase plays a major role in murine acetaminophen hepatotoxicity. *Gastroenterology* **2006**, *131*, 165–178. [CrossRef] [PubMed]
12. Du, K.; Ramachandran, A.; Jaeschke, H. Oxidative stress during acetaminophen hepatotoxicity: Sources, pathophysiological role and therapeutic potential. *Redox. Biol.* **2016**, *10*, 148–156. [CrossRef] [PubMed]
13. Whyte, A.J.; Kehrl, T.; Brooks, D.E.; Katz, K.D.; Sokolowski, D. Safety and effectiveness of acetadote for acetaminophen toxicity. *J. Emerg. Med.* **2010**, *39*, 607–611. [CrossRef] [PubMed]
14. Catarino, M.D.; Silva, A.M.S.; Cardoso, S.M. Phycochemical Constituents and Biological Activities of Fucus spp. *Mar. Drugs* **2018**, *16*, 249. [CrossRef] [PubMed]
15. Hong, S.W.; Lee, H.S.; Jung, K.H.; Lee, H.; Hong, S.S. Protective effect of fucoidan against acetaminophen-induced liver injury. *Arch. Pharm. Res.* **2012**, *35*, 1099–1105. [CrossRef] [PubMed]
16. Dai, H.J.; Li, D.W.; Wang, Y.X.; Sun, A.J.; Lu, Y.X.; Ding, X.; Zhang, M.; Song, Y.G.; Huang, X.D. Induction of heat shock protein 27 by bicyclol attenuates d-galactosamine/lipopolysaccharide-induced liver injury. *Eur. J. Pharmacol.* **2016**, *791*, 482–490. [CrossRef] [PubMed]
17. Yu, H.Y.; Wang, B.L.; Zhao, J.; Yao, X.M.; Gu, Y.; Li, Y. Protective effect of bicyclol on tetracycline-induced fatty liver in mice. *Toxicology* **2009**, *261*, 112–118. [CrossRef]

18. Luo, L.; Xi, C.; Xu, T.; Zhang, G.; Qun, E.; Zhang, W. Muscarinic receptor mediated signaling pathways in hepatocytes from CCL_4—Induced liver fibrotic rat. *Eur. J. Pharmacol.* **2017**, *807*, 109–116. [CrossRef]
19. Luo, L.; Xu, T.; Wang, P.; Mao, L.; Xi, C.; Huang, J.; Zhang, W. Expression of muscarinic acetylcholine receptors in hepatocytes from rat fibrotic liver. *Exp. Toxicol. Pathol.* **2017**, *69*, 73–81. [CrossRef]
20. Ramachandran, A.; Jaeschke, H. Oxidative Stress and Acute Hepatic Injury. *Curr. Opin. Toxicol.* **2018**, *7*, 17–21. [CrossRef]
21. Zhang, J.; Yang, A.; Wu, Y.; Guan, W.; Xiong, B.; Peng, X.; Wei, X.; Chen, C.; Liu, Z. Stachydrine ameliorates carbon tetrachloride-induced hepatic fibrosis by inhibiting inflammation, oxidative stress and regulating MMPs/TIMPs system in rats. *Biomed. Pharmacother.* **2018**, *97*, 1586–1594. [CrossRef] [PubMed]
22. Lu, Y.; Zhang, R.; Liu, S.; Zhao, Y.; Gao, J.; Zhu, L. ZT-25, a new vacuolar H(+)-ATPase inhibitor, induces apoptosis and protective autophagy through ROS generation in HepG2 cells. *Eur. J. Pharmacol.* **2016**, *771*, 130–138. [CrossRef] [PubMed]
23. Saito, C.; Lemasters, J.J.; Jaeschke, H. c-Jun N-terminal kinase modulates oxidant stress and peroxynitrite formation independent of inducible nitric oxide synthase in acetaminophen hepatotoxicity. *Toxicol. Appl. Pharmacol.* **2010**, *246*, 8–17. [CrossRef] [PubMed]
24. Adams, J.M.; Cory, S. The Bcl-2 apoptotic switch in cancer development and therapy. *Oncogene* **2007**, *26*, 1324–1337. [CrossRef] [PubMed]
25. Roh, T.; De, U.; Lim, S.K.; Kim, M.K.; Choi, S.M.; Lim, D.S.; Yoon, S.; Kacew, S.; Kim, H.S.; Lee, B.M. Detoxifying effect of pyridoxine on acetaminophen-induced hepatotoxicity via suppressing oxidative stress injury. *Food Chem. Toxicol.* **2018**, *114*, 11–22. [CrossRef] [PubMed]
26. Yan, X.T.; Sun, Y.S.; Ren, S.; Zhao, L.C.; Liu, W.C.; Chen, C.; Wang, Z.; Li, W. Dietary alpha-Mangostin Provides Protective Effects against Acetaminophen-Induced Hepatotoxicity in Mice via Akt/mTOR-Mediated Inhibition of Autophagy and Apoptosis. *Int. J. Mol. Sci.* **2018**, *19*, 1335. [CrossRef] [PubMed]
27. Bajt, M.L.; Farhood, A.; Lemasters, J.J.; Jaeschke, H. Mitochondrial bax translocation accelerates DNA fragmentation and cell necrosis in a murine model of acetaminophen hepatotoxicity. *J. Pharmacol. Exp. Ther.* **2008**, *324*, 8–14. [CrossRef] [PubMed]
28. Jaeschke, H.; Duan, L.; Akakpo, J.Y.; Farhood, A.; Ramachandran, A. The role of apoptosis in acetaminophen hepatotoxicity. *Food Chem. Toxicol.* **2018**, *118*, 709–718. [CrossRef]
29. Davis, R.J. Signal transduction by the JNK group of MAP kinases. *Cell* **2000**, *103*, 239–252. [CrossRef]
30. Wu, G.; Fang, Y.Z.; Yang, S.; Lupton, J.R.; Turner, N.D. Glutathione metabolism and its implications for health. *J. Nutr.* **2004**, *134*, 489–492. [CrossRef]
31. Fitton, J.H.; Stringer, D.N.; Karpiniec, S.S. Therapies from Fucoidan: An Update. *Mar. Drugs* **2015**, *13*, 5920–5946. [CrossRef] [PubMed]
32. Sanjeewa, K.K.A.; Lee, J.S.; Kim, W.S.; Jeon, Y.J. The potential of brown-algae polysaccharides for the development of anticancer agents: An update on anticancer effects reported for fucoidan and laminaran. *Carbohydr. Polym.* **2017**, *177*, 451–459. [CrossRef] [PubMed]
33. Li, J.; Zhang, Q.; Li, S.; Dai, W.; Feng, J.; Wu, L.; Liu, T.; Chen, K.; Xia, Y.; Lu, J. The natural product fucoidan ameliorates hepatic ischemia-reperfusion injury in mice. *Biomed. Pharmacother.* **2017**, *94*, 687–696. [CrossRef]
34. Liu, S.; Wang, Q.; Song, Y.; He, Y.; Ren, D.; Cong, H.; Wu, L. Studies on the hepatoprotective effect of fucoidans from brown algae Kjellmaniella crassifolia. *Carbohydr. Polym.* **2018**, *193*, 298–306. [CrossRef] [PubMed]
35. Han, M.; Liu, X.; Liu, S.; Su, G.; Fan, X.; Chen, J.; Yuan, Q.; Xu, G. 2,3,7,8-Tetrachlorodibenzo-p-dioxin (TCDD) induces hepatic stellate cell (HSC) activation and liver fibrosis in C57BL6 mouse via activating Akt and NF-kappaB signaling pathways. *Toxicol. Lett.* **2017**, *273*, 10–19. [CrossRef] [PubMed]
36. Wang, Y.; Jiang, Y.; Fan, X.; Tan, H.; Zeng, H.; Wang, Y.; Chen, P.; Huang, M.; Bi, H. Hepato-protective effect of resveratrol against acetaminophen-induced liver injury is associated with inhibition of CYP-mediated bioactivation and regulation of SIRT1-p53 signaling pathways. *Toxicol. Lett.* **2015**, *236*, 82–89. [CrossRef] [PubMed]
37. Nagai, H.; Noguchi, T.; Takeda, K.; Ichijo, H. Pathophysiological roles of ASK1-MAP kinase signaling pathways. *J. Biochem. Mol. Biol.* **2007**, *40*, 1–6. [CrossRef] [PubMed]

38. Nakagawa, H.; Maeda, S.; Hikiba, Y.; Ohmae, T.; Shibata, W.; Yanai, A.; Sakamoto, K.; Ogura, K.; Noguchi, T.; Karin, M. Deletion of apoptosis signal-regulating kinase 1 attenuates acetaminophen-induced liver injury by inhibiting c-Jun N-terminal kinase activation. *Gastroenterology* **2008**, *135*, 1311–1321. [CrossRef]
39. Motohashi, H.; Yamamoto, M. Nrf2-Keap1 defines a physiologically important stress response mechanism. *Trends Mol. Med.* **2004**, *10*, 549–557. [CrossRef]
40. Gum, S.I.; Cho, M.K. Recent updates on acetaminophen hepatotoxicity: The role of nrf2 in hepatoprotection. *Toxicol. Res.* **2013**, *29*, 165–172. [CrossRef]
41. Ni, H.M.; McGill, M.R.; Chao, X.; Du, K.; Williams, J.A.; Xie, Y.; Jaeschke, H.; Ding, W.X. Removal of acetaminophen protein adducts by autophagy protects against acetaminophen-induced liver injury in mice. *J. Hepatol.* **2016**, *65*, 354–362. [CrossRef] [PubMed]

International Journal of *Molecular Sciences*

MDPI

Article

Defined Small Molecules Produced by Himalayan Medicinal Plants Display Immunomodulatory Properties

Phurpa Wangchuk [1,*,†], Simon H. Apte [2,†], Michael J. Smout [1], Penny L. Groves [2], Alex Loukas [1,‡] and Denise L. Doolan [1,‡]

1 Centre for Molecular Therapeutics, Australian Institute of Tropical Health and Medicine, James Cook University, Cairns, QLD 4878, Australia; michael.smout@jcu.edu.au (M.J.S.); alex.loukas@jcu.edu.au (A.L.); denise.doolan@jcu.edu.au (D.L.D.)

2 QIMR Berghofer Medical Research Institute, Brisbane, QLD 4006, Australia; Simon.Apte@health.qld.gov.au (S.H.A.); Penny.Groves@qimrberghofer.edu.au (P.L.G.)

* Correspondence: phurpa.wangchuk@jcu.edu.au; Tel.: +61-07-4232-21249

† These authors contributed equally as first authors to this work.

‡ These authors contributed equally as senior authors to this work.

Received: 20 September 2018; Accepted: 1 November 2018; Published: 6 November 2018

Abstract: Plant-derived compounds that modulate the immune responses are emerging as frontline treatment agents for cancer, infectious diseases and autoimmunity. Herein we have isolated 40 phytochemicals from five Bhutanese *Sowa Rigpa* medicinal plants—*Aconitum laciniatum*, *Ajania nubegina*, *Corydalis crispa*, *Corydalis dubia* and *Pleurospermum amabile*—and tested 14 purified compounds for their immunomodulatory properties using a murine dendritic cell (DC) line, and cytotoxicity against a human cholangiocyte cell line using xCELLigence real time cell monitoring. These compounds were: pseudaconitine, 14-veratryolpseudaconitine, 14-*O*-acetylneoline, linalool oxide acetate, (*E*)-spiroether, luteolin, luteolin-7-*O*-β-D-glucopyranoside, protopine, ochrobirine, scoulerine, capnoidine, isomyristicin, bergapten, and isoimperatorin. Of the 14 compounds tested here, scoulerine had adjuvant-like properties and strongly upregulated *MHC-I* gene and protein expression whereas bergapten displayed immunosuppressive properties and strongly down-regulated gene and protein expression of MHC-I and other co-stimulatory molecules. Both scoulerine and bergapten showed low cytotoxicity against normal healthy cells that were consistent with their immunoregulatory properties. These findings highlight the breadth of immunomodulatory properties of defined compounds from Bhutanese medicinal plants and show that some of these compounds exert their mechanisms of action by modulating DC activity.

Keywords: medicinal plants; phytochemicals; scoulerine; bergapten; immunomodulator; adjuvant; cytoxicity; dendritic cells; immune modulation

---

1. Introduction

The role of plants in preventing and healing ailments has been known since antiquity. Plant-derived natural products are used in both modern and traditional medicines for treating various diseases including but not limited to cancer, malaria, cardiovascular and Alzheimer's diseases [1–3]. The earliest records show that Mesopotamians (2600 B.C.) used *Cupressus* and *Commiphora* species for treating coughs, colds and inflammation, and the plants are still used to this day for treating the same conditions. Ancient Egyptians (*Ebers Papyrus*), Chinese (*Huangdi Neijing*), Indians (*Ayurvedic*), Greeks (*Hippocratic-Galenic*), Romans (*Greco-Roman*), Arabs (*Unani-Tibb*), and Bhutanese (*Sowa Rigpa*) used plants in crude forms as traditional medicines, home remedies, potions and oils [2]. These crude drugs or crude extracts from plants contain many complex compounds with therapeutic properties. For example, the crude bark extract from cinchona tree was used for treating malaria since 1632 and later in 1820, a pure antimalarial compound (quinine) was isolated, which marked the first successful use of a chemical compound in modern medicine to treat infectious diseases [4]. In 1897, aspirin was first manufactured as a synthetic analogue of salicylic acid that was isolated from a willow tree [5], paving the way to the now multi-billion dollar synthetic pharmaceutical industry.

Recent advances in natural product chemistry, spectroscopic and bioscreening technologies have reinvigorated the use of natural products for human health. Today, both naturally-derived and chemically synthesized drugs are used with a tremendous impact on disease prevention and treatment, resulting in the saving of countless lives. Overall, of the 1184 drugs/leads or new chemical entities approved by the U.S Food and Drug Administration between 1981 and 2006, 52% were natural products and their derivatives, and only 30% were of synthetic origin [6]. Moreover, about 11% of the 252 essential drugs currently listed by the World Health Organization (WHO) are exclusively of plant origin, and 80% of those plant-derived drugs were discovered from medicinal plants used in traditional herbal medicines [7]. Some drugs were discovered using biorational strategy, which exploits the knowledge that plants produce various secondary metabolites in response to injury or attack (e.g., by pathogenic bacteria or fungi). With innovation in bioassay screening tools and life science robotic technologies, it is estimated that the global market for plant-derived drugs will grow from $29.4 billion in 2017 to around $39.6 billion by 2022 [8].

Currently, natural products with immune modulating activities are emerging as frontline treatment agents for cancer, infectious diseases and autoimmunity [9]. Of particular interest in immunomodulation is the effect of compounds on dendritic cells (DCs) activity. DCs provide a link between the innate and the adaptive immune responses and are key orchestrators of the adaptive immune response [9,10]. DCs can be subdivided into interferon-producing plasmacytoid (pDC), monocyte-derived (MoDC), and classical/conventional dendritic cell (cDC), which in mice have been further classified into two major subsets as cDC 1 and cDC2 [11]. While cDC1 is specialized in cross-presentation of $CD8^+$ T cells that are critical for immunity against intracellular pathogens, viruses and cancer [12], cDC2 promotes $CD4^+$ T cell differentiation into subsets specializing in antiviral, antifungal or helminth immunity [13]. cDC subset composition in humans depends on the lymph node tissue site with lung-draining lymph nodes (LN) having the highest proportion of mature DC compared to other LN sites, and cDC2 subset exhibits predominant maturation phenotypes within LNs compared to cDC1 [14]. Human $CD141^+$ and $CD1c^+$ cDCs (originally identified in blood) have been ontogenetically aligned to mouse cDC1 and cDC2, respectively [15]. These cDCs have the capacity to acquire antigens in peripheral tissues, deliver them to draining LNs, and undergo maturation through upregulation of major histocompatibility (MHC) and co-stimulatory molecules which are required for T cell activation [14,16].

To become properly activated, T cells require two signals including antigen presentation and costimulatory signals. Antigen presentation requires MHC-I and MHC-II expression on the DC for $CD8^+$ T cell and $CD4^+$ T cell recognition, respectively. The costimulatory signals are provided by the DC to the T cells such as those mediated by CD80, CD86 and CD28. Compounds that can stimulate DCs to upregulate these molecules have therapeutic potential as they can strongly enhance T cell responses and may make good vaccine adjuvants or immunostimulators. Conversely, compounds that can downregulate DC function may be useful to induce immune tolerance and have therapeutic value for treating autoimmune diseases, allergies and to promote transplant tolerance. Several studies have shown that plant products or extracts can affect the behaviour of DCs [17]. For example, pine cone and *Echinacea pupurea* extracts have been demonstrated to modulate the expression of MHC and stimulatory and transmembrane molecules including MHC-II, CD86, and CD54 on DCs [18–20]. Purified secondary metabolites, such as resveratrol isolated from grapes and triptolide isolated from the Chinese medicinal plant *Tripterygium wilfordii* Hook F, have demonstrated suppression of DC maturation and inhibition of the expression of CD80 and CD86 [21,22]. Plant extracts and their secondary metabolites have also been shown to exhibit robust immunomodulatory effects on chronic neuro-inflammation and cognitive aging [23].

We have previously developed a novel high throughput DC-based assay to assess the ability of lipopeptide-based nano-vaccine constructs to modulate DC function [24]. This DC assay utilizes the DC2.4 cell line derived from mouse that is known to present exogenous antigen in the context of both MHC class I and MHC class II molecules and can cross-present antigen to $CD8^+$ T cells [25–27]. Herein we have applied this DC-based screening assay together with a cell-based cytotoxicity assay [28] to investigate the immunomodulatory and cytotoxic properties of plant compounds isolated from five Bhutanese medicinal plants: *Aconitum laciniatum*, *Ajania nubigena*, *Corydalis crispa*, *C. dubia* and *Pleurospermum amabile*. These five medicinal plants grow in an extreme climatic condition of the Himalayan alpine mountains of Bhutan at an altitude between 3900–4700 m above sea level and they are used in the scholarly Bhutanese *Sowa Rigpa* medicine (BSM) for treating various human health disorders (see Table 1 for individual plant uses) [29]. The BSM has been adapted from Tibetan medicine, which is currently practiced worldwide including Nepal, India, China, Mongolia, Russia, Europe and North America [30]. The plants flower between June–September and that is when the farmers collect them from their natural habitat. The plants are either sun-dried or shade-dried before preparing them into multi-ingredient dosage formulations as powders, capsules, tablets, pills, syrup and ointments.

2. Results

2.1. Medicinal Plants, Isolated Phytochemicals and Selected Compounds for In Vitro Assay

Five medicinal plants: *A. laciniatum*, *A. nubigena*, *C. crispa*, *C. dubia*, and *P. amabile* were collected for their roots, aerial parts and whole plant materials from the high altitude Himalayan alpine mountains of Bhutan (3500–4900 m above sea level). These plants were air-dried, sliced, and extracted using methanol/ethanol, and then subjected to repeated column and preparative thin layer chromatography separations. In total, we isolated 40 compounds belonging to alkaloids, flavonoids, terpenoids, phenylpropanoids and furanocoumarins [31–35]. The plant parts used in the Bhutanese medicine, the parts collected for this study, total number of phytochemicals isolated from each plant, the major classes of phytochemicals of isolated compounds, and the phytochemicals selected for the immunoregulatory and cytotoxicity studies are provided in Table 1. Of the 40 isolated compounds, 14 of them including pseudaconitine (**1**), 14-veratryolpseudaconitine (**2**), 14-*O*-acetylneoline (**3**), linalool oxide acetate (**4**), (*E*)-spiroether (**5**), luteolin (**6**), luteolin-7-*O*-β-D-glucopyranoside (**7**), protopine (**8**), ochrobirine (**9**), scoulerine (**10**), capnoidine (**11**), isomyristicin (**12**), bergapten (**13**), and isoimperatorin (**14**) (Figure 1) were obtained in quantities sufficient for bioactivity screening. Compounds **1–3** belong to the phytochemical class of C_{19}-diterpenoid alkaloids. Compounds **4–7** belong to the phytochemical classes of terpenoids and flavonoids. Compounds **8–11** belong to benzylisoquinoline type of alkaloids. Compounds **12–14** belong to the phytochemical classes of phenylpropanoids and furanocoumarins. Their purity was determined by GC-MS and NMR (data on each compound is given in Section 4).

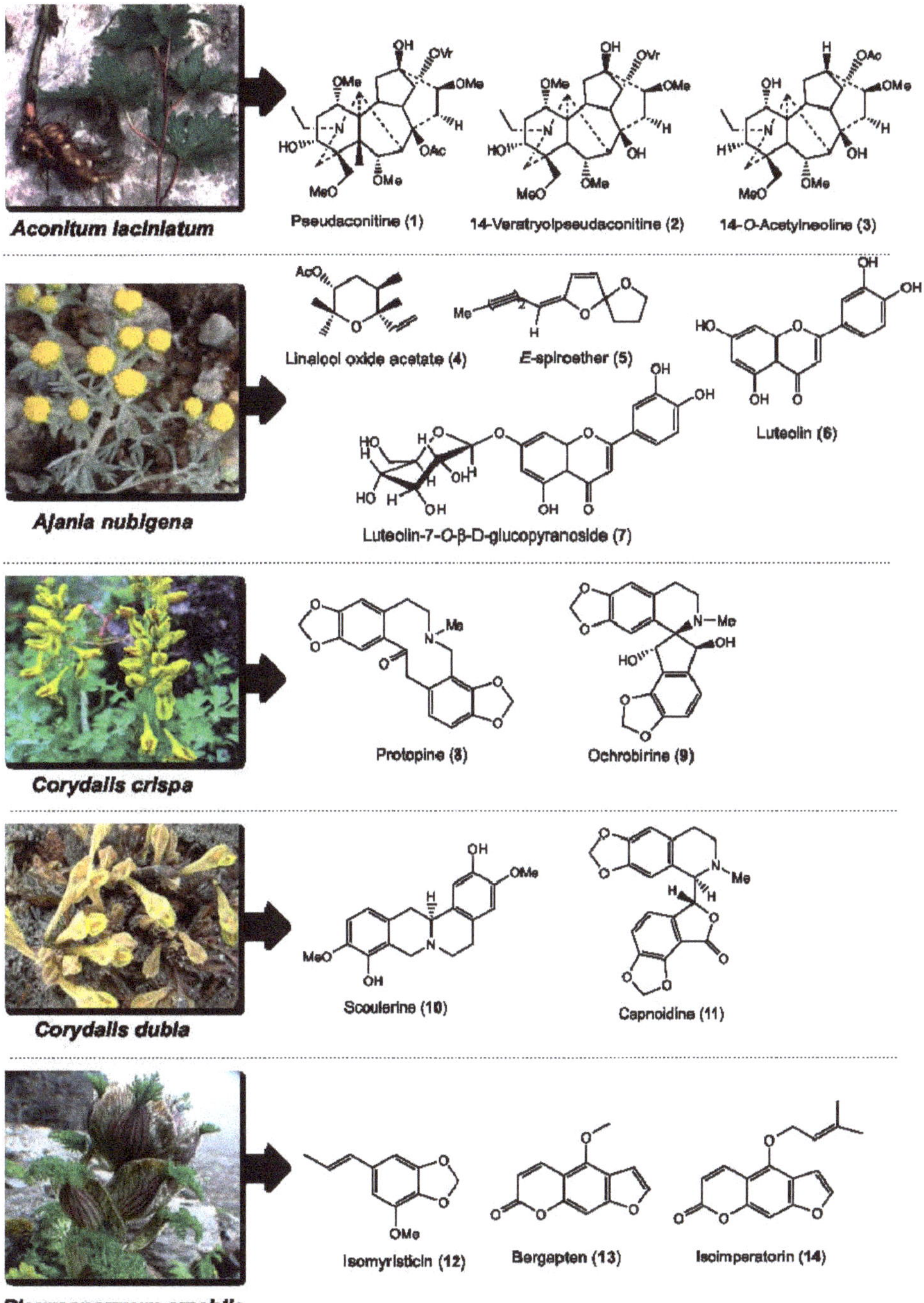

Figure 1. Structures of the compounds isolated from five Bhutanese medicinal plants using methods described by us previously [31–35], which were tested for their immunomodulatory and cytotoxic activities. Representative plant photos of *Aconitum laciniatum*, *Ajania nubigena*, *Corydalis crispa*, *C. dubia*, and *Pleurospermum amabile* are shown.

Table 1. Five medicinal plants and the selected compounds screened for immunomodulatory bioactivity in DC2.4 murine dendritic cell line and cytotoxicity in immortalized non-cancerous H69 human cholangiocyte cell line.

Botanical Name	Voucher Specimen Number	Traditional Uses [36]	Parts Used	Total Compounds Isolated and the Weight Obtained [31–35]	Class of Phytochemical	Major Compounds Selected for DC and Cytotoxicity Assays
Aconitum laciniatum (Ranunculaceae)	93	Parasite infections, leprosy, bone diseases, mumps and gout	Tuber	Pseudaconitine (1.9 g), 14-veratroylpseudaconine (28.7 mg), 14-*O*-acetylneoline (46.9 mg), neoline (428.5 mg), senbusine A (13.8 mg)	Diterpenoid alkaloids	Pseudaconitine (**1**) 14-veratroylpseudaconine (**2**) 14-*O*-acetylneoline (**3**)
Ajania nubigena (Asteraceae)	73	Allays abscess, swelling, tumor, fever, coughs, epistaxis and kidney infection	Aerial	Linalool oxide acetate (1.2 g), chamazulene (2.6 mg), (*E*)-spiroether (87.0 mg), (*Z*)-spiroether (6.7 mg), *p*-hydroxyacetophenone (11.3 mg), oxyanin B (18.6 mg), luteolin (618.0 mg), luteolin-7-*O*-β-D-glucopyranoside (41.3 mg)	Terpenes and flavonoids	Linalool oxide acetate (**4**) (*E*)-spiroether (**5**) luteolin (**6**) luteolin-7-*O*-β-D-glucopyranoside (**7**)
Corydalis crispa (Fumariaceae)	78	Allays blood, liver and bile disorders, and febrifuge	Whole	Protopine (1 g), 13-oxoprotopine (17.6 mg), 13-oxocryptopine (4.5 mg), stylopine (5 mg), coreximine (1 mg), rheagenine (1 mg), ochrobirine (60.6 mg), sibiricine (0.8 mg), bicuculline (8 mg)	Isoquinoline alkaloids	Protopine (**8**) ochrobirine (**9**)
Corydalis dubia (Fumariaceae)	14	Allays neuralgia, tuberculosis, and blood, liver, heart, lung, pancreas and kidney infections	Whole	Dubiamine (6.9 mg), scoulerine (9.4 mg), cheilanthifoline (15.1 mg), protopine (160 g), capnoidine (80.3 mg), bicuculline (18.3 mg), corydecumbine (12.3 mg), hydrastine (1.3 mg)	Isoquinoline alkaloids	Scoulerine (**10**) capnoidine (**11**)
Pleurospermum amabile (Umbelliferae)	29	Anti-dote, febrifuge, and dyspepsia	Aerial	(*E*)-isomyristicin (185.3 mg), (*E*)-isoapiol (30.7 mg), methyl eugenol (44.7 mg), (*E*)-isoelemicin (3.4 mg), psoralen (23.8 mg), bergapten (2.5 g), isoimperatorin (143.1 mg), isopimpinellin (93.8 mg), oxypeucedanin hydrate (109.7 mg), oxypeucedanin methanolate (295.2 mg)	Phenylpropanoids and furanocoumarins	(*E*)-isomyristicin (**12**) bergapten (**13**) isoimperatorin (**14**)

2.2. Plant Compounds Showed Immunomodulatory Activities in Dendritic Cell (DC)-Based Immunoassay

To gain some insight into the immunomodulatory properties of the 14 selected plant compounds, we utilized a dendritic cell (DC)-based immunoassay [24]. Briefly, the 14 selected compounds were prepared in 2% DMSO in cell culture media with 5% FCS (final concentration of 1 mg/mL) and further titrated in cell culture media (6 mid-log dilutions starting) prior to incubation with DC2.4 cells overnight in 96-well plates. The following day, the cells were harvested and prepared for flow cytometric analysis using a panel of defined surface markers including MHC-I, MHC-II, CD40, CD44, CD80, CD86, and CD274 (PDL-1). Dead cells were excluded based on their uptake of a dead cell stain and the potent DC activator cholera toxin (CT) was included as a positive control [37]. In Figure 2A, representative FACS plots for MHC-I expression are shown for all compounds. Notably, the Median Fluorescence Intensity (MFI) showed that compound 13 (bergapten, MFI 304) induced down-regulation of surface MHC-I expression compared to the media only control (MFI 732); this contrasts with compound 10 (scoulerine), which induced an increase in MHC-I expression (MFI 1582). For all compounds and surface markers tested, we calculated the relative fluorescence intensity (RFI) by dividing the MFI of the test sample with the appropriate MFI of the media only control. We next determined the optimal concentration of the compounds by observing the maximal increase (or decrease) in protein expression; for example, for MHC-I, scoulerine (**10**) was maximal at the concentration of 31.6 µg/mL, whereas bergapten (**13**) was most active (with respect to downregulation of MHC-I) at the 100 µg/mL (Figure 2B, Table 2).

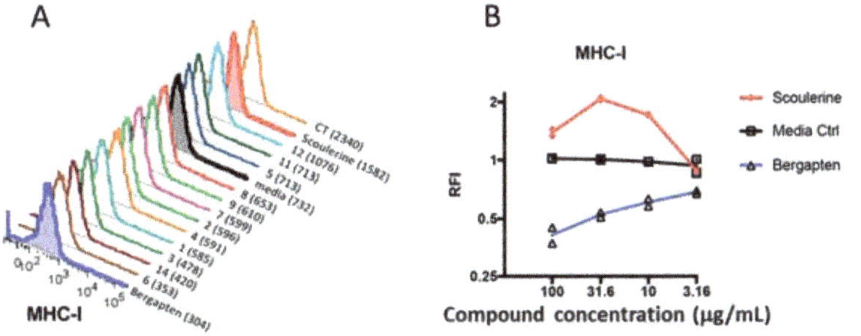

Figure 2. Modulation of immune molecule expression by plant compounds. (**A**) FACS plots showing the median fluorescence intensity (MFI) of MHC-I expression for all selected plant compounds, cells grown in media only, and a control grown with cholera toxin (CT). (**B**) The concentration at which each compound (scoulerine and bergapten) was most active was determined by titrating each compound (four mid-log dilutions starting at 100 µg/mL) and observing the maximal increase (or decrease) in expression of each fluorochrome (Table 2). Data for duplicate assays is presented. Media Ctrl = Media control.

Table 2. Immunomodulatory bioactivity of 14 plant compounds in DC2.4 dendritic cell line (FACS, PCR, SUM and Average).

Comp.	Conc. (μg/mL)	% Live Cell (FACS)	FACS								PCR								SUM FACS + PCR	Ave.
			MHC-I	MHC-II	CD40	CD44	CD80	CD86	CD274	SUM	MHC-I	MHC-II	CD40	CD44	CD80	CD86	CD274	SUM		
1	316.00	99.20	0.90	1.10	1.17	1.09	1.33	0.57	1.22	7.38	0.83	0.57	1.32	1.56	1.86	1.37	1.29	8.80	16.18	1.16
2	1000.00	94.20	0.88	2.60	3.15	0.92	2.64	0.59	3.56	14.34	1.08	0.39	1.04	0.58	1.79	1.87	1.61	8.37	22.71	1.62
3	1000.00	94.20	0.69	2.75	3.68	1.05	3.38	0.96	5.56	18.07	0.81	0.50	2.94	0.69	1.19	2.87	3.01	12.01	30.07	2.15
4	316.00	97.20	0.90	1.29	2.10	1.29	1.71	1.33	1.78	10.39	1.35	0.28	1.52	1.57	2.91	2.36	2.64	12.63	23.02	1.64
5	100.00	94.10	1.08	3.42	1.54	1.78	3.29	1.37	3.24	15.72	0.81	0.45	0.76	1.15	1.48	1.78	1.13	7.57	23.28	1.66
6	10.00	95.70	0.50	1.92	1.11	1.17	1.66	1.25	1.47	9.08	1.05	1.36	0.57	1.30	1.60	1.07	1.82	8.78	17.86	1.28
7	100.00	96.50	0.78	1.64	1.19	1.42	1.24	1.35	1.17	8.80	1.05	0.41	0.71	1.18	1.67	1.00	3.28	9.29	18.09	1.29
8	100.00	93.60	0.94	1.31	1.38	1.53	1.95	1.17	1.67	9.95	0.84	3.35	1.11	0.73	1.64	1.29	1.07	10.01	19.96	1.43
9	100.00	97.90	0.87	1.55	1.16	1.08	1.19	0.91	1.67	8.43	0.79	1.52	1.36	1.45	2.03	1.61	2.64	11.41	19.84	1.42
10	31.60	83.80	2.07	2.03	2.12	2.15	4.89	2.48	3.91	19.64	1.43	1.17	1.40	3.47	5.10	2.19	2.71	17.48	37.12	2.65
11	316.00	96.80	1.08	1.23	2.43	1.78	1.71	1.47	2.99	12.70	0.83	2.66	1.65	1.66	2.09	1.02	2.99	12.89	25.59	1.83
12	100.00	92.00	1.53	1.29	2.90	1.84	1.91	2.46	2.07	14.00	1.05	0.72	1.40	1.43	2.09	1.56	1.03	9.28	23.27	1.66
13	100.00	86.90	0.41	2.08	1.72	1.38	1.12	1.24	2.76	10.70	0.77	0.78	1.30	0.73	0.90	1.08	2.17	7.72	18.41	1.32
14	31.60	95.40	0.61	1.05	1.52	1.51	1.42	1.12	1.44	8.68	0.94	0.50	1.15	1.67	1.83	1.15	2.90	10.13	18.81	1.34
CT	1.00	92.70	2.56	2.32	0.88	1.15	8.25	2.65	3.86	21.67	1.04	0.34	0.31	1.11	6.00	4.32	4.54	17.66	39.33	2.81

Abbreviations: Comp. = Compounds, Conc. = Concentration, Ave. = Average, CT = Cholera toxin.

2.3. Modulation of Gene Expression by Plant Compounds

FACS-based assays give an excellent indication of protein expression, but they do not indicate whether gene expression has been modulated by the compound. Furthermore, possible aberrations associated with this particular case could include potential autofluorescence of the compound itself or cellular autofluorescence induced by the compound. Moreover, protein expression detected by FACS (and particularly surface expression) could be transiently modulated. Hence, measuring changes in gene expression is a very informative accompaniment to FACS-based assays. Accordingly, we co-cultured DC2.4 cells overnight with the most active concentration of the compound as determined above in the FACS-based assay (Table 2). The following day, cells were harvested and 20,000 live cells from each condition were sorted by FACS into RLT buffer and RNA extracted for mRNA analysis by RT-qPCR. The relative gene expression for each gene was calculated for each compound and compared to the media control. We then correlated gene expression with protein expression represented by the FACS RFI (Figure 3). This method allowed us to identify with confidence the compounds that upregulate expression of the genes of interest and the corresponding protein expression, which fall in the upper right quadrant of the mRNA gene expression versus FACS RFI plot. Conversely, compounds that down-regulate the gene and protein of interest fall in the lower left quadrant (Figure 3). The SUM of the changes for all genes and proteins relative to the media-only control is summarized in the bottom right corner of Figure 3 SUM.

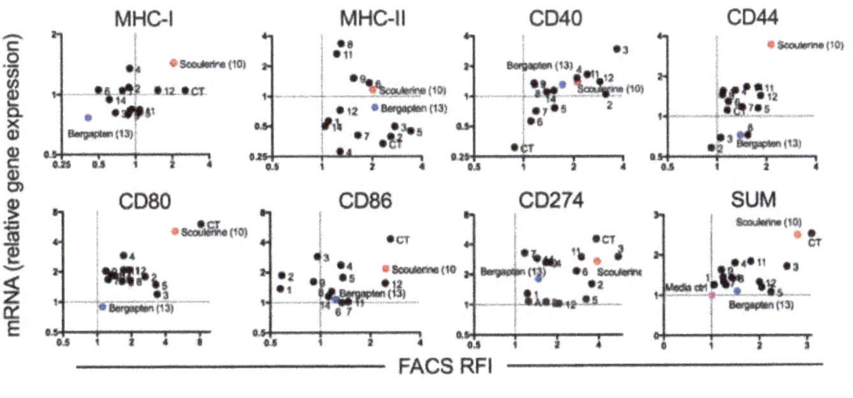

Figure 3. Correlation of modulation of mRNA and protein expression of immune molecules by plant compounds. The up-regulated and down-regulated gene expression induced by compounds falls in the upper right quadrant and the lower left quadrant, respectively. Scoulerine (**10**) and bergapten (**13**) are labeled red and blue circles, respectively. Other compounds tested are labeled as black circles. Culture media is labeled as a pink circle.

Of the 14 compounds tested, scoulerine (**10**) stands out as a strong up-regulator of several important genes including *MHC-I*, *CD80* and *CD86*, suggesting that this compound would make a good potential adjuvant for a CD8$^+$ T cell vaccine. Conversely, compound bergapten (**13**) is highlighted at the other end of the spectrum and it caused suppression of expression of some genes, and notably *MHC-I* at both the gene and protein level. Compound 14-*O*-acetylneoline (**3**) also showed moderate up-regulation of gene expression including *CD40* and *CD274* (*PDL-1*).

2.4. Cytotoxicity of Compounds with the Immortalized Non-Cancerous H69 Human Cholangiocyte Cell Line

Of the 14 compounds tested in the DC assay, 10 of them: linalool oxide acetate (**4**), (*E*)-spiroether (**5**), luteolin (**6**), luteolin-7-*O*-β-D-glucopyranoside (**7**), protopine (**8**), ochrobirine (**9**), capnoidine (**11**), isomyristicin (**12**), bergapten (**13**), and isoimperatorin (**14**), were tested for cytotoxicity against normal bile duct H69 cells using an xCELLigence SP system (ACEA Biosciences Inc., San Diego, CA, USA) as described previously [28]. Quantities of compounds **1**, **2**, **3** and **10** were not sufficient to allow for cytotoxicity testing. Amongst the 10 compounds tested, compound **5** (*E*)-spiroether was the most cytotoxic with almost complete (96.5%) cell death from 6 h with 100 μg/mL and an IC_{50} value that was not able to be calculated with the concentrations assessed (<<<1 μg/mL) (Figure 4). Compound **6** (luteolin) was also reasonably toxic from 6–24 h and showed a 24 h IC_{50} value of 30 μg/mL (95% confidence interval 19–38 μg/mL). Protopine (**8**) showed minor (23%) cell toxicity from 6 h but that increased to 68% at 24 h, generating a more potent but highly variable IC_{50} value of 9 μg/mL (95% confidence interval 1–52 μg/mL).

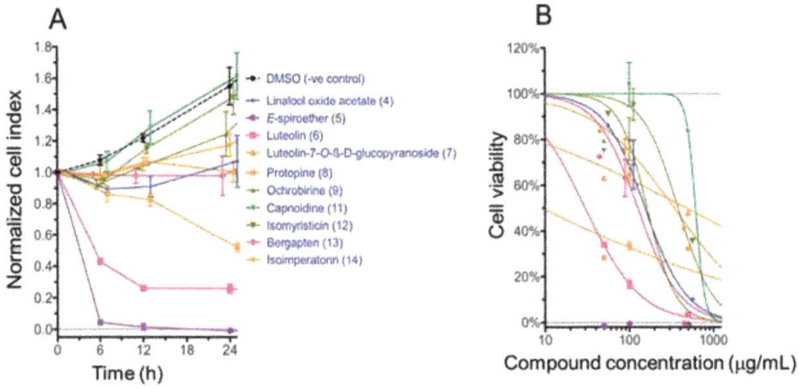

Figure 4. Cytotoxicity of selected plant compounds against immortalized H69 bile duct cells determined by xCELLigence system (ACEA Biosciences Inc.). (**A**) Cell toxicity over time as recorded by normalized cell index when treated with selected compounds. (**B**) Dose response toxicity curves at the 24 h time point show cell viability relative to the untreated control against concentration. Compounds **1–3** and **10** were not tested for cytotoxicity due to insufficient quantities available at the time of the study.

Compound bergapten (**13**) that demonstrated interesting immunomodulatory activity in the DC assay showed far less potent cytotoxicity with the IC_{50} value of 126.4 μg/mL (95% confidence interval 76–248 μg/mL). This was consistent with moderate up-regulation of CD274 (Figure 3), which is the marker for Programmed Death Ligand 1 (PD-L1) known to play a key role in suppressing the immune system. Compound **10**, although not tested in this H69 cell system, has been reported by others to exhibit significant cytotoxic activity against lung carcinoma (A549) and HT-29 cancer cell lines that arrest the proliferation of ovarian carcinoma (A2780) and breast adenocarcinoma (SK-B-3 and MCF-7) cells [38], consistent with its potential adjuvant properties indicated in the DC cell assay.

3. Discussion

Medicinal plants have been an important source of modern drugs for many centuries and are receiving increasing attention worldwide with advancement in drug discovery techniques and technologies [39]. Plants produce various secondary metabolites that belong to different major phytochemical classes including flavonoids, tannins, terpenoids, saponins, triterpenoid saponins, alkaloids, phytosterols, carotenoids, fatty acids and essential oils, which are used for their defense and protection against predators/herbivores. Some of these metabolites display immunomodulatory properties including immunosuppression, immunostimulation and tolerogenicity through dynamic regulation of the target immune systems [40]. While immunostimulators are typically used for remedying infections, immunodeficiency and cancers, immunosuppressants are often used in organ transplantation and for treating autoimmune diseases. Tolerogens on the other hand are known for making the immune system non-responsive to targets [9]. The use of plant-derived secondary metabolites as novel drugs and immunomodulatory agents is a rapidly growing field of investigation [9]. The main categories of plant-derived secondary metabolites which have been transformed into modern drugs include terpenes (34%), glycosides (32%), alkaloids (16%) and others (18%) [41]. These drugs were discovered mostly using three strategies: bio-rational, chemo-rational and random approaches. One promising avenue of the bio-rational approach is ethno-medically directed screening based on the observation of pest-plant analysis, plant characteristics and their ecological adaptations and functions [39]. Among these three search strategies, the ethno-directed bio-rational approach has been proven to offer a higher hit rate of biological activities owing to a long clinical history of medicinal plants use by humans for treating various disorders [42]. Such evidence supports the need to investigate medicinal plant compounds for their usefulness as immunomodulatory agents or immunotherapies.

In the present study, based on the above rationale, we selected five medicinal plants—*A. laciniatum*, *A. nubigena*, *C. crispa*, *C. dubia*, and *P. amabile*—which are used in the scholarly Bhutanese traditional medicines for treating various disorders including fever, inflammation, malaria, tumor, leprosy, gout, mumps, abscess, liver and heart infections (see Table 1 for individual plant uses) [36]. Our initial phytochemical investigation of these plants for major chemotypes showed that their content was primarily alkaloids, terpenoids, tannins, and saponins and that their crude extracts possess antimalarial, antiparasitic, anti-inflammatory and antimicrobial properties [29,36]. To follow up on these findings, we have isolated 40 compounds belonging to different chemotypes (Table 1) using column and preparative thin layer chromatography. Their structures were determined using GC-MS and NMR as described earlier [31–35]. Of these, 14 major compounds were evaluated here for cytotoxicity and immunomodulatory properties using the xCELLigence system and a DC-based immunoassay, respectively. This DC-based immunoassay is an unbiased functional screen and a highly sensitive, high throughput–compatible screening platform for the discovery of DC-targeted small molecule immunomodulators with clinical applicability. Most of the currently known DC-stimulatory agents have been identified by testing rationally selected compounds for their in vitro capacity to induce phenotypic and functional changes that would be expected to accompany DC maturation or by testing a limited array of natural products for their in vivo capacities to augment protective immune responses against cancer or infectious microbes [43]. In this study, we combined FACS-based analysis of immune molecule expression with PCR-based assessment of gene expression. We used this method as we believe concordance in immune molecule regulation at the protein and gene level provides confidence in the actions of the compounds. Perhaps not surprisingly, we noted some discord between the relative effects on gene and protein expression for some compounds [44]. This may be due to several factors, including temporal differences between gene expression and protein expression, or spatial differences such as intracellular protein expression that is not accessible to surface staining by antibodies.

Of the 14 compounds tested here, scoulerine (**10**) strongly up-regulated several important genes and proteins including *MHC-I*, *CD80* and *CD86*, suggesting that this compound would potentially make a good immunologic adjuvant for a $CD8^+$ T cell vaccine. Current vaccines intended for human use incorporate various adjuvants made from proteins, oligonucleotides, liposomes, complex natural products and drug-like small molecules [45]. Among the extant adjuvants, small molecule adjuvants (SMAs) are under-appreciated despite their versatile chemical structures and properties, which can be tailored to specific biological functions, targets and pathways. A review by Flower [45] described a number of SMAs derived from natural products as well as fully-synthetic drug-like molecules and identified as many as 15 natural products that SMAs isolated from plants, fungi, shark oil and marine bryozoans as peptides, lipids, triterpenes, glucosides, saponins, nucleotides, and macrolide lactones. For examples, QS-21 and Quil A are the purified saponin-based plant SMAs (derived from *Quillaja saponaria*) with defined mechanism of action, which are used as adjuvants in vaccines against HIV and cancer [46–48].

Since scoulerine (**10**) is an alkaloid, its mechanism of action may be novel and different to the saponin-based QS-21 and Quil A adjuvants, and therefore it merits further medicinal exploration. Scoulerine (**10**) has been reported from other plants including opium plant (*Croton flavens*) and other *Corydalis* species including *C. calliantha* and *C. cava* [49,50]. Notably, this compound possesses multiple important pharmacological properties. For example, it showed cytotoxicity against lung carcinoma (A549), ovarian carcinoma (A2780), breast adenocarcinoma (SK-B-3 and MCF-7) and gastrointestinal cancer cell lines [38]. It was identified as a potent antimalarial drug lead compound against multi-drug resistant *Plasmodium falciparum* [32]. This compound demonstrated antiemetic, antitussive, antibacterial, antimitotic, antiproliferative, proapoptotic and anti-Alzheimer's activities [50,51]. Scoulerine (**10**) also protects α-adrenoreceptors against irreversible blockades caused by phenoxybenzamine, inhibits [^{3}H]-inositol monophosphate formation caused by noradrenaline, acts as a selective α_{1D}-adrenoreceptor antagonist without affecting the aorta contraction, and it has an affinity for the GABA receptors [52]. With such a diversity of therapeutic properties, scoulerine (**10**) is worthy of further exploration either as an independent drug entity or as an immunomodulator/adjuvant to potentiate other drugs/vaccines, including cancer chemotherapy, malaria vaccine development and Alzheimer's disease.

At the other end of the spectrum, bergapten (**13**) consistently induced down-modulation of MHC-I and MH-II expression, indicative of anti-inflammatory and/or immunosuppressant activity while displaying low cytotoxicity. This compound belongs to the chemical class of furanocoumarins which are also produced by vegetables/herbs/fruits consumed by humans on a daily basis. Indeed, bergapten (**13**) has been used in the cosmetic and pharmaceutical industries for treating inflammatory skin diseases, such as atopic dermatitis, and pigment disorders like vitiligo and psoriasis, which is consistent with our findings about the ability of this compound to down-regulate DC activity [53–55]. In addition, bergapten (**13**) has demonstrated anti-proliferative activity in vitro against HL60 and A431 epithelial cancer cell lines [56] as well as human hepatocellular carcinoma cell line [57]. These reported activities are consistent with the immunosuppressive activity identified herein. To the best of our knowledge, the specific mechanism of action for DC-driven immunomodulation by these two compounds remains unreported. However, Habartova et al. [38] showed that the potent antiproliferative and pro-apoptotic function of scoulerine (**10**) in cancer cells occurs through its action to interfere with the microtubule elements of the cytoskeleton, checkpoint kinase signaling and p53 proteins. The mechanism of action of bergapten (**13**) against breast cancer cells has been illustrated by de Amicis et al. [58], which indicated that this compound drives autophagy through the upregulation of the oncosuppressor gene—phosphatase tension homologue (PTEN) expression.

With such a diversity of therapeutic properties, scoulerine (**10**) and bergapten (**13**) are worthy of further exploration either as an independent drug entity or as an immunomodulator/adjuvant to potentiate other drugs/vaccines, including cancer chemotherapy, malaria vaccines and Alzheimer's disease. For a natural product-based drug discovery, isolating and obtaining enough quantities of the lead compound from natural sources is a big challenge and this has been identified as the bottleneck for advanced large-scale medicinal experimentations including lead optimization, pharmacokinetics and clinical trials. While the lead optimization comprises analogue development, total synthesis, rational drug design and quantitative structure-activity relationship (QSAR); the pharmacokinetics studies include adsorption, distribution, metabolism, excretion and toxicity (ADMET) evaluations. Pharmacodynamics study, which is seldom grouped with pharmacokinetics, provides information on what the drug does to the body and would include dosage formulations. All these drug development studies require large supplies of the drug lead compound and therefore laboratory synthesis of such a compound is very critical. Total synthesis or analogue development of the lead compound could take a synthetic chemist between 1–4 years depending upon the nature and the complexity of the structures. Synthetic chemistry of natural products is often plagued by low success rate of compound synthesis. Even if the compound is successfully synthesized, the synthetic steps may be lengthy, expensive or may afford minute amounts only. Interestingly, both scoulerine (**10**) and bergapten (**13**) had been successfully and efficiently synthesized in the laboratory using a biocatalytic synthetic method and the photochemical aromatic annulation strategy, respectively [59,60]. These make the two new drug lead compounds even more appealing for drug development.

4. Materials and Methods

4.1. Collection and Extraction of Medicinal Plants

As described previously [31–35], we have selected five medicinal plants for this study and their traditional uses are provided in Table 1. The root of *A. laciniatum* (Ranunculaceae) was collected from the opposite site of Lingshi Makhang (altitude: 4183 m; latitude: 27°50′29.9″; longitude: 89°25′41.5″; global positioning system point number (GPSPN): 138; site number: P138; Slope: 25°; aspect: North-East) and was assigned herbarium voucher specimen number (HVSN) 93. The aerial components of *A. nubegina* (Compositae) were collected from Lingzhi and were assigned as HVSN 73. The whole plant of *C. crispa* (Fumariaceae) was collected from Thuphu (altitude: 3962 m; latitude: 27°51′15.4″; longitude: 89°27′12.8″; GPSPN: 187; site number: P187; slope: 40°; aspect: South-East) and was assigned as HVSN 78. The whole plant of *C. dubia* (Fumariaceae) was collected from Thruenchela (altitude: 4651 m; latitude: 27°56′00.1″; longitude: 89°26′11.6″; GPSPN: 167; site number: P167; slope: 30°; aspect: North-West) and was assigned as HVSN 78. The aerial parts of *P. amabile* (Umbelliferae) were collected from Lingzhi (4200 m) and were assigned as HVSN 29. All herbarium specimens were deposited at the Pharmaceutical and Research Unit, Ministry of Health in Bhutan. The dried plant material (2 kg) was chopped and made into powder form and was repeatedly extracted with analytical grade or HPLC grade methanol (5 × 3 L over 48 h). The extract was filtered and then concentrated using a rotary evaporator at 35–50 °C to afford the crude methanol extract of each medicinal plant.

4.2. Isolation and Preparation of Compounds for In Vitro Screening Assays

Since the five target plants contain different phytochemicals, we used two main types of natural product isolation methods as described by us previously [39]. For alkaloid-containing medicinal plants including *A. laciniatum*, *C. crispa* and *C. dubia*, we first used an acid-base fraction method to obtain the total alkaloids present in their MeOH extracts. The MeOH extract of each plant was acidified with HCl (5%) and fractionated successively using hexane (5 × 60 mL) and CH_2Cl_2 (5 × 60 mL) to yield hexane and dichloromethane extracts, respectively. The aqueous solution was then basified (pH 9–11) with NH_4OH solution and fractionated with $CHCl_3$ (5 × 60 mL) to obtain a chloroform extract, which was rich in total alkaloids. Focusing on alkaloids, these $CHCl_3$ extracts were repeatedly separated using flash column chromatography (packed with Merck Kieselgel 60 PF254 (Merck, French Forest, Australia)) and pre-coated silica plates (0.2 mm silica thickness, Merck). Finally, a total of 22 pure alkaloids were obtained from *A. laciniatum*, *C. crispa* and *C. dubia* as amorphous solids or crystals [31,32,35]. Seven major alkaloids were selected for testing in the DC and cytotoxicity bioassays. Specifically, five alkaloids were isolated from *A. laciniatum*, and three of them were selected for bioactivity screening: pseudaconitine (**1**), 14-veratryolpseudaconitine (**2**) and 14-*O*-acetylneoline (**3**). From *C. crispa*, nine alkaloids were isolated and two major compounds—protopine (**8**) and ochrobirine (**9**)—were selected for bioactivity screening. Eight alkaloids were isolated from the related species, *C. dubia*, and two of them—scoulerine (**10**) and capnoidine (**11**)—were selected for DC and cytotoxicity studies.

For non-alkaloidal medicinal plants including *A. nubigena*, we used a solvent-based polarity fractionation method [33]. First, we fractionated the extract using hexane, followed by ethyl acetate, to yield hexane and ethyl acetate extracts, respectively. Repeated separation of ethyl acetate extract using column and preparative thin layer chromatography (Merck, Aluminium backing) resulted in the isolation of seven compounds (Table 1). Four of the seven compounds were selected for the bioactivity assays: linalool oxide acetate (**4**), (*E*)-spiroether (**5**), luteolin (**6**), and luteolin-7-*O*-β-D-glucopyranoside (**7**) (Figure 1). For the isolation of phenylpropanoids and furanocoumarins from *P. amabile*, as reported earlier [34], we dissolved the crude MeOH extract in MeOH/water (1:9) and first fractionated with hexane followed by petroleum spirit. The aqueous portion was acidified with HCl (5%), fractionated with CH_2Cl_2, basified with NH_4OH (at pH 9–12) and then finally fractionated with CH_2Cl_2 to generate the basified CH_2Cl_2 extract. This basified CH_2Cl_2 extract, upon repeated purification using the chromatographic methods described above, yielded 10 compounds (Table 1). Of these 10 compounds, three compounds—isomyristicin (**12**), bergapten (**13**), and isoimperatorin (**14**) (Figure 1)—were obtained in sufficient quantities to carry out the DC and cytotoxicity assays.

The instrumentation for phytochemical identification and structure elucidation were conducted as reported earlier by us [31–35]. Briefly, for determining physiochemical properties including melting point and optical rotation values, we used a Reichert hot-stage apparatus and a JASCO 2000 Series polarimeter, respectively. An average of 10 optical readings were taken to obtain the observed rotation value. For determining the functional group of a compound, we used a Smart Omni-Sampler Avator ESP Nicolet spectrometer. For obtaining the LR-ESI-MS mass and the LR-EI-MS mass of a compound, we used a Micromass Waters Platform LCZ (single quadrupole, MeOH as solvent) and a Shimadzu GCMS-QP-5050 (DI at 70 eV), respectively. A Micromass Waters Q-ToF Ultima (quadrupole time-of-flight) mass spectrometer was used for acquiring the HR-ESI-MS-based molecular formula. GC-MS used NIST and NISTREP mass spectra libraries of GC-MS data for comparing the mass spectra of the plant compounds. For obtaining NMR spectra (^{1}H-NMR, gCOSY, ^{13}C-NMR, APT, gHMBC, gHSQC, and gNOESY, deuterated solvents—CD_3OD or $CDCl_3$) and structure elucidation of a compound, we used a 500 MHz Varian Unity Inova, 500 MHz Varian Premium Shield (VNMRS PS 54), and 300 MHz Varian Mercury spectrometer.

Wherever crystals were obtained for a compound, crystal structures were determined using x-Ray crystallography (PLATON program). Hydrogen atoms were included at calculated positions and were initially refined to regularize their geometry (C–H in the range 0.93–0.98Å) and on U_{iso}(H) (in the range 1.2–1.5 times U_{eg} of the parent atom). Computing details include data collection: COLLECT; cell refinement and data reduction: DENZO/SCALEPACK; program (s) used to solve structure: USER DEFINED STRUCTURE SOLUTION; molecular graphics: ORTEP-II in TEXSAN; and program(s) used to refine structure and prepare material for publication: CRYSTALS [61]. The X-ray diffraction images were measured on a Nonius KappaCCD diffractometer (Mo $K\theta$ radiation, graphite monochromator, θ = 0.71073 Å), data were extracted using the DENZO package and by direct methods (SUPERFLIP, SIR92) [62]. The structures were refined using the CRYSTALS program package. Atomic coordinates, bond lengths and angles and displacement parameters have been deposited at the Cambridge Crystallographic Data Centre (CCDC no. 929725, 929726). These data can be obtained from https://www.ccdc.cam.ac.uk/ or by emailing data_request@ccdc.cam.ac.uk, or by contacting The Cambridge Crystallographic Data Centre, 12 Union Road, Cambridge CB2 1EZ, UK; Fax: +44-1223-336033.

Detailed characterization of each compound using the above equipment and techniques generated the data that shows the level of their purity and distinguishes them from each other as follows.

Pseudaconitine (**1**): Prismic crystals (1.9 g, from $CHCl_3$/MeOH, (1:1)). LR-ESI-MS (m/z): 690 [M + H$^+$]. LR-EI-MS (m/z): 689 [M$^+$], 675, 658, 642, 629, 614, 598, 585, 464, 432, 330, 266, 252, 236, 202, 182, 178, 165, 137, 86, 75, 58, 45. ^{1}H NMR (500 MHz, $CDCl_3$): δ 3.04–3.20 (1H, m, H-1), 1.95–2.11 (1H, m, H$_a$-2), 2.25–2.45 (1H, m, H$_b$-2), 3.79 (1H, m, H-3), 2.10–2.16 (1H, m, H-5), 4.03 (1H, d, J = 6.5 Hz, H-6), 2.90 (1H, m, H-7), 2.89–2.95 (1H, m, H-9), 2.10–2.15 (1H, m, H-10), 2.55–2.63 (2H, m, H-12), 4.87 (1H, d, J = 4.5 Hz, H-14), 2.40–2.55 (1H, m, H$_a$-15), 3.06–3.14 (1H, m, H$_b$-15), 3.38–3.41 (1H, t, J = 7.5, H-16), 3.02 (1H, br s, H-17), 3.51–3.53 (1H, m, H$_a$-18), 3.62–3.65 (1H, m, H$_b$-18), 2.25–2.45 (1H, m, H$_a$-19), 2.90–2.96 (1H, m, H$_b$-19), 2.35–2.60 (2H, m, H-20), 1.13 (3H, t, J = 7.0 Hz, 21-Me), 3.26 (3H, s, 1-OMe), 3.17 (3H, s, 6-OMe), 3.54 (3H, s, 16-OMe), 3.30 (3H, s, 18-OMe), 3.91 (3H, s, 3′-OMe), 3.94 (3H, s, 4′-OMe), 1.34 (3H, s, 8-OAc), 2.10 (1H, s, 3-OH), 3.85 (1H, s, 13-OH), 7.62 (1H, s, H-2′), 6.90 (1H, d, J = 8.5, H-5′), 7.70 (1H, d, J = 8.0, H-6′).

14-Veratroylpseudaconine (**2**): Amorphous white solid (28.7 mg). LR-ESI-MS (m/z): 648 [M + H$^+$]. LR-EI-MS (m/z): 647 [M$^+$], 631, 616, 599, 557, 435, 182, 165, 149, 125, 111, 97, 71, 57, 41. HR-ESI-MS (molecular formula): $C_{34}H_{49}NO_{11}$. ^{1}H NMR (500 MHz, $CDCl_3$): δ 3.13 (1H, dd, J = 6.5 Hz, H-1),

2.04–2.11 (1H, m, H_a-2), 2.26–2.46 (1H, m, H_b-2), 3.64–3.77 (1H, m, H-3), 2.04–2.11 (1H, m, H-5), 4.07 (1H, d, J = 6.5 Hz, H-6), 2.46–2.52 (1H, m, H-7), 2.52–2.57 (1H, m, H-9), 2.04–2.11 (1H, m, H-10), 2.03–2.11 (1H, m, H_a-12), 2.31–2.57 (1H, m, H_b-12), 5.12 (1H, d, J = 5.5 Hz, H-14), 2.27–2.41 (1H, m, H_a-15), 2.51–2.64 (1H, m, H_b-15), 3.33–3.38 (1H, m, H-16), 3.01 (1H, br s, H-17), 3.64–3.77 (2H, m, H-18), 2.43–2.45 (1H, m, H_a-19), 2.88–3.07 (1H, m, H_b-19), 2.39–2.57 (2H, m, H-20), 1.11 (3H, t, J = 7.0 Hz, 21-Me), 3.28 (3H, s, 1-OMe), 3.25 (3H, s, 6-OMe), 3.42 (3H, s, 16-OMe), 3.31 (3H, s, 18-OMe), 3.93 (3H, s, 3′-OMe), 3.94 (3H, s, 4′-OMe), 2.06 (1H, br s, 3-OH), 2.27 (1H, s, 8-OH), 3.67 (1H, s, 13-OH), 7.60 (1H, br s, H-2′), 6.90 (1H, d, J = 8.5, H-5′), 7.67 (1H, d, J = 8.5, H-6′). ^{13}C NMR (125 MHz, $CDCl_3$): δ 82.7 (C-1), 33.7 (C-2), 72.1 (C-4), 42.5 (C-4), 48.0 (C-5), 82.6 (C-6), 53.6 (C-7), 74.0 (C-8), 47.9 (C-9), 42.1 (C-10), 50.4 (C-11), 35.8 (C-12), 76.0 (C-13), 79.9 (C-14), 42.2 (C-15), 83.3 (C-16), 62.0 (C-17), 77.5 (C-18), 47.6 (C-19), 49.1 (C-20), 13.6 (C-21), 56.0 (C-1′), 57.7 (C-6′), 58.5 (C-16′), 59.3 (C-18′), 166.5 (O = C), 122.5 (C-1), 110.5 (C-2), 148.8 (C-3), 153.3 (C-4), 112.3 (C-5), 123.9 (C-6), 56.2 (C-3′), 56.0 (C-4′).

14-*O*-Acetylneoline (**3**): Amorphous white solid (46.9 mg). LR-ESI-MS (*m*/*z*): 690 [M + H$^+$]. HR-EI-MS (molecular formula): $C_{26}H_{41}NO_7$. ^{1}H NMR (500 MHz, $CDCl_3$): δ 3.69 (1H, br s, H-1), 1.50–1.63 (2H, m, H-2), 1.57–1.63 (2H, m, H-3), 2.19 (1H, d, J = 7.0, H-5), 4.11 (1H, d, J = 6.0 Hz, H-6), 2.00 (1H, s, H-7), 2.24 (1H, t, J = 5.5 Hz, H-9), 2.60–2.63 (1H, m, H-10), 1.77–1.81 (2H, m, H-12), 2.30–2.35 (1H, m, H-13), 4.85 (1H, t, J = 4.0 Hz, H-14), 1.88–1.93 (1H, m, H_a-15), 2.30–2.32 (1H, m, H_b-15), 3.29–3.30 (1H, m, H-16), 2.67 (1H, s, H-17), 3.23–3.62 (2H, d, J = 8.0 Hz, H-18), 2.31–2.69 (2H, m, H-19), 2.45–2.58 (2H, m, H-20), 1.13 (3H, t, J = 7.0 Hz, 21-Me), 3.34 (3H, s, 6-OMe), 3.26 (3H, s, 16-OMe), 3.32 (3H, s, 18-OMe), 2.06 (3H, s, OCO-Me). ^{13}C NMR (125 MHz, $CDCl_3$): δ 72.2 (C-1), 29.4 (C-2), 30.0 (C-4), 30.2 (C-4), 44.5 (C-5), 83.4 (C-6), 52.7(C-7), 74.7 (C-8), 46.2 (C-9), 36.7 (C-10), 49.7 (C-11), 29.6 (C-12), 43.4 (C-13), 77.2 (C-14), 42.7 (C-15), 82.0 (C-16), 63.4 (C-17), 80.2 (C-18), 57.1 (C-19), 48.4 (C-20), 13.1 (C-21), 58.1 (6-OMe), 56.2 (16-OMe), 59.3 (18-OMe), 21.3 (OCO-Me), 170.5 (O-C-OMe).

Linalool oxide acetate (**4**): Colourless oil (1.2 g). LR-ESI-MS (*m*/*z*): 213 [M + H$^+$]. LR-EI-MS (*m*/*z*): 212 (100%), 197, 195, 154, 153, 136, 114, 101, 94, 79, 68, 43. ^{1}H-NMR ($CDCl_3$, 500 MHz): δ 4.63 (1H, m, H-3), 2.16–2.09 (2H, m, H-4), 1.59–1.83 (2H, m, H-5), 5.92–6.02 (1H, m, H-7), 4.96–5.02 (2H, m, H-8), 1.17 (3H, s, H-9), 1.15 (3H, s, H-10), 1.20 (3H, s, H-11), 2.02 (3H, s, H-13). ^{13}C-NMR (125 MHz, $CDCl_3$): δ 74.1 (C-2), 76.0 (C-3), 31.8 (C-4), 22.2 (C-5), 73.5 (C-6), 146.0 (C-7), 110.7 (C-8), 31.3 (C-9), 21.9 (C-10), 29.3 (C-11), 170.4 (C-12), 21.2 (C-13).

(*E*)-spiroether (**5**): Colourless liquid (87.0 mg). LR-ESI-MS (*m*/*z*): 201 [M + H$^+$]. LR-EI-MS (*m*/*z*): 200 (M$^+$) (100%), 185, 170, 157, 141, 128, 115, 102, 76. ^{1}H-NMR ($CDCl_3$, 500 MHz): δ 1.98 (3H, s, H-1), 4.92 (1H, br s, H-6), 6.69 (1H, d, J = 5.7, H-8), 6.21 (1H, t, J = 5.0, H-9), 2.00–2.30 (4H, m, H-11/12), 3.87–4.20 (2H, m, H-13). ^{13}C-NMR (125 MHz, $CDCl_3$, APT): δ 4.9 (C-1), 80.8 (C-2), 65.4 (C-3), 79.1 (C-4), 70.9 (C-5), 79.0 (C-6), 167.3 (C-7), 127.6 (C-8), 135.4 (C-9), 121.2 (C-10), 35.8 (C-11), 24.7 (C-12), 69.9 (C-13).

Luteolin (6): White solid (618.0 mg). LR-ESI-MS (*m/z*): 281 [M+H$^+$]. LR-EI-MS (*m/z*): 286 (M$^+$), 277, 258, 229, 153 (100%), 124, 96, 77, 69. ^{1}H NMR (500 MHz, CD_3OD): δ 6.19 (1H, br s), 6.41 (1H, br s), 6.51 (1H, br s), 6.88 (1H, d, J = 9.0 Hz), 7.35 (1H, s), 7.36 (1H, s). ^{13}C NMR (125 MHz, CD_3OD): δ 183.8 (C-4), 166.3 (C-2), 166.1 (C-7), 163.2 (C-5), 159.4 (C-9), 150.9 (C-4), 147.1 (C-3), 123.6 (C-6), 120.2 (C-1), 116.7 (C-5), 114.1 (C-2), 103.8 (C-10), 103.8 (C-3), 100.1 (C-6), 94.9 (C-8).

Luteolin-7-*O*-β-D-glucopyranoside (**7**): Faint yellow powder (41.3 mg). LR-ESI-MS (*m*/*z*): 449 [M + H$^+$]. LR-EI-MS (*m*/*z*): 448, 281, 207, 191, 147, 133, 84, 73, 66, 44. ^{1}H NMR (500 MHz, DMSO): δ 7.44 (1H, dd, J = 8.5, 2.5 Hz, H-6′), 7.40 (1H, s, H-2′), 6.88 (1H, d, J = 8.0 Hz, H-5′), 6.77 (1H, d, J = 2.0 Hz, H-8), 6.74 (1H, s, H-3), 6.43 (1H, d, J = 2.0 Hz, H-6), 5.07 (1H, d, J = 7.0 Hz, glc-1), 3.14–3.70 (6H, m, glc-2 to glc-6). ^{13}C NMR (125 MHz, DMSO): δ 181.9 (C-4), 164.5 (C-2), 162.9 (C-7), 161.1 (C-5), 156.9 (C-9), 150.0 (C-4′), 145.8 (C-3′), 121.3 (C-1′), 119.1 (C-6′), 115.9 (C-5′), 113.5 (C-2′), 105.3 (C-10), 103.1 (C-3), 99.8 (glc-1), 99.5 (C-6), 94.7 (C-8), 77.1 (glc-5), 76.4 (glc-3), 73.1 (glc-2), 69.5 (glc-4), 60.6 (glc-6).

Protopine (**8**): Prisms (MeOH/$CHCl_3$, 1.0 g). mp: 209–211 °C. Optically inactive. LR-ESI-MS (*m*/*z*) 354 [M + H$^+$]. LR-EI-MS (*m*/*z*): 353 [M$^+$], 295, 281, 267, 251, 237, 223, 209, 190, 177, 163, 148 (100%), 134 and this ion fragmentation pattern matched that of protopine reported in the MS library

(NIST08s, Entry # 26245, CAS: 130-86-9, RetIndex: 2943). HR-ESI-MS (molecular formula): $C_{20}H_{19}NO_5$. ^{1}H-NMR (500 MHz, $CDCl_3$): δ 6.90 (1H, s, H-1), 6.64 (1H, s, H-4), 2.65 (2H, br s, H-5), 2.59 (2H, br s, H-6), 3.61 (2H, br s, H-8), 6.68 (1H, d, *J* = 7.5 Hz, H-11), 6.66 (1H, d, *J* = 8.0 Hz, H-12), 3.75 (2H, br s, H-13), 5.94 (2H, s, 2,3-OCH_2O), 5.92 (2H, s, 9,10-OCH_2O), 1.96 (3H, s, 7-NCH_3). ^{13}C-NMR (125 MHz, $CDCl_3$): δ 108.0 (C-1), 145.9 (C-2), 148.0 (C-3), 110.3 (C-4), 132.7 (C-4′), 31.5 (C-5), 57.6 (C-6), 50.9 (C-8), 117.5 (C-8′), 146.2 (C-9), 146.0 (C-10), 106.8 (C-11), 124.9 (C-12), 128.7 (C-12′), 46.1 (C-13), 194.3 (C-14), 136.0 (C-14′), 101.2 (2,3-OCH_2O), 41.5 (7-N-CH_3), 100.9 (9,10-OCH_2O).

Ochrobirine (**9**): Prisms (MeOH/$CHCl_3$, (60.6 mg)); mp: 203–207 °C. $[\alpha]_D^{25}$ + 38.7° (*c* 0.36, $CHCl_3$). LR-ESI-MS (*m*/*z*): 370 [M + H$^+$]. LR-EI-MS (*m*/*z*): 369 [M$^+$], 351, 336, 322 (100%), 293, 264, 204, 190 and this ion fragmentation pattern matched that of ochrobirine in the MS library (NIST08.LIB, Entry # 154984, CAS: 24181-64-4, RetIndex: 3185). HR-ESI-MS (molecular formula): $C_{20}H_{19}NO_6$. ^{1}H-NMR (500 MHz, $CDCl_3$): δ 6.85 (1H, s, H-1), 6.64 (1H, s, H-4), 2.54 (2H, br s, H-5), 3.25 (2H, br s, H-6), 4.87 (2H, s, H-8), 6.03 (1H, s, H-11), 6.87 (1H, s, H-12), 5.42 (2H, d, *J* = 10.5 Hz, H-13), 2.66 (3H, s, N-CH_3), 5.83 (2H, s, 2,3-OCH_2O), 6.01 (2H, s, 9,10-OCH_2O). ^{13}C-NMR (125 MHz, $CDCl_3$): δ 109.4 (C-1), 145.8 (C-2), 146.3 (C-3), 109.8 (C-4), 126.0 (C-4′), 22.5 (C-5), δ 47.4 (C-6), 73.7 (C-8), 121.0 (C-8′), 144.2 (C-9), 148.3 (C-10), 106.7 (C-11), 116.0 (C-12), 140.0 (C-12′), 79.5 (C-13), 75.0 (C-14), 129.5 (C-14′), 37.5 (N-CH_3), 100.8 (2,3-OCH_2O), 101.6 (9,10-OCH_2O).

Capnoidine (**10**): Orthorhombic crystal (80.3 mg). LR-ESI-MS (*m*/*z*): 368 [M + H$^+$]. LR-EI-MS (*m*/*z*): 367 [M$^+$], 207, 190 (100%), 175, 160, 149, 131, 117, 103 and this ion fragmentation pattern matched that of capnoidine reported in the MS library (NIST08.LIB, Entry # 153894, CAS: 485-49-4, RetIndex: 3142. HR-ESI-MS (molecular formula): $C_{20}H_{17}NO_6$. ^{1}H-NMR (500 MHz, $CDCl_3$): δ 4.02 (1H, d, *J* = 3.0 Hz, H-1), 3.05–3.07 (2H, m, H-3), δ 2.44–2.74 (1H, m, H-4), 6.40 (1H, s, H-5), 6.67 (1H, s, H-8), 5.62 (1H, d, *J* = 3.0 Hz, H-9), 6.94 (1H, d, *J* = 7.5 Hz, H-10), 7.14 (1H, d, *J* = 8.0 Hz, H-11), 2.53 (3H, s, N-CH_3), 5.84 (2H, s, OCH_2O), 6.10 (2H, s, OCH_2O). ^{13}C-NMR (125 MHz, $CDCl_3$): δ 66.2 (C-1), 51.4 (C-3), 29.2 (C-4), 125.2 (C-4a), 108.2 (C-5), 146.4 (C-6), 146.0 (C-7), 107.6 (C-8), 130.1 (C-8a), 82.9 (C-9), 140.9 (C-9a), 116.0 (C-10), 113.0 (C-11), 148.9 (12), 144.2 (C-13), 110.0 (C-13a), 45.1 (N-CH_3), 100.9 (OCH_2O) 103.2 (OCH_2O), 167.5 (C = O).

Scoulerine (**11**): Reddish brown solid (9.4 mg). LR-EI-MS: *m/z* 327 [M$^+$], 326, 312, 178 (100%), 176, 163, 150, 150, 135, 121 and 107. HR-EIMS (molecular formula): $C_{19}H_{21}NO_4$. ^{1}H-NMR ($CDCl_3$, 500 MHz): δ 6.82 (1H, s H-1), 6.59 (1H, s, H-4), 2.67–3.14 (2H, m, H-5), 2.61–3.19 (2H, m, H-6), 3.48 (1H, d, *J* = 15.5 Hz, H_a-8) and 4.24 (1H, d, *J* = 15.5 Hz, H_b-8), 6.72 (1H, d, *J* = 8.0 Hz, H-11), 6.67 (1H, d, *J* = 8.0 Hz, H-12), 2.78–2.84 (1H, m, H_a-13) and 3.25 (1H, d, *J* = 16.5, H_b-13), 3.54 (1H, br s, H-13a), 3.86 (3H, s, 3-MeO), 3.87 (3H, s, 10-MeO). ^{13}C-NMR (125 MHz, $CDCl_3$): δ 109.1 (C-1), 145.1 (C-2), 144.1 (C-3), 111.5 (C-4), 130.8 (C-4a), 29.3 (C-5), 51.7 (C-6), 53.6 (C-8), 121.3 (C-8a), 141.6 (C-9), 144.0 (C-10), 110.8 (C-11), 119.5 (C-12), 128.3 (C-12a), 36.4 (C-13), 59.3 (C-13a), 126.2 (C-13b), 56.3 (3-OCH_3), 56.2 (10-OCH_3).

*Isomyristicin (**12**)*: Colourless oil (185.3 mg). LR-ESI-MS (*m/z*): 193 [M+H$^+$]. LR-EI-MS (*m/z*): 192 (100%), 177, 165, 161, 147, 131, 119, 103, 91, 77, 65, 53, 39. ^{1}H NMR (500 MHz, $CDCl_3$): δ 6.45 (1H, s, H-2), 6.55 (1H, s, H-6), 6.29 (1H, d, *J* = 15.6 Hz, H-1′), 6.07 (1H, m, H-2′), 1.84 (3H, d, *J* = 6.6 Hz, H-3′), 5.91 (2H, s), 3.87 (3H, s, OMe). ^{13}C NMR (125 MHz, $CDCl_3$): δ 133.2 (C-1), 99.7 (C-2), 143.7 (C-3), 134.5 (C-4), 149.3 (C-5), 106.2 (C-6), 131.0 (C-1′), 124.8 (C-2′), 18.6 (C-3′), 101.5 (OCH_2O), 56.7 (OMe).

Bergapten (**13**): Clear crystals (2.5 g, from MeOH/$CHCl_3$ (1:1)). LR-ESI-MS (*m*/*z*): 217 [M + H$^+$]. LR-EI-MS (*m*/*z*): 216 [M$^+$], 202 (100%), 192, 173, 158, 145, 131, 118, 102, 89, 74, 69, 63, 51. ^{1}H NMR (500 MHz, $CDCl_3$): δ 6.27 (1H, d, *J* = 9.5 Hz, H-3), 8.15 (1H, d, *J* = 10.0 Hz, H-4), 7.12 (1H, s, H-8), 7.59 (1H, d, *J* = 2.5 Hz, H-2′), 7.02 (1H, d, *J* = 2.0 Hz, H-3′), 4.27 (3H, s, 5-OMe). ^{13}C NMR (125 MHz, $CDCl_3$): δ 161.4 (C-2), 112.7 (C-3), 139.4 (C-4), 106.6 (C-4a), 149.7 (C-5), 112.9 (C-6), 158.5 (C-7), 93.9 (C-8), 152.9 (C-8a), 144.9 (C-2′), 105.2 (C-3′), 60.3 (5-OMe).

Isoimperatorin (**14**): Clear crystals (143.1 mg, from MeOH/$CHCl_3$ (1:3)). LR-ESI-MS (*m*/*z*): 271 [M + H$^+$]. LR-EI-MS (*m*/*z*): 270 [M$^+$], 202 (100%), 174, 158, 145, 131, 118, 103, 89, 69, 51. ^{1}H NMR (500 MHz, $CDCl_3$): δ 6.26 (1H, d, *J* = 10.0 Hz, H-3), 8.15 (1H, d, *J* = 9.5 Hz, H-4), 7.14 (1H, s, H-8), 7.59

(1H, d, J = 2.0, Hz, H-2′), 6.95 (1H, d, J = 1.0 Hz, H-3′), 4.91 (2H, d, J = 7.5 Hz, H-1″), 5.53 (1H, t, J = 7.0 Hz, H-2″), 1.80 (3H, s, 4″-Me), 1.70 (3H, s, 5″-Me). ^{13}C NMR (125 MHz, $CDCl_3$): δ 161.4 (C-2), 112.7 (C-3), 139.6 (C-4), 107.6 (C-4a), 149.1 (C-5), 114.3 (C-6), 158.1 (C-7), 94.3 (C-8), 152.6 (C-9), 145.0 (C-2′), 105.2 (C-3′), 69.9 (C-1″), 119.3 (C-2″), 139.8 (C-3″), 25.9 (C-4″), 18.4 (C-5″).

For immunoregulatory screening, we selected 14 compounds based on their abundance or the quality isolated from each plant (minor compounds were not tested here). The stock solutions of the 14 compounds selected for cytotoxicity and immunoassays were prepared by initially dissolving 1 mg of weighed compounds in 10–20 µL of DMSO and then subsequently diluting them with 980–990 µL of relevant culture media to make the stock concentrations of 1 mg/mL.

4.3. DC Assay Method and Flow Cytometry

DC2.4 cells was a gift of Kenneth L. Rock, University of Massachusetts Medical School and Dana-Farber Cancer Institute (Boston, MA, USA). The DC2.4 cell line was established from bone marrow cells of C57BL/6 mice transduced with murine granulocyte macrophage-colony stimulating factor and retrovirally transfected with *raf* and *myc* oncogenes [25]. DC2.4 cells (4000 cells in exponential phase/200 µL) were cultured in 96-well flat bottom plates overnight with a titration of the test compound in media (stock concentration of 1 mg/mL and further titrated in tissue culture media at 4 mid-log dilutions starting at 100 µg/mL) or media only (modified DMEM, 50 µM 2-mercaptoethanol and 216 mg/L L-glutamine, 10% heat-inactivated FCS). Each compound was tested twice, in replicate assays. The cells were then harvested with trypsin, split in two and transferred to 96-well V-bottom plates, washed and stained on ice with FC-blocking antibody (2.4G2 supernatant) followed by combinations of fluorochrome-conjugated antibodies (all Biolegend except MHC-II) in two panels: (1) MHC-I FITC (H-2K^b), CD86 AF700, MHC-II V500 (BD); (2) CD40 AF647, CD80 FITC, CD44 PeCy7, CD274 BV421 for 10 min on ice. Samples were then washed and resuspended in buffer with sytox blue (panel 1) or propidium iodide (panel 2) for dead cell exclusion and run on a LSRFortessa flow cytometer (BD Biosciences, San Jose, CA, USA). Post-acquisition data analysis was performed with FlowJo software version 9.1 (Treestar, Ashland, OR, USA); calculations were performed using Microsoft Excel (version 12, Microsoft Corporation, Washington, NM, USA). The RFI (relative fluorescence intensity) for each parameter was calculated by dividing the median fluorescence intensity (MFI) of the test sample by that of the control (media-only) samples.

4.4. Gene Expression Analysis

DC2.4 cells were co-cultured overnight with test compounds as described above. The following day, cells were harvested and 20,000 live cells from each condition were sorted by FACS into RLT buffer and stored at −70 °C. On the day of extraction, frozen cell lysates were thawed quickly on ice and mRNA was extracted using the RNEasy micro kit (Qiagen, Chadstone Centre, VIC, Australia) according to the manufacturer's instructions. cDNA was synthesized using oligo-dT and AMVRT (Promega, Sydney, Australia) according to the manufacturer's instructions. Gene expression was measured using individual Taqman gene expression assays (Applied Biosystems, Foster City, CA, USA) and Platinum Taq polymerase (Life Technologies, Carlsbad, CA, USA) in a 15 µL volume reaction using a Rotorgene 3000 PCR machine (Corbett Research, Mortlake, Australia) with the following conditions: 2 min at 50 °C for calibration of fluorescence gain values, then denaturing at for 2 min at 95 °C, followed by 45 cycles of 5 s at 95 °C and 30 s at 60 °C. Gene expression was quantified relative to a standard curve generated from a titration of cloned cDNA and relative gene expression was calculated by dividing the expression value of the test sample by that of the cells grown in media only. All assays were conducted in triplicate.

4.5. Determining Cytotoxicity Using xCELLigence RTCA System

The immortalized non-malignant human cholangiocyte cell line H69 is a SV40-transformed human bile duct epithelial cell line originally derived from a normal liver harvested for transplantation [63,64].

H69s were grown under similar conditions with growth factor-supplemented specialized complete media; DMEM/F12 with high glucose, 10% fetal bovine serum (FBS), 1× antibiotic/antimycotic, 25 μg/mL adenine, 5 μg/mL insulin, 1 μg/mL epinephrine, 8.3 μg/mL holo-transferrin, 0.62 μg/mL, hydrocortisone, 13.6 ng/mL T3 and 10 ng/mL EGF (Life Technologies). Cytotoxicity screening of the test compounds against the H69 cell line was performed using an xCELLigence SP system (ACEA Biosciences Inc., San Diego, CA, USA) as described by us previously [65]. All experiments were carried out as per the manufacturer's instructions with 0.25–60 min read intervals using the real time cell assay (RTCA) software (ACEA Biosciences Inc., USA). All assays were conducted in triplicate. Inter-well spaces were filled with 100 μL of culture medium or PBS to prevent evaporation. The E-plates containing cells were seeded at 5000 cells/well and incubated overnight at 37 °C with 5% CO_2. The cells were then treated with prepared concentrations (50, 100, 500 μg/mL) of the test compounds and the viability of the cells was monitored continually for 24 h.

4.6. IC_{50} Calculations of Cytotoxicity

We determined the IC_{50} values of test compounds based on the normalised cell index (nCI) for cells, as described previously [66]. Briefly, the 24 h nCI relative to the negative DMSO treated controls (deemed 100%) on the y-axis was plotted against the log concentration value x-axis. GraphPad Prism 6.0 used calculated IC_{50} values using the log (test compound concentration) vs normalised response (100–0%) with variable slope formula and the least squares fitting method (i.e., $y = 100/(1 + 10\hat{}((\text{LogIC}_{50} - x) \times \text{HillSlope}))$.

4.7. Research Ethics

All five medicinal plants studied here were collected from Bhutan in 2009 and in a study approved by Menjong Sorig Phamaceuticals of Bhutan and the National Biodiversity Centre of Bhutan (NBCB). A Material Transfer Agreement was signed between Phurpa Wangchuk and the NBCB and the methanol extract samples of these plants were transferred to Australia with approval from Bhutan Agriculture and Food Regulatory Authority and Australian Quarantine Authority. Their voucher specimen number and parts collected are given in Table 1. The DC2.4 cell line was generously provided by Kenneth L. Rock (University of Massachusetts Medical School and Dana-Farber Cancer Institute, USA). The non-malignant cholangiocyte cell line H69 was obtained from Gregory J. Gores, Mayo Clinic, Rochester, MN, USA.

5. Conclusions

Five medicinal plants—*A. laciniatum*, *A. nubigena*, *C. crispa*, *C. dubia*, and *P. amabile*—which grow in extreme Himalayan mountain ecology—are used in the scholarly Bhutanese traditional medicines for treating various disorders that bore relevance to modern disease pathologies including inflammation, tumor and infections. Inspired by the strong bioactivities of their crude extracts, we isolated a total of 40 phytochemicals and tested 14 of them for their capacity to modulate DC activity, and 10 for cytotoxicity. Two of the 14 compounds showed robust immunostimulatory or immunosuppressant activities. Specifically, scoulerine (**10**) showed strong immunostimulatory activity as indicated by upregulation of gene and protein expression of key molecules associated with DC activity, whereas bergapten (**13**) consistently suppressed expression of DC genes involved in T cell signalling and activation. Our data are consistent with reports that these two compounds have broad-ranging therapeutic properties that can be used against cancer, malaria, helminthiasis, inflammation and Alzheimer's disease. Thus, they are worthy of further exploration either as independent drug entities or as immunomodulators to potentiate other drugs/vaccines, including investigating the mechanisms of action of these compounds. Finding a broad-spectrum drug that could treat multiple diseases or potentiate other drugs and vaccines is highly desirable and of great interest to the pharmaceutical industry. This study not only identified potential immunomodulatory compounds from five Bhutanese medicinal plants but also provided molecular and immunological data to support their reported efficacy.

Author Contributions: P.W. isolated plant compounds and wrote the manuscript. S.H.A. and P.L.G. conducted cellular work and wrote the manuscript. M.J.S. performed cytotoxicity assay and wrote the manuscript. A.L. and D.L.D. helped with the experimental design and wrote the manuscript. All authors have read and approved the final manuscript.

Funding: P.W. is supported by an Early Career Fellowship (APP1091011) from the National Health and Medical Research Council (NHMRC) of Australia. D.L.D. and A.L. are supported by an NHMRC Principal Research Fellowship (1137285) and Senior Principal Research Fellowship (1117504), respectively.

Acknowledgments: We thank Samten of Menjong Sorig Pharmaceuticlas and the National Biodiversty Centre in Bhutan for their administrative and technical support for collecting and extracting the plant samples.

Conflicts of Interest: The authors declare no conflict of interest.

References

1. Yuan, H.; Ma, Q.; Ye, L.; Piao, G. The traditional medicine and modern medicine from natural products. *Molecules* **2016**, *21*, 559. [CrossRef] [PubMed]
2. Wangchuk, P. Therapeutic applications of natural products in herbal medicines, biodiscovery programs, and biomedicine. *J. Biol. Active Prod. Nat.* **2018**, *8*, 1–20. [CrossRef]
3. Balunas, M.J.; Kinghorn, A.D. Drug discovery from medicinal plants. *Life Sci.* **2005**, *78*, 431–441. [CrossRef] [PubMed]
4. Achan, J.; Talisuna, A.O.; Erhart, A.; Yeka, A.; Tibenderana, J.K.; Baliraine, F.N.; Rosenthal, P.J.; D'Alessandro, U. Quinine, an old anti-malarial drug in a modern world: Role in the treatment of malaria. *Malar. J.* **2011**, *10*, 144. [CrossRef] [PubMed]
5. Landau, E. From a Tree, a "Miracle" Called Aspirin. CNN Health: Matters of the Heart. 2010. Available online: http://edition.cnn.com/2010/HEALTH/12/22/aspirin.history/index.html (accessed on 18 September 2018).
6. Dias, D.A.; Urban, S.; Roessner, U. A historical overview of natural products in drug discovery. *Metabolites* **2012**, *2*, 303–336. [CrossRef] [PubMed]
7. Amirkia, V.; Heinrich, M. Alkaloids as drug leads—A predictive structural and biodiversity-based analysis. *Phytochem. Lett.* **2014**, *10*, xlviii–liii. [CrossRef]
8. Wood, L. Botanical and Plant Derived Drugs—Analysis, Trends and Forecasts to 201. Research and Markets. 2017. Available online: https://www.businesswire.com/news/home/20171212005666/en/Botanical-Plant-Derived-Drugs-Analysis-Trends-Forecasts (accessed on 19 September 2018).
9. Wen, C.C.; Chen, H.M.; Yang, N.S. Developing phytocompounds from medicinal plants as immunomodulators. *Adv. Bot. Res.* **2012**, *62*, 198–244.
10. Gordon, J.R.; Ma, Y.; Churchman, L.; Gordon, S.A.; Dawicki, W. Regulatory dendritic cells for immunotherapy in immunologic diseases. *Front. Immunol.* **2014**, *5*, 7. [CrossRef] [PubMed]
11. Merad, M.; Sathe, P.; Helft, J.; Miller, J.; Mortha, A. The dendritic cell lineage: Ontogeny and function of dendritic cells and their subsets in the steady state and the inflamed setting. *Annu. Rev. Immunol.* **2013**, *31*, 563–604. [CrossRef] [PubMed]
12. Pooley, J.L.; Heath, W.R.; Shortman, K. Cutting edge: Intravenous soluble antigen is presented to CD4 T cells by CD8 -dendritic cells, but cross-presented to CD8 T Cells by CD8 dendritic cells. *J. Immunol.* **2001**, *166*, 5327–5330. [CrossRef] [PubMed]
13. Plantinga, M.; Guilliams, M.; Vanheerswynghels, M.; Deswarte, K.; Branco-Madeira, F.; Toussaint, W.; Vanhoutte, L.; Neyt, K.; Killeen, N.; Malissen, B.; et al. Conventional and monocyte-derived $CD11b^+$ dendritic cells initiate and maintain T helper 2 cell-mediated immunity to house dust mite allergen. *Immunity* **2013**, *38*, 322–335. [CrossRef] [PubMed]
14. Granot, T.; Senda, T.; Carpenter, D.J.; Matsuoka, N.; Weiner, J.; Gordon, C.L.; Miron, M.; Kumar, B.; Griesemer, A.; Ho, S.H.; et al. Dendritic cells display subset and tissue-specific maturation dynamics over human life. *Immunity* **2017**, *46*, 504–515. [CrossRef] [PubMed]
15. Jongbloed, S.L.; Kassianos, A.J.; McDonald, K.J.; Clark, G.J.; Ju, X.; Angel, C.E.; Chen, C.J.J.; Dunbar, P.R.; Wadley, R.B.; Jeet, V.; et al. Human $CD141^+$ $(BDCA\text{-}3)^+$ dendritic cells (DCs) represent a unique myeloid DC subset that cross-presents necrotic cell antigens. *J. Exp. Med.* **2010**, *207*, 1247–1260. [CrossRef] [PubMed]
16. Worbs, T.; Hammerschmidt, S.I.; Förster, R. Dendritic cell migration in health and disease. *Nat. Rev. Immunol.* **2016**, *17*, 30–48. [CrossRef] [PubMed]

17. Okamoto, M.; Oh-e, G.; Oshikawa, T.; Furuichi, S.; Tano, T.; Ahmed, S.U.; Akashi, S.; Miyake, K.; Takeuchi, O.; Akira, S.; et al. Toll-like receptor 4 mediates the antitumor host response induced by a 55-kilodalton protein isolated from *Aeginetia indica* L., a parasitic plant. *Clin. Diagn. Lab. Immunol.* **2004**, *11*, 483–495. [CrossRef] [PubMed]
18. Aldahlawi, A.M. Modulation of dendritic cell immune functions by plant components. *J. Microsc. Ultrastruct.* **2016**, *4*, 55–62. [CrossRef] [PubMed]
19. Bradley, W.G.; Widen, R.H.; Weiser, A.M.; Powers, J.J.; Fountain, L.B.; Punjwani, P.; Lofgren, S.M.; Hadzic, T.; Klein, R.; Green, W.H.; et al. The novel differentiation of human blood mononuclear cells into CD1a-negative dendritic cells is stimulated in the absence of exogenous cytokines by an extract prepared from pinecones. *Int. Immunopharmacol.* **2003**, *3*, 209–223. [CrossRef]
20. Benson, J.M.; Pokorny, A.J.; Rhule, A.; Wenner, C.A.; Kandhi, V.; Cech, N.B.; Shepherd, D.M. *Echinacea pupurea* extracts modulate murine dendritic cell fate and function. *Food Chem. Toxicol.* **2010**, *48*, 1170–1177. [CrossRef] [PubMed]
21. Kim, G.-Y.; Cho, H.; Ahn, S.-C.; Oh, Y.-H.; Lee, C.-M.; Park, Y.-M. Resveratrol inhibits phenotypic and functional maturation of murine bone marrow-derived dendritic cells. *Int. Immunopharmacol.* **2004**, *4*, 245–253. [CrossRef] [PubMed]
22. Chen, X.; Murakami, T.; Oppenheim, J.J.; Howard, O.M.Z. Triptolide, a constituent of immunosuppressive Chinese herbal medicine, is a potent suppressor of dendritic-cell maturation and trafficking. *Blood* **2005**, *106*, 2409–2416. [CrossRef] [PubMed]
23. Kure, C.; Timmer, J.; Stough, C. The immunomodulatory effects of plant extracts and plant secondary metabolites on chronic neuroinflammation and cognitive aging: A mechanistic and empirical review. *Front. Pharmacol.* **2017**, *8*. [CrossRef] [PubMed]
24. Apte, S.H.; Stephenson, R.J.; Simerska, P.; Groves, P.L.; Aljohani, S.; Eskandari, S.; Toth, I.; Doolan, D.L. Systematic evaluation of self-adjuvanting lipopeptide nano-vaccine platforms for the induction of potent CD8(+) T-cell responses. *Nanomed. Lond.* **2016**, *11*, 137–152. [CrossRef] [PubMed]
25. Shen, Z.; Reznikoff, G.; Dranoff, G.; Rock, K.L. Cloned dendritic cells can present exogenous antigens on both MHC class I and class II molecules. *J. Immunol.* **1997**, *158*, 2723–2730. [PubMed]
26. Gutiérrez-Martínez, E.; Planès, R.; Anselmi, G.; Reynolds, M.; Menezes, S.; Adiko, A.C.; Saveanu, L.; Guermonprez, P. Cross-presentation of cell-associated antigens by MHC Class I in dendritic cell subsets. *Front. Immunol.* **2015**, *6*, 363. [CrossRef] [PubMed]
27. Ichiyanagi, T.; Imai, T.; Kajiwara, C.; Mizukami, S.; Nakai, A.; Nakayama, T.; Udono, H. Essential role of endogenous heat shock protein 90 of dendritic cells in antigen cross-presentation. *J. Immunol.* **2010**, *185*, 2693–2700. [CrossRef] [PubMed]
28. Rinaldi, G.; Yan, H.; Nacif-Pimenta, R.; Matchimakul, P.; Bridger, J.; Mann, V.H.; Smout, M.J.; Brindley, P.J.; Knight, M. Cytometric analysis, genetic manipulation and antibiotic selection of the snail embryonic cell line Bge from Biomphalaria glabrata, the intermediate host of Schistosoma mansoni. *Int. J. Parasitol.* **2015**, *45*, 527–535. [CrossRef] [PubMed]
29. Wangchuk, P.; Keller, P.A.; Pyne, S.G.; Taweechotipatr, M.; Tonsomboon, A.; Rattanajak, R.; Kamchonwongpaisan, S. Evaluation of an ethnopharmacologically selected Bhutanese medicinal plants for their major classes of phytochemicals and biological activities. *J. Ethnopharmacol.* **2011**, *137*, 730–742. [CrossRef] [PubMed]
30. Yeshi, K.; Wangdi, T.; Qusar, N.; Nettles, J.; Craig, S.R.; Schrempf, M.; Wangchuk, P. Geopharmaceuticals of Himalayan *Sowa Rigpa* medicine: Ethnopharmacological uses, mineral diversity, chemical identification and current utilization in Bhutan. *J. Ethnopharmacol.* **2018**, *223*, 99–112. [CrossRef] [PubMed]
31. Wangchuk, P.; Keller, P.A.; Pyne, S.G.; Sastraruji, T.; Taweechotipatr, M.; Rattanajak, R.; Tonsomboon, A.; Kamchonwongpaisan, S. Phytochemical and biological activity studies of the Bhutanese medicinal plant *Corydalis crispa*. *Nat. Prod. Commun.* **2012**, *7*, 575–580. [PubMed]
32. Wangchuk, P.; Keller, P.A.; Pyne, S.G.; Willis, A.C.; Kamchonwongpaisan, S. Antimalarial alkaloids from a Bhutanese traditional medicinal plant *Corydalis dubia*. *J. Ethnopharmacol.* **2012**, *143*, 310–313. [CrossRef] [PubMed]
33. Wangchuk, P.; Keller, P.A.; Stephen, G.P.; Korth, J.; Samten; Taweechotipatr, M.; Rattanajak, R.; Kamchonwongpaisan, S. Antimicrobial, antimalarial and cytoxicity activities of constituents of a Bhutanese variety of *Ajania nubigena*. *Nat. Prod. Commun.* **2013**, *8*, 733–736.

34. Wangchuk, P.; Pyne, S.G.; Keller, P.A.; Taweechotipatr, M.; Kamchonwongpaisan, S. Phenylpropanoids and furanocoumarins as antibacterial and antimalarial constituents of the Bhutanese medicinal plant *Pleurospermum amabile*. *Nat. Prod. Commun.* **2014**, *9*, 957–960. [PubMed]
35. Wangchuk, P.; Navarro, S.; Shepherd, C.; Keller, P.A.; Pyne, S.G.; Loukas, A. Diterpenoid alkaloids of *Aconitum laciniatum* and mitigation of inflammation by 14-*O*-acetylneoline in a murine model of ulcerative colitis. *Sci. Rep.* **2015**, *5*, 1–10. [CrossRef] [PubMed]
36. Wangchuk, P.; Keller, P.A.; Pyne, S.G.; Taweechotipatr, M. Inhibition of TNF-α production in LPS-activated THP-1 monocytic cells by the crude extracts of seven Bhutanese medicinal plants. *J. Ethnopharmacol.* **2013**, *148*, 1013–1017. [CrossRef] [PubMed]
37. Apte, S.H.; Redmond, A.M.; Groves, P.L.; Schussek, S.; Pattinson, D.J.; Doolan, D.L. Subcutaneous cholera toxin exposure induces potent $CD103^+$ dermal dendritic cell activation and migration. *Eur. J. Immunol.* **2013**, *43*, 2707–2717. [CrossRef] [PubMed]
38. Habartova, K.; Havelek, R.; Seifrtova, M.; Kralovec, K.; Cahlikova, L.; Chlebek, J.; Cermakova, E.; Mazankova, N.; Marikova, J.; Kunes, J.; et al. Scoulerine affects microtubule structure, inhibits proliferation, arrests cell cycle and thus culminates in the apoptotic death of cancer cells. *Sci. Rep.* **2018**, *8*, 4829. [CrossRef] [PubMed]
39. Wangchuk, P.; Loukas, A. Techniques and Technologies for the Biodiscovery of Novel Small Molecule Drug Lead Compounds From Natural Products. In *Natural Products and Drug Discovery*; Mandal, S.C., Mandal, V., Konishi, T., Eds.; Elsevier: Amsterdam, The Netherlands, 2018; Chapter 16; pp. 435–465. [CrossRef]
40. Spelman, K.; Burns, J.; Nichols, D.; Winters, N.; Ottersberg, S.; Tenborg, M. Modulation of cytokine expression by traditional medicines: A review of herbal immunomodulators. *Altern. Med. Rev.* **2006**, *11*, 128–150. [PubMed]
41. Wilkinson, J.A.; Wahlqvist, M.L.; Clark, J. *New Food and Pharmaceutical Products from Agriculture*; Rural Industries Research and Development Corporation: Wagga Wagga, Australia, 2002; pp. 1–30.
42. Prance, G.T.; Chadwick, D.J.; Marsh, J. Ethnobotany and the search for new drug discovery. In *Ethnobotany and the Search for New Drugs*; Chadwick, D.J., Marsh, J., Eds.; John Wiley and Sons: England, UK, 1994; p. 185.
43. Mizumoto, N.; Gao, J.; Matsushima, H.; Ogawa, Y.; Tanaka, H.; Takashima, A. Discovery of novel immunostimulants by dendritic-cell–based functional screening. *Blood* **2005**, *106*, 3082–3089. [CrossRef] [PubMed]
44. Liu, Y.; Beyer, A.; Aebersold, R. On the dependency of cellular protein levels on mRNA abundance. *Cell* **2016**, *165*, 535–550. [CrossRef] [PubMed]
45. Flower, D.R. Systematic identification of small molecule adjuvants. *Expert Opin. Drug Discov.* **2012**, *7*, 807–817. [CrossRef] [PubMed]
46. Kensil, C.R.; Kammer, R. QS-21: A water-soluble triterpene glycoside adjuvant. *Expert Opin. Investig. Drugs* **1998**, *7*, 1475–1482. [CrossRef] [PubMed]
47. Evans, T.G.; McElrath, M.J.; Matthews, T.; Montefiori, D.; Weinhold, K.; Wolff, M.; Keefer, M.C.; Kallas, E.G.; Corey, L.; Gorse, G.J.; et al. QS-21 promotes an adjuvant effect allowing for reduced antigen dose during HIV-1 envelope subunit immmunization in humans. *Vaccine* **2001**, *19*, 2080–2091. [CrossRef]
48. Chapman, P.B.; Morrissey, D.M.; Panageas, K.S.; Hamilton, W.B.; Zhan, C.; Destro, A.N.; Williams, L.; Israel, R.J.; Livingston, P.O. Induction of Antibodies against GM2 Ganglioside by Immunizing Melanoma Patients Using GM2-Keyhole Limpet Hemocyanin + QS21 Vaccine: A Dose-Response Study. *Clin. Cancer Res.* **2000**, *6*, 874. [PubMed]
49. Wangchuk, P.; Bremner, J.B.; Samten; Rattanajak, R.; Kamchonwongpaisan, S. Antiplasmodial agents from the Bhutanese medicinal plant *Corydalis calliantha*. *Phytother. Res.* **2010**, *24*, 481–485. [CrossRef] [PubMed]
50. Chlebek, J.; De Simone, A.; Hošťálková, A.; Opletal, L.; Pérez, C.; Pérez, D.I.; Havlíková, L.; Cahlíková, L.; Andrisano, V. Application of BACE1 immobilized enzyme reactor for the characterization of multifunctional alkaloids from *Corydalis cava* (Fumariaceae) as Alzheimer's disease targets. *Fitoterapia* **2016**, *109*, 241–247. [CrossRef] [PubMed]
51. Wangchuk, P.; Sastraruji, T.; Taweechotipatr, M.; Keller, P.A.; Pyne, S.G. Anti-inflammatory, anti-bacterial and anti-acetylcholinesterase activities of two isoquinoline alkaloids-scoulerine and cheilanthifoline. *Nat. Prod. Commun.* **2016**, *11*, 1801–1804.

52. Ko, F.N.; Yu, S.M.; Su, M.J.; Wu, Y.C.; Teng, C.M. Pharmacological activity of (-)-discretamine, a novel vascular alpha-adrenoceptor and 5-hydroxytryptamine receptor antagonist, isolated from Fissistigma glaucescens. *Br. J. Pharmacol.* **1993**, *110*, 882–888. [CrossRef] [PubMed]
53. Chen, Y.; Fan, G.; Zhang, Q.; Wu, H.; Wu, Y. Fingerprint analysis of the fruits of *Cnidium monnieri* extract by high-performance liquid chromatography–diode array detection–electrospray ionization tandem mass spectrometry. *J. Pharm. Biomed. Anal.* **2007**, *43*, 926–936. [CrossRef] [PubMed]
54. Chen, D.; Wang, J.; Jiang, Y.; Zhou, T.; Fan, G.; Wu, Y. Separation and determination of coumarins in *Fructus cnidii* extracts by pressurized capillary electrochromatography using a packed column with a monolithic outlet frit. *J. Pharm. Biomed. Anal.* **2009**, *50*, 695–702. [CrossRef] [PubMed]
55. Bauri, A.K.; Foro, S.; Nhu Do, Q.N. Crystal structure of bergapten: A photomutagenic and photobiologically active furanocoumarin. *Acta Crystallogr. E Crystallogr Commun.* **2016**, *72*, 1194–1196. [CrossRef] [PubMed]
56. Conconi, M.T.; Montesi, F.; Parnigotto, P.P. Antiproliferative activity and phototoxicity of some methyl derivatives of 5-methoxypsoralen and 5-methoxyangelicin. *Pharmacol. Toxicol.* **1998**, *82*, 193–198. [CrossRef] [PubMed]
57. March, K.L.; Patton, B.L.; Wilensky, R.L.; Hathaway, D.R. 8-Methoxypsoralen and longwave ultraviolet irradiation are a novel antiproliferative combination for vascular smooth muscle. *Circulation* **1993**, *87*, 184–191. [CrossRef] [PubMed]
58. De Amicis, F.; Aquila, S.; Morelli, C.; Guido, C.; Santoro, M.; Perrotta, I.; Mauro, L.; Giordano, F.; Nigro, A.; Andò, S.; Panno, M.L. Bergapten drives autophagy through the up-regulation of PTEN expression in breast cancer cells. *Mol. Cancer* **2015**, *14*, 130. [CrossRef] [PubMed]
59. Danheiser, R.L.; Trova, M.P. Synthesis of linear furocoumarins via a photochemical aromatic annulation strategy. An efficient total synthesis of bergapten. *Synlett.* **1995**, *1995*, 573–574. [CrossRef]
60. Oda, K.; Nishizono, N.; Tamai, Y.; Yamaguchi, Y.; Yoshimura, T.; Wada, K.; Machida, M. An efficient synthesis of bergapten. *Heterocycles* **2005**, *65*, 1985–1988. [CrossRef]
61. Betteridge, P.W.; Carruthers, J.R.; Cooper, R.I.; Prout, K.; Watkin, D.J. CRYSTALS version 12: Software for guided crystal structure analysis. *J. Appl. Cryst.* **2003**, *36*, 1487. [CrossRef]
62. Palatinus, L.; Chapuis, G. SUPEFLIP—A computer program for the solution of crystal structures by charge flipping in arbitrary dimensions. *J. Appl. Cryst.* **2007**, *40*, 786–790. [CrossRef]
63. Grubman, S.A.; Perrone, R.D.; Lee, D.W.; Murray, S.L.; Rogers, L.C.; Wolkoff, L.I.; Mulberg, A.E.; Cherington, V.; Jefferson, D.M. Regulation of intracellular pH by immortalized human intrahepatic biliary epithelial cell lines. *Am. J. Physiol. Gastrointest. Liver Physiol.* **1994**, *266*, G1060–G1070. [CrossRef] [PubMed]
64. Reid, L.M.; Jefferson, D.M. Culturing hepatocytes and other differentiated cells. *Hepatology* **1984**, *4*, 548–559. [CrossRef] [PubMed]
65. Dastpeyman, M.; Bansal, P.S.; Wilson, D.; Sotillo, J.; Brindley, P.; Loukas, A.; Smout, M.J.; Daly, N.L. Structural variants of a liver fluke derived granulin peptide potently stimulate wound healing. *J. Med. Chem.* **2018**. [CrossRef] [PubMed]
66. Wangchuk, P.; Giacomin, P.R.; Pearson, M.S.; Smout, M.J.; Loukas, A. Identification of lead chemotherapeutic agents from medicinal plants against blood flukes and whipworms. *Sci. Rep.* **2016**, *6*, 32101. [CrossRef] [PubMed]

International Journal of
Molecular Sciences

MDPI

Article

Spatial Distribution of Glucan Type and Content between Caps and Stalks in *Pleurotus eryngii*: Impact on the Anti-inflammatory Functionality

Vaclav Vetvicka [1], Ofer Gover [2], Hilla Hayby [2], Ofer Danay [3], Nirit Ezov [4], Yitzhak Hadar [5] and Betty Schwartz [2,*]

1 University of Louisville, Department of Pathology, University of Louisville, Louisville, KY 40202, USA; v0vetv01@louisville.edu
2 Institute of Biochemistry, School of Nutritional Sciences, Food Science and Nutrition, The Robert H. Smith Faculty of Agriculture, Food and Environment, The Hebrew University of Jerusalem, Rehovot 76100, Israel; ofer.gover@mail.huji.ac.il (O.G.); hilla.hayby@mail.huji.ac.il (H.H.)
3 Edible Mushrooms, MIGAL, 11016 Kiryat Shmona, and Tel Hai College, 12210 Upper Galilee, Israel; ofer@migal.org.il
4 Edible Mushrooms Development, MIGAL, Kiryat Shmona 11016, Israel; niritezov@walla.co.il
5 Department of Plant Pathology and Microbiology, The Robert H. Smith Faculty of Agriculture, Food and Environment, The Hebrew University of Jerusalem, Rehovot 76100, Israel; yitzhak.hadar@mail.huji.ac.il
* Correspondence: betty.schwartz@mail.huji.ac.il

Received: 8 October 2018; Accepted: 26 October 2018; Published: 28 October 2018

Abstract: *Pleurotus eryngii* is recognized for its prominent nutritional and medicinal value. In our study, we tested the effect of glucans on lipopolysaccharide (LPS)-induced production of TNF-α. We demonstrated that glucan extracts are more effective than mill mushroom preparations. Additionally, the effectiveness of stalk-derived glucans were slightly more pronounced than of caps. Cap and stalk glucans from mill or isolated glucan competed dose-dependently with anti-Dectin-and anti-CR-3 antibodies, indicating that they contain β-glucans recognized by these receptors. Using the dextran sulfate sodium (DSS)-inflammatory bowel disease mice model, intestinal inflammatory response to the mill preparations was measured and compared to extracted glucan fractions from caps and stalks. We found that mill and glucan extracts were very effective in downregulating IFN-γ and MIP-2 levels and that stalk-derived preparations were more effective than from caps. The tested glucans were equally effective in regulating the number of CD14/CD16 monocytes and upregulating the levels of fecal-released IgA to almost normal levels. In conclusion, the most effective glucans in ameliorating some IBD-inflammatory associated symptoms induced by DSS treatment in mice were glucan extracts prepared from the stalk of *P. eryngii*. These spatial distinctions may be helpful in selecting more effective specific anti-inflammatory mushrooms-derived glucans.

Keywords: *P. eryngii*; glucans; inflammation; inflammatory bowel disease

---

1. Introduction

Pleurotus eryngii is generally recognized as the king oyster mushroom. It was originally consumed in Europe but is now widely distributed and consumed in other parts of the world including America, Asia, and Africa [1]. The advantageous nutritional and medicinal properties exerted by *P. eryngii* mushrooms are mediated, at least in part, by potent bioactive constituents such as the polysaccharides fraction (glucans) and other molecules that can confer a variety of health benefits such as strong immunomodulatory effects [2–4].

The notable regulatory effects of glucans present in the fruiting bodies of edible mushrooms on the immune system have received significant attention and extensive studies [5–7]. The regulating activity of the immune system by mushroom glucans appears to be mediated, at least in part, via direct activation of macrophages and dendritic cells, which are essential components of the innate immune system in mammalians [8].

For glucans to induce their biological response, they should bind to their primary targets; i.e., the inflammatory cells. Several studies have established that, at least for β-glucans, biological effects are exerted through specific binding to the lectin-binding site of complement receptor type three (CR3 (CD11b/CD18)) on immune effector cells and NK cells [8]. β-Glucans may also interact with an additional glucan receptor on inflammatory cells, the Dectin-1 receptor expressed in neutrophils, macrophages, dendritic cells, and some T-cells. Following binding of glucans to Dectin-1 or to CR3 (CD11b/CD18) receptor, several specific activities, such as modulation of phagocytosis, variations of release of inflammatory cytokines, and other activities, are modulated [8].

Inflammatory bowel diseases (IBD) are inflammatory disorders of the intestinal tract and bothersome conditions of unknown etiology that are most common in developed countries, distressing the quality of life of the affected population. There are two types of IBD, Crohn's disease and ulcerative colitis, which both feature an overactive immune response. Treatment of IBD symptoms is concentrated on the use of nonspecific immunosuppressive therapies (such as steroids), antibiotics, and some novel biologicals therapies mainly targeting the proinflammatory tumor necrosis factor (TNF) pathway [9]. Altogether, these treatments are not always effective in all patients. We believe that ingestion of purified glucans may exert anti-inflammatory effects similar to those previously reported for *P. pulmonarious* glucans [6] and none of the adverse effects of the aforementioned therapies.

We recently reported that *P. eryngii* has the highest total, β- and α-glucan content compared to other Pleurotus species [10]. We also found that the stalks (stipe) of the fruiting body contained higher glucan content than the caps (pileus) [10]. In the present study, we addressed the question whether this spatial distribution has implications on the extent of the anti-inflammatory effect exerted by the two different parts of *P. eryngii* mushroom. We, therefore, concentrated our efforts on investigating whether glucans extracted from stalks and caps are comparable in their anti-inflammatory effects using a wide variety of experimental designs exemplifying inflammatory disorders such as IBD.

2. Results

2.1. Glucan Content Mushroom Stalk and Cap

The glucan content of the *P. eryngii* was assessed using the Megazyme kit. Total α-glucan and β-glucan content was significantly higher in the stalks of the mushrooms compared to the caps ($p < 0.001$); however, α-glucan content in stalks demonstrated the most significant difference ($p < 0.0001$) (Table 1).

Table 1. Glucan content in cap and stalks from *P. eryngii* mill and glucan extracts. α, β, and total glucan concentrations (g/100 g dried matter) in mills and glucan extracts prepared from cap and stalks harvested from *P. eryngii* mushrooms. * $p < 0.001$, ** $p < 0.0001$ comparison between caps to respective stalks.

P. eryngii Parts and Preparations	α-Glucan (g/100 g)	β-Glucan (g/100 g)	Total Glucans (g/100 g)
Cap whole mill	0.804 ± 0.006	29.519 ± 0.98	30.32 ± 0.5
Stalk whole mill	4.505 ± 0.35 *	38.412 ± 1.2 *	42.92 ± 0.77 *
Cap glucan extract	6.545 ± 1.38	21.804 ± 1.27	28.5 ± 1.32
Stalk glucan extract	16.9851 ± 1.6 **	29.807 ± 2.6 *	46.79 ± 2.12 *

2.2. P. eryngii-Derived Glucans Suppressed TNF-α Secretion from Lipopolysaccharide-Treated J774.2 Cells

TNF-α is an important inflammatory mediator produced from macrophages corresponding to inflammation. Therefore, we used TNF-α as an indicator of macrophage response to lipopolysaccharide (LPS) and glucans. J774.2 cells were incubated with LPS (100 ng/mL) and with/without glucan for 24 h. Supernatant was collected at different intervals (4, 6, 12, and 24 h) and evaluated for TNF-α secretion. Cells were incubated with whole mill or glucan extracts at increasing concentrations. LPS induced TNF-α production in a time-dependent fashion (Figure 1). A significant decrease (~50%) in TNF-α secretion was observed when 0.00025% extract from cap was added after 4 h and at a concentration of 0.025% TNF-α was hardly detected. TNF-α production was suppressed by both glucans in a dose-dependent manner, showing the greatest consistent effect when glucan extracted from stalks was added. Glucans from glucan extracts exerted more notorious effects than glucans from mill preparations.

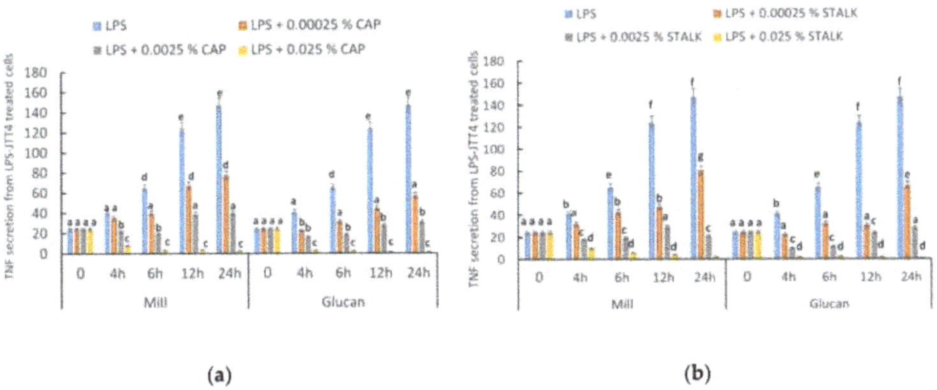

Figure 1. Secretion of lipopolysaccharide (LPS)-stimulated TNF-α by J774.1 (1×10^6 cells/well) macrophages in response to several doses of glucans from mill and isolated glucans from (**a**) caps and (**b**) stalks of *P. eryngii* mushrooms (0.00025%; 0.0025%; 0.025%; i.e., 0.25 or 2.5 or 25 μg/1 mL media). Concentration of TNF-α in the culture supernatants was measured by ELISA and expressed as (pg/mL). Data are expressed as means ± SD. Different letters indicate significantly different values at $p < 0.05$.

2.3. Inhibition of Staining of CR3 and Dectin-1 Receptors by P. eryngii Glucans

Glucans express their immunostimulating activities via interaction with various surface receptors. The most important of these receptors are Dectin-1 and CR3 (CD18/CD11b). In order to establish the affinity of glucans from different parts of the mushroom to these receptors, the next series of experiments focused on binding to CR3 and Dectin-1 receptors. Our results, summarized in Figure 2, demonstrated that glucan extracts had a strong dose-dependent inhibition on both receptors. Glucan extracts competed with both receptors more efficiently than mill. Glucans extracted from the cap had the strongest inhibition profile on Dectin-1 staining (Figure 2a), but for CR3 binding, glucans extracted from caps and stalks had similar inhibitory activity (Figure 2b).

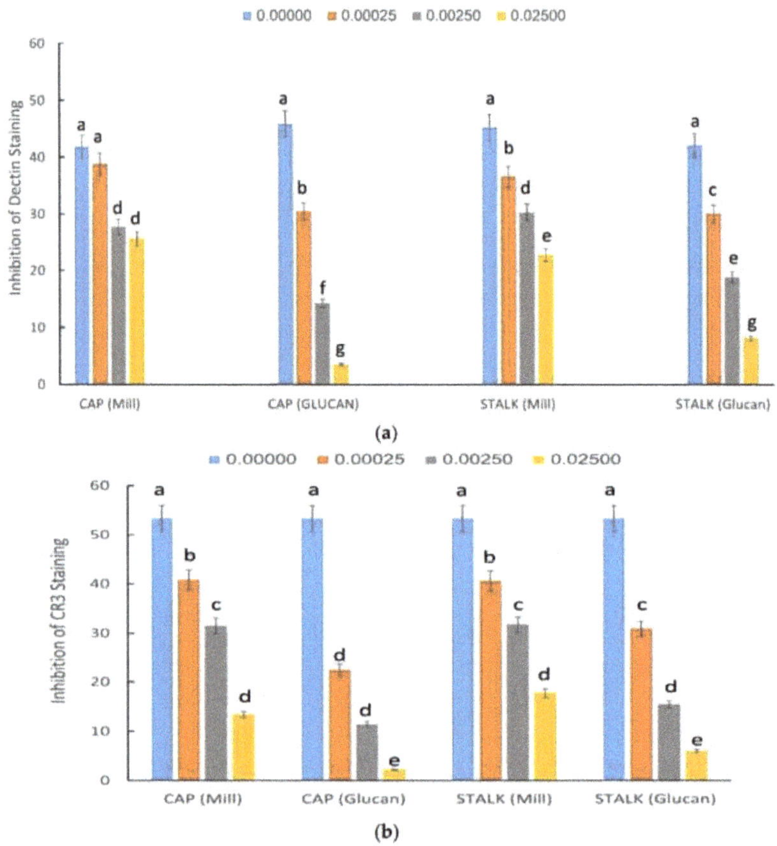

Figure 2. Effect of different concentrations of glucans from mill and isolated glucans from caps and stalks of *P. eryngii* mushrooms (0.00025%; 0.0025%; 0.025%; i.e., 0.25 or 2.5 or 25 μg/1 mL media) on Dectin-1 expressed in human neutrophils (**a**) or CR3 staining expressed in RAW 264.7 cells (**b**). The data shown are the average with error bars indicating the standard deviation. The level of inhibition with increasing concentrations of *P. eryngii* isolated glucans is more potent than that obtained with increasing concentrations of *P. eryngii* mill preparations. No difference between caps and stalks. Different letters indicate significantly different values at $p < 0.05$.

2.4. Effect of Isolated Glucans from Stalk and Cap on Acute Colitis Induction in Mice

Histologic damage is one of the most noticeable results from acute DSS-induced colitis in mice. Figure 3 clearly demonstrates that dextran sulfate sodium (DSS) administration resulted in a high histology score of ~12 that was significantly reduced by administration of glucan extracts. Milled mushrooms had lower effects than glucan extracts, and mill prepared from stalk demonstrated almost complete ineffectiveness.

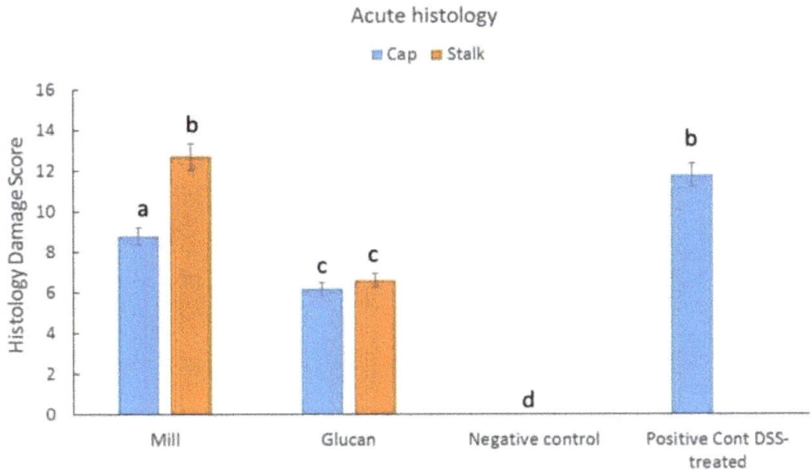

Figure 3. Effect of mill and isolated glucans from caps and stalks of *P. eryngii* mushrooms (1 mg glucan/kg mice BW) on histologic damage score in dextran sulfate sodium (DSS)-induced colitis. DSS was administrated for 7 days and mill and glucan extract treatment started with DSS treatment and continued until day 16 when all mice were sacrificed and tissue samples were taken for analysis. Data represent mean ± SD of six mice per group. Different letters indicate significantly different values at $p < 0.01$.

2.5. CXCL1, MIP-2, and INF-γ mRNA Expression in Large Intestine

Expression levels of genes related to immune response were analyzed in samples of large intestine from mice with experimentally-induced acute colitis. INF-γ showed a strong reduction in gene expression by both whole mill and glucan extracts (Figure 4a); although, there was also a significant difference between cap- and stalk-derived glucans. MIP-2 also showed a decrease in expression in treated mice. Mill preparations were less effective than glucan extracts. Additionally, there was also a difference between cap- and stalk-derived glucans with the latter showing stronger effect (Figure 4b). The chemokine CXCL1 showed a significant decrease in expression compared to positive control when mice were treated with glucan extracts but not with whole mill (Figure 4c).

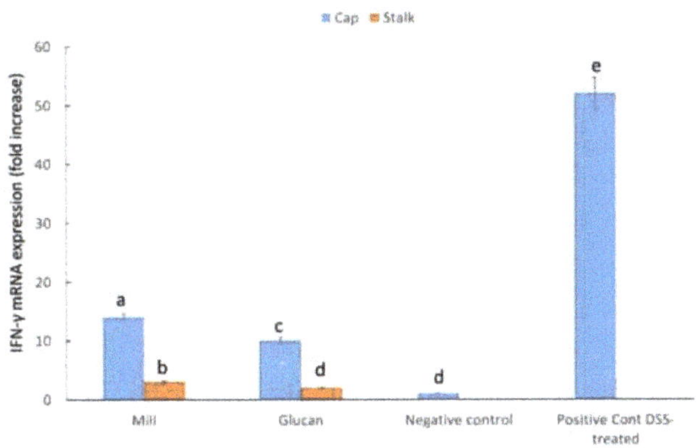

(a)

Figure 4. *Cont.*

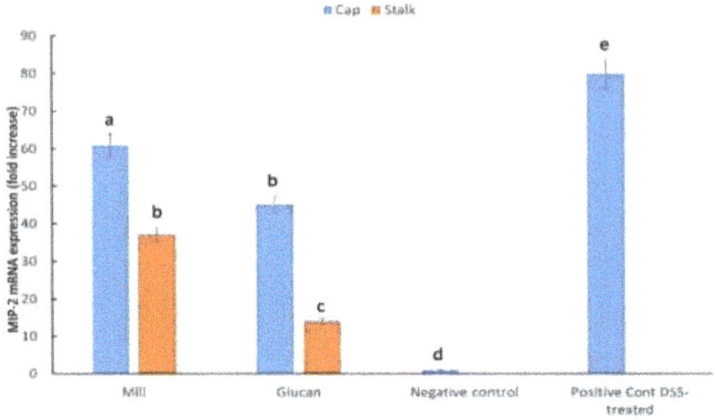

(**b**)

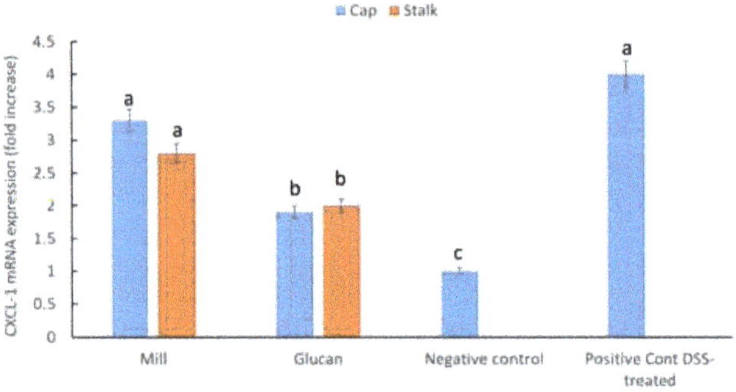

(**c**)

Figure 4. Effect of mill and isolated glucans from caps and stalks of *P. eryngii* mushrooms (1 mg glucan/kg mice BW) on (**a**) INF-γ mRNA levels (**b**) Mip-2 levels mRNA levels and (**c**) CXCL1 mRNA levels in colonic samples relative to negative control (no treatment). DSS was administrated for 7 days and mill and glucan extract treatment started with DSS treatment and continued until day 16 when all mice were sacrificed and tissue samples were taken for analysis. Data represent mean $\pm$ SD of six mice per group. Different letters indicate significantly different values at $p < 0.05$.

2.6. Percentages of CD14/CD16 Monocytes in Colitis

Next, we evaluated the percentages of activated monocytes in circulating blood in the different groups (Figure 5a). The maximum percentage (18.2 $\pm$ 3%) of activated monocytes was observed in the DSS-induced mice, whole mill had no significant effects, while glucan extracts significantly reduced the percentage of activated monocytes. No difference was detected between caps and stalks.

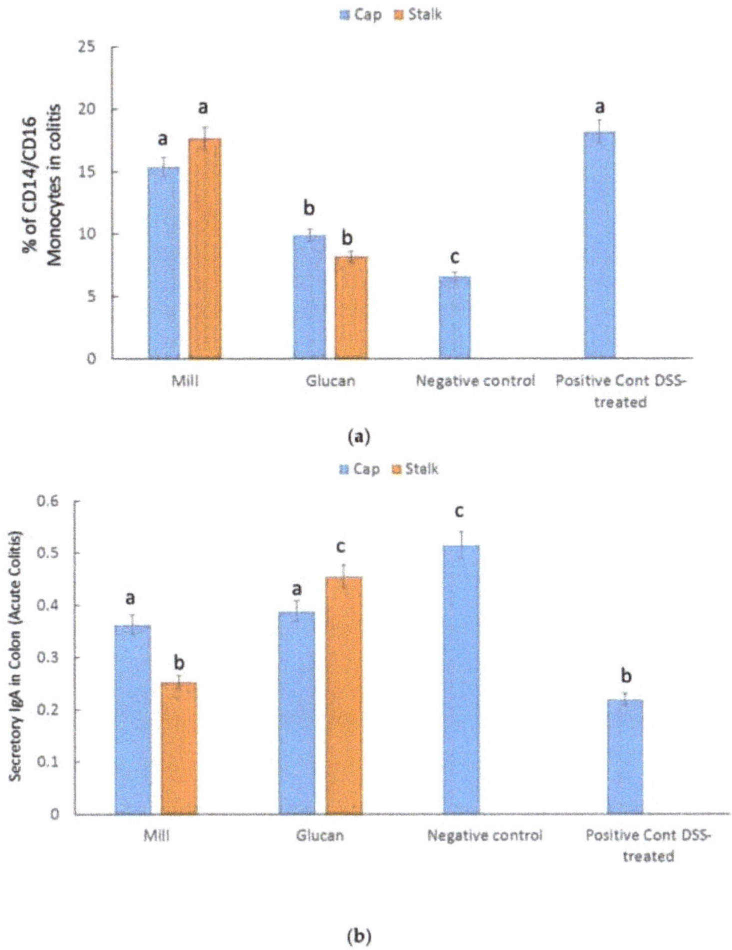

Figure 5. Effect of mill and isolated glucans from caps and stalks of *P. eryngii* mushrooms (1 mg glucan/kg mice BW) on (**a**) percent of $CD14^+/CD16^+$ monocytes and (**b**) on secretory IgA in feces harvested from mice who underwent DSS-induced colitis. Data represent mean ± SD of six mice per group; data were compared between DSS and mill and isolated glucans from caps and stalks of *P. eryngii* mushrooms treated groups. Different letters indicate significantly different values at $p < 0.05$.

2.7. Secretory IgA in the Colon

Secretory IgA is the most important immunoglobulin secreted towards the mucosal surface in most mammals and play a key role in the protection of the intestinal epithelium from bacterial and other pathogens infection. We measured the amount of secretory IgA in the colon of DSS mice in both treated and untreated mice. Secretory IgA increased significantly after treatment with glucan extracts, indicating a higher protective status as is expected in the healthy intestine (Figure 5b). No significant differences were detected in animals treated with whole mill from stalk before DSS and after DSS without pretreatment.

3. Discussion

This study concentrated on evaluating the functional and spatial variation of glucan type and concentration in the edible mushrooms *P. eryngii*. In line with our previous publication [10], we demonstrated that the stalks (stipe) of the fruit body contained higher glucan content than the caps (pileus). Similarly, Park and associates [11] have recently demonstrated that the β-glucan contents were also higher in stipes of *P. eryngii*, claiming that this result is probably associated with the development of the major structural compounds of cell wall in mushrooms allowing for optimal supporting effect of the cap. Since β-glucans were repetitively demonstrated in a myriad of studies [2,12–18] to induce immunostimulatory events in mammalian cells, we hypothesized that this spatial variation may also impinge on the functionality of the different parts of *P. eryngii*.

In the present study, we measured α-glucan, β-glucan, and total glucan concentrations in mill preparations and compared these to extracted glucan lyophilized fractions from caps and stalks prepared from *P. eryngii* mushrooms. Overall, the net α-glucan, β-glucan, and total glucan concentrations were significantly higher in the extracted lyophilized glucan fraction from *P. eryngii* stalks (Table 1). Additionally, the α-glucan concentration was notably higher in extracted glucan fractions. Therefore, we hypothesized that glucan extracts from *P. eryngii* stalks should be significantly more effective than those from *P. eryngii* caps since, per gram of extract, there are more glucans (β-glucans and significantly more α-glucans).

We tested the effect of our glucan samples on LPS-induced production of TNF-α. The results demonstrated that glucan extracts from caps and stalk were more effective than mill mushroom preparations (Figure 1), and the effectiveness of stalks was slightly more pronounced. These results indicated that *P. eryngii* glucans prepared from either part of this edible mushroom could be used as an adequate treatment aimed to control diseases associated with TNF-α overproduction resulting from LPS-mediated inflammation.

In order to demonstrate the putative immunomodulatory effect of *P. eryngii* glucans derived from caps and stalks, we tested whether there are some differential abilities of these glucans to bind to glucan receptors associated with the inflammatory processes expressed on membrane of immune cells. To accomplish this aim, we tested the putative competitive of these glucans towards Dectin-1 and complement-3 (CR-3) receptors. Dectin-1 is a transmembrane protein widely expressed in the cell surface of neutrophils, macrophages, and dendritic cells, and shown to specifically bind β-glucans secreted by edible mushrooms [8]. We demonstrate herein that cap and stalk glucans from mill or isolated glucan dose competed similarly with anti-Dectin-1 antibody, indicating that both structural parts of *P. eryngii* competed for binding. Nonetheless, competition of glucans prepared from glucan extracts were more efficient than glucans from mill preparations (this was strikingly evident at higher concentrations of added glucans). Since the human β-glucan receptor is functionally equivalent to murine Dectin-1 [19] testing the *P. eryngii* derived glucans in human and mouse cell lines broadness the inter-species importance of these molecules.

Similar results were obtained CR-3 receptor. CR3 receptor is a heterodimeric transmembrane glycoprotein receptor consisting of a β2 subunit (CD18), and bound to a αM subunit (CD11b) [8]. The CR3 receptor is expressed on immune-associated cells such as macrophages or NK cells and on leukocytes. Similarly to Dectin-1, stalk and cap glucan preparations from *P. eryngii* did not significantly differ in their binding ability, indicating that glucans from both mushroom parts can compete with the glucan receptor CR3. These results may stress the importance of the interactions between the wide varieties of glucan structures with cells of the immune system. The binding may affect the immune system and keep it alert to fight pathogens or other opportunistic infections.

Next, we tested the effect of glucan preparations as an in vivo anti-inflammatory treatment for IBD. For IBD induction, we used the DSS mice model, which is an important animal research tool that has enormously contributed to our understanding of pathogenetic pathways associated with IBD [20]. Additionally, drugs used to treat human IBD also ameliorate symptoms of DSS-induced mouse IBD [21]. Histologic damage score includes colonic crypt alteration, epithelial cell injury, ulcer formation, and infiltration of inflammatory cells into the colonic lamina propria. Glucan extracts were equally efficient in diminishing histologic damage scores in the DSS-IBD model (Figure 3); however, mill preparations were ineffective. We assume that the concentrations or the specific mix of glucans (especially α-glucans; see Table 1) were more effective and contributed to their impressive ameliorating effect.

We measured the intestinal inflammatory response to the treatment of mill preparations of the DSS-IBD model compared to extracted glucan by assessing pro-inflammatory cytokine transcript levels in the intestinal tissue by RT-PCR. First, we clearly demonstrated that mill and glucan extracts were very effective in downregulating IFN-γ levels; however, glucan extracts were more effective than mill preparations (see Figure 4a). A striking effect was notable following treatment with stalk preparations compared to caps. This is a very interesting and important result if we take into consideration that the significant downregulation of a pro-inflammatory cytokine IFN-γ probably initiated the inflammation in the DSS-IBD model. Ito et al. [22] demonstrated that IFN-γ plays an essential role in the initiation of colitis induced by DSS treatment; additionally, several chemokines are produced in response to triggering in an IFN-γ-dependent manner.

These observations were followed up by measurements of MIP-2 intestinal transcript levels. MIP-2 is specifically expressed in the inflamed areas of the colon in patients with IBD [23] and plays an indispensable role in its development and progression. MIP-2 is produced by a wide variety of cells and plays a role as a powerful chemoattractant for immune cells such as monocytes, T and B cells, and others and thus intensifies the immune-mediated response in colitis. We assumed that MIP-2 is regulated in an IFN-γ-dependent manner and, as such, the effects on the cytokine levels by *P. eryngii* glucan treatment were similar to those exerted on IFN-γ levels. Indeed, mill and glucan extracts were very effective in downregulating MIP-2 levels; and as for IFN-γ, glucan extracts were more effective than mill preparations and stalk glucans were more effective than cap glucans (see Figure 4b).

We also measured the effect on CXCL1 levels. CXCL-1 levels are associated with recruitment of neutrophils into colonic tissues after that the inflammation process is initiated. The response of treatment to mill preparations compared to extracted glucan lyophilized fractions from caps and stalks prepared from *P. eryngii* mushrooms differed to the response of IFN-γ and MIP-2. Mill glucans were ineffective and glucans extracts from both caps and stalks were equally effective (see Figure 4c). We assumed that CXCL1 chemokines participate in later stages of inflammation, therefore controlling their levels was less essential than controlling the effector IFN-γ levels and its downstream response cytokine MIP-2.

CD14/CD16 monocytes represents a major proinflammatory immune cell population in IBD in general and in Crohn's disease specifically [24]. Various researchers have demonstrated that peripheral $CD14^+/CD16^+$ cells play a key role as potential disease indicators and drug targets for anti-inflammatory treatment [25].

In the present study, we demonstrated that mill glucans were ineffective in regulating peripheral $CD14^+/CD16^+$ cell levels similarly to their effects on CXCL1 chemokines intestinal expression. On the other hand, glucan extracts from both caps and stalks were equally effective in regulating the number of $CD14^+/CD16^+$ monocytes, indicating that they induce a systemic anti-inflammatory effect (see Figure 5a). We assumed that $CD14^+/CD16^+$ cells, like CXCL1 chemokines, participated in later stages of inflammation.

One cause of IBD is an abnormally amplified immune response of the intestinal mucosal to the normal intestinal microbiome. IgA is the primary antibody present in intestinal secretions and its role is to stop unwanted pathogenic organisms reaching the intestinal epithelial cell surface. Additionally, IgA deficiency in humans has been closely associated with ulcerative colitis [25]. Our results indicated that intestinal disorders induced by DSS-treatment in mice also involved downregulation of IgA expression (see Figure 5b). Glucan extracts upregulated the levels of IgA to almost normal levels; however, mill preparations were found to be almost ineffective in this regard. We believe that either glucan administration prepared from caps or stalks of *P. eryngii* exerts an important effect in the preservation of the epithelial integrity and greatly contributes to the normal homeostasis phenotype of the intestinal epithelium.

4. Materials and Methods

4.1. Preparation of Whole Mill and Glucan Extractions from Caps and Stalks from *P. eryngii*

P. eryngii mushrooms were grown at the Matityahu Experimental Farm (Upper Galilei, Israel). Fresh mushrooms were harvested when they reached similar cap opening and color. After collection, *P. eryngii* were dissected into caps and stalks, the different parts were weighed, dried and milled to pass a 1.0 mm screen using a Retsch centrifugal mill preparations unit. This preparation provided the whole mill. Dried powder of these whole mill preparations were subsequently used for glucan extraction similarly to the methodology used in our previous publication [10]. Glucan extracts were lyophilized as we previously described [10] and dried pre-weighted glucan extract samples were used for further glucan analyses.

4.2. Glucans Analysis

Glucan concentrations of mill and glucan extracts from *P. eryngii* caps and stalks were determined using a mushroom and yeast-specific β-glucan kit (Megazyme International, Wicklow, Ireland) based on a colorimetric reaction using the previously described method [10]. The absorbance of the resulting color complex was measured using a spectrophotometer (Synergy 2, Multi-Mode Reader, BioTek, Winooski, VT, USA) at 510 nm. Total glucan (% *w*/*w* or g/100 g), α-glucan (% *w*/*w*) and β-glucan content (% *w*/*w*) were measured as we recently described [10].

4.3. TNF-α Secretion from LPS- and Glucan-treated Mouse Macrophage Cell Line J774.2

Mouse macrophage J774.2 cells (1×10^6/well) were incubated with LPS (100 ng/mL) and different concentrations of glucans from mill or isolated glucans (dissolved in PBS under mild heating i.e., 60 °C) for 24 h. Supernatants were collected at different time intervals (4, 6, 12, and 24 h) and evaluated for TNF-α secretion by ELISA employing anti-mouse TNF-α kit (R&D Systems, Minneapolis, MN, USA) and expressed as pg/mL. Glucan treatment did not affect cell viability as determined by MTT (3-(4, 5-dimethylthiazolyl-2)-2,5-diphenyltetrazolium bromide) assay as previously described [5].

4.4. Inhibition of CR3 and Dectin-1 Staining by Mill and Glucan Extracts from *P. eryngii* Caps and Stalks

We evaluated the ability of mill and glucan extracts to compete with specific FITC-labeled antibodies to CR3 (MN-41) or Dectin-1 (CLEC7A) using flow cytometry. To this end, we incubated human neutrophils (in case of CR3) and RAW 264.7 cell lines (in case of Dectin-1) with glucans (0.00025%; 0.0025%; 0.025%; i.e., 0.25 or 2.5 or 25 μg/1 mL media) of each preparation for 45 min at 4 °C then, after washing, we incubated the cells with each of the FITC-labeled antibodies for 30 min on ice. Flow cytometry was performed with a FACScan (Becton Dickinson, San Jose, CA, USA) flow cytometer and the data from over 10,000 cells/sample were analyzed. Results are specified as percentage of inhibition of staining.

4.5. Animals

Female, 8-week-old BALB/c mice (5–10 mice/group) were purchased from the Jackson Laboratory (Bar Harbor, ME, USA). The protocol for the research project was approved by the University of Louisville IACUC Committee and conformed to the provisions of the Declaration of Helsinki (as revised in Edinburgh 2000). Animals were sacrificed by CO_2 asphyxiation followed by cervical dislocation.

4.6. Acute Colitis Induction in Mice

Dextran sodium sulfate (DSS) 3% (*w*/*v*) in water was provided in the drinking water for 7 days essentially as previously described [6]. Glucans were used simultaneously with the start of the treatment at dose 1 mg glucan/kg mice BW dissolved in PBS similarly to in vitro assay. The glucan treatment continued until day 16. Glucans treatment was provided by gavage.

Disease severity was evaluated at the end of the study based on evaluation of histology of the colon (histologic damage score). Histology damage score was performed essentially as we previously described [6]. After killing, the distal third of the colon was transferred to a 4% buffered formalin solution. Histological scoring of the fixed (paraffin-embedded), sectioned and haematoxylin and eosin-stained tissues was performed in a blinded fashion essentially as previously described by Dieleman et al. [26]. Scoring was performed according to the following criteria: inflammation (0 (none) to 4 (severe)), extent (0 (none) to 4 (transmural)) and crypt damage (0 (none) to 4 (entire crypt and epithelium lost)). The three scores were summed to give a total score (0–12). Grading was performed by two investigators blinded to the treatment groups.

4.7. Monocytes Staining

Mice blood samples were obtained from control, DSS-treated, and glucan and DSS-treated mice. Inflammatory monocytes ($CD14^+/CD16^+$) were stained using anti-CD14-FITC and anti-CD16-PE antibodies. 20 μL of whole blood was incubated with the labeled antibodies and washed. Following application of 300 μL erythrocyte lysing buffer, the cells were washed and analyzed by flow cytometry.

4.8. RNA Preparation and Real-time PCR

Total RNA was isolated from colonic tissue (snap frozen in liquid N_2) using the RNeasy Plus Mini Kit (Qiagen, Santa Clarita, CA, USA) as described in the manufacturer's protocol. RNA concentration was quantified by ultraviolet spectrophotometry at 260 nm, and the purity and integrity were determined using a NanoDrop (Thermo Fisher Scientific, Wilmington, DE, USA).

RT real-time PCR assays were performed to quantify steady-state mRNA levels of selected molecules CXCL1, IFN-gamma, and MIP-2. cDNA was synthesized from 0.2 μg of total RNA. Real-time PCR amplification was performed using Primer Express Software (Applied Biosystems, Foster City, CA, USA). Target probe was labeled with fluorescent reporter dye. PreDeveloped TaqMan primers and probes were used for the detection. Reporter dye emission was detected by an automated sequence detector combined with ABI Prism 7700 Sequence Detection System software (Applied Biosystems). Real-time PCR quantification was then performed using TaqMan 18S rRNA controls as described [27]. Gene expression was expressed as fold increase relative to negative control.

The primers used for real-time PCR were as shown in Table 2:

Table 2. Primer sequences used for RT-PCR.

Gene	Forward Primer	Reverse Primer
MIP-2	5′-TGGGTGGGATGTAGCTAGTTCC	5′-AGTTTGCCTTGACCCTGAAGCC
Cxcl1	5′- GCCACACTCAAGAATGGTCG	5′-TGGGGACACCCTTTAGCATC
INF-γ	5′-GTCTCTTCTTGGATATCTGGAGGAACT	5′-GTAGTAATCAGGTGTGATTCAATGACGC

4.9. Secretory Intestinal IgA

Elisa plates were coated with anti-IgA antibodies, incubated with fecal samples from all treatment mice groups, and diluted 1:100 in PBS. IgA was developed using anti-IgA-biotin and HRP-streptavidin as previously reported [28].

4.10. Statistical Analyses

Statistical analyses were performed by one-way repeated-measure ANOVA with Tukey–Kramer or Dunnett's test. Results are presented as mean ± SD. All figures show representative results of at least two independent experiments.

5. Conclusions

We demonstrate that the most effective glucans in ameliorating IBD-associated symptoms induced by DSS treatment in mice were glucan extracts prepared from the stalk of *P. eryngii*. We believe that these spatial distinctions may be helpful in selecting more effectively appropriate medicinal mushrooms.

Author Contributions: V.V.; writing—review and editing, methodology, project administration, O.G.; writing—review and editing, investigation, H.H.; investigation, O.D.; methodology, resources, N.E.; resources, Y.H. writing—review and editing, B.S.; project administration, writing—review and editing.

Funding: This study was supported by BARD (Binational agricultural research and development fund) grant number IS-4851-15 R.

Conflicts of Interest: The authors declare no conflict of interest.

References

1. Ma, G.; Kimatu, B.M.; Zhao, L.; Yang, W.; Pei, F.; Hu, Q. Impacts of Dietary *Pleurotus eryngii* Polysaccharide on Nutrient Digestion, Metabolism, and Immune Response of the Small Intestine and Colon-An iTRAQ-Based Proteomic Analysis. *Proteomics* **2018**, *18*, e1700443. [CrossRef] [PubMed]
2. Kim, Y.H.; Jung, E.G.; Han, K.I.; Patnaik, B.B.; Kwon, H.J.; Lee, H.S.; Kim, W.J.; Han, M.D. Immunomodulatory Effects of Extracellular beta-Glucan Isolated from the King Oyster Mushroom *Pleurotus eryngii* (Agaricomycetes) and Its Sulfated Form on Signaling Molecules Involved in Innate Immunity. *Int. J. Med. Mushrooms* **2017**, *19*, 521–533. [CrossRef] [PubMed]
3. Xu, D.; Wang, H.; Zheng, W.; Gao, Y.; Wang, M.; Zhang, Y.; Gao, Q. Charaterization and immunomodulatory activities of polysaccharide isolated from *Pleurotus eryngii*. *Int. J. Biol. Macromol.* **2016**, *92*, 30–36. [CrossRef] [PubMed]
4. Zhu, F.; Du, B.; Xu, B. A critical review on production and industrial applications of β-glucans. *Food Hydrocoll.* **2016**, *52*, 275–288. [CrossRef]
5. Lavi, I.; Friesem, D.; Geresh, S.; Hadar, Y.; Schwartz, B. An aqueous polysaccharide extract from the edible mushroom *Pleurotus ostreatus* induces anti-proliferative and pro-apoptotic effects on HT-29 colon cancer cells. *Cancer Lett.* **2006**, *244*, 61–70. [CrossRef] [PubMed]
6. Lavi, I.; Levinson, D.; Peri, I.; Nimri, L.; Hadar, Y.; Schwartz, B. Orally administered glucans from the edible mushroom *Pleurotus pulmonarius* reduce acute inflammation in dextran sulfate sodium-induced experimental colitis. *Br. J. Nutr.* **2010**, *103*, 393–402. [CrossRef] [PubMed]
7. Lavi, I.; Nimri, L.; Levinson, D.; Peri, I.; Hadar, Y.; Schwartz, B. Glucans from the edible mushroom *Pleurotus pulmonarius* inhibit colitis-associated colon carcinogenesis in mice. *J. Gastroenterol.* **2012**, *47*, 504–518. [CrossRef] [PubMed]
8. Legentil, L.; Paris, F.; Ballet, C.; Trouvelot, S.; Daire, X.; Vetvicka, V.; Ferrieres, V. Molecular Interactions of β-(1–>3)-Glucans with Their Receptors. *Molecules* **2015**, *20*, 9745–9766. [CrossRef] [PubMed]
9. Yamamoto-Furusho, J.K. Inflammatory bowel disease therapy: Blockade of cytokines and cytokine signaling pathways. *Curr. Opin. Gastroenterol.* **2018**, *34*, 187–193. [CrossRef] [PubMed]
10. Avni, S.; Ezove, N.; Hanani, H.; Yadid, I.; Karpovsky, M.; Hayby, H.; Gover, O.; Hadar, Y.; Schwartz, B.; Danay, O. Olive Mill Waste Enhances α-Glucan Content in the Edible Mushroom *Pleurotus eryngii*. *Int. J. Mol. Sci.* **2017**, *18*. [CrossRef] [PubMed]
11. Earnshaw, S.R.; McDade, C.L.; Chu, Y.; Fleige, L.E.; Sievenpiper, J.L. Cost-effectiveness of Maintaining Daily Intake of Oat β-Glucan for Coronary Heart Disease Primary Prevention. *Clin. Ther.* **2017**, *39*, 804–818. [CrossRef] [PubMed]
12. Chan, G.C.; Chan, W.K.; Sze, D.M. The effects of β-glucan on human immune and cancer cells. *J. Hematol. Oncol.* **2009**, *2*, 25. [CrossRef] [PubMed]
13. Guerra Dore, C.M.; Azevedo, T.C.; De Souza, M.C.; Rego, L.A.; De Dantas, J.C.; Silva, F.R.; Rocha, H.A.; Baseia, I.G.; Leite, E.L. Antiinflammatory, antioxidant and cytotoxic actions of beta-glucan-rich extract from Geastrum saccatum mushroom. *Int. Immunopharmacol.* **2007**, *7*, 1160–1169. [CrossRef] [PubMed]
14. Nosal'ova, V.; Bobek, P.; Cerna, S.; Galbavy, S.; Stvrtina, S. Effects of pleuran (β-glucan isolated from *Pleurotus ostreatus*) on experimental colitis in rats. *Physiol. Res.* **2001**, *50*, 575–581. [PubMed]

15. Soltanian, S.; Stuyven, E.; Cox, E.; Sorgeloos, P.; Bossier, P. Beta-glucans as immunostimulant in vertebrates and invertebrates. *Crit. Rev. Microbiol.* **2009**, *35*, 109–138. [CrossRef] [PubMed]
16. Vetvicka, V.; Vetvickova, J. Glucans and Cancer: Comparison of Commercially Available β-glucans—Part IV. *Anticancer Res.* **2018**, *38*, 1327–1333. [CrossRef] [PubMed]
17. Volman, J.J.; Helsper, J.P.; Wei, S.; Baars, J.J.; Van Griensven, L.J.; Sonnenberg, A.S.; Mensink, R.P.; Plat, J. Effects of mushroom-derived β-glucan-rich polysaccharide extracts on nitric oxide production by bone marrow-derived macrophages and nuclear factor-κB transactivation in Caco-2 reporter cells: Can effects be explained by structure? *Mol. Nutr. Food Res.* **2010**, *54*, 268–276. [CrossRef] [PubMed]
18. Wang, Q.; Sheng, X.; Shi, A.; Hu, H.; Yang, Y.; Liu, L.; Fei, L.; Liu, H. β-Glucans: Relationships between Modification, Conformation and Functional Activities. *Molecules* **2017**, *22*, 257. [CrossRef] [PubMed]
19. Willment, J.A.; Marshall, A.S.; Reid, D.M.; Williams, D.L.; Wong, S.Y.; Gordon, S.; Brown, G.D. The human β-glucan receptor is widely expressed and functionally equivalent to murine Dectin-1 on primary cells. *Eur. J. Immunol.* **2005**, *35*, 1539–1547. [CrossRef] [PubMed]
20. Eichele, D.D.; Kharbanda, K.K. Dextran sodium sulfate colitis murine model: An indispensable tool for advancing our understanding of inflammatory bowel diseases pathogenesis. *World J. Gastroenterol.* **2017**, *23*, 6016–6029. [CrossRef] [PubMed]
21. Wirtz, S.; Neurath, M.F. Mouse models of inflammatory bowel disease. *Adv. Drug Deliv. Rev.* **2007**, *59*, 1073–1083. [CrossRef] [PubMed]
22. Ito, R.; Shin-Ya, M.; Kishida, T.; Urano, A.; Takada, R.; Sakagami, J.; Imanishi, J.; Kita, M.; Ueda, Y.; Iwakura, Y.; et al. Interferon-γ is causatively involved in experimental inflammatory bowel disease in mice. *Clin. Exp. Immunol.* **2006**, *146*, 330–338. [CrossRef] [PubMed]
23. Neurath, M.F. Cytokines in inflammatory bowel disease. *Nat. Rev. Immunol.* **2014**, *14*, 329–342. [CrossRef] [PubMed]
24. Hanai, H.; Iida, T.; Takeuchi, K.; Watanabe, F.; Yamada, M.; Kikuyama, M.; Maruyama, Y.; Iwaoka, Y.; Hirayama, K.; Nagata, S.; et al. Adsorptive depletion of elevated proinflammatory CD14+CD16+DR++ monocytes in patients with inflammatory bowel disease. *Am. J. Gastroenterol.* **2008**, *103*, 1210–1216. [CrossRef] [PubMed]
25. Koch, S.; Kucharzik, T.; Heidemann, J.; Nusrat, A.; Luegering, A. Investigating the role of proinflammatory CD16+ monocytes in the pathogenesis of inflammatory bowel disease. *Clin. Exp. Immunol.* **2010**, *161*, 332–341. [CrossRef] [PubMed]
26. Dieleman, L.A.; Palmen, M.J.; Akol, H.; Bloemena, E.; Pena, A.S.; Meuwissen, S.G.; Van Rees, E.P. Chronic experimental colitis induced by dextran sulphate sodium (DSS) is characterized by Th1 and Th2 cytokines. *Clin. Exp. Immunol.* **1998**, *114*, 385–391. [CrossRef] [PubMed]
27. Vetvicka, V.; Volny, T.; Saraswat-Ohri, S.; Vashishta, A.; Vancikova, Z.; Vetvickova, J. Glucan and resveratrol complex—Possible synergistic effects on immune system. *Biomed. Pap. Med. Fac. Univ. Palacky Olomouc Czech.* **2007**, *151*, 41–46. [CrossRef]
28. Cao, A.T.; Yao, S.; Gong, B.; Elson, C.O.; Cong, Y. Th17 cells upregulate polymeric Ig receptor and intestinal IgA and contribute to intestinal homeostasis. *J. Immunol.* **2012**, *189*, 4666–4673. [CrossRef] [PubMed]

International Journal of
Molecular Sciences

MDPI

Article

Effects of Panax Notoginseng Saponins on Esterases Responsible for Aspirin Hydrolysis In Vitro

Zongxi Sun [1], Yali Wu [1], Song Liu [2], Shaonan Hu [1], Bo Zhao [1], Pengyue Li [1,*] and Shouying Du [1,*]

1 School of Chinese Materia Medica, Beijing University of Chinese Medicine, Beijing 100029, China; zongxisun@126.com (Z.S.); wuyali1993@163.com (Y.W.); hushaonan8980@126.com (S.H.); zhaobowua@163.com (B.Z.)

2 College of Medicine, Wuhan University of Science and Technology, Wuhan 430081, China; liusong@wust.edu.cn

* Correspondence: pengyuelee@126.com (P.L.); dumenzidi123@163.com (S.D.); Tel.: +86-106-428-6426 (P.L. & S.D.)

Received: 27 August 2018; Accepted: 9 October 2018; Published: 12 October 2018

Abstract: Herb–drug interactions strongly challenge the clinical combined application of herbs and drugs. Herbal products consist of complex pharmacological-active ingredients and perturb the activity of drug-metabolizing enzymes. Panax notoginseng saponins (PNS) based drugs are often combined with aspirin in vascular disease treatment in China. PNS was found to exhibit inhibitory effects on aspirin hydrolysis using Caco-2 cell monolayers. In the present study, a total of 22 components of PNS were separated and identified by UPLC-MS/MS. Using highly selective probe substrate analysis, PNS exerted robust inhibitory potency on human carboxylesterase 2 (hCE2), while had a minor influence on hCE1, butyrylcholinesterase (BChE) and paraoxonase (PON). These effects were also verified through molecular docking analysis. PNS showed a concentration-dependent inhibitory effect on hydrolytic activity of aspirin in HepaRG cells. The protein level of hCE2 in HepaRG cells was suppressed after PNS treatment, while the level of BChE or PON1 in the extracellular matrix were elevated after PNS treatment. Insignificant effect was observed on the mRNA expression of the esterases. These findings are important to understand the underlying efficacy and safety of co-administration of PNS and aspirin in clinical practice.

Keywords: Panax notoginseng saponins; aspirin; HepaRG cells; herb–drug interactions

1. Introduction

Herbs have been used for primary health care for thousands of years before the advent of modern medicines. It is estimated that approximately 80% of the population in Asian countries currently uses herbs as complementary or alternative medicine [1]. Patients in these countries with complex diseases use herbs more frequently. However, side effects of herb-drug interactions (HDI) might occur. Some research reported that herbs perturbed the activities of the metabolizing enzymes and/or transporters [2–4]. In the past decades, concerns about HDI have been raised. Liver is the primary drug metabolism site and entails a myriad of chemical reactions. HepaRG cell line, derived from a hepatocellular carcinoma, could express a large panel of liver-specific enzymes [5–7]. Due to the similarity with primary human hepatocytes, HepaRG cell line was found to be a valuable human-relevant in vitro model for testing drug interactions [8].

Panax notoginseng saponins (PNS) are the main biologically active constituents in the roots of Panax notoginseng (family Araliaceae). In China, PNS-based drugs have been developed and widely used to treat cerebral infarction and ischemia [9], coronary heart disease and atherosclerosis [10]. Aspirin (acetylsalicylic acid) is an important member of the therapeutic arsenal for combating the vascular disease. After administration, aspirin is rapidly hydrolyzed in the body with an elimination half-life of approximatly 15 min [11,12]. Aspirin and PNS-based drugs are often taken together to prevent thrombus and clinical benefits have been obtained.

On account of the presence of ester bond, aspirin could be catalyzed by esterases in the intestine, liver, and plasma [13], which mainly include human carboxylesterase 1 (hCE1) and hCE2 in the liver and intestine [14,15], and butyrylcholinesterase (BChE) [16], paraoxonase (PON) [17,18] in plasma. We recently reported that PNS could inhibit aspirin hydrolysis and thereby elevated the level of aspirin through Caco-2 cell monolayers [19]. However, the influence of PNS on the esterases responsible for aspirin hydrolysis has not been fully investigated yet. In the current study, we characterized the effects of PNS on the esterases using highly selective probe substrates and predicted the potential HDI in vivo on the basis of enzyme kinetic parameters of hCE2. The effects toward hCE2 were verified through molecular docking with PNS. Further, we explored the possible HDI using the HepaRG cell line.

2. Results

2.1. UPLC/LTQ-Orbitrap MS/MS Analysis

The main chemical components of PNS were detected with UPLC/LTQ-Orbitrap MS/MS analysis. A total of 22 compounds were identified or tentatively identified (Figure 1). The retention time, m/z values of adduct ions and MS/MS fragment ions in negative ESI modes, mass error, and formula of all the identified compounds were listed in Table 1.

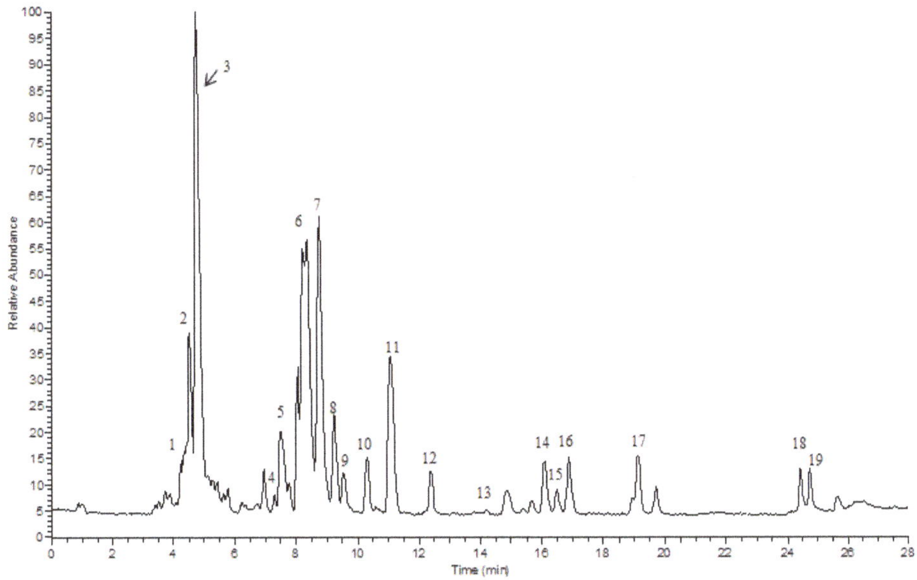

Figure 1. The representative total ion current chromatogram of PNS in negative ESI modes. The corresponding compound names were given in Table 1 (varying from no. 1 to 19).

Table 1. All the identified or tentatively identified components of PNS and their UPLC-MS/MS data.

No.	T_R (min)	Theoretical Mass (*m*/*z*)	Experimental Mass (*m*/*z*)	Mass Error (ppm)	MS^2 Fragment Ions	Formula	Identification
1	4.42	1007.5421	1007.5417	−0.40	799(100), 637(20.49), 475(1.24)	$C_{48}H_{82}O_{19}$	notoginsenoside R_3/R_6
2	4.48	977.5315	977.5316	0.10	799(100), 637(4.13), 475(3.7)	$C_{47}H_{80}O_{18}$	notoginsenoside R_1
3	4.73	845.4891	845.4893	0.24	637(34.70), 475(32.28)	$C_{42}H_{72}O_{14}$	ginsenoside Rg_1
4	7.30	845.4891	845.4890	−0.12	637(10.01), 475(6.54)	$C_{42}H_{72}O_{14}$	ginsenoside F_{11}
5	8.02	815.4787	815.4785	−0.25	637(52.99), 475(100), 391(1.53)	$C_{41}H_{70}O_{13}$	notoginsenoside R_2 or F_3
6	8.30	1107.5946	1107.5994	4.33	945(100), 783(22.44), 621(16.01), 459(3.33)	$C_{54}H_{92}O_{23}$	ginsenoside Rb_1
7	8.62	829.4944	829.4941	−0.36	637(26.69), 475(100), 391(3.34)	$C_{42}H_{72}O_{13}$	ginsenoside Rg_2
8	9.24	683.4365	683.4363	−0.29	945(100), 783(35.03)	$C_{53}H_{90}O_{22}$	ginsenoside Rb_2 or Rb_3
9	9.55	1123.5895	1123.5892	0.27	637(100), 475(16.41)	$C_{36}H_{62}O_9$	ginsenoside Rh_1
10	10.31	683.4365	683.4362	−0.44	637(100), 475(45.43)	$C_{36}H_{62}O_9$	ginsenoside F_1
11	11.08	991.5472	991.5465	−0.71	783(70.63), 675(32.46), 475(3.7)	$C_{48}H_{82}O_{18}$	ginsenoside Re
12	12.36	991.5472	991.5465	−0.71	783(100), 621(7.47), 459(5.62), 375(0.86)	$C_{48}H_{82}O_{18}$	ginsenoside Rd
13	13.76	961.5367	961.5376	0.94	783(0.68), 621(8.38)	$C_{47}H_{80}O_{17}$	notoginsenoside Fd
14	16.09	665.4259	665.4281	3.31	-	$C_{36}H_{60}O_8$	ginsenoside Rh_4
15	16.47	829.4947	829.4944	−0.36	715(100), 621(9.06), 459(18.43), 375(9.79)	$C_{42}H_{72}O_{13}$	ginsenoside Rg_3
16	16.88	665.4259	665.4261	0.30	-	$C_{36}H_{60}O_8$	ginsenoside Rk_3
17	19.11	829.4947	829.4944	−0.36	715(100), 621(9.06), 459(18.43), 375(9.79)	$C_{42}H_{72}O_{13}$	ginsenoside F_2
18	24.17	667.4416	667.4431	2.25	-	$C_{36}H_{62}O_8$	ginsenoside Rh_2
19	24.37	811.4838	811.4843	0.62	603(100)	$C_{42}H_{70}O_{12}$	ginsenoside RK_1

2.2. Enzyme-Specific Probe Substrate Analysis

The chemical analysis was conducted to evaluate the influence on the esterases responsible for aspirin hydrolysis. Compared with the positive inhibitors (bis-p-nitrophenyl phosphate, tetraisopropyl pyrophosphoramide and ethylenediaminetetracetic acid, which are abbreviated as BNPP, iso-OMPA and EDTA in order), PNS exhibited weak or negligible effects on hCE1 (Figure 2A), BChE (Figure 2B), and PON (Figure 2C). In contrast, PNS strikingly reduced hCE2 activity in a concentration-dependent manner (Figure 2D). Further, inhibition kinetic analysis was carried out to investigate the mechanism of PNS toward hCE2. The half inhibition concentration (IC_{50}) of PNS was closed to 23.7 μg/mL (Figure 3). Lineweaver-Burk plots demonstrated that the inhibition type of PNS toward hCE2 was best fit to a non-competitive model (Figure 4A). The inhibition constant K_i of 27.9 was obtained from Dixon plots (Figure 4B).

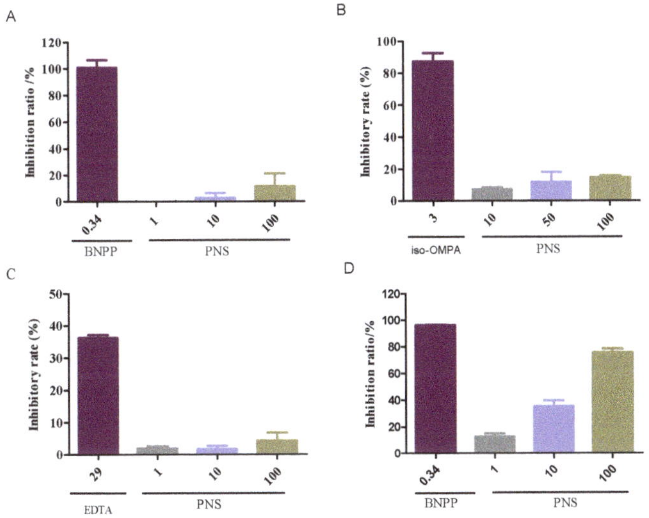

Figure 2. Inhibitory effects of PNS toward the esterases of hCE1, BChE, PON and hCE2 (**A–D** in order) with BMBT (2-(2-benzoyloxy-3-methoxyphenyl)benzothiazole), FD (Fluorescein diacetate), BuSCh (S-Butyrylthiocholine chloride) and PA (phenyl acetate) as a highly selective substrate of each esterase. BNPP, iso-OMPA, and EDTA are well-known inhibitors for hCE1 (hCE2), BChE, and PON, respectively. Data were presented as mean ± SD (n = 3).

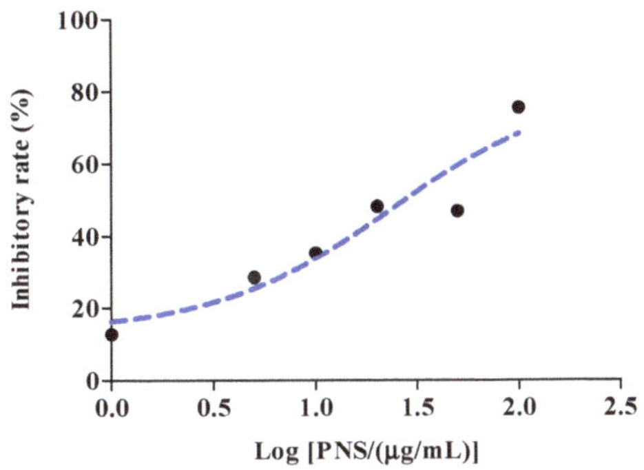

Figure 3. Various concentrations of PNS were used to measure the half inhibition concentration toward hCE2. Each point represents the mean of three independent experiments.

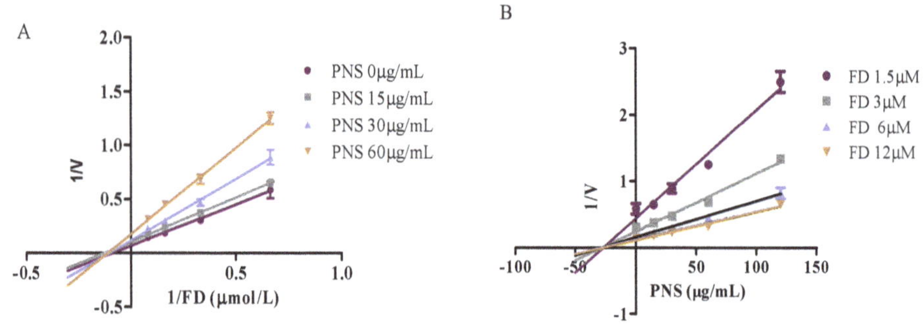

Figure 4. Inhibitory kinetics of PNS toward hCE2 using Lineweaver-Burk plots (**A**) and Dixon plots (**B**). Data were presented as mean ± SD (n = 3).

A clinical study reported that the integrated peak concentration (C_{max}) of the top five high-content compounds (notoginsenoside R_1, ginsenoside Rg_1, Re, Rb_1, and Rd with total amounts over 85%) was 33.2 μg/mL after intravenous infusion of Xuesaitong injection (with PNS as an ingredient) at a dosage of 800 mg/d for two weeks [20]. Thus, we figured out that the ratio of the area under the curve (AUC)(+I)/AUC(control) of Xuesaitong Injection was 2.19, indicating that the AUC(+I) caused by PNS toward hCE2 increased by 119% compared with that of without PNS.

2.3. Molecular Docking Analysis

Molecular docking programs use scoring functions to evaluate the binding energy of predicting ligand-receptor complex. The binding scores between PNS and hCE2 were shown in Table 2. The interaction energy between PNS and the metabolic enzyme varied from −8.8 kJ/mol to −5.5 kJ/mol reflecting the stability of the complex. Among 22 compounds in PNS, the five main compounds (notoginsenoside R_1, ginsenoside Rg_1, Re, Rb_1, and Rd) were screened out and found to bind to a few key amino acid residues in the active pocket of hCE2 (Figure 5). Taking notoginsenoside R_1 as an example, the sugar group formed a conventional hydrogen bond with the residues Glu325 and Met380 to stabilize the space structure of the complex. Moreover, A/B cycle and C-17 side chain were at hydrophobic area and surrounded by residues Leu258, His322, and Leu533.

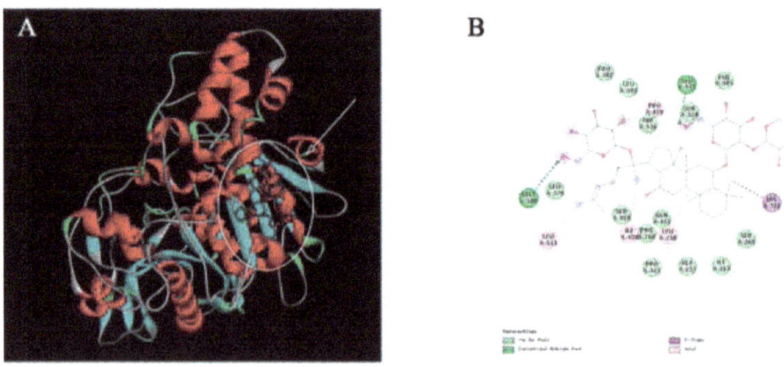

Figure 5. *Cont.*

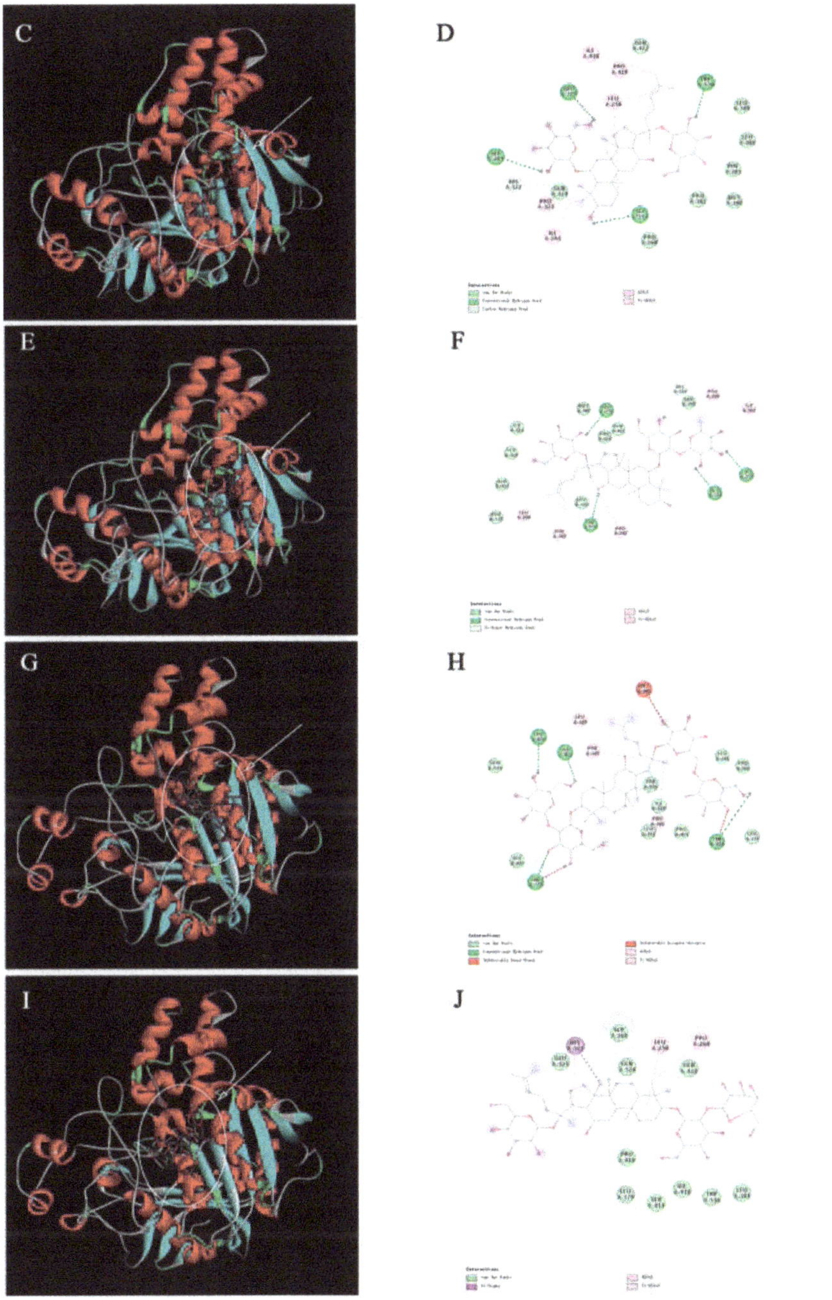

Figure 5. Molecular docking mode and interactions between hCE2 (shown in cartoon representation and colored structure) and notoginsenoside R_1, ginsenoside Rg_1, Re, Rb_1, and Rd (indicated by arrow), respectively. Three-dimensional illustrations show the interactions of hCE2 with notoginsenoside R_1 (**A**), ginsenoside Rg_1 (**C**), Re (**E**), Rb_1 (**G**), and Rd (**I**). Two-dimensional diagrams display interactions of notoginsenoside R_1 (**B**), ginsenoside Rg_1 (**D**), Re (**F**), Rb_1 (**H**), and Rd (**J**) in the active sites of hCE2.

Table 2. Docking scores between the compounds of PNS and hCE2.

Rank	Compound Name	Affinity (kcal/mol)	Rank	Compound Name	Affinity (kcal/mol)
1	ginsenoside Rg_2	−8.8	12	ginsenoside F_2	−6.9
2	ginsenoside Rh_1	−8.7	12	notoginsenoside F_3	−6.9
3	ginsenoside Rh_4	−8.6	14	ginsenoside Fe	−6.8
4	ginsenoside F_1	−8.3	14	ginsenoside Rg_3	−6.8
5	ginsenoside R_2	−8.1	16	notoginsenoside R_1	−6.7
6	notoginsenoside Fd	−7.7	16	ginsenoside Rb_3	−6.7
7	ginsenoside Re	−7.4	18	ginsenoside Rb_1	−6.5
8	notoginsenoside R_6	−7.3	19	ginsenoside Rb_2	−6.1
9	ginsenoside RK_3	−7.2	20	ginsenoside F_{11}	−6.0
10	ginsenoside RK_1	−7.1	20	notoginsenoside R_3	−6.0
10	ginsenoside Rg_1	−7.1	22	ginsenoside Rd	−5.5

2.4. Cytotoxicology of PNS in HepaRG Cells

The effects of PNS exposure in HepaRG cells was conducted by an MTT assay to set the concentrations used in the following trials, using the medium-treated cells group as control. As shown in Figure 6, cell viability of PNS-treated cells changed in a concentration-dependent manner and exhibited no cytotoxicity effect under the concentration of 100 μg/mL.

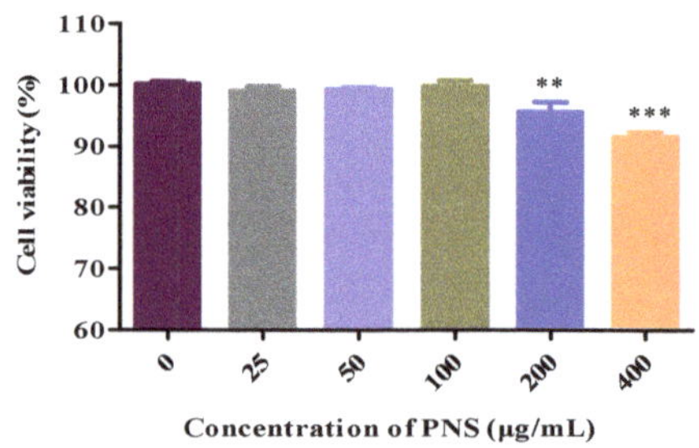

Figure 6. Cytotoxicity tests of PNS on HepaRG cells. Data were presented as mean ± SD (n = 5). ** and *** denoted result significantly different from that of the control group ($p < 0.01$ and $p < 0.001$, respectively).

2.5. Aspirin Hydrolysis after PNS Treatment

The property of esterases responsible for aspirin hydrolysis in HepaRG cells was investigated in an inhibition experiment. The results were presented in Figure 7. The hydrolase activity was significantly inhibited by the addition of BNPP, a specific inhibitor of hCE1 or hCE2. However, there was no significant inhibition on aspirin hydrolysis when treated with iso-OMPA or EDTA, hydrolase inhibitors for BChE and PON, respectively.

Meaningfully, PNS significantly decreased the hydrolase activity of aspirin in a concentration-dependent manner. There was no significant difference between BNPP (68 μg/mL) and PNS (150 μg/mL). These data indicated that PNS exhibited an appreciating efficiency in inhibiting aspirin hydrolysis.

2.6. ELISA Analysis for Esterases

We further explored the role of PNS in the protein expression in HepaRG cells. The results of the expression of hCE1, hCE2, BChE, and PON1 in HepaRG cells after PNS treatment were presented in Figure 8. There was no significant influence on hCE1 expression compared to the control (Figure 8A), while PNS (100 μg/mL) significantly reduced hCE2 protein level ($p < 0.05$) (Figure 8B). Though BChE levels intracelluar was not significantly changed compared to the control, PNS (100 μg/mL) led to the great rise in the extracelluler medium (Figure 8C,D). The same situation was also seen in PON1 (Figure 8E,F).

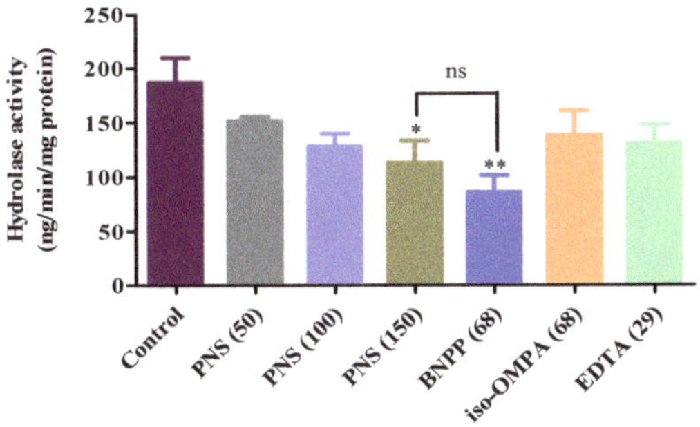

Figure 7. Hydrolysis of aspirin (ASA) in HepaRG cell homogenates treated with PNS. HepaRG cells homogenates were prepared and then diluted with 50 mM HEPES buffer (pH 7.4). Hydrolysis of ASA (1.8 μg/mL) in cell homogenates was conducted in the presence/absence of PNS. No significance (ns) was detected between BNPP (68 μg/mL) and PNS (150 μg/mL) treated group. Data were presented as mean ± SD (n = 3). *, and ** denoted results significantly different compared with the control group ($p < 0.05$, $p < 0.01$, respectively).

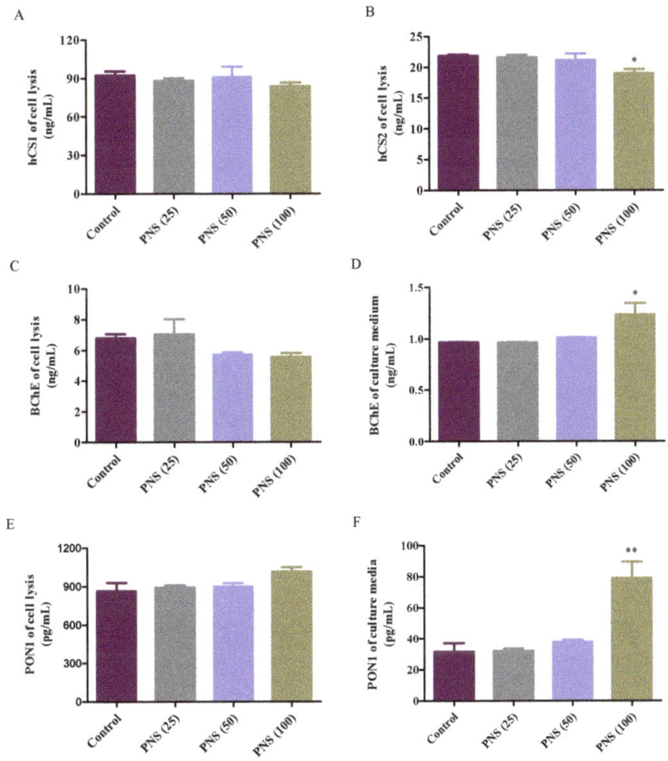

Figure 8. Effects on human carboxylesterase 1 (hCE1) (**A**), hCE2 (**B**), BChE (**C**,**D**), and PON1 (**E**,**F**) protein level after PNS treatment. Cells were incubated with PNS for up to 24 h. After the removal of PNS, cell lysates were prepared for ELISA analysis. Data were presented as mean ± SD (n = 3). * and ** denote results significantly different from those of the control group ($p < 0.05$, $p < 0.01$, respectively).

2.7. qRT-PCR Analysis

To elucidate the effect of PNS on the transcription factor contributed to the change of the protein level of esterases, we also explored mRNA expression in HepaRG cells with PNS treatment. Compared with the control, there was no significant difference on the mRNA expression of hCE1, hCE2, BChE, and PON1 (Figure 9).

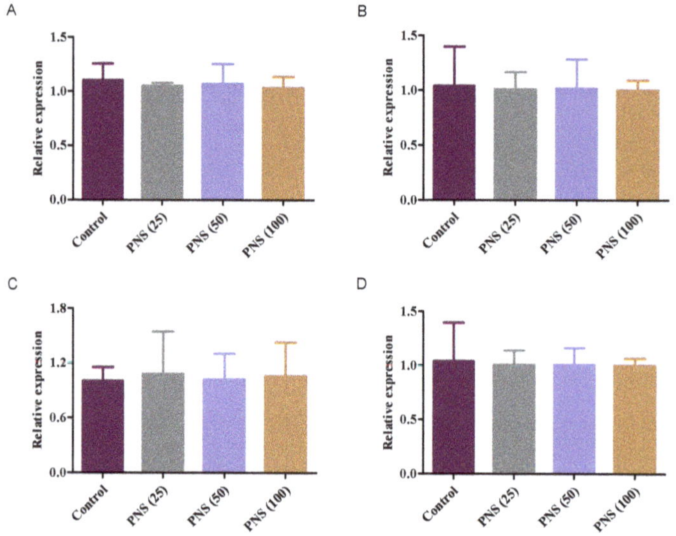

Figure 9. Effects on mRNA expression of human carboxylesterase 1 (hCE1) (**A**), hCE2 (**B**), BChE (**C**), and PON1 (**D**) with PNS treatment. Cells were incubated with PNS for up to 24 h. After the removal of PNS, total mRNA was prepared for qRT-PCR. Data were presented as mean ± SD (n = 3).

3. Discussion

Multi-drug therapy is now a common therapeutic practice for patients due to their therapeutic benefits, in both developed and developing countries. As a consequence, drug interactions are sometimes unavoidable. Apart from cytochrome P450, esterases is an important class of phase I metabolic enzymes, and plays a vital role in the biotransformation of ester-linked compounds. Drugs with the ability to inhibit the catalytic activity of esterases in the body might improve systemic exposure of the drug which is primarily cleared via the esterases. Except for synthetic compounds, many natural triterpenoids have been reported to exhibit the potent inhibitory effects on esterases in recent years [21–23].

Aspirin is one of the oldest antiplatelet agents used for antithrombotic therapy. It is rapidly hydrolyzed to salicylic acid by esterases in the body. Compared with other esterases, it has been reported that aspirin was primarily hydrolyzed by hCE2 [15]. In China, aspirin and PNS-based drugs are often taken together under many conditions and produce enhanced therapeutic effects. In our previous study, the plasma concentration of salicylic acid was highly increased when PNS and aspirin were co-administrated in SD rats, indicating that the HDI in vivo definitely existed in both drugs [24]. In addition, using Caco-2 cell monolayers model, we demonstrated that PNS exhibited appreciative inhibitory ability on the activity of the esterases responsible for aspirin hydrolysis, resulting in the elevated level of aspirin across Caco-2 cell monolayers [19].

Highly-selective probe substrate analysis is extensively used for determination of the inhibitory potential of a test compound. The basic premise of the methodology is that if test compounds cannot inhibit a particular metabolic enzyme, the probe substrate will be metabolized to its product (metabolite) which can then be measured. Conversely, if test compounds inhibit the enzyme, the substrate will not be metabolized or the rate of biotransformation and the formation of product declines [25]. In the study, we used probe substrate analysis to explore the inhibitory effects of PNS toward esterases. The results demonstrated that PNS exhibited strong inhibitory influence toward hCE2, whereas displayed weak inhibition toward hCE1, BChE, and PON with IC_{50} higher than 100 μg/mL, along with well-known inhibitors for verification. We provided convincing evidence that the activity of esterases responsible for aspirin hydrolysis could be directly inhibited by PNS treatment with varying potency. Lineweaver–Burk plot analysis showed that the inhibitory pattern of PNS toward hCE2 could be attributed to a non-competitive model. Hence, we speculated that PNS could bind to some specific sites of hCE2 and might alter its original spatial conformation, resulting in the reduced enzymatic activity.

Theoretically, significant enzyme inhibition occurs when the concentration of the inhibitor at the metabolic site is not lower than the K_i [26]. An apparent K_i value established in vitro defines the affinity of an inhibitor toward a particular enzyme. The likelihood of an in vivo interactions is projected on the basis of the $[I]/K_i$ ratio. Generally, the likelihood of interactions in vivo increases along with the ratio increases. The interactions in vivo were considered significant when the ratio of $[I]/K_i > 1$ [27]. In the study, we predicted the likelihood of HDI in vivo for Xuesaitong injection based on the inhibitory kinetics data obtained from in vitro studies. High possibility of HDI was found to exist in vivo via moderating hCE2 by PNS. However, since the effect of other metabolic pathways on drug elimination is not taken into account, and the drug clearance is assumed to be mediated only by inhibiting hCE2, the possibility of drug interactions between PNS and aspirin might be overestimated. Applied C_{max} as a substitute for [I] might also overestimate the actual HDI effects. Though $[I]/K_i$ can predict the occurrence of drug interactions, in vivo quantitative prediction on the basis of in vitro investigations should be further confirmed, and studies should be carried out to explore the potential pharmacokinetic interactions in vivo.

Molecular docking is the widely used methods to investigate structure-activity relationships owing to the predictive ability of the conformation of small-molecule ligands within receptor binding sites [28]. By executing quantitative predictions of binding energetics, molecular docking provided rankings of docked compounds on the basis of the binding affinity of complexes [29,30]. The main saponins presented in PNS include notoginsenoside R_1 and ginsenosides Rg_1, Re, Rb_1, and Rd [31]. These ginsenosides contain two to five sugars. The presence of key molecular interactions and the calculated binding free energy were usually used to evaluate the reliability of the predicting enzyme-inhibitor complexes. In the current study, the compounds in PNS demonstrated high binding affinity for hCE2 with the Gibbs free energy. The molecular interactions induced these compounds to anchor in the binding sites of hCE2. Thus, we speculated that some active sites of hCE2 were occupied by these compounds and could alter the original catalytic activity of hCE2. These results provided valuable information on structure-activity relationships between hCE2 and PNS.

Almost all herbal drugs undergo phase I and/or phase II metabolism to yield inactive or active metabolites. Herbal drugs are made of a complex mixture of pharmacological active phytochemicals [32]. This complexity may act as inhibitors or inducers of liver drug enzymes, thus altering the other drug's concentration in target sites and influencing therapeutic effects [2]. Liver drug enzymes are the common sites of drug interaction in human. HepaRG cell line can express esterases responsible for aspirin hydrolysis. In the inhibition experiment, we observed an interesting phenomenon that the hydrolysis of aspirin was inhibited by PNS. Thus, it is possible that the inhibitory effects of aspirin hydrolysis triggered by PNS occurred as it travels through human liver. The results further support our studies above and are consistent with our earlier finding that PNS is an effective inhibitor of esterases.

We further explored the potential effects of PNS on the major esterases expressed in the human liver. PNS reduced the protein level of hCE2 in HepaRG cells, indicating together regulation of protein expression other than the catalytic activity. PON1 has been reported to be beneficial in preventing atherosclerosis, attributing to its ability to reduce lipid hydroperoxides [33]. Blatter–Garin et al. reported that aspirin application can increase the PON1 activity in plasma [34]. In this study, PNS increased the release of PON1 out of the HepaRG cells. Considering PON1 catalyzing the hydrolysis of aspirin, this may balance the harmful and beneficial actions of PNS. Notably, PNS had insignificant effects on mRNA expression of four tested esterases. Taken together, it was conceived that the effects of PNS might be related to the translation, processing, and stability of the esterases.

The findings from our study clearly indicated that PNS possess high potency in the inhibition of esterases, in particular hCE2. Aspirin hydrolysis inhibited by PNS also had been confirmed on the cellular level. It is likely that PNS could result in HDI in the clinical practice when combined with aspirin. In many case, however, the effects of some drug in vitro and in vivo have no inevitable correlation. A further study is warranted to investigate the HDI of PNS and aspirin in large test animals.

4. Materials and Methods

4.1. Chemicals

Aspirin was obtained from the National Institute for the Control of Pharmaceutical and Biological Products (Beijing, China). PNS was obtained from Yunnan Sanqi Technology Co., Ltd. (Wenshan, China). PNS contents were determined as: notoginsenoside R_1, 7.4%; ginsenoside Rg_1, 26.3%; ginsenoside Re, 3.7%; ginsenoside Rb_1, 27.7%; ginsenoside Rd, 7.6%. All chemicals were of the highest quality available.

4.2. UPLC/LTQ-Orbitrap MS/MS Analysis

UPLC-MS/MS analysis was conducted on an Ultimate 3000 UPLC system (Thermo Fisher Scientific, Waltham, MA, USA) equipped with an LTQ-Orbitrap Elite mass spectrometer (Thermo Fisher Scientific, Waltham, MA, USA). The chromatographic column used was an ACQUICTY UPLC®BEH C_{18} column (1.7 μm, 2.1 × 100 mm). A linear gradient elution of 0.1% formic acid aqueous solution (A) and acetonitrile (B) was employed in the analysis (5–30% solvent B for 2 min, 30–50% solvent B for 18 min, and 50–100% solvent B for 8 min). The flow rate and injection volume were maintained at 0.3 mL/min and 3 μL, respectively. The MS conditions were set as follows: sheath gas flow, 40 arb; auxiliary gas flow, 20 arb; spray voltage, 3 kV; source heater temperature, 300 °C; capillary temperature, 350 °C; capillary voltage, 35 V; tube lens voltage, 110 V, and scan range (m/z), 50 to 2000.

4.3. Enzyme-Specific Probe Substrate Analysis

4.3.1. Enzyme Inhibition Experiments

The highly selectively probe substrates were used to evaluate the influence of PNS on esterases responsible for aspirin hydrolysis. The chemical assays for hCE1 and hCE2 were performed according to the methods reported by Wang et al. [35] and Wang et al. [36], respectively. The study on the effects of BChE was conducted using the method by Gulcin et al. [37]. The influence test for PON was conducted by the method of Furlong et al. [38] with some modifications. Briefly, the reaction system contained fresh plasma and freshly prepared paraoxon substrate solution (1 mM) in a total of 200 μL of assay buffer (pH 8.0, 20 mM Tris-HCl, 1 mM $CaCl_2$), in the presence/absence of PNS. The assay was conducted at 37 °C and initiated by adding the substrate solution, and the absorbance was continuously monitored at 270 nm for 5 min. A molar extinction coefficient of 1.31×10^3 was used to calculate the activity.

Known inhibitors were run in triplicate as positive controls: BNPP for hCE1 or hCE2, iso-OMPA for BChE, and EDTA for PON. The K_i value of PNS was further determined with low IC_{50} value (<100 μg/mL).

4.3.2. Inhibitory Kinetics Evaluation and In Vitro-In Vivo Extrapolation

The likelihood of HDI in vivo was predicted based on the [I] and K_i according to the following equation [27]:

$$AUC(+I)/AUC(control) = 1 + [I]/K_i$$

in which AUC(+I) and AUC(control) represent the area under the concentration–time curve in the presence/absence of inhibitor, respectively; [I] represents C_{max} of inhibitor in the systemic blood.

4.4. Molecular Docking Analysis

Molecular docking studies were performed to investigate the binding mode of PNS to hCE2 by using AutodockVina 1.1.2 (http://autodock.scripps.edu/). To date, there is no complete crystal structure of hCE2. Thus, we constructed the model with homology modeling method. The three-dimensional (3D) coordinates of hCE1 (PDB ID, 1MX9; resolution, 2.9 Å) were downloaded from the Protein Data Bank (http://www.rcsb.org/pdb/home/home.do). The 3D structures of PNS were drawn using the ChemBio3D Ultra 12.0 software (Cambridge Soft Corporation, Cambridge, MA, USA). The AutoDock Tools 1.5.6 package (http://mgltools.scripps.edu/documentation/links/autodock) was employed to generate docking input files. The search grid of hCE2 was identified as center_*x*: −1.27, center_*y*: 32.939, and center_*z*: 27.6, with dimensions of size_*x*: 15, size_*y*: 21, and size_*z*: 19. For Vina docking, the default parameters were used unless otherwise stated. The best-scoring pose as judged by the Vina docking score was selected and visually analyzed using the PyMOL 1.5 software (http://www.pymol.org/).

4.5. Cell Culture

HepaRG cells were generously provided by Du Yanan (Tsinghua University, Beijing, China). Cells were cultured in growth medium composed of Williams' E medium supplemented with 12% fetal bovine serum (FBS), 100 U/mL penicillin, 100 μg/L streptomycin, 5 mg/mL insulin, 2 mM glutamax-I, and 50 μM hydrocortisone hemisuccinate under 5% CO_2/95% humidified air at 37 °C.

4.6. Cell Viability Assay

The cell viability was examined by the methyl thiazolyl tetrazolium (MTT) assay. HepaRG cells were seeded into 96-well plates at 5×10^3 cells per well. After 48 h of incubation, the medium was replaced with a fresh medium containing increasing concentrations of PNS. After 24 h, 20 μL MTT (5 mg/mL) solution was added to each well. The MTT solution was discarded and 150 μL DMSO was added after 4 h. The plates were gently shaken for 5 min and the optical density was measured at 490 nm using a microplate reader (Thermo, USA). The cell viability of the untreated control was arbitrarily considered as 100%.

4.7. Hydrolysis Experiments

The changes of aspirin hydrolysis in HepaRG cell homogenates after the addition of PNS was investigated. The harvested cells were suspended in ice-cold buffer and then homogenized using an ultrasonic homogenizer under the ice-cold condition. The cell homogenate was diluted with HEPES buffer to the appropriate protein concentrations. PNS was added to the reaction solution and pre-incubated for 5 min. The reaction was then started by adding aspirin and terminated by adding ice-cold methanol. After centrifugation, the supernatants containing acetic acid (final concentration of 2%) were determined using HPLC. The chromatographic separation was achieved using a C_{18} column (4.6 mm × 250 mm, 5 μm). The mobile phase comprised of acetonitrile-water-acetic (29:69:2, *v*/*v*) at a flow rate of 1.0 mL/min. An injection volume of 10 μL was used, and the detection wavelength was set at 276 nm.

4.8. ELISA Analysis for Esterases

The expression level of hCE1, hCE2, PON1, and BChE in HepaRG cells treated by PNS was quantitatively measured using ELISA Kit according to the manufacturer's protocol. Briefly, 2×10^5 cells/well were seeded in a six-well plate for 48 h and then incubated with different concentrations of PNS for another 24 h. The analyzed cells were washed with cold PBS, resuspended in the RIPA lysis buffer, and then centrifuged at 10,000 rpm for 5 min. The resulting supernatants, together with the conditional media collected from HepaRG cells were assayed, and the enzymatic reaction was determined at 450 nm using an automatic microplate reader.

4.9. qRT-PCR Analysis

Total RNA was extracted from the cells using the Trizol (CW0581, CWbio, Beijing, China). One microgram of RNA was used to synthesize cDNA using a reverse transcription reagents Kit (CW0744, CWbio, Beijing, China). The qRT-PCR analysis was then carried out using UltraSYBR (with ROX) on Line Gene 9600 Plus qRT-PCR Detection system (Bioer Technology, Hangzhou, China) in the one-step protocol. Reactions were initiated at 95 °C for 10 min, followed by 45 cycles of 95 °C for 15 s and 60 °C for 60 s. Melting curve analysis was performed to confirm the specificity of primers. The relative mRNA expressions of hCE1, hCE2, BChE, and PON1 mRNA were normalized to GAPDH and calculated using the $2^{-\Delta\Delta Ct}$ method. The primers used in the study were listed in Table 3.

Table 3. Primer sequences for qRT-PCR.

Gene	Forward Sequences 5′–3′	Reverse Sequences 5′–3′
hCE1	GGGCACTGTGATTGATGGGA	CCTTCGGAGAGTGGATAGCTC
hCE2	TCAGAAGTTTCTTTGGGGGCA	GCAGGTATTGCTCCTCCTGG
BChE	GCTGGCCTGTCTTCAAAAGC	TCCTGCTTTCCACTCCCATTC
PON1	AAGTTCGAGTGGTGGCAGAA	TGGCATCCAACCCAAAGGTC
GAPDH	CTCCTCCACCTTTGACGCTG	TCCTCTTGTGCTCTTGCTGG

4.10. Statistical Analysis

Statistical analysis was performed using Prism v5.0 (GraphPad Software Inc., San Diego, CA, USA). Data were presented in the format of the mean ± SD from at least three independent measurements. ANOVA was run to determine significance between groups in the different experiments. A value of $p < 0.05$ was considered to be significant.

5. Conclusions

In conclusion, we provided the comprehensive in vitro data that enable us to understand and predict HDI with PNS. PNS could directly affect the activity of esterases in vitro with varying potency with hCE2 being the most susceptible to inhibition. Molecular docking revealed that PNS targeted hCE2 thus leading to its inhibition. We further confirmed the inhibitory potential at the cellular level. Our data also showed that PNS lead to the alteration of the esterase expression level, while exhibited insignificant effects on mRNA expression. The present work provides an insight into the mechanism exploration governing HDI between aspirin and PNS. We hope that the findings will urge us to pay more attention to the underlying safety and efficiency of combined drugs in the clinic.

Author Contributions: S.D. and P.L. conceived and designed the whole experiments. Z.S. and Y.W. performed the experiments; S.L. and S.H. analyzed the data; and B.Z. wrote the paper.

Funding: This work was supported by the Fundamental Research Funds for the Central Universities (No. 2017-JYB-XS-071).

Conflicts of Interest: The authors declare no conflict of interest.

References

1. Choi, Y.H.; Chin, Y.; Kim, Y.G. Herb-drug interactions: Focus on metabolic enzymes and transporters. *Arch. Pharm. Res.* **2011**, *34*, 1843–1863. [CrossRef] [PubMed]
2. Brantley, S.J.; Argikar, A.A.; Lin, Y.S.; Nagar, S.; Paine, M.F. Herb-drug interactions: Challenges and opportunities for improved predictions. *Drug Metab. Dispos.* **2013**, *12*, 301–317. [CrossRef] [PubMed]
3. Li, C.; Wang, Q.; Ren, T.; Zhang, Y.; Lam, C.W.K.; Chow, M.S.S.; Zuo, Z. Non-linear pharmacokinetics of piperine and its herb-drug interactions with docetaxel in Sprague-Dawley rats. *J. Pharm. Biomed. Anal.* **2016**, *128*, 286–293. [CrossRef] [PubMed]
4. Murray, J.; Picking, D.; Lamm, A.; McKenzie, J.; Hartley, S.; Watson, C.; Williams, L.; Lowe, H.; Delgoda, R. Significant inhibitory impact of dibenzyl trisulfide and extracts of Petiveria alliacea on the activities of major drug-metabolizing enzymes in vitro: An assessment of the potential for medicinal plant-drug interactions. *Fitoterapia* **2016**, *111*, 138–146. [CrossRef] [PubMed]
5. Aninat, C.; Piton, A.; Glaise, D.; Le Charpentier, T.; Langouet, S.; Morel, F.; Guguen-Guillouzo, C.; Guillouzo, A. Expression of cytochromes P450, conjugating enzymes and nuclear receptors in human hepatoma HepaRG cells. *Drug Metab. Dispos.* **2006**, *34*, 75–83. [CrossRef] [PubMed]
6. Kanebratt, K.P.; Andersson, T.B. Evaluation of HepaRG cells as an in vitro model for human drug metabolism studies. *Drug Metab. Dispos.* **2008**, *36*, 1444–1452. [CrossRef] [PubMed]
7. Hart, S.N.; Ye, L.; Nakamoto, K.; Subileau, E.; Steen, D.; Zhong, X. A comparison of whole genome gene expression profiles of HepaRG cells and HepG2 cells to primary human hepatocytes and human liver tissues. *Drug Metab. Dispos.* **2010**, *38*, 988–994. [CrossRef] [PubMed]
8. Andersson, T.B.; Kanebratt, K.P.; Kenna, J.G. The HepaRG cell line: A unique in vitro tool for understanding drug metabolism and toxicology in human. *Expert. Opin. Drug. Metab. Toxicol.* **2012**, *8*, 909–920. [CrossRef] [PubMed]
9. Liu, L.; Zhu, L.; Zou, Y.; Liu, W.; Zhang, X.; Wei, X.; Hu, B.; Chen, J. Panax notoginseng saponins promotes stroke recovery by influencing expression of Nogo-A, NgR and p75NGF, in vitro and in vivo. *Biol. Pharm. Bull.* **2014**, *37*, 560–568. [CrossRef] [PubMed]
10. Wan, J.; Lee, S.M.; Wang, J.D.; Wang, N.; He, C.W.; Wang, Y.T.; Kang, J.X. Panax notoginseng reduces atherosclerotic lesions in apoE-deficient mice and inhibits TNF-α-Induced endothelial adhesion molecule expression and monocyte adhesion. *J. Agric. Food Chem.* **2009**, *57*, 6692–6697. [CrossRef] [PubMed]
11. Levy, G. Clinical pharmacokinetics of aspirin. *Pediatrics* **1978**, *62*, 867–872. [PubMed]
12. Levy, G. Comparative pharmacokinetics of aspirin and acetaminophen. *Arch. Intern. Med.* **1981**, *141*, 279–281. [CrossRef] [PubMed]
13. Williams, F.M.; Mutch, E.M.; Nicholson, E.; Wynne, H.; Wright, P.; Lambert, D.; Rawlins, M.D. Human liver and plasma aspirin esterase. *J. Pharm. Pharmacol.* **1989**, *41*, 407–409. [CrossRef] [PubMed]
14. Inoue, M.; Morikawa, M.; Tsuboi, M.; Ito, Y.; Sugiura, M. Comparative study of human intestinal and hepatic esterases as related to enzymatic properties and hydrolizing activity forester-type drugs. *Jpn. J. Pharmacol.* **1980**, *30*, 529–535. [CrossRef] [PubMed]
15. Tang, M.; Mukundan, M.; Yang, J.; Charpentier, N.; LeCluyse, E.L.; Black, C.; Yang, D.; Shi, D.; Yan, B. Antiplatelet agents aspirin and clopidogrel are hydrolyzed by distinct carboxylesterases, and clopidogrel is transesterificated in the presence of ethyl alcohol. *J. Pharmacol. Exp. Ther.* **2006**, *319*, 1467–1476. [CrossRef] [PubMed]
16. Zhou, G.; Marathe, G.K.; Hartiala, J.; Hazen, S.L.; Allayee, H.; Tang, W.H.; McIntyre, T.M. Aspirin hydrolysis in plasma is a variable function of butyrylcholinesterase and PAF acetylhydrolase 1b2. *J. Biol. Chem.* **2013**, *288*, 11940–11948. [CrossRef] [PubMed]
17. Santanam, N.; Parthasarathy, S. Aspirin is a substrate for paraoxonase-like activity: Implications in atherosclerosis. *Atherosclerosis* **2007**, *191*, 272–275. [CrossRef] [PubMed]
18. Jaichander, P.; Selvarajan, K.; Garelnabi, M.; Parthasarathy, S. Induction of paraoxonase 1 and apolipoprotein A-I gene expression by aspirin. *J. Lipid. Res.* **2008**, *49*, 2142–2148. [CrossRef] [PubMed]

19. Sun, Z.X.; Wu, Y.L.; Yang, B.; Zhu, B.C.; Hu, S.N.; Lu, Y.; Zhao, B.; Du, S.Y. Inhibitory influence of Panax notoginseng saponins on aspirin hydrolysis in human intestinal Caco-2 cells. *Molecules* **2018**, *23*, 455. [CrossRef]
20. Li, X.; Wang, G.; Xiong, Y.; Sun, J.; Hao, H.; Zou, L.; Zheng, Y.; Yan, B.; Xia, C.; Liu, G. Population pharmacokinetic and pharmacodynamic evaluation of Xuesaitong Injection, a typical multiple constituent tradition Chinese medicine in patients with cerebral ischemia. *Chin. J. Clin. Pharmacol. Ther.* **2007**, *12*, 1183–1184.
21. Zou, L.W.; Dou, T.Y.; Wang, P.; Lei, W.; Weng, Z.M.; Hou, J.; Wang, D.D.; Fan, Y.M.; Zhang, W.D.; Ge, G.B.; et al. Structure-activity relationships of pentacyclic triterpenoids as potent and selective inhibitors against human carboxylesterase 1. *Front. Pharmacol.* **2017**, *8*, 435. [CrossRef] [PubMed]
22. Mai, Z.P.; Zhou, K.; Ge, G.B.; Wang, C.; Huo, X.K.; Dong, P.P.; Deng, S.; Zhang, B.J.; Zhang, H.L.; Huang, S.S.; et al. Protostane triterpenoids from the rhizome of *Alisma orientale* exhibit inhibitory effects on human carboxylesterase 2. *J. Nat. Prod.* **2015**, *78*, 2372–2380. [CrossRef] [PubMed]
23. Jamila, N.; Khairuddean, M.; Yeong, K.K.; Osman, H.; Murugaiyah, V. Cholinesterase inhibitory triterpenoids from the bark of *Garcinia hombroniana*. *J. Enzyme Inhib. Med. Chem.* **2015**, *30*, 133–139. [CrossRef] [PubMed]
24. Tian, Z.H.; Pang, H.H.; Du, S.Y.; Lu, Y.; Zhang, L.; Wu, H.C.; Guo, S.; Wang, M.; Zhang, Q. Effect of Panax notoginseng saponins on the pharmacokinetics of aspirin in rats. *J. Chromatogr. B* **2017**, *1040*, 136–143. [CrossRef] [PubMed]
25. Wienkers, L.C.; Heath, T.G. Predicting in vivo drug interactions from in vitro drug design data. *Nat. Rev. Drug Discov.* **2005**, *4*, 825–833. [CrossRef] [PubMed]
26. Li, T.; Li, N.; Guo, Q.; Ji, H.; Zhao, D.; Xie, S.; Li, X.; Qiu, Z.; Han, D.; Chen, X.; et al. Inhibitory effects of wogonin on catalytic activity of cytochrome P450 enzyme in human liver microsomes. *Eur. J. Drug Metab. Pharmacokinet.* **2011**, *36*, 249–256. [CrossRef] [PubMed]
27. Blanchard, N.; Richert, L.; Coassolo, P.; Lavé, T. Qualitative and quantitative assessment of drug-drug interaction potential in man, based on Ki, IC_{50} and inhibitor concentration. *Curr. Drug Metab.* **2004**, *5*, 147–156. [CrossRef] [PubMed]
28. Ferreira, L.G.; Santos, R.N.D.; Oliva, G.; Andricopulo, A.D. Molecular docking and structure-based drug design strategies. *Molecules* **2015**, *20*, 13384–13421. [CrossRef] [PubMed]
29. López-Vallejo, F.; Caulfield, T.; Martínez-Mayorga, K.; Giulianotti, M.A.; Houghten, R.A.; Nefzi, A.; Nefzi, A.; Houghten, R.A.; Medina-Franco, J.L. Integrating virtual screening and combinatorial chemistry for accelerated drug discovery. *Comb. Chem. High Scr.* **2011**, *14*, 475–487. [CrossRef]
30. Huang, S.Y.; Zou, X. Advances and challenges in protein-ligand docking. *Int. J. Mol. Sci.* **2010**, *11*, 3016–3034. [CrossRef] [PubMed]
31. Liu, H.F.; Yang, J.; Du, F.J.; Gao, X.M.; Ma, X.T.; Huang, Y.H.; Xu, F.; Niu, W.; Wang, F.; Mao, Y.; et al. Absorption and disposition of ginsenosides after oral administration of Panax notoginseng extract to rats. *Drug Metab. Dispos.* **2009**, *37*, 2290–2298. [CrossRef] [PubMed]
32. Hermann, R.; von Richter, O. Clinical evidence of herbal drugs as perpetrators of pharmacokinetic drug interactions. *Planta Med.* **2012**, *78*, 1458–1477. [CrossRef] [PubMed]
33. Durrington, P.N.; Mackness, B.; Mackness, M.I. Paraoxonase and atherosclerosis. *Arterioscl. Throm. Vas.* **2001**, *21*, 473–480. [CrossRef]
34. Blatter-Garin, M.C.; Kalix, B.; De Pree, S.; James, R.W. Aspirin use is associated with higher serum concentrations of the anti-oxidant enzyme, paraoxonase-1. *Diabetologia* **2003**, *46*, 594–595. [CrossRef] [PubMed]
35. Wang, D.D.; Jin, Q.; Hou, J.; Feng, L.; Li, N.; Li, S.Y.; Zhou, Q.; Zou, L.W.; Ge, G.B.; Wang, J.G.; et al. Highly sensitive and selective detection of human carboxylesterase 1 activity by liquid chromatography with fluorescence detection. *J. Chromatogr. B* **2016**, *1008*, 212–218. [CrossRef] [PubMed]
36. Wang, J.; Williams, E.T.; Bourgea, J.; Wong, Y.N.; Patten, C.J. Characterization of recombinant human carboxylesterases: fluorescein diacetate as a probe substrate for human carboxylesterase 2. *Drug Metab. Dispos.* **2011**, *39*, 1329–1333. [CrossRef] [PubMed]

37. Gulcin, I.; Scozzafava, A.; Supuran, C.T.; Koksal, Z.; Turkan, F.; Cetinkaya, S.; Bingöl, Z.; Huyut, Z.; Alwasel, S.H. Rosmarinic acid inhibits some metabolic enzymes including glutathione S-transferase, lactoperoxidase, acetylcholinesterase, butyrylcholinesterase and carbonic anhydrase isoenzymes. *J. Enzyme Inhib. Med. Chem.* **2016**, *31*, 1698–1702. [CrossRef] [PubMed]
38. Furlong, C.E.; Richter, R.J.; Seidel, S.L.; Motulsky, A.G. Role of genetic polymorphism of human plasma paraoxonase/arylesterase in hydrolysis of the insecticide metabolites chlorpyrifos oxon and paraoxon. *Am. J. Hum. Genet.* **1988**, *43*, 230–238. [PubMed]

International Journal of *Molecular Sciences*

MDPI

Article

Dihydromyricetin Attenuates Myocardial Hypertrophy Induced by Transverse Aortic Constriction via Oxidative Stress Inhibition and SIRT3 Pathway Enhancement

Yun Chen [1,2,†], Hui-Qin Luo [1,†], Lin-Lin Sun [1,†], Meng-Ting Xu [1], Jin Yu [1], Lu-Lu Liu [1], Jing-Yao Zhang [1], Yu-Qin Wang [1], Hong-Xia Wang [1], Xiao-Feng Bao [1] and Guo-Liang Meng [1,2,*]

1 Department of Pharmacology, School of Pharmacy and Key Laboratory of Inflammation and Molecular Drug Target of Jiangsu Province, Nantong University, Nantong 226001, China; cytina1012@163.com (Y.C.); luohuiqin23@163.com (H.-Q.L.); linlin_sun1991@sina.com (L.-L.S.); xumengting0222@163.com (M.-T.X.); yujin_yancheng@163.com (J.Y.); guiqulaixi214@163.com (L.-L.L.); zjingyao1994@163.com (J.-Y.Z.); wangyuqin@ntu.edu.cn (Y.-Q.W.); whxyc1711@163.com (H.-X.W.); baoxi@ntu.edu.cn (X.-F.B.)

2 School of Medicine, Nantong University, Nantong 226001, China

* Correspondence: mengguoliang@ntu.edu.cn; Tel.: +86-513-8505-1726; Fax: +86-513-8505-1728

† These authors contributed equally to this work.

Received: 31 July 2018; Accepted: 29 August 2018; Published: 31 August 2018

Abstract: Dihydromyricetin (DMY), one of the flavonoids in vine tea, exerts several pharmacological actions. However, it is not clear whether DMY has a protective effect on pressure overload-induced myocardial hypertrophy. In the present study, male C57BL/6 mice aging 8–10 weeks were subjected to transverse aortic constriction (TAC) surgery after 2 weeks of DMY (250 mg/kg/day) intragastric administration. DMY was given for another 2 weeks after surgery. Blood pressure, myocardial structure, cardiomyocyte cross-sectional area, cardiac function, and cardiac index were observed. The level of oxidative stress in the myocardium was assessed with dihydroethidium staining. Our results showed that DMY had no significant effect on the blood pressure. DMY decreased inter ventricular septum and left ventricular posterior wall thickness, relative wall thickness, cardiomyocyte cross-sectional areas, as well as cardiac index after TAC. DMY pretreatment also significantly reduced arterial natriuretic peptide (ANP), brain natriuretic peptide (BNP) mRNA and protein expressions, decreased reactive oxygen species production and malondialdehyde (MDA) level, while increased total antioxidant capacity (T-AOC), activity of superoxide dismutase (SOD), expression of sirtuin 3 (SIRT3), forkhead-box-protein 3a (FOXO3a) and SOD2, and SIRT3 activity in the myocardium of mice after TAC. Taken together, DMY ameliorated TAC induced myocardial hypertrophy in mice related to oxidative stress inhibition and SIRT3 pathway enhancement.

Keywords: dihydromyricetin; myocardial hypertrophy; oxidative stress; sirtuin 3

1. Introduction

Myocardial hypertrophy includes physiological hypertrophy and pathological hypertrophy [1]. Sustained pathologic myocardial hypertrophy may lead to congestive heart failure, arrhythmia, and sudden death. It is one of the vital causes of many cardiovascular diseases [2]. The exact mechanism of myocardial hypertrophy has not been elucidated, which might be related to oxidative stress, energy metabolism, hemodynamic factors, neurohumoral factors, cardiovascular autocrine/paracrine regulation, insulin secretion, heredity, and so on [3–6]. Oxidative stress is the state that redox balance of the cell is broken, which means the reactive oxygen species (ROS) levels exceed the scavenging capacity of the antioxidant defense system [7]. ROS directly or indirectly activate hypertrophy-related signal kinases, transcription factors, and extracellular factors to induce and promote cardiac hypertrophy [8]. Paradoxically, clinical studies have found that the use of antioxidants vitamin C and vitamin E is ineffective or even detrimental to cardiovascular diseases [9], while the detailed reason is unknown.

Dihydromyricetin (DMY, the chemical structure of DMY is shown in Figure 1) is a kind of dihydroflavonol flavonoid compound, which is widely found in vine tea [10]. It shows a variety of pharmacological effects including free radical scavenging, anti-oxidation, anti-inflammatory, anti-thrombotic, anti-lipid peroxidation, anti-microbial, liver protection, anti-carcinogenesis, and so on [11–16]. Our previous study suggested that DMY pretreatment significantly inhibited angiotensin II (Ang II) induced proliferation of cardiac fibroblasts, decreased collagen I and collagen III levels, suppressed α-smooth muscle actin expression, and attenuated oxidative stress [17]. We also found that DMY inhibited phosphorylation of mitogen-activated protein kinases but increased phosphorylation of endothelial nitric oxide synthase to antagonize Ang II-induced cardiomyocyte hypertrophy [18]. However, whether DMY attenuated myocardial hypertrophy in vivo is unknown.

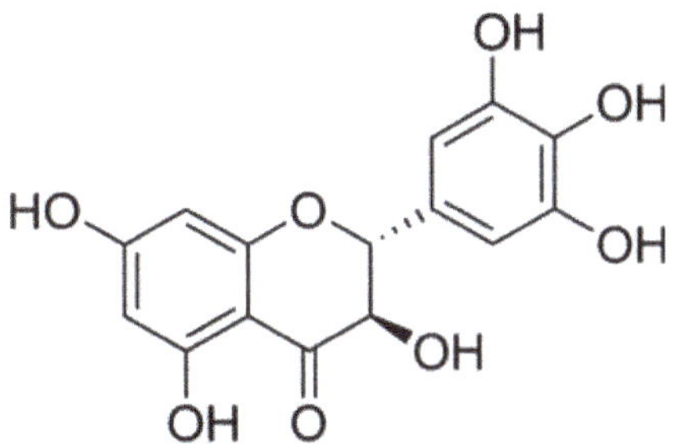

Figure 1. Chemical structure of dihydromyricetin (DMY).

Sirtuin 3 (SIRT3), a member of the sirtuins' family, is regarded as the key mediator of mitochondrial biogenesis, and is of great importance on alleviating oxidative stress related diseases [19–21]. Previous study suggested that SIRT3 promoted autophagy by forkhead-box-protein 1 (FOXO1) deacetylation, thereby ameliorating Ang II induced myocardial hypertrophy [22]. It is noteworthy that DMY improved hypoxic hypoxia-induced memory loss via a SIRT3 signal pathway [23]. The latest study indicated that DMY ameliorated nonalcoholic fatty liver disease through a SIRT3-depedent mechanism [24]. These studies suggested that DMY was able to regulate a SIRT3 signal pathway to perform potential protective effects.

However, the effects of DMY on myocardial hypertrophy in vivo are not clear. Additionally, whether the SIRT3 signal pathway is involved in the possible protection against myocardial hypertrophy by DMY remains unknown. In the present study, we explored the role of DMY on myocardial hypertrophy induced by transverse aortic constriction (TAC) and investigated the SIRT3-related signal molecules to elucidate possible mechanisms.

2. Results

2.1. DMY Had No Significant Effects on Blood Pressure in Mice after TAC

DMY (250 mg/kg/day) was administrated by gavage for 2 weeks followed by TAC. Then DMY was given for another 2 weeks. No mice were dead after TAC operation in our study. For systolic blood pressure (SBP) measured by non-invasive tail-cuff method, the two-way Analysis of Variance (ANOVA) revealed significant effects for TAC, but not for drug treatment or for TAC × drug treatment interaction. For SBP, diastolic blood pressure (DBP) and average mean artery pressure (MAP) measured by invasive artery catheterization, the two-way ANOVA indicated significant effects for TAC, but there were no marked effects for drug treatment or for TAC × drug treatment interaction. Post hoc analysis showed that there was no significant difference in SBP in mice of all the groups at the beginning of experiments. SBP measured by both non-invasive tail-cuff method increased after TAC. SBP, DBP, and MAP measured by invasive artery catheterization also elevated significantly after TAC surgery. However, DMY pre-treatment had no significant effects on both non-invasive and invasive blood pressure (Figure 2).

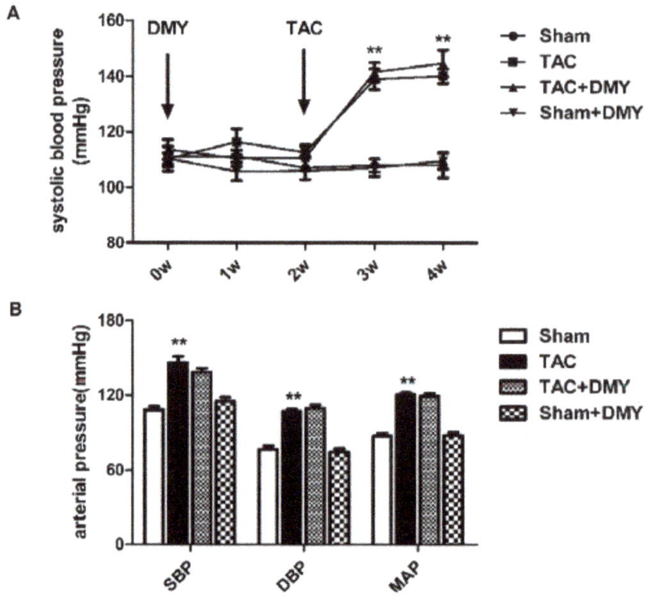

Figure 2. Effect of DMY on blood pressure in mice after transverse aortic constriction (TAC). Male C57BL/6 mice were given DMY (250 mg/kg/day) or carboxymethylcellulose (CMC) (0.5%) by gavage for 2 weeks followed by TAC or sham operation. Then DMY was administered for another 2 weeks. (**A**) Systolic blood pressure (SBP) was measured by tail-cuff method weekly; (**B**) SBP, diastolic blood pressure (DBP) and average mean artery pressure (MAP) were measured via carotid artery cannulation 2 weeks after TAC. ** $p < 0.01$ versus Sham ($n = 8$).

2.2. DMY Improved Myocardial Structure in Mice after TAC

To determine the effect of DMY on myocardial structure and cardiac function after TAC, we compared the myocardial structure in each group with echocardiography. For the thickness of inter ventricular septum (IVS) and left ventricular posterior wall (LVPW) as well as relative wall thickness (RWT), the two-way ANOVA showed marked effects for TAC, drug treatment and TAC × drug treatment interaction. However, for ejection fraction (EF) and fraction shortening (FS), there were no significant effects for TAC or drug treatment or TAC × drug treatment interaction. Post hoc analysis revealed that mice with DMY pre-treatment exhibited considerable improved myocardial structure, as IVS, LVPW, and RWT increased significantly after TAC (Figure 3A–D). There was no significant difference of ejection fraction (EF) and fraction shortening (FS) in each group (Figure 3E). Additionally, no significant alternation on myocardial structure and cardiac function were found in DMY-treated sham mice (Figure 3).

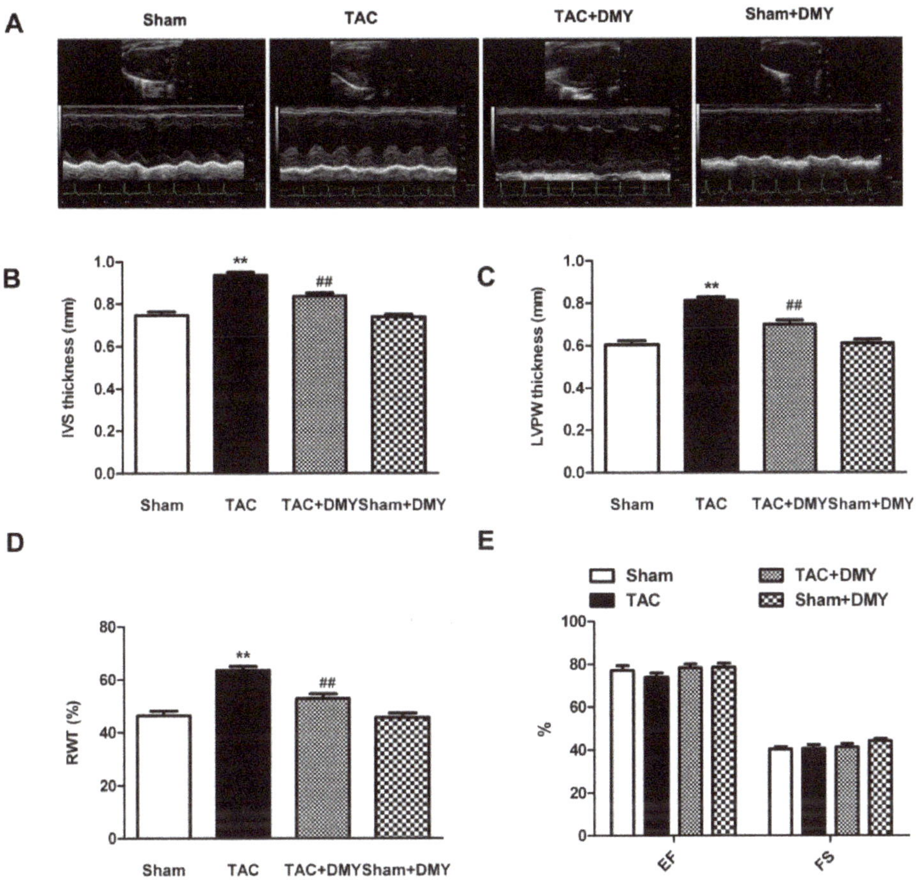

Figure 3. Effect of DMY on myocardial structure in mice after TAC. (**A**) Representative M-mode echocardiograms were shown; (**B–E**) Inter ventricular septum (IVS) thickness, left ventricular posterior wall (LVPW) thickness, relative wall thickness (RWT), ejection fraction (EF) and fraction shortening (FS) were quantified by echocardiography. ** $p < 0.01$ versus Sham, ## $p < 0.01$ versus TAC ($n = 8$).

2.3. DMY Reduced Cardiomyocyte Cross-Sectional Area and Cardiac Index in Mice after TAC

Myocardial tissue sections with hematoxylin and eosin (HE) staining were observed under the microscope (Figure 4A). Wheat germ agglutinin (WGA) staining was also used to measure the cross-sectional areas of cardiomyocytes. Compared with the sham group [(205.4 ± 23.1) μm^2], the cardiomyocyte cross-sectional area after TAC [(317.9 ± 27.6) μm^2] increased significantly, which was significantly suppressed by DMY-pretreatment [(254.3 ± 17.23) μm^2]. There is no significant alternation on cardiomyocyte cross-sectional area in DMY-treated sham mice [(206.6 ± 21.2) μm^2]. It suggested cell areas were increased after TAC, while DMY reduced the areas markedly (Figure 4B). For cardiac index, including heart weight (HW), heart mass index (HMI) and left ventricular mass index (LVMI), and the ratio of left ventricular weight (LVW) to tibia length (TL), two-way ANOVA showed significant effects of TAC, drug treatment and TAC × drug treatment interaction. Post hoc analysis exhibited a significant increase in HW, HMI, LVMI, and the ratio of LVM to TL in mice after TAC, suggesting that TAC successfully induced myocardial hypertrophy. All these elevated cardiac indexes after TAC were reduced in the DMY group, indicating that DMY attenuated TAC-induced myocardial hypertrophy (Figure 4C–F). No significant alternation on cardiac index was found in DMY-treated sham mice (Figure 4).

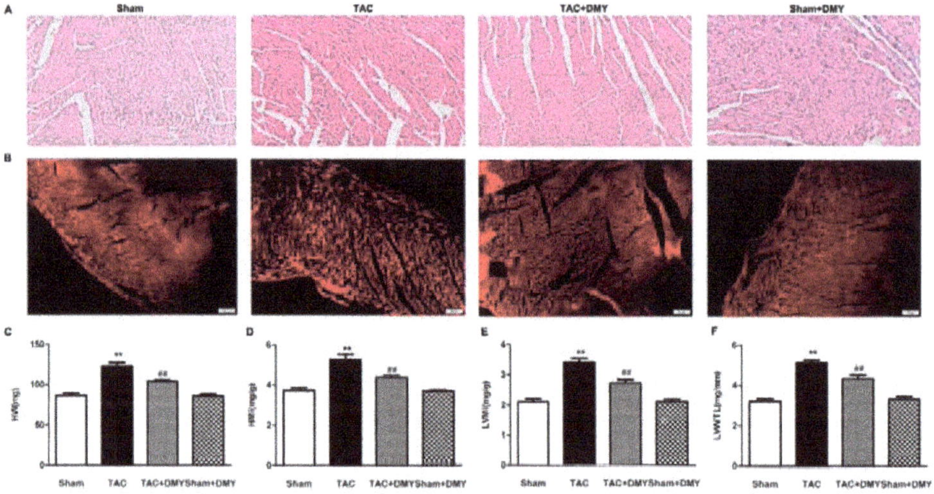

Figure 4. Effect of DMY on cardiomyocyte cross-sectional area and cardiac index in mice after TAC. (**A**) Representative images of hematoxylin and eosin (HE) staining of the myocardium were shown. Bar = 300 μm; (**B**) Representative images of wheat germ agglutinin (WGA) staining of the mice myocardium were shown. Bar = 50 μm. (**C–F**) Heart weight (HW), heart mass index (HMI), left ventricular mass index (LVMI) and LVW/TL were calculated. ** $p < 0.01$ versus Sham, ## $p < 0.01$ versus TAC ($n = 8$).

2.4. DMY Suppressed the Hypertrophic Genes Expression in the Myocardium of Mice after TAC

In order to further evaluate the effect of DMY on TAC-induced myocardial hypertrophy, atrial natriuretic peptides (ANP) and brain natriuretic peptides (BNP), two hypertrophic genes, expressions were assessed. For ANP and BNP expression at mRNA and protein level, two-way ANOVA revealed significant effects for TAC, drug treatment and TAC treatment interaction. Post hoc analysis showed that TAC markedly increased expression of ANP and BNP at both mRNA and protein level, but this increase could be suppressed by DMY (Figure 5).

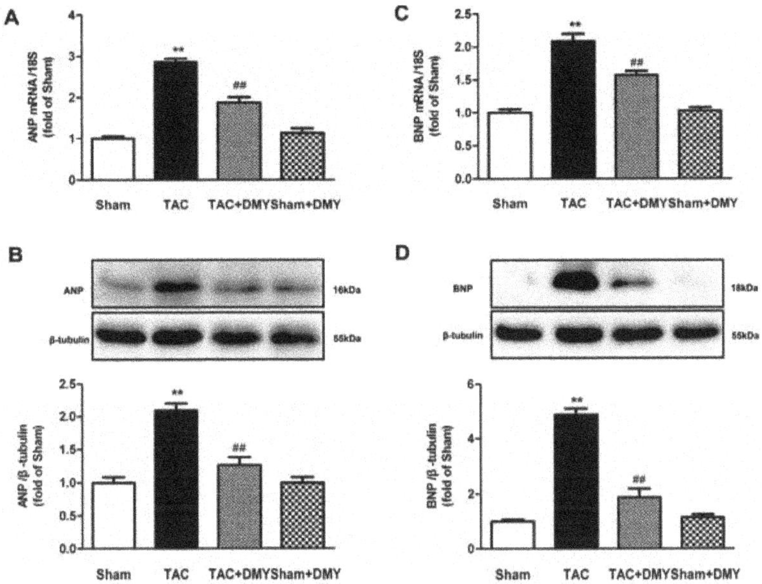

Figure 5. Effect of DMY on hypertrophic gene expression in the myocardium of mice after TAC. (**A**,**B**) Atrial natriuretic peptide (ANP) mRNA and protein expression were respectively quantified by real-time PCR and western blot. (**C**,**D**) Brain natriuretic peptide (BNP) mRNA and protein expression were respectively quantified by real-time PCR and western blot. 18S was used as a housekeeping gene. β-tubulin was used as a loading control. ** $p < 0.01$ versus Sham, ## $p < 0.01$ versus TAC (n = 5–8).

2.5. DMY Attenuated Oxidative Stress in the Myocardium of Mice after TAC

Oxidative stress plays a vital role in the pathogenesis of myocardial hypertrophy. Dihydroethidium (DHE) staining was performed to verify the effect of DMY on oxidative stress during myocardial hypertrophy. For DHE fluorescence, the ANOVA indicated remarked effects for TAC, drug treatment and TAC × drug treatment interaction. Post hoc analysis indicated that there was stronger DHE fluorescence in the myocardium after TAC, which was attenuated by DMY pre-treatment (Figure 6). These data suggested that DMY inhibited excessive oxidative stress in the myocardium of mice after TAC.

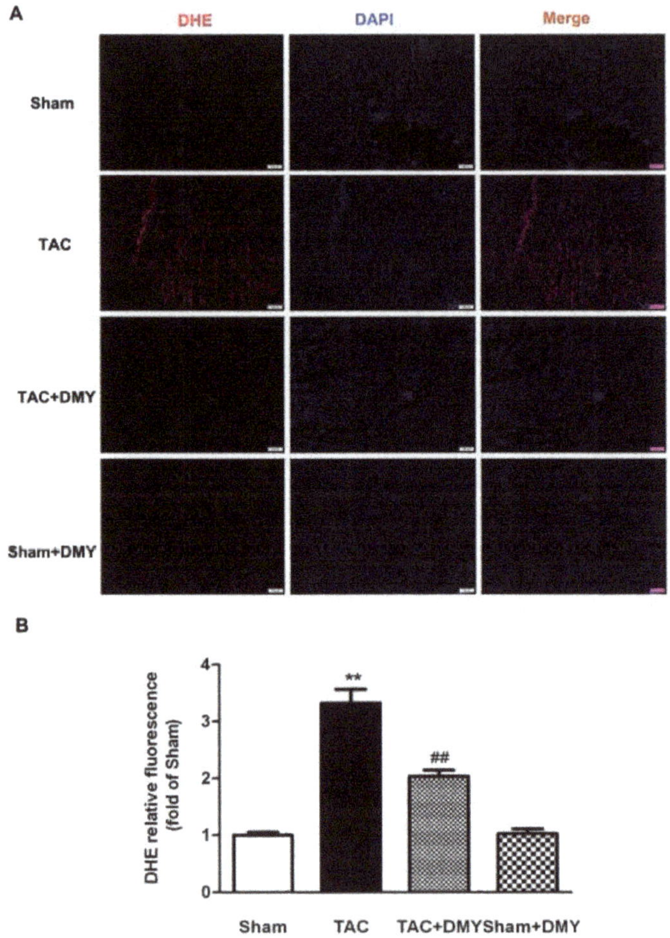

Figure 6. Effect of DMY on oxidative stress in the myocardium of mice after TAC. (**A**) Representative images of dihydroethidium (DHE) staining (Red) of the myocardium were shown. The nuclei were counter-stained with 4′,6-diamidino-2-phenylindole, dihydrochloride (DAPI) (Blue). Bar = 100 μm (Figure 6A); (**B**) Quantification of DHE fluorescence intensity was shown. ** $p < 0.01$ versus Sham, ## $p < 0.01$ versus TAC ($n = 8$).

2.6. DMY Reduced Myocardial MDA Levels but Enhanced T-AOC and SOD Activity in Mice after TAC

Malondialdehyde (MDA) is one of the most important products of membrane lipid peroxidation, which represents the damage of membrane and the degree of oxidative stress. In the present study, two-way ANOVA revealed significant effect for TAC, drug treatment and TAC × drug treatment on myocardial MDA levels, total antioxidant capacity (T-AOC), activity of superoxide dismutase (SOD) (mainly SOD2 in mitochondria, but not SOD1 in the cytoplasm). Post hoc analysis indicated that TAC increased myocardial MDA levels, which were reduced by DMY pre-treatment (Figure 7A). Our results showed T-AOC and activity of SOD2, but not SOD1, decreased in TAC group, which was restored by DMY pre-treatment (Figure 7B–C). There was no significant change on MDA level, T-AOC, and SOD activity in the myocardium of DMY-treated sham mice (Figure 7).

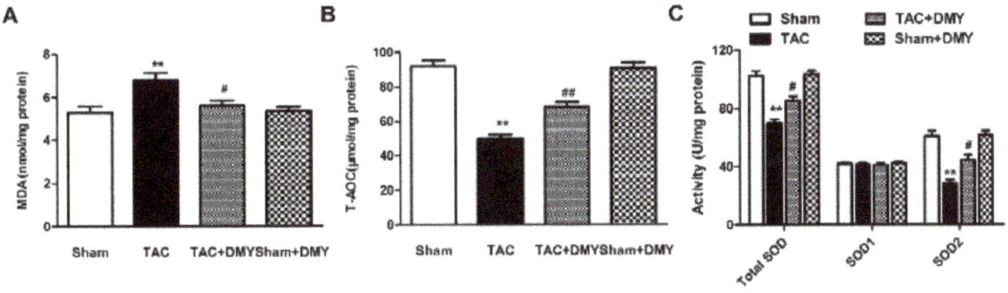

Figure 7. Effect of DMY on myocardial malondialdehyde (MDA) levels, total antioxidant capacity (T-AOC), and superoxide dismutase (SOD) activity in mice after TAC. (**A**) Myocardial MDA levels were detected; (**B**) Total myocardial antioxidant capacity (T-OAC) was measured; (**C**) SOD activity in the myocardium was measured. ** $p < 0.01$ versus Sham; $^{\#}$ $p < 0.05$, $^{\#\#}$ $p < 0.01$ versus TAC ($n = 8$).

2.7. DMY Increased SIRT3 Expression and Activity in the Myocardium of Mice after TAC

Previous studies have found that SIRT3 has a close relationship with oxidative stress and myocardial hypertrophy [25,26]. To investigate whether SIRT3 is involved in the anti-myocardial hypertrophy of DMY, SIRT3 gene and protein expression in the myocardium were determined. The two-way ANOVA showed significant effects for TAC, drug treatment and TAC × drug treatment on SIRT3 gene and protein expression, as well as SIRT3 activity. Post hoc analysis showed a significant decrease on SIRT3 expression in the myocardium of mice after TAC, which was reversed by DMY pre-treatment (Figure 8A,B). Moreover, SIRT3 activity was reduced after TAC, which was restored by DMY pre-treatment (Figure 8C). No significant change on SIRT3 expression and activity was found in the myocardium of DMY-treated sham mice.

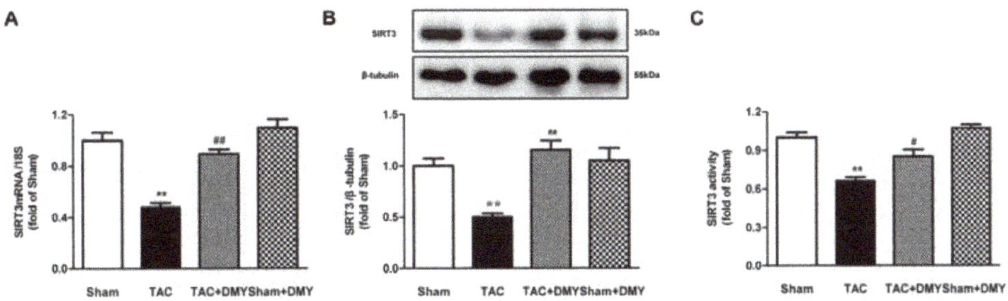

Figure 8. Effect of DMY on sirtuin 3 (SIRT3) expression in the myocardium of mice after TAC. (**A**) SIRT3 mRNA expression was quantified by real-time PCR. 18S was used as a housekeeping gene; (**B**) SIRT3 protein expression was quantified by western blot. β-tubulin was used as a loading control; (**C**) SIRT3 activity was quantified with fluorimetry. ** $p < 0.01$ versus Sham; $^{\#}$ $p < 0.05$, $^{\#\#}$ $p < 0.01$ versus TAC ($n = 5$–8).

2.8. DMY Elevated FOXO3a and SOD2 Protein Expression in the Myocardium of Mice after TAC

The above results indicated that DMY increased SIRT3 expression during the preventive effects on myocardial hypertrophy. However, the downstream mechanism of SIRT3 involved in this process is not clear. As we know, forkhead-box-protein 3a (FOXO3a) is a transcription factor which suppresses ROS production. SOD2 is also one of the important anti-oxidative stress enzymes to alleviate ROS. More importantly, FOXO3a and SOD2 are important downstream molecules of SIRT3 [19,27]. The two-way ANOVA showed that there were significant effects for TAC, drug treatment and TAC × drug treatment on FOXO3a and SOD2 protein expression. Results of post hoc analysis showed there was a decrease of FOXO3a and SOD2 protein expression in the myocardium of mice after TAC. DMY pre-treatment elevated FOXO3a and SOD2 protein expression (Figure 9). No significant change on FOXO3a and SOD2 expression was found in the myocardium of DMY-treated sham mice.

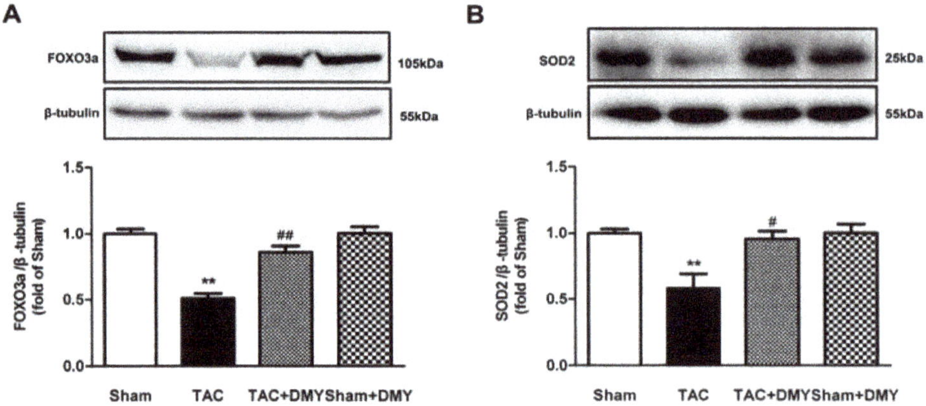

Figure 9. Effect of DMY on forkhead-box-protein 3a (FOXO3a) and SOD2 protein expression in the myocardium of mice after TAC. (**A**,**B**) FOXO3a and SOD2 protein expression were quantified by western blot. β-tubulin was used as a loading control. ** $p < 0.01$ versus Sham; # $p < 0.05$, ## $p < 0.01$ versus TAC ($n = 5$).

3. Discussion

Pathological hypertrophy is characterized by ventricular wall thickening, myocardial infraction, cardiomyopathy, or structural heart disease caused by long-term hypertension, which is often accompanied by cardiac systolic dysfunction and myocardial interstitial fibrosis, the re-expression of fetal genes such as ANP, BNP, myosin heavy chain β, and so on [28–31].

DMY, a kind of flavonoid compound, was isolated from stems and leaves of vine tea. Several studies suggested that DMY had multiple cardiovascular protective effects [17,18,32–34]. It was found that DMY protected cardiac function, inhibited oxidative stress, reduced inflammatory reaction, alleviated pathological damage, improved mitochondrial function, decreased apoptosis, suppressed autophagy and protected against diabetic cardiomyopathy [32]. DMY reduced serum low density lipoprotein (LDL), interleukin-6 (IL-6), and tumor necrosis factor α (TNF-α) levels in the fat-diet-fed LDLR$^{-/-}$ mice and exhibited anti-atherosclerotic effects [35]. Previous research has demonstrated that DMY alleviated myocardial injury and decreased mortality in doxorubicin-induced myocardial injury in mice [36]. Another study indicated that DMY attenuated atherosclerosis by improving endothelial dysfunction, inhibiting macrophage foam cell formation and ameliorating lipid profiles [37]. Our previous study found that DMY inhibited Ang II-induced cardiomyocyte hypertrophy and myocardial fibroblast proliferation in vitro [17,18]. In this study, we explored the effects of DMY on myocardial hypertrophy in vivo.

It is well documented that blood pressure is one of the most vital factors affecting myocardial hypertrophy [38]. Sustained hypertension is more likely to lead to myocardial hypertrophy. Effective control of blood is an ideal strategy to alleviate myocardial hypertrophy [4]. In order to clarify whether the effect of DMY on myocardial hypertrophy is related to regulation of blood pressure, invasive blood pressure and noninvasive blood pressure were determined. Additionally, our results showed DMY attenuated TAC-induced myocardial hypertrophy without blood pressure lowering effect, which suggested that the protective effect of DMY on myocardial hypertrophy was independent of blood pressure reduction.

Several studies had demonstrated that DMY exerted pharmacological effects via its antioxidant ability. DMY protected neuronal cells against pyruvate-induced oxidative stress in AMP-activated protein kinase/glucose transporter 4 (AMPK/GLUT4)-dependent signal pathway [13]. DMY prevented endothelial cells from hydrogen peroxide-induced oxidative injury by regulating mitochondrial function [39]. DMY also inhibited lipid production and oxidative stress to lessen oleic acid-induced lipid accumulation in L02 cells and HepG2 cells [40]. Previous study proved that DMY suppressed caspase activation but elevated Bcl-2 expression to exhibit a powerful anti-apoptosis effect on osteosarcoma cells [41]. Our previous research demonstrated that DMY suppressed Ang II-induced cardiac fibroblast proliferation via decreasing ROS production [17]. One recent study verified that DMY delayed atherosclerosis process by enhancing the activity of antioxidant enzymes in the liver and aorta [35]. In addition, the improvement on diabetic cardiomyopathy by DMY was also ascribed to oxidative stress inhibition [32]. However, our present study only confirmed that DMY significantly reduced ROS production in global cells but not of the mitochondria of the myocardium, which might be detected in further study. Moreover, we confirmed that DMY significantly decreased MDA levels, suggesting that DMY effectively attenuated oxidative stress in mice after TAC.

The exact mechanisms involved in the antioxidant stress effect of DMY have not been well clarified. We found that decreased SIRT3 expression of the myocardium in mice after TAC was restored by DMY. Sirtuins are highly conserved NAD^+-dependent deacetylases involved in many cellular processes, including oxidative stress regulation, genomic stability maintaining, and DNA repair [41,42]. Deletion of SIRT3 promoted protein acetylation, cyclophilin D rearrangement, and mitochondrial permeability transition pore opening, thereby resulting in severe oxidative damage [43]. Low expression of SIRT3 resulted in myocardial NAD^+ depletion, mitochondrial enzyme acetylation, and heart failure, indicating that SIRT3 is pivotal for the maintenance of mitochondrial homeostasis [44–48]. Previous study demonstrated DMY unregulated SIRT3 in HT22 cell in a dose-dependent manner [23]. The latest studies demonstrated that DMY elevated SIRT3 expression to improve hypoxic hypoxia-induced memory and to attenuate the hepatic injury in nonalcoholic fatty liver disease [23,24]. The present results revealed that DMY up-regulated SIRT3 expression, enhanced antioxidant capacity, suppressed oxidative stress, and inhibited myocardial hypertrophy in mice after TAC. These results indicated that elevated SIRT3 expression may be one of the important mechanisms of anti-oxidation during the protective effect of DMY on myocardial hypertrophy. However, the detailed mechanism of how DMY increased SIRT3 expression was unknown. One latest study found that DMY increased SIRT3 expression by activating the adenosine monophosphate-activated protein kinase (AMPK)-peroxisome proliferator-activated receptor-γ coactivator-1 alpha (PGC1α)/estrogen-related receptor-α (ERRα) signaling pathway [24]. Our previous study also found that NaHS increased SIRT3 expression by enhancing PGC-1α expression or increasing activator protein 1 (AP-1) binding activity with SIRT3 promoter [49,50]. It indicated that DMY might also regulate above signaling pathway to increases SIRT3 expression.

SIRT3 is mainly located in mitochondria and deacetylates acetylated mitochondrial proteins, such as acetyl-CoA synthetase, glutamate dehydrogenase, isocitrate dehydrogenase 2 (IDH2), FOXO3a, and SOD2, thereby modulating their activities. SIRT3 increased FOXO3a-dependent gene expression by interacting with daf-16 homolog in mitochondria [51]. Confocal microscopy images clearly showed that there was an interaction between SIRT3 and FOXO3a, indicating that SIRT3 may be a monitoring factor for mitochondrial metabolism. FOXO3a played a vital role in controlling mitochondrial metabolism and redox balance [52]. Environmental stimuli, such as insulin, nutrition, and oxidative stress, regulate longevity genes by altering FOXO activity, protein subcellular localization, DNA-binding properties, and transcriptional activity [53]. FOXO3a and other cellular antioxidant molecules constituted the first line of defense against oxidative stress. FOXO3a was a ROS-sensitive transcription factor that regulated the expression of several important antioxidant genes such as the peroxidase family, glutathione peroxidase, SOD, and so on [54]. FOXO3a regulated the expression of antioxidant enzymes such as SOD2 by deacetylating the acetylation site of the DNA-binding region, regulating its intracellular shift, and binding to DNA. Over-expression of SIRT3 increased the binding force between FOXO3a DNA and SOD2 promoter, thereby increasing the activity of SOD2 promoter [27,55]. The deacetylation effect of SIRT3 on SOD2 increased its enzymatic activity, thereby enhancing mitochondrial ROS scavenging [56]. Our study firstly demonstrated that DMY effectively increased SIRT3 expression and activity during myocardial hypertrophy. Both FOXO3a and SOD2 are important downstream proteins in the SIRT3 signal pathway. Previous study suggested that the HKL-treatment increased SIRT3 levels, which was associated with reduced acetylation of SOD2 [57]. Another study found that overexpression of exogenous SIRT3 protein lowered the acetylation levels of SOD2K68 in diabetic oocytes [58]. FOXO3a was also able to be deacetylated by SIRT3 [59]. Altogether, our present findings suggested that DMY might decrease FOXO3a and SOD2 acetylation to exhibit anti-hypertrophic function, which needs to be elucidated in further study.

In conclusion, DMY attenuates myocardial hypertrophy induced by transverse aortic constriction via oxidative stress inhibition and SIRT3 pathway enhancement in mice. We propose novel evidence that DMY is a potential agent for prevention and treatment of myocardial hypertrophy.

4. Materials and Methods

4.1. Animals

Male C57BL/6 mice aged 8–10 (8 per group) were provided by Experimental Animal Center of Nantong University (Nantong, China). The experimental procedures were conducted according to NIH Guidelines for Care and Use of Laboratory Animals. The study was approved by the Institutional Animal Ethical Committee of Nantong University (approval no. NTU-20160812, 12 August 2016). The mice were randomized to intragastric administration of DMY (250 mg/kg/day) ((2R,3R)-3,5,7-trihydroxy-2-(3,4,5-trihydroxyphenyl)-2,3-dihydrochromen-4-one, $C_{15}H_{12}O_8$, PubChem identifier: 161557, Standard Center of China, Beijing, China) dissolved in carboxymethylcellulose (CMC, Sinopharm Chemical Reagent Co., Ltd., Shanghai, China) once daily. CMC was used as vehicle for DMY [35]. Two weeks later, anaesthesia was induced with 3% isoflurane in oxygen (3 L/min) and maintained with 1.5% isoflurane. Then mice were subjected to TAC or sham operation.

4.2. Transverse Aortic Constriction (TAC)

Mice were anesthetized and artificially ventilated with a respirator and were kept warm on a heating pad. Then left chest of the mouse was opened and the transverse aortic arch was ligated between the innominate artery and the left carotid artery with a 6-0 silk suture ligature tied firmly against a 26-gauge needle, followed by quick withdrawal of the needle to establish a rat model of TAC induced myocardial hypertrophy [60]. Mice in the sham group were underwent the same operation without the constriction.

4.3. Blood Pressure Measurement

SBP in mice was monitored by tail-cuff method with a small animal non-invasive blood pressure analysis system once a week (Vistech System, Apex, NC, USA). After echocardiography, a polyethylene catheter filled with heparin saline was inserted into the common carotid artery of anesthetized mice. The pressure transducer was connected with a biological signal acquisition system (MedLab-U/4C501, Nanjing, China) to record carotid SBP, DBP, and MAP.

4.4. Echocardiography

Two weeks after surgery, the mice were anaesthetized with isoflurane (1.5%). Myocardial configuration and cardiac function were measured by echocardiography (Visual Sonic Vevo 2100,

Toronto, ON, Canada). IVS and LVPW thickness, EF, and FS, left ventricular internal diastolic diameter (LVIDD) were measured. Relative wall thickness was calculated by 2× LVPW/LVIDD.

4.5. Cardiac Index Determination

After blood pressure measurement via carotid artery cannulation, the heart was isolated quickly, washed to remove residual blood as much as possible, and dried with a filter paper. Then HW was measured with an electronic balance. LVW including ventricular septum was weighed after atrium and right ventricle had been removed. HW/BW and LVW/BW were calculated, which represent HMI and LVMI respectively. TL from the tibial plateau to the medial malleolus was measured and the ratio of LVW to TL was calculated.

4.6. Wheat Germ Agglutinin (WGA) Staining

Heart tissue sections were reconstituted with different concentrations of ethanol (100%, 95%, 85%, 75%, 50% for 1 min respectively), then was washed in distilled water for 1 min. Tissue sections were washed with 0.1M PBS on a shaker 3 times for 5 min. After dry, the sections were put in a dark box, and were incubated with working solution containing WGA-FITC (100 μg/mL; Sigma-Aldrich, St. Louis, MO, USA) and $CaCl_2$ (1 mM) for 60 min. After washing carefully for 3 times with PBS, tissue sections were photographed with a fluorescence microscope. Cardiomyocyte area was quantified by morphometric analysis.

4.7. Histological Analysis

The myocardium from left ventricular was fixed in 4% paraformaldehyde for 24 h, embedded in paraffin, and cut transversely into 4 μm thickness. Slides were deparaffinized with xylene and rehydrated with graded alcohol and then stained with HE (Beyotime, Shanghai, China). The pathological structure of the myocardium was measured with an inverted phase contrast microscope (Olympus, Tokyo, Japan). Image analysis software was used to calculate the cardiomyocyte cross-sectional area.

4.8. Oxidative Stress Evaluation

Production of ROS was evaluated by observing the red fluorescence intensity with DHE (Beyotime, Shanghai, China) staining. In brief, frozen heart tissue was cut into 4 μm sections, followed by DHE (0.2 μM) incubation at 37 °C for 30 min in dark and DAPI incubation at room temperature for 5 min. Intracellular reactive oxygen species, represented as fluorescence, was measured by fluorescence microscopy (Leica, Wetzlar, Germany) at 488 nm excitation and 525 nm emission wavelength. The DHE fluorescence intensity was quantified using Image J software.

As an indicator of lipid peroxidation, levels of MDA in the myocardium were detected using the thiobarbituric acid method (Beyotime, Shanghai, China). T-AOC of the myocardium was measured by the T-AOC Assay Kit with ferric reducing ability of plasma method (Beyotime, Shanghai, China). Concentration of total SOD, SOD1, and SOD2 in the myocardium was evaluated using the WST-1 (2-(4-iodophenyl)-3-(4-nitrophenyl)-5-(2,4-disulfophenyl)-2H-tetrazolium, Beyotime, Shanghai, China) method, in accordance with the manufacturer's instructions.

4.9. SIRT3 Activity

SIRT3 enzymatic activity was assayed using a fluorometric kit (Enzo Life Sciences Inc., New York, NY, USA) according to the manufacturer's instructions. Protein (40 mg) was incubated at 37 °C or 45 min with specific substrates. Next, 25 mL of developer was added, and samples were incubated for an additional 45 min. SIRT3 activity was measured using a Microplate reader at 350 nm/450 nm.

4.10. Quantitative Real-Time PCR

Total RNA from the myocardium was extracted using Trizol reagent (Takara, Kyoto, Japan), and first-stand cDNA was synthesized using PrimeScript™ RT Master Mix Kit (Takara, Kyoto, Japan). Quantitative real-time PCR was performed with SYBR Green (Takara, Kyoto, Japan) Fast qPCR mix (Takara, Kyoto, Japan) with ABI 7500 Real Time PCR System (ABI, Carlsbad, CA, USA). 18S was served as a housekeeping gene. Comparative cycle threshold (CT) ($2^{-\Delta\Delta Ct}$) method was used. The primers used are listed as: ANP, sense, 5′-GAGAAGATGCCGGTAGAAGA-3′ and antisense, 5′-AAGCACTGCCGTCTCTCAGA-3′; BNP, sense, 5′-CTGCTGGAGCTGATAAGAGA-3′ and antisense, 5′-TGCCCAAAGCAGCTTGAGAT-3′, SIRT3, sense, 5′-CTGGATGGACAGGACAGATAAG-3′ and antisense, 5′-TCTTGCTGGACATAGGATGATC-3′; 18S, sense, 5′-AGTCCCTGCCCTTTGTACACA-3′ and antisense, 5′-CGATCCGAGGGCCTCACTA-3′.

4.11. Western Blot

Proteins were extracted with radioimmunoprecipitation assay (RIPA) buffer (150 mM NaCl, 1% Triton X-100, 1% sodium deoxycholate, 50 mM Tris-HCl, 2 mM ethylenediamine tetraacetic acid, 1 mM phenylmethylsulfonylfluoride, 1 mM dithiothreitol, 10 mM Na_3VO_4 and 20 mM NaF, pH 7.5). Homogenates were centrifuged at 4 °C for 15 min, and the supernatant was used for western blot. Proteins of 20–50 μg were separated with sodium dodecyl sulfate polyacrylamide gel electrophoresis (SDS-PAGE, Beyotime, Shanghai, China) and then transferred to a polyvinylidene fluoride (PVDF) membrane (Millipore, Billerica, MA, USA). After blocking with 5% non-fat milk for 2 h at room temperature, the membranes were incubated with anti-SIRT3 (1:1000, Santa Cruz Biotechnology Inc., San Diego, CA, USA), anti-ANP, anti-BNP, anti-forkhead-box-protein 3a (FOXO3a), anti-SOD2 (1:1000, Abcam, Cambridge, UK), or anti-β-tubulin (1:3000, Bioworld Technology, St. Louis, MO, USA) primary antibodies overnight at 4 °C. After washing with TBST, the membranes were incubated with a horseradish peroxidase-conjugated secondary antibody (Santa Cruz Biotechnology Inc., San Diego, CA, USA) for 2 h at room temperature. Finally, the membrane was exposed to enhanced chemiluminescence substrate (ECL, Thermo Fisher Scientific Inc., Rockford, IL, USA) reagent for determination of protein expression.

4.12. Statistical Analysis

The data were expressed on mean ± standard error of mean (SEM) and analyzed with two-way ANOVA followed by Bonferroni post-hoc test using Stata 13.0 software (StataCorp LLC, Texas, USA), GraphPad Software (San Giego, CA, USA). A value of p less than 0.05 was considered statistically significant.

Author Contributions: Conceptualization, Y.C. and G.-L.M.; Data curation, Y.C. and G.-L.M.; Formal analysis, Y.C. and G.-L.M.; Methodology, Y.C., H.-Q.L., L.-L.S., M.-T.X., J.Y., L.-L.L., J.-Y.Z., Y.-Q.W., H.-X.W., X.-F.B. and G.-L.M.; Writing–original draft, Y.C.; Writing–review & editing, G.-L.M.

Funding: This research was funded by the National Natural Science Foundation of China (81770279, 31500649), a major project of Natural Science Research in Jiangsu Higher Education Institutions (18KJA310005), a project funded by China Postdoctoral Science Foundation (2017M610342), a Postgraduate Research & Practice Innovation Program of Jiangsu Province (1701050A), a Research and Innovation Project of Graduate Students in Jiangsu Province (KYCX18_2401), grants from the Natural Science Foundation of Nantong City (MS12015015, MS12015101), and the Nantong University Cooperative Innovation Program of Small Molecular Compound R&D-NTU2016-1.

Conflicts of Interest: The authors declare no conflict of interest.

Abbreviations

ANP	Atrial natriuretic peptides
BNP	Brain natriuretic peptides
DBP	Diastolic blood pressure
DHE	Dihydroethidium
FOXO3a	Forkhead-box-protein 3a
HMI	Heart mass index
HW	Heart weight
IVS	Inter ventricular septum
LVMI	Left ventricular mass index
LVPW	Left ventricular posterior wall
MAP	Average mean artery pressure
RWT	Relative wall thickness
SBP	Systolic blood pressure
SOD	Superoxide dismutase
T-AOC	Total antioxidant capacity
WGA	Wheat germ agglutinin

References

1. Pagliaro, P.; Penna, C. Hypertension, hypertrophy, and reperfusion injury. *J. Cardiovasc. Med. (Hagerstown)* **2017**, *18*, 131–135. [CrossRef] [PubMed]
2. Lazzeroni, D.; Rimoldi, O.; Camici, P.G. From left ventricular hypertrophy to dysfunction and failure. *Circ. J.* **2016**, *80*, 555–564. [CrossRef] [PubMed]
3. Guan, Y.; Zhao, X.; Liu, S.; Ji, Y.; Yao, J.; Xu, H. Knockout of the prostaglandin E-2 receptor subtype 3 promotes eccentric cardiac hypertrophy and fibrosis in mice. *J. Cardiovasc. Pharmacol.* **2017**, *22*, 71–82.
4. Liao, R.J.; Tong, L.J.; Huang, C.; Cao, W.W.; Wang, Y.Z.; Wang, J.; Chen, X.F.; Zhu, W.Z.; Zhang, W. Rescue of cardiac failing and remodelling by inhibition of protein phosphatase 1 gamma is associated with suppression of the alternative splicing factor-mediated splicing of Ca^{2+}/calmodulin-dependent protein kinase delta. *Clin. Exp. Pharmacol. Physiol.* **2014**, *41*, 976–985. [CrossRef] [PubMed]
5. Woo, A.Y.; Song, Y.; Xiao, R.P.; Zhu, W. Biased (2)-adrenoceptorsignalling in heart failure: pathophysiology and drug discovery. *Br. J. Pharmacol.* **2015**, *172*, 5444–5456. [CrossRef] [PubMed]
6. Zhao, L.; Wu, D.; Sang, M.; Xu, Y.; Liu, Z.; Wu, Q. Stachydrine ameliorates isoproterenol-induced cardiac hypertrophy and fibrosis by suppressing inflammation and oxidative stress through inhibiting NF-kappa B and JAK/STAT signaling pathways in rats. *Int. Immunopharmacol.* **2017**, *48*, 102–109. [CrossRef] [PubMed]
7. Cervantes Gracia, K.; Llanas-Cornejo, D.; Husi, H. CVD and oxidative stress. *J. Clin. Med.* **2017**, *6*, E22. [CrossRef] [PubMed]
8. Maulik, S.K.; Kumar, S. Oxidative stress and cardiac hypertrophy: a review. *Toxicol. Mech. Methods* **2012**, *22*, 359–366. [CrossRef] [PubMed]
9. Tsutsui, H.; Kinugawa, S.; Matsushima, S. Oxidative stress and heart failure. *Am. J. Physiol. Heart Circ. Physiol.* **2011**, *301*, H2181–H2190. [CrossRef] [PubMed]
10. Jin, M.Y.; Ding, Y.; Zhang, T.; Cai, Z.; Tao, J. Simultaneous determination of dihydromyricetin and resveratrol in ampelopsis sinica (Miq.) W.T. Wang by high-performance liquid chromatography coupled with a diode array detection method. *J. Chromatogr. Sci.* **2014**, *52*, 339–343. [CrossRef] [PubMed]
11. Chen, S.; Zhao, X.; Wan, J.; Ran, L.; Qin, Y.; Wang, X.; Gao, Y.; Shu, F.; Zhang, Y.; Liu, P.; et al. Dihydromyricetin improves glucose and lipid metabolism and exerts anti-inflammatory effects in nonalcoholic fatty liver disease: arandomized controlled trial. *Pharmacol. Res.* **2015**, *99*, 74–81. [CrossRef] [PubMed]
12. Huang, H.; Hu, M.; Zhao, R.; Li, P.; Li, M. Dihydromyricetin suppresses the proliferation of hepatocellular carcinoma cells by inducing G2/M arrest through the Chk1/Chk2/Cdc25C pathway. *Oncol. Rep.* **2013**, *30*, 2467–2475. [CrossRef] [PubMed]
13. Jiang, B.; Le, L.; Pan, H.; Hu, K.; Xu, L.; Xiao, P. Dihydromyricetin ameliorates the oxidative stress response induced by methylglyoxal via the AMPK/GLUT4 signal pathway in PC12 cells. *Brain Res. Bull.* **2014**, *109*, 117–126. [CrossRef] [PubMed]

14. Wang, Y.; Fu, L.; Wang, L.; Xu, L.; Yang, B. Electrophysiological study on the antiarrhythmic mechanism of ampelopsin in rats. *Zhonghua Xin Xue Guan Bing Za Zhi* **2014**, *42*, 675–679. (In Chinese) [PubMed]
15. Liao, S.F.; Wang, H.T.; Yan, F.X.; Zheng, Y.X.; Zeng, Z.W.; Zheng, W.H. Protective effect and mechanisms of dihydromyricetin on PC12 cells induced by oxidative injury. *Zhongyaocai* **2014**, *37*, 1014–1020. (In Chinese) [PubMed]
16. Wong, I.L.; Wang, B.C.; Yuan, J.; Duan, L.X.; Liu, Z.; Liu, T.; Li, X.M.; Hu, X.; Zhang, X.Y.; Jiang, T.; et al. Potent and nontoxic chemosensitizer of P-glycoprotein-mediated multidrug resistance in cancer: synthesis and evaluation of methylated epigallocatechin, gallocatechin, and dihydromyricetin derivatives. *J. Med. Chem.* **2015**, *58*, 4529–4549. [CrossRef] [PubMed]
17. Song, Q.; Liu, L.; Yu, J.; Zhang, J.; Xu, M.; Sun, L.; Luo, H.; Feng, Z.; Meng, G. Dihydromyricetin attenuated Ang II induced cardiac fibroblasts proliferation related to inhibitory of oxidative stress. *Eur. J. Pharmacol.* **2017**, *807*, 159–167. [CrossRef] [PubMed]
18. Meng, G.; Yang, S.; Chen, Y.; Yao, W.; Zhu, H.; Zhang, W. Attenuating effects of dihydromyricetin on angiotensin II-induced rat cardiomyocyte hypertrophy related to antioxidative activity in a NO-dependent manner. *Pharm. Biol.* **2015**, *53*, 904–912. [CrossRef] [PubMed]
19. Xie, L.; Feng, H.; Li, S.; Meng, G.; Liu, S.; Tang, X.; Ma, Y.; Han, Y.; Xiao, Y.; Gu, Y.; et al. SIRT3 mediates the antioxidant effect of hydrogen sulfide in endothelial cells. *Antioxid. Redox Signal.* **2016**, *24*, 329–343. [CrossRef] [PubMed]
20. Rangarajan, P.; Karthikeyan, A.; Lu, J.; Ling, E.A.; Dheen, S.T. Sirtuin 3 regulatesFoxo3a-mediated antioxidant pathway in microglia. *Neuroscience* **2015**, *311*, 398–414. [CrossRef] [PubMed]
21. Yue, Z.; Ma, Y.; You, J.; Li, Z.; Ding, Y.; He, P.; Lu, X.; Jiang, J.; Chen, S.; Liu, P. NMNAT3 is involved in the protective effect of SIRT3 in Ang II-induced cardiac hypertrophy. *Exp. Cell Res.* **2016**, *347*, 261–273. [CrossRef] [PubMed]
22. Li, J.; Chen, T.; Xiao, M.; Li, N.; Wang, S.; Su, H.; Guo, X.; Liu, H.; Yan, F.; Yang, Y.; et al. Mouse SIRT3 promotes autophagy in Ang II-induced myocardial hypertrophy through the deacetylation of FoxO1. *Oncotarget* **2016**, *7*, 86648–86659. [CrossRef] [PubMed]
23. Liu, P.; Zou, D.; Chen, K.; Zhou, Q.; Gao, Y.; Huang, Y.; Zhu, J.; Zhang, Q.; Mi, M. Dihydromyricetin improves hypobaric hypoxia-induced memory impairment via modulation of SIRT3 signaling. *Mol. Neurobiol.* **2016**, *53*, 7200–7212. [CrossRef] [PubMed]
24. Zeng, X.; Yang, J.; Hu, O.; Huang, J.; Ran, L.; Chen, M.; Zhang, Y.; Zhou, X.; Zhu, J.; Zhang, Q.; et al. Dihydromyricetin ameliorates nonalcoholic fatty liver disease by improving mitochondrial respiratory capacity and redox homeostasis through modulation of SIRT3 signaling. *Antioxid. Redox Signal.* **2018**. [CrossRef] [PubMed]
25. Koentges, C.; Bode, C.; Bugger, H. SIRT3 in cardiac physiology and disease. *Front. Cardiovasc. Med.* **2016**, *3*, 38. [CrossRef] [PubMed]
26. Tham, Y.K.; Bernardo, B.C.; Ooi, J.Y.; Weeks, K.L.; McMullen, J.R. Pathophysiology of cardiac hypertrophy and heart failure: signaling pathways and novel therapeutic targets. *Arch. Toxicol.* **2015**, *89*, 1401–1438. [CrossRef] [PubMed]
27. Sundaresan, N.R.; Gupta, M.; Kim, G.; Rajamohan, S.B.; Isbatan, A.; Gupta, M.P. SIRT3 blocks the cardiac hypertrophic response by augmenting Foxo3a-dependent antioxidant defense mechanisms in mice. *J. Clin. Investig.* **2009**, *119*, 2758–2771. [CrossRef] [PubMed]
28. Goh, V.J.; Le, T.T.; Bryant, J.; Wong, J.I.; Su, B.; Lee, C.H.; Pua, C.J.; Sim, C.P.Y.; Ang, B.; Aw, T.C.; Cook, S.A.; Chin, C.W.L. Novel index of maladaptive myocardial remodeling in hypertension. *Circ. Cardiovasc. Imaging* **2017**, *10*, e006840. [CrossRef] [PubMed]
29. Froese, N.; Wang, H.; Zwadlo, C.; Wang, Y.; Grund, A.; Gigina, A.; Hofmann, M.; Kilian, K.; Scharf, G.; Korf-Klingebiel, M.; et al. Anti-androgenic therapy with finasteride improves cardiac function, attenuates remodeling and reverts pathologic gene-expression after myocardial infarction in mice. *J. Mol. Cell. Cardiol.* **2018**, *122*, 114–124. [CrossRef] [PubMed]
30. Peng, Y.; Zeng, Y.; Xu, J.; Huang, X.L.; Zhang, W.; Xu, X.L. PPAR-gamma is involved in the protective effect of 2,3,4′,5-tetrahydroxystilbene-2-*O*-beta-D-glucoside against cardiac fibrosis in pressure-overloaded rats. *Eur. J. Pharmacol.* **2016**, *791*, 105–114. [CrossRef] [PubMed]

31. Protsenko, Y.L.; Balakin, A.A.; Kuznetsov, D.A.; Kursanov, A.G.; Lisin, R.V.; Mukhlynina, E.A.; Lookin, O.N. Contractility of right ventricular myocardium in male and female rats during physiological and pathological hypertrophy. *Bull. Exp. Biol. Med.* **2017**, *162*, 303–305. [CrossRef] [PubMed]
32. Wu, B.; Lin, J.; Luo, J.; Han, D.; Fan, M.; Guo, T.; Tao, L.; Yuan, M.; Yi, F. Dihydromyricetin Protects against Diabetic Cardiomyopathy in Streptozotocin-Induced Diabetic Mice. *Biomed. Res. Int.* **2017**, *2017*, 3764370. [CrossRef] [PubMed]
33. Zhou, M.Q.; Shao, L.; Wu, J.; Peng, N.; Jin, L.P.; Wei, G.Z.; Cheng, W.; Deng, C.J. Dihydromyricetin protects against lipopolysaccharide-induced cardiomyocyte injury through the toll-like receptor-4/nuclear factor-κB pathway. *Mol. Med. Rep.* **2017**, *16*, 8983–8988. [CrossRef] [PubMed]
34. Liu, S.; Ai, Q.; Feng, K.; Li, Y.; Liu, X. The cardioprotective effect of dihydromyricetin prevents ischemia-reperfusion-induced apoptosis in vivo and in vitro via the PI3K/Akt and HIF-1α signaling pathways. *Apoptosis* **2016**, *21*, 1366–1385. [CrossRef] [PubMed]
35. Liu, T.T.; Zeng, Y.; Tang, K.; Chen, X.; Zhang, W.; Xu, X.L. Dihydromyricetin ameliorates atherosclerosis in LDL receptor deficient mice. *Atherosclerosis* **2017**, *262*, 39–50. [CrossRef] [PubMed]
36. Zhu, H.; Luo, P.; Fu, Y.; Wang, J.; Dai, J.; Shao, J.; Yang, X.; Chang, L.; Weng, Q.; Yang, B.; et al. Dihydromyricetin prevents cardiotoxicity and enhances anticancer activity induced by adriamycin. *Oncotarget* **2015**, *6*, 3254–3267. [CrossRef] [PubMed]
37. Zeng, Y.; Peng, Y.; Tang, K.; Wang, Y.Q.; Zhao, Z.Y.; Wei, X.Y.; Xu, X.L. Dihydromyricetin ameliorates foam cell formation via LXRα-ABCA1/ABCG1-dependent cholesterol efflux in macrophages. *Biomed. Pharmacother.* **2018**, *101*, 542–552. [CrossRef] [PubMed]
38. Xu, X.L.; Zhu, Q.Y.; Zhao, C.; Wang, F.; Zhou, Z.Y.; Hu, Y.E.; Zhang, W. The Effect of 2,3,4′,5-Tetrahydroxystilbene-2-*O*-beta-D-Glucoside on pressure overload-induced cardiac remodeling in rats and its possible mechanism. *Planta Med.* **2014**, *80*, 130–138. [PubMed]
39. Hou, X.; Tong, Q.; Wang, W.; Xiong, W.; Shi, C.; Fang, J. Dihydromyricetin protects endothelial cells from hydrogen peroxide-induced oxidative stress damage by regulating mitochondrial pathways. *Life Sci.* **2015**, *130*, 38–46. [CrossRef] [PubMed]
40. Xie, C.; Chen, Z.; Zhang, C.; Xu, X.; Jin, J.; Zhan, W.; Han, T.; Wang, J. Dihydromyricetin ameliorates oleic acid-induced lipid accumulation in L02 and HepG2 cells by inhibiting lipogenesis and oxidative stress. *Life Sci.* **2016**, *157*, 131–139. [CrossRef] [PubMed]
41. Wang, Y.; Wang, W.; Qiu, E. Protection of oxidative stress induced apoptosis in osteosarcoma cells by dihydromyricetin through down-regulation of caspase activation and up-regulation of BcL-2. *Saudi J. Biol. Sci.* **2017**, *24*, 837–842. [CrossRef] [PubMed]
42. Elhassan, Y.S.; Philp, A.A.; Lavery, G.G. Targeting NAD^+ in metabolic disease: new insight into an old molecule. *J. Endocr. Soc.* **2017**, *1*, 816–825. [CrossRef] [PubMed]
43. Fan, D.; Yang, Z.; Liu, F.Y.; Jin, Y.G.; Zhang, N.; Ni, J.; Yuan, Y.; Liao, H.H.; Wu, Q.Q.; Xu, M.; et al. Sesamin Protects Against Cardiac Remodeling via SIRT3/ROS Pathway. *Cell. Physiol. Biochem.* **2017**, *44*, 2212–2227. [CrossRef] [PubMed]
44. Hafner, A.V.; Dai, J.; Gomes, A.P.; Xiao, C.Y.; Palmeira, C.M.; Rosenzweig, A.; Sinclair, D.A. Regulation of the mPTP by SIRT3-mediated deacetylation of CypD at lysine 166 suppresses age-related cardiac hypertrophy. *Aging* **2010**, *2*, 914–923. [CrossRef] [PubMed]
45. Hsu, C.P.; Oka, S.; Shao, D.; Hariharan, N.; Sadoshima, J. Nicotinamide phosphoribosyltransferase regulates cell survival through NAD+ synthesis in cardiac myocytes. *Circ. Res.* **2009**, *105*, 481–491. [CrossRef] [PubMed]
46. Lu, Y.; Wang, Y.D.; Wang, X.Y.; Chen, H.; Cai, Z.J.; Xiang, M.X. SIRT3 in cardiovascular diseases: emerging roles and therapeutic implications. *Int. J. Cardiol.* **2016**, *220*, 700–705. [CrossRef] [PubMed]
47. Osborne, B.; Bentley, N.L.; Montgomery, M.K.; Turner, N. The role of mitochondrial sirtuins in health and disease. *Free Radic. Biol. Med.* **2016**, *100*, 164–174. [CrossRef] [PubMed]
48. Pillai, V.B.; Bindu, S.; Sharp, W.; Fang, Y.H.; Kim, G.; Gupta, M.; Samant, S.; Gupta, M.P. SIRT3 protects mitochondrial DNA damage and blocks the development of doxorubicin-induced cardiomyopathy in mice. *Am. J. Physiol. Heart Circ. Physiol.* **2016**, *310*, H962–H972. [CrossRef] [PubMed]
49. Tanno, M.; Kuno, A.; Horio, Y.; Miura, T. Emerging beneficial roles of sirtuins in heart failure. *Basic Res. Cardiol.* **2012**, *107*, 273. [CrossRef] [PubMed]

50. Meng, G.; Liu, J.; Liu, S.; Song, Q.; Liu, L.; Xie, L.; Han, Y.; Ji, Y. Hydrogen sulfide pretreatment improves mitochondrial function in myocardial hypertrophy via a SIRT3-dependent manner. *Br. J. Pharmacol.* **2018**, *175*, 1126–1145. [CrossRef] [PubMed]
51. Jacobs, K.M.; Pennington, J.D.; Bisht, K.S.; Aykin-Burns, N.; Kim, H.S.; Mishra, M.; Sun, L.; Nquyen, P.; Ahn, B.H.; Leclerc, J.; et al. SIRT3 interacts with the daf-16 homolog FOXO3a in the mitochondria, as well as increases FOXO3a dependent gene expression. *Int. J. Biol. Sci.* **2008**, *4*, 291–299. [CrossRef] [PubMed]
52. Das, S.; Mitrovsky, G.; Vasanthi, H.R.; Das, D.K. Antiaging properties of a grape-derived antioxidant are regulated by mitochondrial balance of fusion and fission leading to mitophagy triggered by a signaling network of Sirt1-SIRT3-Foxo3-PINK1-PARKIN. *Oxid. Med. Cell Longev.* **2014**, *2014*, 345105. [CrossRef] [PubMed]
53. Queiroz, E.A.; Puukila, S.; Eichler, R.; Sampaio, S.C.; Forsyth, H.L.; Lees, S.J.; Barbosa, A.M.; Dekker, R.F.; Fortes, Z.B.; Khaper, N. Metformin induces apoptosis and cell cycle arrest mediated by oxidative stress, AMPK and FOXO3a in MCF-7 breast cancer cells. *PLoS ONE* **2014**, *9*, e98207. [CrossRef] [PubMed]
54. Tothova, Z.; Kollipara, R.; Huntly, B.J.; Lee, B.H.; Castrillon, D.H.; Cullen, D.E.; McDowell, E.P.; Lazo-Kallanian, S.; Williams, I.R.; Sears, C.; et al. FoxOs are critical mediators of hematopoietic stem cell resistance to physiologic oxidative stress. *Cell* **2007**, *128*, 325–339. [CrossRef] [PubMed]
55. Song, C.; Zhao, J.; Fu, B.; Li, D.; Mao, T.; Peng, W.; Wu, H.; Zhang, Y. Melatonin-mediated upregulation of SIRT3 attenuates sodium fluoride-induced hepatotoxicity by activating the MT1-PI3K/AKT-PGC-1α signaling pathway. *Free Radic. Biol. Med.* **2017**, *112*, 616–630. [CrossRef] [PubMed]
56. Chen, Y.; Zhang, J.; Lin, Y.; Lei, Q.; Guan, K.L.; Zhao, S.; Xiong, Y. Tumour suppressor SIRT3 deacetylates and activates manganese superoxide dismutase to scavenge ROS. *EMBO Rep.* **2011**, *12*, 534–541. [CrossRef] [PubMed]
57. Pillai, V.B.; Samant, S.; Sundaresan, N.R.; Raghuraman, H.; Kim, G.; Bonner, M.Y.; Arbiser, J.L.; Walker, D.; Jones, D.P.; Gius, D.; et al. Honokiol blocks and reverses cardiac hypertrophy in mice by activating mitochondrial SIRT3. *Nat. Commun.* **2015**, *6*, 6656. [CrossRef] [PubMed]
58. Liu, X.; Zhang, L.; Wang, P.; Li, X.; Qiu, D.; Li, L.; Zhang, J.; Hou, X.; Han, L.; Ge, J.; et al. SIRT3-dependent deacetylation of SOD2 plays a protective role against oxidative stress in oocytes from diabetic mice. *Cell Cycle* **2017**, *16*, 1302–1308. [CrossRef] [PubMed]
59. Valdecantos, M.P.; Pérez-Matute, P.; González-Muniesa, P.; Prieto-Hontoria, P.L.; Moreno-Aliaga, M.J.; Martínez, J.A. Lipoic acid improves mitochondrial function in nonalcoholic steatosis through the stimulation of sirtuin 1 and sirtuin 3. *Obesity* **2012**, *20*, 1974–1983. [CrossRef] [PubMed]
60. De Almeida, A.C.; van Oort, R.J.; Wehrens, X.H. Transverse aortic constriction in mice. *J. Vis. Exp.* **2010**, *38*, 172.

International Journal of
Molecular Sciences

MDPI

Article

Flavonones from *Penthorum chinense* Ameliorate Hepatic Steatosis by Activating the SIRT1/AMPK Pathway in HepG2 Cells

Wei-Wei Guo, Xing Wang, Xiao-Qing Chen, Yin-Ying Ba, Nan Zhang, Rong-Rong Xu, Wen-Wen Zhao and Xia Wu *

Beijing Key Lab of TCM Collateral Disease Theory Research, School of Traditional Chinese Medicine, Capital Medical University, 10 Youanmen, Xitoutiao, Beijing 100069, China; gww1023@163.com (W.-W.G.); kingstar1016@sina.com (X.W.); cxqcpu@163.com (X.-Q.C.); byy3333@sina.com (Y.-Y.B.); nan623@126.com (N.Z.); xrr9515@163.com (R.-R.X.); wenwenzhao1994@163.com (W.-W.Z.)

* Correspondence: wuxia6710@ccmu.edu.cn; Tel.: +86-10-8391-1671; Fax: +86-10-8391-1627

Received: 11 July 2018; Accepted: 22 August 2018; Published: 28 August 2018

Abstract: Pinocembrin-7-*O*-*β*-D-glucoside (PCBG), pinocembrin (PCB), and 5-methoxy-pinocembrin-7-*O*-*β*-D-glucoside (MPG) are three flavonones isolated from *Penthorum chinense* Pursh (*P. chinense*). The effects of the three flavonones on hepatic steatosis and their molecular mechanisms in HepG2 cells were investigated in this study for the first time. A model of hepatic steatosis in HepG2 cells was induced by free fatty acid (FFA), and co-treated with the three flavonones as mentioned. Intracellular lipid droplets were detected by Oil Red O staining. PCB, PCBG, and MPG suppressed oxidative stress by decreasing malondialdehyde (MDA) levels and increasing superoxide dismutase (SOD) and glutathione peroxidase (GSH-Px) activities. The levels of aspartate aminotransferase (AST) and alanine aminotransferase (ALT) were ameliorated. Moreover, these flavonones enhanced the phosphorylation of AMP-activated protein kinase (AMPK) and the expression of silent mating type information regulation 2 homolog 1 (SIRT1) and peroxisome proliferator-activated receptor α (PPARα), and reduced the expression of sterol regulatory element binding protein-1c (SREBP1c) and the downstream targets fatty acid synthase (FAS), acetyl-CoA carboxylase (ACC), and stearoyl-CoA desaturase 1 (SCD1). Molecular docking was used to predict the interaction and combination patterns between the three flavonones and the enzymes above. The results revealed that the SIRT1/AMPK pathway is involved in the functions of the three flavonones, and the most effective flavonone against hepatic steatosis might be PCBG, followed by MPG and PCB. Therefore, the three flavonones from *P. chinense* were found to exert preventive effects against hepatic steatosis by regulating the SIRT1/AMPK pathway.

Keywords: *Penthorum chinense* Pursh; NAFLD; hepatic steatosis; flavonoids; SIRT1; AMPK

1. Introdution

Non-alcoholic fatty liver disease (NAFLD) is now the most common chronic liver disease in the world [1]. Currently, the prevalence of NAFLD in Asia is around 25%, similar to that in many Western countries [2]. NAFLD is characterized as a metabolic syndrome, which is associated with insulin resistance, obesity, and dyslipidemia [3]. NAFLD ranges from simple steatosis, steatohepatitis, and fibrosis to cirrhosis, and the prevalence of non-alcoholic steatohepatitis (NASH), developed from NAFLD, is estimated at 3–5% in the general population [4,5]. People with NASH have a much higher risk of liver fibrosis, cirrhosis, and even hepatocellular carcinoma [6,7].

Several studies concluded that weight loss, dietary interventions, and physical activity could potentially ameliorate biochemical, histological, and structural abnormalities of NAFLD, whereas drugs, such as statins, vitamin E, glitazones, and metformin are used to reduce the amelioration [5,8,9]. The pathogenesis of NAFLD is complex and not completely understood, although increased visceral adiposity and insulin resistance with increased free fatty acid (FFA) release are confirmed to play an important role in the development of liver steatosis [10]. AMP-activated protein kinase (AMPK) and silent mating type information regulation 2 homolog 1 (SIRT1) are the key enzymes responsible for longevity and energy homeostasis by regulating glucose and lipid metabolism in a finely tuned network [11–13]. AMPK stimulation during fatty acid metabolism is presented as AMPK phosphorylation, and it is known as a critical regulator for sterol regulatory element binding protein-1 (SREBP1) activation and lipogenesis [14,15]. Sterol regulatory element binding protein-1c (SREBP1c) regulates gene expression related to glucose metabolism, fatty acid, and lipid production, and its activity is regulated by insulin [16]. Moreover, SREBP1c can up-regulate the transcription of fatty acid synthase (FAS), stearoyl-CoA desaturase 1 (SCD1), and acetyl-CoA carboxylase (ACC) [17,18], which primarily catalyzes the synthesis of long-chain fatty acids from acetyl-CoA and malonyl-CoA [19,20].

Penthorum chinense Pursh (*P. chinense*), a Chinese medicine in the family of Saxifragaceage, is used as folk medicine and a functional drink with antioxidant, anti-complement, and liver-protecting effects [21,22]. A previous study showed that *P. chinense* extract has effects on NAFLD treatment [23]. Gansu granules, made from *P. chinense* extract, are widely used in the clinic for various ailments of the liver, such as chronic hepatitis B and NAFLD [24,25]. Pinocembrin-7-*O*-β-D-glucoside (PCBG), pinocembrin (PCB), and 5-methoxy-pinocembrin-7-*O*-β-D-glucoside (MPG) are three flavonones with similar nuclear structures isolated from the extract of *P. chinense*. PCBG and PCB were reported to possess hepatoprotective, antioxidant, anti-inflammatory, and anti-hepatocarcinoma activities [26,27]. Moreover, our previous studies identified MPG as a new flavonone [28], and PCBG can be degraded into PCB rapidly not only in pharmacokinetic studies in vivo, but also in biotransformation in vitro [29]. However, there is no report on NAFLD treatment using these three ingredients.

To investigate the resistant effects of PCBG, PCB, and MPG on NAFLD and their possible therapeutic mechanism, targets on the SIRT1/AMPK/SREBP1c pathway related to lipid metabolism were evaluated in a nonalcoholic injured HepG2 cell model induced by FFA in the present study. Moreover, molecular docking of the binding of the three flavonones to several targets in the lipid metabolic pathway was performed to determine the ligand–protein binding interaction in silico. We hypothesized that the flavonones in *P. chinense* produced their hepatoprotective action via the regulation of lipid generation and metabolism, and in vivo research will be performed in our group.

2. Results

2.1. FFA-Induced Cytotoxicity and Concentration Screening of PCB, PCBG, and MPG

The effects of FFA and drugs on the viability of HepG2 cells were assessed. As shown in Figure 1E,F, 0.8 mM FFA reduced cell viability to approximately 70%, and concentrations of 10, 50, and 100 μM PCB and MPG were not cytotoxic to HepG2 cells. A concentration range below 10 μM of PCBG was not cytotoxic. Thus, FFA (0.8 mM) and co-treatment with PCB, MPG (1, 10, and 100 μM), and PCBG (0.1, 1, and 10 μM) were used to evaluate drug effects in HepG2 cells in this study.

2.2. PCB, PCBG, and MPG Inhibited Intracellular Lipid Accumulation in HepG2 Cells

To verify the inhibition of FFA-induced lipid accumulation by PCB, PCBG, and MPG, the cells were stained with Oil Red O, then observed under the microscope and quantified by measuring the absorbance at 510 nm. Oil Red O staining showed more lipid droplets in HepG2 cells after FFA treatment compared to the control group (Figure 2). The lipids accumulated in the presence of FFA (0.8 mM); however, co-treatment of FFA with PCB, PCBG, and MPG significantly declined the number of lipid droplets in a dose-dependent manner ($p < 0.01$). Quantitative measurements also showed that treatment with PCB, PCBG, and MPG alleviated the FFA-induced accumulation of triglycerides.

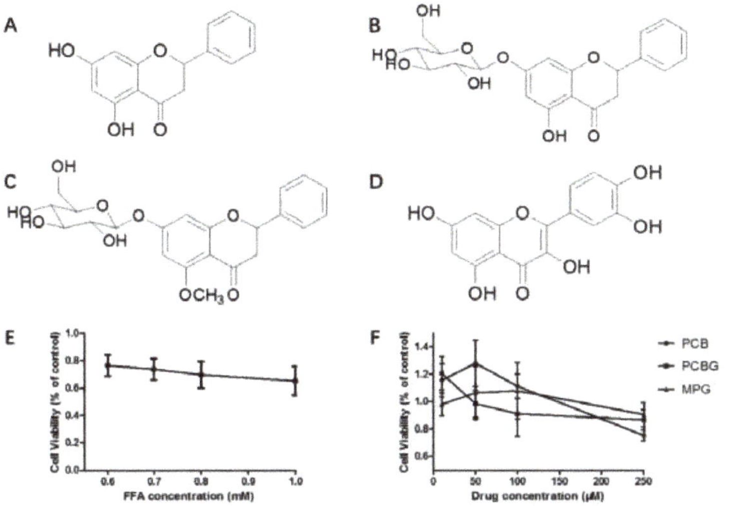

Figure 1. Structures of pinocembrin (PCB; **A**), pinocembrin-7-*O*-*β*-D-glucoside (PCBG; **B**), fcg 5-methoxy-pinocembrin-7-*O*-*β*-D-glucoside (MPG; **C**), and reference quercetin (QCT; **D**). The cytotoxicity of free fatty acid (FFA; **E**) and the three compounds (**F**) toward HepG2 cells. The experiments were performed at least three times independently, and the results are displayed as mean ± SD.

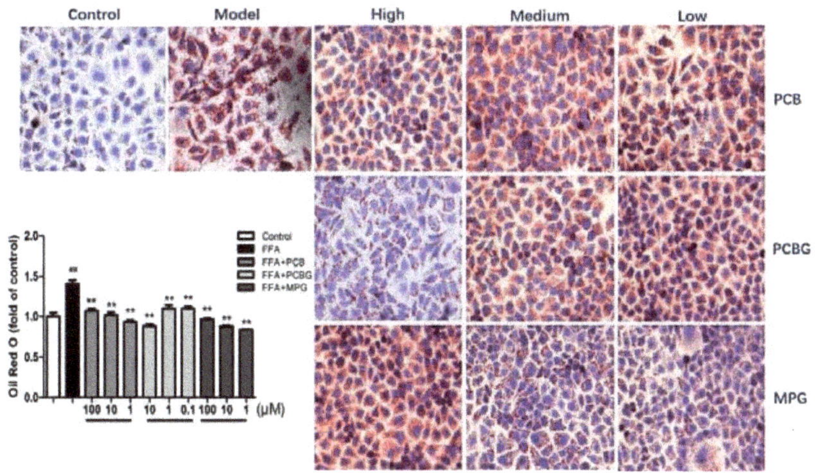

Figure 2. Qualitive and quantitative measurements of hepatic lipid accumulation in the HepG2 cells as observed by Oil Red O staining (original magnification 400×). Data represent the mean ± SD of five independent experiments. ## $p < 0.01$ versus control; ** $p < 0.01$ versus FFA group.

2.3. PCB, PCBG, and MPG Weakened Lipid Levels and Up-Regulated Antioxidant Enzymes

To evaluate the effect of PCB, PCBG, and MPG on liver function, an enzymatic method was used to evaluate liver function. FFA treatment caused severe liver function injury in HepG2 cells, as indicated by the increase in alanine aminotransferase (ALT) and aspartate aminotransferase (AST) activities ($p < 0.01$). Treatment with PCB, PCBG, and MPG at three doses significantly blocked the increase in ALT and AST activities in the presence of FFA. Analysis of hepatic total cholesterol (TC) and triglyceride (TG) contents confirmed hepatic steatosis by FFA. Intracellular TG and TC levels were increased by FFA treatment, but this effect was blocked by PCB, PCBG, and MPG (Figure 3).

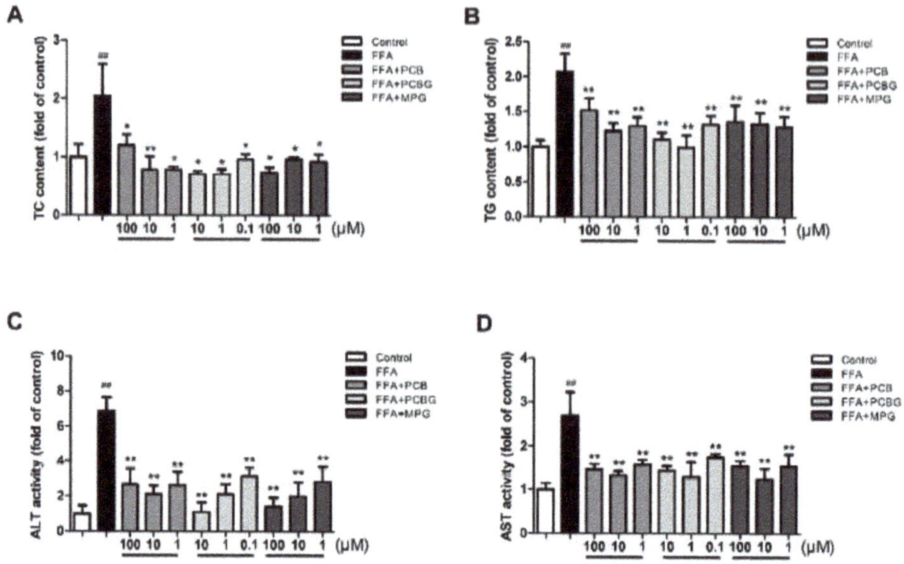

Figure 3. The effects of PCB, PCBG, and MPG on total cholesterol (TC; **A**), triglyceride (TG; **B**), alanine aminotransferase (ALT; **C**), and aspartate aminotransferase (AST; **D**) levels in HepG2 cells. The experiments were performed at least three times independently, and the results are displayed as mean ± SD. ## $p < 0.01$ versus control; * $p < 0.05$ versus FFA group; ** $p < 0.01$ versus FFA group.

The effects of each treatment on the levels of oxidative stress are shown in Figure 4. Compared to the control group, the activities of superoxide dismutase (SOD) and glutathione peroxidase (GSH-Px) in FFA-treated HepG2 cells were significantly reduced, while malondialdehyde (MDA) levels were increased, indicating that antioxidant activity was reduced, but lipid peroxidation was increased. Furthermore, PCB, PCBG, and MPG treatments significantly enhanced SOD ($p < 0.05$) and GSH-Px ($p < 0.05$) activities, and decreased MDA ($p < 0.01$) levels when compared with FFA-treated cells. The beneficial role of MPG on the level of oxidative stress was stronger than PCB and PCBG, and presented a dose-dependent manner.

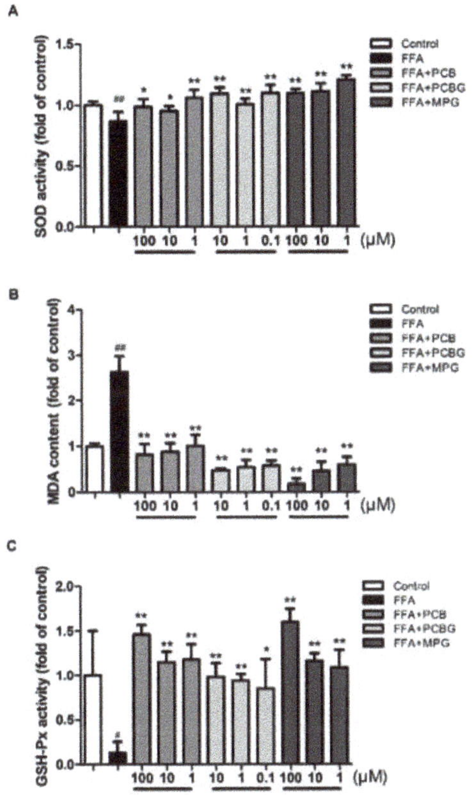

Figure 4. The effects of PCB, PCBG, and MPG on superoxide dismutase (SOD; **A**), malondialdehyde (MDA; **B**), and glutathione peroxidase (GSH-Px; **C**) levels in HepG2 cells. The experiments were performed at least three times independently and the results are displayed as mean ± SD. # $p < 0.05$ versus control; ## $p < 0.01$ versus control; * $p < 0.05$ versus FFA group; ** $p < 0.01$ versus FFA group.

2.4. *Effects of PCB, PCBG, and MPG on the Expression of Factors Associated with Hepatic Lipid Accumulation*

To determine the alternation of de novo lipogenesis in response to FFA and the three flavonones, the mRNA expressions of SREBP1c and its target enzymes, FAS, ACC, and SCD1 were examined using qRT-PCR and compared with the mRNA expression of quercetin (QCT). As shown in Figure 5, FFA enhanced their mRNA expressions in HepG2 cells, which were attenuated by PCB, PCBG, and MPG treatment, particularly by high and medium concentrations of PCBG and MPG. The protein expressions of peroxisome proliferator-activated receptor α (PPARα), SREBP1c, FAS, ACC, and SCD1 were assessed using Western blot. Compared to the control group, FFA treatment enhanced the protein expressions of SREBP1c, FAS, ACC, and SCD1 (Figure 5E–G). Moreover, FFA induced a remarkable decrease in PPARα protein expression. When co-treated with PCB, PCBG, and MPG, the FFA-induced alternations in the proteins for de novo lipogenesis were ameliorated significantly. More specifically, PCB, PCBG, and MPG at medium concentration down-regulated SREBP1c protein levels by 30.64%, 27.67% and 30.81% (Figure 5C), respectively, and recovered PPARα protein expression by 46.65%, 47.12% and 50.04% (Figure 5D), respectively. The results suggest that PCB, PCBG, and MPG attenuated HepG2 cells induced by FFA via the de novo lipogenesis pathway.

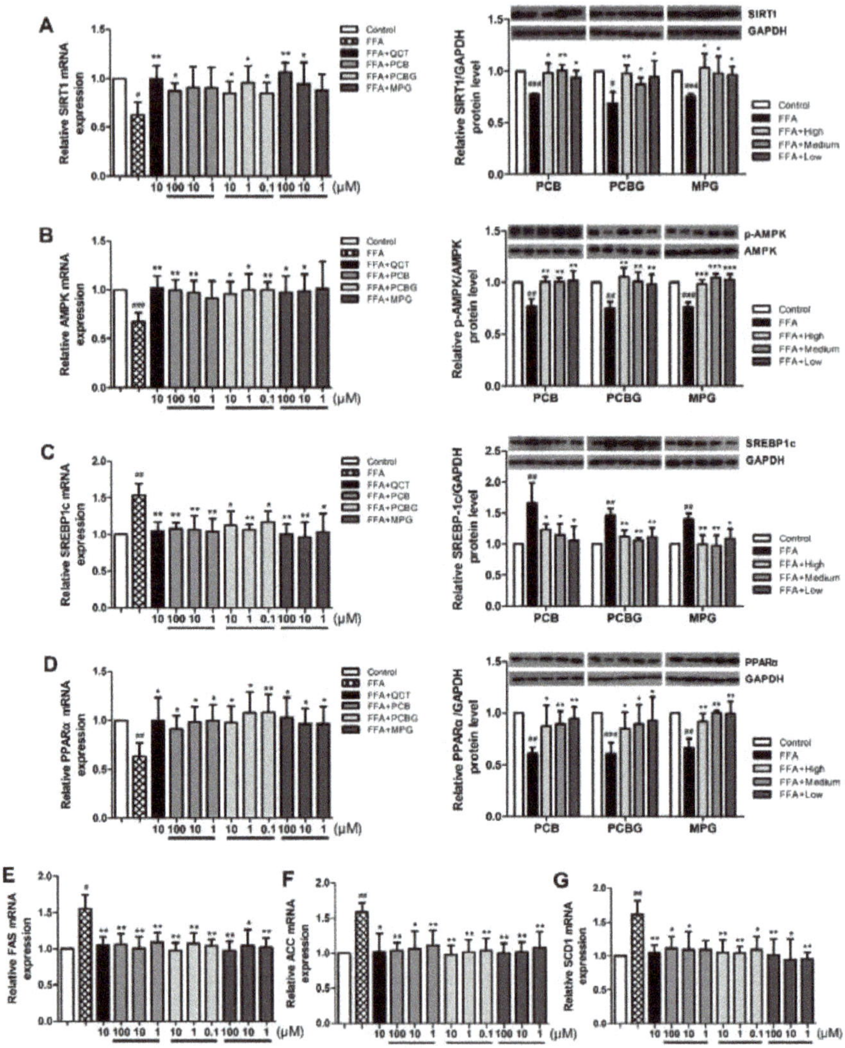

Figure 5. The effects of PCB, PCBG, and MPG on hepatic steatosis depends on the silent mating type information regulation 2 homolog 1/AMP-activated protein kinase (SIRT1/AMPK) pathway. (**A**) Effect on mRNA and protein expressions of SIRT1. (**B**) Effect on AMPK mRNA expression and phosphorylated (p)-AMPK/AMPK protein levels. (**C**) Effect on mRNA and protein expressions of sterol regulatory element binding protein-1c (SREBP1c). (**D**) Effect on mRNA and protein expressions of peroxisome proliferator-activated receptor α (PPARα). (**E–G**) Effects on fatty acid synthase (FAS), acetyl-CoA carboxylase (ACC), and stearoyl-CoA desaturase 1 (SCD1) protein levels. The experiments were performed at least four times independently and the results are displayed as mean ± SD. $^{\#}$ $p < 0.05$ versus control; $^{\#\#}$ $p < 0.01$ versus control; $^{\#\#\#}$ $p < 0.001$ versus control; * $p < 0.05$ versus FFA group; ** $p < 0.01$ versus FFA group; *** $p < 0.001$ versus FFA group.

2.5. Effects of PCB, PCBG, and MPG on AMPK and SIRT1 Activities in HepG2 Cells

Activated AMPK reduces lipogenesis and lipid accumulation by suppressing SREBP1c cleavage and nuclear translocation [30,31]. To further evaluate the mechanism for the roles of PCB, PCBG, and MPG in relieving fatty liver, we assessed the phosphorylation of AMPK and SIRT1 using qRT-PCR and Western blot. The expression of phosphorylated (p)-AMPK decreased significantly in the FFA group compared with the control group, and this effect was blocked in the presence of PCB and MPG at 100 and 10 μM, and at all three concentrations of PCBG. SIRT1 and AMPK are two key enzymes responsible for longevity and energy homeostasis. The expression and deacetylation activities of SIRT1 are enhanced by the increase in oxidized nicotinamide adenine dinucleotide (NAD^+) levels or the ratio of NAD^+ to reduced nicotinamide adenine dinucleotide (NADH), which was suggested by the activation of AMPK to some extent [32]. Therefore, we studied the mRNA and protein expressions of SIRT1, and found that FFA treatment reduced SIRT1 expression, which was recovered by PCB and MPG at 100 and 10 μM, and was significantly up-regulated by PCBG.

2.6. Docking Studies

Molecular docking studies were performed to investigate the interactions between targets including SIRT1, AMPK, PPARα, FAS, ACC1, and SCD1 and ligands including PCB, PCBG, MPG and the reference compound, QCT. The docking score and binding mode were evaluated with docking studies (Table 1), and images of the compounds with amino acids involved in binding poses are shown in Figure 6. PCBG showed a higher docking score for binding with AMPK, FAS, and ACC1 than QCT. MPG showed better AMPK, PPARα, and FAS binding action than QCT. However, PCB showed weak binding with the selected proteins.

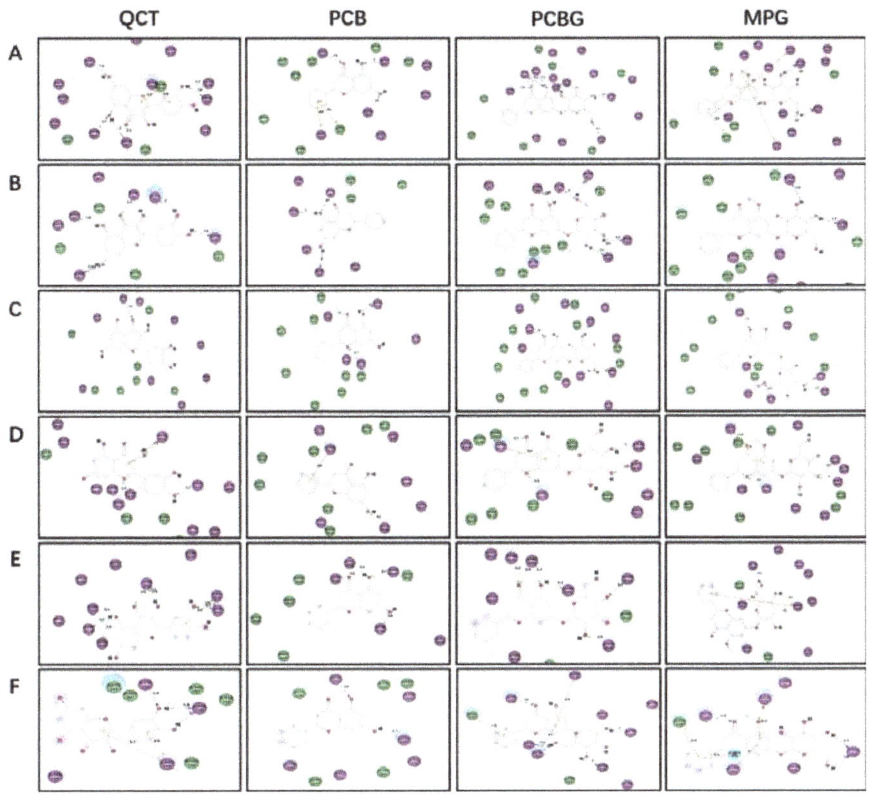

Figure 6. Molecular interactions of PCB, PCBG, MPG, and QCT binding with (**A**) SIRT1, (**B**) AMPK, (**C**) PPARα, (**D**) FAS, (**E**) ACC1, and (**F**) SCD1. Sharper images are in Supplementary Figure S1.

Table 1. Docking Results of Pinocembrin (PCB), Pinocembrin-7-*O*-*β*-D-Glucoside (PCBG), 5-Methoxy-Pinocembrin-7-*O*-*β*-D-Glucoside (MPG), and Quercetin (QCT).

Targets	Ligand	Docking Score	H-Bonds	Residue of Hydrogen Bond	Targets	Ligand	Docking Score	H-Bonds	Residue of Hydrogen Bond
SIRT1 (4ZZJ)	QCT	7.4850	6	GLY263, ASN465, GLU467, ARG276, GLU656	AMPK (4ZHX)	QCT	5.1547	6	GLU94, MET93, VAL96, LEU22, GLU100
	PCB	5.0529	3	ALA262, SER442, GLN294		PCB	3.7372	3	SER97, TYR95, ASP103
	PCBG	7.2696	9	ARG466, GLU467, ASN465, GLY263, ALA262, GLN345, GLN294		PCBG	5.6765	7	VAL96, TYR95, SER97, ASP103, GLU100
	MPG	7.0478	4	SER442, ASP272, ARG274		MPG	6.3571	2	GLU100, ASN144
PPARα (3KDU)	QCT	5.7407	1	THR279	FAS (5C37)	QCT	5.3856	3	ARG1917, ASN1945
	PCB	3.1022	3	ALA333, THR279, CYS275		PCB	4.4753	1	ILE1946
	PCBG	4.8008	4	TYR464, PHE273, PHE351, MET355		PCBG	7.2480	4	ARG1917, VAL1973, GLY1895, PHE1896
	MPG	6.5830	5	TYR464, MET355, CYS276, GLU269, PHE273		MPG	8.1074	5	ARG1917, VAL1973, PHE1896, GLY1895, GLY1897
ACC1 (3TVU)	QCT	4.6247	8	SER1999, ARG1954, ARG1996, PHE1956, GLY1958, MET1963	SCD1 (4ZYO)	QCT	5.5432	3	LYS189, ASP156
	PCB	3.3302	4	ARG1996, GLY1998, SER1999, PHE1956		PCB	5.5185	2	LYS189, ARG155
	PCBG	4.8381	6	PHE1956, SER1999, ARG1996, ARG1954, GLU2026		PCBG	5.8544	5	LYS194, ASP156, LYS189, ASN75, ASN148
	MPG	4.5763	2	PHE1956, ARG1954		MPG	4.9069	4	LYS194, LYS189, GLU152

SIRT1—silent mating type information regulation 2 homolog 1; PPARα—peroxisome proliferator-activated receptor α; ACC1—acetyl-CoA carboxylase; AMPK—AMP-activated protein kinase; FAS—fatty acid synthase; SCD1—stearoyl-CoA desaturase 1.

3. Discussion

NAFLD, a metabolic syndrome, is a major health problem. The reported prevalence of NAFLD is up to 20% in the general population worldwide [5]. NAFLD is characterized by increased fatty-acid uptake, de novo lipogenesis, reduced fatty-acid oxidation, and very-low-density lipoprotein (VLDL) secretion. Flavonoids were reported to exert multiple benefits on the disorders associated with NAFLD [33]. *P. chinense* was reported to possess antioxidant and hepatoprotective activities [21,22]. Previous studies revealed that *P. chinense* is rich in flavonoids [34] and that these flavonoids play roles in protecting the liver [26,27]. The three selected compounds had the same structure in the nucleus. MPG is a new flavonone, while PCBG is the highest-level flavonone in *P. chinense*. In this study, the effects and mechanisms of PCB, PCBG, and MPG on a nonalcoholic injured HepG2 cell model were investigated for the first time.

FFA-induced lipid accumulation in hepatocytes is a commonly used model to study hepatic steatosis [35,36]. These fatty acids may be converted into other lipid species, such as glycerolipids, glycerophospholipids, and sterols. Fatty-acid oxidation damages the mitochondrial function of cells [37]. The HepG2 cells were co-treated with FFA and three doses of PCB, PCBG, and MPG, and the doses were decided upon screening cell cytotoxicity. The results of Oil Red O staining showed that PCB, PCBG, and MPG declined the number of lipid droplets in a dose-dependent manner. FFA treatment increased the concentrations of TC and TG, as well as the levels of AST and ALT, which reflected the extent of hepatocyte damage and hepatic steatosis [38]. Flavonoids significantly reduced FFA-induced changes in TC, TG, AST, and ALT, indicating their protective effects on liver. These results suggest that PCB, PCBG, and MPG inhibited FFA-induced lipid accumulation. PCBG inhibited the activity of ALT in a dose-dependent manner (high vs. medium, $p < 0.05$; medium vs. low, $p < 0.01$; high vs. low, $p < 0.001$).

Free radicals may lead to cell damage not only by lipid peroxidation, but also through decomposition products of lipid hydroperoxides, while flavonoids show good antioxidative effects [39]. Therefore, parameters including MDA, SOD, and GSH-Px were measured to evaluate the oxidative stress. MDA, as the product of lipid peroxidation, indirectly reflects the severity of attack by free radicals. SOD is in charge of catalytic dismutation of free radicals and reducing superoxide levels, which reflects the ability to scavenge free radicals [40]. GSH-Px specifically catalyzes the decomposition of hydrogen peroxide to protect the integrity of cell membrane structure and function. The increased concentration of SOD levels and the decreased levels of MDA and GSH-Px in flavonoid-treated cells proved their protective effect. Furthermore, the effect of MPG occurred in a dose-dependent manner with significant differences between high and low levels of MPG ($p < 0.01$).

The SIRT1/AMPK-SREBP1c pathway is key in regulating lipid metabolism [41]. Both SIRT1 and AMPK are known to regulate each other and share many common target molecules, and the interaction between SIRT1 and AMPK could be reciprocal [42]. AMPK is a protein that regulates mitochondrial biogenesis, fatty-acid synthesis, and oxidative metabolism in response to energy deprivation. SIRT1 was shown to be the primary mediator for regulating the expression levels of mitochondrial metabolism genes and lipid metabolism, as well as the consumption of O_2. Both AMPK and SIRT1 act in concert with the master regulator of mitochondrial biogenesis to regulate energy homeostasis in response to environmental and nutritional stimuli [11,43,44]. AMPK inhibits the rate-limiting enzyme, SREBP1c, in lipogenesis, which leads to decreased lipid deposition [45,46]. SREBP1c is located in the upstream promoter region up-regulating the transcriptions of FAS, ACC, and SCD1, which directly catalyze lipogenesis [18,47]. Moreover, PPARα, known as the ligand-activated nuclear receptor, regulates lipid homeostasis genes [48]. We detected the expression of these genes after treatment with PCB, PCBG, MPG, and the reference compound, QCT, which was reported to exert a preventive effect against hepatic steatosis probably through SIRT1/AMPK and PPARα pathways [49,50]. Our data showed that PCBG (0.1, 1, and 10 μM) and MPG (10 and 100 μM) significantly enhanced SIRT1 and AMPK gene expression, but only 100 μM PCB showed significant improvement on SIRT1 expression, which led to a significant reduction in SREBP1c levels, followed by reduced FAS, ACC, and SCD1 expressions. From the results, it was observed that PCBG (0.1, 1, and 10 μM) and MPG (10 and 100 μM) had appreciably similar hypolipidemic effects to reference QCT (10 μM), while PCB (100 μM) had a visible effect on hepatic steatosis, but weaker than that of QCT (10 μM). A series of recent studies showed that the effects of the active components in traditional Chinese herbs on NAFLD are associated with activating the AMPK signaling pathway, improving insulin resistance, modulating the activity and expression of peroxisome proliferator-activated receptor γ, antioxidant and anti-inflammatory activities, and regulating intestinal flora [51]. These three flavonones might have effects on different potential therapeutic targets. The docking results suggested that binding with polyhydroxy ligands might get higher scores by forming hydrogen-bond interactions with side chains. The C3 carbonyl group and C5 hydroxyl or methoxy group of flavonoids acted as the key hydrogen-bond acceptors by interacting with the amino-acid residues in the active-site region of proteins. The docking score of the compounds was in the order of PCBG, QCT, MPG, and PCB. Finally, this is of great significance to study the pharmacodynamic basis of *P. chinense* and mechanisms on ameliorating hepatic steatosis which was not reported before now. The potency against hepatic steatosis on targets of these flavonoids via molecular docking was consistent with the pharmacophoric features from the cell model (Figure 7).

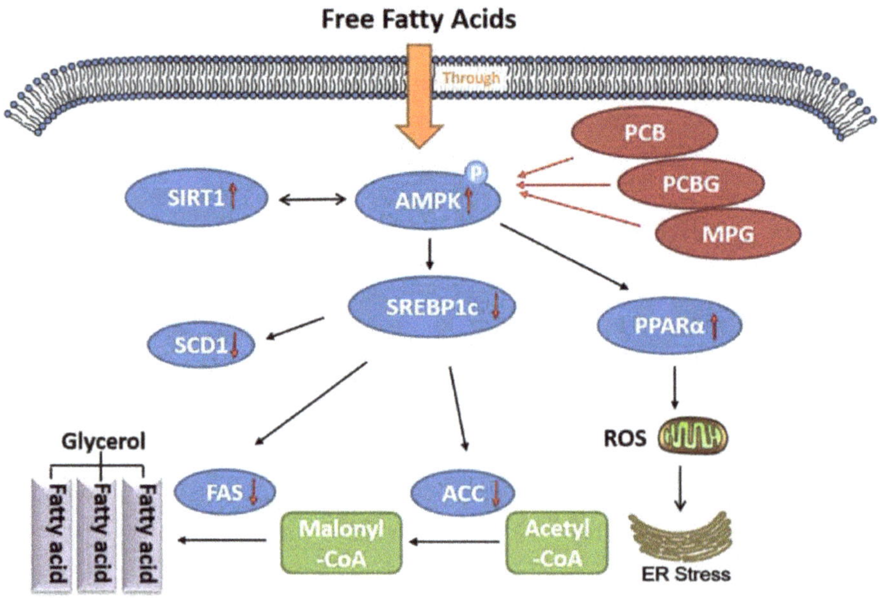

Figure 7. Schematic diagram presenting pathways via which PCB, PCBG, and MPG ameliorate hepatic steatosis by activating the SIRT1/AMPK pathway. Red arrows upward present increased protein expression; Red arrows downward present decreased protein expression.

4. Materials and Methods

4.1. Cell Culture

HepG2 cells were obtained from the American Type Culture Collection (ATCC; Manassas, VA, USA). Cells were cultured in Dulbecco's modified Eagle's medium (DMEM) (Gibco Invitrogen Corporation, Carlsbad, CA, USA) supplemented with 10% fetal bovine serum (FBS) (Gibco Invitrogen Corporation, Carlsbad, CA, USA) in an incubator with 5% CO_2 at 37 °C. The cells were seeded at 70% confluence in six-well plates and were grown in serum-free DMEM containing 0.5% bovine serum albumin (BSA) (Sigma-Aldrich Co., St. Louis, MO, USA) for 12 h before treatment. Cells of the control group were incubated in DMEM containing 0.5% BSA, and model cells were treated with FFA (oleic acid:palmic acid = 2:1) (Sigma-Aldrich Co., St. Louis, MO, USA)dissolved in DMEM containing 0.5% BSA.

4.2. Measurement of Cell Viability

HepG2 cells were seeded at a density of 5×10^3 cells/well in a 96-well plate. PCBG, PCB, and MPG (purity ≥98%; Figure 1) were isolated by the chemistry department of the Chinese Material Medicine Laboratory at the Capital Medical University (Beijing, China) and QCT was purchased from National Institutes for Food and Drug Control (purity = 97.3%; Figure 1D). They were dissolved in dimethyl sulfoxide (DMSO) (Sigma-Aldrich, St. Louis, MO, USA) and diluted to suitable concentrations in DMEM containing 0.5% BSA (DMSO < 0.1%). To determine the modeling concentration and the non-toxic concentration for the cells, FFA (0.6, 0.7, 0.8, and 1 mM), in addition to PCB, PCBG, and MPG (10, 50, 100, and 250 μM) were then added to each well. The plates were then incubated for 24 h at 37 °C under 5% CO_2. Then, 10 μL of 3-(4,5-dimethylthiazol-2-yl)-2,5-diphenyltetrazolium bromide (MTT) solution (5 mg/mL) (Sigma-Aldrich Co., St. Louis, MO, USA) was added to each well and the cells were cultured for another 4 h. The supernatant was removed and 100 μL of DMSO/well was added to dissolve the intracellular crystalline formazan product. Cell viability was determined by measuring the absorbance at 490 nm using a SpectraMax Plus 384 Microplate Reader (Molecular Devices, Sunnyvale, CA, USA).

4.3. Oil Red O Staining

The fat accumulation in the HepG2 cells was determined by Oil Red O staining using a commercial kit (Nanjing Jiancheng Bioengineering Institute, Nanjing, China). The cells were treated for 24 h with 0.8 mM FFA and various concentrations of PCBG (0.1, 1, and 10 μM), PCB, and MPG (1, 10, and 100 μM). Cells were rinsed with cold phosphate-buffered saline (PBS) (Hyclone, South Logan, UT, USA), then stained with fresh Oil Red O working solution for 20 min. Stained cells were washed with PBS prior to microscopic observation using a Nikon 80i upright microscope (Nikon, Tokyo, Japan). To quantify, 250 μL of DMSO was added to the dried plates, and the optical density was measured at 510 nm.

4.4. Biochemical Assay

HepG2 cells were seeded into six-well plates at 2×10^5 cells per well. After 24 h of incubation, the culture medium was removed and treated with 0.8 mM FFA and various concentrations of PCBG (0.1, 1, and 10 μM), PCB, and MPG (1, 10, and 100 μM). Cells were collected and made into a homogenate with PBS. The levels of TC, TG, ALT, AST, MDA, SOD, and GSH-Px were determined with commercial kits (Nanjing Jiancheng Bioengineering Institute, Nanjing, China) and normalized by protein content (mg/mL).

4.5. Western Blots Analysis

To detect the proteins of cells, cells (2×10^6) were plated into 100-mm dishes and incubated overnight, before being starved for 12 h in DMEM with 0.5% BSA and submitted to different treatments as described above. After each 24-h treatment, cells were collected and washed with PBS and lysed on ice in Radio-Immunoprecipitation Assay (RIPA) buffer with a protease and phosphatase inhibitor cocktail for 15 min. Cell lysates were centrifuged at 12,000 rpm for 10 min, before the supernatant was collected and the protein content of each lysate was measured using a bicinchoninic (BCA) protein assay kit (Beijing Biosynthesis Biotechnology Co., Ltd., Beijing, China). Proteins (20 μg/lane) were subjected to SDS-PAGE with 10% resolving gel. The separated proteins on gels were then transferred onto a polyvinylidene difluoride (PVDF) membrane (Merch/Millipore, Schwalbach, Germany). After blocking nonspecific binding with 5% fat-free milk or 2% BSA solution, the membranes were incubated with antibodies against SIRT1 (sc-74465), AMPK (sc-25792), p-AMPK (sc-33524), SREBP1c (sc-365513), PPARα (sc-130640), and glyceraldehyde 3-phosphate dehydrogenase (GAPDH; sc-32233)

(Santa Cruz, CA, USA) at 4 °C overnight. After being washed with Tris-buffered saline/Tween (TBST) four times, the membranes were incubated with horseradish peroxidase (HRP)-conjugated goat anti-rabbit immunoglobulin G (IgG) or rabbit anti-mouse IgG (Zhongshan Goldenbridge, Beijing, China) for 1 h at room temperature. The blots were incubated in Immobilon Western Chemiluminescent HRP Substrate and exposed to an X-film to form an image. The protein bands were quantitated using the Image J software. (Version 1.51k, National Institutes of Health, Bethesda, MD, USA)

4.6. Quantitative Real-Time Polymerase Chain Reaction (qRT-PCR)

HepG2 cells were plated at a density of 3×10^5 cells/well in a six-well plate and incubated overnight, before being starved for 12 h in DMEM with 0.5% BSA and used for different treatments as described above; one group was treated with QCT (10 μM) as a comparison. Total RNA from HepG2 cells was extracted using an RNAprep pure Cell/Bacteria Kit (Tiangen Biotech Co., Beijing, China). The purity and concentration of RNA were determined with a Genova Nano spectrophotometer (BIBBY JENWAY, Staffordshire, UK). Complementary DNA (cDNA) was synthesized with a FastQuant RT Kit (With gDNase) (Tiangen Biotech Co., Beijing, China) according to the manufacturer's protocols. The relative levels of mRNA to *GAPDH* were analyzed using an SYBR fast universal qPCR kit (KAPA Biosystems, MA, USA) and specific primers. The primer sequences are shown in Table 2. The qRT-PCR was performed on an ABI Quant 5 PCR system using the $2^{-\Delta\Delta Ct}$ method. *GAPDH* was used as the normalized reference gene.

Table 2. The Primers Used for qRT-PCR.

Gene Name	Forward Primer (5′–3′)	Reverse Primer (5′–3′)	Reference
SIRT1	GCCAGAGTCCAAGTTTAGAAGA	CCATCAGTCCCAAATCCAG	[52]
AMPK	CAGGCATATGGTGGTCCATAGAG	TCATGGGATCCACCTGCAGC	[18]
SREBP1c	ATACCACCAGCGTCTACC	CACCAACAGCCCATTGAG	[48]
PPARα	AGCAAGGAAGGGTTGTGGCAAA	ATGGACTCGGAAGCAGGAAGGT	[53]
FAS	CGGCTCGCCCACCT	CGGGCCGCAAAGC	[48]
ACC	GCTGCTCGGATCACTAGTGAA	TTCTGCTATCAGTCTGTCCAG	[54]
SCD1	CCTCTACTTGGAAGACGACATTCGC	GCAGCCGAGCTTTGTAAGAGCGGT	[54]
GAPDH	TGCACCACCAACTGCTTAGC	GGCATGGACTGTGGTCATGAG	[55]

4.7. Molecular Docking

The docking studies of PCB, PCBG, MPG, and reference compound, QCT, were performed with energy-metabolism-related molecular targets, including SIRT1 (Protein Data Bank identifier (PDB ID): 4ZZJ), AMPK (PDB ID: 4ZHX), PPARα (PDB ID: 3KDU), FAS (PDB ID: 5C37), ACC1 (PDB ID: 3TVU), and SCD1 (PDB ID: 4ZYO). The crystal structures were obtained from the Research Collaboratory for Structural Bioinformatics Protein Data Bank (RCSB PDB; http://www.rcsb.org), and were protonated and energy minimized using the AMBER FF99 force field [56]. The structures of compounds were drawn using ChemDraw Ultra 7.0 (CambridgeSoft, Perkin Elmer Inc., Waltham, MA, USA) and converted to three-dimensional (3D) structures with all proton and tripos force charges added to optimize the minimum energy conformation using SYBYL-X 1.2. The optimized conformation was used for the analysis of docking events with Surflex-Dock, which is a well-recognized method in the field of molecular docking. In this way, the virtual screening and ligand–receptor interaction were evaluated.

4.8. Statistics

Data were shown as mean ± standard deviation of at least three independent experiments. One-way ANOVA and a Student's *t*-test were used to evaluate statistical significance with the SPSS statistics 23.0 software. Values of $p < 0.05$ were considered as statistically significant.

Supplementary Materials: The following are available online at http://www.mdpi.com/1422-0067/19/9/2555/s1, Figure S1: Molecular interactions of PCB, PCBG, MPG, and QCT binding with SIRT1, AMPK, PPARα, FAS, ACC1 and SCD1.

Author Contributions: Data curation, Y.-Y.B. and N.Z. Formal analysis, X.-Q.C. Funding acquisition, X.W. Investigation, W.-W.G. and X.W. Project administration, X.W. Writing—original draft, W.-W.G. Writing—review and editing, R.R.X. and W.-W.Z.

Acknowledgments: This work was supported by the grants of National Natural Science Foundation of China (No. 81773999).

Conflicts of Interest: The authors declare no conflict of interest.

References

1. Younossi, Z.M.; Koenig, A.B.; Abdelatif, D.; Fazel, Y.; Henry, L.; Wymer, M. Global epidemiology of nonalcoholic fatty liver disease-Meta-analytic assessment of prevalence, incidence, and outcomes. *Hepatology* **2016**, *64*, 73–84. [CrossRef] [PubMed]
2. Fan, J.G.; Kim, S.U.; Wong, V.W. New trends on obesity and nafld in asia. *J. Hepatol.* **2017**, *67*, 862–873. [CrossRef] [PubMed]
3. Reccia, I.; Kumar, J.; Akladios, C.; Virdis, F.; Pai, M.; Habib, N.; Spalding, D. Non-alcoholic fatty liver disease: A sign of systemic disease. *Metabolism* **2017**, *72*, 94–108. [CrossRef] [PubMed]
4. Abenavoli, L. Non-alcoholic fatty liver disease: Today and tomorrow. *Rev. Recent Clin. Trials* **2014**, *9*, 125. [CrossRef] [PubMed]
5. Chalasani, N.; Younossi, Z.; Lavine, J.E.; Diehl, A.M.; Brunt, E.M.; Cusi, K.; Charlton, M.; Sanyal, A.J. The diagnosis and management of non-alcoholic fatty liver disease: Practice guideline by the American Gastroenterological Association, American Association for the Study of Liver Diseases, and American College of Gastroenterology. *Gastroenterology* **2012**, *142*, 1592–1609. [CrossRef] [PubMed]
6. Dyson, J.; Jaques, B.; Chattopadyhay, D.; Lochan, R.; Graham, J.; Das, D.; Aslam, T.; Patanwala, I.; Gaggar, S.; Cole, M.; et al. Hepatocellular cancer: The impact of obesity, type 2 diabetes and a multidisciplinary team. *J. Hepatol.* **2014**, *60*, 110–117. [CrossRef] [PubMed]
7. Musso, G.; Gambino, R.; Cassader, M.; Pagano, G. Meta-analysis: Natural history of non-alcoholic fatty liver disease (NAFLD) and diagnostic accuracy of non-invasive tests for liver disease severity. *Ann. Med.* **2011**, *43*, 617–649. [CrossRef] [PubMed]
8. Nascimbeni, F.; Pais, R.; Bellentani, S.; Day, C.P.; Ratziu, V.; Loria, P.; Lonardo, A. From NAFLD in clinical practice to answers from guidelines. *J. Hepatol.* **2013**, *59*, 859–871. [CrossRef] [PubMed]
9. Than, N.N.; Newsome, P.N. A concise review of non-alcoholic fatty liver disease. *Atherosclerosis* **2015**, *239*, 192–202. [CrossRef] [PubMed]
10. Stanković, M.N.; Mladenović, D.R.; Đuričić, I.; Šobajić, S.S.; Timić, J.; Jorgačević, B.; Aleksić, V.; Vučević, D.B.; Ješić-Vukićević, R.; Radosavljević, T.S. Time-dependent changes and association between liver free fatty acids, serum lipid profile and histological features in mice model of nonalcoholic fatty liver disease. *Arch. Med. Res.* **2014**, *45*, 116–124. [CrossRef] [PubMed]
11. Cantó, C.; Gerharthines, Z.; Feige, J.N.; Lagouge, M.; Noriega, L.; Milne, J.C.; Elliott, P.J.; Puigserver, P.; Auwerx, J. AMPK regulates energy expenditure by modulating NAD^+ metabolism and SIRT1 activity. *Nature* **2009**, *458*, 1056–1060. [CrossRef] [PubMed]
12. Lan, F.; Cacicedo, J.M.; Ruderman, N.; Ido, Y. SIRT1 modulation of the acetylation status, cytosolic localization, and activity of LKB1. Possible role in AMP-activated protein kinase activation. *J. Biol. Chem.* **2008**, *283*, 27628–27635. [CrossRef] [PubMed]
13. Lim, C.T.; Kola, B.; Korbonits, M. AMPK as a mediator of hormonal signalling. *J. Mol. Endocrinol.* **2010**, *44*, 87–97. [CrossRef] [PubMed]
14. You, M.; Matsumoto, M.; Pacold, C.M.; Cho, W.K.; Crabb, D.W. The role of AMP-activated protein kinase in the action of ethanol in the liver. *Gastroenterology* **2004**, *127*, 1798–1808. [CrossRef] [PubMed]
15. Zhou, G.; Myers, R.; Li, Y.; Chen, Y.; Shen, X.; Fenykmelody, J.; Wu, M.; Ventre, J.; Doebber, T.; Fujii, N.; et al. Role of AMP-activated protein kinase in mechanism of metformin action. *J. Clin. Investg.* **2001**, *108*, 1167–1174. [CrossRef] [PubMed]

16. Ferre, P.; Foufelle, F. Hepatic steatosis: A role for de novo lipogenesis and the transcription factor SREBP-1c. *Diabetes Obes. Metab.* **2010**, *12*, 83–92. [CrossRef] [PubMed]
17. Fortin, É.; Blouin, R.; Lapointe, J.; Petit, H.V.; Palin, M.F. Linoleic acid, α-linolenic acid and enterolactone affect lipid oxidation and expression of lipid metabolism and antioxidant-related genes in hepatic tissue of dairy cows. *Br. J. Nutr.* **2017**, *117*, 1199–1211. [CrossRef] [PubMed]
18. Kohjima, M.; Higuchi, N.; Kato, M.; Kotoh, K.; Yoshimoto, T.; Fujino, T.; Yada, M.; Yada, R.; Harada, N.; Enjoji, M.; et al. SREBP-1c, regulated by the insulin and AMPK signaling pathways, plays a role in nonalcoholic fatty liver disease. *Int. J. Mol. Med.* **2008**, *21*, 507–511. [CrossRef] [PubMed]
19. Chirala, S.S.; Jayakumar, A.; Gu, Z.W.; Wakil, S.J. Human fatty acid synthase: Role of interdomain in the formation of catalytically active synthase dimer. *Proc. Natl. Acad. Sci. USA* **2001**, *98*, 3104–3108. [CrossRef] [PubMed]
20. Huang, C.H.; Shiu, S.M.; Wu, M.T.; Chen, W.L.; Wang, S.G.; Lee, H.M. Monacolin K affects lipid metabolism through SIRT1/AMPK pathway in HepG2 cells. *Arch. Pharm. Res.* **2013**, *36*, 1541–1551. [CrossRef] [PubMed]
21. Wang, M.; Wu, X.; Jiang, Y.; Zhang, D.Y. The research progress of *Penthorum chinense* Pursh. *Food Drug* **2013**, *15*, 202–205.
22. Zeng, Q.H.; Zhang, X.W.; Xu, X.L.; Jiang, M.H.; Xu, K.P.; Piao, J.H.; Zhu, L.; Chen, J.; Jiang, J.G. Antioxidant and anticomplement functions of flavonoids extracted from *Penthorum chinense* Pursh. *Food Funct.* **2013**, *4*, 1811–1818. [CrossRef] [PubMed]
23. Xiao, L.P.; Song, Y.Y.; Zhou, Y.X.; Liu, J.L.; He, S.; Zhang, D.Y. Experiment research about resistant effects of *Penthorum chinense* on nonalcoholic fatty liver. *Chin. J. Exp. Tradit. Med. Form.* **2014**, *20*, 125–129.
24. Chen, X.R.; Yao, H.; Jiang, Y.; Wu, S.M.; Zhu, X.F.; Zhou, X.Q.; Cai, Y.M.; Zhou, Y.H.; Chen, J.J.; Wang, L.T. Evaluate of the therapeutic efficiency of the Chinese traditional medicine Gansu granule on chronic hepatitis B. *Chin. J. Hepatol.* **2004**, *12*, 50.
25. Xu, C.X.; Ni, X.Y. Clinic observation of treatment on NAFLD using Gansu granule with polyenophosphorylcholine. *J. Pract. Tradit. Chin. Med.* **2014**, *30*, 857.
26. Kapoor, S. Comment on isolation and identification of compounds from Penthorum chinense Pursh with antioxidant and antihepatocarcinoma properties: Pinocembrin and its rapidly emerging neuroprotective effects. *J. Agric. Food. Chem.* **2013**, *61*, 1416. [CrossRef] [PubMed]
27. Rasul, A.; Millimouno, F.M.; Ali, E.W.; Ali, M.; Li, J.; Li, X. Pinocembrin: A novel natural compound with versatile pharmacological and biological activities. *Biomed. Res. Int.* **2013**, *2013*, 379850. [CrossRef] [PubMed]
28. Wang, M.; Jiang, Y.; Liu, H.L.; Chen, X.Q.; Wu, X.; Zhang, D.Y. A new flavanone from the aerial parts of *Penthorum chinense*. *Nat. Prod. Res.* **2014**, *28*, 70–73. [CrossRef] [PubMed]
29. Guo, W.W.; Qiu, F.; Chen, X.Q.; Ba, Y.Y.; Wang, X.; Wu, X. In-vivo absorption of pinocembrin-7-*O*-*β*-D-glucoside in rats and its in-vitro biotransformation. *Sci. Rep.* **2016**, *6*, 29340. [CrossRef] [PubMed]
30. Kang, O.H.; Kim, S.B.; Seo, Y.S.; Joung, D.K.; Mun, S.H.; Choi, J.G.; Lee, Y.M.; Kang, D.G.; Lee, H.S. Kwon DY Curcumin decreases oleic acid-induced lipid accumulation via AMPK phosphorylation in hepatocarcinoma cells. *Eur. Rev. Med. Pharmacol. Sci.* **2013**, *17*, 2578–2586. [PubMed]
31. Li, Y.; Xu, S.; Mihaylova, M.; Zheng, B.; Hou, X.; Jiang, B.; Park, O.; Luo, Z.; Lefai, E.; Shyy, J.Y.J.; et al. AMPK Phosphorylates and Inhibits SREBP Activity to Attenuate Hepatic Steatosis and Atherosclerosis in Diet-Induced Insulin-Resistant Mice. *Cell Metab.* **2007**, *13*, 376–388. [CrossRef] [PubMed]
32. Sinclair, D.A.; Guarente, L. Unlocking the secrets of longevity genes. *Sci. Am.* **2006**, *294*, 48–51, 54–57. [CrossRef] [PubMed]
33. Pisonero-Vaquero, S.; González-Gallego, J.; Sánchez-Campos, S.; García-Mediavilla, M.V. Flavonoids and related compounds in non-alcoholic fatty liver disease therapy. *Curr. Med. Chem.* **2015**, *22*, 2991–3012. [CrossRef] [PubMed]
34. Guo, W.; Jiang, Y.; Chen, X.; Yu, P.; Wang, M.; Wu, X.; Zhang, D. Identification and quantitation of major phenolic compounds from *Penthorum chinense* Pursh. by HPLC with tandem mass spectrometry and HPLC with diode array detection. *J. Sep. Sci.* **2015**, *38*, 2789–2796. [CrossRef] [PubMed]
35. Kwan, H.Y.; Fong, W.F.; Yang, Z.; Yu, Z.L.; Hsiao, W.L. Inhibition of DNA-dependent protein kinase reduced palmitate and oleate-induced lipid accumulation in HepG2 cells. *Eur. J. Nutr.* **2013**, *52*, 1621–1630. [CrossRef] [PubMed]

36. Wang, H.; Chan, P.K.; Pan, S.Y.; Kwon, K.H.; Ye, Y.; Chu, J.H.; Fong, W.F.; Tsui, W.M.; Yu, Z.L. ERp57 is up-regulated in free fatty acids-induced steatotic L-02 cells and human nonalcoholic fatty livers. *J. Cell. Biochem.* **2010**, *110*, 1447–1456. [CrossRef] [PubMed]
37. Kawano, Y.; Cohen, D.E. Mechanisms of hepatic triglyceride accumulation in non-alcoholic fatty liver disease. *J. Gastroenterol.* **2013**, *48*, 434–441. [CrossRef] [PubMed]
38. Kasetti, R.B.; Rajasekhar, M.D.; Kondeti, V.K.; Fatima, S.S.; Swapna, S.; Ramesh, B.; Rao, C.A. Antihyperglycemic and antihyperlipidemic activities of methanol:water (4:1) fraction isolated from aqueous extract of Syzygium alternifolium seeds in streptozotocin induced diabetic rats. *Food Chem. Toxicol.* **2010**, *48*, 1078–1084. [CrossRef] [PubMed]
39. Ruskovska, T.; Bernlohr, D.A. Oxidative stress and protein carbonylation in adipose tissue-implications for insulin resistance and diabetes mellitus. *J. Proteomics* **2013**, *92*, 323–334. [CrossRef] [PubMed]
40. Keshari, A.K.; Kumar, G.; Kushwaha, P.S.; Bhardwaj, M.; Kumar, P.; Rawat, A.; Kumar, D.; Prakash, A.; Ghosh, B.; Saha, S. Isolated flavonoids from Ficus racemosa stem bark possess antidiabetic, hypolipidemic and protective effects in albino Wistar rats. *J. Ethnopharmacol.* **2016**, *181*, 252–262. [CrossRef] [PubMed]
41. Chen, W.L.; Kang, C.H.; Wang, S.G.; Lee, H.M. Alpha-Lipoic acid regulates lipid metabolism through induction of sirtuin 1 (SIRT1) and activation of AMP-activated protein kinase. *Diabetologia* **2012**, *55*, 1824–1835. [CrossRef] [PubMed]
42. Park, E.J.; Kim, Y.M.; Kim, H.J.; Jang, S.Y.; Oh, M.H.; Lee, D.H.; Chang, K.C. (S)YS-51, a novel isoquinoline alkaloid, attenuates obesity-associated non-alcoholic fatty liver disease in mice by suppressing lipogenesis, inflammation and coagulation. *Eur. J. Pharmacol.* **2016**, *788*, 200–209. [CrossRef] [PubMed]
43. Chau, M.D.; Gao, J.; Yang, Q.; Wu, Z.; Gromada, J. Fibroblast growth factor 21 regulates energy metabolism by activating the AMPK-SIRT1-PGC-1α pathway. *Proc. Natl. Acad. Sci. USA* **2010**, *107*, 12553–12558. [CrossRef] [PubMed]
44. Price, N.L.; Gomes, A.P.; Ling, A.J.; Duarte, F.V.; Martinmontalvo, A.; North, B.J.; Agarwal, B.; Ye, L.; Ramadori, G.; Teodoro, J.S.; et al. Sirt1 is required for ampk activation and the beneficial effects of resveratrol on mitochondrial function. *Cell Metab.* **2012**, *15*, 675–690. [CrossRef] [PubMed]
45. Lv, Q.; Zhen, Q.; Liu, L.; Gao, R.; Yang, S.; Zhou, H.; Goswami, R.; Li, Q. AMP-kinase pathway is involved in tumor necrosis factor alpha-induced lipid accumulation in human hepatoma cells. *Life Sci.* **2015**, *131*, 23–29. [CrossRef] [PubMed]
46. Scott, J.W.; Hawley, S.A.; Green, K.A.; Anis, M.; Stewart, G.; Scullion, G.A.; Norman, D.G.; Hardie, D.G. CBS domains form energy-sensing modules whose binding of adenosine ligands is disrupted by disease mutations. *J. Clin. Investig.* **2004**, *113*, 274–284. [CrossRef] [PubMed]
47. Quan, H.Y.; Kim, D.Y.; Kim, S.J.; Jo, H.K.; Kim, G.W.; Chung, S.H. Betulinic acid alleviates non-alcoholic fatty liver by inhibiting SREBP1 activity via the AMPK-mTOR-SREBP signaling pathway. *Biochem. Pharmacol.* **2013**, *85*, 1330–1340. [CrossRef] [PubMed]
48. Berger, J.P.; Akiyama, T.E.; Meinke, P.T. PPARs: Therapeutic targets for metabolic disease. *Trends Pharmacol. Sci.* **2005**, *26*, 244–251. [CrossRef] [PubMed]
49. Dong, J.; Zhang, X.; Zhang, L.; Bian, H.X.; Xu, N.; Bao, B.; Liu, J. Quercetin reduces obesity-associated ATM infiltration and inflammation in mice: A mechanism including AMPKalpha1/SIRT1. *J. Lipid Res.* **2014**, *55*, 363–374. [CrossRef] [PubMed]
50. Yin, J.; Luo, Y.; Deng, H.; Qin, S.; Tang, W.; Zeng, L.; Zhou, B. Hugan Qingzhi medication ameliorates hepatic steatosis by activating AMPK and PPARalpha pathways in L02 cells and HepG2 cells. *J. Ethnopharmacol.* **2014**, *154*, 229–239. [CrossRef] [PubMed]
51. Pan, Y.T.; Xu, F.Y.; Yu, X.Z.; Shang, W.B. Research progress on therapeutic targets of active components in Chinese herbs for treatment of nonalcoholic fatty liver disease. *China J. Chin. Mater. Med.* **2017**, *42*, 1109–1112.
52. Li, Z.; Feng, S.; Zhou, L.; Liu, S.; Cheng, J. NS5ATP6 modulates intracellular triglyceride content through FGF21 and independently of SIRT1 and SREBP1. *Biochem. Biophys. Res. Commun.* **2016**, *475*, 133–139. [CrossRef] [PubMed]
53. Zeng, L.; Tang, W.; Yin, J.; Feng, L.; Li, Y.; Yao, X.; Zhou, B. Alisol A 24-Acetate Prevents Hepatic Steatosis and Metabolic Disorders in HepG2 Cells. *Cell. Physiol. Biochem.* **2016**, *40*, 453–464. [CrossRef] [PubMed]
54. Jin, S.H.; Yang, J.H.; Shin, B.Y.; Seo, K.; Shin, S.M.; Cho, I.J.; Ki, S.H. Resveratrol inhibits LXRalpha-dependent hepatic lipogenesis through novel antioxidant Sestrin2 gene induction. *Toxicol. Appl. Pharmacol.* **2013**, *271*, 95–105. [CrossRef] [PubMed]

55. Wu, Z.S.; Wu, Q.; Wang, C.Q.; Wang, X.N.; Huang, J.; Zhao, J.J.; Mao, S.S.; Zhang, G.H.; Xu, X.C.; Zhang, N. miR-340 inhibition of breast cancer cell migration and invasion through targeting of oncoprotein c-Met. *Cancer* **2011**, *117*, 2842–2852. [CrossRef] [PubMed]
56. Spasic, A.; Serafini, J.; Mathews, D.H. The Amber ff99 Force Field Predicts Relative Free Energy Changes for RNA Helix Formation. *J. Chem. Theory. Comput.* **2012**, *8*, 2497–2505. [CrossRef] [PubMed]

International Journal of
Molecular Sciences

MDPI

Article

Prenylated Flavonoids from Roots of *Glycyrrhiza uralensis* Induce Differentiation of B16-F10 Melanoma Cells

Yunfeng Zheng [1], Huaiyou Wang [2,3], Min Yang [1], Guoping Peng [1], Tina Ting Xia Dong [2,3], Miranda Li Xu [2,3] and Karl Wah Keung Tsim [2,3,*]

1 School of Pharmacy, Nanjing University of Chinese Medicine, Nanjing 210023, China; zyunfeng88@126.com (Y.Z.); yangmingnj90@163.com (M.Y.); guopingpeng@sohu.com (G.P.)

2 Division of Life Science and Center for Chinese Medicine, The Hong Kong University of Science and Technology, Hong Kong 999077, China; hyw@ust.hk (H.W.); botina@ust.hk (T.T.X.D.); lxuae@connect.ust.hk (M.L.X.)

3 Shenzhen Key Laboratory of Edible and Medicinal Bioresources, The Hong Kong University of Science and Technology Shenzhen Research Institute, Hi-Tech Park, Shenzhen 518057, China

* Correspondence: botsim@ust.hk; Tel.: +86-852-2358-7332

Received: 12 July 2018; Accepted: 8 August 2018; Published: 16 August 2018

Abstract: Roots of *Glycyrrhiza uralensis* have been used as herbal medicine and natural sweetener. By activity-guided phytochemical investigation of the extracts from *G. uralensis* root, ten flavonoids, namely GF-1–GF-10, of which five were prenylated flavonoids, were found to show antiproliferative effects in melanoma B16-F10 cells. Three of the prenylated flavonoids, namely GF-1, GF-4 and GF-9, significantly induced the differentiation of B16-F10 cells; the inductions included increase of tyrosinase activity, tyrosinase protein, and melanin content. In GF-1 and GF-9 induced melanoma differentiation, the phosphorylation of p38 MAPK (mitogen activated potein kinase) was identified; while GF-4 could trigger the phosphorylation of PI3K/AKT (phosphatidylinositol 3-kinase/Protein Kinase B) signaling. However, application of GF-6 to the melanoma cells did not induce differentiation; but which promoted cell apoptotic signaling, i.e., increase levels of cleaved-PRAP, cleaved-caspase 3, and cleaved-caspase 9. These results suggested that different types of prenylated flavonoids from *G. uralensis* might have potential anticancer effects against melanoma cells by acting through different signaling pathways.

Keywords: *Glycyrrhiza uralensis*; prenylated flavonoids; antiproliferation; differentiation; melanoma cell

1. Introduction

The roots of *Glycyrrhiza uralensis* Fisch (GlycyrrhizaeUralensis Radix; GUR), named as licorice or gancao, have been extensively used as a herbal drug in both Eastern and Western countries [1]. Clinical studies have shown GUR is highly effective in the treatment of respiratory, gastrointestinal, cardiovascular and genitourinary conditions [2]. According to traditional Chinese medicine (TCM) theory, GUR is described as a beneficial herb to enhance therapeutic effects; meanwhile, this herb is being employed commonly to detoxify potential adverse effects in many herbal mixtures during clinical application. Phytochemical studies revealed that triterpene saponins and flavonoid glycosides were two major active substances in GUR [3]. In the extractive of GUR, the nonpolar fraction of GUR is rich in various types of prenylated flavonoids, e.g., flavones, isoflavones, flavanones, chalcones, and coumestans [4]. These flavonoids are being considered to be active ingredients of GUR, and indeed which have been commonly used in food industries. In recent pharmacological studies, GUR flavonoids have been proposed to have anti-oxidation [5], anti-inflammatory [6], antiproliferative, and cytotoxic effects in various cells [7]. Despite the aforementioned proposed actions, the roles of GUR prenylated flavonoids in cancer cells have not been extensively investigated.

Malignant melanoma is a highly aggressive and invasive skin cancer with high metastatic potential and extraordinary resistance to cytotoxic agents [8]. The occurrence of melanoma is related to different factors, e.g., sun exposure, fair pigmentation, and genetic mutation [9]. In recent years, the incidence of melanoma is rapidly increasing throughout the world, especially in America and Europe [10]. Although drug therapy for this cancer has been developed rapidly, e.g., immunotherapies with PD-1 inhibition drugs (ipilimumab and nivolumab) and T-cell checkpoint blockade therapies [11,12], the usage of herbal products is still one of the alternative approaches for melanoma cancer treatment.

Considering the pathogenesis and clinical treatment of melanoma, the recent targets in cancer therapy is focusing on discovery of natural products that are able to suppress cancer cell proliferation and promote cell differentiation [13,14]. Here, the CH_2Cl_2 extract of GUR (GUR_{CH2Cl2}) was shown to exhibited potent effect in antiproliferation and inducing differentiation of cultured melanoma B16-F10 cells: these effects were significant higher than that deriving from water extract (GUR_{water}) and ethanol extract of GUR (GUR_{EtOH}). To explore the possible underlying mechanism for anticancer effect of GUR, ten flavonoids (GF1-GF10) of which five were prenylated flavonoids, were isolated. The roles of these flavonoids in inducing the differentiation of cultures B16-F10 cells were illustrated, and subsequently the signaling cascades, triggered by various flavonoids, were revealed and compared.

2. Results

2.1. *G. uralensis* Extracts in Proliferation and Differentiation of Melanoma Cells

Different extractives of GUR, i.e., GU_{water}, GU_{EtOH}, and GU_{CH2Cl2}, were subjected to HPLC analyses. As shown in HPLC chromatograms (Figure 1A), saponins and flavonoid glycosides were the major constituents in both GU_{water} (water extract) and GU_{EtOH} (ethanol extract). Besides, a small amount of free flavonoids could be detected in GU_{EtOH}. In comparison with GU_{water} and GU_{EtOH}, GU_{CH2Cl2} (dichloromethane extract) exhibited a comparable enrichment of free flavonoids. To a certain extent, difference in chemicals might cause possible difference in their biological capacities.

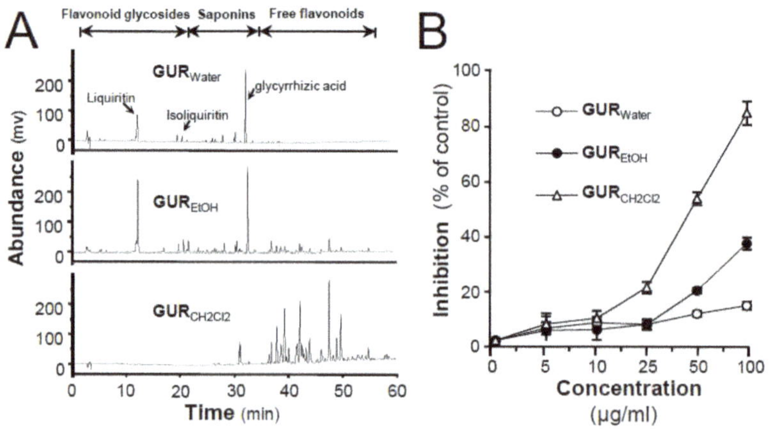

Figure 1. *Cont.*

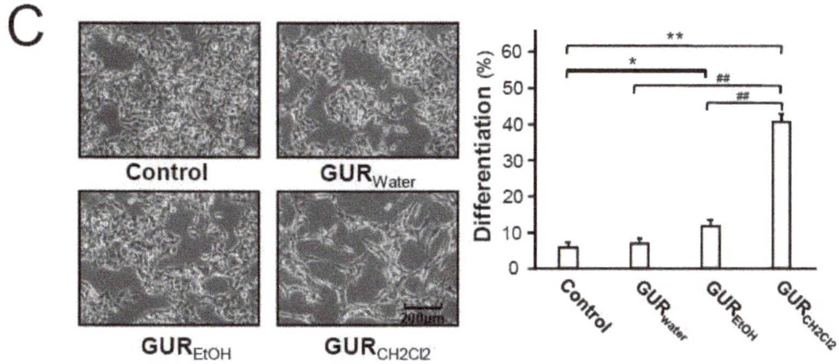

Figure 1. Effects of different extracts of *G. uralensis* root in antiproliferation and differentiation-inducing activities in B16-F10 cells. (**A**) HPLC chromatograms of different extracts, all at 1 mg/mL, from GUR, i.e., GU_{water} (water extract of GUR), GU_{EtOH} (EtOH extract of GUR), and GU_{CH2Cl2} (CH_2Cl_2 extract of GUR). (**B**) Melanoma B16-F10 cells were treated with different extracts of GUR or with medium of 0.1% DMSO (dimethylsulphoxide) for 48 h, after which cells were counted under MTT (3-(4,5-dimethyl-2-thiazolyl)-2,5-diphenyl-2-H-tetrazolium bromide) assay. (**C**) Melanoma B16-F10 cells were treated with GU_{water}, GU_{EtOH}, and GU_{CH2Cl2} (50 μg/mL, respectively) for 48 h (left panel). At least 150 cells were counted for cells with dendrite longer than 3× cellular body, as differentiated cells (right panel). Data are expressed as percentage of control, in means ± SEM of 3 independent experiments. * $p < 0.05$, ** $p < 0.01$, compared with control; ## $p < 0.01$, compared with other extracts.

To investigate the effect of *G. uralensis* extracts, cultured B16-F10 melanoma cells were treated with different extracts at indicated concentrations for 48 h. As shown in Figure 1B, GU_{CH2Cl2} inhibited the proliferation of B16-F10 cells with an IC_{50} value of 48.7 ± 2.5 μg/mL, whereas GU_{water} and GU_{EtOH} exhibited little effects (IC_{50} > 100 μg/mL). In addition to the differentiation induction, as shown in Figure 1C, the GU_{CH2Cl2}-treated (50 μg/mL) cells showed typical dendrite-like cellular protrusions, as compared with control cells. Although GU_{EtOH} had a certain degree of differentiation-inducing activity, as compared with the control group, its effect was far lower than that of GU_{CH2Cl2}. Over 40% cells were induced to differentiate under the treatment of GU_{CH2Cl2} (Figure 1C). Similar to antiproliferative activity, GU_{water} showed little morphological changes towards cultured B16-F10 cells. These results suggested that free flavonoid content in the extract could be responsible for differentiation and antiproliferation of B16-F10 cells.

2.2. Structure Identification of Isolated Compounds

To explore active compounds in GUR extracts corresponding for activitieson cell differentiation, phytochemical investigation of GU_{CH2Cl2} was performed, and there after 10 compounds were isolated. Their structures and types were elucidated on the basic of ESI-Q-TOF/MS and ^{1}H and ^{13}C NMR and by comparison with the literatures. The ^{13}C NMR data were presented in Table 1, and the MS and ^{1}H NMR data of each compound were available in the supplementary information.

As shown in Figure 2, all isolated compounds were identified as free flavonoids, including three isoflavones, three flavones, two chalcones, one coumarin, and one flavanone, namely GF-1–GF-10. Compounds GF-1, 2, and 5 were isoflavones, identified as licoisoflavone B, glabrone, and formononetin, respectively. Compounds GF-3, 9, and 10 were classified as flavones and elucidated successively as 7, 4′-dihydroxyflavone, licoflavone, and kumatakenin A, respectively. With the data of NMR and MS, two chalcones, GF-6 and GF-8 were established as licochalcone A and isoliquiritigenin, respectively. GF-4 was identified as a coumarin namely as neoglycyrol, which could be regarded as an isoflavone derivative with methoxyl, hydroxyl, and prenyl groups. GF-7 was identified as a common flavanone, namely as liquiritigenin. The HPLC of isolated flavonoids and dichloromethane extract of *G. uralensis* were available in the supplementary information. The purities of these ten flavonoids were tested to be higher than 95% by HPLC-UV area normalization method.

Table 1. Table of ^{13}C NMR Spectroscopic data of 10 flavonoid compounds in DMSO-d6.

	GF-1	GF-2	GF-3	GF-4	GF-5	GF-6	GF-7	GF-8	GF-9	GF-10
C-1						113.5		125.7		
C-2	155.7	155.1	162.5	157.9	153.0	158.2	78.9	131.1	162.2	155.8
C-3	120.5	122.1	104.4	102.7	124.2	99.9	43.1	115.8	104.4	137.7
C-4	180.6	176.0	176.2	158.6	174.5	159.6	190.0	160.3	176.2	178.0
C-4a	104.6	116.2	16.1	100.2	127.2		113.5		115.8	105.1
C-5	161.8	127.2	126.4	154.3	116.6	126.5	128.3	115.8	124.5	160.9
C-6	98.8	115.3	114.7	120.1	115.0	127.7	110.5	131.1	127.2	97.6
C-7	164.1	162.8	160.6	160.0	162.5		164.6		160.3	165.0
C-8	93.6	102.0	102.4	99.7	102.0		102.5		101.7	92.2
C-8a	157.7	157.5	157.3	153.4	158.9		163.1		155.6	160.2
C-α						117.8		144.2		
C-β						138.7		117.4		
C-γ						187.3		191.5		
C-1′	111.2	112.7	121.7	114.7	123.1	129.6	129.3	112.9	121.9	120.4
C-2′	151.2	151.3	128.0	156.6	130.0	130.6	128.2	165.8	127.9	130.1
C-3′	109.7	110.1	115.8	99.0	113.5	115.2	115.1	102.5	115.8	115.6
C-4′	153.6	153.5	162.4	157.4	157.4	161.6	157.6	165.4	160.5	156.2
C-5′	107.4	107.6	115.8	114.5	113.5	115.2	115.1	108.0	115.8	115.6
C-6′	131.3	130.9	128.0	120.9	130.0	130.6	128.2	132.7	127.9	130.1
C-1″				22.5		39.5			27.5	
C-2″	75.4	75.4		122.9		147.5			121.8	
C-3″	128.8	128.8		131.4		109.9			132.3	
C-4″	116.9	117.0		18.2		26.9			25.5	
C-5″	27.4	27.5		25.9		26.9			17.6	
C-6″	27.4	27.5								
2-OCH_3						55.4				
3-OCH_3										56.0
4′-OCH_3					55.1					
5-OCH_3				62.8						
7-OCH_3										59.6

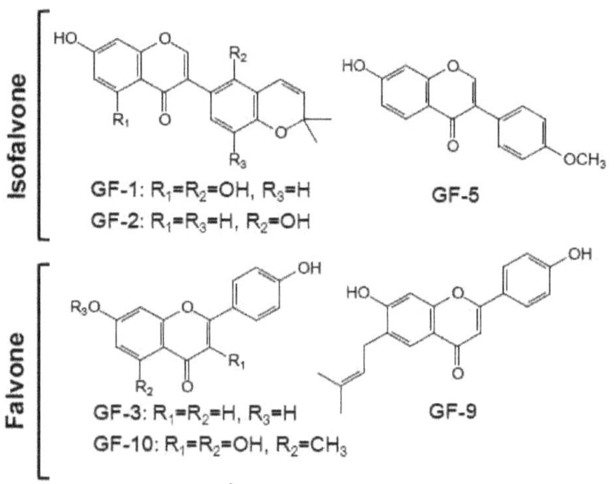

Figure 2. *Cont.*

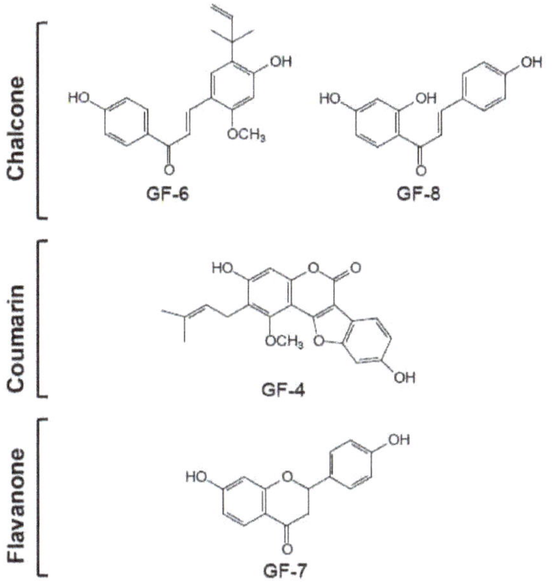

Figure 2. Structures of flavonoids isolated from CH_2Cl_2 extract of *G. uralensis* root.

In recent years, flavonoids, especially the prenylated ones, have attracted extensive attention because of its resulting radicals can enhance their biological activities [15]. In this study, several flavonoids, including GF-1, 2, 4, 6, and 9, were found to contain a substituent of prenyl moiety or dimethylpyran (formation from prenyl) in their structures.

2.3. Isolated Flavonoidsin Proliferation and Differentiation of Melanoma Cells

The isolated flavonoids were tested for their antiproliferative capacity using MTT bioassay on cultured B16-F10 cells (Figure 3A). In cell inhibition, the most active component was GF-4 (neoglycyrol), with an IC_{50} of 17.5 μM, while compounds GF-1, 2, 6, and 9 showed good activities in the range of 26.0–35.8 μM. The other nonprenyl flavonoids, GF-3, 5, 7, 8, and 10, possessed low activities of cell inhibition. Thus, the prenyl could be an important group for inhibition activity of licorice flavonoids in cancer cell growth.

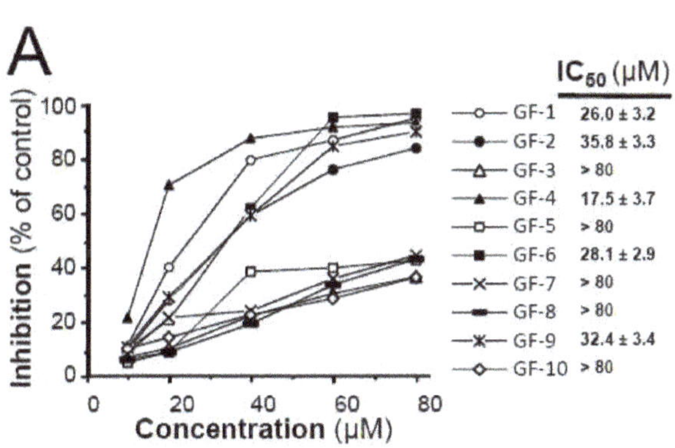

Figure 3. *Cont.*

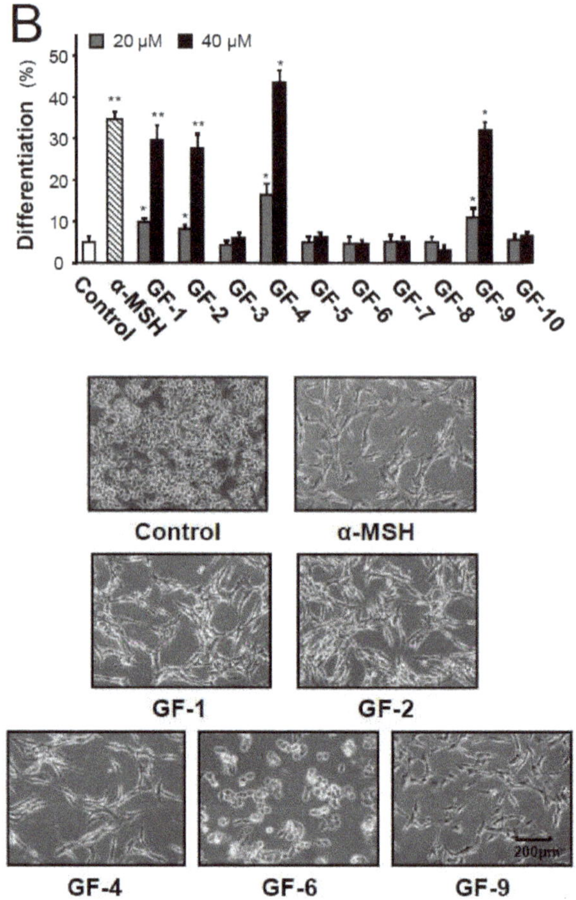

Figure 3. Antiproliferation and differentiation activity of *G. uralensis* flavonoids on B16-F10 cells. (**A**) Melanoma B16-F10 cells were treated with 10 flavonoids (GF-1–GF-10) at different concentrations or with medium (0.1% DMSO) for 48 h, after which the cells were assayed under MTT assay. IC_{50} value was calculated using SPSS statistics software. (**B**) Melanoma B16-F10 cells were treated with 10 flavonoids (GF-1–GF-10) at 20 or 40 μM, positive drug (α-MSH) at 20 nM or medium (0.1% DMSO) for 48 h. At least 150 cells were counted for dendrite longer than 3× cell body, as differentiated cell (upper panel). Data are expressed as percentage of control, as means ± SEM (n = 3) * $p < 0.05$, ** $p < 0.01$, compared with control. Morphological of B16-F10 cells treated with selected flavonoids at 40 μM (lower panel).

In order to evaluate the differentiating effect of isolated flavonoids, cultured B16-F10 cells were treated with α-MSH (positive drug) or these compounds at two concentrations for 48 h. Accordingly, typical dendrite-like cellular protrusions of cells, induced by GF-1, 2, 4, and 9, were similar with those induced by 20 nM α-melanocyte-stimulating hormone(α-MSH) (Figure 3B) [16]. Surprisingly, GF-6 had no such phenotype induction regardless of its role in cell inhibition (Figure 3B). After comparison of structures of above compounds, the opening of central C-ring in GF-6 could be a possible domain in inducing differentiation in cultured B16-F10 cells.

2.4. Isolated Flavonoids in Melanogenesis

Melanoma cell differentiation is generally accepted to be related to inhibition of cell proliferation, dendritic-like morphology, increased tyrosinase activity, and melanin production [17]. To validate the implications of morphological observations, the amounts of intracellular melanin content, tyrosinase activity and protein were evaluated in B16-F10 cells with the treatment of α-MSH or selected prenylated flavonoids, i.e., GF-1, 4, 6, and 9. The application of α-MSH (positive drug) at 20nM, GF-1, 4, and 9 at 40 μM significantly increased the melanin amounts by about 2-fold, as compared to the control (Figure 4A). However, GF-6 showed no effect. Except for GF-6, the prenylated flavoniods could induce tyrosinase activity in a dose-dependent manner in cultured B16-F10 cells (Figure 4A). The level of tyrosinase protein in the melanoma cells was measured by Western blot analysis. The expression of tyrosinase protein was enhanced to about 2-fold in GF-1, 4, and 9 treated cells (Figure 4B), demonstrating that the melanogenesis promotion was partly mediated by increased tyrosinase in melanoma cells.

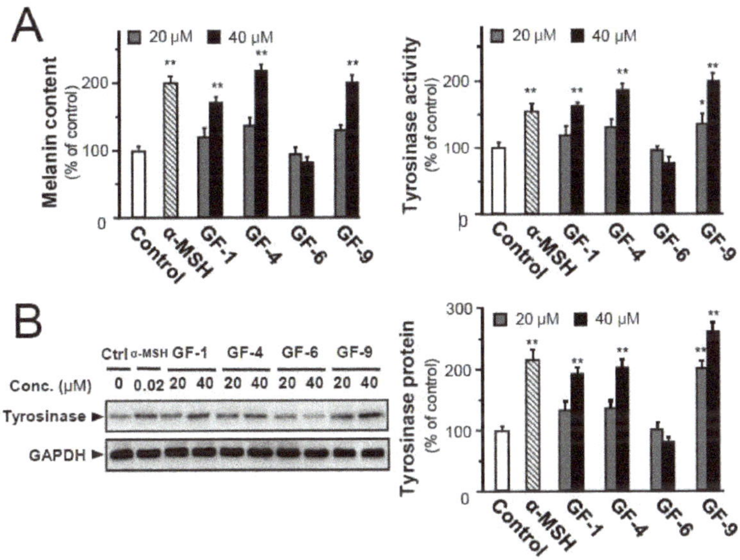

Figure 4. The *G. uralensis* flavonoids induce the amounts of melanin content, tyrosinase activity, and tyrosinase expression of B16-F10 melanoma cells. (**A**) B16-F10 cells were treated with indicated concentrations of selected flavonoids (GF-1, 4, 6, and 9) or with α-MSH at 20 nM for 48 h. The amounts of melanin (left panel) and tyrosinase activity (right panel) were determined. (**B**) The level of tyrosinase protein (~91 kDa) in the melanoma cells was measured by Western blot (left panel). The amount of tyrosinase was qualified against GAPDH (~37 kDa) (right panel). Data are expressed as percentage of control, in means ± SEM (n = 3). * $p < 0.05$, ** $p < 0.01$, compared with control.

To explore potential mechanism of the four prenylated flavonoids (GF-1, 4, 6, and 9) on antiproliferation and differentiation-inducing activities in B16 cells, the activations of MAPKs (ERK 1/2, JNK, and p38), AKT (Protein Kinase B), and PARP (poly ADP-ribose polymerase) signaling pathwayswere probed in the treated B16-F10 cells. These signaling pathways have been identified as important regulators of cell proliferation, differentiation, and tumor development of the malignant phenotype of tumor [18]. The levels of phospho-ERK1/2 (p-ERK1/2) and phospho-JNK (p-JNK) remained unchanged after treatment with the four prenylated flavonoids (Figure 5). However, the level of phospho-p38 (p-p38) was significantly induced by treatment of GF-1 and GF-9, with ~16- and ~13-fold of increase, in respect to the control. In the phosphorylation of p-AKT, only GF-4 showed a reduction (Figure 5). In the cultures, GF-6 showed cell inhibition, but not in cell differentiation, and did not cause phosphorylation of p-ERK1/2, p-JNK, p38, and p-AKT. In contrast, GF-6 application in B16-F10 cells induced the phosphorylation of Cl-PRAP by ~30-fold (Figure 5). Thus, the four tested prenylated flavonoids showed distinction in inducing the signaling cascades, i.e., p-ERK1/2 and p-JNK triggered by GF-1 and GF-9, p-AKT triggered by GF-4, and Cl-PARP triggered by GF-9.

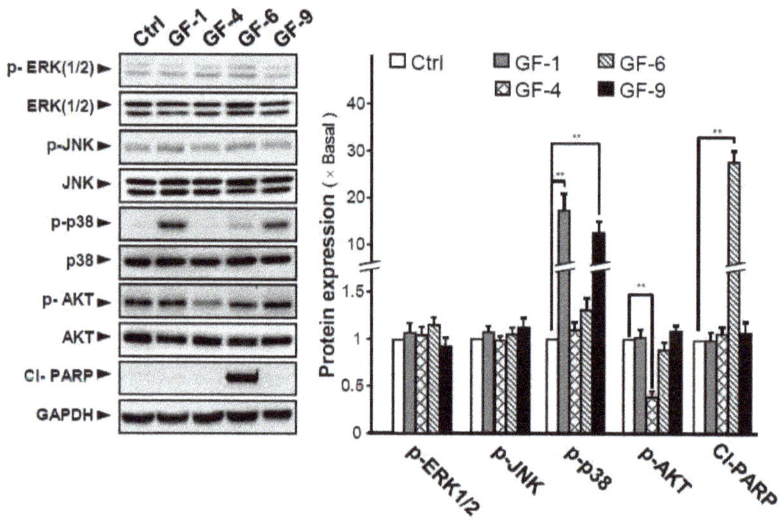

Figure 5. The *G. uralensis* flavoniods induce signaling of ERK (1/2), JNK, p38, AKT, and PARP. B16-F10 cells were treated with selected flavonoids (GF-1, 4, 6,and 9) at concentration of 40 μM or with medium (0.1% DMSO) for 48 h. Cell lysates were analyzed by Western blotting with the indicated antibodies (left panel). Photographs of the chemiluminescent detection of the blots, which were representative of three independent experiments, are shown (right panel). The relative abundance of each band to their own GAPDH was quantified, and the control levels were set at 1.0. Data are expressed as percentage of control, in means ± SEM (n = 3). ** $p < 0.01$, compared with control.

The phosphorylation of p38 could lead to activation of cAMP response element binding protein (CREB) and induction of microphthalmia associated transcription factor (MITF) expression [19]. MITF is a known downstream effector that is required for melanoblast survival, as well as a key regulator to induce genes associated with the differentiation, e.g., tyrosinase [20]. Here, GF-1 and GF-9 markedly increased the phosphorylations of p-p38 and p-CREB, as well as promoting the expression of MITF in dose-dependent manners (Figure 6A).

The PI3K/AKT signaling pathway is another crucial pathway involved in melanoma cell differentiation. Application of GF-4 down-regulated the phosphorylation of p-AKT and PI3K in cultured B16-F10 cells, and this suppression was in a dose-dependent manner (Figure 6B). Glycogen synthase kinase 3 β, a direct downstream target of AKT, phosphorylates MITF and regulates expression of tyrosinase [21]. Therefore, the protein expression of MITF was determined under the treatment of GF-4 in cultured B16-F10 cells. As expected, the level of MITF was induced by 50% after the treatment of GF-4 (Figure 6B). The GF-6-induced Cl-PRAP expression suggested that apoptosis could be involved in the inhibition of B16-F10 cells, triggered by GF-6. In line with an increase of Cl-PRAP, the levels of cleaved caspase-3 and cleaved caspase-9 were markedly induced by treatment of GF-6: the maximal induction over 5-fold and 15-fold could be revealed in cleaved caspase-3 and cleaved caspase-9, respectively (Figure 6C). The increase of apoptotic biomarkers strongly suggested the possible anticancer function of GF-6.

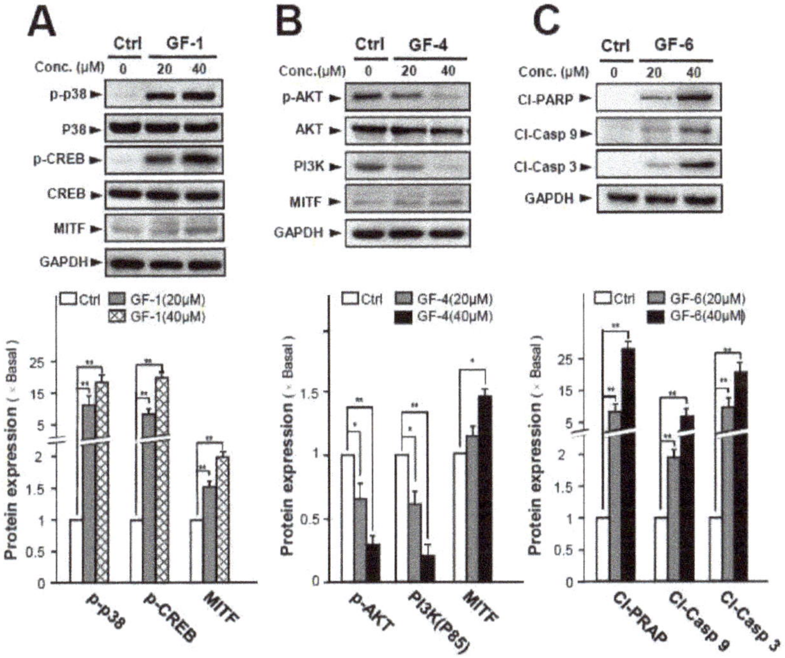

Figure 6. *G. uralensis* flavonoids induce differentiation or apoptosis via different signaling pathways in B16-F10 cells. B16-F10 cells were treated with various concentrations of selected flavonoids at concentration of 20 and 40 μM for 48 h, after which protein expression in total cells were assayed by Western blot analysis. (**A**) GF-1 and GF-9 induced phosphorylations of p 38 (~38 kDa) and p-CREB (~43 kDa), as well as expression of and MITF (~60 kDa). (**B**) GF-4 induced protein expression of p-AKT (~60 kDa), PI3K(~85 kDa), and MITF (~60 kDa). (**C**) GF-6 induced expression of Cl-PARP(~89 kDa), Cl-Casp 9(~37 kDa), and Cl-Casp 3(~19 kDa). The relative abundance of each band to their own GAPDH was quantified, and the control levels were set at 1.0 (lower panel). Data are expressed as percentage of control, in means ± SEM (n = 3).* $p < 0.05$, ** $p < 0.01$, compared with control.

3. Discussion

It has been estimated that 30–40% of cancers can be prevented by dietary or lifestyle condition [22]. Some anticancer drugs currently used in clinics, such as paclitaxel and camptothecin, are derived from natural products. Thus, the search for natural products having anticancer activity represents an interesting area, probably due to its diversity and distinct action mechanism. Flavonoids, commonly found in foods or herbal medicines, are a group of compounds with potential antitumor activities. According to their variations of backbone and substitution, flavonoids can be classified into different subclasses, providing an extremely diverse range of derivatives. Among them, prenylated flavonoids have attracted considerable attention due to their promising and diverse bioactivities [15]. For example, the prenylated substituted chalcones were shown to be cytotoxic in MCF-7, HT-29, and A-2780 cancer cells, whereas the conversion of a chalcone to a favanone resulted in reduced antiproliferative activity [23]. In addition, a prenylated flavonoid, artonol A, exhibited cytotoxic activity against human lung cancer cells [24]. Thus, the substitution in flavonoid structure might possess a profound influence on their antiproliferative effect on cancer cells. As shown here, the proliferation of B16-F10 cells could be significantly inhibited by CH_2Cl_2 extract of GUR. From this extract, ten flavonoids were isolated, of which five flavonoids with a prenylated group, i.e., GF-1, 2, 4, 6, and 9, displayed effectively cytotoxic activity: these results suggested that the prenyl group could be an indispensable moiety for licorice flavonoids to inhibit B16-F10 cell growth. Considering the structure-activity relationship, the free isoprene flavonoids, e.g., deprenylated compound of GF-9 and kumatakenin B, are showing low antiproliferative effect on B16-F10 cells.

The differentiation process represents a crucial point in progression of many types of cancer. A potential cancer treatment is to promote cancer cell differentiation, and thereafter, to reduce its proliferative capacity: this approach is a novel therapeutic method aiming to modify tumor cells to a slower rate of proliferation, and thus which leads to the loss of its earlier neoplastic attributes [25,26]. In melanoma, the differentiation status of cells could be monitored by melanogenesis, which resulted in the conversion of L-tyrosine to L-dopa by tyrosinase [27]. Indeed, the levels of melanin and tyrosinase are being considered as indicators of differentiated melanoma cells. Our current results supported the contrary action of differentiation against proliferation in melanoma. Here, we have shown the prenylated flavonoids GF-1, 4, and 9 inhibited B16-F10 cell growth, and subsequently which induced cell differentiation. The differentiation, induced by the prenylated flavonoids, was illustrated by morphological change and increase of melanin and tyrosinase. Having a distinction here, GF-6 (licochalcone A) showed inhibitory effect only on cell growth but not differentiation. The GF-6-inhibited cell growth was revealed to be mediated by its apoptotic role. In line to this observation, licochalcone A was shown to activate apoptotic processes in both in vitro and in vivo [28]. Thus, different backbone structure of flavonoids, as revealed here for *G.uralensis* flavonoids, might have distinct mechanisms to inhibit growth of tumor cells.

Numerous studies have shown that the MAPKs and AKT signaling pathways could play role in survival, proliferation, and differentiation of melanoma [18]. The MAPKs include three well characterized sub-families, i.e., extra cellular signal-regulated kinases -1/2(ERK 1/2), c-jun N-terminal or stress-activated protein kinases (JNK), and p38 mitogen activated protein kinase (p38 MAPK). The activations of ERK (1/2) and JNK were shown to relate with suppression of melanogenesis [20]. Activation of p38 MAPK signaling could upregulate melanin synthesis and induce differentiation by promoting expressions of MITF and tyrosinase [19]. In addition, the activation of AKT could inhibit melanogenesis and differentiation of melanoma [29]. These different lines of evidence support the antiproliferation and differentiation-inducing effects of natural products on melanoma, and the regulation of MAPKs and AKT signaling could be one of key mediators. For example, 5, 7-dimethoxycoumarin, from *Citrus limon* L., showed potential antigrowth and differentiation-inducing effect on melanoma cell, involving Ras/Raf/MEK/ERK pathway [30]. Lupeol, a lupine-type triterpene from Danelion root, showed significant inhibition on melanoma cell growth both in vitro and in vivo: the effect was trigged by its induction on cell differentiation [31]. Ye [27] reported that three sesquiterpenes, isolated from the largehead atractylode rhizome, induced melanoma cell differentiation and inhibited cell migration through inactivating the signals of Ras/ERK MAPK (for AT-I and AT-II) and PI3K/AKT. Here, we isolated and identified several prenylated flavonoids including isoflavone, flavone, chalcone, and coumarin. Interestingly, prenylatedflavone (GF-1) and prenylatedisoflavone (GF-9) could induce activation of p38 MAPK pathway, while prenylated coumarin (GF-4) showed inhibition on PI3K/AKT signaling. The prenylated chalcone GF-6 did not affect cell differentiation, but which induced melanoma cell apoptosis with activation of proteins in caspase-mediated signaling pathway. This result was in good agreement with recent literature [32]. However, a more detailed mechanism by which the prenylated flavonoids in melanoma cell differentiation and cell proliferation are waiting for further elucidation.

4. Material and Methods

4.1. Plant Material

The roots of *G. uralensis* (GUR) were collected in Minqin County, Gansu province, China in September 2016. Voucher specimen (No. 20160919) was stored in a dry and dark room and deposited at Jiangsu Collaborative Innovation Center of Chinese Medicinal Resources Industrialization (Nanjing

University of Chinese Medicine). The authentication of GUR was carried out by Prof. Qinan Wu from Nanjing University of Chinese Medicine, Nanjing, China.

4.2. Extraction and Isolation

4.2.1. Phytochemical Extractions of *G. uralensis* Roots

The water extract of GUR (GUR_{water}) was prepared by boiling GUR crude materials (100 g of fine powder) with water (1000 mL, 1 h) at 100 °C, extracted twice. Likewise, 100 g GUR powder was extracted with ethanol (1000 mL, 1 h) at 80 °C, extracted twice to obtain the ethanol extract (GU_{EtOH}). To prepare GUR dichloromethane extract (GUR_{CH2Cl2}), 100 g of GUR powder was boiled at 50 °C (1000 mL, 1 h) with CH_2Cl_2, extracted twice. The fractions were concentrated in vacuumand then freeze-dried to obtain loose fine powder.

HPLC chromatograms of different GUR extracts (GUR_{water}, GUR_{EtOH}, and GUR_{CH2Cl2}) were carried out using an Agilent 1100 HPLC system (Agilent Technologies, Santa Clara, CA, USA). An Agilent RP C_{18} column (250 × 4.6 mm id, 5 μm) was used. Samples were separated using a gradient mobile phase consisting of 0.2% (*v*/*v*) formic acid water (A) and acetonitrile (B). The gradient conditions were: 18–25% B at 0–10 min, 25–45% B at 10–30 min, 45–70% B at 30–45 min, and 70% B at 45–60 min. The flow rate was set at 1.0 mL/min. The detection wavelength was 254 nm. The sample concentration was 1 mg/mL, and injection volume was 10 μL.

4.2.2. Isolation and Identification of Flavonoids

GUR (dry weight, 5 kg) were exhaustively extracted two times with dichloromethane (30 L × 2, each extraction for 1 h). The extractives were combined and concentrated in vacuo. The residue (a total of about 105 g) was then separated to three fractions (Fr. A–C) by normal-phase silica gel CC (800 g, 200–300 mesh Silica) using a step-wise gradient elution of CH_2Cl_2-MeOH (100:0–80:20, *v*/*v*).Fr. A (about 6.5g) applied to middle pressure liquid chromatography (MPLC, BUCHI Chromatography B-688, Switzerland) on ODS column with a gradient solution of MeOH-H_2O (60:40–70:30, *v*/*v*) as elution to give GF-1 (43 mg) and GF-2 (18 mg). Fr. B (about 31.6 g) was subjected to MPLC silica gel using a stepwise gradient elution of CH_2Cl_2-MeOH (95:5–90:10, *v*/*v*) to provide the two sub-fractions Fr. B1 and Fr. B2. Fr. B1 was subsequently purified by MPLC chromatography over RP-18 silica gel column (400 g, 25–50 μm, 4.5 × 50 cm) eluted with MeOH-H_2O (70:30) to afford GF-3 (55 mg), GF-4 (102 mg) and GF-5 (31 mg). Fr. B2 was subjected to MPLC with a ODS column (400 g, 25–50 μm, 4.5×50 cm) to give GF-6 (26 mg) and GF-7 (34 mg). Fr. C (about 9.4 g) was applied to MPLC chromatography on ODS column with a gradient solution of MeOH-H_2O (60:40–70:30, *v*/*v*) as elution to afford GF-8 (23 mg), GF-9 (42 mg), and GF-10 (67 mg). The purified compounds were characterized by LC-MS and NMR analyses. The MS spectra were recorded on an Agilent 1200 HPLC/Q-TOF mass spectrometer instrument (Agilent) in positive ion mode. The specimens were dissolved in DMSO-d_6 (dimethylsulphoxide), and ^1H NMR and ^{13}C NMR were assayed with ASR-500 or ASR-300 NMR spectrometer, nuclear magnetic resonance, TMS was used as an internal standard.

4.3. Cell Culture

The melanoma B16-F10 cell line was obtained from American Type Culture Collection (ATCC, Manassas, Virginia, VA, USA). The cells were maintained in Dulbecco's modified Eagle's medium containing 10% fetal bovine serum, 100 units/mL penicillin and 100 μg/mL streptomycin in a humidified CO_2 (5%) incubator at 37 °C. All reagents for cell cultures were purchased from Invitrogen (Carlsbad, California, CA, USA).

4.4. Antiproliferative Activity Assay

The antiproliferative activities of GUR extracts and flavonoids were investigated using the MTT assay [14]. Firstly, B16-F10 cells were cultured in 96-well plates at approximately 7.5 × 10^3 cells per well and incubated for 12 h. Then cells were treated with different concentrations of GUR extracts (5, 10, 25, 50, and 100 μg/mL) or GUR flavonoids (10, 20, 40, 60, and 80 μM). After incubation of 48 h, MTT solution (5 mg/mL in PBS) was added to each well, and cells were incubated at 37 °C for 4 h. Subsequently, 150 μL DMSO was added to each well, and the plate was put on a shaker for 5 min, the absorbance were measured at 570 nm using a fluorescence plate reader (Thermo scientific, Waltham, MA, USA). Inhibition percentage (%) was calculated according to the following formula: Inhibition percentage of cell viability (%) = [1−(OD treated well/OD control well)] × 100%. The IC_{50} value was calculated using the SPSS v. 22.0 Statistics Software (IBM Corp., Armonk, New York, NY, USA).

4.5. Morphological and Differentiation Analysis

B16-F10 cellswere cultured in 35-mm dishes (2×10^5 cells/well) and treatedwith different concentration of GUR extracts (0, 50 μg/mL), its flavonoids(0, 20, 40 μM), or α-MSH (20 nM) for 48 h.Afterthe treatment, the morphological changes were observed under a microscope (Olympus, Japan). Differentiation and mature phenotypes were characterized by formation of dendrite-like cellular protrusions. Differentiation ratio (%) was expressed as the percentage of cells with cytoplasmic extension longer than three cellular bodies in relation tothe total number of cells [33,34].

4.6. Measurement of Tyrosinase Activity

Measurement of tyrosinase activity was performed according to a previously published method with slight modifications [27]. In brief, cells were cultured in 6-wells/plate at a density of 2×10^5 cells/well, and treated with different concentrations of GUR flavonoids (0, 20, and 40 μM, respectively) or α-MSH (20 nM) for 48 h. After the treatment, the cells were washed with ice-cold PBS twice, lysed at 4 °C for 30 min in RIPA lysis buffer (150 mMNaCl, 1 mM EDTA, 1 mM EGTA, 50 mM Tris–Cl, 0.35% *w*/*v* sodium-deoxycholate, 1 mM phenylmethylsulfonyl fluoride, 1% *v*/*v* NP-40, 1 mM NaF, 1 mM Na_3VO_4, pH 7.4) containing a protease-inhibitor cocktail. Each lysate was centrifuged at 15,000× *g* for 30 min. Then, 50 μL of supernatant was added to 100 μL of 0.1% L-DOPA in PBS (pH = 6.8) in a well on a 96-well plate. After 2 h of incubation at 37 °C, the absorbance at 475 nm was measured. Meanwhile, the protein concentration of each lysate was determined by Bio-Rad protein assay. Tyrosinase activity was normalized with protein amount.

4.7. Determination of Melanin Content

Cellular melanin content was measured as described previously with a slight modification [14]. B16-F10 cells (2×10^5 cells) were placed in 6-well/plate and treated with different concentrations of GUR flavonoids (0, 20, and 40 μM, respectively) or α-MSH (20 nM) to determinate melanin content of B16-F10 cells. After incubation for 48 h, the cells were washed twice with PBS, then cells were collected after digestion with 0.05% Trypsin-EDTA for cell counting. Then 1×10^5 cells per well were dissolved in 150 μL of 1 M NaOH containing 10% DMSO for 1 h at 80 °C. The lysate was centrifuged at 16,000× *g* for 20min. Then, 100 μL supernatant was transferred to 96-well plates. The absorbance of each well was measured at 490 nm by fluorescence plate reader.

4.8. Western Blot Analysis

Western blot was performed as previously described [35]. B16-F10 Cells cultured in 100-mm dishes were treated with the required GUR flavonoids concentration of 0, 20, and 40 μM or α-MSH (20 nM) for 48 h. Then, cells were collected and proteins were extracted with RIPA lysis buffer containing a protease-inhibitor cocktail. The total protein concentrations were measured using the Bradford method, and the normalized protein samples were added to 4× sample buffer, then boiled and denatured. Equal amounts of proteins were separated by SDS-PAGE and then transferred to nitrocellulose membranes. The membranes were blocked and then probed with indicated primary antibodies, respectively, with anti-GAPDH (1:5000), anti-tyrosinase (1:200), anti-ERK1/2 (1:2500), anti-p-ERK1/2 (1:1000), anti-JNK (1:2500), anti-p-JNK (1:1000), anti-p38 (1:2500), anti-p-p38 (1:1000), anti-AKT (1:2500), anti-p-AKT (1:1000), anti-cleaved-PARP (1:1000), anti-P-CREB (1:1000), anti-CREB (1:1000), anti-MITF (1:200), anti-PI3K(P85) (1:1000), anti-caspase 3 (1:2500), anti-caspase 9 (1:2500), anti-cleaved-caspase 3 (1:1000), anti-cleaved-caspase 9 (1:1000), at 4 °C overnight. Anti-tyrosinase and anti-MITF antibodies were purchased from Santa Cruz. Biotech (Santa Cruz, California, CA, USA), others were from Cell Signaling Technology (Cell Signaling, Danvers, Massachusetts, MA, USA). All antibodies were diluted with 5% BSA in TBST buffer. The blots were rinsed and then incubated with secondary antibodies (anti-mouse antibody or anti-rabbit antibody, 1:5000, Cell Signaling Technology). Reactive bands were visualized using ECL (Thermo Fisher Scientific; Waltham, MA, USA) and then calibrated by Chemidoc Imaging System (Bio-Rad; Hercules, California, CA, USA).

4.9. Statistical Analysis

The significant difference among groups was statistically performed by one-way analysis of variance (ANOVA) combined with Tukey'stest by SPSS v. 22.0 program (IBM Corp., Armonk, New York, NY, USA). Probability value less than 0.05 ($p < 0.05$) was considered to be statistically significant. Data are expressed as the means±standard error of mean (SEM) of at least three independent experiments.

5. Conclusions

Here, we provided different lines of evidence that the dichloromethane extract of *G. uralensis* roots has potential antiproliferation and differentiation-inducing activities in cultured B16-F10 melanoma cells. Prenylated flavoniods were isolated and demonstrated to be the active constituents within the extract of *G. uralensis* roots. These prenylated flavonoids have different backbone structures, and thus each of them has distinct activity in inhibiting cancer cell growth. The present results provided the molecular basis for using nonpolar extract of *G. uralensis* roots, and the identified bioactive prenylated flavonoids could be further developed for the prevention and/or treatment of melanoma cancer.

Supplementary Materials: Supplementary materials can be found at http://www.mdpi.com/1422-0067/19/8/2422/s1.

Author Contributions: K.W.K.T. and T.T.X.D. conceived and designed the experiments; Y.Z. performed the experiments, analyzed the results, and made figures and tables; M.Y. and M.X.L. performed the experiments; H.W. and G.P. contributed to designing the experiments; K.W.K.T. and Y.Z. wrote the paper.

Acknowledgments: This work was supported by A Project Funded by the Priority Academic Program Development of Jiangsu Higher Education Institutions (PAPD), the Priority Academic Program Development of Jiangsu Higher Education Institutions, and Jiangsu Oversea Research & Training Program. Shenzhen Science and Technology Committee Research Grant (CKFW2,016,082,916,015,476; JCYJ20,170,413,173,747,440; JCYJ20,160,229,205,726,699; JCYJ20, 160,229,205,812,004; JCYJ20,160,229,210,027,564; ZDSYS201,707,281,432,317 and 20,170,326). We also thank Qinan Wu of Nanjing University of Chinese Medicine for identification of the plant material.

Conflicts of Interest: The authors declare no conflicts of interest.

References

1. Birari, R.B.; Gupta, S.; Mohan, C.G.; Bhutani, K.K. Antiobesity and lipid lowering effects of *Glycyrrhiza* chalcones: Experimental and computational studies. *Phytomedicine.* **2011**, *18*, 795–801. [CrossRef] [PubMed]
2. Fiore, C.; Eisenhut, M.; Ragazzi, E.; Zanchin, G.; Armanini, D. A history of the therapeutic use of liquorice in Europe. *J. Ethnopharmacol.* **2005**, *99*, 317–324. [CrossRef] [PubMed]
3. Kuang, Y.; Lin, Y.; Li, K.; Song, W.; Ji, S.; Qiao, X.; Zhang, Q.Y.; Ye, M. Screening of hepatoprotective compounds from licorice against carbon tetrachloride and acetaminophen induced HepG2 cells injury. *Phytomedicine.* **2017**, *34*, 59–66. [CrossRef] [PubMed]
4. Fang, S.Q.; Qu, Q.Y.; Zheng, Y.F.; Zhong, H.H.; Shan, C.X.; Wang, F.; Li, C.Y.; Guo, P.P. Structural characterization and identification of flavonoid aglycones in three *Glycyrrhiza* species by liquid chromatography with photodiode array detection and quadrupole time-of-flight mass spectrometry. *J. Sep. Sci.* **2016**, *39*, 2068–2078. [CrossRef] [PubMed]

5. Fu, Y.; Chen, J.; Li, Y.J.; Zheng, Y.F.; Li, P. Antioxidant and anti-inflammatory activities of six flavonoids separated from licorice. *Food Chem.* **2013**, *141*, 1063–1071. [CrossRef] [PubMed]
6. Cho, H.J.; Lim, S.S.; Lee, Y.S.; Kim, J.S.; Lee, C.H.; Kwon, D.Y.; Park, J.H.Y. Hexane/ethanol extract of *Glycyrrhiza uralensis* licorice exerts potent anti-inflammatory effects in murine macrophages and in mouse skin. *Food Chem.* **2010**, *141*, 959–966. [CrossRef]
7. Huo, X.W.; Liu, D.Y.; Gao, L.; Li, L.Y.; Cao, L. Flavonoids extracted from licorice prevents Colitis-associated carcinogenesis in AOM/DSS mouse model. *Int. J. Mol. Sci.* **2016**, *17*, 1343. [CrossRef] [PubMed]
8. Hoang, M.T.; Echenfield, L.F. The rising incidence of melanoma in children and adolescents. *Dermatol. Nurs.* **2000**, *121*, 192–193.
9. Lo, J.A.; Fisher, D.E. Melanoma pathogenesis. *Cancer Drug Discov. Develop.* **2015**, *82*, 25–45.
10. Parka, H.J.; Hana, E.S.; Park, D.K. The ethyl acetate extract of PGP (*Phellinuslinteus* grown on *Panax ginseng*) suppresses B16F10 melanoma cell proliferation through inducing cellular differentiation and apoptosis. *J. Ethnopharmacol.* **2010**, *132*, 115–121. [CrossRef] [PubMed]
11. Van den, B.; Verdegaal, E.M.; De Miranda, N.F. Cancer immunotherapy: Broadening the scope of targetable tumours. *Open Biol.* **2018**. [CrossRef] [PubMed]
12. Thomas, K.; Rebecca, W.K.; Rafael, C.; Brian, G. Malignant melanoma: Diagnostic and management—-Update. *Plast. Reconstr. Surg.* **2018**, *142*, 202–216.
13. Skandrani, P.A.; Simon, A.; Ghedira, K.; Chekir-Ghedira, L. Chloroform extract from *Moricandiaarvensis* inhibits growth of B16-F0 melanoma cells and promotes differentiation in vitro. *Cell Prolif.* **2010**, *43*, 471–479. [CrossRef] [PubMed]
14. Wang, D.; Xu, W.; Chen, X.; Han, J.; Yu, L.; Gao, C.; Hao, W.; Liu, X.; Zheng, Q.; Li, D. Icariin induces cell differentiation and cell cycle arrest in mouse melanoma B16 cells via Erk1/2-p38-JNK-dependent pathway. *Oncotarget.* **2017**, *8*, 99504–99513. [CrossRef] [PubMed]
15. Chen, X.; Mukwaya, E.; Wong, M.; Zhang, Y.A. systematic review on biological activities of isoprenyl flavonoids. *Pharm. Biol.* **2013**, *52*, 655–660. [CrossRef] [PubMed]
16. Keishi, H.; Kyoko, I.; Kazuyuki, H.; Tomokazu, K. Differentiation-inducing activity of lupeol, a lupine-type triterpene from Chinese Dandelion root (Hokouei-kon), on a mouse melanoma cell line. *Biol. Pharm. Bull.* **2000**, *23*, 962–967.
17. Puri, N.; Eller, M.S.; Byers, H.R.; Dykstra, S.; Kubera, J.; Gilchrest, B.A. Telomere-based DNA damage responses: A new approach to melanoma. *FASEB J.* **2004**, *18*, 1373–1381. [CrossRef] [PubMed]
18. Russo, AE.; Torrisi, E.; Bevelacqua, Y.; Perrotta, R.; Libra, M.; Mccubrey, JA.; Spandidos, DA.; Stivala, F.; Malaponte, G. Melanoma: Molecular pathogenesis and emerging target therapies (Review). *Int. J. Oncol.* **2009**, *34*, 1481–1489. [PubMed]
19. Hata, K.; Hori, K.; Takahashi, S. Role of p38 MAPK in lupeol-induced B16 2F2 mouse melanoma cell differentiation. *J. Biochem.* **2003**, *134*, 441–445. [CrossRef] [PubMed]
20. Jin, M.L.; Park, S.Y.; Kim, Y.H.; Park, G.; Son, H.J.; Lee, S.J. Suppression of α-MSH and IBMX-induced melanogenesis by cordycepin via inhibition of CREB and MITF, and activation of PI3K/Akt and ERK-dependent mechanisms. *Int. J. Mol. Sci.* **2012**, *29*, 119–124.
21. Takeda, K. Ser298 of MITF, a mutation site in Waardenburg syndrome type 2, is a phosphorylation site with functional significance. *Hum. Mol. Genet.* **2000**, *9*, 125–132. [CrossRef] [PubMed]
22. Neuhouser, M.L. Review: Dietary flavonoids and cancer risk: Evidence from human population studies. *Nutr. Cancer.* **2004**, *50*, 1–7. [CrossRef] [PubMed]
23. Miranda, C.; Stevens, J.; Helmrich, A.; Henderson, M.; Rodriguez, R.; Yang, Y.; Deinzer, M.; Barnes, D.; Buhler, D. Antiproliferative and cytotoxic effects of prenylated flavonoids from hops (*Humuluslupulus*) in human cancer cell lines. *Food Chem. Toxicol.* **1999**, *37*, 271–285. [CrossRef]
24. Ko, H.; Lu, Y.; Yang, S.; Won, S.; Lin, C. Cytotoxic prenyl flavonoids from *Artocarpuselasticus*. *J. Nat. Prod.* **2005**, *68*, 1692–1695. [CrossRef] [PubMed]
25. Leszczyniecka, M.; Roberts, T.; Dent, P.; Grant, S.; Fisher, P.B. Differentiation therapy of human cancer: Basic science and clinical applications. *Pharmacol. Ther.* **2001**, *90*, 105–156. [CrossRef]
26. Serafino, A.; Sinibaldi, V.P.; Lazzarino, G.; Tavazzi, B.; Rasi, G.; Pierimarchi, P.; Andreola, F.; Moroni, G.; Galvano, G.; Galvano, F.; et al. Differentiation of human melanoma cells induced by cyanidin-3-O-β-glucopyranoside. *FASEB J.* **2004**, *18*, 1940–1942. [CrossRef] [PubMed]

27. Ye, Y.; Chou, G.X.; Wang, H.; Chu, J.H.; Fong, W.F.; Yu, Z.L. Effects of sesquiterpenes isolated from *LargeheadAtractylodes* Rhizome on growth, migration, and differentiation of B16 melanoma cells. *Integr. Cancer Ther.* **2010**, *10*, 92–100.
28. Tsai, J.; Lee, C.; Ying, T.; Lin, C.; Lin, C.; Hsueh, J.; Hsieh, Y. Licochalcone A induces autophagy through PI3K/Akt/mTOR inactivation and autophagy suppression enhances Licochalcone A-induced apoptosis of human cervical cancer cells. *Oncotarget* **2015**, *6*, 28851–28866. [CrossRef] [PubMed]
29. Jeong, H.; Gu, G.E.; Jo, A.R.; Bang, J.S.; Yun, H.; Baek, K.J.; Kwon, N.S.; Park, K.C.; Kim, D.S. Baicalin-induced Akt activation decreases melanogenesis through downregulation of microphthalmia-associated transcription factor and tyrosinase. *Eur. J. Pharmacol.* **2015**, *761*, 19–27. [CrossRef] [PubMed]
30. Alesiani, D.; Cicconi, R.; Mattei, M.; Montesano, C.; Bei, R.; Canini, A. Cell cycle arrest and differentiation induction by 5, 7-dimethoxycoumarin in melanoma cell lines. *Int. J. Oncol.* **2008**, *32*, 425–434. [CrossRef] [PubMed]
31. Ogihara, K.; Naya, Y.; Okamoto, Y.; Hata, K. Differentiation-inducing and antiproliferative activities of lupeol on canine melanoma cells. *SpringerPlus.* **2014**, *3*, 632–638. [CrossRef] [PubMed]
32. Yuan, X.; Li, D.; Zhao, H.; Jiang, J.; Wang, P.; Ma, X.; Sun, X.; Zheng, Q. Licochalcone A-Induced Human Bladder Cancer T24 Cells apoptosis triggered by mitochondria dysfunction and endoplasmic reticulum stress. *BioMed. Res. Int.* **2013**, *2013*, 474272. [CrossRef] [PubMed]
33. Ren, K.K.; Wang, H.Z.; Xie, L.P.; Chen, D.W.; Liu, X.; Sun, J.; Nie, Y.C.; Zhang, R.Q. The effects of oridonin on cell growth, cell cycle, cell migration and differentiation in melanoma cells. *J. Ethnopharmacol.* **2006**, *103*, 176–180. [CrossRef] [PubMed]
34. Naliwaiko, K.; Luvizon, A.C.; Donatti, L.; Chammas, R.; Mercadante, A.F.; Zanata, S.M.; Nakao, L.S. Guanosine promotes B16F10 melanoma cell differentiation through PKC–ERK 1/2 pathway. *Chem. Biol. Interact.* **2008**, *173*, 122–128. [CrossRef] [PubMed]
35. Lou, J.S.; Yan, L.; Bi, C.W.; Chan, G.K.; Wu, Q.Y.; Liu, Y.; Wang, H.Y.; Yao, P.; Du, C.Y.; Dong, T.T.; et al. Yu Ping Feng San reverses cisplatin-induced multi-drug resistance in lung cancer cells via regulating drug transporters and p62/TRAF6 signalling. *Sci. Rep.* **2016**, *6*, 31926. [CrossRef] [PubMed]

International Journal of *Molecular Sciences*

MDPI

Article

Novel Therapeutic Agent against Platelet Activation In Vitro and Arterial Thrombosis In Vivo by Morin Hydrate

Chih-Wei Hsia [1,†], Ming-Ping Wu [1,2,†], Marappan Velusamy [3], Chih-Hsuan Hsia [1], Duen-Suey Chou [4], Cheng-Lin Tsai [5], Chia-Yuan Hsu [1], Thanasekaran Jayakumar [1,4], Chi-Li Chung [6,*] and Joen-Rong Sheu [1,4,*]

1 Graduate Institute of Medical Sciences, College of Medicine, Taipei Medical University, Taipei 110, Taiwan; d119106003@tmu.edu.tw (C.-W.H.); mpwu@mail.chimei.org.tw (M.-P.W.); d119102013@tmu.edu.tw (C.-H.H.); gordanmike1003@gmail.com (C.-Y.H.); tjaya_2002@yahoo.co.in (T.J.)
2 Department of Obstetrics and Gynecology, Chi-Mei Medical Center, Tainan 710, Taiwan
3 Department of Chemistry, North Eastern Hill University, Shillong 793022, India; mvelusamy@gmail.com
4 Department of Pharmacology, School of Medicine, College of Medicine, Taipei Medical University, Taipei 110, Taiwan; fird@tmu.edu.tw
5 Graduate Institute of Metabolism and Obesity Sciences, College of Nutrition, Taipei Medical University, Taipei 110, Taiwan; ma48106001@tmu.edu.tw
6 Division of Pulmonary Medicine, Department of Internal Medical, Taipei Medical University Hospital, Taipei 110, Taiwan
* Correspondence: clchung@tmu.edu.tw (C.-L.C.); sheujr@tmu.edu.tw (J.-R.S.); Tel.: +886-2-27372181 (C.-L.C.); +886-2-27361661-3199 (J.-R.S.)
† All the authors contributed equally to this work.

Received: 31 July 2018; Accepted: 13 August 2018; Published: 13 August 2018

Abstract: Morin hydrate, a bioactive flavonoid, has been proven to prevent inflammation and apoptosis of cells. Flavonoids can reduce the risk of cardiovascular diseases, in which platelet activation plays a major role. This study investigated the effect of morin hydrate on platelet activation in vitro and in vivo. Morin hydrate markedly inhibited platelet aggregation stimulated by collagen in human platelets but not that stimulated by other agonists. In collagen-activated platelets, morin hydrate inhibited adenosine triphosphate (ATP) release; intracellular Ca^{2+} mobilization; P-selectin expression; and phosphorylation of phospholipase Cγ2 (PLCγ2), protein kinase C (PKC), and Akt. In mitogen-activated protein kinase (MAPK) activation, morin hydrate evidently diminished ERK2 or JNK1 activation, except for p38 MAPK. Additionally, morin hydrate markedly reduced the OH· signals in platelet suspensions but not in the cell-free system (Fenton reaction solution). Moreover, morin hydrate substantially increased the occlusion time of thrombotic platelet plug formation but had no effect on bleeding time in mice. In conclusion, morin hydrate crucially inhibits platelet activation through inhibition of the PLCγ2–PKC cascade and subsequent suppression of Akt and MAPK activation, thereby ultimately inhibiting platelet aggregation. Therefore, this paper suggests that morin hydrate constitutes a novel and potential natural therapeutic product for preventing or treating thromboembolic disorders.

Keywords: bleeding time; flavonoid; morin hydrate; OH· free radical; platelet activation; protein kinase; thromboembolism

1. Introduction

Flavonoids are naturally occurring compounds that contain a number of phenolic hydroxyl groups attached to ring structures designated as A, B, and C (Figure 1A). The structure of flavonoids is usually characterized by two aromatic rings (A and B) joined by a three-carbon linked C-pyrone ring (C) to form a C6–C3–C6 skeletal unit (Figure 1A). The bioactivity of flavonoids has attracted academic interest because of its potential health benefits for humans. Diets rich in fruits and vegetables exert protective effects against cardiovascular diseases (CVDs) and certain forms of cancer [1]. Flavonoids have been used as valuable therapeutic agents in modern and traditional medicine.

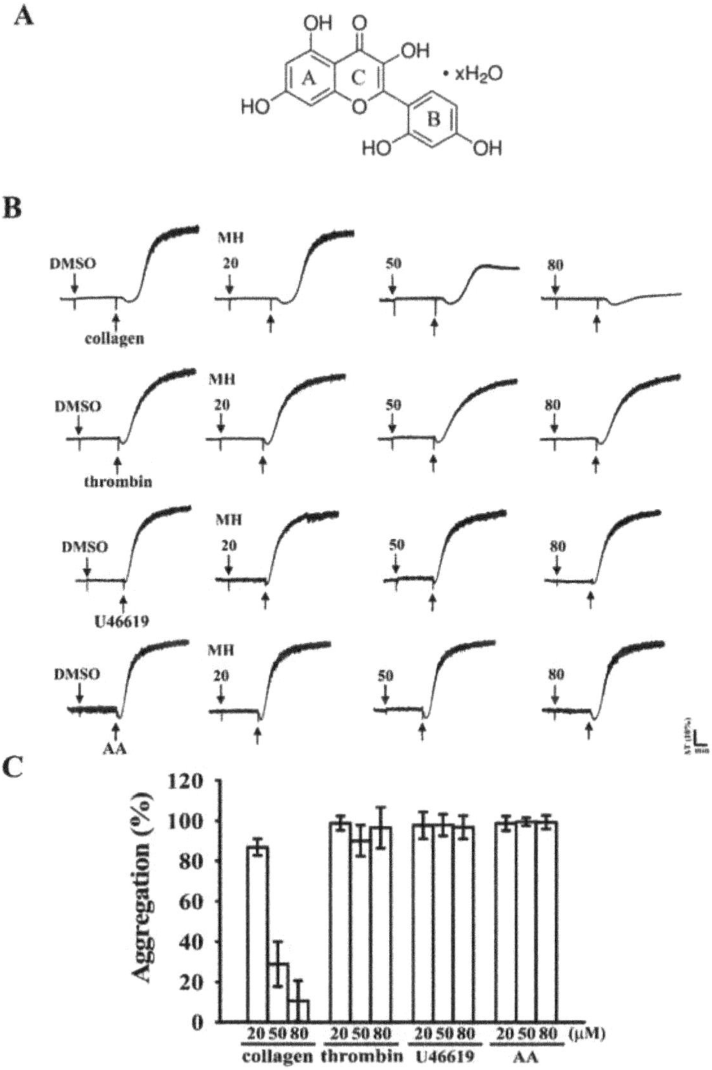

Figure 1. Inhibitory activity of morin hydrate in platelet aggregation stimulated by various agonists in washed human platelets. (**A**) Chemical structure of morin hydrate; (**B**) washed human platelets (3.6×10^8 cells/mL) were preincubated with the solvent control (0.1% dimethyl sulfoxide, DMSO) or morin hydrate (20, 50, and 80 μM) and subsequently treated with 1 μg/mL of collagen, 0.01 U/mL of thrombin, 1 μM of U46619, and 60 μM of arachidonic acid (AA) to stimulate platelet aggregation; (**C**) concentration–response histograms of morin hydrate in inhibition of platelet aggregation (%). All data are presented as means ± standard errors of means (n = 4).

Morin is a well-known bioactive constituent belonging to the flavonol group and is found in old fustic (*Chlorophora tinctoria*), Osage orange (*Maclura pomifera*), almond, mill (*Prunus dulcis*), fig (*Chlorophora tinctoria*), onion, apple, and other Moraceae, which are used as dietary agents and herbal medicines [2,3]. Morin exhibits various biological activities such as antimutagenesis, anti-inflammation, antiarthritis, and cardioprotective activities, and inhibits xanthine oxidase activity and cell proliferation [4–6]. Morin has attracted considerable interest because of its antitumor activity in vitro and in vivo [7].

Dietary factors play key roles in the development and prevention of various human diseases, such as myocardial infarction and ischemic stroke. The risk of CVDs have been reduced with intake of dietary flavonoids [8]. Platelet adherence and aggregation is believed to be initiated intraluminal thrombosis and thus, these events may play a crucial role in atherothrombotic processes in addition to mediating hemostasis [9]. Moreover, platelets are the first-line defense against hemorrhage and important for maintaining the integrity of the vascular system. Upon platelet activation, several mediators such as adenosine triphosphate (ATP) and thromboxane A_2 are released in conjunction with intracellular Ca^{2+} ($[Ca^{2+}]i$) mobilization. These processes further attract other platelets toward the injured endothelium and therefore cause the thickening of the initial platelet monolayer. Finally, fibrinogen binds to its specific platelet receptor of integrin $\alpha_{IIb}\beta_3$, thereby completing the final common pathway for platelet aggregation.

Tzeng et al. [10] demonstrated that morin hydrate exhibited potent bioactivity in the inhibition of rabbit platelet aggregation stimulated by arachidonic acid (AA). In our preliminary study, we observed that 20 μM of morin hydrate significantly inhibited platelet aggregation in washed human platelets. However, the effect of morin hydrate on platelet activation remained to be thoroughly investigated. Therefore, in the current study, we systematically examined in vitro and in vivo effects of morin hydrate on washed human platelets and experimental mice to further characterize the detailed mechanisms of morin hydrate–mediated inhibition of platelet activation.

2. Results

2.1. Effect of Morin Hydrate on Aggregation of Washed Human Platelets Stimulated by Various Agonists

Morin hydrate (20, 50, and 80 μM; Figure 1B,C) strongly inhibited platelet aggregation stimulated by 1 μg/mL of collagen but not by 0.01 U/mL of thrombin, 1 μM of U46619, a prostaglandin endoperoxide, or AA (60 μM). At 80 μM, morin hydrate almost inhibited platelet aggregation stimulated by collagen. The 50% inhibitory concentration (IC_{50}) of morin hydrate for collagen-stimulated aggregation was approximately 40 μM. Therefore, in subsequent experiments, the IC_{50} (40 μM) and maximal concentration (80 μM) of morin hydrate were used to explore the possible mechanisms in human platelets. In addition, the solvent control (0.1% dimethyl sulfoxide, DMSO) did not significantly affect platelet aggregation (Figure 1B).

2.2. Regulatory Role of Morin Hydrate in ATP Release, Relative $[Ca^{2+}]i$ Mobilization, and Surface P-Selectin Expression in Washed Human Platelets

Platelet activation is associated with release of granular contents (e.g., ATP and Ca^{2+} from dense granules and P-selectin expression from α-granules). In the present study, morin hydrate (40 and 80 μM) markedly and concentration-dependently hindered ATP release (Figure 2A) and relative $[Ca^{2+}]i$ mobilization (resting control, 75.4 ± 25.5 nM; collagen stimulated, 444.9 ± 35.7 nM; 40 μM, 125.9 ± 17.6 nM; 80 μM, 69.1 ± 12.7 nM; $n = 4$; Figure 2B) in platelets stimulated by collagen (1 μg/mL). In resting platelets, P-selectin is located on the inner walls of α-granules. Platelet activation exposes the inner walls of the granules to the outer parts of the cell [11]. Treatment with morin hydrate markedly reduced collagen-induced surface P-selectin expression (resting control, 55.0 ± 22.5; collagen activated, 591.7 ± 44.9; 40 μM, 197.3 ± 30.8; 80 μM, 149.7 ± 27.0; $n = 4$; Figure 2C). The corresponding statistical data are presented on the right panels of Figure 2A–C.

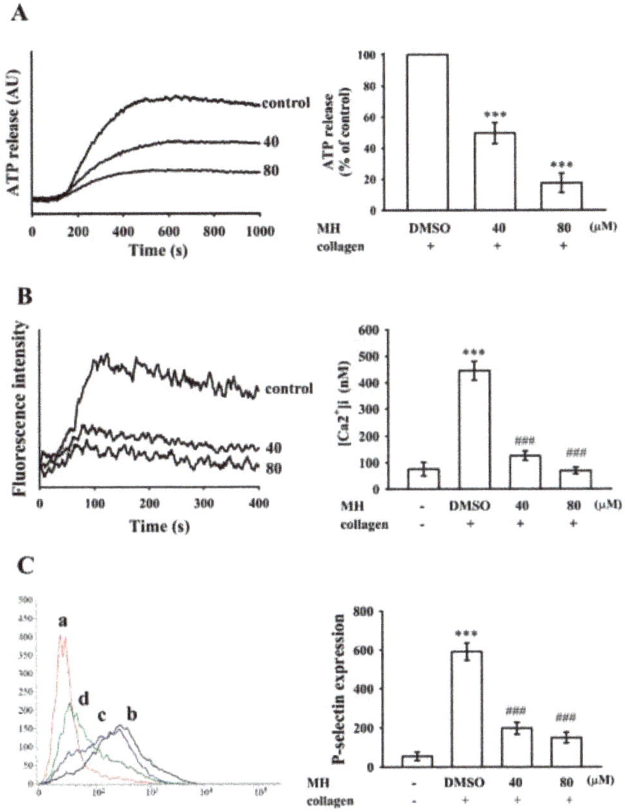

Figure 2. Effects of morin hydrate on adenosine triphosphate (ATP) release, relative intracellular Ca^{2+} ($[Ca^{2+}]i$) mobilization, and surface P-selectin expression in human platelets. Washed platelets (3.6×10^8 cells/mL) were preincubated with the solvent control (0.1% DMSO), morin hydrate (40 and 80 μM), or fluorescein isothiocyanate (FITC)–P-selectin (2 μg/mL); collagen (1 μg/mL) was then added to trigger either: (**A**) ATP release (AU; arbitrary unit), (**B**) relative $[Ca^{2+}]i$ mobilization, or (**C**) the fluorescence profiles of (a) FITC only as a resting control; washed platelets were preincubated with the (b) solvent control (0.1% DMSO) or morin hydrate (c, 40 μM; d, 80 μM) for 3 min, followed by the addition of FITC–P-selectin and subsequently treated with collagen to induce platelet activation. The corresponding statistical data are shown on the right panel of each figure (**A–C**). Data are presented as means ± standard errors of means (n = 4). *** $p < 0.001$ compared with the (**A**) DMSO-treated group or (**B**,**C**) resting control; ### $p < 0.001$ compared with the DMSO-treated group.

2.3. Effects of Morin Hydrate on Cytotoxicity, the PLCγ2–PKC Cascade, and Akt Activation

The aggregation curves of platelets preincubated with morin hydrate (100 μM) for 10 min and successively washed with Tyrode's solution were not significantly different from those of platelets preincubated with the solvent control (0.1% DMSO) under equivalent conditions (Figure 3A). This result primarily indicated that the inhibitory effects of morin hydrate on platelet aggregation are reversible and noncytotoxic. In addition, the lactate dehydrogenase (LDH) study revealed that morin hydrate (40, 80, and 100 μM) incubated with platelets for 20 min did not significantly increase the LDH activity in the platelets (Figure 3B); these findings demonstrated that morin hydrate does not affect platelet permeability or induce platelet cytolysis.

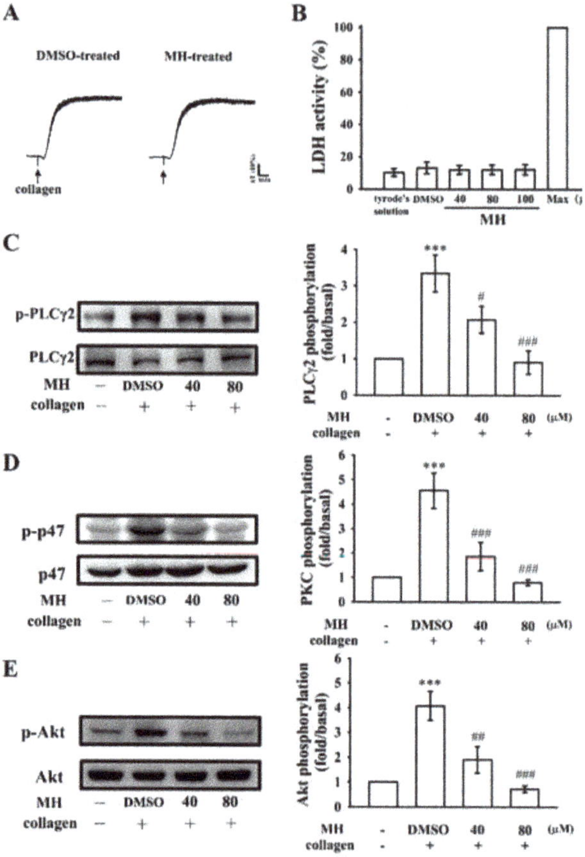

Figure 3. Effects of morin hydrate on cytotoxicity, lactate dehydrogenase (LDH) release, and PLCγ2, PKC, and Akt activation in human platelets. (**A**) Washed platelets (3.6×10^8 cells/mL) were preincubated with the solvent control (0.1% DMSO) or morin hydrate (100 μM) for 10 min and consequently washed twice with Tyrode's solution; collagen (1 μg/mL) was then added to trigger platelet aggregation; (**B**) washed platelets were preincubated with the solvent control (0.1% DMSO) or morin hydrate (40, 80, and 100 μM) for 20 min and a 10-μL aliquot of the supernatant was deposited on a Fuji Dri-Chem slide LDH-PIII, as described in Materials and Methods. (**C–E**) For the other experiments, washed platelets were preincubated with the solvent control (0.1% DMSO) or morin hydrate (40 and 80 μM) and subsequently treated with collagen (1 μg/mL) to induce (**C**) PLCγ2 and (**D**) PKC activation (p47, pleckstrin phosphorylation) and (**E**) Akt phosphorylation. Data are presented as means ± standard errors of means (n = 4). *** $p < 0.001$ compared with the resting control; # $p < 0.05$, ## $p < 0.01$, and ### $p < 0.001$ compared with the DMSO-treated group.

Phospholipase C (PLC) hydrolyzes phosphatidylinositol 4,5-bisphosphate to produce the secondary messengers inositol 1,4,5-trisphosphate (IP_3) and diacylglycerol (DAG). IP_3 activates relative [Ca^{2+}]i mobilization and DAG stimulates protein kinase C (PKC), giving an approximately 47 kDa protein that is principally phosphorylated (p47 protein; pleckstrin) and causes ATP release [12]. As specified, morin hydrate markedly reduced relative [Ca^{2+}]i mobilization (Figure 2B). We further examined the effect of morin hydrate on the phosphorylation of the PLCγ2–PKC signaling cascade. As shown in Figure 3C, D, morin hydrate (40 and 80 μM) markedly reduced both PLCγ2 and PKC activation (p47) phosphorylation in collagen-activated platelets. Moreover, Akt is a serine/threonine-specific protein kinase that plays a key role in multiple cellular processes such as cell proliferation, apoptosis, cell migration, and platelet activation [13]. Morin hydrate (40 and 80 μM) evidently inhibited collagen-induced Akt phosphorylation (Figure 3E).

2.4. Effect of Morin Hydrate on p38 MAPK, ERK2, and JNK1 Activation

To further examine the inhibitory mechanisms of morin hydrate, several signaling molecules associated with MAPKs were evaluated. The major kinases, including p38 MAPK, ERKs, and JNKs, regulate cellular responses in eukaryotic organisms and contribute to cell proliferation, migration, differentiation, and apoptosis. ERK2, JNK1, and p38 MAPK have been identified in platelets [14]. As shown in Figure 4A–C, morin hydrate (40 and 80 μM) evidently inhibited ERK2 and JNK1 phosphorylation except for p38 MAPK.

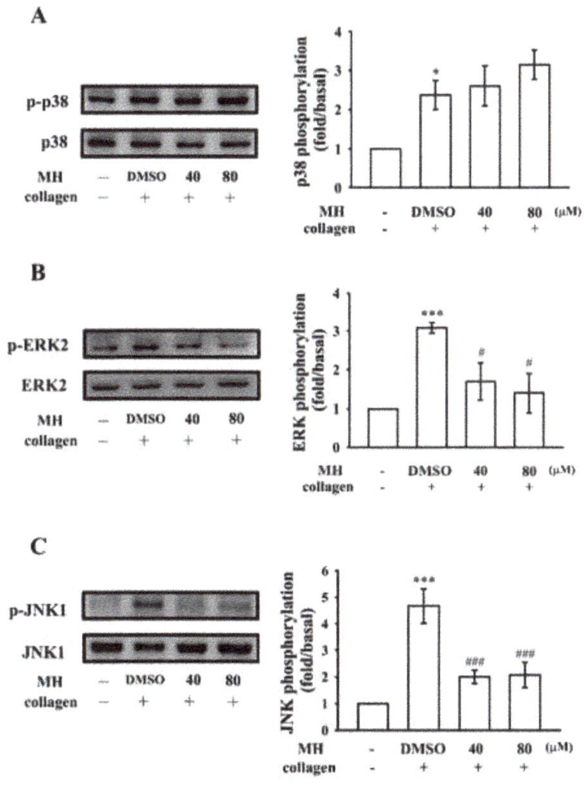

Figure 4. Morin hydrate inhibits p38 MAPK, ERK2, and JNK1 phosphorylation in collagen-activated platelets. Washed platelets were preincubated with the solvent control (0.1% DMSO) or morin hydrate (40 and 80 μM) and subsequently treated with collagen (1 μg/mL) to trigger (**A**) p38 MAPK, (**B**) ERK2, and (**C**) JNK1 activation. Data are presented as means ± standard errors of means ($n = 4$). * $p < 0.05$ and *** $p < 0.001$ compared with the resting control; # $p < 0.05$ and ### $p < 0.001$ compared with the DMSO-treated group.

2.5. Evaluation of OH·-Scavenging Activity of Morin Hydrate through Electron Spin Resonance (ESR) Spectrometry

Signals from the ESR study are the indicative of OH· radical formation, which was increased in collagen-stimulated platelet suspensions (Figure 5Ab) and the Fenton reaction solution (cell-free system; Figure 5Bb) when compared with the resting control (Figure 5Aa,Ba). Morin hydrate (80 μM) markedly reduced collagen-induced OH• signals in the platelet suspensions (Figure 5Ad) but not in the Fenton reaction solution (Figure 5Bd). This result indicated that morin hydrate reduced intracellular OH• radical formation but had no significant effect on the cell-free system.

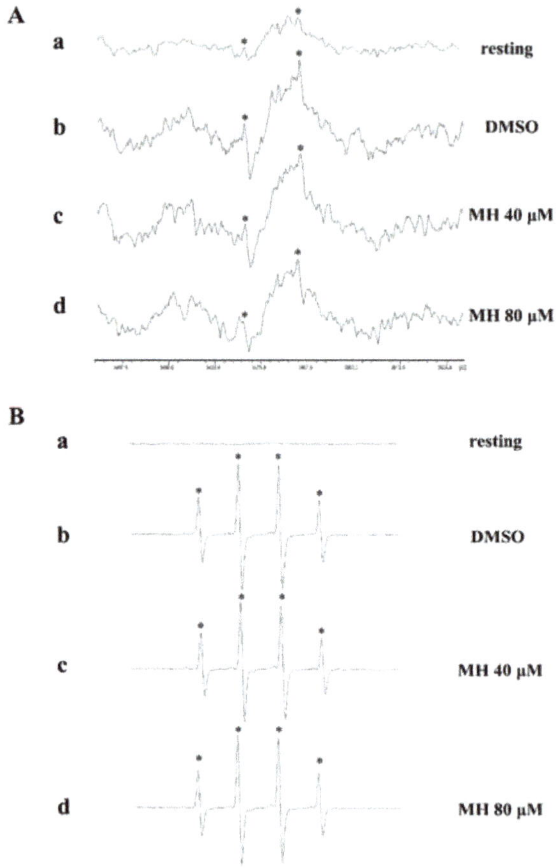

Figure 5. Activities of morin hydrate on OH• formation in human platelet suspensions or the Fenton reaction solution. (**A**) Washed platelet suspensions or (**B**) the Fenton reaction solution was preincubated with (a) Tyrode's solution (resting control), (b) 0.1% DMSO, or morin hydrate at (c) 40 μM or (d) 80 μM. Collagen (1 μg/mL) was then added for the Electron Spin Resonance (ESR) experiments, as described in Materials and Methods. Profiles are representative of four independent experiments, and an asterisk (*) indicates OH• formation.

2.6. *Effects of Morin Hydrate on Platelet Thrombi in Mesenteric Microvessels and Bleeding Time In Vivo*

We investigated the effect of morin hydrate on thrombus formation in vivo. The occlusion time in microvessels pretreated with 15 μg/kg of fluorescein sodium was approximately 150 s. When morin hydrate was administered at 10 mg/kg but not 5 mg/kg after pretreatment with fluorescein sodium, the occlusion times were significantly prolonged compared with those of the DMSO-treated controls (DMSO: 144.5 ± 16.1 s vs. 5 mg/kg: 133.9 ± 12.2 s, $n = 6$, $p > 0.05$; DMSO: 133.0 ± 17.9 s vs. 10 mg/kg: 478.4 ± 27.9 s, $n = 6$, $p < 0.001$; Figure 6A). The thrombotic platelet plug was observed in mesenteric microvessels at 150 s (black arrow) but not at 5 s after irradiation in the DMSO-treated group (Figure 6Ba,Bb). When 5 mg/kg morin hydrate was administered, platelet plug formation was also observed at 150 s (black arrow) but not at 5 s after irradiation (Figure 6Bc,Bd). However, upon administration of 10 mg/kg of morin hydrate, the thrombotic platelet plug was not observed at 5 or 150 s (Figure 6Be,Bf). The blood flow rate of the DMSO-treated venule was lower than that of the morin hydrate–treated venule because the platelet plug appeared at 150 s (Figure 6Bb). We also investigated the tail transection model of mice 30 min after administration of 5 or 10 mg/kg morin hydrate intraperitoneally; the bleeding times recorded were 191.3 ± 37.6 s (DMSO-treated group; n = 6), 260.7 ± 41.9 s (group treated with morin hydrate, 5 mg/kg; n = 6), and 271.3 ± 66.7 s (group treated with morin hydrate, 10 mg/kg; n = 6) (Figure 6C). Each mouse was monitored for 15 min after bleeding had stopped to detect any re-bleeding. The results suggested that morin hydrate markedly diminished the platelet plug formation in vivo but had no significant effect on bleeding time.

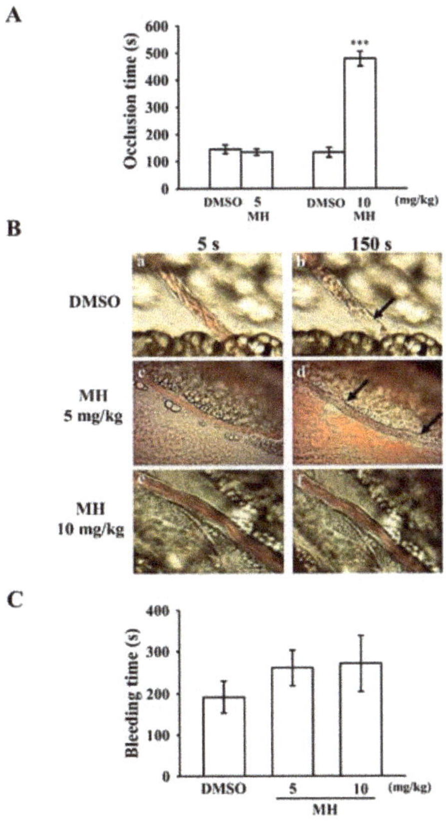

Figure 6. In vivo activities of morin hydrate on thrombotic platelet plug formation in the mesenteric venules and bleeding time in the tail veins of mice. (**A**) Mice were given an intravenous bolus of the solvent control (0.1% DMSO) or morin hydrate (5 and 10 mg/kg) and the mesenteric venules were irradiated to induce microthrombus formation (occlusion time); (**B**) microscopic images (400× magnification) of 0.1% DMSO-treated controls (a and b); the 5 mg/kg (c and d) and 10 mg/kg (e and f) morin hydrate–treated groups were recorded at 5 s (a, c, and e) and 150 s (b, d, and f) after irradiation. The photographs are representative of six similar experiments. The black arrows indicate platelet plug formation; (**C**) bleeding time was measured through transection of the tail in mice after 30 min of administration of 5 or 10 mg/kg of morin hydrate intraperitoneally. Data are presented as means ± standard errors of means (**A**–**C**, n = 6). *** $p < 0.001$ compared with the 0.1% DMSO-treated group.

3. Discussion

Our study was the first to demonstrate that morin hydrate shows in vitro antiplatelet effect and effectively inhibit arterial thrombosis in vivo. In general, dietary intake from the natural sources is likely insufficient for attaining plasma concentrations that can inhibit platelet activation in vivo, however, several nontoxic prophylactic agents such as food products and nutritional supplements is ideal for stopping atherothrombotic events. Thus, morin hydrate may signify a novel antithrombotic agent for use in humans.

In the present study, morin hydrate effectively inhibited platelet aggregation stimulated by collagen but not that stimulated by thrombin, AA, or U46619, indicating that this compound inhibits platelet aggregation through a markedly PLC-dependent mechanism. Various physiological stimuli (e.g., thrombin, collagen, ADP, and epinephrine) activate platelets, and these stimulators are believed to exert their effects via interaction with specific receptors on platelet membranes. The matrix protein collagen is present in the vascular subendothelium and vessel wall and acts as a substrate for platelet adhesion; it is also an endogenous platelet activator. Among the platelet receptors known to interact directly with collagen, integrin $\alpha_2\beta_1$ and glycoprotein (GP) VI [15] appear to play a key role and have recently gained academic attention. GP VI is widely recognized as a requisite factor for formation of platelet aggregates on collagen surfaces under blood flow [16]. Integrin $\alpha_2\beta_1$ is another major collagen receptor on endothelial cells and platelets. In cells expressing integrin $\alpha_2\beta_1$, many signals (including tyrosine phosphorylation and matrix remodeling) are activated after cell adhesion to collagen [17]. Recent findings have suggested that integrin $\alpha_2\beta_1$ and GP VI might contribute to the overall processes of platelet adhesion and activation [18].

Activation of platelets by collagen substantially alters phospholipase activation. PLC activation is an early event in response to numerous extracellular stimuli. Upon activation, PLC produces two crucial second messengers, namely DAG and inositol trisphosphate (IP_3), both of which play key roles in many signaling pathways, including activation of protein kinase C (PKC) and protein kinase D (PKD) and induction of calcium influx [19]. The signaling axis of PLC/PKC/PKD was shown to play a key role in many signaling pathways [20]. In response to various extracellular stimuli, there are 13 phosphatidylinositide-specific PLCs that are divided into six subgroups: PLCβ, PLCγ, PLCδ, PLCε, PLCξ, and PLCη [21]. The PLCγ family comprises isozymes 1 and 2. PLCγ2 is involved in collagen-dependent signaling on platelets [21]. In our study, morin hydrate diminished the activation of the PLCγ2–PKC cascade stimulated by collagen, suggesting that the morin hydrate–mediated inhibition of platelet activation involves PLCγ2 downstream signaling; moreover, this result explains why morin hydrate was more efficacious in inhibiting collagen induced platelet aggregation than that induced by thrombin, U46619, or AA.

Platelets adhere to the subendothelial matrix protein collagen, which alters their shape and releases granular contents of ATP, Ca^{2+}, and P-selectin. P-selectin is an adhesion molecule kept in the platelets α-granules, upon activation it is expressed on a platelet surface membrane and successively expressed on the external membrane through membrane flipping. P-selectin mediates the initial formation of platelet aggregates and simplifies the development of large platelet aggregates [22]. Agonists such as collagen, thrombin, and AA activate $[Ca^{2+}]$i to phosphorylate the Ca^{2+}/calmodulin-dependent myosin light chain (20 kDa), which is involved in the secretion of granule contents such as serotonin and ATP [23], as well as platelet aggregation. So, suppression of $[Ca^{2+}]$i mobilization and ATP production is critical for assessing the antiplatelet effects of a compound.

Specific MAPK kinases (MEKs), specifically, MEK1/2, MEK3/6, and MEK4/7 activate MAPKs, such as ERKs, p38 MAPK, and JNKs, respectively [24]. ERK2 activation is involved in platelet aggregation needing prior ATP release, which triggers P_2X_1-mediated Ca^{2+} influx and activates ERK2, thereby increasing the phosphorylation of myosin light chain kinase [25]. JNK1 is recently identified in platelets and it activated by several agonists, including collagen, thrombin, and ADP [26], however its role in platelets is poorly recognized. Furthermore, a reduced integrin $\alpha_{IIb}\beta_3$ activation and severe granule secretion impairment was proved in $JNK^{-/-}$ platelets [25]. Additionally, cytosolic phospholipase A_2 ($cPLA_2$), a substrate of p38 MAPK activity is induced by agonists such as von Willebrand factor and thrombin [25]. Therefore, p38 MAPK is consider important for $cPLA_2$ stimulation [27]. These literatures revealed reasonable explanation is why morin hydrate inhibited ERK2 and JNK1 activation largely than p38 MAPK activation.

Akt is a downstream effector of phosphoinositide 3 (PI3)-kinase. A defective agonist-induced platelet activation was found in Akt-knockout mice, proposing that Akt regulates platelet activation and such regulation may have consequences related to thrombosis [13]. Among the three mammalian Akt isoforms of Akt 1, 2, and 3, the first two isoforms were detected in human platelets [28]. Akt inhibitors have usually reported similar roles of Akt 1 and 2 in human platelet activation. Therefore, protein kinases for Akt activation, particularly PI3-kinase β, may be appropriate targets for the development of antithrombotic therapies. Our previous study found PI3-kinase/Akt and MAPKs are mutually activated as upstream regulators of PKC in activated platelets [29].

Reactive oxygen species (ROS) produced through platelet activation (i.e., H_2O_2 and OH•) might affect cells that they come into contact with such as endothelial cells, thereby enhancing platelet reactivity during thrombus formation. Free radicals act as secondary signals that increase $[Ca^{2+}]i$ levels during the initial phase of platelet activation, and PKC is involved in receptor-mediated production of free radicals in platelets [30]. In addition, H_2O_2 produced by platelets is converted into OH• because platelet aggregation is inhibited by OH• scavengers [30]. Morin was reported to scavenge ROS and free radicals of oxygen in an indirect analysis study [31]. Our ESR spectrometry results provided direct evidence that morin hydrate significantly reduced OH• formation in platelet suspensions but had no effect in a cell-free system.

In this study on thrombosis, mesenteric venules were continuously irradiated by fluorescein sodium throughout the experimental period, leading to strong damage to the endothelial cells. Here, 10 mg/kg of morin hydrate significantly prolonged the occlusion times; this effect may be mediated, at least partially, by inhibition of platelet activation. In addition, we used the tail transection mouse model to examine the effects of morin hydrate on bleeding time in vivo. Although aspirin is the most effective antiplatelet drug prescribed for preventing or treating cardiovascular and cerebrovascular diseases, it causes unwanted prolongation of bleeding time. In this model, the bleeding time of the morin hydrate–treated mice was not significantly different to the solvent control, indicating that morin hydrate possesses antiplatelet activity in vivo but had no effect on bleeding time. Liu et al. [32] reported that treatment with 20 mg/kg of morin hydrate markedly reduced myocardial ischemia-reperfusion injury (MIRI) in rats. Although results in animal species and experimental models have differed, morin hydrate evidently possesses a more potent ability to inhibit arterial thrombosis than protect against MIRI.

The findings of the present study revealed that morin hydrate plays a novel role in inhibiting platelet activation in vitro and in vivo, suggesting that it can be used in prophylactic applications. Generally, a nutritional or dietary supplement is required to produce a prophylactic effect in humans. However, selection of doses for time-course treatments may be confounded by variation in responses among users. This study provided new insights into the role of morin hydrate in blocking collagen-specific signaling events involved in platelet activation. However, the involvement of other mechanisms yet to be identified in morin hydrate–mediated inhibition of platelet activation requires investigation.

4. Materials and Methods

4.1. Chemicals and Reagents

Morin hydrate, thrombin, collagen, AA, luciferin–luciferase, U46619, heparin, prostaglandin E_1 (PGE_1), 5,5-dimethyl-1-pyrroline N-oxide (DMPO), and bovine serum albumin (BSA) were purchased from Sigma (St. Louis, MO, USA). Fura-2AM was obtained from Molecular Probes (Eugene, OR, USA). An anti-phospho-p38 mitogen-activated protein kinase (MAPK) Ser^{182} monoclonal antibody (mAb) was purchased from Santa Cruz Biotechnology (Santa Cruz, CA, USA). Anti-p38 MAPK, anti-phospho-c-Jun N-terminal kinase (JNK) (Thr^{183}/Tyr^{185}), and anti-p44/42 extracellular signal-regulated kinase (ERK) mAbs, as well as anti-phospholipase Cγ2 (PLCγ2), anti-phospho (Tyr^{759}) PLCγ2, anti-phospho-(Ser) protein kinase C (PKC) substrate (pleckstrin; p-p47), anti-JNK, and anti-phospho-p44/p42 ERK (Thr^{202}/Tyr^{204}) polyclonal antibodies (pAbs) were purchased from Cell Signaling (Beverly, MA, USA). Anti-phospho-protein kinase B (Akt) (Ser^{473}) and anti-Akt mAbs were purchased from Biovision (Mountain View, CA, USA). An anti-pleckstrin (p47) pAb was purchased from GeneTex (Irvine, CA, USA). A Hybond-P polyvinylidene fluoride (PVDF) membrane, an enhanced chemiluminescence Western blotting detection reagent, horseradish peroxidase (HRP)-conjugated donkey anti-rabbit immunoglobulin G (IgG), and sheep anti-mouse IgG were purchased from Amersham (Buckinghamshire, UK). A fluorescein isothiocyanate (FITC) anti-human CD42P (P-selectin) mAb was obtained from BioLegend (San Diego, CA, USA). Morin hydrate was dissolved in 0.1% dimethyl sulfoxide (DMSO) and stored at 4 °C.

4.2. Platelet Aggregation

This study was approved by the Institutional Review Board of Taipei Medical University (N201612050; 20/January/2017) and conformed to the directives of the Declaration of Helsinki. All human volunteers involved in this study provided informed consent. Human platelet suspensions were prepared as described previously [9]. Human blood samples were obtained from adult volunteers who refrained from use of drugs or other substances that could have interfered with the experiment for at least 14 days before sample collection; the collected blood samples were mixed with an acid-citrate-dextrose solution. After centrifugation, platelet-rich plasma (PRP) was supplemented with 0.5 μM of PGE_1 and 6.4 IU/mL of heparin. Tyrode's solution containing 3.5 mg/mL of BSA was used to prepare the final suspension of washed human platelets. The final Ca^{2+} concentration in the Tyrode's solution was 1 mM. A platelet aggregation study was conducted using a lumi-aggregometer (Payton Associates, Scarborough, ON, Canada), as described previously [9]. An isovolumetric solvent control (0.1% DMSO) or morin hydrate was preincubated with platelet suspensions (3.6×10^8 cells/mL) for 3 min before the addition of the agonists (i.e., collagen). The extent of platelet aggregation was calculated as the percentage compared with individual control (without morin hydrate) expressed in light transmission units after the reaction had proceeded for 6 min. For an ATP release assay, 20 μL of luciferin–luciferase was added 1 min before the addition of collagen (1 μg/mL), and the amount of ATP released was compared with that released by the control (without morin hydrate).

4.3. Measurement of Relative [Ca^{2+}]i Mobilization

The relative [Ca^{2+}]i concentration was determined using Fura-2AM, as described previously [9]. Concisely, citrated whole blood was centrifuged at 120× *g* for 10 min and the PRP was collected and incubated with Fura-2AM (5 μM) for 1 h. The Fura-2AM-loaded platelets were preincubated with morin hydrate (40 and 80 μM) in the presence of 1 mM of $CaCl_2$ and then stimulated with collagen (1 μg/mL). The Fura-2 fluorescence was measured using a spectrofluorometer (Hitachi FL Spectrophotometer F-4500, Tokyo, Japan) at excitation wavelengths of 340 and 380 nm and an emission wavelength of 510 nm.

4.4. Flow Cytometric Analysis of Surface P-selectin Expression

Washed platelets were prepared as described in the preceding subsection and aliquots of platelet suspensions (3.6×10^8 cells/mL) were preincubated with the solvent control (0.1% DMSO) or morin hydrate (40 and 80 μM) and FITC-P-selectin (2 μg/mL) for 3 min; collagen (1 μg/mL) was added to trigger platelet activation. The suspensions were then assayed for fluorescein-labeled platelets by using a flow cytometer (FACScan System, Becton Dickinson, San Jose, CA, USA). Data were collected from 50,000 platelets per experimental group. All experiments were repeated at least four times to ensure reproducibility.

4.5. Detection of Lactate Dehydrogenase

Washed platelets (3.6×10^8 cells/mL) were preincubated with the solvent control (0.1% DMSO) or morin hydrate (40, 80, 100 μM) for 20 min at 37 °C. An aliquot of the supernatant (10 μL) was deposited on a Fuji Dri-Chem slide LDH-PIII (Fuji, Tokyo, Japan) and the absorbance wavelength was read at 540 nm by using an ultraviolet–visible spectrophotometer (UV-160; Shimadzu, Japan). A maximal value of lactate dehydrogenase (LDH) was recorded in the sonicated platelets (Max).

4.6. Immunoblotting of Protein Phosphorylation

Washed platelets (1.2×10^9 cells/mL) were preincubated with the solvent control (0.1% DMSO) or morin hydrate (40 and 80 μM) for 3 min. Subsequently, collagen (1 μg/mL) was added to trigger platelet activation. The reaction was then stopped and the platelets were immediately resuspended in 200 μL of lysis buffer. Samples containing 80 μg of protein were separated through 12% sodium dodecyl sulfate gel electrophoresis, and the proteins were electrotransferred to PVDF membranes by using a Bio-Rad semidry transfer unit (Bio-Rad, Hercules, CA, USA). The blots were then blocked through treatment with Tris-buffered saline in Tween 20 (TBST; 10 mM of Tris-base, 100 mM of NaCl, and 0.01% Tween 20) containing 5% BSA for 1 h and were probed with various primary antibodies. The membranes were incubated with HRP-conjugated anti-mouse IgG or anti-rabbit IgG (diluted 1:3000 in TBST) for 1 h. An enhanced chemiluminescence system was used to detect immunoreactive bands, whose optical density was quantified using Bio-profil Biolight (version V2000.01; Vilber Lourmat, Marne-la-Vallée, France).

4.7. Measurement of OH· Formation in the Platelet Suspensions or Fenton Reaction Solution Through Electron Spin Resonance Spectrometry

Electron spin resonance (ESR) spectrometry was performed using a Bruker EMX ESR spectrometer (Bruker, Billerica, MA, USA), as described previously [33]. Suspensions of washed platelets (3.6×10^8 cells/mL) or the Fenton reagent (50 μM $FeSO_4$ + 2 mM H_2O_2) were preincubated with 0.1% DMSO or morin hydrate (40 and 80 μM) for 3 min. Subsequently, collagen (1 μg/mL) was added into platelet suspensions to trigger platelet activation for 5 min. Before ESR spectrometry, 100 μM of DMPO was added to both solutions. ESR spectra were recorded using a quartz flat cell designed for aqueous solutions. The spectrometer was operated under the following conditions: power, 20 mW; frequency, 9.78 GHz; scan range, 100 G; and receiver gain, 5×10^4. The modulation amplitude was 1G, the time constant was 164 ms, and scanning was performed for 42 s; each ESR spectrum obtained was the sum of four scans.

4.8. Measurement of Sodium Fluorescein-Induced Thrombus Formation in Mouse Mesenteric Microvessels

Male ICR mice (aged 6 weeks) were anesthetized using a mixture containing 75% air and 3% isoflurane maintained in 25% oxygen; the mice's external jugular veins were then cannulated with a PE-10 tube for administration of dye and drugs intravenously [34]. Venules (30–40 μm) were irradiated at wavelengths of <520 nm to produce a microthrombus. Two morin hydrate doses (5 and 10 mg/kg) were administered 1 min following sodium fluorescein (15 μg/kg) administration, and the time required for the thrombus to occlude the microvessel (occlusion time) was recorded. In this experiment, the method applied to the thrombogenic animal model conformed to the Guide for the Care and Use of Laboratory Animals (8th edition, 2011), and we received an affidavit of approval for the animal use protocol from Taipei Medical University (LAC-2016-0276; 01/August/2017).

4.9. Measurement of Bleeding Time in Mouse Tail Vein

Bleeding time was measured through transection of the tails of the male ICR mice. In brief, after 30 min of administration of 5 or 10 mg/kg of morin hydrate intraperitoneally, the tails of the mice were cut 3 mm from the tip. The tails were then immediately placed into a tube filled with normal saline at 37 °C to measure the bleeding time, which was recorded until the bleeding completely stopped. In the animal experiments, the method applied to the animal model conformed to the Guide for the Care and Use of Laboratory Animals (8th edition, 2011), and we received an affidavit of approval for the animal use protocol from Taipei Medical University (LAC-2016-0276; 01/August/2017).

4.10. Statistical Analysis

The experimental results are expressed as means ± standard errors of means alongside the number of observations (n); n refers to the number of experiments; each experiment was performed using different blood donors. The unpaired Student's t test was used to determine the significance of differences between control and experimental mice. Differences between groups in other experiments were assessed using an analysis of variance (ANOVA). When the ANOVA results indicated significant differences among group means, the groups were compared using the Student–Newman–Keuls method. A p value of <0.05 indicated statistical significance. Statistical analyses were performed using SAS (version 9.2; SAS Inc., Cary, NC, USA).

5. Conclusions

This paper reports that morin hydrate inhibits collagen-stimulated platelet activation by hindering the PLCγ2–PKC cascade and hydroxyl radical generation and consequently by inhibiting Akt and MAPKs activation. Together these alterations reduce the level of [Ca^{2+}]i and eventually inhibit platelet aggregation. Moreover, morin hydrate does not affect platelet permeability or induce platelet cytolysis. These findings may recommend that morin hydrate establish a novel therapeutic agent for treating thromboembolic disorders.

Author Contributions: J.-R.S. and C.-L.C. perceived the work and planned the experiments. C.-W.H. and M.-P.W. conducted most of the experiments. M.V., C.-H.H., D.-S.C., C.-L.T., C.-Y.H., and T.J. contributed to interpretations and assisted with the manuscript. All authors were involved in editing the manuscript.

Funding: This work was supported by grants from the Ministry of Science and Technology of Taiwan (MOST 104-2622-B-038-003, MOST 104-2320-B-038-045-MY2, MOST 106-2320-B-038-012, MOST 107-2320-B-038-035-MY2), Chi-Mei Medical Center–Taipei Medical University (105CM-TMU-14), and the University Grants Commission of India (MRP-MAJOR-CHEM-2013-5144; 69/2014 F. No. 10-11/12UGC).

Conflicts of Interest: The authors have no competing financial interests to declare.

References

1. Brown, J.; O'Prey, J.; Harrison, P.R. Enhanced sensitivity of human oral tumours to the flavonol, morin, during cancer progression: Involvement of the Akt and stress kinase pathways. *Carcinogenesis* **2003**, *24*, 171–177. [CrossRef] [PubMed]
2. Aggarwal, B.B.; Shishodia, S. Molecular targets of dietary agents for prevention and therapy of cancer. *Biochem. Pharmacol.* **2006**, *7*, 1397–1421. [CrossRef] [PubMed]
3. Lotito, S.B.; Frei, B. Consumption of flavonoid-rich foods and increased plasma antioxidant capacity in humans: Cause, consequence, or epiphenomenon? *Free Radic. Biol. Med.* **2006**, *41*, 1727–1746. [CrossRef] [PubMed]
4. Hanasaki, Y.; Ogawa, S.; Fukui, S. The correlation between active oxygens scavenging and antioxidative effects of flavonoids. *Free Radic. Biol. Med.* **1994**, *16*, 845–850. [CrossRef]
5. Kempuraj, D.; Madhappan, B.; Christodoulou, S.; Boucher, W.; Cao, J.; Papadopoulou, N.; Cetrulo, C.L.; Theoharides, T.C. Flavonols inhibit proinflammatory mediator release, intracellular calcium ion levels and protein kinase C theta phosphorylation in human mast cells. *Br. J. Pharmacol.* **2005**, *145*, 934–944. [CrossRef] [PubMed]
6. Zeng, N.; Tong, B.; Zhang, X.; Dou, Y.; Wu, X.; Xia, Y.; Dai, Y.; Wei, Z.F. Antiarthritis effect of morin is associated with inhibition of synovial angiogenesis. *Drug Dev. Res.* **2015**, *76*, 463–473. [CrossRef] [PubMed]
7. Kawabata, T.; Tanaka, T.; Honjo, S.; Kakumoto, M.; Hara, A.; Makita, H.; Tatematsu, N.; Ushida, T.; Tsuda, H.; Mori, H. Chemopreventive effect of dietary flavonoid morin on chemically induced rat tongue carcinogenesis. *Int. J. Cancer* **1999**, *83*, 381–386. [CrossRef]

8. Peluso, M.R. Flavonoids attenuate cardiovascular disease, inhibit phosphodiesterase, and modulate lipid homeostasis in adipose tissue and liver. *Exp. Biol. Med. (Maywood)* **2006**, *231*, 1287–1299. [CrossRef] [PubMed]
9. Sheu, J.R.; Lee, C.R.; Lin, C.H.; Hsiao, G.; Ko, W.C.; Chen, Y.C. Mechanisms involved in the antiplatelet activity of Staphylococcus aureus lipoteichoic acid in human platelets. *Thromb. Haemost.* **2000**, *83*, 777–784. [PubMed]
10. Tzeng, S.H.; Ko, W.C.; Ko, F.N.; Teng, C.M. Inhibition of platelet aggregation by some flavonoids. *Thromb. Res.* **1991**, *64*, 91–100. [CrossRef]
11. Harrison, P.; Cramer, E.M. Platelet α-granules. *Blood Rev.* **1993**, *7*, 52–62. [CrossRef]
12. Singer, W.D.; Brown, H.A.; Sternweis, P.C. Regulation of eukaryotic phosphatidylinositol-specific phospholipase C and phospholipase D. *Annu. Rev. Biochem.* **1997**, *6*, 475–509. [CrossRef] [PubMed]
13. Woulfe, D.S. Akt signaling in platelet and thrombosis. *Expert Rev. Hematol.* **2010**, *3*, 81–91. [CrossRef] [PubMed]
14. Bugaud, F.; Nadal-Wollbold, F.; Levy-Toledano, S.; Rosa, J.P.; Bryckaert, M. Regulation of c-jun-NH2 terminal kinase and extracellular-signal regulated kinase in human platelets. *Blood* **1999**, *94*, 3800–3805. [PubMed]
15. Niedergang, F.; Alcover, A.; Knight, C.G.; Farndale, R.W.; Barnes, M.J.; Francischetti, I.M.; Bon, C.; Leduc, M. Convulxin binding to platelet receptor GPVI: Competition with collagen related peptides. *Biochem. Biophys. Res. Commun.* **2000**, *273*, 246–250. [CrossRef] [PubMed]
16. Chang, C.H.; Chung, C.H.; Kuo, H.L.; Hsu, C.C.; Huang, T.F. The highly specific platelet glycoprotein (GP) VI agonist trowaglerix impaired collagen-induced platelet aggregation ex vivo through matrix metalloproteinase-dependent GPVI shedding. *J. Thromb. Haemost.* **2008**, *6*, 669–676. [CrossRef] [PubMed]
17. Chung, C.H.; Wu, W.B.; Huang, T.F. Aggretin, a snake venom-derived endothelial integrin alpha 2 beta 1 agonist, induces angiogenesis via expression of vascular endothelial growth factor. *Blood* **2004**, *103*, 2105–2113. [CrossRef] [PubMed]
18. Nieswandt, B.; Watson, S.P. Platelet-collagen interaction: Is GPVI the central receptor? *Blood* **2003**, *102*, 449–461. [CrossRef] [PubMed]
19. Li, Z.; Jiang, H.; Xie, W.; Zhang, Z.; Smrcka, A.V.; Wu, D. Roles of PLC-beta2 and -beta3 and PI3Kgamma in chemoattractant-mediated signal transduction. *Science* **2000**, *287*, 1046–1049. [CrossRef] [PubMed]
20. Wang, Q.J. PKD at the crossroads of DAG and PKC signaling. *Trends Pharmacol. Sci.* **2006**, *27*, 317–323. [CrossRef] [PubMed]
21. Ragab, A.; Séverin, S.; Gratacap, M.P.; Aguado, E.; Malissen, M.; Jandrot-Perrus, M.; Malissen, B.; Ragab-Thomas, J.; Payrastre, B. Roles of the C-terminal tyrosine residues of LAT in GP VI-induced platelet activation: Insights into the mechanism of PLC gamma 2 activation. *Blood* **2007**, *110*, 2466–2474. [CrossRef] [PubMed]
22. Borsig, L.; Wong, R.; Feramisco, J.; Nadeau, D.R.; Varki, N.M.; Varki, A. Heparin and cancer revisited: Mechanistic connections involving platelets, P-selectin, carcinoma mucins, and tumor metastasis. *Proc. Natl. Acad. Sci. USA* **2001**, *98*, 3352–3357. [CrossRef] [PubMed]
23. Kaibuchi, K.; Sano, K.; Hoshijima, M.; Takai, Y.; Nishizuka, Y. Phosphatidylinositol turnover in platelet activation; calcium mobilization and protein phosphorylation. *Cell Calcium* **1982**, *3*, 323–335. [CrossRef]
24. Chang, L.; Karin, M. Mammalian MAP kinase signaling cascades. *Nature* **2001**, *410*, 37–40. [CrossRef] [PubMed]
25. Adam, F.; Kauskot, A.; Rosa, J.P.; Bryckaert, M. Mitogen-activated protein kinases in hemostasis and thrombosis. *J. Thromb. Haemost.* **2008**, *6*, 2007–2016. [CrossRef] [PubMed]
26. Adam, F.; Kauskot, A.; Nurden, P.; Sulpice, E.; Hoylaerts, M.F.; Davis, R.J.; Rosa, J.P.; Bryckaert, M. Platelet JNK1 is involved in secretion and thrombus formation. *Blood* **2010**, *115*, 4083–4092. [CrossRef] [PubMed]
27. Canobbio, I.; Reineri, S.; Sinigaglia, F.; Balduini, C.; Torti, M. A role for p38 MAP kinase in platelet activation by von Willebrand factor. *Thromb. Haemost.* **2004**, *91*, 102–110. [CrossRef] [PubMed]
28. Chen, J.; De, S.; Damron, D.S.; Chen, W.S.; Hay, N.; Byzova, T.V. Impaired platelet responses to thrombin and collagen in AKT-1-deficient mice. *Blood* **2004**, *104*, 1703–1710. [CrossRef] [PubMed]
29. Jayakumar, T.; Chen, W.F.; Lu, W.J.; Chou, D.S.; Hsiao, G.; Hsu, C.Y.; Sheu, J.R.; Hsieh, C.Y. A novel antithrombotic effect of sulforaphane via activation of platelet adenylate cyclase: Ex vivo and in vivo studies. *J. Nutr. Biochem.* **2013**, *24*, 1086–1095. [CrossRef] [PubMed]

30. Wachowicz, B.; Olas, B.; Zbikowska, H.M.; Buczyński, A. Generation of reactive oxygen species in blood platelets. *Platelets* **2002**, *13*, 175–182. [CrossRef] [PubMed]
31. Zhang, R.; Kang, K.A.; Piao, M.J.; Maeng, Y.H.; Lee, K.H.; Chang, W.Y.; You, H.J.; Kim, J.S.; Kang, S.S.; Hyun, J.W. Cellular protection of morin against the oxidative stress induced by hydrogen peroxide. *Chem. Biol. Interact.* **2009**, *177*, 21–27. [CrossRef] [PubMed]
32. Liu, S.; Wu, N.; Miao, J.; Huang, Z.; Li, X.; Jia, P.; Guo, Y.; Jia, D. Protective effect of morin on myocardial ischemia/reperfusion injury in rats. *Int. J. Mol. Med.* **2018**, *42*, 1379–1390. [CrossRef] [PubMed]
33. Chou, D.S.; Hsiao, G.; Shen, M.Y.; Tsai, Y.J.; Chen, T.F.; Sheu, J.R. ESR spin trapping of a carbon-centered free radical from agonist-stimulated human platelets. *Free Radic. Biol. Med.* **2005**, *39*, 237–248. [CrossRef] [PubMed]
34. Hsiao, G.; Lin, K.H.; Chang, Y.; Chen, T.L.; Tzu, N.H.; Chou, D.S.; Sheu, J.R. Protective mechanisms of inosine in platelet activation and cerebral ischemic damage. *Arterioscler. Thromb. Vasc. Biol.* **2005**, *25*, 1998–2004. [CrossRef] [PubMed]

International Journal of
Molecular Sciences

MDPI

Article

Synthesis and Spectrum of Biological Activities of Novel *N*-arylcinnamamides

Sarka Pospisilova [1,2], Jiri Kos [1,*], Hana Michnova [1,2], Iva Kapustikova [1], Tomas Strharsky [1], Michal Oravec [3], Agnes M. Moricz [4], Jozsef Bakonyi [4], Tereza Kauerova [5], Peter Kollar [5], Alois Cizek [2] and Josef Jampilek [1]

1 Department of Pharmaceutical Chemistry, Faculty of Pharmacy, Comenius University, Odbojarov 10, 83232 Bratislava, Slovakia; sharka.pospisilova@gmail.com (S.P.); michnova.hana@gmail.com (H.M.); kapustikova@fpharm.uniba.sk (I.K.); strharsky2@uniba.sk (T.S.); josef.jampilek@gmail.com (J.J.)

2 Department of Infectious Diseases and Microbiology, Faculty of Veterinary Medicine, University of Veterinary and Pharmaceutical Sciences, Palackeho 1, 61242 Brno, Czech Republic; cizeka@vfu.cz

3 Global Change Research Institute CAS, Belidla 986/4a, 60300 Brno, Czech Republic; oravec.m@czechglobe.cz

4 Plant Protection Institute, Centre for Agricultural Research, Hungarian Academy of Sciences, Herman Otto Str. 15, 1022 Budapest, Hungary; moricz.agnes@agrar.mta.hu (A.M.M.); bakonyi.jozsef@agrar.mta.hu (J.B.)

5 Department of Human Pharmacology and Toxicology, Faculty of Pharmacy, University of Veterinary and Pharmaceutical Sciences, Palackeho 1, 61242 Brno, Czech Republic; tereza.kauerova@gmail.com (T.K.); kollarp@vfu.cz (P.K.)

* Correspondence: jirikos85@gmail.com; Tel.: +421-2-5011-7224

Received: 9 July 2018; Accepted: 3 August 2018; Published: 7 August 2018

Abstract: A series of sixteen ring-substituted *N*-arylcinnamamides was prepared and characterized. Primary in vitro screening of all the synthesized compounds was performed against *Staphylococcus aureus*, three methicillin-resistant *S. aureus* strains, *Mycobacterium tuberculosis* H37Ra, *Fusarium avenaceum*, and *Bipolaris sorokiniana*. Several of the tested compounds showed antistaphylococcal, antitubercular, and antifungal activities comparable with or higher than those of ampicillin, isoniazid, and benomyl. (2*E*)-*N*-[3,5-bis(trifluoromethyl)phenyl]-3-phenylprop-2-enamide and (2*E*)-3-phenyl-*N*-[3-(trifluoromethyl)phenyl]prop-2-enamide showed the highest activities (MICs = 22.27 and 27.47 µM, respectively) against all four staphylococcal strains and against *M. tuberculosis*. These compounds showed an activity against biofilm formation of *S. aureus* ATCC 29213 in concentrations close to MICs and an ability to increase the activity of clinically used antibiotics with different mechanisms of action (vancomycin, ciprofloxacin, and tetracycline). In time-kill studies, a decrease of CFU/mL of >99% after 8 h from the beginning of incubation was observed. (2*E*)-*N*-(3,5-Dichlorophenyl)- and (2*E*)-*N*-(3,4-dichlorophenyl)-3-phenylprop-2-enamide had a MIC = 27.38 µM against *M. tuberculosis*, while a significant decrease (22.65%) of mycobacterial cell metabolism determined by the MTT assay was observed for the 3,5-dichlorophenyl derivative. (2*E*)-*N*-(3-Fluorophenyl)- and (2*E*)-*N*-(3-methylphenyl)-3-phenylprop-2-enamide exhibited MICs = 16.58 and 33.71 µM, respectively, against *B. sorokiniana*. The screening of the cytotoxicity of the most effective antimicrobial compounds was performed using THP-1 cells, and these chosen compounds did not shown any significant lethal effect. The compounds were also evaluated for their activity related to the inhibition of photosynthetic electron transport (PET) in spinach (*Spinacia oleracea* L.) chloroplasts. (2*E*)-*N*-(3,5-dichlorophenyl)-3-phenylprop-2-enamide (IC_{50} = 5.1 µM) was the most active PET inhibitor. Compounds with fungicide potency did not show any in vivo toxicity against *Nicotiana tabacum* var. Samsun. The structure–activity relationships are discussed.

Keywords: cinnamamides; antistaphylococcal activity; time-kill assay; biofilm; antitubercular activity; MTT assay; antifungal activity; PET inhibition; toxicity; structure–activity relationship

1. Introduction

Cinnamic acids and other hydroxy- or phenyl-substituted derivatives of cinnamic acids have been widely investigated by scientists due to their significant and varied biological effects. Cinnamic acids occur naturally in all plants [1]. They are formed in the biochemical pathway providing phenyl-propanoids, coumarins, lignans, isoflavonoids, flavonoids, stilbenes, aurones, anthocyanins, spermidines, and tannins [2]. The spectrum of their biological activities include anti-inflammatory, antioxidant, hepatoprotective, antidiabetic, antidepressant/anxiolytic, antifungal, antibacterial, antiviral, and anticancer effects [3–16]. Derivatives of cinnamic acids are used as agriculture fungicides as well [17].

The adaptation of microorganisms to external influences and, thus, the development of their resistance against antimicrobial agents is not a surprise; unfortunately, this process is faster and faster. Thus, the emerging resistance of microbial pathogens to clinically used drugs, including second- and third-choice drugs, and the development of cross-resistant or multidrug-resistant strains are alarming. Microbial pathogens have developed a number of mechanisms to adapt to the effects of the environment. In addition, the increase in the number of infections and the occurrence of new, especially opportunistic species are also caused by the general immunosuppression of patients, and this fact makes these diseases extremely serious. Since the 1990s, only an inconsiderable number of really new drugs for systemic administration have been marketed for the treatment of infections, although the discovery of new molecules has been a priority [18].

Thus, in the light of the above mentioned facts, new simple anilides of cinnamic acid were designed as antimicrobial multitarget agents, synthesized using a modern microwave-assisted method and screened against a battery of bacterial/mycobacterial and fungal pathogens. These compounds were designed based on the experience with naphthalenecarboxamides—simple molecules with a number of biological activities, and in fact, the new ring-substituted (2*E*)-*N*-phenyl-3-phenylprop-2-enamides can be considered as open analogues of recently described naphthalene-2-carboxanilides [19,20].

As an amide moiety is able to affect photosystem II (PS II) by reversible binding [21], resulting in the interruption of the photosynthetic electron transport (PET) [22–24], and can be found in many herbicides acting as photosynthesis inhibitors [25–30], these *N*-arylcinnamamides were additionally tested on the inhibition of PET in spinach (*Spinacia oleracea* L.) chloroplasts using the Hill reaction. The idea of this screening is based on the fact that both drugs and pesticides are designed to target particular biological functions. These functions/effects may overlap at the molecular level, which causes a considerable structural similarity between drugs and pesticides. Since different classes of herbicides are able to bind to different mammalian cellular receptors, the majority of pharmaceutical companies have pesticide divisions, and developed biologically active agents are investigated as both pesticides and drugs. Previously, several successful pesticides became pharmaceuticals and vice versa [31–35].

2. Results and Discussion

2.1. Chemistry and Physicochemical Properties

All the studied compounds **1–16** were prepared according to Scheme 1. The carboxyl group of starting cinnamic acid was activated with phosphorus trichloride. In the reaction with an appropriate ring-substituted aniline, the generated acyl chloride subsequently gave the final amide in dry chlorobenzene via microwave-assisted synthesis. All the compounds were recrystallized from ethanol.

Many different molecular parameters/descriptors are used to determine structure-activity relationships (SAR). Lipophilicity and electronic properties are among the most frequent ones. Hammett's σ parameters were used for the description of electronic properties. They were calculated for the whole substituted anilide ring using ACD/Percepta ver. 2012 (Advanced Chemistry Development Inc., Toronto, ON, Canada, 2012), see Table 1. The lipophilicity of the studied compounds was predicted as log *P* using ACD/Percepta software and Clog *P* using ChemBioDraw Ultra 13.0 (CambridgeSoft, PerkinElmer Inc., Cambridge, MA, USA). Log *P* is the logarithm of the partition coefficient for *n*-octanol/water. Clog *P* is the logarithm of *n*-octanol/water partition coefficient based on the established chemical interactions. In addition, the lipophilicity of studied compounds **1–16** was investigated by means of reversed-phase high-performance liquid chromatography (RP-HPLC) determination of capacity factors *k* with the subsequent calculation of log *k* [36]. The analysis was made under isocratic conditions with methanol as an organic modifier in the mobile phase using an end-capped nonpolar C18 stationary RP column. The results are shown in Table 1.

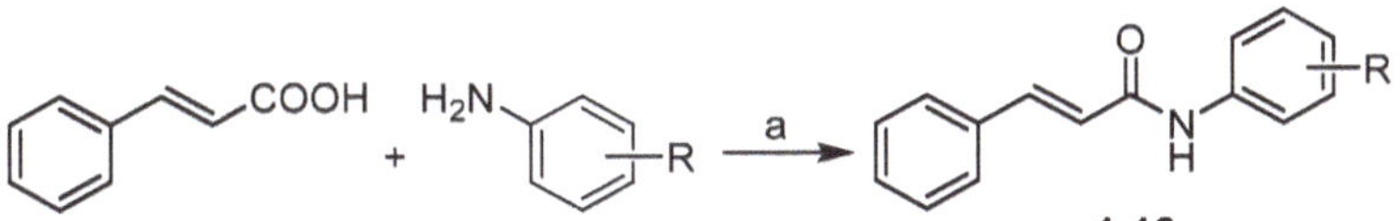

Scheme 1. Synthesis of (2*E*)-*N*-aryl-3-phenylprop-2-enamides **1–16**. Reagents and conditions: (a) PCl_3, chlorobenzene, and MW.

Table 1. Structure of ring-substituted (2*E*)-*N*-aryl-3-phenylprop-2-enamides **1–16**, experimentally determined values of lipophilicity log *k*, calculated values of log *P*/Clog *P*, and electronic Hammett's σ parameters.

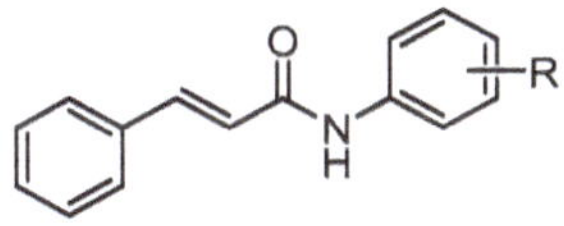

Comp.	R	log *k*	Clog *P* [a]	log *P* [b]	σ_{Ar} [b]
1	H	0.1146	3.6640	3.18	0.60
2	3-CH_3	0.2729	4.1630	3.40	0.48
3	4-CH_3	0.2640	4.1630	3.40	0.46
4	2-F	0.1330	3.4646	3.17	1.02
5	3-F	0.2327	4.0646	3.32	0.82
6	3-CF_3	0.4859	4.9978	4.26	0.89
7	2,5-CH_3	0.2691	4.0120	3.57	0.59
8	2,5-Cl	0.5799	4.5878	4.65	1.22
9	2,6-Cl	0.0632	3.7378	4.56	1.33
10	3,4-Cl	0.6821	5.3178	4.70	1.19
11	3,5-Cl	0.8155	5.4378	4.79	1.11
12	2,6-Br	0.0992	3.9778	4.80	1.33
13	3,5-CF_3	0.9814	6.0386	5.68	1.05
14	2-F-5-Br	0.4875	4.4178	4.07	1.28
15	2-Br-5-F	0.4588	4.1378	4.12	1.19
16	2-Cl-5-CF_3	0.6178	4.9509	4.88	1.19

[a] calculated using ChemBioDraw Ultra 13.0; [b] calculated using ACD/Percepta ver. 2012.

The results obtained with the discussed compounds show that the experimentally-determined lipophilicities (log *k*) are in accordance with the calculated Clog *P* values as illustrated in Figure 1A; correlation coefficient $r = 0.9513$, $n = 16$. On the other hand, log *P* values calculated by ACD/Percepta show differences for compounds **9** (2,6-Cl) and **12** (2,6-Br), see Figure 1B. When these two compounds are excluded, $r = 0.9774$ ($n = 14$) is observed. This poor match for 2,6-disubstituted anilides **9** and **12** may be caused by intramolecular interactions that are probably caused by the steric effect of spatially-close moieties, which was not included in prediction by ACD/Percepta. The proximity of the di-*ortho*-substituents to the carboxamide group on the aniline ring leads to the twist of the aniline ring plane towards the carboxamide group, i.e., to the plane of the benzene ring of cinnamic acid. The described process resulted in the planarity violation of the molecule. Otherwise, (2*E*)-*N*-[3,5-bis(trifluoromethyl)phenyl]-3-phenylprop-2-enamide (**13**) is the most lipophilic, while compounds **9**, **12** and *N*-phenylcinnamamide (**1**) are characterized by the lowest lipophilicity. It can be stated that log *k* values specify lipophilicity within the series of the studied compounds.

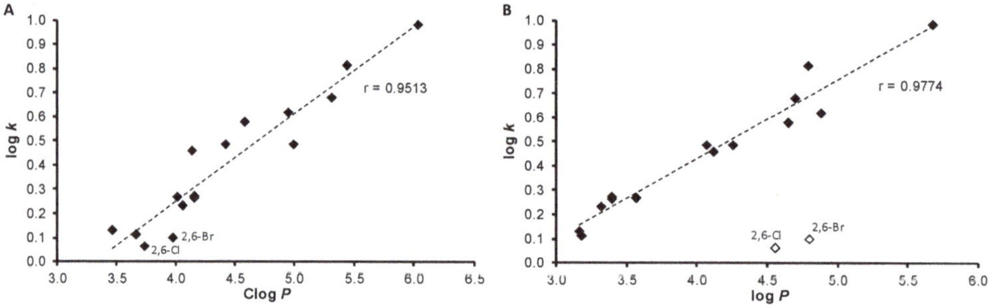

Figure 1. Comparison of experimentally found log *k* values of ring-substituted *N*-arylcinnamamides **1–16** with Clog *P* calculated using ChemBioDraw Ultra (**A**) and log *P* calculated using ACD/Percepta (**B**).

2.2. *In Vitro Antibacterial Susceptibility Testing*

All the cinnamanilides were tested on their antistaphylococcal activity against three clinical isolates of methicillin-resistant *Staphylococcus aureus* (MRSA) [37,38] and *S. aureus* ATCC 29213 as the reference and quality control strain. Although various derivatives of cinnamic acid were described as promising antibacterial agents [4–6,8,9,14,15], the compounds showed only limited activity (MICs > 256 µg/mL), except for (2*E*)-3-phenyl-*N*-[3-(trifluoromethyl)phenyl]prop-2-enamide (**6**) and 3,5-bis(trifluoromethyl)phenyl derivative **13**, see Table 2. As minimum inhibitory concentrations (MICs) of these compounds are the same against the reference and the MRSA strains (27.47 and 22.27 µM, respectively), it can be speculated about the specific effectivity against *Staphylococcus* sp. These compounds were also tested against *Enterococcus faecalis* ATCC 29212 as the reference strain and three isolates from American crows of vanA-carrying vancomycin-resistant *E. faecalis* (VRE) [39] but without any effect in the tested concentrations, which may indicate a specific mechanism of action [37,40]. From Table 2 it is obvious that compounds **6** and **13** exhibited activities comparable with those of the standards. Due to the small number of active compounds, no SAR could be established.

2.2.1. Synergy Effect with Clinically Used Drugs against MRSA

The most effective compounds **6** and **13** were tested for their ability of synergic activity with clinically used antibacterial drugs tetracycline, ciprofloxacin, and vancomycin. These antibiotics have different mechanisms of actions and different mechanisms of resistance to them, thus the prospective synergism could give an idea of the mechanism of action of the cinnamic derivatives. The investigation of synergistic activity was performed according to the methodology [41]. The method of fractional inhibitory concentration (FIC) was used [42]. For all the wells of the microtitration plates that corresponded to a MIC value, the sum of the FICs (ΣFIC) was calculated for each well, using the equation $\Sigma FIC = FIC_A + FIC_B = (C_A/MIC_A) + (C_B/MIC_B)$, where MIC_A and MIC_B are the MICs of drugs A and B alone, respectively, and C_A and C_B are the concentrations of the drugs in the combination, respectively [42]. Synergy was defined as a ΣFIC ≤ 0.5; additivity was defined as 0.5 < ΣFIC < 1; indifference was defined as 1 ≤ ΣFIC < 4; and antagonism was defined as ΣFIC ≥ 4 [41]. As the FIC index was evaluated for every single well corresponding to the MIC value, the results are presented as a range. The test was made with all 3 methicillin-resistant isolates, MRSA 63718, SA 3202, and SA 630. The isolates were also resistant to used antibiotics. Note that isolate MRSA SA 630 is susceptible to tetracycline. The results are mentioned in Table 3.

Table 2. Structure of ring-substituted (2*E*)-*N*-aryl-3-phenylprop-2-enamides **1–16**, IC_{50} (μM) values related to PET inhibition in spinach chloroplasts in comparison with 3-(3,4-dichlorophenyl)-1,1-dimethylurea (DCMU) standard, in vitro anti-*Staphylococcus* activities MIC (μM) in comparison with standard ampicillin (AMP), in vitro antitubercular activity MIC (μM (μg/mL)) in comparison with standard isoniazid (INH), in vitro antifungal activity MIC (μM (μg/mL)) of compounds **1–16** compared to standard benomyl (BNM), and in vitro antiproliferative (Tox) assay (IC_{50} (μM)) of chosen compounds compared to standard camptothecin (CMP).

Comp.	R	MIC (μM (μg/mL))							Tox IC_{50} (μM)	PET IC_{50} (μM)
		SA	MRSA 63718	MRSA SA 630	MRSA SA 3202	Mtb	FA	BS		
1	H	>1146 (>256)	>1146 (>256)	>1146 (>256)	>1146 (>256)	286 (64)	1146 (256)	143 (32)	–	250
2	3-CH_3	>1078 (>256)	>1078 (>256)	>1078 (>256)	>1078 (>256)	67.43 (16)	270 (64)	33.71 (8)	>30	343
3	4-CH_3	>1078 (>256)	>1078 (>256)	>1078 (>256)	>1078 (>256)	134 (32)	1078 (256)	539 (128)	–	320
4	2-F	>1061 (>256)	>1061 (>256)	>1061 (>256)	>1061 (>256)	265 (64)	1061 (256)	66.32 (16)	–	223
5	3-F	>1061 (>256)	>1061 (>256)	>1061 (>256)	>1061 (>256)	66.31 (16)	531 (128)	16.58 (4)	>30	165
6	3-CF_3	27.47 (8)	27.47 (8)	27.47 (8)	27.47 (8)	27.47 (8)	54.93 (16)	54.93 (16)	22.72 ± 1.73	189
7	2,5-CH_3	>1018 (>256)	>1018 (>256)	>1018 (>256)	>1018 (>256)	254 (64)	1019 (256)	1019 (256)	–	338
8	2,5-Cl	>876 (>256)	>876 (>256)	>876 (>256)	>876 (>256)	876 (256)	876 (256)	876 (256)	–	67.1
9	2,6-Cl	>876 (>256)	>876 (>256)	>876 (>256)	>876 (>256)	876 (256)	876 (256)	876 (256)	–	1380
10	3,4-Cl	438 (128)	876 (256)	438 (128)	876 (256)	27.38 (8)	219 (64)	110 (32)	29.81 ± 0.31	54.9
11	3,5-Cl	438 (128)	876 (256)	109 (64)	438 (128)	27.38 (8)	219 (64)	110 (32)	29.44 ± 1.73	5.1
12	2,6-Br	>671 (256)	>671 (256)	>671 (256)	>671 (256)	167 (64)	671 (256)	671 (256)	–	732
13	3,5-CF_3	22.27 (8)	22.27 (8)	22.27 (8)	22.27 (8)	22.27 (8))	713 (256)	356 (128)	22.59 ± 1.88	111
14	2-F-5-Br	>799 (>256)	>799 (>256)	>799 (>256)	>799 (>256)	199 (64)	799 (256)	49.98 (16)	–	188
15	2-Br-5-F	>799 (>256)	>799 (>256)	>799 (>256)	>799 (>256)	199 (64)	799 (256)	799 (256)	–	205
16	2-Cl-5-CF_3	>785 (>256)	>785 (>256)	>785 (>256)	>785 (>256)	785 (256)	785 (256)	785 (256)	–	63.2
AMP	–	5.72 (2)	45.81 (16)	45.81 (16)	45.81 (16)	–	–	–	–	–
INH	–	–	–	–	–	36.55 (5)	–	–	–	–
BNM	–	–	–	–	–	–	1.94 (0.5)	17.22 (5)	–	–
CMP	–	–	–	–	–	–	–	–	0.16 ± 0.07	–
DCMU	–	–	–	–	–	–	–	–	–	2.1

SA = *Staphylococcus aureus* ATCC 29213; MRSA = clinical isolates of methicillin-resistant *S. aureus* 63718, SA 630, and SA 3202 (National Institute of Public Health, Prague, Czech Republic); Mtb = *Mycobacterium tuberculosis* H37Ra; FA = *Fusarium avenaceum* (Fr.) Sacc. IMI 319947; BS = *Bipolaris sorokiniana* (Sacc.) Shoemaker H-299 (NCBI GenBank accession No. MH697869).

Table 3. Combined effect of most potent *N*-arylcinnamamides and tetracycline (TET), ciprofloxacin (CPX), and vancomycin (VAN).

Isolate	Combination of Compds.	Separate MIC (µg/mL)	FIC Index	Concentration (µg/mL) Causing Synergistic Effect	Concentration (µg/mL) Causing Additive Effect
MRSA 63718	**6**/TET	8/128	1.004–2.250	–	2/64; 8/32
	6/CPX	16/16	0.75–1.125	–	8/4; 4/8
	6/VAN	32/2	1.000–1.250	–	–
MRSA SA 3202	**6**/TET	16/64	1.002–1.25	–	–
	6/CPX	8/8	1.000–1.250	–	–
	6/VAN	8/1	0.750–1.256	–	4/0.25
	13/TET	32/64	0.500–1.125	8/16	16/16; 4/32; 2/64
	13/CPX	32/8	0.375–1.250	8/1	2/4
	13/VAN	32/1	0.750–1.25	–	16/0.25
MRSA SA 630	**6**/CPX	8/256	0.625–1.125	–	4/64; 1/128
	6/VAN	8/1	0.750–1.250	–	2/0.5
	13/CPX	8/256	0.375–1.004	2/32; 1/64	4/8
	13/VAN	4/1	0.562–1.250	–	0.25/0.5

Although the activity of cinnamic acid derivatives is known for a long time, the exact mechanism of action is still unknown. The most reported mechanism of action is interaction with plasmatic membrane. The compounds can cause disruption of the membrane, damage the membrane proteins, etc. [43–46]. There are also specific targets for cinnamic acid derivatives [46]. Nevertheless, it is possible that the wide spectrum of effects to cells is caused by the primary activity of the compounds, which is membrane destabilization [46].

Both compounds 6 and 13 tested for synergy showed additivity with vancomycin against MRSA SA 630 and SA 3202. A similar effect was reported by Hemaiswarya et al. [47]; compound 13 had synergistic effect with ciprofloxacin against both tested strains. The effect of derivative 13 was also synergistic with tetracycline against MRSA SA 3202. The rest combinations with compound 13 had additive effect. Whereas compound 13 had a potential to increase the activity of all tested antibiotics, which have different mechanisms of actions and to which bacteria develop different resistance mechanisms, it can be expected that compound 13 acts by its own mechanism of action or increases the availability of the antibiotics by interaction with the membrane.

2.2.2. Dynamics of Antibacterial Activity

Within the pre-test subcultivation aliquots on agar, antistaphylococcal-effective compounds **6** and **13** showed bactericidal activity, i.e., minimal bactericidal concentrations were $\leq 4\times$ MIC. These facts were verified using the time-kill curve assay for testing the bactericidal effect. The dynamics of antibacterial activity was tested against *S. aureus* ATCC 29213 for the most active compounds **6** (Figure 2A) and **13** (Figure 2B). Both compounds showed concentration-dependent activity that was bactericidal in concentration $4\times$ MIC in the case of compound **13** or very close to the bactericidal level for compound **6** after 8 h from the beginning of incubation. The increase of bacterial growth at 24 h could be caused by the selection of resistant mutants, as observed previously [37].

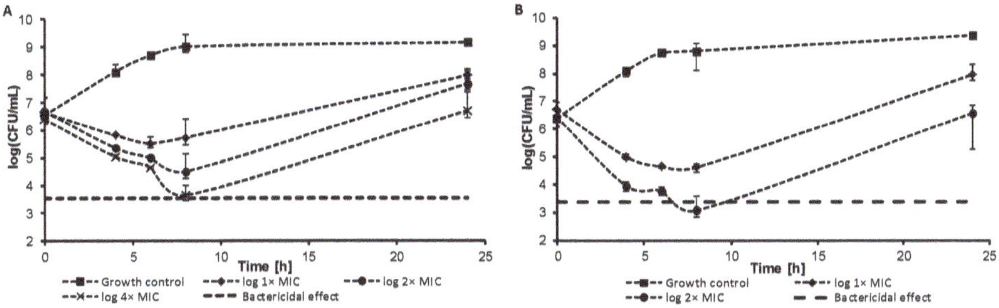

Figure 2. Time-kill curve of compound **6** (**A**) and compound **13** (**B**) against *S. aureus* ATCC 29213.

2.2.3. Inhibition of Bofilm Formation

There are many evidences in literature that cinnamic acid derivatives are inhibitors of biofilm formation [47–51]. The most studied derivate is cinnamaldehyde that interacts with quorum sensing system in bacterial biofilms [46,52,53]. Thus, selected compounds were also tested for their ability to inhibit biofilm formation. Compounds **6** and **13** were tested as inhibitors of biofilm formation against *S. aureus* ATCC 29213. MRSA strains were not producers of biofilm.

The activity of compound **6** does not depend on concentration in concentrations above 8 μg/mL; only the highest concentration showed lower inhibition effect. This could be caused the higher lipophilicity of the compound and potential formation of precipitates, which could decrease the antibacterial activity of the compound. The lowest concentration of the compound, which inhibited ≥80% of biofilm formation, was 8 μg/mL, then the activity sharply decreased. Interestingly, on the other hand, concentrations of compound **13** close to MIC against planktonic cells had the lowest inhibition activities against biofilm forming, and the activity increased for sub-MIC values. These conditions could be potentially toxic for planktonic cells, but they can induce biofilm formation [54]. In general, the inhibition activity against biofilm formation was comparable with the activity against planktonic cells. Despite many studies reported a higher resistance of biofilm, there were also studies that proved a similar or only little lower antibiofilm activity of tested compounds compared to planktonic cells. [13,55]. Budzynska et al. [55] described high antibiofilm activity of plant essential oils compared to MICs. De Vita et al. [13] studied the activity of cinnamic acid derivatives against candida biofilm. These compounds had good effect against biofilm formation, and the effective concentrations were lower than 10× MIC. Thus, the high activity of our compounds can be explained due to their structure, based on cinnamic acid.

Ampicillin (16–0.125 μg/mL), vancomycin (32–0.25 μg/mL), and ciprofloxacin (8–0.063 μg/mL) were used as positive controls. Ciprofloxacin and vancomycin caused the induction of biofilm formation in sub-MIC concentrations, which is in line with already published results [56,57]. All the results are shown in Figure 3.

2.3. *In Vitro Antitubercular Activity*

The evaluation of the in vitro antitubercular activity of the compounds was performed against *Mycobacterium tuberculosis* ATCC 25177/H37Ra, see Table 2. In order to reduce risks, a replacement of model pathogens is commonly used in basic laboratory screening. For *M. tuberculosis*, avirulent strain H37Ra is used that has a similar pathology as *M. tuberculosis* strains infecting humans and, thus, represents a good model for testing antitubercular agents [58]. The potency of the compounds was expressed as the MIC that is defined for mycobacteria as 90% or greater (IC_{90}) reduction of growth in comparison with the control.

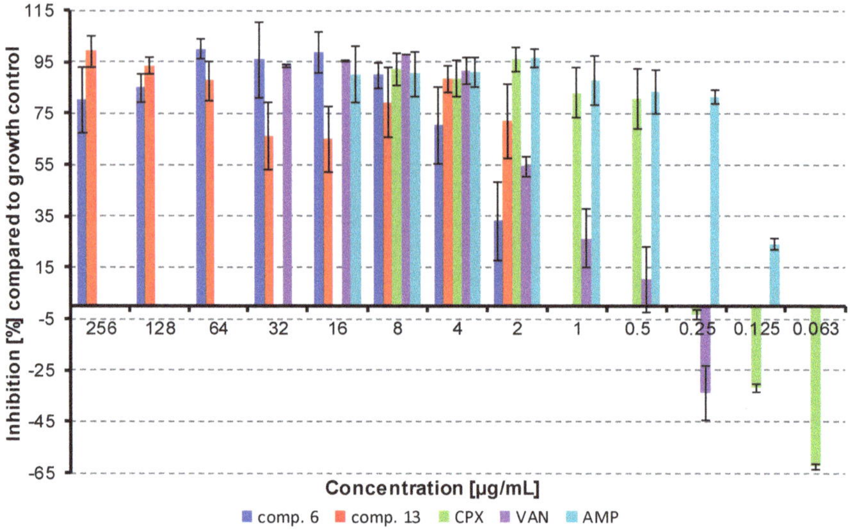

Figure 3. Inhibition of bacterial film formation. (CPX = ciprofloxacin, AMP = ampicillin, VAN = vancomycin).

In comparison with antibacterial activities, the investigated compounds exhibited much higher effect against *M. tuberculosis*. Compounds **13** (R = 3,5-CF_3), **10** (R = 3,4-Cl), **11** (R = 3,5-Cl), and **6** (R = 3-CF_3) were the most effective; their activity ranged from 22.27 to 27.47 µM. The dependences of the antitubercular activity of the compounds against *M. tuberculosis* expressed as log (1/MIC (M)) on lipophilicity expressed as log *k* are illustrated in Figure 4A. When inactive compounds **8** (R = 2,5-Cl), **9** (R = 2,6-Cl), and **16** (R = 2-Cl-5-CF_3) are eliminated from the SAR study (illustrated by empty symbols), two different dependences in relation to the position and the type of substituents can be observed. Based on Figure 4A, it can be stated that compounds substituted in positions $C_{(3)}'$, $C_{(3,4)}'$, $C_{(3,5)}'$, or $C_{(2,6)}'$ showed an increasing trend of activity with the lipophilicity increase up to compound **6** (R = 3-CF_3), at which the activity achieved plateau and from approximately $\log k \approx 0.5$ had an insignificant increase. The second, in fact, a linear, insignificantly increasing dependence can be found for the compounds substituted in positions $C_{(2)}'$ and $C_{(2,5)}'$. It is important to note that the antitubercular activity of the discussed cinnamanilides is also dependent on electronic σ parameters, see Figure 4B. As mentioned above, the linear insignificantly increasing dependence can be found for the derivatives substituted on the anilide in positions $C_{(2)}'$ and $C_{(2,5)}'$, while a bilinear dependence of activity on σ (for derivatives substituted in positions $C_{(3)}'$, $C_{(3,4)}'$, $C_{(3,5)}'$, and $C_{(2,6)}'$) can be observed. The activity increases with the increasing electron-withdrawing effect with $r = 0.8803$ ($n = 5$) to optimum σ_{Ar} ca. 1 (compound **13**, R = 3,5-CF_3) and then decreases ($r = 0.9162$, $n = 4$) with increasing values of the electron-withdrawing parameter.

Additionally, a standard MTT (3-(4,5-dimethylthiazol-2-yl)-2,5-diphenyltetrazolium bromide) assay was performed on selected compounds that were the most effective against *M. tuberculosis* H37Ra and the MICs of which were previously determined, see Table 2. The MTT test can be used to assess cell growth by measuring respiration. The MTT measured viability of *M. tuberculosis* H37Ra less than 70% after exposure to the MIC values for each test agent is considered as a positive result of this assay. This low level of cell viability indicates inhibition of cell growth by inhibition of respiration [59]. All the selected compounds, i.e., **6** (R = 3-CF_3, 40.99%), **10** (R = 3,4-Cl, 59.65%), **11** (R = 3,5-Cl, 22.65%), and **13** (R = 3,5-CF_3, 66.09%) showed less than 70% viability of *M. tuberculosis* H37Ra at the tested concentration equal to MICs (i.e., 8 µg/mL or 22 and 27 µM). At MIC = 16 µg/mL (33 µM) compound

2 (R = 3-CH_3) showed inhibition of viability 13.23%, and compound **5** (R = 3-F) showed inhibition of viability 11.04% at MIC = 32 μg/mL (33 μM).

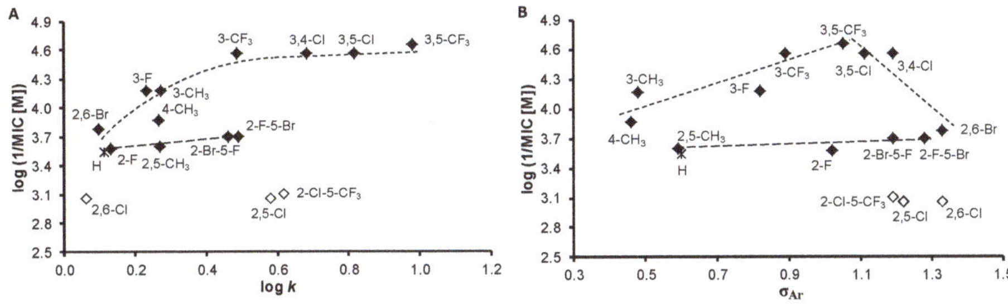

Figure 4. Relationships between in vitro antitubercular activity against *M. tuberculosis* log (1/MIC (M)) and lipophilicity expressed as log *k* (**A**) and electronic Hammett's σ parameters of ring-substituted anilide ring (**B**) of studied compounds. (Derivatives excluded from SAR are illustrated by empty symbols.).

Similar effects were observed previously, for example, with ring-substituted 6-hydroxynaphthalene-2-carboxanilides, where 3-Cl, 4-Cl, 3-Br, and 3-CF_3 substituted derivatives decreased the viability of *M. tuberculosis* H37Ra in the range from 41.2% to 46.5% at the lowest tested concentration (MICs = 8 μg/mL) [20], with 8-hydroxy-*N*-(3-trifluoromethylphenyl)quinoline-2-carboxamide, where the decrease of the viability of *M. tuberculosis* H37Ra was to 18.8% at MIC = 8 μg/mL [60], and with *N*-alkoxyphenylhydroxynaphthalenecarboxanilides substituted in $C_{(3)}'$ position of the anilide core by a longer alkoxy tail [61,62]. Since the MTT assay was positive, it can be stated that the tested compounds caused a decrease of mycobacterial cell metabolism. Thus, based on the structure analogy of (2*E*)-*N*-aryl-3-phenylprop-2-enamides with naphthalene-2-carboxanilides, it may be hypothesized that the mechanism of action of these ring-substituted anilides of cinnamic acid could be connected with the affection of mycobacterial energy metabolism [59,63–66]; nevertheless, another possible site of action of the studied compounds in the mycobacteria cannot be excluded [67–70].

2.4. *In Vitro Activity against Plant Pathogenic Fungi*

Fungal infections are not only a problem in human and veterinary medicine, but also an important problem in agriculture. Plants diseases in general are a major factor limiting the crop quality. Fungal pathogens cause production losses and also can product mycotoxins, which are dangerous for consumers. The widespread use of fungicides increases food availability and safety, but it can leads to the selection of resistant pathogens and an increase of the production of mycotoxins [71]. As cinnamic acid and its derivatives do not have only antibacterial and antimycobacterial activity, but also activity against plant pathogens [7,72], all the prepared compounds were tested for their potency against *Fusarium avenaceum* (Fr.) Sacc. IMI 319947 and *Bipolaris sorokiniana* (Sacc.) Shoemaker H-299. *B. sorokiniana* is a wide-spread wheat and barley pathogen. It causes many diseases, such as head blight, seedling blight, common root rot, spot blotch, etc. [73]. The last one is a big problem, especially in Southern Asia, where 20% of crop yield is lost because of leaf blight disease [74]. *F. avenaceum* is one of the most common *Fusarium* species causing head blight disease of cereals. It can be isolated from cereal seeds and feed products [75]. *Fusarium* spp. produces a wide spectrum of mycotoxins. The most important are the trichothecenes, zearalenone, moniifromin, and the fumonisins. These compounds have toxic effect on humans and animals [76].

Only compound **6** (R = 3-CF_3) showed moderate activity (MIC = 54.93 μM) against *F. avenaceum* within the series of compounds, see Table 2. On the other hand, the investigated compounds demonstrated higher effect against *B. sorokiniana*. (2*E*)-*N*-(3-Fluorophenyl)- (**5**) and (2*E*)-*N*-(3-methylphenyl)-3-phenylprop-2-enamide (**2**) had MICs = 16.58 and 33.71 μM, respectively, which is comparable with the benomyl standard. Also compounds **6**, **4** (R = 2-F), and **14** (2-F-5-Br) demonstrated moderate activity (MIC range 49.98–66.32 μM) against *B. sorokiniana*. Surprising was the inactivity of compound **13** (R = 3,5-CF_3) against both fungal pathogens.

The dependences of the antifungal activity of the compounds against *B. sorokiniana* expressed as log (1/MIC (M)) on lipophilicity expressed as log *k* are illustrated in Figure 5. In general, effective compounds are preferentially substituted in positions $C_{(3)}'$, $C_{(3,5)}'$, or $C_{(3,4)}'$. When inactive compounds (illustrated by empty symbols) substituted in $C_{(4)}'$, $C_{(2,6)}'$, or $C_{(2,5)}'$ are eliminated from the SAR study, a bilinear dependence can be found. The activity increases with increasing lipophilicity from unsubstituted derivative **1** to compound **5** (R = 3-F) with the supposed lipophilicity optimum log $k = 0.23$ and then decreases to derivative **13** (R = 3,5-CF_3); $r = 0.9678$, $n = 7$. It can be stated that it is an opposite trend in comparison with antitubercular findings, which can be caused by differences in the composition and structure of mycobacterial and fungal cell walls [77]. A similar trend can be found for electronic properties of substituents in individual derivatives. The activity increases with an increase of electron-withdrawing effect from compound **2** (R = 3-CH_3, $\sigma_{Ar} = 0.48$) to an optimum $\sigma_{Ar} = 0.82$ (compound **5**, R = 3-F) and then decreases with increasing electron-withdrawing effect as follows: $\sigma_{Ar} = 0.89$ (compound **6**, R = 3-CF_3), 1.02 (compound **4**, R = 2-F), 1.11 (compound **11**, R = 3,5-Cl), and 1.19 (compound **10**, R = 3,4-Cl).

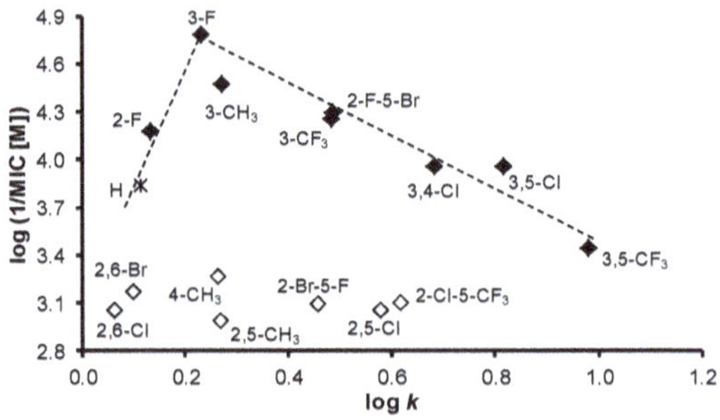

Figure 5. Relationships between in vitro antifungal activity against *B. sorokiniana* log (1/MIC (M)) and lipophilicity expressed as log *k* of studied compounds. (Derivatives excluded from SAR are illustrated by empty symbols.).

Inhibition of *B. sorokiniana* Germination

All the compounds were additionally evaluated for the inhibition of *B. sorokiniana* conidium germination at two concentrations (128 and 256 μg/mL), see results in Table 4. It can be stated that at both concentrations, the compounds showed the inhibition of germination. The effect was concentration-dependent for compounds **7**, **10**, **15**, and **16**, and the rest of compounds had concentration-independent effect on the germination. Interestingly, compound **6** that was one of the most active against all bacterial cells including *M. tuberculosis* and displayed strong inhibition on the mycelial growth of both investigated fungi (*F. avenaceum* and *B. sorokiniana*) (Table 2), showed the weakest effect in the germination test. Apart from compound **6**, compounds **2**, **4**, **5**, and **14** exerted the highest *B. sorokiniana* mycelial growth inhibitory effect and had characteristic anti-germination activity. Moreover, compound **5** was the most effective in both assays (IC_{50} = 16.58 μM in mycelial growth test and 95.4% germination inhibition at 128 μg/mL).

2.5. In Vitro Antiproliferative Assay

The preliminary in vitro screening of the antiproliferative activity of the most effective antimicrobial compounds was performed using a Water Soluble Tetrazolium salts-1 (WST-1) assay kit [78] and the human monocytic leukemia THP-1 cell line by means of the method described recently [20,79]. The principle of the WST-1 assay kit is that antiproliferative compounds inhibit mitochondrial dehydrogenases. The activity of this enzyme directly correlates with the number of metabolically active cells in the culture. Antiproliferative effect was evaluated as IC_{50} value (concentration of compound causing 50% inhibition of cell proliferation). It can be stated that a compound is considered cytotoxic if it shows a toxic effect on cells up to 10 μM [80]. The highest compound concentration used for the toxicity test was 3-fold higher than this.

IC_{50} values of the most effective compounds **2** (R = 3-CH_3), **5** (R = 3-F), **6** (R = 3-CF_3), **10** (R = 3,4-Cl), **11** (R = 3,5-Cl), and **13** (R = 3,5-CF_3) ranged from ca. 22 to >30 μM, see Table 2. For comparison, the IC_{50} of camptothecin was 0.16 ± 0.07 μM. Both compounds **5** and **2** effective against *B. sorokiniana* as well as compounds **10** and **11** potent against *M. tuberculosis* showed IC_{50} approximately 30 μM and higher, and compounds **6** and **13** showed IC_{50} = 22 μM, i.e., the treatment with these concentrations did not lead to significant antiproliferative effect on THP-1 cells, and these compounds inhibited selectively vital processes in *B. sorokiniana*, *M. tuberculosis*, or *Staphylococcus* strains. Based on these observations, it can be concluded that all the tested compounds can be considered as nontoxic agents for subsequent design of novel therapeutic agents.

Table 4. Inhibition (%) of *Bipolaris sorokiniana* conidium germination by compounds **1–16** in comparison to negative control. Benomyl (BNM) was used as positive control.

Comp.	Concentration (μg/mL)	Inhibition (%) Compared to Negative Control	Comp.	Concentration (μg/mL)	Inhibition (%) Compared to Negative Control
1	256	59.6	9	256	82.5
	128	74.2		128	76.3
2	256	64.7	10	256	84.3
	128	59.1		128	51.3
3	256	88.7	11	256	84.8
	128	89.1		128	82.6
4	256	60.8	12	256	91.3
	128	58.7		128	82.1
5	256	93.6	13	256	76.3
	128	95.4		128	75.5
6	256	18.4	14	256	81.8
	128	26.7		128	77.6
7	256	73.5	15	256	100
	128	35.1		128	60.9
8	256	92.7	16	256	86.2
	128	88.7		128	61.2
BNM	10	100	BNM	10	100
	5	100		5	100

2.6. Inhibition of Photosynthetic Electron Transport (PET) in Spinach Chloroplasts

The activity of the evaluated cinnamamides related to the inhibition of photosynthetic electron transport (PET) in spinach (*Spinacia oleracea* L.) chloroplasts was moderate or low relative to the standard, see Table 2, except for compound **11** (R = 3,5-Cl) that expressed the highest PET-inhibiting activity comparable with the Diuron® standard (IC_{50} = 5.1 μM). With respect to these low activities, no detailed SAR study can be proposed; nevertheless, from the results listed in Table 2, bilinear trends for both PET inhibition vs. lipophilicity and PET inhibition vs. electronic properties of the anilide core can be suggested. Thus, PET inhibition activity increases with the lipophilicity (log *k*) increase as follows: 0.063 (**9**, R = 2,6-Cl) < 0.264 (**3**, R = 4-CH_3) < 0.487 (**14**, R = 2-F-5-Br) < 0.682 (**10**, R = 3,4-Cl) <<< 0.815 (**11**, R = 3,5-Cl) and then decreases to 0.981 (**13**, R = 3,5-CF_3). Also PET inhibition activity increases with the increase of electron-withdrawing (σ_{Ar}) properties as follows: 0.46 (**3**, R = 4-CH_3) < 1.05 (**13**, 3,5-CF_3) <<< 1.11 (**11**, R = 3,5-Cl) and decreases as follows: >>> 1.19 (**10**, R = 3,4-Cl) > 1.28 (**14**,

R = 2-F-5-Br) >> 1.33 (**9**, R = 2,6-Cl). It can be concluded, as mentioned above, that the substitution of the anilide core in $C_{(3,5)}'$ or $C_{(3,4)}'$ positions is preferable for high PET-inhibiting activity.

The inhibition of electron transport in PS II at the Q_B site plastoquinone, i.e., at the acceptor side of PS II was observed for ring-substituted salicylanilides and carbamoylphenylcarbamates [26,28], ring-substituted hydroxynaphthalene-2-carboxanilides [27,30], *N*-alkoxyphenylhydroxynaphthalene-carboxamides [29], 8-hydroxyquinoline-2-carboxamides [81], and *N*-substituted 2-aminobenzothiazoles [82]. Based on the structural analogy and the presence of the amide bond, it can be hypothesized that the mechanism of action of the investigated compounds is not different from the mechanism of action of the above compounds. Moreover, as mentioned previously [26–29,83,87], a good correlation between antimycobacterial activity and herbicidal effect was found.

2.7. *In Vivo Toxicity against Plant Cells*

The most potent antifungal compounds **2**, **5**, **6**, and **14** were tested for in vivo toxicity against plant cells. *Nicotiana tabacum* var. Samsun was used for this test [88]. The results of treatment of plant leaves with injected water solutions of each compound as well as dimethyl sulfoxide (DMSO) are illustrated in Figure 6, where photographs of leaves are shown. The negative DMSO control did not have any toxic effect to the plant cells as well. On the other hand, the 5% aqueous solution of DMSO showed a significant toxic effect on the leaves demonstrated as a loss of chlorophyll in the injected area (Figure 6A). Based on Figure 6B,C, it can be concluded that the most effective antifungal compounds had no visible influence on the plant tissue.

These results correspond to above-mentioned PET-inhibiting activity, when all the tested compounds showed no PET inhibition, and thus, they will not be toxic for plants at their prospective application as a plant fungicide.

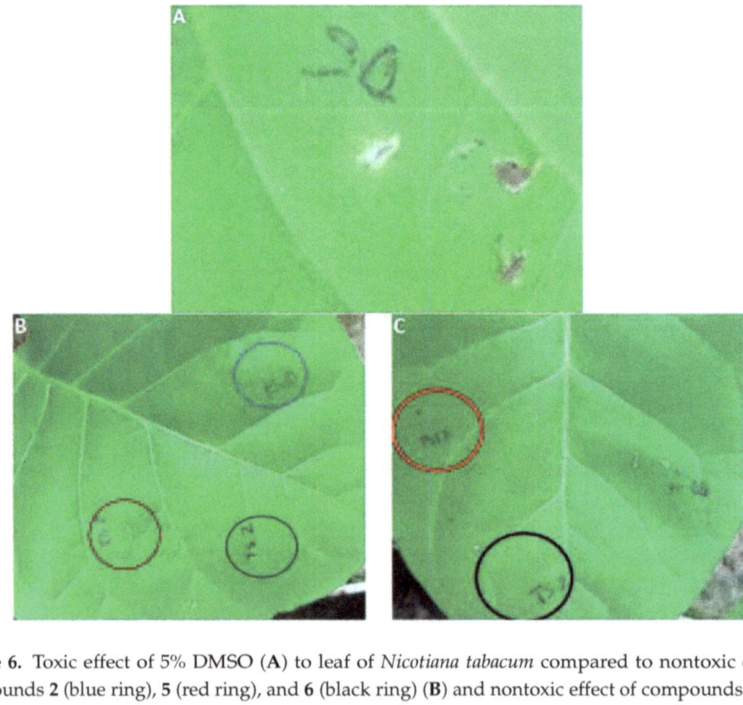

Figure 6. Toxic effect of 5% DMSO (**A**) to leaf of *Nicotiana tabacum* compared to nontoxic effect of compounds **2** (blue ring), **5** (red ring), and **6** (black ring) (**B**) and nontoxic effect of compounds **6** (black ring) and **14** (red ring) (**C**). The black spots in the injected area of compound **5** in Figure 6B are damages of the leaf tissue caused by a needle.

3. Materials and Methods

3.1. Chemistry—General Information

All reagents were purchased from Merck (Sigma-Aldrich, St. Louis, MO, USA) and Alfa (Alfa-Aesar, Ward Hill, MA, USA). Reactions were performed using a CEM Discover SP microwave reactor (CEM, Matthews, NC, USA). Melting points were determined on an apparatus Stuart SMP10 (Stone, UK) and are uncorrected. Infrared (IR) spectra were recorded on an UATR Zn/Se for a Spectrum Two™ Fourier-transform IR spectrometer (PerkinElmer, Waltham, MA, USA). The spectra were obtained by the accumulation of 32 scans with 4 cm^{-1} resolution in the region of 4000–400 cm^{-1}. All ^{1}H- and ^{13}C-NMR spectra were recorded on a JEOL ECZR 400 MHz NMR spectrometer (400 MHz for ^{1}H and 100 MHz for ^{13}C, Jeol, Tokyo, Japan) in dimethyl sulfoxide-d_6 (DMSO-d_6). ^{1}H and ^{13}C chemical shifts (δ) are reported in ppm. High-resolution mass spectra were measured using a high-performance liquid chromatograph Dionex UltiMate® 3000 (Thermo Scientific, West Palm Beach, FL, USA) coupled with an LTQ Orbitrap XL™ Hybrid Ion Trap-Orbitrap Fourier Transform Mass Spectrometer (Thermo Scientific) equipped with a HESI II (heated electrospray ionization) source in the positive mode.

Synthesis

Cinnamic acid (3.37 mM) was suspended at room temperature in dry chlorobenzene (20 mL) inside a microwave tube, where phosphorus trichloride (1.7 mM) and the corresponding aniline (3.37 mM) were added dropwise. Then a magnetic stirrer was used, and the reaction mixture was transferred to the microwave reactor at 120 °C for 20 min, where the synthesis at elevated pressure was performed. After the mixture was cooled to 60 °C, and solvent was evaporated in vacuum. A solid was washed with 2 M HCl, and a crude product was recrystallized, first using 96% ethanol and then using 50% ethanol.

(2E)-N-Phenyl-3-phenylprop-2-enamide (**1**) [89]. Yield 91%; Mp 116–118 °C; IR (cm^{-1}): 3062, 3028, 1661, 1626, 1594, 1578, 1543, 1493, 1442, 1347, 1288, 1248, 1188, 976, 904, 864, 759, 737, 704, 690, 676, 620, 592, 553, 512, 484, 454; ^{1}H-NMR (DMSO-d_6), δ: 10.22 (s, 1H), 7.72 (d, J = 7.3 Hz, 2H), 7.64–7.59 (m, 3H), 7.47–7.36 (m, 3H), 7.34 (t, J = 8 Hz, 2H), 7.09–7.05 (m, 1H), 6.85 (d, J = 16 Hz, 1H); ^{13}C-NMR (DMSO-d_6), δ: 163.53, 140.16, 139.28, 134.73, 129.77, 129.03, 128.81, 127.72, 123.36, 122.29, 119.23; HR-MS: for $C_{15}H_{14}NO$ $[M + H]^+$ calculated 224.1070 m/z, found 224.1065 m/z.

(2E)-N-(3-Methylphenyl)-3-phenylprop-2-enamide (**2**) [89]. Yield 80%; Mp 113–115 °C; IR (cm^{-1}): 3259, 3136, 3082, 3064, 3028, 2918, 1658, 1620, 1541, 1488, 1447, 1408, 1342, 1292, 1201, 987, 978, 864, 775, 763, 729, 714, 685, 676, 556, 487; ^{1}H-NMR (DMSO-d_6), δ: 10.14 (s, 1H), 7.64–7.60 (m, 2H), 7.58 (d, J = 15.6 Hz, 1H), 7.53 (m, 1H), 7.5 (d, J = 8.2 Hz, 1H), 7.47–7.40 (m, 3H), 7.21 (t, J = 7.8 Hz, 1H), 6.89 (d, J=7.8 Hz, 1H), 6.84 (d, J = 15.6 Hz, 1H), 2.3 (s, 3H); ^{13}C-NMR (DMSO-d_6), δ: 163.48, 140.06, 139.23, 137.99, 134.75, 129.78, 129.04, 128.67, 127.73, 124.11, 122.38, 119.73, 116.45, 21.25; HR-MS: for $C_{16}H_{16}NO$ $[M + H]^+$ calculated 238.1226 m/z, found 238.1222 m/z.

(2E)-N-(4-Methylphenyl)-3-phenylprop-2-enamide (**3**) [89]. Yield 82%; Mp 166–168 °C; IR (cm^{-1}): 3240, 3187, 3128, 3085, 3028, 2954, 1660, 1622, 1597, 1538, 1493, 1448, 1405, 1342, 1252, 1187, 984, 973, 813, 781, 762, 720, 674, 533, 510, 485; ^{1}H-NMR (DMSO-d_6) δ: 10.14 (s, 1H), 7.63–7.55 (m, 5H), 7.47–7.40 (m, 3H), 7.15–7.13 (m, 2H), 6.83 (d, J = 16 Hz, 1H), 2.26 (s, 3H); ^{13}C-NMR (DMSO-d_6) δ: 163.33, 139.90, 136.81, 134.79, 132.32, 129.73, 129.22, 129.03, 127.70, 122.40, 119.22, 20.51; HR-MS: for $C_{16}H_{16}NO$ $[M + H]^+$ calculated 238.1226 m/z, found 238.1222 m/z.

(2E)-N-(2-Fluorophenyl)-3-phenylprop-2-enamide (**4**) [89]. Yield 85%; Mp 114–116 °C; IR (cm^{-1}): 3238, 3182, 3126, 3085, 3059, 3020, 1661, 1627, 1539, 1491, 1448, 1342, 1257, 1188, 1105, 973, 760, 731, 719, 701, 687, 659, 557, 535, 495, 479; ^{1}H-NMR (DMSO-d_6) δ: 9.69 (s, 1H), 8.11 (td, J = 7.9 Hz, 2.1 Hz, 1H), 7.64–7.57 (m, 3H), 7.48–7.40 (m, 4H), 7.31–7.26 (m, 1H), 7.20–7.16 (m, 1H), 7.09 (d, J=15.6 Hz, 1H);

^{13}C-NMR (DMSO-d_6) δ: 163.96, 153.34 (d, *J* = 244.7 Hz), 140.72, 134.74, 129.90, 129.05, 127.82, 126.41 (d, *J* = 10.6 Hz), 125.09 (d, *J* = 7.7 Hz), 124.44 (d, *J* = 2.9 Hz), 121.88, 119.23, 115.47 (d, *J* = 19.3 Hz); HR-MS: for $C_{15}H_{13}FNO$ $[M + H]^+$ calculated 242.0976 *m/z*, found 242.0971 *m/z*.

(2E)-N-(3-Fluorophenyl)-3-phenylprop-2-enamide (**5**). Yield 84%; Mp 112–114 °C; IR (cm^{-1}): 3298, 3061, 3031, 2979, 1625, 1596, 1529, 1489, 1420, 1334, 1186, 974, 943, 858, 777, 768, 756, 727, 714, 688, 679, 658, 556, 492; ^{1}H-NMR (DMSO-d_6) δ: 10.44 (s, 1H), 7.76–7.72 (m, 1H), 7.65–7.61 (m, 3H), 7.48–7.34 (m, 5H), 6.92–6.88 (m, 1H), 6.82 (d, *J* = 15.6 Hz, 1H); ^{13}C-NMR (DMSO-d_6) δ: 163.87, 162.23 (d, *J* = 241.8 Hz), 141.00 (d, *J* = 10.6 Hz), 140.80, 134.61, 130.44 (d, *J* = 9.6 Hz), 129.95, 129.06, 127.85, 121.87, 115.02 (d, J=2.9 Hz), 109.83 (d, *J* = 21.2 Hz), 106.07 (d, *J* = 27.3 Hz); HR-MS: for $C_{15}H_{13}FNO$ $[M + H]^+$ calculated 242.0976 *m/z*, found 242.0972 *m/z*.

(2E)-3-Phenyl-N-[3-(trifluoromethyl)phenyl]prop-2-enamide (**6**) [90]. Yield 75%; Mp 109–111 °C; IR (cm^{-1}): 3400, 2905, 2360, 1678, 1630, 1526, 1491, 1331, 1154, 1112, 1100, 1072, 982, 886, 808; ^{1}H-NMR (DMSO-d_6) δ: 10.57 (s, 1H), 8.22 (s, 1H), 7.87 (d, *J* = 8.2 Hz, 1H), 7.66–7.62 (m, 3H), 7,58 (t, *J* = 7.8 Hz, 1H), 7.48–7.40 (m, 4H), 6.82 (d, *J* = 15.6 Hz, 1H); ^{13}C-NMR (DMSO-d_6) δ: 164.05, 140.98, 140.07, 134.54, 130.04, 129.99, 129.58 (q, *J* = 30.8 Hz), 129.05, 127.88, 124.16 (q, *J* = 272.6 Hz), 122.76, 121.72, 119.65 (q, *J* = 3.9 Hz), 115.29 (q, *J* = 3.9 Hz); HR-MS: for $C_{16}H_{13}F_3NO$ $[M + H]^+$ calculated 292.0944 *m/z*, found 292.0938 *m/z*.

(2E)-N-(2,5-Dimethylphenyl)-3-phenylprop-2-enamide (**7**). Yield 91%; Mp 174–176 °C; IR (cm^{-1}): 3242, 3056, 3028, 2977, 2918, 1657, 1621, 1579, 1544, 1494, 1449, 1417, 1343, 1286, 1266, 1199, 1159, 990, 978, 878, 780, 764, 746, 734, 724, 707, 681, 624, 560, 492; ^{1}H-NMR (DMSO-d_6) δ: 9.42 (s, 1H), 7.63 (d, *J* = 6.9 Hz, 2H), 7.58 (d, *J* = 16 Hz, 1H), 7.47–7.39 (m, 4H), 7.10 (d, *J* = 7.8 Hz, 1H), 6.99 (d, *J* = 16 Hz, 1H), 6.90 (d, *J* = 7.3 Hz, 1H), 2.26 (s, 3H), 2.20 (s, 3H); ^{13}C-NMR (DMSO-d_6) δ: 163.58, 139.88, 136.17, 134.97, 134.85, 130.15, 129.67, 128.99, 127.94, 127.68, 125.70, 124.97, 122.36, 20.67, 17.54; HR-MS: for $C_{17}H_{18}NO$ $[M + H]^+$ calculated 252.1383 *m/z*, found 252.1378 *m/z*.

(2E)-N-(2,5-Dichlorophenyl)-3-phenylprop-2-enamide (**8**). Yield 83%; Mp 173–175 °C; IR (cm^{-1}): 3234, 3108, 3062, 3026, 1662, 1622, 1582, 1528, 1463, 1449, 1406, 1341, 1261, 1182, 1093, 1055, 992, 979, 917, 872, 856, 806, 761, 718, 693, 675, 580, 559, 488; ^{1}H-NMR (DMSO-d_6) δ: 9.77 (s, 1H), 8.15 (d, *J* = 2.3 Hz, 1H), 7.66–7.62 (m, 3H), 7.54 (d, *J* = 8.7 Hz, 1H), 7.45–7.41 (m, 3H), 7.24 (dd, *J* = 8.7 Hz, 2.7 Hz, 1H), 7.18 (d, *J* = 15.6 Hz, 1H); ^{13}C-NMR (DMSO-d_6) δ: 164.20, 141.47, 136.28, 134.60, 131.61, 130.83, 130.05, 129.03, 127.94, 125.40, 124.11, 123.61, 121.51; HR-MS: for $C_{18}H_{12}Cl_2NO$ $[M + H]^+$ calculated 292.0290 *m/z*, found 292.0289 *m/z*.

(2E)-N-(2,6-Dichlorophenyl)-3-phenylprop-2-enamide (**9**). Yield 85%; Mp 212–214 °C; IR (cm^{-1}): 3256, 1661, 1630, 1569, 1522, 1449, 1428, 1338, 1183, 971, 782, 758, 712, 697, 508; ^{1}H-NMR (DMSO-d_6) δ: 10.09 (s, 1H), 7.67–7.62 (m, 3H), 7.58–7.56 (m, 2H), 7.48–7.41 (m, 3H), 7.39–7.35 (m, 1H), 6.89 (d, *J* = 16 Hz, 1H); ^{13}C-NMR (DMSO-d_6) δ: 163.67, 140.98, 134.51, 133.69, 133.03, 129.97, 129.19, 129.05, 128.56, 127.85, 120.72; HR-MS: for $C_{15}H_{12}Cl_2NO$ $[M + H]^+$ calculated 292.0290 *m/z*, found 292.0288 *m/z*.

(2E)-N-(3,4-Dichlorophenyl)-3-phenylprop-2-enamide (**10**). Yield 78%; Mp 173–175 °C; IR (cm^{-1}): 3269, 3095, 3025, 1663, 1627, 1585, 1526, 1474, 1378, 1339, 1289, 1229, 1182, 1126, 1025, 974, 863, 810, 761, 699, 677, 579, 564, 515, 484; ^{1}H-NMR (DMSO-d_6) δ: 10.52 (s, 1H), 8.12–8.11 (m, 1H), 7.64–7.61 (m, 3H), 7.58 (s, 2H), 7.46–7.40 (m, 3H), 6.79 (d, *J* = 16 Hz, 1H); ^{13}C-NMR (DMSO-d_6) δ: 163.63, 141.08, 139.38, 134.49, 131.09, 130.72, 130.03, 129.05, 127.88, 124.78, 121.55, 120.39, 119.25; HR-MS: for $C_{15}H_{12}Cl_2NO$ $[M + H]^+$ calculated 292.0290 *m/z*, found 292.0288 *m/z*.

(2E)-N-(3,5-Dichlorophenyl)-3-phenylprop-2-enamide (**11**) [89]. Yield 79%; Mp 139–141 °C; IR (cm^{-1}): 3246, 3177, 3085, 2967, 1663, 1622, 1584, 1532, 1442, 1408, 1338, 1180, 1109, 969, 937, 844, 802, 760,717, 668, 556, 484; ^{1}H-NMR (DMSO-d_6) δ: 10.56 (s, 1H), 7.76 (d, *J* = 1.8 Hz, 2H), 7.65–7.61 (m, 3H), 7.48–7.40 (m, 3H), 7.29 (t, *J* = 2,1 Hz, 1H), 6.76 (d, J = 15.6 Hz, 1H); ^{13}C-NMR (DMSO-d_6) δ: 164.06, 141.60, 141.35, 134.41, 134.12, 130.06, 129.02, 127.90, 122.48, 121.37, 117.30; HR-MS: for $C_{15}H_{12}Cl_2NO$ $[M + H]^+$ calculated 292.0290 *m/z*, found 292.0288 *m/z*.

(2E)-N-(2,6-Dibromophenyl)-3-phenylprop-2-enamide (**12**). Yield 81%; Mp 240–242 °C; IR (cm^{-1}): 3251, 3180, 3028, 2902, 1660, 1627, 1558, 1516, 1441, 1422, 1337, 1263, 1180, 970, 781, 766, 759, 721, 710, 694, 686, 626, 561, 501; ^{1}H-NMR (DMSO-d_6) δ: 10.12 (s, 1H), 7.75 (d, J = 7.8 Hz, 2H), 7.67–7.64 (m, 2H), 7.60 (d, J = 16 Hz, 1H), 7.48–7.40 (m, 3H), 7.21 (t, J = 8 Hz, 1H), 6.87 (d, J = 15.6 Hz, 1H); ^{13}C-NMR (DMSO-d_6) δ: 163.50, 140.85, 135.77, 134.50, 132.24, 130.19, 129.94, 129.05, 127.80, 124.33, 120.86; HR-MS: for $C_{15}H_{12}Br_2NO$ $[M + H]^+$ calculated 379.9280 *m/z*, found 379.9288 *m/z*.

(2E)-N-[3,5-bis(Trifluoromethyl)phenyl]-3-phenylprop-2-enamide (**13**). Yield 75%; Mp 143–145 °C; IR (cm^{-1}): 3272, 3085, 2967, 2938, 2879, 1663, 1622, 1575, 1472, 1440, 1377, 1276, 1168, 1129, 1110, 1096, 974, 937, 886, 859, 841, 728, 680, 627, 557, 486; ^{1}H-NMR (DMSO-d_6) δ: 10.89 (s, 1H), 8.36 (s, 2H), 7.77 (s, 1H), 7.70–7.65 (m, 3H), 7.48–7.40 (m, 3H), 6.78 (d, J = 16 Hz, 1H); ^{13}C-NMR (DMSO-d_6) δ: 164.42, 141.78, 141.13, 134.28, 130.80 (q, J = 32.8 Hz), 130.22, 129.08, 127.98, 123.23 (q, J = 272.6 Hz), 121.07, 118.93–118.78 (m), 116.12–115.98 (m); HR-MS: for $C_{17}H_{12}F_6NO$ $[M + H]^+$ calculated 360.0818 *m/z*, found 360.0811 *m/z*.

(2E)-N-(2-Fluoro-5-bromophenyl)-3-phenylprop-2-enamide (**14**). Yield 83%; Mp 161–164 °C; IR (cm^{-1}): 3280, 2967, 2936, 2879, 1660, 1613, 1529, 1474, 1448, 1411, 1345, 1254, 1174, 985, 870, 800, 762, 722, 676, 617, 600, 564, 484; ^{1}H-NMR (DMSO-d_6) δ: 10.13 (s, 1H), 8.44 (dd, J = 7.1 Hz, 2.5 Hz, 1H), 7.65–7.60 (m, 3H), 7.48–7.40 (m, 3H), 7.35–7.27 (m, 2H), 7.11 (d, J = 15.6 Hz, 1H); ^{13}C-NMR (DMSO-d_6) δ: 164.22, 152.03 (d, J = 245.6 Hz), 141.30, 134.60, 130.02, 129.04, 128.25 (d, J = 12.5 Hz), 127.88, 127.10 (d, J = 7.7 Hz), 125.10, 121.50, 117.41 (d, J = 21.2 Hz), 115.91 (d, J = 2.9 Hz); HR-MS: for $C_{15}H_{12}FBrNO$ $[M + H]^+$ calculated 320.0081 *m/z*, found 320.0077 *m/z*.

(2E)-N-(2-Bromo-5-fluorophenyl)-3-phenylprop-2-enamide (**15**). Yield 81%; Mp 164–166 °C; IR (cm^{-1}): 3230, 3072, 3045, 2967, 2937, 2880, 1661, 1623, 1591, 1538, 1420, 1342, 1198, 1155, 991, 977, 869, 854, 804, 761, 715, 668, 598, 589, 559, 482; ^{1}H-NMR (DMSO-d_6) δ: 9.64 (s, 1H), 7.83 (dd, J = 11 Hz, 3.2 Hz, 1H), 7.72 (dd, J = 8.7 Hz, 5.9 Hz, 1H), 7.67–7.62 (m, 3H), 7.48–7.42 (m, 3H), 7.15 (d, J = 15.6 Hz, 1H), 7.04 (ddd, J = 8.9 Hz, 8 Hz, 3.2 Hz, 1H); ^{13}C-NMR (DMSO-d_6) δ: 164.12, 161.05 (d, J = 243.7 Hz), 141.44, 137.74 (d, J = 11.6 Hz), 134.61, 133.85 (d, J = 8.7 Hz), 130.05, 129.04, 127.95, 121.55, 113.41 (d, J = 23.1 Hz), 112.44 (d, J = 27 Hz), 110.6 (d, J = 2.9 Hz); HR-MS: for $C_{15}H_{12}FBrNO$ $[M + H]^+$ calculated 320.0081 *m/z*, found 320.0077 *m/z*.

(2E)-N-[2-Chloro-5-(trifluoromethyl)phenyl]-3-phenylprop-2-enamide (**16**). Yield 77%; Mp 144–146 °C; IR (cm^{-1}): 3280, 2967, 2936, 2879, 1528, 1329, 1262, 1165, 1116, 1080, 964, 892, 814, 758, 707, 686, 668, 644, 605, 560, 534, 490, 452; ^{1}H-NMR (DMSO-d_6) δ: 9,22 (s, 1H), 8.40 (d, J = 1.8 Hz, 1H), 7.79–7.77 (m, 1H), 7.68–7.64 (m, 3H), 7.55–7.53 (m, 1H), 7.49–7.40 (m, 3H), 7.19 (d, J = 15.6 Hz, 1H); ^{13}C-NMR (DMSO-d_6) δ: 164.42, 141.66, 135.99, 134.60, 130.70, 130.06, 129.02, 128.98, 128.09 (q, J = 38.2 Hz), 127.96, 123.69 (q, J = 272.6 Hz), 121.98 (q, J = 3.9 Hz), 121.46, 120.95 (q, J = 3.9 Hz); HR-MS: for $C_{16}H_{12}ClF_3NO$ $[M + H]^+$ calculated 326.0554 *m/z*, found 326.0547 *m/z*.

3.2. Lipophilicity Determination by HPLC (Capacity Factor k/Calculated log k)

A HPLC separation module Waters® e2695 equipped with a Waters 2996 PDA Detector (Waters Corp., Milford, MA, USA) were used. A chromatographic column Symmetry® C_{18} 5 μm, 4.6 × 250 mm, Part No. W21751W016 (Waters Corp.) was used. The HPLC separation process was monitored by the Empower™ 3 Chromatography Data Software (Waters Corp.). Isocratic elution by a mixture of MeOH p.a. (72%) and H_2O-HPLC Mili-Q grade (28%) as a mobile phase was used. The total flow of the column was 1.0 mL/min, injection 5 μL, column temperature 40 °C, and sample temperature 10 °C. The detection wavelength 214 nm was chosen. The KI methanolic solution was used for the determination of dead time (t_D). Retention times (t_R) were measured in minutes. The capacity factors k were calculated using the Empower™ 3 Chromatography Data Software according to the formula $k = (t_R - t_D)/t_D$, where t_R is the retention time of the solute, while t_D is the dead time obtained using an unretained analyte. Each experiment was repeated three times. Log k, calculated from the capacity factor k, is used as the lipophilicity index converted to log P scale [36]. The log k values of individual compounds are shown in Table 1.

3.3. Biological Testing

3.3.1. In Vitro Antibacterial Evaluation

The synthesized compounds were evaluated for in vitro antibacterial activity against representatives of multidrug-resistant bacteria and clinical isolates of methicillin-resistant *Staphylococcus aureus* (MRSA) 63718, SA 630, and SA 3202 [37,38] that were obtained from the National Institute of Public Health (Prague, Czech Republic). *S. aureus* ATCC 29213 was used as a reference and quality control strain. In addition, all the compounds were tested for their activity against vancomycin-susceptible *Enterococcus faecalis* ATCC 29212 as a reference strain and three isolates from American crows of vanA-carrying vancomycin-resistant *E. faecalis* (VRE) 342B, 368, and 725B [39]. Ampicillin (Sigma) was used as the standard. Prior to testing, each strain was passaged onto nutrient agar (Oxoid, Basingstoke, UK) with 5% of bovine blood, and bacterial inocula were prepared by suspending a small portion of bacterial colony in sterile phosphate buffered saline (pH 7.2–7.3). The cell density was adjusted to 0.5 McFarland units using a densitometer (Densi-La-Meter, LIAP, Riga, Latvia). This inoculum was diluted to reach the final concentration of bacterial cells 5×10^5 CFU/mL in the wells. The compounds were dissolved in DMSO (Sigma), and the final concentration of DMSO in the Cation Adjusted Mueller-Hinton (CaMH) broth (Oxoid) or Brain-Heart Infusion for enterococci did not exceed 2.5% of the total solution composition. The final concentrations of the evaluated compounds ranged from 256 to 0.008 μg/mL. The broth dilution micro-method, modified according to the NCCLS (National Committee for Clinical Laboratory Standards) guidelines [91] in Mueller–Hinton (MH) broth, was used to determine the minimum inhibitory concentration (MIC). Drug-free controls, sterility controls, and controls consisting of MH broth and DMSO alone were included. The determination of results was performed visually after 24 h of static incubation in the darkness at 37 °C in an aerobic atmosphere. The results are shown in Table 2.

3.3.2. Synergy Effect with Clinically Used Drugs

For synergy effect study, a method of fractional inhibitory concentration was used. The tested compounds (A) and conventional used antibiotic (B) (tetracycline, ciprofloxacin, and vancomycin (purchased from Sigma)) were diluted in the microtitration plate in CaMH broth (Oxoid) to get an original combination of concentration in every well. The raw H was used for evaluation of $MIC_{(A)}$; column 12 was used for evaluation of $MIC_{(B)}$. The plate was inoculated by the bacterial suspension to reach final concentration 5×10^5 CFU/mL in the wells. The fractional inhibitory concentration (FIC) index was calculated using the concentrations in the first nonturbid (clear) well found in each row and column along the turbidity/nonturbidity interface [42]. A $\Sigma FIC \leq 0.5$ means synergy; $0.5 < \Sigma FIC < 1$ is additivity; $1 \leq \Sigma FIC < 4$ is indifference; and $\Sigma FIC \geq 4$ is antagonism [41]. The tests were made in duplicate, and the results were averaged. The results are summarized in Table 3.

3.3.3. Dynamics of Antibacterial Effect

The most active antistaphylococcal compounds were studied for their dynamics of antibacterial effect. The method of time-kill curves were used [37,40]. Compound **6** was diluted in CaMH to reach the final concentration equal to 1× MIC, 2× MIC, and 4× MIC. For the compound **13**, only concentrations 1× MIC and 2× MIC were used, due to the higher MIC and dissolution problems in the concentration equal to 4× MIC. The tubes were inoculated with the culture of *S. aureus* ATTC 29213 diluted to 1 McFarland in the exponential phase of growth. The final concentration of bacteria was 7.5×10^6 CFU/mL. Tubes were stored in an incubator at 37 °C without shaking. Immediately after 4, 6, 8, and 24 h of inoculation, 100 μL of sample was serially diluted 1:10 in phosphate buffered saline (PBS). From each dilution 2 × 20 μL were put onto MH agar plates. The plates were incubated at 37 °C for 24 h, and the colonies were counted. Bactericidal effect is defined as a −3log decrease of CFU/mL compared to the growth control in time 0. The test was made in duplicate on 2 separate occasions, and the results were averaged. The results are illustrated in Figure 2.

3.3.4. Biofilm Inhibition Assay

The most active antistaphylococcal compounds were studied for their ability to inhibit biofilm formation. The compounds were diluted in a 96-well plate in tryptic soy broth (TSB) containing 2% of glucose to reach concentrations 256–2 μg/mL. *S. aureus* ATCC 29213 cultivated overnight on blood agar was used for preparing the inoculum. A few colonies were put in a tube with 5 mL of TSB + 2% glucose and cultivated to reach the exponential phase of growth. The inoculum was diluted to 1 McFarland and then 1:1000 in TSB + 2% glucose. The final concentration of bacteria in each well was 1×10^5. As positive controls, ampicillin, vancomycin, ciprofloxacin, and tetracycline (Sigma) were used. As the compounds were dissolved in DMSO (up to 5%), the growth control included 5% of DMSO for verification that the applied DMSO concentration did not possess bacterial growth-inhibiting activity. The plate was cultivated for 48 h at 37 °C without shaking. After incubation, the content of the wells was removed and the wells were washed 3-fold by PBS. After drying, 125 μL of 0.1% crystal violet was put to every well. The plane was stained for 20 min at room temperature, the content was removed, and the plate was again washed by PBS 3-fold. The coloured biofilm was taken off from the wells by 33% acetic acid, and absorbance in 595 nm was measured. As a blank, non-inoculated plate treated in the same way was used. The test was made in triplicates in 3 separated occasions. The ability to inhibit biofilm formation was evaluated as a percentage inhibition of growth compared to the growth control. The results are illustrated in Figure 3.

3.3.5. In Vitro Antimycobacterial Evaluation

Mycobacterium tuberculosis ATCC 25177/H37Ra was grown in Middlebrook broth (MB), supplemented with Oleic-Albumin-Dextrose-Catalase (OADC) supplement (Difco, Lawrence, KS, USA). At log phase growth, a culture sample (10 mL) was centrifuged at 15,000 rpm/20 min using a bench top centrifuge (MPW-65R, MPW Med Instruments, Warszawa, Poland). Following the removal of the supernatant, the pellet was washed in fresh Middlebrook 7H9GC broth and resuspended in fresh, ODAC-supplemented MB (10 mL). The turbidity was adjusted to match McFarland standard No. 1 (3×10^8 CFU) with MB broth. A further 1:10 dilution of the culture was then performed in MB broth. The antimicrobial susceptibility of *M. tuberculosis* was investigated in a 96-well plate format. In these experiments, sterile deionised water (300 μL) was added to all outer-perimeter wells of the plates to minimize evaporation of the medium in the test wells during incubation. Each evaluated compound (100 μL) was incubated with *M. tuberculosis* (100 μL). Dilutions of each compound were prepared in duplicate. For all synthesized compounds, final concentrations ranged from 128 to 4 μg/mL. All compounds were dissolved in DMSO, and subsequent dilutions were made in supplemented MB. The plates were sealed with Parafilm and incubated at 37 °C for 14 days. Following incubation, a 10% addition of alamarBlue (Difco) was mixed into each well, and readings at 570 nm and 600 nm were taken, initially for background subtraction and subsequently after 24 h reincubation. The background subtraction is necessary for strongly coloured compounds, where the colour may interfere with the interpretation of any colour change. For noninterfering compounds, a blue colour in the well was interpreted as the absence of growth, and a pink colour was scored as growth. Isoniazid (Sigma) was used as the positive control, as it is a clinically used antitubercular drug. The results are shown in Table 2.

3.3.6. MTT Assay

Compounds were prepared as previously stated and diluted in Middlebrook media to achieve the desired final concentration 128–1 μg/mL. *Mycobacterium tuberculosis* ATCC 25177/H37Ra was suspended in ODAC supplemented Middlebrook broth at a MacFarland standard of 1.0 and then diluted 1:10, using Middlebrook broth as a diluent. The diluted mycobacteria (50 μL) were added to each well containing the compound to be tested. Diluted mycobacteria in broth free from inhibiting compounds were used as a growth control. As positive controls, ciprofloxacin and rifampicin were used. All compounds and controls were prepared in duplicate. Plates were incubated at 37 °C for 7 days. After the incubation period, 10% well volume of MTT (3-(4,5-dimethylthiazol-2-yl)-2,5-diphenyl-tetrazolium bromide) reagent (Sigma) was mixed into each well and incubated at 37 °C for 4 h in dark. Then 100 μL of 17% Sodium dodecyl sulfate in 40% dimethylformamide was added to each well. The plates were read at 570 nm. The absorbance readings from the cells grown in the presence of the tested compounds were compared with uninhibited cell growth to determine the relative percent viability. The percent viability was determined through the MTT assay. The percent viability is calculated through comparison of a measured value against that of the uninhibited control: % viability = $OD_{570E}/OD_{570P} \times 100$, where OD_{570E} is the reading from the compound-exposed cells, while OD_{570P} is the reading from the uninhibited cells (positive control). Cytotoxic potential is determined by a percent viability of <70% [59,92]. Rifampicin a ciprofloxacin (Sigma) were used as positive controls.

3.3.7. In Vitro Antifungal Activity

96-Well microplates were used for testing the inhibitory effect of compounds against mycelial growth of *Fusarium avenaceum* (Fr.) Sacc. IMI 319947 and *Bipolaris sorokiniana* (Sacc.) Shoemaker H-299 (NCBI GenBank accession No. MH697869). The compounds were diluted in DMSO to reach the concentration of 10 mg/mL and then diluted in the microtiter plates in supplemented lysogeny broth (LB, 10 g/L tryptone (Microtrade, Budapest, Hungary), 5 g/L yeast extract (Scharlau, Barcelona, Spain), and 10 g/L NaCl (Reanal, Budapest, Hungary)) to get the final concentration of 256–2 μg/mL. Positive (benomyl, Chinoin Fundazol 50WP®, Chinoin, Budapest, Hungary) and negative (solvents of the compounds) controls were used. 50 mL LB medium was inoculated with the fungal culture grown in an agar plate and shaken at 100 rpm at 22 °C for 3 days in dark; then mycelium was cut with a sterile blender to small parts. The mycelium suspension was diluted to set OD_{600} = 0.2. This inoculum was diluted 2-fold with the content of the wells. The absorbance at 600 nm was measured by a spectrophotometer (Labsystems Multiscan MS 4.0, Thermo Scientific) immediately, and the plates were incubated at 22 °C. The absorbance was measured again after 24, 48, and 72 h. The MIC was counted in the time, when absorbance in the negative control tripled. The experiment was repeated on 3 separated occasions, and the results were averaged. The results are summarized in Table 2.

3.3.8. Inhibition of *Bipolaris sorokiniana* Germination

The inhibitory effect on the conidium germination was tested according to De Lucca et al. [93] with some modifications. The tested compounds were diluted in a 96-well microplate in 45 μL sterile distilled water to reach the final concentrations of 256 and 128 μg/mL. As a positive control, benomyl (10 and 5 μg/mL) was used. As a negative control, nontreated wells with 5% DMSO were used. Conidium suspension was prepared from sporulating culture grown on an agar plate. 5 μL of the aliquot was added to each well. The final concentration of conidia in each well was 3000 conidia in 1 mL. The plate was incubated at 22 °C for 48 h in dark. After the incubation, the aliquot from each well was observed microscopically (400×) for germination. A total of 50 conidia from each well were observed. Germination was defined as the development of germ tube(s) of any size from a conidium. The inhibition effect was counted as a ratio of nongerminated conidia compared to the negative control. The experiment was performed in duplicate. The results are summarized in Table 4.

3.3.9. In Vitro Antiproliferative Assay

Human monocytic leukemia THP-1 cells were used for in vitro antiproliferative assay. Cells were obtained from the European Collection of Cell Cultures (ECACC, Salisbury, UK) and routinely cultured in RPMI (Roswell Park Memorial Institute) 1640 medium supplemented with 10% fetal bovine serum, 2% L-glutamine, 1% penicillin, and streptomycin at 37 °C with 5% CO_2. Cells were passaged at approximately one-week intervals. The antiproliferative activity of the compounds was determined using a Water Soluble Tetrazolium Salts-1 (WST-1, 2-(4-iodophenyl)-3-(4-nitrophenyl)-5-(2,4-disulfophenyl)-2*H*-tetrazolium) assay kit (Roche Diagnostics, Mannheim, Germany) according to the manufacturer's instructions. The tested compounds were dissolved in DMSO and added in five increasing concentrations (0.37, 1.1, 3.3, 10, and 30 μM) to the cell suspension in the culture RPMI 1640 medium. The maximum concentration of DMSO in the assays never exceeded 0.1%. Subsequently, the cells were incubated at 37 °C with 5% CO_2 for 24 h. For WST-1 assays, cells were seeded into 96-well plates (5×10^4 cells/well in 100 μL culture medium) in triplicate in serum-free RPMI 1640 medium, and measurements were taken 24 h after the treatment with the compounds. The median inhibition concentration values, IC_{50}, were deduced through the production of a dose-response curve. All data were evaluated using GraphPad Prism 5.00 software (GraphPad Software, San Diego, CA, USA). The results are shown in Table 2.

3.3.10. Study of Inhibition of Photosynthetic Electron Transport (PET) in Spinach Chloroplasts

Chloroplasts were prepared from spinach (*Spinacia oleracea* L.) according to Masarovicova and Kralova [94]. The inhibition of photosynthetic electron transport (PET) in spinach chloroplasts was determined spectrophotometrically (Genesys 6, Thermo Scientific), using an artificial electron acceptor 2,6-dichlorophenol-indophenol (DCIPP) according to Kralova et al. [95], and the rate of photosynthetic electron transport was monitored as a photoreduction of DCPIP. The measurements were carried out in phosphate buffer (0.02 mol/L, pH 7.2) containing sucrose (0.4 mol/L), $MgCl_2$ (0.005 mol/L), and NaCl (0.015 mol/L). The chlorophyll content was 30 mg/L in these experiments, and the samples were irradiated (~100 W/m^2 with 10 cm distance) with a halogen lamp (250 W) using a 4 cm water filter to prevent warming of the samples (suspension temperature 22 °C). The studied compounds were dissolved in DMSO due to their limited water solubility. The applied DMSO concentration (up to 4%) did not affect the photochemical activity in spinach chloroplasts. The inhibitory efficiency of the studied compounds was expressed by IC_{50} values, i.e., by molar concentration of the compounds causing a 50% decrease in the oxygen evolution rate relative to the untreated control. The comparable IC_{50} value for the selective herbicide 3-(3,4-dichlorophenyl)-1,1-dimethylurea, DCMU (Diuron®) was about 2.1 μmol/L. The results are shown in Table 2.

3.3.11. In Vivo Toxicity against Plant Cells

Nicotiana tabacum var. Samsun was used for this test. The compounds were diluted in water to reach concentrations equal to 1× MIC and 4× MIC. As the negative control, solutions of DMSO in the same concentration were used. The positive control was 5% DMSO, which should be toxic to the plant cells. The aqueous solutions were injected into the plant leaves by a syringe (needle 27G × ¾") to fill area approx. 1 cm^2 [88]. The test was made in triplicates in three different plants. The plants were kept in a greenhouse on direct sunlight. The effect of the compounds was visually checked every day for 5 weeks. In the presence of tested compounds, no visible changes in the plant tissues were observed. The results are illustrated in Figure 6.

4. Conclusions

A series of sixteen ring-substituted *N*-arylcinnamamides was prepared, characterized, and evaluated against *Staphylococcus aureus*, three methicillin-resistant *S. aureus* strains, *Mycobacterium tuberculosis* H37Ra, *Fusarium avenaceum*, and *Bipolaris sorokiniana*. Additionally, the compounds were tested for their activity related to the inhibition of photosynthetic electron transport in spinach chloroplasts. (2*E*)-3-Phenyl-*N*-[3-(trifluoromethyl)phenyl]prop-2-enamide (**6**) and (2*E*)-*N*-[3,5-bis(tri-fluoromethyl)phenyl]-3-phenylprop-2-enamide (**13**) showed the highest activity (MIC = 27.47 and 22.27 μM, respectively) against all four staphylococcal strains as well as against *M. tuberculosis*. These compounds also showed activity against bacterial biofilm forming, the ability to increase the effect of clinically used antibiotics such as tetracycline, vancomycin, and ciprofloxacin and concentration-dependent antibacterial effect, which led to killing >99% of bacteria. On the other hand, (2*E*)-*N*-(3-fluorophenyl)- (**5**) and (2*E*)-*N*-(3-methylphenyl)-3-phenylprop-2-enamide (**2**) had MICs = 16.58 and 33.71 μM, respectively, against *B. sorokiniana*, while both compounds did not show any in vivo toxicity against *Nicotiana tabacum* var. Samsun. (2*E*)-*N*-(3,5-dichlorophenyl)-3-phenylprop-2-enamide (**11**, IC_{50} = 5.1 μM) was the most active PET inhibitor. These compounds showed activities comparable with or higher than those of standards. A significant decrease of mycobacterial cell metabolism (viability of *M. tuberculosis* H37Ra) was observed using the MTT assay. The screening of the cytotoxicity of the selected compounds was performed using THP-1 cells, and no significant lethal effect was observed for the most potent compounds. The position of substituents on the anilide ring seems to be crucial for both antitubercular and antifungal activity; positions $C_{(3)}'$, $C_{(3,4)}'$, and $C_{(3,5)}'$ are preferable. Lipophilicity is another important factor; antitubercular activity increases with increasing lipophilicity, while antifungal activity, to the contrary, decreases from the most effective compound **5** (R = 3-F) with lipophilicity log k = 0.23 with increasing lipophilicity. The activity is also dependent on the electronic parameters of substituents on the anilide core. Bilinear trends for effective compounds can be observed for both antitubercular and antifungal dependences; nevertheless, for antitubercular effectivity, rather more electron-withdrawing properties are preferred ($\sigma_{Ar} \approx 1$, compound **13**, R = 3,5-CF_3), while for antifungal activity against *B. sorokiniana*, less electron-withdrawing properties are preferred (σ_{Ar} = 0.82, compound **5**, R = 3-F). Also the dependences of PET-inhibiting activity on lipophilicity and electronic properties showed bilinear trends, as mentioned above, where $C_{(3,5)}'$ or $C_{(3,4)}'$ substitution of the anilide core is preferable.

Author Contributions: J.K. and T.S.—synthesis and characterization of the compounds and study of PET inhibition. I.K. and M.O.—analysis of the compounds. S.P., H.M., A.C., A.M.M., and J.B.—antimicrobial and pesticide evaluation and in vivo toxicity test. T.K. and P.K.—in vitro cytotoxicity assay. J.J.—conceived and designed the experiments, SAR, and the writing of the paper.

Acknowledgments: This contribution was supported by grant of the Comenius University in Bratislava No. UK/229/2018, grants of the Faculty of Pharmacy of Comenius University in Bratislava FaF UK/9/2018 and FaF UK/37/2018, VEGA project No.1/0040/17 and partially by SANOFI-AVENTIS Pharma Slovakia, s.r.o. and the National Research, Development, and Innovation Office (NKFIH) of Hungary (grant no. K119276). The HPLC/HRMS system forms a part of the National Infrastructure CzeCOS ProCES CZ.02.1.01/0.0/0.0/16_013/0001609; Michal Oravec was supported by the National Sustainability Program (NPU I; Grant No. LO1415).

Conflicts of Interest: The authors declare no conflicts of interest.

References

1. Lichtenthaler, H.K.; Schweiger, J. Cell wall bound ferulic acid, the major substance of the blue-green fluorescence emission of plants. *J. Plant Physiol.* **1998**, *152*, 272–282. [CrossRef]
2. Vogt, T. Phenylpropanoid biosynthesis. *Mol. Plant* **2010**, *3*, 2–20. [CrossRef] [PubMed]
3. Adisakwattana, S.; Chantarasinlapin, P.; Thammarat, H.; Yibchok-Anun, S. A series of cinnamic acid derivatives and their inhibitory activity on intestinal alpha-glucosidase. *J. Enzyme Inhib. Med. Chem.* **2009**, *24*, 1194–1200. [CrossRef] [PubMed]
4. Berrin, O.; Murat, K.; Ilkay, O. Cytotoxicity, antiviral and antimicrobial activities of alkaloids, flavonoids, and phenolic acids. *Pharm. Biol.* **2011**, *49*, 396–402.
5. Sharma, P. Cinnamic acid derivatives: A new chapter of various pharmacological activities. *J. Chem. Pharm. Res.* **2011**, *3*, 403–423.
6. Sova, M. Antioxidant and antimicrobial activities of cinnamic acid derivatives. *Mini Rev. Med. Chem.* **2012**, *12*, 749–767. [CrossRef] [PubMed]
7. Korosec, B.; Sova, M.; Turk, S.; Krasevec, N.; Novak, M.; Lah, L.; Stojan, J.; Podobnik, B.; Berne, S.; Zupanec, N.; et al. Antifungal activity of cinnamic acid derivatives involves inhibition of benzoate 4-hydroxylase (CYP53). *J. Appl. Microbiol.* **2014**, *116*, 955–966. [CrossRef] [PubMed]
8. Guzman, J.D. Natural cinnamic acids, synthetic derivatives and hybrids with antimicrobial activity. *Molecules* **2014**, *19*, 19292–19349. [CrossRef] [PubMed]

9. Peperidou, A.; Kapoukranidou, D.; Kontogiorgis, C.; Hadjipavlou-Litina, D. Multitarget molecular hybrids of cinnamic acids. *Molecules* **2014**, *19*, 20197–20226. [CrossRef] [PubMed]
10. Pontiki, E.; Hadjipavlou-Litina, D.; Litinas, K.; Geromichalos, G. Novel cinnamic acid derivatives as antioxidant and anticancer agents: Design, synthesis and modeling studies. *Molecules* **2014**, *19*, 9655–9674. [CrossRef] [PubMed]
11. Hadjipavlou-Litina, D.; Pontiki, E. Aryl-acetic and cinnamic acids as lipoxygenase inhibitors with antioxidant, anti-inflammatory, and anticancer activity. *Methods Mol. Biol.* **2015**, *1208*, 361–377. [PubMed]
12. Su, P.; Shi, Y.; Wang, J.; Shen, X.; Zhang, J. Anticancer agents derived from natural cinnamic acids. *Anticancer Agents Med. Chem.* **2015**, *15*, 980–987. [CrossRef] [PubMed]
13. De Vita, D.; Simonetti, G.; Pandolfi, F.; Costi, R.; Di Santo, R.; D'Auria, F.D.; Scipione, L. Exploring the anti-biofilm activity of cinnamic acid derivatives in Candida albicans. *Bioorg. Med. Chem. Lett.* **2016**, *26*, 5931–5935. [CrossRef] [PubMed]
14. Peperidou, A.; Pontiki, E.; Hadjipavlou-Litina, D.; Voulgari, E.; Avgoustakis, K. Multifunctional cinnamic acid derivatives. *Molecules* **2017**, *22*, 1247. [CrossRef] [PubMed]
15. Lima, T.C.; Ferreira, A.R.; Silva, D.F.; Lima, E.O.; de Sousa, D.P. Antifungal activity of cinnamic acid and benzoic acid esters against *Candida albicans* strains. *Nat. Prod. Res.* **2018**, *32*, 572–575. [CrossRef] [PubMed]
16. Dolab, J.G.; Lima, B.; Spaczynska, E.; Kos, J.; Cano, N.H.; Feresin, G.; Tapia, A.; Garibotto, F.; Petenatti, E.; Olivella, M.; et al. Antimicrobial activity of Annona emarginata (Schltdl.) H. Rainer and most active isolated compound against clinically important bacteria. *Molecules* **2018**, *23*, 1187. [CrossRef] [PubMed]
17. FRAC Code List 2018. Available online: http://www.frac.info/docs/default-source/publications/frac-code-list/frac_code_list_2018-final.pdf?sfvrsn=6144b9a_2 (accessed on 18 June 2018).
18. WHO. *Global Antimicrobial Resistance Surveillance System (GLASS) Report*; HO Press: Geneva, Switzerland, 2017.
19. Gonec, T.; Bobal, P.; Sujan, J.; Pesko, M.; Guo, J.; Kralova, K.; Pavlacka, L.; Vesely, L.; Kreckova, E.; Kos, J.; et al. Investigating the spectrum of biological activity of substituted quinoline-2-carboxamides and their isosteres. *Molecules* **2012**, *17*, 613–644. [CrossRef] [PubMed]
20. Kos, J.; Nevin, E.; Soral, M.; Kushkevych, I.; Gonec, T.; Bobal, P.; Kollar, P.; Coffey, A.; O'Mahony, J.; Liptaj, T.; et al. Synthesis and antimycobacterial properties of ring-substituted 6-hydroxynaphthalene-2-carboxanilides. *Bioorg. Med. Chem.* **2015**, *23*, 2035–2043. [CrossRef] [PubMed]
21. Tischer, W.; Strotmann, H. Relationship between inhibitor binding by chloroplasts and inhibition of photosynthetic electron-transport. *Biochim. Biophys. Acta* **1977**, *460*, 113–125. [CrossRef]
22. Trebst, A.; Draber, W. Structure activity correlations of recent herbicides in photosynthetic reactions. In *Advances in Pesticide Science*; Greissbuehler, H., Ed.; Pergamon Press: Oxford, UK, 1979; pp. 223–234.
23. Bowyer, J.R.; Camilleri, P.; Vermaas, W.F.J. *Herbicides, Topics in Photosynthesis*; Baker, N.R., Percival, M.P., Eds.; Elsevier: Amsterdam, The Netherlands, 1991; Volume 10, pp. 27–85.
24. Izawa, S. Acceptors and donors for chloroplast electron transport. In *Methods in Enzymology*; Colowick, P., Kaplan, N.O., Eds.; Academic Press: New York, NY, USA; London, UK, 1980; Volume 69, Part C; pp. 413–434.
25. Good, N.E. Inhibitors of the Hill reaction. *Plant Physiol.* **1961**, *36*, 788–803. [CrossRef] [PubMed]
26. Otevrel, J.; Mandelova, Z.; Pesko, M.; Guo, J.; Kralova, K.; Sersen, F.; Vejsova, M.; Kalinowski, D.; Kovacevic, Z.; Coffey, A.; et al. Investigating the spectrum of biological activity of ring-substituted salicylanilides and carbamoylphenylcarbamates. *Molecules* **2010**, *15*, 8122–8142. [CrossRef] [PubMed]
27. Gonec, T.; Kos, J.; Zadrazilova, I.; Pesko, M.; Keltosova, S.; Tengler, J.; Bobal, P.; Kollar, P.; Cizek, A.; Kralova, K.; et al. Antimycobacterial and herbicidal activity of ring-substituted 1-hydroxynaphthalene-2-carboxanilides. *Bioorg. Med. Chem.* **2013**, *21*, 6531–6541. [CrossRef] [PubMed]
28. Kralova, K.; Perina, M.; Waisser, K.; Jampilek, J. Structure-activity relationships of *N*-benzylsalicylamides for inhibition of photosynthetic electron transport. *Med. Chem.* **2015**, *11*, 156–164. [CrossRef] [PubMed]
29. Gonec, T.; Kralova, K.; Pesko, M.; Jampilek, J. Antimycobacterial *N*-Alkoxyphenylhydroxynaphthalenecarboxamides Affecting Photosystem II. *Bioorg. Med. Chem. Lett.* **2017**, *27*, 1881–1885. [CrossRef] [PubMed]
30. Gonec, T.; Kos, J.; Pesko, M.; Dohanosova, J.; Oravec, M.; Liptaj, T.; Kralova, K.; Jampilek, J. Halogenated 1-Hydroxynaphthalene-2-carboxanilides Affecting Photosynthetic Electron Transport in Photosystem II. *Molecules* **2017**, *22*, 1709. [CrossRef] [PubMed]
31. Shaner, D.L. Herbicide safety relative to common targets in plants and mammals. *Pest. Manag. Sci.* **2004**, *60*, 17–24. [CrossRef] [PubMed]

32. Delaney, J.; Clarke, E.; Hughes, D.; Rice, M. Modern agrochemical research: A missed opportunity for drug discovery? *Drug Discov. Today* **2006**, *11*, 839–845. [CrossRef] [PubMed]
33. Duke, S.O. Herbicide and pharmaceutical relationships. *Weed Sci.* **2010**, *58*, 334–339. [CrossRef]
34. Myung, K.; Klittich, C.J. Can agricultural fungicides accelerate the discovery of human antifungal drugs? *Drug Discov. Today* **2015**, *20*, 7–10. [CrossRef] [PubMed]
35. Jampilek, J. Potential of agricultural fungicides for antifungal drug discovery. *Expert Opin. Drug Dis.* **2016**, *11*, 1–9. [CrossRef] [PubMed]
36. Pliska, V. Methods and Principles in Medicinal Chemistry. In *Lipophilicity in Drug Action and Toxicology*, 1st ed.; Pliska, V., Testa, B., van der Waterbeemd, H., Eds.; Wiley-VCH: Weinheim, Germany, 1996; Volume 4.
37. Zadrazilova, I.; Pospisilova, S.; Pauk, K.; Imramovsky, A.; Vinsova, J.; Cizek, A.; Jampilek, J. In vitro bactericidal activity of 4- and 5-chloro-2-hydroxy-N-[1-oxo-1-(phenylamino)alkan-2-yl]benzamides against MRSA. *Biomed Res. Int.* **2015**, *2015*, 349534. [CrossRef] [PubMed]
38. Zadrazilova, I.; Pospisilova, S.; Masarikova, M.; Imramovsky, A.; Monreal-Ferriz, J.; Vinsova, J.; Cizek, A.; Jampilek, J. Salicylanilide carbamates: Promising antibacterial agents with high in vitro activity against methicillin-resistant *Staphylococcus aureus*. *Eur. J. Pharm. Sci.* **2015**, *77*, 197–207. [CrossRef] [PubMed]
39. Oravcova, V.; Zurek, L.; Townsend, A.; Clark, A.B.; Ellis, J.C.; Cizek, A. American crows as carriers of vancomycin-resistant enterococci with vanA gene. *Environ. Microbiol.* **2014**, *16*, 939–949. [CrossRef] [PubMed]
40. Pospisilova, S.; Michnova, H.; Kauerova, T.; Pauk, K.; Kollar, P.; Vinsova, J.; Imramovsky, A.; Cizek, A.; Jampilek, J. In vitro activity of salicylamide derivatives against vancomycin-resistant enterococci. *Bioorg. Med. Chem. Lett.* **2018**, *28*, 2184–2188. [CrossRef] [PubMed]
41. Schwalbe, R.; Steele-Moore, L.; Goodwin, A.C. *Antimicrobial Susceptibility Testing Protocols*; CRC Press: Boca Raton, FL, USA, 2007.
42. Bonapace, C.R.; Bosso, J.A.; Friedrich, L.V.; White, R.L. Comparison of methods of interpretation of checkerboard synergy testing. *Diagn. Microbiol. Infect. Dis.* **2002**, *44*, 363–366. [CrossRef]
43. Helander, I.M.; Alakomi, H.L.; Latva-Kala, K.; Mattila-Sandholm, T.; Pol, I.; Smid, E.J.; Gorris, L.G.M.; von Wright, A. Characterization of the action of selected essential oil components on gram negative bacteria. *J. Agric. Food Chem.* **1998**, *46*, 3590–3595. [CrossRef]
44. Ultee, A.; Bennik, M.H.J.; Moezelaar, R. The phenolic hydroxyl group of carvacrol is essential for action against the food-borne pathogen Bacillus cereus. *Appl. Environ. Microbiol.* **2002**, *68*, 1561–1568. [CrossRef] [PubMed]
45. Gill, A.O.; Holley, R.A. Inhibition of membrane bound ATPases of Escherichia coli and Listeria monocytogenes by plant oil aromatics. *Int. J. Food Microbiol.* **2006**, *3*, 170–174. [CrossRef] [PubMed]
46. Langeveld, W.T.; Veldhuizen, E.J.; Burt, S.A. Synergy between essential oil components and antibiotics: A review. *Crit. Rev. Microbiol.* **2014**, *40*, 76–94. [CrossRef] [PubMed]
47. Hemaiswarya, S.; Doble, M. Synergistic interaction of phenylpropanoids with antibiotics against bacteria. *J. Med. Microbiol.* **2010**, *59*, 1469–1476. [CrossRef] [PubMed]
48. Kim, Y.G.; Lee, J.H.; Kim, S.I.; Baek, K.H.; Lee, J. Cinnamon bark oil and its components inhibit biofilm formation and toxin production. *Int. J. Food Microbiol.* **2015**, *195*, 30–39. [CrossRef] [PubMed]
49. Brackman, G.; Defoirdt, T.; Miyamoto, C.; Bossier, P.; Van Calenbergh, S.; Nelis, H.; Coenye, T. Cinnamaldehyde and cinnamaldehyde derivatives reduce virulence in Vibrio spp. by decreasing the DNA-binding activity of the quorum sensing response regulator LuxR. *BMC Microbiol.* **2008**, *8*, 149. [CrossRef] [PubMed]
50. Zodrow, K.R.; Schiffman, J.D.; Elimelech, M. Biodegradable polymer (PLGA) coatings featuring cinnamaldehyde and carvacrol mitigate biofilm formation. *Langmuir* **2012**, *28*, 13993–13999. [CrossRef] [PubMed]
51. Jia, P.; Xue, Y.J.; Duan, X.J.; Shao, S.H. Effect of cinnamaldehyde on biofilm formation and sarA expression by methicillin-resistant *Staphylococcus aureus*. *Lett. Appl. Microbiol.* **2011**, *53*, 409–416. [CrossRef] [PubMed]
52. Brackman, G.; Coenye, T. Quorum sensing inhibitors as anti-biofilm agents. *Curr. Pharm. Des.* **2015**, *21*, 5–11. [CrossRef] [PubMed]
53. Niu, C.; Afre, S.; Gilbert, E.S. Subinhibitory concentrations of cinnamaldehyde interfere with quorum sensing. *Lett. Appl. Microbiol.* **2006**, *43*, 489–494. [CrossRef] [PubMed]

54. Nuryastuti, T.; van der Mei, H.C.; Busscher, H.J.; Iravati, S.; Aman, A.T.; Krom, B.P. Effect of cinnamon oil on icaA expression and biofilm formation by Staphylococcus epidermidis. *Appl. Environ. Microbiol.* **2009**, *75*, 6850–6855. [CrossRef] [PubMed]
55. Budzynska, A.; Wieckowska-Szakiel, M.; Sadowska, B.; Kalemba, D.; Rozalska, B. Antibiofilm activity of selected plant essential oils and their major components. *Pol. J. Microbiol.* **2011**, *60*, 35–41. [PubMed]
56. Kaplan, J.B. Antibiotic-induced biofilm formation. *Int. J. Artif. Organs* **2011**, *34*, 737–751. [CrossRef] [PubMed]
57. Mirani, Z.A.; Jamil, N. Effect of sub-lethal doses of vancomycin and oxacillin on biofilm formation by vancomycin intermediate resistant *Staphylococcus aureus*. *J. Basic Microbiol.* **2011**, *51*, 191–195. [CrossRef] [PubMed]
58. Zheng, H.; Lu, L.; Wang, B.; Pu, S.; Zhang, X.; Zhu, G.; Shi, W.; Zhang, L.; Wang, H.; Wang, S.; et al. Genetic basis of virulence attenuation revealed by comparative genomic analysis of Mycobacterium tuberculosis strain H37Ra versus H37Rv. *PLoS ONE* **2008**, *3*, e2375. [CrossRef] [PubMed]
59. Bueno, J. Antitubercular in vitro drug discovery: Tools for begin the search. In *Understanding Tuberculosis-New Approaches to Fighting against Drug Resistance*; Cardona, P.J., Ed.; InTech: Rijeka, Croatia, 2012; pp. 147–168.
60. Kos, J.; Zadrazilova, I.; Nevin, E.; Soral, M.; Gonec, T.; Kollar, P.; Oravec, M.; Coffey, A.; O'Mahony, J.; Liptaj, T.; et al. Ring-substituted 8-Hydroxyquinoline-2-carboxanilides as potential antimycobacterial agents. *Bioorg. Med. Chem.* **2015**, *23*, 4188–4196. [CrossRef] [PubMed]
61. Gonec, T.; Zadrazilova, I.; Nevin, E.; Kauerova, T.; Pesko, M.; Kos, J.; Oravec, M.; Kollar, P.; Coffey, A.; O'Mahony, J.; et al. Synthesis and biological evaluation of *N*-alkoxyphenyl-3-hydroxynaphthalene-2-carbox-anilides. *Molecules* **2015**, *20*, 9767–9787. [CrossRef] [PubMed]
62. Gonec, T.; Pospisilova, S.; Kauerova, T.; Kos, J.; Dohanosova, J.; Oravec, M.; Kollar, P.; Coffey, A.; Liptaj, T.; Cizek, A.; et al. *N*-Alkoxyphenylhydroxynaphthalenecarboxamides and their antimycobacterial activity. *Molecules* **2016**, *21*, 1068. [CrossRef] [PubMed]
63. Zumla, A.; Nahid, P.; Cole, S.T. Advances in the development of new tuberculosis drugs and treatment regimens. *Nat. Rev. Drug Discov.* **2013**, *12*, 388–404. [CrossRef] [PubMed]
64. Upadhayaya, R.S.; Vandavasi, J.K.; Kardile, R.A.; Lahore, S.V.; Dixit, S.S.; Deokar, H.S.; Shinde, P.D.; Sarmah, M.P.; Chattopadhyaya, J. Novel quinoline and naphthalene derivatives as potent antimycobacterial agents. *Eur. J. Med. Chem.* **2010**, *45*, 1854–1867. [CrossRef] [PubMed]
65. Wang, Z.; Li, L.; Zhou, Z.; Geng, Y.; Chen, Y.; Sun, T. Design, synthesis, configuration research, and in vitro antituberculosis activities of two chiral naphthylamine substituted analogs of bedaquiline. *J. Heterocycl. Chem.* **2017**, *54*, 1024–1030. [CrossRef]
66. Tong, A.S.T.; Choi, P.J.; Blaser, A.; Sutherland, H.S.; Tsang, S.K.Y.; Guillemont, J.; Motte, M.; Cooper, C.B.; Andries, K.; van den Broeck, W.; et al. 6-Cyano analogues of bedaquiline as less lipophilic and potentially safer diarylquinolines for tuberculosis. *ACS Med. Chem. Lett.* **2017**, *8*, 1019–10242. [CrossRef] [PubMed]
67. Chen, Y.L.; Huang, S.T.; Sun, F.M.; Chiang, Y.L.; Chiang, C.J.; Tsai, C.M.; Weng, C.J. Transformation of cinnamic acid from trans- to cis-form raises a notable bactericidal and synergistic activity against multiple-drug resistant Mycobacterium tuberculosis. *Eur. J. Pharm. Sci.* **2011**, *43*, 188–194. [CrossRef] [PubMed]
68. De, P.; Koumba, Y.G.; Constant, P.; Bedos-Belval, F.; Duran, H.; Saffon, N.; Daffe, M.; Baltas, M. Design, synthesis, and biological evaluation of new cinnamic derivatives as antituberculosis agents. *J. Med. Chem.* **2011**, *54*, 1449–1461. [CrossRef] [PubMed]
69. De, P.; Veau, D.; Bedos-Belval, F.; Chassaing, S.; Baltas, M. Cinnamic derivatives in tuberculosis. In *Understanding Tuberculosis-New Approaches to Fighting against Drug Resistance*; Cardona, P.J., Ed.; InTech: Rijeka, Croatia, 2012; pp. 337–362.
70. Adeniji, S.E.; Uba, S.; Uzairu, A. Quantitative structure–activity relationship and molecular docking of 4-alkoxy-cinnamic analogues as anti-mycobacterium tuberculosis. *J. King Saud Uni. Sci.* **2018**. [CrossRef]
71. Degola, F.; Morcia, C.; Bisceglie, F.; Mussi, F.; Tumino, G.; Ghizzoni, R.; Pelosi, G.; Terzi, V.; Buschini, A.; Restivo, F.M.; et al. In vitro evaluation of the activity of thiosemicarbazone derivatives against mycotoxigenic fungi affecting cereals. *Int. J. Food Microbiol.* **2015**, *200*, 104–111. [CrossRef] [PubMed]
72. Zhou, K.; Chen, D.; Li, B.; Zhang, B.; Miao, F.; Zhou, L. Bioactivity and structure-activity relationship of cinnamic acid esters and their derivatives as potential antifungal agents for plant protection. *PLoS ONE* **2017**, *12*, e0176189. [CrossRef] [PubMed]

73. Krishnendu, A.; Dutta, A.K.; Pradhan, P. Bipolaris sorokiniana'(Sacc.) Shoem.: The most destructive wheat fungal pathogen in the warmer areas. *Aust. J. Crop Sci.* **2011**, *5*, 1064–1071.
74. Saari, E.E. Leaf blight disease and associated soil borne fungal pathogens of wheat in South and Southeast Asia. In *Helminthosporium Blights of Wheat: Spot Blotch and Tan Spot*; Duveiller, E., Dubin, H.J., Reeves, J., McNab, A., Eds.; CIMMYT: Texcoco de Mora, Mexico, 1998; pp. 37–51.
75. Sundheim, L.; Brodal, G.; Hofgaard, I.S.; Rafoss, T. Temporal variation of mycotoxin producing fungi in norwegian cereals. *Microorganisms* **2013**, *1*, 188–198. [CrossRef] [PubMed]
76. Placinta, C.M.; D'Mello, J.P.F.; MacDonald, A.M.C. A review of worldwide contamination of cereal grains and animal feed with Fusarium mycotoxins. *Anim. Feed Sci. Technol.* **1999**, *78*, 21–37. [CrossRef]
77. Tortora, G.J.; Funke, B.R.; Case, C.L. *Microbiology: An introduction*, 10th ed.; Benjamin Cummings: San Francisco, CA, USA, 2010.
78. ROCHE. Cell proliferation reagent WST-1. Roche Diagnostics GmbH, Mannheim, Germany. 2011. Available online: https://www.sigmaaldrich.com/content/dam/sigma-aldrich/docs/Roche/Bulletin/1/cellprorobul.pdf (accessed on 26 June 2018).
79. Kauerova, T.; Kos, J.; Gonec, T.; Jampilek, J.; Kollar, P. Antiproliferative and pro-apoptotic effect of novel nitro-substituted hydroxynaphthanilides on human cancer cell lines. *Int. J. Mol. Sci.* **2016**, *17*, 1219. [CrossRef] [PubMed]
80. Suffness, M.; Douros, J. Current status of the NCI plant and animal product program. *J. Nat. Prod.* **1982**, *45*, 1–14. [CrossRef] [PubMed]
81. Jampilek, J.; Kralova, K.; Pesko, M.; Kos, J. Ring-substituted 8-hydroxyquinoline-2-carboxanilides as photosystem II inhibitors. *Bioorg. Med. Chem. Lett.* **2016**, *26*, 3862–3865. [CrossRef] [PubMed]
82. Fajkusova, D.; Pesko, M.; Keltosova, S.; Guo, J.; Oktabec, Z.; Vejsova, M.; Kollar, P.; Coffey, A.; Csollei, J.; Kralova, K.; et al. Anti-infective and herbicidal activity of *N*-substituted 2-aminobenzothiazoles. *Bioorg. Med. Chem.* **2012**, *20*, 7059–7068. [CrossRef] [PubMed]
83. Gonec, T.; Kos, J.; Zadrazilova, I.; Pesko, M.; Govender, R.; Keltosova, S.; Kollar, B.; Imramovsky, A.; O'Mahony, J.; Coffey, A.; et al. Antibacterial and herbicidal activity of ring-substituted 2-hydroxynaphthalene-1-carboxanilides. *Molecules* **2013**, *18*, 9397–9419. [CrossRef] [PubMed]
84. Kralova, K.; Sersen, F.; Cizmarik, J. Inhibitory effect of piperidinoethylesters of alkoxyphenylcarbamic acids on photosynthesis. *Gen. Physiol. Biophys.* **1992**, *11*, 261–267.
85. Kralova, K.; Bujdakova, H.; Kuchta, T.; Loos, D. Correlation between biological activity and the structure of 6-amino-2-*R*-thiobenzothiazoles. Anti-yeast activity and inhibition of photochemical activity of chloroplasts. *Pharmazie* **1994**, *49*, 460–461. [PubMed]
86. Kralova, K.; Kallova, J.; Loos, D.; Devinsky, F. Correlation between biological activity and the structure of *N,N'*-bis(alkyldimethyl)-1,6-hexanediammonium dibromides. Antibacterial activity and inhibition of photochemical activity of chloroplasts. *Pharmazie* **1994**, *49*, 857–858. [PubMed]
87. Kralova, K.; Bujdakova, H.; Cizmarik, J. Antifungal and antialgal activity of piperidinopropyl esters of alkoxy substituted phenylcarbamic acids. *Pharmazie* **1995**, *50*, 440–441. [PubMed]
88. Szabo, E. Isolation and characterization of EBR specific induced chitinases from tobacco (*Nicotiana tabacum*). *Acta Biol. Szeged.* **2008**, *52*, 251–252.
89. Zhang, M.; Lu, X.; Zhang, H.J.; Li, N.; Xiao, Y.; Zhu, H.L.; Ye, Y.H. Synthesis, structure, and biological assay of cinnamic amides as potential EGFR kinase inhibitors. *Med. Chem. Res.* **2013**, *22*, 986–994. [CrossRef]
90. Lee, C.C.; Lo, Y.; Ho, L.J.; Lai, J.H.; Lien, S.B.; Lin, L.C.; Chen, C.L.; Chen, T.C.; Liu, F.C.; Huang, H.S. A new application of parallel synthesis strategy for discovery of amide-linked small molecules as potent chondroprotective agents in TNF-α-stimulated chondrocytes. *PLoS ONE* **2016**, *11*, e0149317. [CrossRef] [PubMed]
91. Clinical and Laboratory Standards Institute. *Performance Standards for Antimicrobial Susceptibility Testing*; The 8th Informational Supplement Document; CLSI: Wayne, PA, USA, 2012; M100-S22.
92. Abate, G.; Mshana, R.N.; Miorner, H. Evaluation of a colorimetric assay based on 3-(4,5-dimethylthiazol-2-yl)-2,5-diphenyl tetrazolium bromide (MTT) for rapid detection of rifampicin resistance in Mycobacterium tuberculosis. *Int. J. Tuberc. Lung Dis.* **1998**, *2*, 1011–1016. [PubMed]
93. De Lucca, A.J.; Walsh, T.J.; Daigle, D.J. *N*-acetylcysteine inhibits germination of conidia and growth of Aspergillus spp. and Fusarium spp. *Antimicrob. Agents Chemother.* **1996**, *40*, 1274–1276. [PubMed]

94. Masarovicova, E.; Kralova, K. Approaches to Measuring Plant Photosynthesis Activity. In *Handbook of Photosynthesis*, 2nd ed.; Pessarakli, M., Ed.; Taylor & Francis Group: Boca Raton, FL, USA, 2005; pp. 617–656.
95. Kralova, K.; Sersen, F.; Sidoova, E. Photosynthesis inhibition produced by 2-alkylthio-6-*R*-benzothiazoles. *Chem. Pap.* **1992**, *46*, 348–350.

International Journal of
Molecular Sciences

MDPI

Article

Polyphenols Derived from Lychee Seed Suppress Aβ (1-42)-Induced Neuroinflammation

Yong Tang [1], Rui Xiong [1], An-Guo Wu [1,2], Chong-Lin Yu [3], Ya Zhao [1], Wen-Qiao Qiu [1], Xiu-Ling Wang [1], Jin-Feng Teng [1], Jian Liu [1], Hai-Xia Chen [1], Jian-Ming Wu [1,2] and Da-Lian Qin [1,2,*]

1 Laboratory of Chinese Materia Medica, Department of Pharmacology, School of Pharmacy, Southwest Medical University, Luzhou 646000, China; tangy1989@yeah.net (Y.T.); rxiong2017@sina.com (R.X.); wag1114@foxmail.com (A.-G.W.); zhaoya129@126.com (Y.Z.); fanny.qiu@outlook.com (W.-Q.Q.); wangxiulinbest@gmail.com (X.-L.W.); 18883178848@163.com (J.-F.T.); belkn@icloud.com (J.L.); dna0805001@163.com (H.-X.C.); jianmingwu@swmu.edu.cn (J.-M.W.)

2 Institute of Cardiovascular Research, the Key Laboratory of Medical Electrophysiology, Ministry of Education of China, Collaborative Innovation Center for Prevention and Treatment of Cardiovascular Disease of Sichuan Province, Southwest Medical University, Luzhou 646000, China

3 Department of Human Anatomy, School of Preclinical Medicine, Southwest Medical University, Luzhou 646000, China; 8056ycl@swmu.edu.cn

* Correspondence: dalianqin@swmu.edu.cn; Tel.: +86-0830-316-2291

Received: 11 May 2018; Accepted: 17 July 2018; Published: 20 July 2018

Abstract: Amyloid-β (Aβ) is commonly recognized as the most important factor that results in neuronal cell death and accelerates the progression of Alzheimer's disease (AD). Increasing evidence suggests that microglia activated by Aβ release an amount of neurotoxic inflammatory cytokines that contribute to neuron death and aggravate AD pathology. In our previous studies, we found that lychee seed fraction (LSF), an active fraction derived from the lychee seed, could significantly improve the cognitive function of AD rats and inhibit Aβ-induced neuroinflammation in vitro, and decrease neuronal injuries in vivo and in vitro. In the current study, we aimed to isolate and identify the specific components in LSF that were responsible for the anti-neuroinflammation effect using preparative high performance liquid chromatography (pre-HPLC), liquid chromatography-mass spectrometry (LC-MS), and nuclear magnetic resonance (NMR) methods. To this end, we confirmed two polyphenols including catechin and procyanidin A2 that could improve the morphological status of BV-2 cells and suppress the release, mRNA levels, and protein expression of pro-inflammatory cytokines such as tumor necrosis factor-α (TNF-α), interleukin-1β (IL-1β), and interleukin-6 (IL-6) through downregulating the nuclear factor-κB (NF-κB) signaling pathway using ELISA, RT-PCR, and Western blotting methods. Furthermore, catechin and procyanidin A2 could inhibit Aβ-induced apoptosis in BV-2 cells by upregulating Bcl-2 and downregulating Bax protein expression. Therefore, the current study illustrated the active substances in lychee seed, and first reported that catechin and procyanidin A2 could suppress neuroinflammation in Aβ-induced BV-2 cells, which provides detailed insights into the molecular mechanism of catechin and procyanidin A2 in the neuroprotective effect, and their further validations of anti-neuroinflammation in vivo is also essential in future research.

Keywords: Aβ; AD; lychee seed; neuroinflammation; catechin; procyanidin A2; apoptosis

1. Introduction

Alzheimer's disease (AD) is the most common type of late-onset dementia, which is characterized by dysfunction in cognition and behavior. Senile plaques (SPs) and neurofibrillary tangles (NFTs) are recognized as two key pathological features of AD, and amyloid-β (Aβ) and hyperphosphorylated tau are the two main aggregated proteins in SPs and NFTs, respectively. These aggregated proteins accumulate in neurons, which lead to neuronal death and ultimately dementia. Therefore, AD patients exhibit an extensive loss of synapses and neurons in the cortex and hippocampus [1,2].

AD pathogenesis is not the only Aβ- and tau-induced neuronal injury, but is also a kind of neuroinflammation activated by Aβ and tau [3–6]. Microglia are a special form of macrophage, which are involved in the innate immune system of the central nervous system (CNS) and mediate the key neuroinflammatory cytokines [7–9]. In general, aggregated proteins such as Aβ, α-synuclein, and mHtt associated with AD, Parkinson's disease (PD), and Huntington's disease (HD) respectively, can activate microglia and release amounts of pro-inflammatory cytokines such as tumor necrosis factor alpha (TNF-α), interleukin-1β (IL-1β), interleukin-6 (IL-6), nitric oxide (NO), and reactive oxygen species (ROS). These toxic inflammatory cytokines then induce microglial activation and neuronal death, which in turn further aggravate the inflammatory response. In AD patients, the morphology of microglia has been found to be abnormal and over-activated by oligomeric Aβ [9,10].

With the improvements in the material standards of people's lives, the aging population is becoming an important issue. More and more age-related diseases—such as dementia, diabetes, hypertension, coronary heart disease, etc.—are accelerating, of which, dementia with dysfunction in cognition and behavior brings a heavy spirit and economic burdens to the patients, their families, and countries. However, up until now, there are still no effective drugs that can be used for the treatment of AD owing to its complicated mechanisms [11]. Traditional Chinese medicines (TCMs) have a long usage history in the prevention and treatment of diverse diseases. There are many Chinese medical herbs and formulas—such as *Radix polygalae*, *Radix ginseng*, *Ginkgo biloba*, *Salvia miltiorrhiza*, *Ginseng*, Dangguishaoyao San, Tiaoxin Fang, and Zhiling Tang—that have been proven to modulate neurodegenerative disease [12–18].

Lychee seed (lizhihe in Chinese) is from the dried mature seeds of *Litchi chinensis Sonn*, which is a Chinese folk medicine recorded in "Ben cao gang mu". Its traditional efficacies include promoting the circulation of Qi to resolve stagnation and treating hernia. Modern pharmacological studies have proven that lychee seed exerts the following bioactivities including improving blood sugar concentration, liver-protection, anti-oxidation, anti-virus, and anti-tumor effects. In our previous studies, we found that LSF, a bioactive fraction derived from lychee seed, could improve cognitive function of AD rats, suppress apoptosis in Aβ-induced PC-12 cells, and reduce Aβ and tau proteins in T2DM rats [19,20]. Recently, we have characterized the detailed components in LSF and proven that LSF could suppress Aβ-induced neuroinflammation in BV-2 cells. In the present study, we aimed to isolate and identify the components in LSF that are responsible for the anti-neuroinflammation effect in Aβ-induced BV-2 cells. Through its isolation, purification, identification, and elucidation using column chromatography, preparative high performance liquid chromatography (Pre-HPLC), and nuclear magnetic resonance (NMR) technologies, two polyphenols including catechin and procyanidin A2 were proven to suppress Aβ-induced neuroinflammation and apoptosis in Aβ-induced BV-2 cells. These findings in the current study provide evidences for the action substances and mechanism of lychee seed in the improvement of the cognition and behavior of AD rats, and further investigation of their pharmacokinetics in rat brain and the validation of their anti-inflammation effect in vivo are also essential for future therapeutic approaches.

2. Results

2.1. Isolation, Purification, Identification, and Elucidation of Catechin and Procyanidin A2 in LSF

LSF was prepared according to the previous study [19,20] and first analyzed using RP-HPLC monitored at 280 nm. A total of 12 main peaks were collected using AKTA protein purification system (Figure S1A,B). The purity of 12 collected peaks were measured by using RP-HPLC (Figure S1C). Through the preliminary evaluation of the anti-neuroinflammation effect of these 12 fractions using Wright–Giemsa staining and ELISA methods, Fractions 3 and 9 were found to improve the morphological status, decrease the ratio of activated BV-2 cells, increase cell density, and decrease the release of pro-inflammatory cytokines in Aβ(1-42)-induced BV-2 cells (Figures S2 and S3), suggesting that the compounds in Fraction 3 and 9 could be the major bioactive components that are responsible for the anti-inflammation effect. Therefore, we applied pre-HPLC to further purify the compounds in Fractions 3 and 9, and obtained compounds **1** and **2** from Fractions 3 and 9, respectively. Through the elucidation using ultra-high-performance liquid chromatography with diode array detector coupled with electrospray ionization-tandem mass spectrometry (UHPLC-DAD-ESI-/MS/MS) and NMR instruments (Figures S4–S6), Compounds **1** and **2** were confirmed to be catechin and procyanidin A2, respectively. Their structures, DAD chromatograms, and MS spectrums are displayed in Figure 1 and Figure S7.

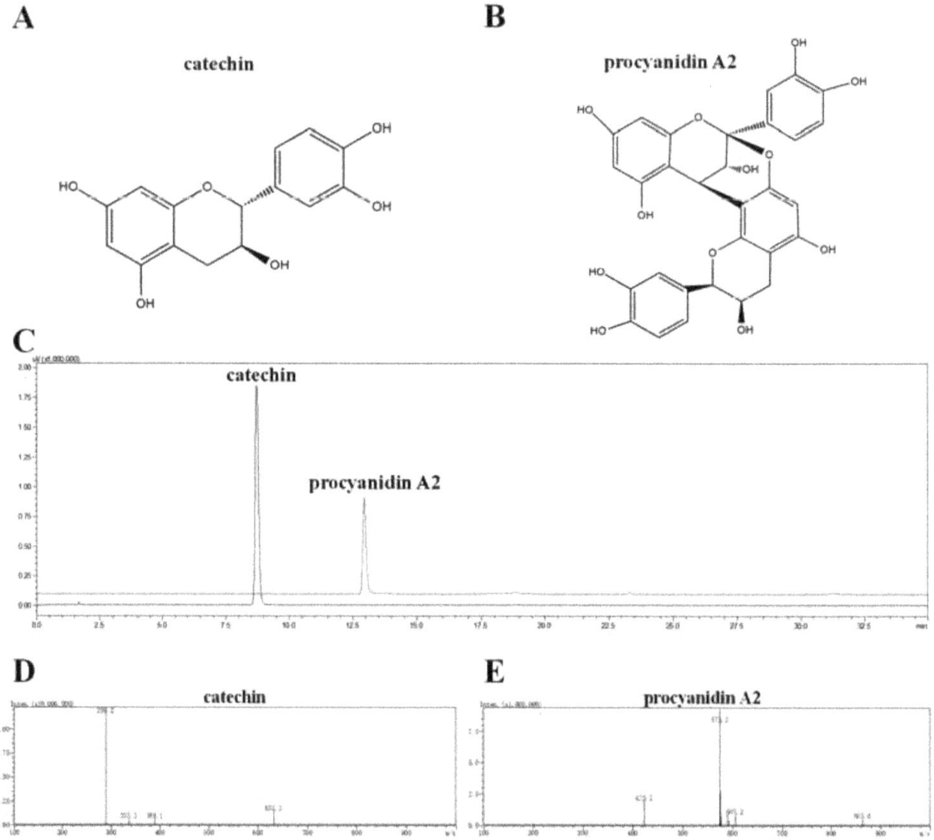

Figure 1. UHPLC-DAD-ESI-MS/MS chromatograms of catechin and procyanidin A2. The structures of (**A**) catechin and (**B**) procyanidin A2. (**C**) DAD chromatograms of catechin and procyanidin A2 recorded at 280 nm, MS spectrum of (**D**) catechin and (**E**) procyanidin A2 in negative mode.

Compound **1**: UV λmax: 215, 276 nm, LC-ESI-MS/MS: *m/z* 289.2 $[M-H]^-$, ^{1}H-NMR (400 MHz, DMSO): d 9.22 (s, 1H, 5-OH), 8.97 (s, 1H, 7-OH), 8.90 (s, 1H, 3′-OH), 8.85 (s, 1H, 4′-OH), 6.71 (m, 1H, 2′-H), 6.67 (d, *J* = 1.9 Hz, 1H, 5′-H), 6.60 (d, *J* = 1.9 Hz, 1H, 6′-H), 5.88 (d, *J* = 2.3 Hz, 1H, 6-H), 5.68 (d, *J* = 2.2 Hz, 1H, 8-H), 4.90 (d, *J* = 5.1 Hz, 1H, 3-OH), 4.48 (d, *J* = 7.5 Hz, 1H, 2-H), 3.81 (m, 1H, 3-H), 2.63 (dd, *J* = 16.1, 5.3 Hz, 1H, 4-H), 2.35 (dd, *J* = 16.0, 8.0 Hz, 1H, 4-H); ^{13}C-NMR (101 MHz, DMSO): d 156.90 (C-7), 156.62 (C-5), 155.80 (C-8a), 145.28 (C-39, 49), 131.00 (C-19), 118.88 (C-69), 115.49 (C-29), 114.94 (C-59), 99.47 (C-4a), 95.49 (C-6), 94.24 (C-8), 81.44 (C-2), 66.73 (C-3), 28.34 (C-4). The above data were consistent with the reported papers and identified as catechin [21,22].

Compound **2**: UV λmax: 215, 276 nm, LC-MS/MS: *m/z* 575.2 $[M-H]^-$, ^{1}H-NMR (400 MHz, MeOD) δ 7.14 (1H, d, *J* = 2.0 Hz, H-2″), 7.13 (1H, d, *J* = 2.0 Hz, H-2′″), 7.01 (1H, dd, *J* = 8.3, 2.2 Hz, H-6″), 6.97 (1H, dd, *J* = 8.3, 2.0 Hz, H-6′″), 6.81 (1H, d, *J* = 1.7 Hz, H-5″), 6.79 (1H, d, *J* = 1.8 Hz, H-5′″), 6.08 (1H, s, H-6′), 6.06 (1H, d, *J* = 2.3 Hz, H-8), 5.99 (1H, d, *J* = 2.4 Hz, H-6), 4.92 (1H, s, H-2′), 4.40 (1H, d, *J* = 3.4 Hz, H-4), 4.23 (1H, m, H-3′), 4.05 (1H, d, *J* = 3.4 Hz, H-3), 2.94 (1H, dd, *J* = 17.2, 4.9 Hz, H-4′α), 2.75 (1H, dd, *J* = 17.2, 2.3 Hz, H-4′β); ^{13}C-NMR (101 MHz, MeOD) δ 158.29 (C-7), 157.15 (C-5), 156.76 (C-5′), 154.42 (C-9), 152.46 (C-7′), 152.30 (C-9′), 146.93 (C-3′″), 146.47 (C-3″), 146.16 (C-4′″), 145.82 (C-4″), 132.63 (C-1″), 131.36 (C-1′″), 120.57 (C-6″), 119.97 (C-6′″), 116.23 (C-5″), 116.1 (C-5′″), 115.85 (C-2″), 115.82 (C-2′″), 107.39 (C-8′), 104.45 (C-10), 102.62 (C-10′), 100.36 (C-2), 98.50 (C-6), 96.82 (C-8), 96.70 (C-6′), 81.94 (C-2′), 68.24 (C-3), 67.14 (C-3′), 30.06 (C-4′), 29.43 (C-4). The above data were consistent with the reported papers and identified as procyanidin A2 [23].

2.2. Catechin and Procyanidin A2 Improve the Morphology of BV-2 Cells

The cellular morphology of BV-2 cells can reflect the inflammatory response [24]. In this part, we first examined the cytotoxicity of catechin and procyanidin A2 against BV-2 cells using a CCK-8 kit, and there no cytotoxicity was observed under 80 μM (Figure 2A). Figure 2B showed the morphologic changes of BV-2 cells treated with Aβ(1-42) alone and Aβ(1-42) co-treated with LSF, catechin, and procyanidin A2, which were detected by the Wright–Giemsa staining method. As shown in Figure 2B–D, LSF, catechin and procyanidin A2 could reduce the ratio of activated BV-2 cells that displayed ameboid shape, fusiform, more synapse and obvious nucleus fragmentations, and increase cell density in Aβ(1-42)-induced BV-2 cells, suggesting that LSF and its derived compounds could suppress Aβ(1-42) induced neuroinflammation. Therefore, catechin and procyanidin A2 could be the bioactive components that are responsible for the anti-neuroinflammation effect.

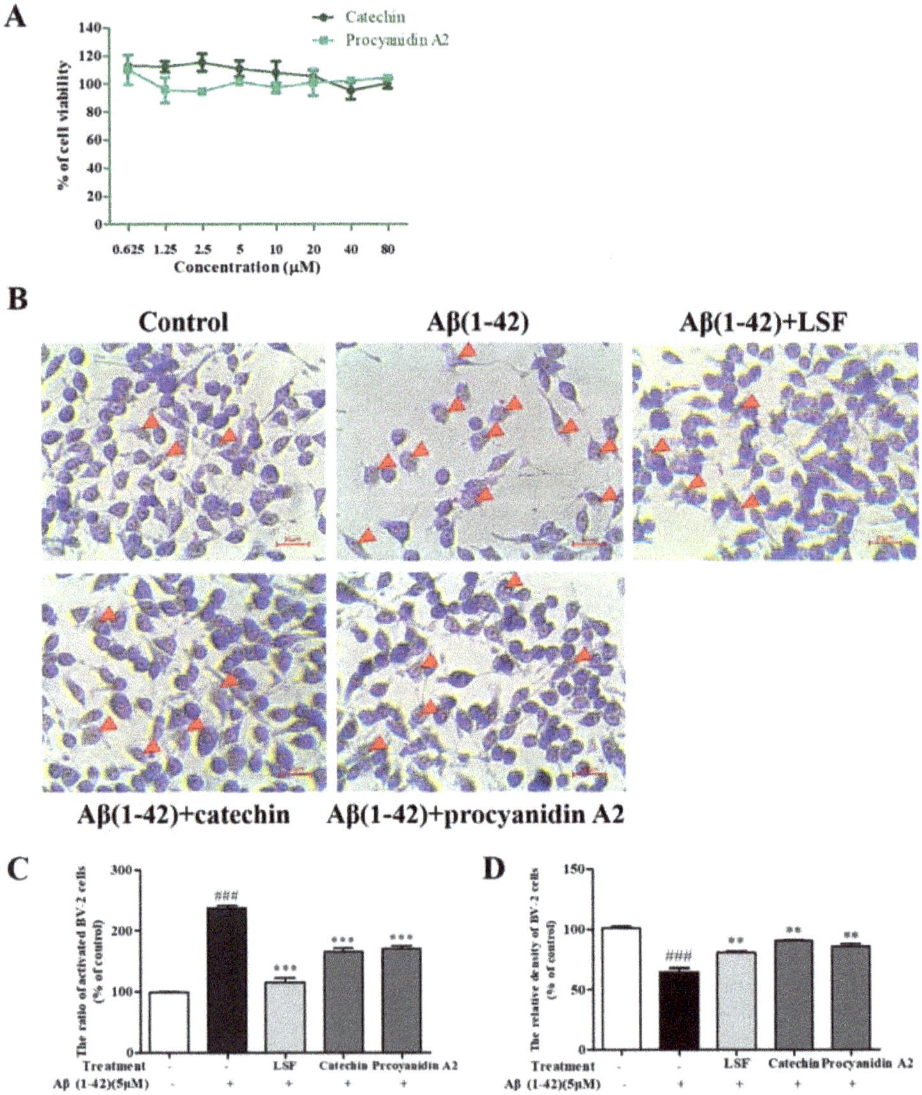

Figure 2. Morphological changes of BV-2 cells. (**A**) Cytotoxicity of catechin and procyanidin A2 against BV-2 cells for 48 h using CCK-8 kit; (**B**) BV-2 cells were pretreated with 5 μM Aβ(1-42) for 12 h, followed by incubations of LSF (0.469 μg/mL), catechin (10 μM), and procyanidin A2 (10 μM), respectively. The red arrows indicate the activated BV-2 cells with ameboid shape. Magnification: ×100; Scale bar: 50 μm. (**C**) The ratio of activated BV-2 cells, which was calculated by counting the number of activated BV-2 cells in all of the BV-2 cells views; (**D**) The density of BV-2 cells, which was quantified by counting the number of all the BV-2 cells, and a minimum of 150 cells from three randomly selected fields were scored. BV-2 cells treated with medium alone were set as the control group, and BV-2 cells treated with 5 μM Aβ(1-42) alone were set as the Aβ group. ### $p < 0.001$ vs. Control group; ** $p < 0.005$, *** $p < 0.001$ vs. Aβ group.

2.3. Catechin and Procyanidin A2 Inhibit Pro-Inflammatory Cytokines in Aβ(1-42)-Induced BV-2 Cells

Our previous study proved that LSF could inhibit the release, mRNA levels, and protein expressions of TNF-α, IL-1β, COX-2, and iNOS. Based on the preliminary screen result of the anti-neuroinflammation effect of the 12 isolated fractions, we further validated the anti-neuroinflammation effect of catechin and procyanidin A2 in Fractions 3 and 9 in the current experiment. As shown in Figure 3, LSF, catechin and procyanidin A2 could significantly decrease the release of TNF-α, IL-1β, and IL-6 levels in cell culture supernatants using an ELISA kit in Aβ(1-42)-induced BV-2 cells. Additionally, the mRNA levels of TNF-α, IL-1β, and iNOS were measured using RT-PCR. Figure 4 shows that LSF, catechin, and procyanidin A2 could significantly reduce the mRNA levels in Aβ(1-42)-induced BV-2 cells. Correspondingly, the protein expressions of TNF-α, IL-1β, and iNOS in Aβ(1-42)-induced BV-2 cells under the treatments of LSF, catechin, and procyanidin A2 were detected by Western blotting. As shown in Figure 5, LSF, catechin, and procyanidin A2 dramatically reduced the protein content of TNF-α, IL-1β, and iNOS. In summary, catechin and procyanidin A2 could inhibit the inflammatory response in Aβ(1-42)-induced BV-2 cells, suggesting that catechin and procyanidin A2 could be the key active components in LSF.

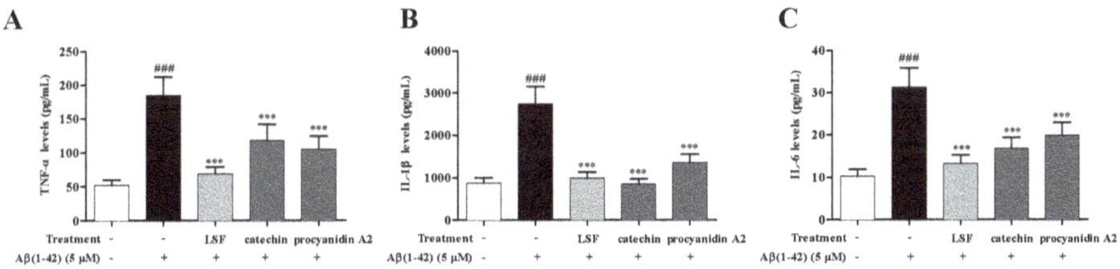

Figure 3. The release of TNF-α, IL-1β, and IL-6 in Aβ(1-42)-induced BV-2 cells under the treatments of LSF, catechin, and procyanidin A2. BV-2 cells were pretreated with 5 μM Aβ(1-42) for 12 h, followed by incubations of LSF (0.469 μg/mL), catechin (10 μM), and procyanidin A2 (10 μM) for another 12 h. After treatment, the cell free supernatants were subsequently employed for TNF-α (**A**), IL-1β (**B**), and IL-6 (**C**) assays using ELISA kit. BV-2 cells treated with medium alone were set as the control group, and BV-2 cells treated with 5 μM Aβ(1-42) alone were set as the Aβ group. ### $p < 0.001$ vs. control group; *** $p < 0.001$ vs. Aβ group. Data are the mean value ± S.D. of ten independent experiments.

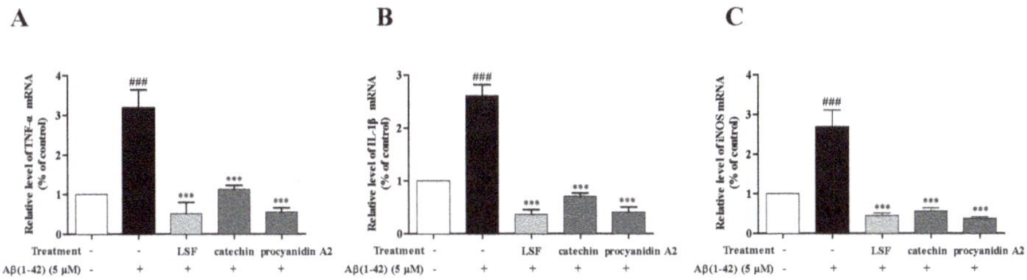

Figure 4. The mRNA levels of TNF-α, IL-1β, and iNOS in Aβ(1-42)-induced BV-2 cells under the treatments of LSF, catechin, and procyanidin A2. BV-2 cells were pretreated with 5 μM Aβ(1-42) for 12 h, followed by incubations of LSF (0.469 μg/mL), catechin (10 μM), and procyanidin A2 (10 μM) for another 12 h. After treatment, total mRNA were extracted and subsequently employed for TNF-α (**A**), IL-1β (**B**), and iNOS (**C**) measurements using RT-PCR. BV-2 cells treated with medium alone were set as the control group, and BV-2 cells treated with 5 μM Aβ(1-42) alone were set as the Aβ(1-42) group. ### $p < 0.001$ vs. control group; *** $p < 0.001$ vs. Aβ group. Data are the mean value ± S.D. of five independent experiments.

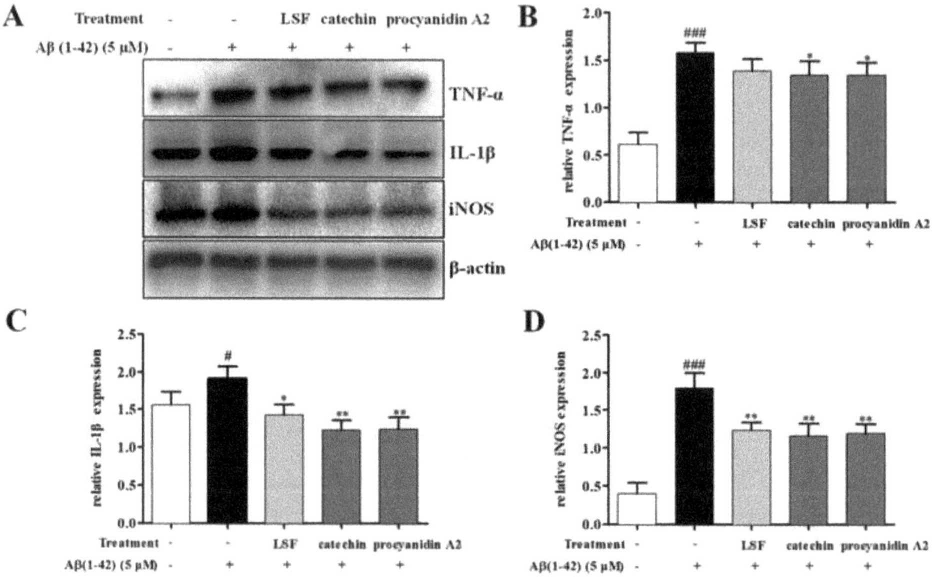

Figure 5. The protein expressions of TNF-α, IL-1β, and iNOS in Aβ(1-42)-induced BV-2 cells under the treatments of LSF (0.469 μg/mL), catechin (10 μM), and procyanidin A2 (10 μM). BV-2 cells were pretreated with 5 μM Aβ(1-42) for 12 h, followed by incubations of LSF, catechin, and procyanidin A2 for another 12 h. (**A**) After treatment, cell lysates were harvested and subsequently employed for TNF-α, IL-1β, and iNOS measurements using Western blotting. Band intensities of TNF-α (**B**), IL-1β (**C**), and iNOS (**D**) were quantified using Image J software and normalized to β-actin. Bars are representatives of three independent experiments. BV-2 cells treated with medium alone were set as the control group, and BV-2 cells treated with 5 μM Aβ(1-42) alone were set as the Aβ group. # $p < 0.05$, ### $p < 0.001$ vs. control group; * $p < 0.05$, ** $p < 0.01$ vs. Aβ group. The full-length Western blotting images are shown in Figure S8.

2.4. Catechin and Procyanidin A2 Inhibit the Activation of NF-κB Signaling Pathway

Emerging evidence implies that the NF-κB signaling pathway is activated in AD pathogenesis. This pathway can regulate the release and expression of pro-inflammatory cytokines, and its function is related to its inhibitory factor, IκBα. Aβ can activate the NF-κB signaling pathway then release the pro-inflammatory cytokines. In this study, we investigated the inhibition effect of LSF and the isolated components, catechin and procyanidin A2 in neuroinflammation in Aβ(1-42)-induced BV-2 cells. As shown in Figure 6, LSF, catechin, and procyanidin A2 could significantly suppress the protein expression of NF-κB and the ratio of p-IκBα/IκBα, suggesting that LSF, catechin, and procyanidin A2 suppressed the neuroinflammation via inhibiting the NF-κB signaling pathway in Aβ(1-42)-induced BV-2 cells.

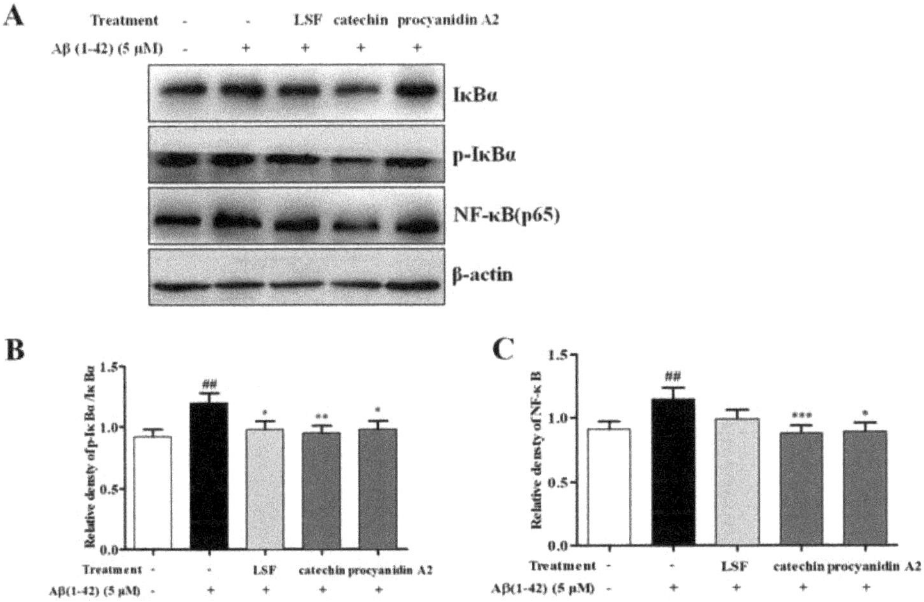

Figure 6. Catechin and procyanidin A2 inhibit the activation of the NF-κB signaling pathway. BV-2 cells were pretreated with 5 μM Aβ(1-42) for 12 h, followed by incubations of LSF (0.469 μg/mL), catechin (10 μM), and procyanidin A2 (10 μM) for another 12 h. (**A**) After treatment, the cell lysates were harvested and subsequently employed for IκBα, p-IκBα, and NF-κB detections using Western blotting. Band intensities of p-IκBα/IκBα (**B**) and NF-κB (**C**) were quantified using Image J software and normalized to β-actin. Bars are representatives of three independent experiments. BV-2 cells treated with medium alone were set as the control group, and BV-2 cells treated with 5 μM Aβ(1-42) alone were set as the Aβ group. ## $p < 0.01$ vs. control group; * $p < 0.05$, ** $p < 0.01$, *** $p < 0.001$ vs. Aβ group. The full-length Western blotting images are shown in Figure S8.

2.5. Catechin and Procyanidin A2 Inhibit Cell Apoptosis in Aβ(1-42)-Induced BV-2 Cells

As is known to us, over-expression of pro-inflammatory cytokines can induce the microglial activation and lead to neuronal death. Our previous study have proved that LSF could inhibit cell apoptosis in Aβ(1-42)-induced BV-2 cells. In this current experiment, we also investigated the suppression effect of cell apoptosis in Aβ(1-42)-induced BV-2 cells under the treatments of LSF and the isolated components, catechin and procyanidin A2. As shown in Figure 7, LSF, catechin and procyanidin A2 could inhibit Aβ(1-42)-induced BV-2 cells apoptosis by reducing Bax/Bcl-2 ratio and attenuating the proportion of cleaved-PARP in total PARP. These results suggested that the decreased cell apoptosis could relate to the inhibition of inflammatory response in Aβ(1-42)-induced BV-2 cells with the treatments of catechin and procyanidins A2.

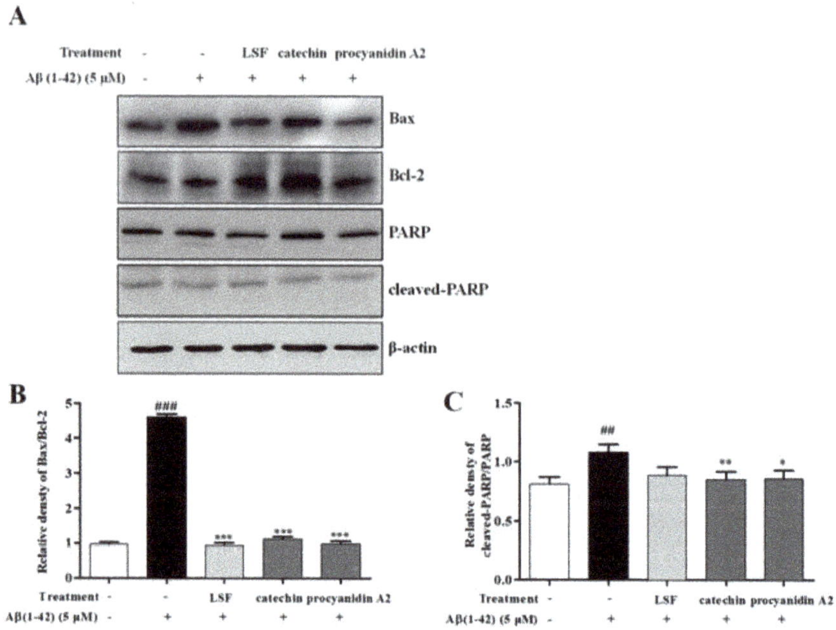

Figure 7. Catechin and procyanidin A2 inhibit cell apoptosis in the Aβ(1-42)-induced BV-2 cells. BV-2 cells were pretreated with 5 μM Aβ(1-42) for 12 h, followed by incubations of LSF (0.469 μg/mL), catechin (10 μM), and procyanidin A2 (10 μM) for another 12 h. (**A**) After treatment, cell lysates were harvested and subsequently employed for Bax, Bcl-2 PARP, and cleaved-PARP detections using Western blotting. Band intensities of Bax/Bcl-2 (**B**) and cleaved-PARP/PARP (**C**) were quantified using Image J software and normalized to β-actin. Bars are representatives of three independent experiments. BV-2 cells treated with medium alone were set as the control group, and BV-2 cells treated with 5 μM Aβ(1-42) alone were set as the Aβ group. $^{##}$ $p < 0.01$, $^{###}$ $p < 0.001$ vs. control group; * $p < 0.05$, ** $p < 0.01$, *** $p < 0.001$ vs. Aβ group. The full-length Western blotting images are shown in Figure S8.

3. Discussion

AD is the most common type of dementia worldwide. Its pathological hallmarks are recognized as the accumulated Aβ in SPs and the hyperphosphorylation of tau in NFTs [25,26]. The inactivated microglia can improve Aβ clearance and promote anti-inflammatory effects, and also protect the CNS from injury and invading pathogens [27]. However, it has recently been shown that microglial depletion for 2–4 weeks in the mouse model at advanced stage cannot reduce Aβ plaque, suggesting that the aged microglia is inactivated in clearing plaques in the AD brain [28]. It has been reported that immune activation early in life could trigger the onset of AD, while exposing microglia to Aβ could induce sustained chronic neuroinflammation, tau hyperphosphorylation, and a loss of synapses and neurons [7,29–31]. Therefore, the timing of Aβ pathogenesis is recognized to be critical for microglia to form a physical barrier to limit neurotoxicity [32], and a potent inhibitor of microglia activation is essential for inhibiting neuroinflammation. Lychee seed, a commonly used TCM, has been reported to exert many biological activities such as anti-oxidation, anti-virus, and improving insulin resistance (IR) [33–36]. In our previous study, LSF, a bioactive fraction from lychee seed, was first proven to improve the cognitive function of AD rats, protect PC12 cells against Aβ-induced injury, and suppress neuroinflammation in Aβ(1-42)-induced BV-2 cells [19,20]. However, the specific components being responsible for this effect are still unknown. In this experiment, we isolated and identified two bioactive components from LSF that are responsible for these neuroprotective effects.

It has been reported that SP is surrounded by a cluster of reactive microglia as phagocytic cells. These microglia can remove Aβ in brain and protect neurons [29,37,38]. On the other hand, studies have shown that the content of Aβ in microglia was remarkably increased in AD patients and model animals' brains, suggesting that the microglia are over activated and then contribute to the occurrence of AD [39,40]. Therefore, the over-activated microglia induced by accumulated Aβ or tau will induce neuroinflammation and accelerate AD progression. Based on this evidence, we used Aβ(1-42)-induced BV-2 cells to simulate the over activated microglia in AD patients or rats. With persistent activation of BV-2 cells by Aβ(1-42), many cytotoxic factors including TNF-α, IL-1β, IL-6, nitric oxide (NO), and superoxide are released from the over-activated microglia [29,41–43]. The released toxic inflammatory cytokines induce microglial activation and lead to neuronal death, and ultimately dementia [44]. In the present study, we symmetrically isolated and identified two polyphenols including catechin and procyanidin A2 from LSF using column chromatography, pre-HPLC, and NMR technologies. The bioactive validation proved that catechin and procyanidin A2 could suppress Aβ-induced neuroinflammation in Aβ(1-42)-induced BV-2 cells by inhibiting the release, mRNA levels, and protein expressions of TNF-α, IL-1β, IL-6, and iNOS.

Polyphenols widely exist in most natural plants such as *Radix et Rhizoma Rhei*, *Radix Scutellariae*, *Rhizoma et Radix Polygoni Cuspidati*, etc. As is known to us, polyphenols exert a potent anti-oxidative effect and protect cells or tissue against oxidative damage, which results in improved immunity, anti-cancer, and anti-aging effects. Recently, many polyphenols such as resveratrol from *Rhizoma et Radix Polygoni Cuspidati* [45]; epigallocatechin gallate (EGCG) from green tea [46]; curcumin from the spice turmeric [47]; and the flavonoids—including baicalin, baicalein, wogonoside, wogonin, oroxylin A, etc.—from *Radix Scutellariae* [48] have been proved to inhibit Aβ aggregation. Catechin and procyanidin A2 widely exist in fruit seed and skin including grape seed, apple seed, and the skin from *Hylocereus undatus 'Foo-Lon'*. Catechin has been reported to stimulate antioxidant activity by scavenging free radicals, inhibiting pro-oxidant enzymes, and stimulating antioxidant enzymes. In this study, our data suggested that catechin inhibited neuroinflammation, which is consistent with previous studies that claimed that catechin possessed a neuroprotective effect [49]. Procyanidins are members of the proanthocyanidin (or condensed tannins) class of flavonoids. They are oligomeric compounds composed of catechin and epicatechin. It has been reported that procyanidins have an extremely strong antioxidant and free radical clearing effect. At the same time, catechin and procyanidins have also been proved to inhibit Aβ-induced apoptosis in PC12 cells and inhibit Aβ aggregation, respectively [50,51]. However, up to now, there have been no reports on the inhibition effect of catechin and procyanidin A2 in Aβ-induced neuroinflammation.

In this study, we identified the key active components of LSF to inhibit Aβ(1-42)-mediated neuroinflammation. In general, morphological appearance is often related to functional properties, and we found the appearance of BV-2 cells treated with Aβ(1-42) were ameboid shaped, indicating a fully activated state [52,53]. Furthermore, the proportion of ameboid-shaped cells in Aβ(1-42) pre-treated BV-2 cells was decreased after the treatment of LSF, catechin, or procyanidin A2, suggesting that LSF, catechin, and procyanidin A2 can inhibit BV-2 cells activation.

NF-κB is a protein complex that regulates the transcription of DNA, pro-inflammatory cytokine release, and cell survival [54–58]. Pro-inflammatory mediators such as TNF-α, IL-1, IL-6, iNOS, and cyclooxygenase-2 (COX-2) are released from cells as NF-κB is activated [59]. NF-κB usually exists in the cytoplasm in the form of homo- and/or heterodimers, and forms an inactive complex with its inhibitory factor IκBα [60,61]. IκBα is phosphorylated by IκB kinase (IKK) and releases the NF-κB dimer when the pathway is activated. Our previous studies proved that LSF could inhibit neuronal and BV-2 cells apoptosis, which could be associated with the inhibition of the NF-κB pathways [20]. In the current study, catechin and procyanidin A2 in LSF were found to inhibit the NF-κB pathway by downregulating the p-IκBα/IκBα and NF-κB expressions.

Aβ also induces microglial apoptosis and further aggravates the inflammatory response. The Bcl-2 family plays an important role in the regulation of apoptosis. It consists of anti-apoptotic proteins such as Bcl-2, Bcl-xl, Bcl-w, and Mcl-1, and pro-apoptotic proteins including Bax, Bak, Bad, Bid, and Bim. In the present study, we found that catechin and procyanidin A2 could decrease the Bax/Bcl-2 ratio in Aβ(1-42)-induced BV-2 cells. Additionally, another apoptosis related protein, the poly (ADP-ribose) polymerase (PARP) protein family, is associated with many cellular processes such as DNA repair, genomic stability, and programmed cell death. The cleaved-PARP is generally considered to be an important indicator of apoptosis and caspase 3 activation [62,63]. Similarly, catechin and procyanidin A2 could reduce the proportion of cleaved-PARP in total PRAP in Aβ(1-42)-induced BV-2 cells. Taken together, all of the above results indicated that catechin and procyanidin A2 could suppress apoptosis in Aβ-induced BV-2 cells.

The blood–brain barrier (BBB) permeability of the drugs acting on CNS is becoming an important issue to which we should pay attention. The permeability of dietary polyphenols across the blood–brain barrier (BBB) is selective, has poor absorption, and rapid metabolism, which limits their bioavailability and neuroprotective effect. Most polyphenols have been proven to have a neuroprotective effect in vitro and vivo. Recently, a study found that the bioavailable polyphenol metabolites could transport across the BBB endothelium and protect brain endothelial cells and neuronal cells, and reduce neuroinflammation [64]. Although the polyphenols intracellular concentrations in neurons and microglial cells are limited, such concentrations are in fact beneficial [65]. Catechin, the compound identified from LSF in the current study, has previously been reported to pass through BBB after intravenous (iv) administration [66]. In addition, nanosystems could be a promising strategy for delivering resveratrol, a polyphenol, into the brain, which can protect it from degradation in the blood stream [67]. Therefore, a rational administration or formulation could avoid the first pass effect, protect degradation, and improve the BBB permeability of the polyphenols.

Collectively, our study confirmed that the two key active substances of LSF, catechin and procyanidin A2, could inhibit Aβ-induced neuroinflammation. In future study, we will try to investigate the concentration of catechin and procyanidin A2 passed through BBB by selecting the optimal administration route and formulation, which are expected to be developed as novel drugs for AD.

4. Materials and Methods

4.1. Reagent and Instrument

LSF was prepared according to our previous method [19,20]. HPLC-grade acetonitrile and methanol, sodium dodecyl sulfate (SDS), and Aβ(1-42) were purchased from Sigma-Aldrich (St. Louis, MO, USA). Roswell Park Memorial Institute 1640 medium (RPMI 1640) was obtained from Gibco (Grand Island, NY, USA). Fetal bovine serum (FBS), RT-PCR kit, and PCR kit were purchased from TransGen Biotech Inc. (Beijing, China). The Wright–Giemsa stain kit was purchased from Nanjing Jiancheng Bioengineering Institute (Nanjing, China). Primary antibodies such as TNF-α, IL-1β, inducible nitric oxide synthase (iNOS), nuclear factor kappa-light-chain-enhancer of activated B (NF-κB), inhibitor of NF-κB alpha (IκBα), phosphorylate-IκBα (p-IκBα), poly ADP-ribose polymerase (PARP), cleaved-PARP, Bax, Bcl-2, and β-actin were obtained from Cell Signaling Technology (CST) (Beverly, MA, USA). Enzyme linked immunosorbent assay (ELISA) kits of TNF-α, IL-1β, and IL-6 were purchased from Beijing Cheng Lin Biological Technology Co., Ltd. (Beijing, China).

4.2. Instrument and Chromatograph Condition for the Separation of the Components in LSF

The separation and purification of the components in LSF was performed using AKAT protein purification system equipped with a UV–vis detector at 280 nm on an amethyst C_{18}–H column (21.2 × 250 mm, 5 μm) which was purchased from Sepax Technologies Inc. (Suzhou, China) at a flow rate of 10 mL/min. The parameters of the gradient elution program were applied as follows: the ratio of mobile phase B (acetonitrile) to mobile phase A (0.1% formic acid in water) changed from 15% to

35% in 45 min. The peaks displaying in the chromatograms were collected according to their retention time. All the collected solutions were concentrated by rotary evaporator.

4.3. Cell Culture

BV-2 cells, an immortalized mouse microglia cell line, was purchased from the Kunming Institute of Zoology, Chinese Academy of Science (Kunming, China). It was cultured in RPMI 1640 medium supplemented with 20% fetal bovine serum and 1% penicillin/streptomycin at 37 °C with CO_2 (5%) [8].

4.4. Cell Viability

Twelve isolated fractions were dissolved with dimethyl sulfoxide (DMSO) to make a final concentration of 80 g/L. Cell viability of Fractions 1–12 against BV-2 cells was measured with a CCK-8 kit according to the manufacture's protocols. In brief, BV-2 cells were plated on 96-well plates (100 μL, 1×10^5 cells/well) one day before LSF treatment under the indicated concentrations. After 48 h treatment, 10 μL of CCK-8 solution was added into each well and incubated for another 2 h. Colorimetric reading of the solute mixture was then determined at OD 450 nm using a standard plate-reader (DG5032, Hua Dong, Nanjing, China). The percentage of cell viability was calculated using the following formula: Cell viability (%) = Cells number $_{\text{treated}}$/Cells number $_{\text{DMSO control}}$ × 100. Data were obtained from three independent experiments.

4.5. Identification of the Components in LSF

Reverse phase ultra-high-performance liquid chromatography (RP-UHPLC) (Shimadzu Corporation, Hadano, Japan) equipped with DGU-20A5R degasser, two LC-20ADXR pumps, a SIL-20ACXR autosampler, a CTO-20AC column oven, a SPD-M20A diode array detector, and a Shimadzu CBM-20A system controller was used for analysis in the current study. All the samples dissolved in methanol were separated by a C18 column (4.6 × 250 mm, 5.0 μm particle size) (GL Science, Torrance, CA, USA) at a flow rate of 1 mL/min. The gradient elution system consisting of mobile phase A (acetonitrile) and mobile phase B (0.1% acetic acid, *v*/*v*) was set as follows: 0–10 min, 5–24% (A); 10–11 min, 24–24% (A); 11–11.01 min, 24–28% (A); 11.01–12 min, 28–28% (A); 12–12.01 min, 28–36% (A); 12.01–13 min, 36–36% (A); 13–13.01 min, 36–40% (A); 13.01–14 min, 40–40% (A); 14–14.01 min, 40–45% (A); 14.01–15 min, 55–55% (A); 15–15.01 min, 55–50% (A); 15.01–16 min, 50–50% (A); 16–18 min, 50–60% (A); 18–30 min, 60–70% (A). The column temperature was maintained at 25 °C and the injection volume was 20 μL of each sample. The UV–vis absorption spectra were recorded on-line from 190 to 800 nm during the analysis and the components in LSF were monitored at 280 nm. Data analysis was carried out using Shimadzu LabSolutions software B.01.03 (Shimadzu Corporation, Hadano, Japan).

Ultra-high-performance liquid chromatography (UHPLC) (Shimadzu Corporation, Hadano, Japan) equipped with DGU-30A5R degasser, two LC-30ADXR pumps, a SIL-30ACXR autosampler, a CTO-30AC column oven, a SPD-M30A diode array detector, a Shimadzu CBM-30A system controller, and a 8045 electrospray ionization tandem mass spectroscopic (ESI-MS/MS) was used to identify the isolated components from LSF in negative and positive modes. Data were acquired in scan mode from m/z 100 to 1000 Da with 2.0 spectra/s. Data analysis was carried out using Shimadzu LabSolutions software B.01.03 (Shimadzu Corporation, Hadano, Japan).

4.6. Wright–Giemsa Staining

BV-2 cells were seeded on coverslips in a 6-well plate a day before treatments. The cells were pretreated with 5 μM Aβ(1-42) for 12 h, followed by incubations of the test fractions or compounds for another 12 h. After treatments, these coverslips were air-dried and stained with Giemsa solution as described previously [68]. In brief, slides stained in the diluted Giemsa solution (1:20) in PBS for 15–20 min were washed with PBS to remove the excess stain and air-dried at room temperature. The air-dried slides were mounted with FluorSave™ mounting media (Calbiochem, San Diego, CA, USA), and the optical microscope images were observed and taken with an optical microscope (Leica DM750 optical microscope, Leica, Germany). The ratio of activated BC-2 cells was calculated by counting the number of the activated BV-2 cells in all of the BV-2 cells. In addition, the density of BV-2 cells was quantified by counting the number of all of the BV-2 cells. A minimum of 150 cells from three randomly selected fields were scored.

4.7. Cytokines ELISA

BV-2 cells were plated on a 96-well plate (100 μL, 1 × 10^5 cells/well) a day before treatments. The cells were pretreated with 5 μM Aβ(1-42) for 12 h, followed by an incubation of the fractions or compounds for another 12 h. The cell-free supernatants were subsequently employed for TNF-α, IL-1β, and IL-6 assays using the ELISA kits according to the manufacturer's instructions.

4.8. Quantitative Reverse Transcription PCR (qRT-PCR)

The total RNA of BV-2 cells was extracted by TRIZOL reagent, and its reverse transcription into cDNA were performed according to the manufacture's protocol for the Prime Script RT reagent kit (Trans Serum, Beijing, China). The primers are listed as follows

TNF-α	Forward: 5′-GAGCACAGAAAGCATGATCC-3′ Reverse: 5′-GAGAAGAGGCTGAGACATAG-3′
IL-1β	Forward: 5′-CTAGGGACTTAGGTGCTGTC-3′ Reverse: 5′-CTCTGCCTTTGCTTCCAAGC-3′
iNOS	Forward: 5′-CGTTGGATTTGGAGCAGAAG-3′ Reverse: 5′-CCTCTTTCAGGTCACTTTGG-3′
GAPDH	Forward: 5′-GACAGTCGGAAACTGGGAAG-3′ Reverse: 5′-CATCACGTCCTCCATCATCC-3′

4.9. Western Blotting

After treatment, cells were washed with pre-cooled PBS and lysed by RIPA lysis buffer (Beyotime, Shanghai, China) containing 20 mM Tris-HCl (pH 7.4), 1% Triton X-100, 140 mM NaCl, and 1 mM phenylmethylsulfonyl fluoride (PMSE). Protein concentrations were measured by BCA kit (Beyotime, Shanghai, China) as per the previous report [20]. Equal amounts of each protein (50 μg/well) were loaded onto SDS-PAGE and the separated proteins on the gel were transferred onto a polyvinylidene difluoride (PVDF) membrane, which was then blocked with 5% non-fat milk in Tris-buffered saline and Tween 20 (TBST) for 1 h. The membrane was then washed with TBST three times and incubated with the primary antibodies including β-actin, TNF-α, IL-1β, iNOS, NF-κB, IκBα, p-IκBα, PARP, cleaved-PARP, Bax, and Bcl-2 overnight at 4 °C. After the membrane was washed with TBST three times, it was followed with a further incubation for 1 h at room temperature with horseradish peroxidase (HRP) conjugated secondary antibodies. The protein expression bands were revealed by the ultra ECL Detection Reagent ECL (4A Biotech Co., Ltd., Beijing, China) and detected by the ChemiDoc MP Imaging System (Bio-Rad, Hercules, CA, USA). Band intensity was quantified using Image J software (National Institutes of Health, Bethesda, MD, USA) and the ratio of the interest proteins to β-actin was calculated.

4.10. Statistical Analysis

All data were presented as the mean ± standard deviation (S.D.) and were analyzed using GraphPad Prism 5.0 statistical analytical software (GraphPad Software, San Diego, CA, USA). The data were considered to have significant difference as $p < 0.05$. One-way ANOVA followed by the post-Tukey test was applied for statistical analysis to compare all the different groups in the current study.

5. Conclusions

In the current study, two polyphenols—catechin and procyanidin A2—were isolated and identified in LSF derived from lychee seed; they were proven to be the bioactive components responsible for the inhibition effect of neuroinflammation in Aβ(1-42)-induced BV-2 cells by modulating the NF-κB signaling pathway. Furthermore, catechin and procyanidin A2 could also inhibit cell apoptosis in Aβ(1-42)-induced BV-2 cells. This study illuminated the action substances and molecular mechanism of LSF in anti-neuroinflammation. Further studies on brain pharmacokinetics and the pharmacological activity in vivo are also essential.

Supplementary Materials: Supplementary materials can be found at http://www.mdpi.com/xxx/s1.

Author Contributions: Y.T., R.X., and A.-G.W. performed the data analysis and draft writing; Y.T., R.X., Y.Z., W.-Q.Q., J.-F.T., H.-X.C., and X.-L.W. contributed to the experiments and data analysis; Y.T., R.X., A.-G.W., and C.-L.Y. contributed to the data analysis and interpretation; A.-G.W., J.-M.W., and D.-L.Q. contributed to modifying the article language; Y.T., J.-M.W., and D.-L.Q. designed the experiments and revised the manuscript. All authors reviewed the manuscript.

Funding: This research was funded by "The Science and Technology Program of Luzhou" (grant numbers 2016LZXNYD-T03 and 2017LZXNYD-J28), the "Educational Commission of Sichuan Province" (grant numbers 18ZA0528 and 18TD0051), the "Science and Technology Planning Project of Sichuan Province" (grant numbers 2018JY0474 and 2018JY0237), and the "Traditional Chinese Medicines Commission of Sichuan Province" (grant number 2018QN070).

Acknowledgments: The authors thank Can Tang of the Department of Chinese Materia Medica, School of Pharmacy, Southwest Medical University (Luzhou, Sichuan, China), for authenticating the lychee seed used in this study, and also thank Jiang Pi of the Department of Microbiology and Immunology, University of Illinois at Chicago, (Chicago, IL, USA), for polishing the English writing of this manuscript.

Conflicts of Interest: The authors declare no conflict of interest.

Abbreviations

Aβ	Amyloid-β
AD	Alzheimer's disease
LSF	Lychee seed fraction
pre-HPLC	Preparation of high performance liquid chromatography
NMR	Nuclear magnetic resonance
TNF-α	Tumor necrosis factor-α
IL-1β	Interleukin-1β
IL-6	Interleukin-6
NF-κB	Nuclear factor-κB
ELISA	Enzyme linked immunosorbent assay
RT-PCR	Real time-PCR
SPs	Senile plaques
NFTs	Neurofibrillary tangles
CNS	Central nervous system
PD	Parkinson's disease
HD	Huntington's disease
NO	Nitric oxide
ROS	Reactive oxygen species
TCMs	Traditional Chinese medicines
T2DM	Type 2 diabetes mellitus
COX-2	Cyclooxygenase 2
iNOS	Inducible nitric oxide synthase
IκBα	NF-κB inhibitor α
PARP	Poly ADP-ribose polymerase

IR	Insulin resistance
EGCG	Epigallocatechin gallate
IKK	IκB kinase
BBB	Blood–brain barrier

References

1. Wang, X.; Wang, W.; Li, L.; Perry, G.; Lee, H.; Zhu, X. Oxidative stress and mitochondrial dysfunction in Alzheimer's disease. *BBA Mol. Basis Dis.* **2014**, *1842*, 1240–1247. [CrossRef] [PubMed]
2. Scheff, S.W.; Price, D.A.; Schmitt, F.A.; Mufson, E.J. Hippocampal synaptic loss in early Alzheimer's disease and mild cognitive impairment. *Neurobiol. Aging* **2006**, *27*, 1372–1384. [CrossRef] [PubMed]
3. Varnum, M.M.; Ikezu, T. The Classification of Microglial Activation Phenotypes on Neurodegeneration and Regeneration in Alzheimer's Disease Brain. *Arch. Immunol. Ther. Exp.* **2012**, *60*, 251–266. [CrossRef] [PubMed]
4. Heneka, M.T.; Carson, M.J.; Khoury, J.E.; Landreth, G.E. Neuroinflammation in Alzheimer's disease. *Lancet Neurol.* **2015**, *14*, 388–405. [CrossRef]
5. Ferreira, S.T.; Clarke, J.R.; Bomfim, T.R.; de Felice, F.G. Inflammation, defective insulin signaling, and neuronal dysfunction in Alzheimer's disease. *Alzheimers Dement.* **2014**, *10*, S76–S83. [CrossRef] [PubMed]
6. Hung, A.S.M.; Liang, Y.; Chow, T.C.H.; Tang, H.C.; Wu, S.L.Y.; Wai, M.S.M.; Yew, D.T. Mutated tau, amyloid and neuroinflammation in Alzheimer disease—A brief review. *Prog. Histochem. Cytochem.* **2016**, *51*, 1–8. [CrossRef] [PubMed]
7. Streit, W.J.; Mrak, R.E.; Griffin, W.S. Microglia and neuroinflammation: A pathological perspective. *J. Neuroinflamm.* **2004**, *1*, 14. [CrossRef] [PubMed]
8. Yuan, L.; Wu, Y.; Ren, X.; Liu, Q.; Wang, J.; Liu, X. Isoorientin attenuates lipopolysaccharide-induced pro-inflammatory responses through down-regulation of ROS-related MAPK/NF-κB signaling pathway in BV-2 microglia. *Mol. Cell. Biochem.* **2014**, *386*, 153–165. [CrossRef] [PubMed]
9. Song, S.; Jung, Y.Y.; Hwang, C.J.; Lee, H.P.; Sok, C.H.; Kim, J.H.; Lee, S.M.; Seo, H.O.; Hyun, B.K.; Choi, D.Y.; et al. Inhibitory effect of ent-Sauchinone on amyloidogenesis via inhibition of STAT3-mediated NF-κB activation in cultured astrocytes and microglial BV-2 cells. *J. Neuroinflamm.* **2014**, *11*, 118. [CrossRef] [PubMed]
10. Bhaskar, K.; Maphis, N.; Xu, G.; Varvel, N.H.; Kokiko-Cochran, O.N.; Weick, J.P.; Staugaitis, S.M.; Cardona, A.; Ransohoff, R.M.; Herrup, K.; et al. Microglial derived tumor necrosis factor-α drives Alzheimer's disease-related neuronal cell cycle events. *Neurobiol. Dis.* **2014**, *62*, 273–285. [CrossRef] [PubMed]
11. Beauchet, O.; Launay, C.P.; Allali, G.; Annweiler, C. Changes in Gait Variability with Anti-dementia Drugs: A Systematic Review and Meta-analysis. *CNS Drugs* **2014**, *28*, 513–518. [CrossRef] [PubMed]
12. Wei, S. Potential therapeutic action of natural products from traditional Chinese medicine on Alzheimer's disease animal models targeting neurotrophic factors. *Fund. Clin. Pharmacol.* **2016**, *30*, 490–501. [CrossRef] [PubMed]
13. Yuan, Q.; Wang, C.; Shi, J.; Lin, Z. Effects of Ginkgo biloba on dementia: An overview of systematic reviews. *J. Ethnopharmacol.* **2017**, *195*, 1–9. [CrossRef] [PubMed]
14. Zhou, Y.; Li, W.; Xu, L.; Chen, L. In Salvia miltiorrhiza, phenolic acids possess protective properties against amyloid beta-induced cytotoxicity, and tanshi-nones act as acetylcholinesterase inhibitors. *Environ. Toxicol. Pharmacol.* **2011**, *31*, 443–452. [CrossRef] [PubMed]
15. Wu, A.; Zeng, W.; Wong, V.K.; Zhu, Y.; Lo, A.C.Y.; Liu, L.; Law, B.Y. Hederagenin and α-hederin promote degradation of proteins in neurodegenerative diseases and improve motor deficits in MPTP-mice. *Pharmacol. Res.* **2017**, *115*, 25–44. [CrossRef] [PubMed]
16. Wu, A.; Kam-Wai Wong, V.; Zeng, W.; Liu, L.; Yuen-Kwan Law, B. Identification of novel autophagic Radix Polygalae fraction by cell membrane chromatography and UHPLC-(Q)TOF-MS for degradation of neurodegenerative disease proteins. *Sci. Rep.* **2015**, *5*, 17199. [CrossRef] [PubMed]
17. Wu, A.; Wong, V.K.; Xu, S.; Chan, W.; Ng, C.; Liu, L.; Law, B.Y. Onjisaponin B Derived from Radix Polygalae Enhances Autophagy and Accelerates the Degradation of Mutant α-Synuclein and Huntingtin in PC-12 Cells. *Int. J. Mol. Sci.* **2013**, *14*, 22618–22641. [CrossRef] [PubMed]

18. Wong, V.K.; Wu, A.G.; Wang, J.R.; Liu, L.; Law, B.Y. Neferine Attenuates the Protein Level and Toxicity of Mutant Huntingtin in PC-12 Cells via Induction of Autophagy. *Molecules* **2015**, *20*, 3496–3514. [CrossRef] [PubMed]
19. Wang, X.; Wu, J.; Yu, C.; Tang, Y.; Liu, J.; Chen, H.; Jin, B.; Mei, Q.; Cao, S.; Qin, D. Lychee Seed Saponins Improve Cognitive Function and Prevent Neuronal Injury via Inhibiting Neuronal Apoptosis in a Rat Model of Alzheimer's Disease. *Nutrients* **2017**, *9*, 105. [CrossRef] [PubMed]
20. Wang, X.; Zhang, H.; Liu, J.; Chen, R.; Tang, Y.; Chen, H.; Gu, L.; Li, M.; Cao, S.; Qin, D.; et al. Inhibitory Effect of Lychee Seed Saponins on Apoptosis Induced by Aβ25-35 through Regulation of the Apoptotic and NF-κB Pathways in PC12 Cells. *Nutrients* **2017**, *9*, 337. [CrossRef] [PubMed]
21. Miketova, P.; Schram, K.H.; Whitney, J.; Li, M.; Huang, R.; Kerns, E.; Valcic, S.; Timmermann, B.N.; Rourick, R.; Klohr, S. Tandem mass spectrometry studies of green tea catechins. Identification of three minor components in the polyphenolic extract of green tea. *J. Mass Spectrom.* **2000**, *35*, 860–869. [CrossRef]
22. Porter, L.J.; Newman, R.H.; Foo, L.Y.; Wong, H.; Hemingway, R.W. Polymeric Proanthocyanidins. I3C Nmr Studies of Procyanidins. *J. Chem. Soc. Perkin Trans.* **1982**, *1*, 1217–1221. [CrossRef]
23. Koerner, J.L.; Hsu, V.L.; Lee, J.; Kennedy, J.A. Determination of proanthocyanidin A2 content in phenolic polymer isolates by reversed-phase high-performance liquid chromatography. *J. Chromatogr. A* **2009**, *1216*, 1403–1409. [CrossRef] [PubMed]
24. Latta, C.H.; Sudduth, T.L.; Weekman, E.M.; Brothers, H.M.; Abner, E.L.; Popa, G.J.; Mendenhall, M.D.; Gonzalez-Oregon, F.; Braun, K.; Wilcock, D.M. Determining the role of IL-4 induced neuroinflammation in microglial activity and amyloid-β using BV2 microglial cells and APP/PS1 transgenic mice. *J. Neuroinflamm.* **2015**, *12*, 41. [CrossRef] [PubMed]
25. Godyń, J.; Jończyk, J.; Panek, D.; Malawska, B. Therapeutic strategies for Alzheimer's disease in clinical trials. *Pharmacol. Rep.* **2016**, *68*, 127–138. [CrossRef] [PubMed]
26. Sevigny, J.; Chiao, P.; Bussière, T.; Weinreb, P.H.; Williams, L.; Maier, M.; Dunstan, R.; Salloway, S.; Chen, T.; Ling, Y.; et al. The antibody aducanumab reduces Aβ plaques in Alzheimer's disease. *Nature* **2016**, *537*, 50–56. [CrossRef] [PubMed]
27. Alarcón, R.; Fuenzalida, C.; Santibáñez, M.; Bernhardi, R. Expression of Scavenger Receptors in Glial Cells: Comparing the adhesion of astrocytes and microglia from neonatal rats to surface-bound β-amyloid. *J. Biol. Chem.* **2005**, *280*, 30406–30415. [CrossRef] [PubMed]
28. Grathwohl, S.A.; Kälin, R.E.; Bolmont, T.; Prokop, S.; Winkelmann, G.; Kaeser, S.A.; Odenthal, J.; Radde, R.; Eldh, T.; Gandy, S.; et al. Formation and maintenance of Alzheimer's disease β-amyloid plaques in the absence of microglia. *Nat. Neurosci.* **2009**, *12*, 1361–1363. [CrossRef] [PubMed]
29. Jantzen, P.T.; Connor, K.E.; DiCarlo, G.; Wenk, G.L.; Wallace, J.L.; Rojiani, A.M.; Coppola, D.; Morgan, D.; Gordon, M.N. Microglial Activation and β-Amyloid Deposit Reduction Caused by a Nitric Oxide-Releasing Nonsteroidal Anti-Inflammatory Drug in Amyloid Precursor Protein Plus Presenilin-1 Transgenic Mice. *J. Neurosci.* **2002**, *22*, 2246–2254. [CrossRef] [PubMed]
30. Lull, M.E.; Block, M.L. Microglial Activation and Chronic Neurodegeneration. *Neurotherapeutics* **2010**, *7*, 354–365. [CrossRef] [PubMed]
31. Dheen, S.T.; Kaur, C.; Ling, E.A. Microglial Activation and its Implications in the Brain Diseases. *Curr. Med. Chem.* **2007**, *14*, 1189–1197. [CrossRef] [PubMed]
32. Condello, C.; Yuan, P.; Schain, A.; Grutzendler, J. Microglia constitute a barrier that prevents neurotoxic protofibrillar Aβ42 hotspots around plaques. *Nat. Commun.* **2015**, *6*, 6176. [CrossRef] [PubMed]
33. Liu, S.; Lin, J.; Wang, C.; Chen, H.; Yang, D. Antioxidant properties of various solvent extracts from lychee (*Litchi chinenesis* Sonn.) flowers. *Food Chem.* **2009**, *114*, 577–581. [CrossRef]
34. Sakurai, T.; Nishioka, H.; Fujii, H.; Nakano, N.; Kizaki, T.; Radak, Z.; Iizawa, T.; Haga, S.; Ohno, H. Antioxidative Effects of a New Lychee Fruit-Derived Polyphenol Mixture, Oligonol, Converted into a Low-Molecular Form in Adipocytes. *Biosci. Biotechnol. Biochem.* **2008**, *72*, 463–476. [CrossRef] [PubMed]
35. Xu, X.; Xie, H.; Wang, Y.; Wei, X. A-Type Proanthocyanidins from Lychee Seeds and Their Antioxidant and Antiviral Activities. *J. Agric. Food Chem.* **2010**, *58*, 11667–11672. [CrossRef] [PubMed]
36. Qi, S.; Huang, H.; Huang, J.; Wang, Q.; Wei, Q. Lychee (*Litchi chinensis* Sonn.) seed water extract as potential antioxidant and antiobese natural additive in meat products. *Food Control.* **2015**, *50*, 195–201. [CrossRef]
37. Heneka, M.T.; Golenbock, D.T.; Latz, E. Innate immunity in Alzheimer's disease. *Nat. Immunol.* **2015**, *16*, 229–236. [CrossRef] [PubMed]

38. Tarasoff-Conway, J.M.; Carare, R.O.; Osorio, R.S.; Glodzik, L.; Butler, T.; Fieremans, E.; Axel, L.; Rusinek, H.; Nicholson, C.; Zlokovic, B.V.; et al. Clearance systems in the brain-implications for Alzheimer disease. *Nat. Rev. Neurol.* **2015**, *11*, 457–470. [CrossRef] [PubMed]
39. Rajmohan, R.; Reddy, P.H. Amyloid-Beta and Phosphorylated Tau Accumulations Cause Abnormalities at Synapses of Alzheimer's disease Neurons. *J. Alzheimers Dis.* **2017**, *57*, 975–999. [CrossRef] [PubMed]
40. Ferreira, S.T.; Lourenco, M.V.; Oliveira, M.M.; De Felice, F.G. Soluble amyloid-β oligomers as synaptotoxins leading to cognitive impairment in Alzheimer's disease. *Front. Cell. Neurosci.* **2015**, *9*, 191. [CrossRef] [PubMed]
41. Couturier, J.; Paccalin, M.; Morel, M.; Terro, F.; Milin, S.; Pontcharraud, R.; Fauconneau, B.; Page, G. Prevention of the b-amyloid peptide-induced inflammatory process by inhibition of double-stranded RNA-dependent protein kinase in primary murine mixed co-cultures. *J. Neuroinflamm.* **2011**, *8*, 72–89. [CrossRef] [PubMed]
42. Zujovic, V.; Benavides, J.; Vige, X.; Carter, C.; Taupin, V. Fractalkine Modulates TNF-α Secretion and Neurotoxicity Induced by Microglial Activation. *Glia* **2000**, *29*, 305–315. [CrossRef]
43. Faro, M.L.L.; Fox, B.; Whatmore, J.L.; Winyard, P.G.; Whiteman, M. Hydrogen sulfide and nitric oxide interactions in inflammation. *Nitric Oxide* **2014**, *41*, 38–47. [CrossRef] [PubMed]
44. Tian, M.; Deng, Y.Y.; Hou, D.R.; Li, W.; Feng, X.L.; Yu, Z.L. Association of IL-1, IL-18, and IL-33 gene polymorphisms with late-onset Alzheimer's disease in a Hunan Han Chinese population. *Brain Res.* **2015**, *1596*, 136–145. [CrossRef] [PubMed]
45. Jia, Y.; Wang, N.; Liu, X. Resveratrol and Amyloid-Beta: Mechanistic Insights. *Nutrients* **2017**, *9*, 1122. [CrossRef] [PubMed]
46. Ehrnhoefer, D.E.; Bieschke, J.; Boeddrich, A.; Herbst, M.; Masino, L.; Lurz, R.; Engemann, S.; Pastore, A.; Wanker, E.E. EGCG redirects amyloidogenic polypeptides into unstructured, off-pathway oligomers. *Nat. Struct. Mol. Biol.* **2008**, *15*, 558–566. [CrossRef] [PubMed]
47. Yang, F.; Lim, G.P.; Begum, A.N.; Ubeda, O.J.; Simmons, M.R.; Ambegaokar, S.S.; Chen, P.P.; Kayed, R.; Glabe, C.G.; Frautschy, S.A.; et al. Curcumin Inhibits Formation of Amyloid β Oligomers and Fibrils, Binds Plaques, and Reduces Amyloid In Vivo. *J. Biol. Chem.* **2005**, *280*, 5892–5901. [CrossRef] [PubMed]
48. Kook, Y. The inhibitory effect of Scutellaria baicalensis on type 1 interferon production in Raw 264.7 cells. *Herb. Formula Sci.* **2008**, *16*, 219–228.
49. Pervin, M.; Unno, K.; Ohishi, T.; Tanabe, H.; Miyoshi, N.; Nakamura, Y. Beneficial Effects of Green Tea Catechins on Neurodegenerative Diseases. *Molecules* **2018**, *23*, 1297. [CrossRef] [PubMed]
50. Toda, T.; Sunagawa, T.; Kanda, T.; Tagashira, M.; Shirasawa, T.; Shimizu, T. Apple Procyanidins Suppress Amyloid β-Protein Aggregation. *Biochem. Res. Int.* **2011**, *2011*, 784698. [CrossRef] [PubMed]
51. Heo, H.J.; Lee, C.Y. Epicatechin and Catechin in Cocoa Inhibit Amyloid β Protein Induced Apoptosis. *J. Agric. Food Chem.* **2005**, *53*, 1445–1448. [CrossRef] [PubMed]
52. Laurenzi, M.A.; Arcuri, C.; Rossi, R.; Marconi, P.; Bocchini, V. Effects of Microenvironment on Morphology and Function of the Microglial Cell Line BV-2. *Neurochem. Res.* **2001**, *26*, 1209–1216. [CrossRef] [PubMed]
53. Liu, X.; Wu, J.Y.; Zhou, F.; Sun, X.L.; Yao, H.H.; Yang, Y.; Ding, J.H.; Hu, G. The regulation of rotenone-induced inflammatory factor production by ATP-sensitive potassium channel expressed in BV-2 cells. *Neurosci. Lett.* **2006**, *394*, 131–135. [CrossRef] [PubMed]
54. Mincheva-Tasheva, S.; Soler, R.M. NF-κB Signaling Pathways. *Neuroscientist* **2013**, *19*, 175–194. [CrossRef] [PubMed]
55. Alawdi, S.H.; El-Denshary, E.S.; Safar, M.M.; Eidi, H.; David, M.; Abdel-Wahhab, M.A. Neuroprotective Effect of Nanodiamond in Alzheimer's Disease Rat Model: A Pivotal Role for Modulating NF-κB and STAT3 Signaling. *Mol. Neurobiol.* **2017**, *54*, 1906–1918. [CrossRef] [PubMed]
56. Zhong, Z.; Umemura, A.; Sanchez-Lopez, E.; Liang, S.; Shalapour, S.; Wong, J.; He, F.; Boassa, D.; Perkins, G.; Ali, S.R.; et al. NF-κB Restricts Inflammasome Activation via Elimination of Damaged Mitochondria. *Cell* **2016**, *164*, 896–910. [CrossRef] [PubMed]
57. Liu, B.; Sun, L.; Liu, Q.; Gong, C.; Yao, Y.; Lv, X.; Lin, L.; Yao, H.; Su, F.; Li, D.; et al. A Cytoplasmic NF-κB Interacting Long Noncoding RNA Blocks IκB Phosphorylation and Suppresses Breast Cancer Metastasis. *Cancer Cell* **2015**, *27*, 370–381. [CrossRef] [PubMed]
58. Seo, E.; Fischer, N.; Efferth, T. Phytochemicals as inhibitors of NF-κB for treatment of Alzheimer's disease. *Pharmacol. Res.* **2018**, *129*, 262–273. [CrossRef] [PubMed]

59. Park, S.; Kim, M.; Kim, Y.J.; Lee, Y.; Bae, D.; Kim, S.; Na, Y.; Yoon, H. Selective PCAF inhibitor ameliorates cognitive and behavioral deficits by suppressing NF-κB-mediated neuroinflammation induced by Aβ in a model of Alzheimer's disease. *Int. J. Mol. Med.* **2015**, *35*, 1109–1118. [CrossRef] [PubMed]
60. Shi, Z.; Han, Y.; Han, X.; Zhang, K.; Chang, Y.; Hu, Z.; Qi, H.; Ting, C.; Zhen, Z.; Hong, W. Upstream regulators and downstream effectors of NF-κB in Alzheimer's disease. *J. Neurol. Sci.* **2016**, *366*, 127–134. [CrossRef] [PubMed]
61. Lian, H.; Yang, L.; Cole, A.; Sun, L.; Chiang, A.C.A.; Fowler, S.W.; Shim, D.J.; Rodriguez-Rivera, J.; Taglialatela, G.; Jankowsky, J.L.; et al. NF-κB-Activated Astroglial Release of Complement C3 Compromises Neuronal Morphology and Function Associated with Alzheimer's Disease. *Neuron* **2015**, *85*, 101–115. [CrossRef] [PubMed]
62. Martire, S.; Mosca, L.; d'Erme, M. PARP-1 involvement in neurodegeneration: A focus on Alzheimer's and Parkinson's diseases. *Mech. Ageing Dev.* **2015**, *146*, 53–64. [CrossRef] [PubMed]
63. Zeng, J.; Libien, J.; Shaik, F.; Wolk, J.; Hernández, A.I. Nucleolar PARP-1 Expression Is Decreased in Alzheimer's Disease: Consequences for Epigenetic Regulation of rDNA and Cognition. *Neural Plast.* **2016**, *2016*, 8987928. [CrossRef] [PubMed]
64. Figueira, I.; Garcia, G.; Pimpão, R.C.; Terrasso, A.P.; Costa, I.; Almeida, A.F.; Tavares, L.; Pais, T.F.; Pinto, P.; Ventura, M.R.; et al. Polyphenols journey through blood-brain barrier towards neuronal protection. *Sci. Rep.* **2017**, *7*, 11456. [CrossRef] [PubMed]
65. Schaffer, S.; Halliwell, B. Do polyphenols enter the brain and does it matter? Some theoretical and practical considerations. *Genes Nutr.* **2012**, *7*, 99–109. [CrossRef] [PubMed]
66. Wu, L.; Zhang, Q.L.; Zhang, X.Y.; Lv, C.; Li, J.; Yuan, Y.; Yin, F.X. Pharmacokinetics and Blood-Brain Barrier Penetration of (+)-Catechin and (−)-Epicatechin in Rats by Microdialysis Sampling Coupled to High-Performance Liquid Chromatography with Chemiluminescence Detection. *J. Agric. Food Chem.* **2012**, *60*, 9377–9383. [CrossRef] [PubMed]
67. Neves, A.R.; Queiroz, J.F.; Reis, S. Brain-targeted delivery of resveratrol using solid lipid nanoparticles functionalized with apolipoprotein E. *J. Nanobiotechnol.* **2016**, *14*, 27. [CrossRef] [PubMed]
68. Jain, A.; Rani, V. Mode of treatment governs curcumin response on doxorubicin-induced toxicity in cardiomyoblasts. *Mol. Cell. Biochem.* **2018**, *442*, 81–96. [CrossRef] [PubMed]

International Journal of
Molecular Sciences

MDPI

Article

Pharmacokinetic Comparisons of Multiple Triterpenic Acids from *Jujubae Fructus* Extract Following Oral Delivery in Normal and Acute Liver Injury Rats

Yao Li [1], Sheng Guo [1,*], Quanjin Ren [2], Dandan Wei [1], Ming Zhao [1], Shulan Su [1], Zhishu Tang [3] and Jin-Ao Duan [1,*]

1. Jiangsu Collaborative Innovation Center of Chinese Medicinal Resources Industrialization/State Key Laboratory Cultivation Base for Traditional Chinese Medicine Quality and Efficacy, Nanjing University of Chinese Medicine, Nanjing 210023, China; liyaonjutcm@163.com (Y.L.); wei.dandan@njucm.edu.cn (D.W.); mingzhao@njucm.edu.cn (M.Z.); sushulan@njucm.edu.cn (S.S.)
2. Institute of Botany, Jiangsu Province and Chinese Academy of Science, Nanjing 210014, China; renquanjin@cnbg.net
3. Shaanxi Collaborative Innovation Center of Chinese Medicinal Resources Industrialization, Shaanxi University of Chinese Medicine, Xianyang 712046, China; tzs6565@163.com

* Correspondence: guosheng@njucm.edu.cn (S.G.); dja@njucm.edu.cn (J.-A.D.); Tel./Fax: +86-25-8581-1916 (S.G.); +86-25-8581-1291 (J.-A.D.)

Received: 2 July 2018; Accepted: 11 July 2018; Published: 13 July 2018

Abstract: *Jujubae Fructus*, the dried fruit of *Ziziphus jujuba*, has been used as Chinese medicine and food for centuries. Triterpenic acids have been found to be the major bioactive constituents in *Jujubae Fructus* responsible for their hepatoprotective activity in previous phytochemical and biological studies, while few pharmacokinetic studies have been conducted. To reveal the kinetics of the triterpenic acids under the pathological liver injury state, an established ultra-performance liquid chromatography coupled with a mass spectrometry method was applied for the simultaneous quantitation of seven triterpenic acids (ceanothic acid, epiceanothic acid, pomonic acid, alphitolic acid, maslinic acid, betulinic acid, and betulonic acid) in plasma samples of normal and acute liver injury rats induced by CCl_4. The results showed that there were significant differences ($p < 0.05$) in the pharmacokinetic parameters of seven triterpenic acids between model and normal groups. The AUC_{0-t} and $AUC_{0-\infty}$ of epiceanothic acid (5227 ± 334 μg·h/L vs. 1478 ± 255 μg·h/L and 6127 ± 423 μg·h/L vs. 1482 ± 255 μg·h/L, respectively) and pomonic acid (4654 ± 349 μg·h/L vs. 1834 ± 225 μg·h/L and 4776 ± 322 μg·h/L vs. 1859 ± 230 μg·h/L, respectively) in model rats were significantly higher than those in normal rats, and the CLz/F of them were significantly decreased (0.28 ± 0.02 L/h/kg vs. 1.36 ± 0.18 L/h/kg and 19.96 ± 1.30 L/h/kg vs. 53.15 ± 5.60 L/h/kg, respectively). In contrast, the above parameters for alphitolic acid, betulinic acid and betulonic acid exhibited the quite different trend. This pharmacokinetic research might provide useful information for the clinical usage of triterpenic acids from *Jujubae Fructus*.

Keywords: *Ziziphus jujuba*; triterpenic acids; pharmacokinetic study; acute liver injury

1. Introduction

Jujubae Fructus, the fruit of *Ziziphus jujuba* Mill., has been used as herb medicine and food for centuries in China [1,2]. According to traditional Chinese medicine theory, *Jujubae Fructus* could reinforce spleen and stomach, and is commonly used for the treatment of anorexia, fatigue and loose stools related to deficiency syndromes of the spleen and hysteria in women [3]. The controlled clinical trials also showed that *Jujubae Fructus* extract is an effective treatment for chronic constipation [4] and type 2 diabetes [5]. In addition, in northern China, the decoction of *Jujubae Fructus* are claimed as useful remedies for the management and/or control of hepatitis in folk [6].

In support of its traditional efficacy, modern researches have revealed that *Jujubae Fructus* has pharmacological properties including hepatoprotective [6], gastrointestinal protective [7], anti-inflammatory [8], immunomodulating [9] and hematopoiesis effects [10]. Among them, ethanolic extract of *Jujubae Fructus* with a dose of 200 mg/kg could significantly decrease ALT and AST, and attenuate histopathology of hepatic injury induced by carbon tetrachloride (CCl_4), and the results indicated that hepatic protective effects of *Jujubae Fructus* were relevant to modulate the oxidative stress in hepatic injury [6,11]. These results further confirmed the traditional efficacy of *Jujubae Fructus* on the hepatoprotective effect. Phytochemical and biological studies showed that these multiple bioactivities of *Jujubae Fructus* could be attributed to its various constituents, such as triterpenic acids [12], polysaccharides [2], phenolic acids [13], flavonoids [14], nucleoside and amino acids [15,16]. Among these components, triterpenic acids, such as betulinic acid, alphitolic acid, maslinic acid, etc., have been reported to possess biological effects of hepatoprotective, anti-inflammatory, antimicrobial and antioxidant activities [6,8,17,18], which have attracted great attention from researchers.

The liver is a crucial organ for metabolism and detoxification in the human body, and liver disease has nowadays become one of the most common causes of death [19]. There are reports that acute liver injury is the main initiating factor and pathological basis for liver fibrosis, hepatitis, cirrhosis and even liver cancer, which could result in terminal liver failure [20,21]. The previous studies have reported the hepatoprotective effect of *Jujubae Fructus*, and triterpenic acids have been considered as the main bioactive compounds for the above activity [6,11]. However, there were few reports on the pharmacokinetic studies of triterpenic acids from *Jujubae Fructus* in liver injury model animals, and relevant pharmacokinetic studies of *Jujubae Fructus* in humans were also rare. It is well known that under the pathological condition of liver injury, pharmacokinetic and metabolic behaviors of drugs are often altered [20,22,23]. Thus, based on the ultra-performance liquid chromatography coupled with mass spectrometry (UHPLC-MS/MS) method established in the previous study [24], the pharmacokinetics of triterpenic acids from *Jujubae Fructus* in normal and acute liver injury rats were compared in this paper for the purpose of providing clinical reference for *Jujubae Fructus*.

2. Results and Discussion

2.1. Validation of the Acute Liver Injury Rats Model

To verify whether the rat model of acute liver injury was successful, peripheral blood routine, levels of alanine aminotransferase (ALT), aspartate aminotransferase (AST) and histopathological characteristics were analyzed. All the results are presented in Figures 1 and 2. It was shown that the liver injury score and the levels of white blood cell count (WBC), neutrophil (NEU) count and ratio, erythrocyte mean corpuscular volume (MCV), mean corpuscular hemoglobin (MCH), AST and ALT of the model group after being injected intraperitoneally with CCl_4 increased significantly ($p < 0.05$) compared to control group. Lymphocyte (LYM) ratios of the model group decreased significantly. It was known that the levels of AST and ALT were all related to liver function. Besides, it has reported that liver injury induced by CCl_4 could cause inflammation [19,25], which could be presented with the increases of WBC and NEU. Thus, the above results indicated that the acute liver injury rat model was successful, and could be used for the following experiment.

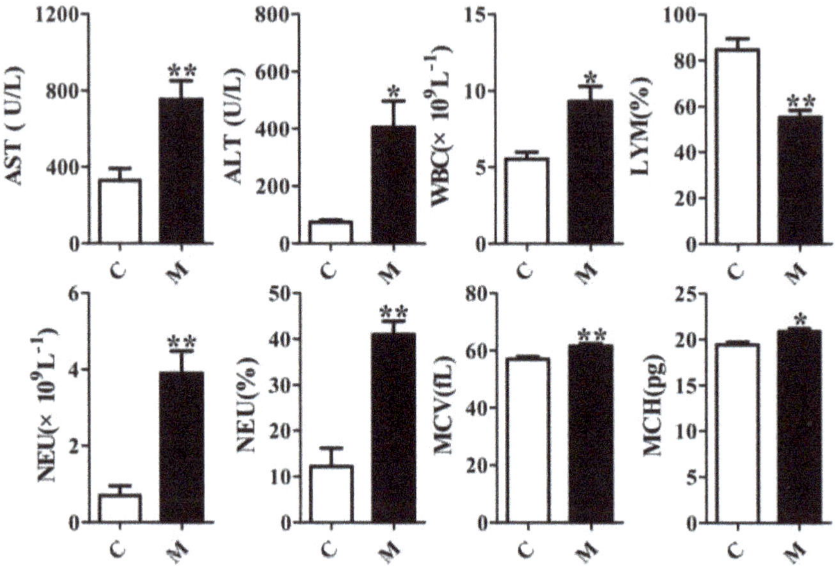

Figure 1. Changes in alanine aminotransferase (ALT), aspartate aminotransferase (AST), and peripheral blood routine between control group (C) and model group of acute liver injury (M). WBC: white blood cell count, LYM: lymphocyte ratio, NEU: neutrophil count/ratio, MCV: erythrocyte mean corpuscular volume, MCH: mean corpuscular hemoglobin (means ± SEM, n = 6, * $p < 0.05$, ** $p < 0.01$ vs. control group).

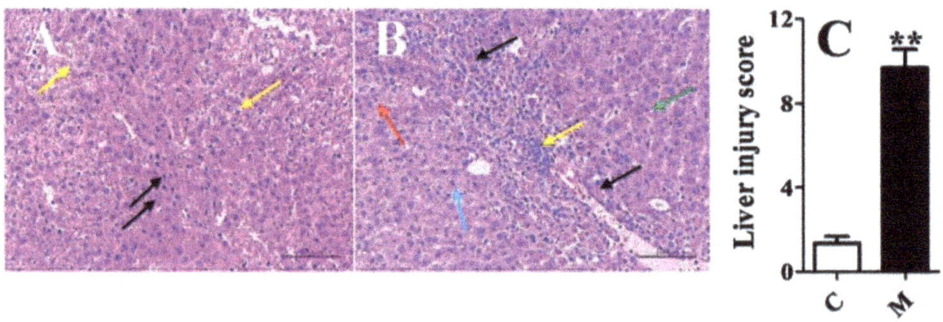

Figure 2. Pathological sections of liver, means ± SEM, n = 6, ** $p < 0.01$ vs. control group. (**A**) blank group: Local hepatocellular necrosis, nucleus fragmentation dissolves or pyknosis, and eosinophilic cytoplasm can be seen as shown by **black** arrows; degeneration of hepatocytes, swelling of cell bodies, irregular vacuoles and eosinophilic particles in the cytoplasm were shown by **yellow** arrows; (**B**) acute liver injury group: hepatocyte necrosis, nucleus fragmentation or dissolution, and eosinophilic cytoplasmic enhancement were shown by the **black** arrow; inflammatory cell infiltration was indicated by the **yellow** arrow; hepatic cell vesicle steatosis was shown by the **green** arrow; some hepatocytes in the vicinity of the necrotic lesions are degenerated, as indicated by the **red** arrow; pathological mitoses can be seen, as indicated by the **blue** arrows; and (**C**) Column chart of liver injury score.

2.2. Method Validation

The method for separation and detection of analytes was performed in the established UHPLC-MS/MS method previously [24] with appropriate adjustments.

2.2.1. Selectivity

Figure 3 showed the chromatograms obtained from the blank plasma of a rat, blank plasma spiked with the standards of seven mixed triterpenic acids and internal standard (IS), and rat plasma acquired at 6 h after oral administration of triterpenic acids extract (TAE). No significant endogenous interference or metabolites were found in the blank plasma at the retention times of standards and IS, which revealed that the selectivity of the method was acceptable.

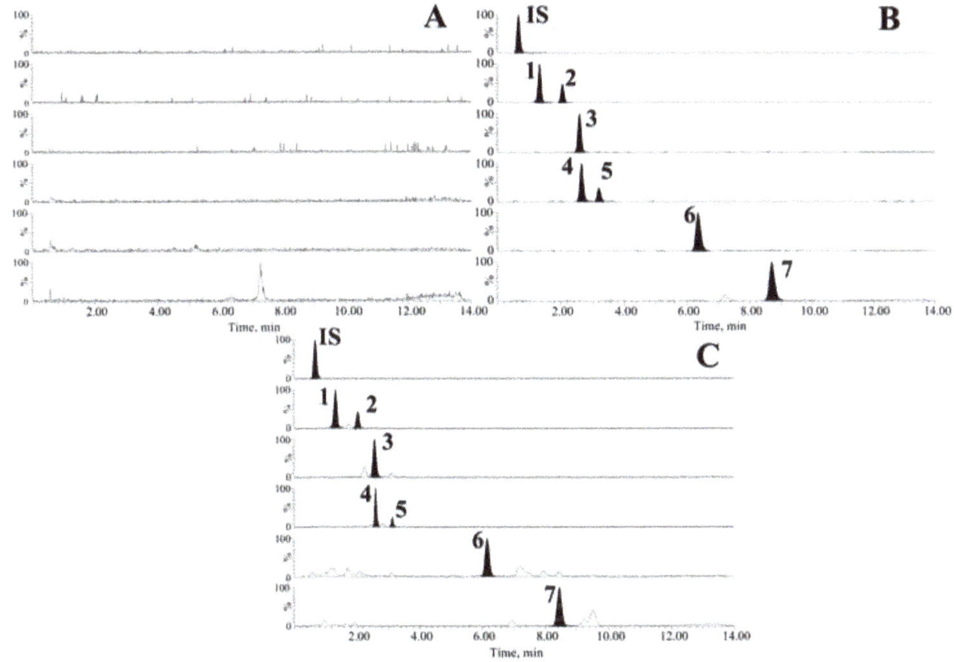

Figure 3. Typical UHPLC-MS/MS chromatograms of (**A**) blank plasma, (**B**) blank plasma spiked with the analytes and IS, and (**C**) plasma sample from a normal rat at 6 h after oral administration of TAE, which were detected with multiple reaction monitoring mode.; ceanothic acid (1), epiceanothic acid (2), pomonic acid (3), alphitolic acid (4), maslinic acid (5), betulinic acid (6), betulonic acid (7).

2.2.2. Linearity and Lower Limit of Quantification (LLOQ)

The linearity of the proposed method was evaluated by means of representative calibration curves, correlation coefficients and a linear range of the seven standards, and LLOQs were used for determining the sensitivity of the method. As shown in Table 1, all the correlation coefficients (R^2) are $\geq$0.9930, which indicated the good linearity of all analytes and the LLOQs of the seven triterpenic acids in plasma were suitable for quantitative detection.

2.2.3. Precision and Accuracy

As shown in Table 2, the deviation in intra- and inter-day precision of all the analytes in QC samples were $\leq$10.11% and $\leq$14.29%, respectively, and the accuracies (RE) of those analytes ranged from −2.03% to 14.87%. The results indicated that the method was accurate, precise and was acceptable for analysis of biological samples due to the values being within the acceptable criteria.

Table 1. Regression equation and LLOQ of seven compounds.

Compound	Linear Regression Equation	R^2	Range (ng/mL)	LLOQ (ng/mL)
Ceanothic acid	$y = 2.347 \times 10^{-3} x + 8.488 \times 10^{-2}$	0.9982	4.61–2951	2.93
Epiceanothic acid	$y = 1.832 \times 10^{-3} x - 3.799 \times 10^{-2}$	0.9987	2.35–3009	0.92
Pomonic acid	$y = 2.989 \times 10^{-4} x - 1.377 \times 10^{-3}$	0.9997	22.82–2922	6.47
Alphitolic acid	$y = 4.411 \times 10^{-3} x + 4.185 \times 10^{-1}$	0.9930	22.60–2892	7.34
Maslinic acid	$y = 1.657 \times 10^{-3} x + 1.111 \times 10^{-1}$	0.9968	22.94–2936	15.02
Betulinic acid	$y = 6.084 \times 10^{-3} x + 9.910 \times 10^{-2}$	0.9996	23.62–3023	17.23
Betulonic acid	$y = 3.058 \times 10^{-3} x + 1.718 \times 10^{-2}$	0.9999	23.51–3009	22.68

Table 2. Precision and accuracy for the determination of the seven compounds.

Compound	Concentration (ng/mL)	Intra-Day		Inter-Day	
		Accuracy (RE, %)	Precision (RSD, %)	Accuracy (RE, %)	Precision (RSD, %)
Ceanothic acid	23.05	14.39	1.98	9.85	6.29
	368.8	14.12	1.68	8.64	7.18
	2951	5.62	8.49	4.77	8.03
Epiceanothic acid	23.51	10.40	3.94	5.66	11.33
	376.1	9.97	1.33	5.95	5.43
	3009	5.04	7.30	2.74	6.52
Pomonic acid	22.82	−2.03	10.11	9.02	9.31
	365.2	13.73	6.63	11.33	12.443
	2922	9.42	9.49	11.09	9.75
Alphitolic acid	22.60	12.42	1.38	10.95	13.39
	361.6	12.18	2.39	9.76	5.14
	2892	5.87	7.69	1.19	5.90
Maslinic acid	22.94	12.03	4.88	14.61	14.29
	367.0	14.87	1.17	12.99	9.18
	2936	12.44	6.58	8.21	5.77
Betulinic acid	23.62	12.86	7.05	11.93	8.80
	377.9	13.93	3.97	10.59	7.69
	3023	4.42	5.63	2.43	4.96
Betulonic acid	23.51	13.50	7.82	10.31	12.88
	376.1	12.88	2.14	10.52	8.78
	3009	8.41	8.57	5.52	8.75

2.2.4. Extraction Recovery and Matrix Effect

The results of extraction recovery and the matrix effect are shown in Table 3. It was shown that the extraction recoveries ranged from 78.98% to 103.8%, and the matrix effects were between 75.28% and 109.3% with the RSD values less than 15.0% for the seven analytes at three QC concentrations. As for IS, the extraction recoveries and matrix effects were 87.37–98.45% and 75.52–80.31%, respectively. All the results suggested the reliable extraction recoveries of these analytes and no significant matrix effect in this experiment.

2.2.5. Stability

The QC samples with different conditions (three freeze-thaw cycles; 12 h at room temperature; 24 h at 4 °C; 20 days at −20 °C) were used to investigate the stability of the seven triterpenic acids, and the results (Table 4) showed that the RSD values were all less than 13.59%, which indicated that all analytes were stable throughout the whole test.

Table 3. Recoveries and matrix effects of the seven compounds in rat plasma.

Compound	Concentration (ng/mL)	Recovery (%, Mean ± S.D.)	Matrix Effect (%, Mean ± S.D.)
Ceanothic acid	23.05	87.77 ± 3.88	94.42 ± 4.37
	368.8	89.99 ± 6.08	91.57 ± 12.23
	2951	83.88 ± 2.30	82.64 ± 1.67
Epiceanothic acid	23.51	91.06 ± 13.06	91.71 ± 8.25
	376.1	90.87 ± 6.21	108.4 ± 15.8
	3009	82.01 ± 1.28	105.9 ± 1.6
Pomonic acid	22.82	78.98 ± 2.93	75.28 ± 9.39
	365.2	89.32 ± 5.73	94.82 ± 12.17
	2922	83.31 ± 3.72	109.3 ± 3.9
Alphitolic acid	22.60	90.09 ± 3.62	85.95 ± 6.71
	361.6	93.48 ± 5.93	82.60 ± 7.93
	2892	85.33 ± 0.80	77.22 ± 0.67
Maslinic acid	22.94	94.67 ± 8.49	89.02 ± 8.68
	367.0	93.23 ± 5.66	93.72 ± 8.65
	2936	83.58 ± 2.24	89.37 ± 1.33
Betulinic acid	23.62	103.8 ± 11.3	89.83 ± 10.73
	377.9	100.5 ± 8.9	101.8 ± 14.8
	3023	89.34 ± 1.81	91.10 ± 0.28
Betulonic acid	23.51	101.0 ± 8.1	92.62 ± 7.51
	376.1	101.7 ± 7.2	100.4 ± 13.5
	3009	85.79 ± 2.10	102.0 ± 2.0

Table 4. Stabilities of the seven compounds in rat plasma.

Compound	Concentration (ng/mL)	Three Freeze-Thaw Cycles (RSD%)	12 h at Room Temperature (RSD%)	24 h at 4 °C (RSD%)	20 Days at −20 °C (RSD%)
Ceanothic acid	23.05	9.10	12.59	10.45	8.57
	368.8	2.56	10.12	5.91	2.04
	2951	3.41	11.68	8.14	7.15
Epiceanothic acid	23.51	9.22	13.33	9.92	6.33
	376.1	3.05	9.67	6.30	1.65
	3009	5.46	12.27	8.07	6.30
Pomonic acid	22.82	13.42	13.59	12.50	11.71
	365.2	5.33	10.54	7.15	7.01
	2922	4.17	12.67	8.42	7.72
Alphitolic acid	22.60	9.78	11.32	11.99	1.82
	361.6	3.06	8.64	6.14	2.88
	2892	4.28	11.39	9.52	4.90
Maslinic acid	22.94	10.21	9.47	13.61	10.65
	367.0	3.10	7.76	5.34	1.17
	2936	5.54	11.54	9.72	6.31
Betulinic acid	23.62	10.49	11.32	9.31	5.82
	377.9	3.61	6.96	5.46	3.35
	3023	5.32	11.95	8.62	4.50
Betulonic acid	23.51	11.18	10.50	4.53	7.47
	376.1	3.44	6.99	4.08	2.48
	3009	6.47	11.46	6.13	8.51

2.3. Pharmacokinetic Study

The pharmacokinetics of seven triterpenic acids in plasma after a single oral administration of TAE in normal and acute liver injury rats were analyzed by the validated UHPLC-MS/MS method. The pharmacokinetic parameters obtained with the non-compartment module of Drug and Statistic (DAS) 3.2.8 pharmacokinetic software are listed in Table 5. The mean concentration-time profiles are presented in Figure 4.

Table 5. Pharmacokinetic parameters of seven compounds after an oral administration in normal and model rats (means ± SEM, n = 6).

Compound	Group	C_{max} (μg/L)	CLz/F (L/h/kg)	T_{max} (h)	$T_{1/2z}$ (h)	AUC_{0-t} (μg·h/L)	$AUC_{0-\infty}$ (μg·h/L)
Ceanothic acid	C	326.9 ± 67.4	1.25 ± 0.08	6.67 ± 0.47	2.06 ± 0.26	2474 ± 168	2479 ± 171
	M	286.5 ± 21.1	0.87 ± 0.06	8.67 ± 1.25	4.11 ± 0.48	3431 ± 171 *	3567 ± 232
Epiceanothic acid	C	169.7 ± 34.4	1.36 ± 0.18	7.33 ± 0.47	2.45 ± 0.03	1478 ± 255	1482 ± 255
	M	371.9 ± 19.9 *	0.28 ± 0.02 *	7.33 ± 0.47	7.00 ± 1.33	5227 ± 334 **	6127 ± 423 **
Pomonic acid	C	304.9 ± 53.8	53.15 ± 5.60	6.00 ± 0.00	2.88 ± 0.54	1834 ± 225	1859 ± 230
	M	495.2 ± 60.9	19.96 ± 1.30 *	6.00 ± 0.82	3.87 ± 0.58	4654 ± 349 **	4776 ± 322 **
Alphitolic acid	C	526.7 ± 45.6	3.53 ± 0.27	6.67 ± 0.47	3.72 ± 0.46	5446 ± 346	5580 ± 379
	M	171.0 ± 21.9 **	10.25 ± 0.59 **	4.67 ± 0.47	4.18 ± 0.65	1855 ± 126 **	1912 ± 112 **
Maslinic acid	C	899.5 ± 144.4	13.50 ± 0.67	6.00 ± 0.00	2.17 ± 0.36	5026 ± 245	5040 ± 239
	M	578.7 ± 78.6	11.96 ± 1.24	6.00 ± 0.82	3.06 ± 0.13	5879 ± 702	5931 ± 715
Betulinic acid	C	189.5 ± 20.5	33.90 ± 3.03	8.00 ± 1.41	3.58 ± 0.57	1951 ± 180	1995 ± 192
	M	69.8 ± 7.8 *	70.09 ± 4.33 **	1.33 ± 0.24 *	9.00 ± 2.20	774 ± 42 *	945 ± 54 *
Betulonic acid	C	522.7 ± 65.6	13.65 ± 0.61	6.00 ± 0.00	3.74 ± 0.92	3939 ± 98	4107 ± 190
	M	133.2 ± 14.8 *	22.80 ± 0.78 **	3.33 ± 0.47 *	10.49 ± 1.56	1928 ± 205 **	2450 ± 88 **

* $p < 0.05$, ** $p < 0.01$ vs. control group.

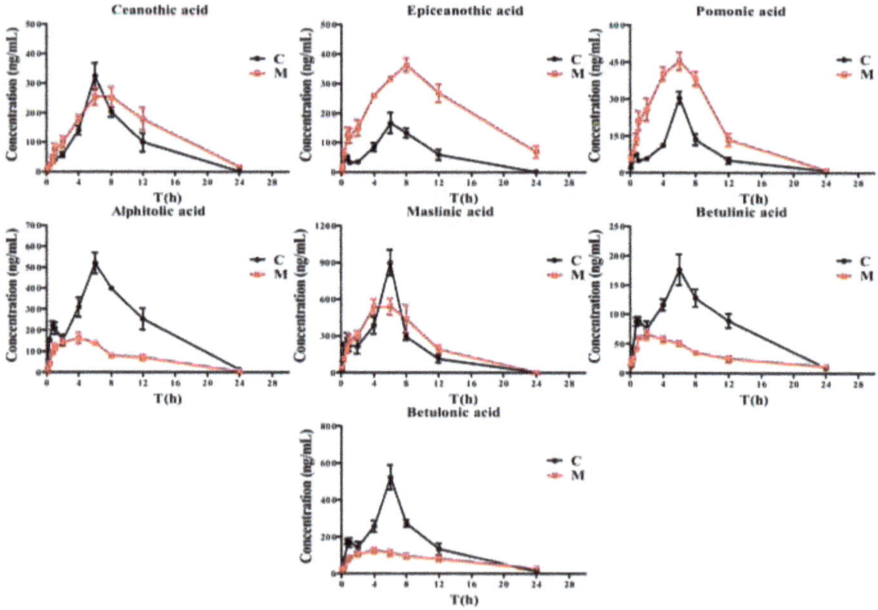

Figure 4. Mean plasma concentration–time curves of seven triterpenic acids after oral administration of TAE for control (C) and acute liver injury model groups (M) (means ± SEM, n = 6).

As shown in Figure 4, the consistent plasma concentration-time profiles in normal rats were found for these seven analytes, which may be attributed to their similar chemical structures. However, this phenomenon was not found in the acute liver injury model, which could be ascribed to the pathological changes of the liver. Moreover, certain pharmacokinetic parameters for these triterpenic acids in acute liver injury rats showed significant differences from those in normal rats, especially for the area under the time curve (AUC_{0-t} and $AUC_{0-\infty}$) and the apparent plasma clearance (CLz/F). The AUC_{0-t} and $AUC_{0-\infty}$ of epiceanothic acid and pomonic acid achieved from the drug concentration-time in acute liver injury rats after oral administration of TAE were significantly higher than those in normal rats, and the CLz/F of them were significantly decreased. These indicated that the acute liver injury could increase the bioavailiability of epiceanothic acid and pomonic acid, and decrease their elimination. In contrast, the mean AUC_{0-t}, $AUC_{0-\infty}$ and the mean peak concentration (C_{max}) of alphitolic acid, betulinic acid and betulonic acid in acute liver injury rats were achieved with relatively lower values compared to those in normal rats. The obvious higher CLz/Fs of alphitolic acid, betulinic acid and betulonic acid compared to normal rats were also found. The above results suggested that the systemic exposure of alphitolic acid, betulinic acid and betulonic acid were weakened and the elimination increased under the liver injury pathological condition. Additionally, the T_{max} of betulinic acid and betulonic acid of the model group were lower than those of the normal group ($p < 0.05$), and the AUC_{0-t} of ceanothic acid and the C_{max} of epiceanothic acid were significantly higher in acute liver injury rats. The other pharmacokinetic parameters in the model rats were found to be different but not significant compared with the normal rats.

It is well known that the liver plays important roles in drug biotransformation, metabolism, detoxification and so on [19]. It contains various enzymes involved in drug metabolism, including cytochrome P450 which converts the drug to active metabolites and directly affects the rate of metabolism [26]. Liver injury might lead to liver cell degeneration, necrosis and changes in cytochrome P450 isoenzyme contents, which could alter the disposition of drugs in the body [22,27]. There have been reports on changes in biotransformation, clearance and pharmacokinetics of drugs in liver injury [28].

Besides, the influence of intestinal drug transport and its microbiota might be an important factor in the absorption and bioavailability of the orally administered medicines. It has been reported that liver injury often causes the increase in intestinal permeability and endotoxin, and the disorder of the intestinal microbiota [29–31]. The increased endotoxin could further cause liver injury more severely and might be a vicious cycle [30]. All the above reasons might synthetically result in differences in pharmacokinetic behavior between acute liver injury and normal rats after oral administration of TAE. However, the hypotheses are still undefined and need further validation.

It is worth noting that the plasma concentration–time profiles of epiceanothic acid and pomonic acid were markedly different from alphitolic acid, betulinic acid and betulonic acid in acute liver injury rats administered TAE from Jujubae Fructus. The AUC_{0-t} and $AUC_{0-\infty}$ of epiceanothic acid and pomonic acid achieved from the drug concentration-time in acute liver injury rats were significantly higher than those in normal rats, and the CLz/F of them were significantly decreased. In contrast, the mean AUC_{0-t}, $AUC_{0-\infty}$ and CLz/F of alphitolic acid, betulinic acid and betulonic acid in acute liver injury rats showed quite a different trend. This phenomenon might be attributed to their subtle difference in chemical structures which could lead to different metabolic pathways. Therefore, further studies for the investigation of triterpenic acids metabolism and distribution in vivo are warranted.

At present, there are some clinical reports about the liver protection of *Jujubae Fructus*, but there is little relevant pharmacokinetic study of *Jujubae Fructus* in humans. Thus, the depth clinical studies to validate the proposed hypothesis need to be conducted in the future.

3. Materials and Methods

3.1. Chemicals and Reagents

Acetonitrile and methanol were purchased from Merck KGaA (Darmstadt, Germany). Chloramphenicol used as the internal standard (IS) was obtained from Aladdin reagent Co., Ltd. (Shanghai, China). Ammonium acetate and CCl_4 were purchased from Sinopharm Chemical Reagent Co., Ltd. (Shanghai, China). Deionized water was prepared by a Milli-Q system (Millipore, Bedford, MA, USA). *Jujubae Fructus* was gathered at Liuling, Shanxi Province, China. The standards (>98% purity) including ceanothic acid, epiceanothic acid, pomonic acid, alphitolic acid, maslinic acid, betulinic acid and betulonic acid were isolated from *Z. jujuba* fruits in our laboratory, and their structures were identified by NMR, HPLC and MS. Other reagents used were of analytical grade.

TAE of *Jujubae Fructus* prepared in our previous experiment [24] was used in this experiment, which contains ceanothic acid, epiceanothic acid, pomonic acid, alphitolic acid, maslinic acid, betulinic acid, and betulonic acid with the contents of 0.78, 0.44, 24.08, 4.97, 17.31, 16.79 and 14.29 mg/g, respectively.

3.2. Instrumentation and Chromatographic Conditions

A Waters Acquity™ UPLC system (Waters Corp., Milford, MA, USA) equipped with a Waters Xevo™ TQ/MS (Waters Corp.) was used. Separation and detection of analytes was performed with the established method described previously [24]. Data acquired was analyzed by MassLynx V4.1 workstation (Waters Corp.).

3.3. Animals and Induction of Acute Liver Injury

Male Sprague-Dawley rats (SPF, 220-240 g) were bought from Experimental Animal Center of Zhejiang Province and the permit number was SCXK (zhe) 2014-0001 (project identification code: No1703300021, 31/03/2017). Animals were housed in Drug Safety Evaluation Center of Nanjing University of Chinese Medicine, Nanjing, China. Animal welfare and all experimental protocols were performed in accordance with the Regulations of Experimental Animal Administration (State Committee of Science and Technology of the People's Republic of China) and approved by the Animal Ethics Committee of Nanjing University of Chinese Medicine. These rats were housed under standard environment with food and water provided ad libitum. After adaptation for 7 days, the 12 rats were randomly divided into 2 groups: control group (C) and acute liver injury group (model group, M). Rats of M group were injected intraperitoneally with 50% CCl_4 once at a dose of 2 mL/kg. CCl_4 used for injection was dissolved in peanut oil. To verify whether the model was successful, whole blood and serum samples were collected from the retro-orbital plexus of rats after modeling for measuring the peripheral blood routine parameters using ADVIA120 fully automatic blood analyzer (Bayer, Germany) and the levels of ALT and AST with Dimension Xpand automatic biochemical analyzer (Bayer, Germany). Furthermore, after the final collection of blood, the rats were anesthetized and sacrificed with 10% choral hydrate (350 mg/kg *ip*) and the liver samples were taken and fixed in formaldehyde solution for histopathological analysis.

3.4. Sample Preparation

After being thawed at room temperature (18–25 °C), each plasma sample (100 μL) was precipitated with 300 μL acetonitrile and 20 μL IS. The mixture was vortexed for 1 min and centrifuged at 15,000× *g* for 15 min. Then, 2 μL of supernatant was injected for UHPLC-MS/MS analysis.

3.5. Preparation of Standard Solutions, Calibration Standards and Quality Control (QC) Samples

A mixed stock solution containing 126.9 μg/mL of ceanothic acid, 129.4 μg/mL of epiceanothic acid, 125.6 μg/mL of pomonic acid, 124.4 μg/mL of alphitolic acid, 126.3 μg/mL of maslinic acid, 130.0 μg/mL of betulinic acid and 129.4 μg/mL of betulonic acid was prepared with methanol as a solvent. A series of working standard solutions were prepared from the mixed stock solution by sequential dilution with methanol. Calibration solutions were prepared by spiking 10 μL of working solution into 100 μL blank plasma to obtain a mixed final dilution of 2.31–2951 ng/mL ceanothic acid, 2.35–3009 ng/mL epiceanothic acid, 2.28–2922 ng/mL pomonic acid, 2.26–2892 ng/mL alphitolic acid, 2.29–2936 ng/mL maslinic acid, 2.36–3023 ng/mL betulinic acid, and 2.35–3009 ng/mL betulonic acid. The quality control (QC) samples were prepared at low, medium, and high concentrations (23.05, 368.8, and 2951 ng/mL ceanothic acid, 23.51, 376.1, and 3009 ng/mL epiceanothic acid, 22.82, 365.2, and 2922 ng/mL pomonic acid, 22.60, 361.6, and 2892 ng/mL alphitolic acid, 22.94, 367.0, and 2936 ng/mL maslinic acid, 23.62, 377.9, and 3023 ng/mL betulinic acid, and 23.51, 376.1, and 3009 ng/mL betulonic acid) in the same way as calibration solutions. The stock solution of IS (9.76 μg/mL chloramphenicol) was also prepared in methanol.

3.6. Method Validation

This proposed method was validated according to US-FDA Bioanalytical Method Validation Guidance [32], and selectivity, linearity, precision, extraction recovery, matrix effect and stability were assessed.

3.6.1. Selectivity

The chromatograms of the rat blank plasma, blank plasma spiked with the seven standards and IS, and rat plasma acquired at 6 h after gavage of TAE, were analyzed and compared to investigate the selectivity of the method [33].

3.6.2. Linearity and LLOQ

The peak area ratio (y) of the analyte to the IS vs. the nominal concentration (x, ng/mL) was used to plot the calibration curve and determine the linearity with weighted ($1/x^2$) least square linear regression [34]. LLOQ of the method was determined based on the signal to noise ratio of 10:1 with the acceptable precision in six replicates of blank plasma (RSD $\leq$ 20%) [35].

3.6.3. Accuracy and Precision

The intra-day and inter-day accuracy and precision were assessed by determining the concentration of six replicates of QC samples (as described in section '3.5') at three concentration levels (low, medium and high) on the same day and on three consecutive days, respectively. The accuracy was described as relative error (RE, %) and precision was expressed as relative standard deviation (RSD, %) [36]. The acceptability criteria for accuracy and precision were required within $\pm$15% according to the guidelines of FDA.

3.6.4. Recovery and Matrix Effect

Extraction recovery and matrix effect were evaluated with six replicates of QC samples at three concentrations. Extraction recovery of the seven triterpenic acids were performed by comparing the peak area of every analyte extracted from plasma samples with that of post-extraction spiked plasma blank [24]. For evaluation of the matrix effect, the peak areas of the analytes in post-extraction standard plasma samples (B) were compared with those of pure methanol containing an equivalent amount of standards at QC levels (A) [37].

3.6.5. Stability

The stability of analytes in rat plasma were assessed by analyzing six replicates of QC samples at three concentration levels. The QC samples in different storage conditions including three freeze-thaw cycles (from −80 °C to room temperature), 12 h at room temperature, and 20 days at −20 °C, were used to evaluate the freeze-thaw, short-term, and long-term stability, respectively. In addition, the autosampler stability was also evaluated after samples were stored in the autosampler at 4 °C for 24 h [38].

3.7. Pharmacokinetic Study in Rat and Statistical Analysis

After fasting for 12 h with free access to water, rats in both C and M groups were intragastrically administered TAE (dissolved in water with 10% tween-80) at a dose of 4.0 g/kg. The administered volume was 10 mL/kg for each rat, each time. Serial blood samples (about 500 μL for each) were collected into heparinized tubes from the retro-orbital plexus at 0, 5, 10, 20, 45, 60, 120, 240, 360, 480, 720 and 1440 min after oral administration. All blood samples were centrifuged at 3500 rpm at 4 °C for 10 min, then the supernatants were separated and stored at −80 °C until analysis. The pharmacokinetic parameters were calculated by Drug and Statistic (DAS) 3.2.8 pharmacokinetic software in a non-compartment model. The experimental data were expressed as mean ± SEM. Independent Samples *t*-test via the software SPSS 22.0 (IBM SPSS, Chicago, IL, USA) was used for evaluation of statistical significance.

4. Conclusions

A rapid, sensitive, and simple UHPLC-MS/MS method was used for the determination of seven triterpenic acids in the plasma of acute liver injury and normal rats after oral administration of TAE. The results demonstrated that acute liver injury induced by CCl_4 could alter the pharmacokinetic parameters of seven triterpenic acids, such as AUC_{0-t}, $AUC_{0-\infty}$, CLz/F and C_{max}. And the differences might be due to the changes in liver function, intestinal permeability and intestinal microbiome in the acute liver injury pathological state. These pharmacokinetic results in the pathological state of acute liver injury might provide more useful information for the application of *Jujubae Fructus* in treating liver disease.

Author Contributions: S.G. and J.-A.D. designed the study. Y.L., S.G. and Q.R. performed the laboratory work. Y.L., S.G. and D.W. analyzed the data and wrote the paper. M.Z., S.S. revised the manuscript. J.-A.D., Z.T. and Q.R. contributed reagents/materials/analysis tools.

Funding: This research was funded by National Natural Science Foundation of China (No. 81473538), Six Talent Peaks Project in Jiangsu Province (No. YY-026) and Henry Fok Education Foundation (No. 141040).

Conflicts of Interest: The authors declare no conflict of interest.

References

1. Lam, C.T.W.; Gong, A.G.W.; Lam, K.Y.C.; Zhang, L.M.; Chen, J.-P.; Dong, T.T.X.; Lin, H.-Q.; Tsim, K.W.K. Jujube-containing herbal decoctions induce neuronal differentiation and the expression of anti-oxidant enzymes in cultured PC12 cells. *J. Ethnopharmacol.* **2016**, *188*, 275–283. [CrossRef] [PubMed]
2. Ji, X.; Peng, Q.; Yuan, Y.; Shen, J.; Xie, X.; Wang, M. Isolation, structures and bioactivities of the polysaccharides from jujube fruit (*Ziziphus jujuba* Mill.): A review. *Food Chem.* **2017**, *227*, 349–357. [CrossRef] [PubMed]
3. Gao, Q.-H.; Wu, C.-S.; Wang, M. The Jujube (*Ziziphus Jujuba* Mill.) Fruit: A review of current knowledge of Fruit composition and health benefits. *J. Agric. Food Chem.* **2013**, *61*, 3351–3363. [CrossRef] [PubMed]
4. Naftali, T.; Feingelernt, H.; Lesin, Y.; Rauchwarger, A.; Konikoff, F.M. *Ziziphus jujuba* extract for the treatment of chronic idiopathic constipation: a controlled clinical trial. *Digestion* **2008**, *78*, 224–228. [CrossRef] [PubMed]
5. Yazdanpanah, Z.; Ghadiri-Anari, A.; Mehrjardi, A.V.; Dehghani, A.; Zardini, H.Z.; Nadjarzadeh, A. Effect of *Ziziphus jujube* fruit infusion on lipid profiles, glycaemic index and antioxidant status in type 2 diabetic patients: a randomized controlled clinical trial. *Phytother. Res.* **2017**, *31*, 755–762. [CrossRef] [PubMed]
6. Shen, X.; Tang, Y.; Yang, R.; Yu, L.; Fang, T.; Duan, J.A. The protective effect of *Zizyphus jujube* fruit on carbon tetrachloride-induced hepatic injury in mice by anti-oxidative activities. *J. Ethnopharmacol.* **2009**, *122*, 555–560. [CrossRef] [PubMed]
7. Huang, Y.-L.; Yen, G.-C.; Sheu, F.; Chau, C.F. Effects of water-soluble carbohydrate concentrate from Chinese jujube on different intestinal and fecal indices. *J. Agric. Food Chem.* **2008**, *56*, 1734–1739. [CrossRef] [PubMed]
8. Yu, L.; Jiang, B.P.; Luo, D.; Shen, X.C.; Guo, S.; Duan, J.A.; Tang, Y. P. Bioactive components in the fruits of *Ziziphus jujuba* Mill. against the inflammatory irritant action of Euphorbia plants. *Phytomedicine* **2012**, *19*, 239–244. [CrossRef] [PubMed]
9. Chen, J.; Du, C.Y.; Lam, K.Y.; Zhang, W.L.; Lam, C.T.; Yan, A.L.; Yao, P.; Lau, D.T.; Dong, T.T.; Tsim, K.W. The Standardized extract of *Ziziphus jujuba* Fruit (Jujube) regulates pro-inflammatory cytokine expression in cultured murine macrophages: suppression of lipopolysaccharide-stimulated NF-κB Activity. *Phytother. Res.* **2014**, *28*, 1527–1532. [CrossRef] [PubMed]
10. Chen, J.; Lam, C.T.; Kong, A.Y.; Zhang, W.L.; Zhan, J.Y.; Bi, C.W.; Chan, G.K.; Lam, K.Y.; Yao, P.; Dong, T.T.; et al. The Extract of *Ziziphus jujuba* fruit (Jujube) induces expression of erythropoietin via hypoxia-inducible factor-1 alpha in cultured Hep3B Cells. *Planta Med.* **2014**, *80*, 1622–1627. [PubMed]

11. Rajopadhye, A.; Upadhye, A.S. Estimation of bioactive compound, maslinic acid by HPTLC, and evaluation of hepatoprotective activity on fruit pulp of *Ziziphus jujuba* Mill. cultivars in India. *eCAM* **2016**, *2016*, 4758734. [PubMed]
12. Lee, S.M.; Min, B.S.; Lee, C.G.; Kim, K.S.; Kho, Y.H. Cytotoxic triterpenoids from the fruits of *Zizyphus jujuba*. *Planta Med.* **2003**, *69*, 1051–1054. [PubMed]
13. Wang, B.N.; Liu, H.F.; Zheng, J.B.; Fan, M.T.; Cao, W. Distribution of phenolic acids in different tissues of jujube and their antioxidant activity. *J. Agric. Food Chem.* **2011**, *59*, 1288–1292. [CrossRef] [PubMed]
14. Chen, J.P.; Li, Z.G.; Maiwulanjiang, M.; Zhang, W.L.; Zhan, J.Y.; Lam, C.T.; Zhu, K.Y.; Yao, P.; Choi, R.C.; Lau, D.T.; et al. Chemical and biological assessment of *Ziziphus jujuba* fruits from China: different geographical sources and developmental stages. *J. Agric. Food Chem.* **2013**, *61*, 7315–7324. [CrossRef] [PubMed]
15. Guo, S.; Duan, J.A.; Qian, D.; Tang, Y.; Wu, D.; Su, S.; Wang, H.; Zhao, Y. Content variations of triterpenic acid, nucleoside, nucleobase, and sugar in jujube (*Ziziphus jujuba*) fruit during ripening. *Food Chem.* **2015**, *167*, 468–474. [CrossRef] [PubMed]
16. Guo, S.; Duan, J.A.; Qian, D.; Tang, Y.; Qian, Y.; Wu, D.; Su, S.; Shang, E. Rapid determination of amino acids in fruits of *Ziziphus jujuba* by hydrophilic interaction ultra-high-performance liquid chromatography coupled with triple-quadrupole mass spectrometry. *J. Agric. Food Chem.* **2013**, *61*, 2709–2719. [CrossRef] [PubMed]
17. Fujiwara, Y.; Hayashida, A.; Tsurushima, K.; Nagai, R.; Yoshitomi, M.; Daiguji, N.; Sakashita, N.; Takeya, M.; Tsukamoto, S.; Ikeda, T. Triterpenoids isolated from *Zizyphus jujuba* inhibit foam cell formation in macrophages. *J. Agric. Food Chem.* **2011**, *59*, 4544–4552. [CrossRef] [PubMed]
18. Guo, S.; Duan, J.A.; Tang, Y.P.; Zhu, Z.H.; Qian, Y.F.; Yang, N.Y.; Shang, E.X.; Qian, D.W. Characterization of nucleosides and nucleobases in fruits of *Ziziphus jujuba* by UPLC-DAD-MS. *J. Agric. Food Chem.* **2010**, *58*, 10774–10780. [CrossRef] [PubMed]
19. Chiu, Y.J.; Chou, S.C.; Chiu, C.S.; Kao, C.P.; Wu, K.C.; Chen, C.J.; Tsai, J.C.; Peng, W.H. Hepatoprotective effect of the ethanol extract of *Polygonum orientale* on carbon tetrachloride-induced acute liver injury in mice. *J. Food Drug Anal.* **2018**, *26*, 369–379. [CrossRef] [PubMed]
20. Zhang, Y.; Li, H.; Hu, T.; Li, H.; Jin, G.; Zhang, Y. Metabonomic profiling in study hepatoprotective effect of polysaccharides from *Flammulina velutipes* on carbon tetrachloride-induced acute liver injury rats using GC-MS. *Int. J. Biol. Macromol.* **2018**, *110*, 285–293. [CrossRef] [PubMed]
21. Xie, J.; Wang, W.; Dong, C.; Huang, L.; Wang, H.; Li, C.; Nie, S.; Xie, M. Protective effect of flavonoids from *Cyclocarya paliurus* leaves against carbon tetrachloride-induced acute liver injury in mice. *Food Chem. Toxicol.* **2018**. [CrossRef] [PubMed]
22. Li, P.; Lu, Q.; Jiang, W.; Pei, X.; Sun, Y.; Hao, H.; Hao, K. Pharmacokinetics and pharmacodynamics of rhubarb anthraquinones extract in normal and disease rats. *Biomed. Pharmacother.* **2017**, *91*, 425–435. [CrossRef] [PubMed]
23. Kropeit, D.; McCormick, D.; Erb-Zohar, K.; Moiseev, V.S.; Kobalava, Z.D.; Stobernack, H.P.; Zimmermann, H.; Rubsamen-Schaeff, H. Pharmacokinetics and safety of the anti-human cytomegalovirus drug letermovir in subjects with hepatic impairment. *Br. J. Clin. Pharmacol.* **2017**, *83*, 2678–2686. [CrossRef] [PubMed]
24. Li, Y.; Guo, S.; Hua, T.T.; Wang, Y.Y.; Wei, D.D.; Zhao, M.; Su, S.L.; Duan, J.A. Comparative pharmacokinetics of triterpenic acids in normal and immunosuppressed rats after oral administration of Jujubae Fructus extract by UPLC-MS/MS. *J. Chromatogr. B* **2018**, *1077*, 13–21. [CrossRef] [PubMed]
25. Geier, A.; Kim, S.K.; Gerloff, T.; Dietrich, C.G.; Lammert, F.; Karpen, S.J.; Stieger, B.; Meier, P.J.; Matern, S.; Gartung, C. Hepatobiliary organic anion transporters are differentially regulated in acute toxic liver injury induced by carbon tetrachloride. *J. Hepatol.* **2002**, *37*, 198–205. [CrossRef]
26. Wang, W.; Wang, S.; Liu, J.; Cai, E.; Zhu, H.; He, Z.; Gao, Y.; Li, P.; Zhao, Y. Sesquiterpenoids from the root of Panax Ginseng protect CCl4-induced acute liver injury by anti-inflammatory and anti-oxidative capabilities in mice. *Biomed. Pharmacother.* **2018**, *102*, 412–419. [CrossRef] [PubMed]
27. Xie, Y.; Hao, H.P.; Wang, H.; Guo, C.; Kang, A.; Wang, G.J. Reversing effects of lignans on CCl4-induced hepatic CYP450 down regulation by attenuating oxidative stress. *J. Ethnopharmacol.* **2014**, *155*, 213–221. [CrossRef] [PubMed]

28. Schrieber, S.J.; Wen, Z.M.; Vourvahis, M.; Smith, P.C.; Fried, M.W.; Kashuba, A.D.M.; Hawke, R.L. Pharmacokinetics of silymarin is altered in patients with hepatitis C virus and nonalcoholic fatty liver disease and correlates with plasma caspase-3/7 activity. *Drug Metab. Dispos.* **2008**, *36*, 1909–1916. [CrossRef] [PubMed]
29. Fouts, D.E.; Torralba, M.; Nelson, K.E.; Brenner, D.A.; Schnabl, B. Bacterial translocation and changes in the intestinal microbiome in mouse models of liver disease. *J. Hepatol.* **2012**, *56*, 1283–1292. [CrossRef] [PubMed]
30. Jiang, F.J.; Zhao, Y.L.; Wang, J.B.; Wei, S.S.; Wei, Z.M.; Li, R.S.; Zhu, Y.; Sun, Z.Y.; Xiao, X.H. Comparative pharmacokinetic study of paeoniflorin and albiflorin after oral administration of Radix Paeoniae Rubra in normal rats and the acute cholestasis hepatitis rats. *Fitoterapia* **2012**, *83*, 415–421. [CrossRef] [PubMed]
31. Li, Y.T.; Wang, L.; Chen, Y.; Chen, Y.B.; Wang, H.Y.; Wu, Z.W.; Li, L.J. Effects of gut microflora on hepatic damage after acute liver injury in rats. *J. Trauma* **2010**, *68*, 76–83. [CrossRef] [PubMed]
32. US Department of Health and Human Services; Food and Drug Administration&Center for Drug Evaluation and Research. Guidance for industry: Bioanalytical method validation. *Fed. Regist.* **2001**, *66*, 206–207.
33. Liu, Y.; Pu, Y.; Zhang, T.; Ding, Y.; Wang, B.; Cai, Z. Rapid and sensitive determination of timosaponin AIII in rat plasma by LC-MS/MS and its pharmacokinetic application. *Int. J. Mol. Sci.* **2013**, *14*, 3656–3670. [CrossRef] [PubMed]
34. Zhao, M.; Qian, D.; Shang, E.X.; Jiang, S.; Guo, J.; Liu, P.; Su, S.L.; Duan, J.A.; Du, L.; Tao, J. Comparative pharmacokinetics of the main compounds of Shanzhuyu extract after oral administration in normal and chronic kidney disease rats. *J. Ethnopharmacol.* **2015**, *173*, 280–286. [CrossRef] [PubMed]
35. Liu, J.H.; Cheng, Y.Y.; Hsieh, C.H.; Tsai, T.H. The Herb-drug pharmacokinetic interaction of 5-fluorouracil and its metabolite 5-fluoro-5,6-dihydrouracil with a traditional Chinese medicine in rats. *Int. J. Mol. Sci.* **2018**, *19*, 25. [CrossRef] [PubMed]
36. Du, P.; Lei, M.; Liu, Y.; Yang, S. Simultaneous determination and pharmacokinetic study of six components in rat plasma by HPLC-MS/MS after oral administration of *Acanthopanax sessiliflorus* fruit extract. *Int. J. Mol. Sci.* **2017**, *18*, 45. [CrossRef] [PubMed]
37. Zhao, M.; Tao, J.H.; Qian, D.W.; Liu, P.; Shang, E.X.; Jiang, S.; Guo, J.M.; Su, S.L.; Duan, J.A.; Du, L.Y. Simultaneous determination of loganin, morroniside, catalpol and acteoside in normal and chronic kidney disease rat plasma by UPLC-MS for investigating the pharmacokinetics of *Rehmannia glutinosa* and *Cornus officinalis* Sieb drug pair extract. *J. Chromatogr. B* **2016**, *1009*, 122–129. [CrossRef] [PubMed]
38. Pang, H.Q.; Tang, Y.P.; Cao, Y.J.; Tan, Y.J.; Jin, Y.; Shi, X.Q.; Huang, S.L.; Sun, D.Z.; Sun, J.; Tang, Z.S.; et al. Comparatively evaluating the pharmacokinetic of fifteen constituents in normal and blood deficiency rats after oral administration of Xin-Sheng-Hua Granule by UPLC-MS/MS. *J. Chromatogr. B* **2017**, *1061*, 372–381. [CrossRef] [PubMed]

International Journal of
Molecular Sciences

MDPI

Article

Asperuloside and Asperulosidic Acid Exert an Anti-Inflammatory Effect via Suppression of the NF-κB and MAPK Signaling Pathways in LPS-Induced RAW 264.7 Macrophages

Jingyu He [1], Xianyuan Lu [2], Ting Wei [1], Yaqian Dong [2], Zheng Cai [2], Lan Tang [2] and Menghua Liu [2,*]

1 Bioengineering Research Centre, Guangzhou Institute of Advanced Technology, Chinese Academy of Sciences, Guangzhou 511458, China; jy.he@giat.ac.cn (J.H.); ting.wei@siat.ac.cn (T.W.)

2 Guangdong Provincial Key Laboratory of New Drug Screening, School of Pharmaceutical Sciences, Southern Medical University, Guangzhou 510515, China; luxianyuan_211723@163.com (X.L.); yqdongchn@163.com (Y.D.); caizheng2002@sina.com (Z.C.); tl405@smu.edu.cn (L.T.)

* Correspondence: liumenghua@smu.edu.cn; Tel.: +86-20-6164-8597

Received: 6 June 2018; Accepted: 10 July 2018; Published: 12 July 2018

Abstract: *Hedyotis diffusa* is a folk herb that is used for treating inflammation-related diseases in Asia. Previous studies have found that iridoids in *H. diffusa* play an important role in its anti-inflammatory activity. This study aimed to investigate the anti-inflammatory effect and potential mechanism of five iridoids (asperuloside (ASP), asperulosidic acid (ASPA), desacetyl asperulosidic acid (DAA), scandoside methyl ester (SME), and *E*-6-*O*-*p*-coumaroyl scandoside methyl ester (CSME)) that are presented in *H. diffusa* using lipopolysaccharide (LPS)—induced RAW 264.7 cells. ASP and ASPA significantly decreased the production of nitric oxide (NO), prostaglandin E_2 (PGE_2), tumor necrosis factor-α (TNF-α), and interleukin-6 (IL-6) in parallel with the inhibition of inducible nitric oxide synthase (iNOS), cyclooxygenase-2 (COX-2), TNF-α, and IL-6 mRNA expression in LPS-induced RAW 264.7 cells. ASP treatment suppressed the phosphorylation of the inhibitors of nuclear factor-kappaB alpha (IκB-α), p38, extracellular signal-regulated kinase (ERK), and c-Jun N-terminal kinase (JNK). The inhibitory effect of ASPA was similar to that of ASP, except for p38 phosphorylation. In summary, the anti-inflammatory effects of ASP and ASPA are related to the inhibition of inflammatory cytokines and mediators via suppression of the NF-κB and mitogen-activated protein kinase (MAPK) signaling pathways, which provides scientific evidence for the potential application of *H. diffusa*.

Keywords: iridoids; nuclear factor-kappaB; mitogen-activated protein kinase; anti-inflammation

1. Introduction

Inflammation is a natural defense response against bacteria, viral, and fungal infections [1]. During the development of inflammation, macrophages can be recruited to inflammatory sites and play an essential role by stimulating intracellular cascades of cytokines and chemokines via various signals [2,3]. Lipopolysaccharide (LPS) is one of the most common inflammatory triggers derived from Gram-negative bacteria. It can cause multiple inflammatory reactions by activating macrophages [4] and results in the increase of inflammatory mediators, such as nitric oxide (NO) and prostaglandin E_2 (PGE_2), and inflammatory cytokines, such as tumor necrosis factor-α (TNF-α) and interleukin-6 (IL-6) [5–7]. There is good evidence that nuclear factor-kappaB (NF-κB) and mitogen-activated protein kinases (MAPKs) are two crucial signaling pathways in the inflammatory process induced by LPS [5,8,9]. Once activated, the gene expression of pro-inflammatory cytokine is induced collaboratively by NF-κB and MAPKs, subsequently releasing cytokines under inflammatory conditions [10]. Therefore, chemicals targeting NF-κB and/or MAPK signaling pathways are supposed to be anti-inflammatory candidates for the treatment of inflammation related disorders.

Hedyotis diffusa Willd (*Rubiaceae*) is a famous folk herb that is widely distributed in China, Indonesia, Nepal, and other Asian regions [11]. Generally, *H. diffusa* is used as a single herb or in Chinese traditional medicine prescription for the treatment of nephritis, arthritis, bronchitis, and appendicitis [12]. Modern pharmacological studies have confirmed that *H. diffusa* possesses multiple effects, such as anti-inflammatory, anti-cancer, neuroprotective, hepatoprotective, and immunemodulating activities [13]. Iridoids, flavonoids, and anthraquinones are the main constituents responsible for the multiple bioactivities of *H. diffusa* [14,15]. Scandoside, an iridoid isolated from *H. diffusa*, has been proven to be an anti-inflammatory compound [16]. Previously, we confirmed that the aqueous extract of *H. diffusa*, mainly containing asperuloside (ASP), asperulosidic acid (ASPA), desacetyl asperulosidic acid (DAA), scandoside methyl ester (SME), and *E*-6-*O*-*p*-coumaroyl scandoside methyl ester (CSME), showed a protective effect on LPS-induced renal inflammation in mice (Figure 1) [17]. However, the contribution of these five iridoids to the anti-inflammatory effect and their anti-inflammatory mechanisms is still unclear.

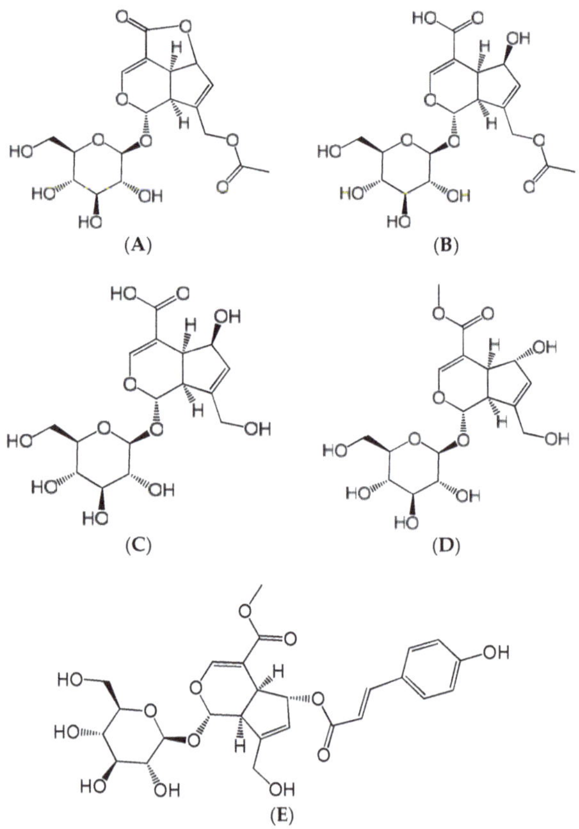

Figure 1. Chemical structures of the five iridoids. (**A**) Asperuloside (ASP); (**B**) Asperulosidic acid (ASPA); (**C**) Desacetyl asperulosidic acid (DAA); (**D**) Scandoside methyl ester (SME); and (**E**) *E*-6-*O*-*p*-Coumaroyl scandoside methyl ester (CSME).

In this study, the anti-inflammatory effect of five iridoids found in *H. diffusa* was investigated using LPS-induced RAW 264.7 cells. The underlying mechanisms of the anti-inflammatory compounds were further illustrated.

2. Results

2.1. Effects of Five Iridoids on RAW 264.7 Cell Viability

As shown in Figure 2, the percentages of cell viability for the five iridoids were from 94.83 to 105.52%. Cell viability was not significantly affected by the five iridoids at various concentrations (0–200 μg/mL) after 24 h of treatment in the presence of 50 ng/mL LPS. These data indicated that ASP, ASPA, DAA, SME, and CSME had no toxic effect on RAW 264.7 cells at concentrations below 200 μg/mL. Subsequent experiments were performed at the concentrations of 40, 80, and 160 μg/mL.

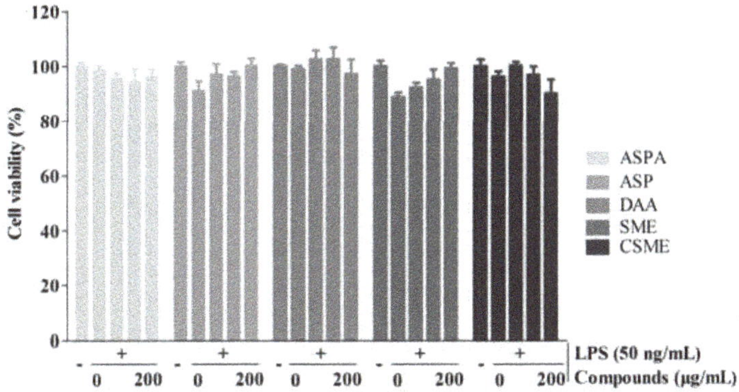

Figure 2. Effects of five iridoids on the viability of RAW 264.7 cells. RAW 264.7 cells were treated with asperuloside (ASP), asperulosidic acid (ASPA), desacetyl asperulosidic acid (DAA), scandoside methyl ester (SME) and *E*-6-*O*-*p*-coumaroyl scandoside methyl ester (CSME) at the concentration of 0, 50, 100, and 200 μg/mL, respectively, for 1 h, and then induced with 50 ng/mL lipopolysaccharide (LPS) for 24 h. Cell viability was measured by the Cell Counting Kit-8 (CCK-8) assay ($n = 3$).

2.2. Effects of Five Iridoids on Inflammatory Mediators and Inflammatory Cytokines in RAW 264.7 Cells

As shown in Figure 3, the levels of inflammatory mediators (NO and PGE_2) and inflammatory cytokines (TNF-α and IL-6) in the LPS-treatment group were significantly increased when compared with the control group. However, the groups treated with the five iridoids showed different behaviors. ASP and ASPA treatment significantly reduced the level of NO ($p < 0.05$), whereas no significant difference was observed in the CSME group at any concentration. The effects on NO in the DAA- and SME-treated groups were only found at higher concentration levels. Furthermore, all iridoids, except SME, inhibited the production of PGE_2 and TNF-α at 80 and 160 μg/mL ($p < 0.05$). In addition, ASP and ASPA treatment significantly decreased the level of IL-6 in concentration-dependent manners. SME and CSME treatment significantly reduced the production of IL-6 at 80 and 160 μg/mL. Conversely, no inhibitory effect of DAA on the production of IL-6 was observed. Considering the strongly potential bioactivities, ASP and ASPA were selected for further investigation.

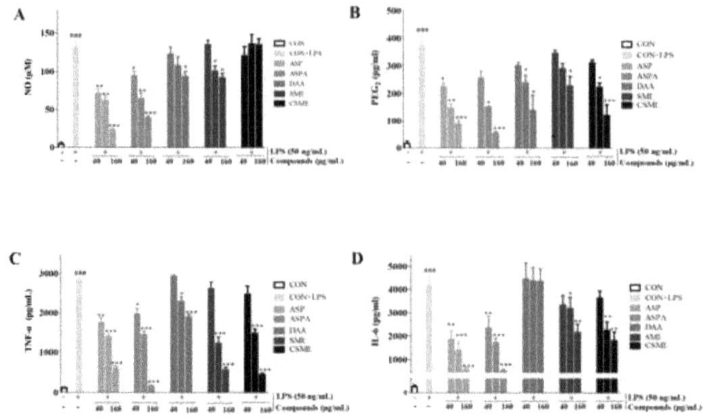

Figure 3. Effects of five iridoids on the productions of nitric oxide (NO), prostaglandin E_2 (PGE_2), tumor necrosis factor-α (TNF-α), and interleukin-6 (IL-6). RAW 264.7 cells were treated with ASP, ASPA, DAA, SME, and CSME at the concentration of 40, 80, and 160 μg/mL, respectively, for 1 h, and then induced with 50 ng/mL LPS for 24 h. The levels of NO (**A**), PGE_2 (**B**), TNF-α (**C**), and IL-6 (**D**) in the cell-free culture were measured by ELISA. * $p < 0.05$, ** $p < 0.01$ and *** $p < 0.001$ versus LPS-only treatment group; ### $p < 0.001$ versus control group ($n = 3$).

2.3. Effects of ASP and ASPA on TNF-α and IL-6 mRNA Expression in LPS-Induced RAW 264.7 Cells

The mRNA expression of TNF-α and IL-6 was tested to determine whether ASP and ASPA regulated their transcriptional levels. As shown in Figure 4, ASP and ASPA treatment significantly down-regulated the mRNA levels of TNF-α and IL-6 in LPS-induced RAW 264.7 cells compared with the group treated with LPS alone. Similarly, the protein levels of TNF-α and IL-6 were also reduced by treatment with ASP and ASPA.

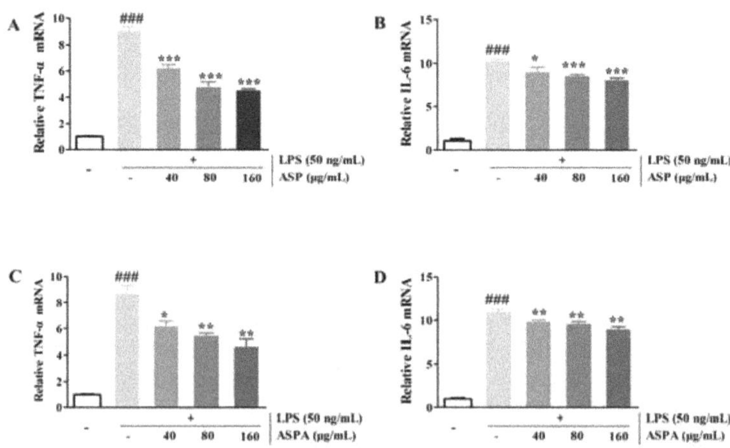

Figure 4. Effects of ASP and ASPA on TNF-α and IL-6. RAW 264.7 cells were treated with ASPA and ASP (40, 80, and 160 μg/mL) for 1 h and then induced with LPS (50 ng/mL) for 24 h. The TNF-α and IL-6 mRNA were analyzed by real-time PCR. (**A**) The TNF-α levels in ASP treatment groups. (**B**) The IL-6 levels in ASP treatment groups. (**C**) The TNF-α mRNA levels in ASPA treatment groups. (**D**) The IL-6 levels in ASPA treatment groups. * $p < 0.05$, ** $p < 0.01$ and *** $p < 0.001$ versus LPS-only treatment group; ### $p < 0.001$ versus control group ($n = 3$).

2.4. Effects of ASP and ASPA on iNOS and COX-2 Protein and mRNA Expression in LPS-Induced RAW 264.7 Cells

To investigate whether ASP and ASPA suppressed NO and PGE_2 via inhibition of their corresponding synthases, the protein and mRNA expression of inducible nitric oxide synthase (iNOS) and cyclooxygenase-2 (COX-2) was measured. LPS induced a significant up-regulation of the mRNA transcript levels of iNOS and COX-2, while ASP and ASPA treatment significantly down-regulated their mRNA transcript levels, in a concentration-dependent manner (Figure 5A–D). Western blot analysis showed that ASP and ASPA treatment reduced the protein levels of iNOS and COX-2 induced by LPS in a concentration-dependent manner (Figure 5E,F). The reduction of iNOS and COX-2 mRNA and protein levels correlated with the reduced production of NO and PGE_2, respectively.

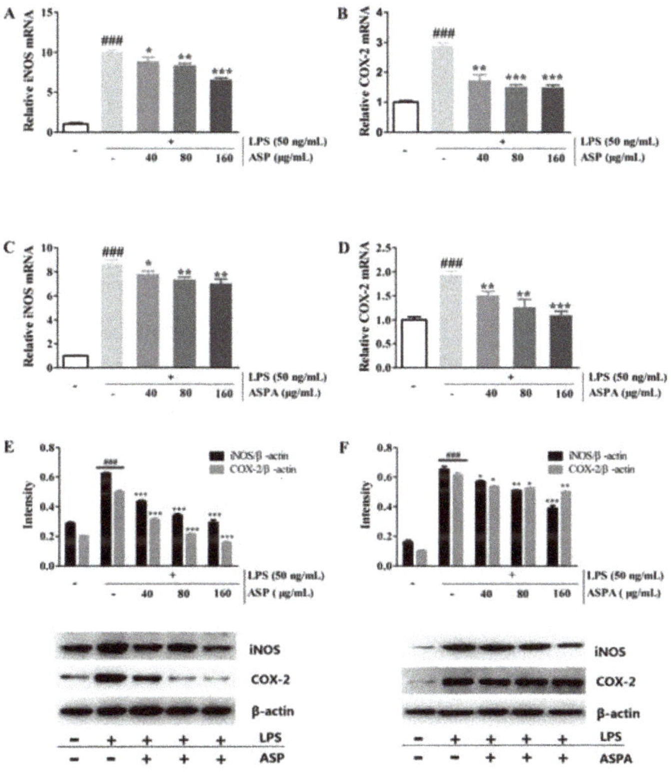

Figure 5. Effects of ASP and ASPA on inducible nitric oxide synthase (iNOS) and cyclooxygenase-2 (COX-2) mRNA and protein expression. RAW 264.7 cells were treated with ASP and ASPA (40, 80, and 160 μg/mL) for 1 h and then induced with LPS (50 ng/mL) for 24 h. mRNA levels were analyzed by real-time PCR. (**A**) The levels of iNOS mRNA in ASP treatment groups. (**B**) The levels of COX-2 mRNA in ASP treatment groups. (**C**) The levels of iNOS mRNA in ASPA treatment groups. (**D**) The levels of COX-2 mRNA in ASPA treatment groups. The proteins were analyzed by Western blot. The quantitative evaluation of protein band by densitometry was shown. (**E**) The expression levels of iNOS and COX-2 in ASP treatment groups. (**F**) The expression levels of iNOS and COX-2 in ASPA treatment groups. * $p < 0.05$, ** $p < 0.01$ and *** $p < 0.001$ versus LPS-only treatment group; ### $p < 0.001$ versus control group ($n = 3$).

2.5. Effects of ASP and ASPA on NF-κB and MAPK Pathways in LPS-Induced RAW 264.7 Cells

To study the potential anti-inflammatory mechanism, we examined the effects of ASP and ASPA on nuclear factor-kappaB alpaha (IκB-α) phosphorylation and degradation in LPS-induced RAW 264.7 cells. As shown in Figure 6, LPS-induced IκB-α phosphorylation was significantly decreased after pretreatment with ASP and ASPA in a concentration-dependent manner. The potential involvement of MAPKs was also investigated by testing the modulatory effects of ASP and ASPA on MAPK signaling pathways. In LPS-induced RAW 264.7 cells, p38, extracellular signal-regulated protein kinases 1/2 (Erk1/2), and c-Jun N-terminal kinase (JNK) were triggered high phosphorylation, whereas the phosphorylation of p38, Erk1/2, and JNK was inhibited by ASP in a concentration-dependent manner. For the effect of ASPA on MAPKs, ASPA treatment decreased Erk1/2 phosphorylation at all concentration levels, but there was no effect on p-p38.

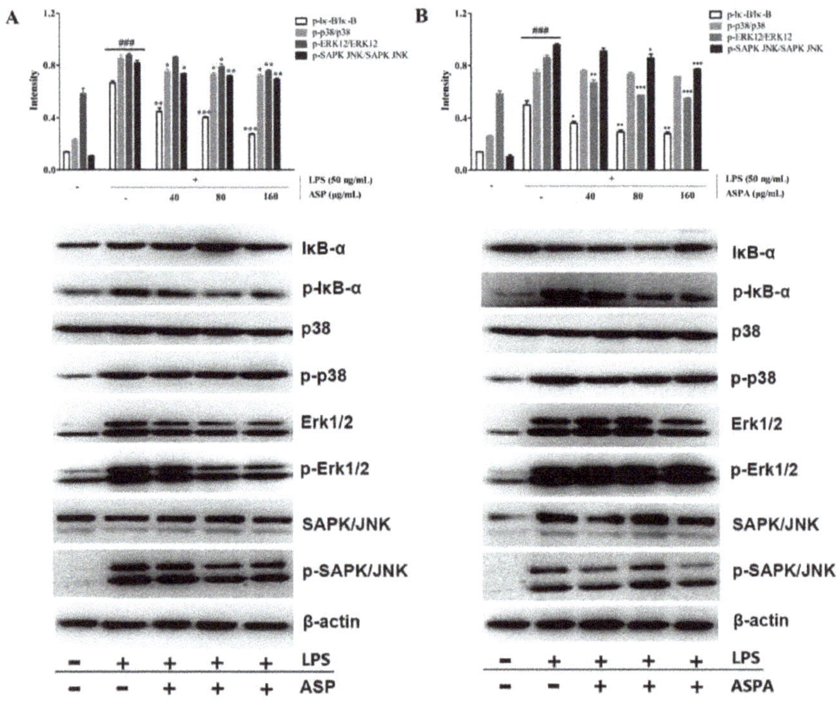

Figure 6. Effects of ASP and ASPA on nuclear factor-kappaB alpaha (IκBα), p38, extracellular signal-regulated protein kinases 1/2 (Erk1/2), and stress-activated protein kinase (SAPK)/c-Jun N-terminal kinase (JNK) phosphorylation. RAW 264.7 cells were treated with ASP and ASPA (40, 80, and 160 μg/mL) for 1 h and then induced with LPS (50 ng/mL) for 24 h. The protein was analyzed by Western blot. The quantitative evaluation of protein bands by densitometry is shown. (**A**) The phosphorylation levels of IκBα, p38, Erk1/2, and SAPK/JNK in ASP treatment groups. (**B**) The phosphorylation levels of IκBα, p38, Erk1/2, and SAPK/JNK in ASPA treatment groups. * $p < 0.05$, ** $p < 0.01$ and *** $p < 0.001$ versus LPS-only treatment group; ### $p < 0.001$ versus control group ($n = 3$).

3. Discussion

To date, numerous natural products have been identified as potential anti-inflammatory agents that can scavenge inflammatory mediators [18–22]. Among them, iridoids play an important role in inflammatory treatment and are considered as the major bioactive constituents of *H. diffusa* [16,17]. In a phytochemical analysis, ASP, ASPA, DAA, SME, and CSME were found by ultra performance liquid chromatography-electrospray ionization-quadrupole-time of flight-mass spectrometry (UPLC-ESI-Q-TOF-MS) methods and identified by comparison with their reference substances [17]. Moreover, these five iridoids were also found in various medicinal plants [23–25]. However, there is still a lack of further pharmacological studies on these iridoids, especially their anti-inflammatory mechanism. In this study, the results indicated that the five iridoids could inhibit inflammation related factors at particular concentrations. Importantly, ASP and ASPA were the target compounds that had the greatest anti-inflammatory effects among the five compounds.

NO is one of the most important inflammatory mediators. When activated by inflammatory inducers, the immune cells will produce NO, which is catalyzed by iNOS [26,27]. A high concentration of NO can cause oxidative damage or even inflammatory and autoimmune diseases [28,29]. COX enzymes produce prostaglandins involved in the inflammatory process. Actually, two distinct cyclooxygenase isoforms, namely COX-1 and COX-2, are commonly used as molecular targets for non-steroidal anti-inflammatory drugs (NSAIDs) [30]. COX-1 is expressed ubiquitously and constitutively, which plays a housekeeping role in processes, such as gastrointestinal mucosa protection, while COX-2 is not constitutively expressed in the cell, but can be activated by inducers, such as endotoxins, cytokines, and growth factors [31]. In LPS-induced macrophages, COX-2 can convert arachidonic acid to PGG_2 and, finally, to PGE_2 [32–34]. Selective inhibition of COX-2 expression can block PGE_2 production induced by inflammation and alleviate inflammation. Thus, COX-2 is regarded as a target for anti-inflammatory treatment. The results demonstrated that ASP and ASPA significantly decreased the levels of NO and PGE_2 by suppressing iNOS and COX-2, respectively. Moreover, pro-inflammatory cytokines, such as TNF-α and IL-6, play crucial roles in the development of inflammatory diseases and are involved in the innate immunity and autoimmune diseases [35,36]. The levels of inflammatory-related factors are considered to be indicators of the degree of inflammation. Thus, the expression of TNF-α and IL-6 mRNA in LPS-induced RAW 264.7 cells was measured. ASPA and ASP significantly suppressed TNF-α and IL-6 mRNA expression. These results suggested that ASPA and ASP exerted an anti-inflammatory effect through the inhibition of iNOS, COX-2, TNF-α, and IL-6 mRNA expression.

NF-κB is a key signaling pathway that stimulates the expression of inflammatory mediators and cytokines, including iNOS, COX-2, TNF-α, and IL-6 [5,9]. The IκBα proteins are phosphorylated and degraded, leading to activation of NF-κB, which triggers the transcription of inflammatory-related factors [37]. When activated, p65 translocates into the nucleus and then promotes the transcription of corresponding pro-inflammatory genes [38,39]. ASP and ASPA were found to significantly inhibit the NF-κB activation via decreasing the phosphorylation of IκB. MAPKs, including ERK, JNK, and p38, also take part in the regulation of the expression of inflammation-related genes, leading to the overproduction of pro-inflammatory cytokines [40,41]. Western blot analysis showed that ASP inhibited LPS-induced phosphorylation of p38, ERK, and JNK in RAW 264.7 cells, thus, displaying an anti-inflammatory effect consistent with a previous report [42]. ASPA also exerted an anti-inflammatory effect via suppression of the MAPK signaling pathway, though it did not inhibit the phosphorylation of p38. This data demonstrated that the anti-inflammatory mechanisms of ASP and ASPA were likely via the inhibition of NF-κB and MAPK signaling pathways. The results also indicated that ASPA and ASP were the main compounds responsible for the anti-inflammatory effect of *H. diffusa*. Given the relationship between inflammation and tumors [43], the anti-tumor effect and mechanism of ASPA and ASP are worthy to be studied since *H. diffusa* is widely used for treating tumors. Additionally, ASPA and ASP were useful markers for the quality control of *H. diffusa* and its herbal formula, and even the other plant materials containing these two compounds. In view of the results achieved in vitro, the in vivo anti-inflammatory effects and mechanisms of ASP and ASPA require further elucidation in a further study. Importantly, for the development of ASPA and ASP, research on the distribution in tissues, pharmacokinetic properties, and the safety after administration is necessary.

4. Materials and Methods

4.1. Chemicals, Reagents, and Cell Line

Asperulosidic acid (PubChem CID: 11968867, ASPA), asperuloside (PubChem CID: 84298, ASP), desacetyl asperulosidic acid (PubChem CID: 12315349, DAA), scandoside methyl ester (PubChem CID: 442433, SME), and *E*-6-*O*-*p*-coumaroyl scandoside methyl ester (PubChem CID: 44584784, CSME) were purchased from Shanghai Yuanye Biotechnology Co., Ltd. (Shanghai, China). Dulbecco's Modified Eagle's Medium (DMEM) and fetal bovine serum (FBS) were purchased from Gibco (Thermo Scientific, Waltham, MA, USA). The Cell Counting Kit-8 (CCK-8) was purchased from Dojindo (Kumamoto, Japan). LPS obtained from *Escherichia coli* O111:B4 was purchased from Sigma-Aldrich Co. (St. Louis, MO, USA). The antibodies against iNOS, COX-2, IκB-α, p38, and Erk1/2 were obtained from Proteintech Group, Inc. (Chicago, IL, USA). The antibodies against p-IκB-α, p-p38, p-Erk1/2, SAPK/JNK, and p-SAPK/JNK were purchased from Cell Signaling Technology, Inc. (Danvers, MA, USA). The ELISA kits for IL-6, IL-1β, and TNF-α were purchased from Neobioscience Technology Company (Shenzhen, China). The NO ELISA and bicinchoninic acid (BCA) assay kits were purchased from Beyotime Biotechnology (Shanghai, China). The PGE_2 ELISA kit was from Enzo Life Sciences (New York, NY, USA). RAW 264.7 murine macrophages were purchased from the Cell Bank of the Chinese Academy of Science (Shanghai, China). All other reagents were of an analytical grade.

4.2. Cell Culture

RAW 264.7 cells were cultured in DMEM supplemented with 10% FBS, 100 units/mL penicillin, and 100 μg/mL streptomycin, and maintained in a carbon dioxide incubator (Thermo Fisher Scientific, Waltham, MA, USA) at 37 °C in 5% CO_2 with a humidified atmosphere of 95% air. RAW 264.7 cells were induced with LPS (50 ng/mL) for 24 h after being incubated with iridoids for 1 h [16].

4.3. Cell Viability Assay

The cytotoxicity of the five iridoids on RAW 264.7 cells was measured using the CCK-8 assay. After being incubated for 24 h in 96-well plates at a density of 1×10^4 cells/well, the cells were treated with serial concentrations of five iridoids (0, 50, 100, and 200 μg/mL) in triplicate for 1 h, and then induced with 50 ng/mL LPS for 24 h. Finally, 10 μL of CCK-8 was added to each plate and incubated for 1 h at 37 °C. The absorption wavelength was read at 450 nm using a Tecan microplate reader (Tecan Group Ltd., Männedorf, Switzerland). The cell viability was evaluated by comparing the absorbance values between the treatment groups and the control group, which was considered as 100%.

4.4. ELISA Assay of NO, PGE_2, TNF-α, and IL-6

Briefly, after being incubated for 24 h at a density of 1×10^4 cells/well in 96-well plates, RAW 264.7 cells were pretreated with five iridoids (0, 40, 80, and 160 μg/mL) in triplicate for 1 h. Then, the cells were induced with 50 ng/mL LPS for 24 h. Subsequently, the cell supernatant was collected and the concentration of NO, PGE_2, TNF-α, and IL-6 was measured according to the ELISA manufacturer's instructions using a Tecan microplate reader. The absorption wavelengths were set at 540, 450, 450, and 450 nm for NO, PGE_2, TNF-α, and IL-6, respectively.

4.5. Real-Time PCR Assay

RAW 264.7 cells were incubated at 37 °C for 24 h in six-well plates at a density of 2×10^5 cells/well. The cells were treated with ASP and ASPA at three concentrations (40, 80, and 160 μg/mL) for 1 h and induced with LPS (50 ng/mL) for 24 h. Total RNA was extracted from the RAW 264.7 cells using the RNAprep Pure Cell kit (Qiagen, Valencia, CA, USA) according to the manufacturer's protocol. RNA (3 μL) concentration and purity was measured by the ratio of 260/280 nm absorbance and the remaining RNA solution was stored at −80 °C for reverse transcription. The total RNA was converted into the first-strand complementary DNA (cDNA) with a reverse transcription system as follows: 4 μL 5x prime Script RT Master MIX (Takara Bio INC., Kusatsu, Japan), 0.5 μg total RNA, and RNase-free water in a 20-μL reaction. The cDNA was used for real-time PCR (RT-PCR) and the reaction system contained 10 μL SYBR Premix EX Taq (2x) (Promega Corporation, Madison, USA), 1 μL forward primer (10 μM), 1 μL reverse primer (10 μM, iNOS, TNF-α, IL-6, and COX-2; Table 1), and 8 μL cDNA, which was amplified in an Applied Biosystems 7500 Fast Real-time PCR System version v2.3 (Thermo Fisher Scientific, Waltham, MA, USA) under the following reaction conditions: 50.0 °C for 3 min and 95.0 °C for 3 min, followed by 40 cycles of 95.0 °C for 10 s and 60.0 °C for 30 s. The threshold cycle (C_t) was analyzed by the instrument's software and fold changes in the mRNA expression were calculated according to the comparative C_t method ($2^{-\Delta\Delta C_t}$).

Table 1. The primers used for RT-PCR analysis.

Genes	Sense Primer Sequence 5′–3′	Antisense Primer Sequence 5′–3′
TNF-α	GCGACGTGGAACTGGCAGAA	CAGTAGACAGAAGAGCGTGGTG
IL-6	GTTGCCTTCTTGGGACTGAT	CATTTCCACGATTTCCCAGA
iNOS	TGGAGCGAGTTGTGGATTGT	CTCTGCCTATCCGTCTCGTC
COX-2	ACCTGGTGAACTACGACTGC	TGGTCGGTTTGATGTTACTG
β-actin	TGCTGTCCCTGTATGCCTCTG	GCTGTAGCCACGCTCGGTCA

4.6. Western Blot Analysis

RAW 264.7 cells were incubated at 37 °C for 24 h in six-well plates at a density of 2×10^5 cells/well. The cells were treated with ASP and ASPA at three concentrations (40, 80, and 160 μg/mL) for 1 h and induced with LPS (50 ng/mL) for 24 h. Subsequently, 100 μL cell lysis buffer (10 mM Tris-HCl, 0.15 M NaCl, 5 mM ethylenediaminetetraacetic acid (EDTA), 1% Triton×100, 5 mM dithiothreitol (DTT), and 0.1 mM phenylmethanesulfonyl fluoride (PMSF)) was added and incubated for 30 min at 4 °C and then centrifuged at 12,000 rpm for 10 min to collect the supernatant for protein analysis using the BCA assay kit after adding 5× loading buffer for Western blotting. All protein samples were loaded onto 12% sodium dodecyl sulfate-polyacrylamide gel electrophoresis (SDS-PAGE) and transferred onto a polyvinylidene fluoride (PVDF) membrane. The membrane was blocked for 2 h with 10% non-fat milk at room temperature and then incubated overnight with the primary antibodies, including those against iNOS (1:1000), COX-2 (1:1000), IκB-α (1:1000), p-IκB-α (1:1000), p38 (1:1000), p-p38 (1:1000), Erk1/2 (1:1000), p-Erk1/2 (1:1000), SAPK/JNK (1:1000), p-SAPK/JNK (1:1000), and β-Actin (1:1000), at 4 °C. The membranes were washed three times and incubated with the secondary antibody (1:10,000) at room temperature for 1 h. Finally, the blots were measured by an ECL chemiluminescence method and a Western blotting detection System (FluorChem R, ProteinSimple, San Jose, CA, USA).

4.7. Statistical Analyses

All experiments were performed in triplicate. Data were analyzed using IBM SPSS Statistics 20.0 (IBM SPSS Statistics, Chicago, IL, USA) and are presented as the mean ± standard deviation (SD). One-way ANOVA followed by Tukey's multiple comparison test was used to assess the statistical differences among groups. $p < 0.05$ was considered significant.

5. Conclusions

The present study compared the anti-inflammatory effects of the five iridoids found in *H. diffusa* and shows that ASP and ASPA have an anti-inflammatory effect. ASP and ASPA could significantly decrease the levels of PGE_2, NO, TNF-α, and IL-6 in LPS-induced RAW 264.7 cells. The possible mechanism involved the down-regulation of the expressions of inflammatory mediators and pro-inflammatory cytokines via the inhibition of NF-κB and MAPK signaling pathways. Taken together, ASP and ASPA may be potent bioactive iridoids to treat inflammatory diseases.

Author Contributions: J.H. and M.L. conceived and designed the experiments; J.H., X.L., T.W., Y.D., and M.L. performed the experiments; J.H., Z.C., L.T., and M.L. analyzed the data; J.H. and M.L. wrote the paper.

Funding: This research was funded by National Natural Science Foundation of China (Nos. 81503376 and 31500104), Applied Science and Technology Research Foundation of Guangdong Province (Nos. 2017A030303005 and 2016B020237005), Guangdong Natural Science Foundation (Nos. 2016A030313562 and 2017A030313149), Student Innovation Training Program (No. 201612121195) and Open Project of Guangdong Provincial Key Laboratory of New Drug Screening.

Conflicts of Interest: The authors declare no conflict of interest.

References

1. Tall, A.R.; Yvan-Charvet, L. Cholesterol, inflammation and innate immunity. *Nat. Rev. Immunol.* **2015**, *15*, 104–116. [CrossRef] [PubMed]
2. Fernandez, M.I.; Pedron, T.; Tournebize, R.; Olivo-Marin, J.C.; Sansonetti, P.J.; Phalipon, A. Anti-inflammatory role for intracellular dimeric immunoglobulin a by neutralization of lipopolysaccharide in epithelial cells. *Immunity* **2003**, *18*, 739–749. [CrossRef]
3. Mancino, A.; Termanini, A.; Barozzi, I.; Ghisletti, S.; Ostuni, R.; Prosperini, E.; Ozato, K.; Natoli, G. A dual *cis*-regulatory code links IRF8 to constitutive and inducible gene expression in macrophages. *Genes Dev.* **2015**, *29*, 394–408. [CrossRef] [PubMed]
4. Voll, R.E.; Herrmann, M.; Roth, E.A.; Stach, C.; Kalden, J.R.; Girkontaite, I. Immunosuppressive effects of apoptotic cells. *Nature* **1997**, *390*, 350–351. [CrossRef] [PubMed]
5. Kiemer, A.K.; Hartung, T.; Huber, C.; Vollmar, A.M. *Phyllanthus amarus* has anti-inflammatory potential by inhibition of iNOS, COX-2, and cytokines via the NF-κB pathway. *J. Hepatol.* **2003**, *38*, 289–297. [CrossRef]
6. Kawahara, K.; Hohjoh, H.; Inazumi, T.; Tsuchiya, S.; Sugimoto, Y. Prostaglandin E 2-induced inflammation: Relevance of prostaglandin E receptors. *BBA-Mol. Cell Biol. Lipids* **2015**, *1851*, 414–421. [CrossRef] [PubMed]
7. Blaser, H.; Dostert, C.; Mak, T.W.; Brenner, D. TNF and ROS crosstalk in inflammation. *Trends Cell Biol.* **2016**, *26*, 249–261. [CrossRef] [PubMed]
8. Zhai, X.T.; Zhang, Z.Y.; Jiang, C.H.; Chen, J.Q.; Ye, J.Q.; Jia, X.B.; Yang, Y.; Ni, Q.; Wang, S.X.; Song, J.; et al. *Nauclea officinalis* inhibits inflammation in LPS-mediated RAW 264.7 macrophages by suppressing the NF-κB signaling pathway. *J. Ethnopharmacol.* **2016**, *183*, 159–165. [CrossRef] [PubMed]
9. Tak, P.P.; Firestein, G.S. NF-κB: A key role in inflammatory diseases. *J. Clin. Investig.* **2001**, *107*, 7–11. [CrossRef] [PubMed]
10. Craig, R.; Larkin, A.; Mingo, A.M.; Thuerauf, D.J.; Andrews, C.; McDonough, P.M.; Glembotski, C.C. p38 MAPK and NF-κB collaborate to induce interleukin-6 gene expression and release evidence for a cytoprotective autocrine signaling pathway in a cardiac myocyte model system. *J. Biol. Chem.* **2000**, *275*, 23814–23824. [CrossRef] [PubMed]
11. Editorial Board of Flora of China. *The Chinese Academy of Sciences, Flora of China*; Science Press: Beijing, China, 1999; Volume 71, p. 75.
12. Nanjing University of Chinese Medicine. *Dictionary of Chinese Traditional Medicine (Zhong Yao Da Ci Dian)*, 2nd ed.; Shanghai Scientific & Technical Publishers: Shanghai, China, 2006; pp. 1039–1041.
13. Chen, R.; He, J.; Tong, X.; Tang, L.; Liu, M. The *Hedyotis diffusa* Willd (Rubiaceae): A review on phytochemistry, pharmacology, quality control and pharmacokinetics. *Molecules* **2016**, *21*, 710. [CrossRef] [PubMed]
14. Kim, Y.; Park, E.J.; Kim, J.; Kim, Y.B.; Kim, S.R.; Kim, Y.C. Neuroprotective constituents from *Hedyotis diffusa*. *J. Nat. Prod.* **2001**, *64*, 75–78. [CrossRef] [PubMed]
15. Li, M.; Jiang, R.W.; Hon, P.M.; Cheng, L.; Li, L.L.; Zhou, J.R.; Shaw, P.C.; But, P.P.H. Authentication of the anti-tumor herb Baihuasheshecao with bioactive marker compounds and molecular sequences. *Food Chem.* **2010**, *119*, 1239–1245. [CrossRef]
16. He, J.Y.; Li, J.F.; Liu, H.; Yang, Z.C.; Zhou, F.H.; Wei, T.; Dong, Y.Q.; Xue, H.J.; Tang, L.; Liu, M.H. Scandoside exerts anti-Inflammatory effect via suppressing NF-κB and MAPK signaling pathways in LPS-induced RAW 264.7 macrophages. *Int. J. Mol. Sci.* **2018**, *19*, 457. [CrossRef] [PubMed]
17. Ye, J.H.; Liu, M.H.; Zhang, X.L.; He, J.Y. Chemical profiles and protective effect of *Hedyotis diffusa* Willd in lipopolysaccharide-induced renal inflammation mice. *Int. J. Mol. Sci.* **2015**, *16*, 27252–27269. [CrossRef] [PubMed]

18. Lin, C.W.; Hwang, T.L.; Chen, F.A.; Huang, C.H.; Hung, H.Y.; Wu, T.S. Chemical constituents of the rhizomes of *Bletilla formosana* and their potential anti-inflammatory activity. *J. Nat. Prod.* **2016**, *79*, 1911–1921. [CrossRef] [PubMed]
19. Li, D.; Chen, J.; Ye, J.; Zhai, X.; Song, J.; Jiang, C.; Wang, J.; Zhang, H.; Jia, X.; Zhu, F. Anti-inflammatory effect of the six compounds isolated from *Nauclea officinalis* Pierrc ex Pitard, and molecular mechanism of strictosamide via suppressing the NF-κB and MAPK signaling pathway in LPS-induced RAW 264.7 macrophages. *J. Ethnopharmacol.* **2017**, *196*, 66–74. [CrossRef] [PubMed]
20. Shen, D.Y.; Kuo, P.C.; Huang, S.C.; Hwang, T.L.; Chan, Y.Y.; Shieh, P.C.; Ngan, N.T.; Thang, T.D.; Wu, T.S. Constituents from the leaves of *Clausena lansium* and their anti-inflammatory activity. *J. Nat. Med.* **2017**, *71*, 96–104. [CrossRef] [PubMed]
21. Saravanan, S.; Islam, V.I.; Babu, N.P.; Pandikumar, P.; Thirugnanasambantham, K.; Chellappandian, M.; Raj, C.S.D.; Paulraj, M.G.; Ignacimuthu, S. Swertiamarin attenuates inflammation mediators via modulating NF-κB/Iκb and JAK2/STAT3 transcription factors in adjuvant induced arthritis. *Eur. J. Pharm. Sci.* **2014**, *56*, 70–86. [CrossRef] [PubMed]
22. Shi, Q.; Cao, J.; Fang, L.; Zhao, H.; Liu, Z.; Ran, J.; Zheng, X.; Li, X.; Zhou, Y.; Ge, D.; et al. Geniposide suppresses LPS-induced nitric oxide, PGE_2 and inflammatory cytokine by downregulating NF-κB, MAPK and AP-1 signaling pathways in macrophages. *Int. Immunopharmacol.* **2014**, *20*, 298–306. [CrossRef] [PubMed]
23. Tran, P.H.; Le, V.D.; Do, T.H.; Nquyen, T.L.; Nquyen, P.T.; Nquyen, T.T.; Nquyen, T.D. Anti-inflammatory constituents from *Psychotria prainii* H. Lév. *Nat. Prod. Res.* **2017**. [CrossRef] [PubMed]
24. Li, C.; Dong, J.; Tian, J.; Deng, Z.; Song, X. LC/MS/MS determination and pharmacokinetic study of iridoid glycosides monotropein and deacetylasperulosidic acid isomers in rat plasma after oral administration of *Morinda officinalis* extract. *Biomed. Chromatogr.* **2015**, *30*, 163–168. [CrossRef] [PubMed]
25. Qu, K.; Dai, J.; Zhao, L.; Lu, Y.; Li, B.; Zhao, X.; Hou, P.; Zhang, Y.; Bi, K.; Chen, X. A sensitive liquid chromatographic-mass spectrometric method for simultaneous quantification of six iridoid glycosides from Zhi-zi-chi decoction in rat plasma and its application to a pharmacokinetic study. *J. Pharm. Biomed. Anal.* **2013**, *78–79*, 83–91. [CrossRef] [PubMed]
26. Minc-Golomb, D.; Tsarfaty, I.; Schwartz, J.P. Expression of inducible nitric oxide synthase by neurones following exposure to endotoxin and cytokine. *Brit. J. Pharm.* **1994**, *112*, 720–722. [CrossRef]
27. Bogdan, C. Nitric oxide and the immune response. *Nat. Immunol.* **2001**, *2*, 907–916. [CrossRef] [PubMed]
28. Reuter, S.; Gupta, S.C.; Chaturvedi, M.M.; Aggarwal, B.B. Oxidative stress, inflammation, and cancer: How are they linked? *Free Radic. Biol. Med.* **2010**, *49*, 1603–1616. [CrossRef] [PubMed]
29. Simmons, D.L.; Botting, R.M.; Hla, T. Cyclooxygenase isozymes: The biology of prostaglandin synthesis and inhibition. *Pharmacol. Rev.* **2004**, *56*, 387–437. [CrossRef] [PubMed]
30. Sun, L.L.; Wu, H.; Zhang, Y.Z.; Wang, R.; Wang, W.Y.; Wang, W.; Li, S.P.; Dai, L.; Zhang, Z.R. Design, synthesis and preliminary evaluation of the anti-inflammatory of the specific selective targeting druggable enzymome cyclooxygenase-2 (cox-2) small molecule. *Pharm. Biol.* **2016**, *54*, 2505–2514. [CrossRef] [PubMed]
31. Choi, Y.K.; Ye, B.R.; Kim, J.; Kim, M.S.; Lee, W.W.; Ahn, G.N.; Kang, N.; Jung, W.K.; Heo, S.J. Bis (3-bromo-4, 5-dihydroxybenzyl) ether, a novel bromophenol from the marine red alga *Polysiphonia morrowii* that suppresses LPS-induced inflammatory response by inhibiting ROS-mediated ERK signaling pathway in RAW 264.7 macrophages. *Biomed. Pharmacother.* **2018**, *103*, 1170–1177. [CrossRef] [PubMed]
32. Yayeh, T.; Oh, W.J.; Park, S.C.; Kim, T.H.; Cho, J.Y.; Park, H.J.; Lee, I.K.; Kim, S.K.; Hong, S.B.; Yun, B.S.; et al. *Phellinus baumii* ethyl acetate extract inhibits lipopolysaccharide-induced iNOS, COX-2, and proinflammatory cytokine expression in RAW264. 7 cells. *J. Nat. Med.* **2012**, *66*, 49–54. [CrossRef] [PubMed]
33. Pan, M.H.; Lai, C.S.; Wang, Y.J.; Ho, C.T. Acacetin suppressed LPS-induced up-expression of iNOS and COX-2 in murine macrophages and TPA-induced tumor promotion in mice. *Biochem. Pharmacol.* **2006**, *72*, 1293–1303. [CrossRef] [PubMed]
34. Varfolomeev, E.E.; Ashkenazi, A. Tumor necrosis factor: An apoptosis JuNKie? *Cell* **2004**, *116*, 491–497. [CrossRef]
35. De Gonzalo-Calvo, D.; Neitzert, K.; Fernández, M.; Vega-Naredo, I.; Caballero, B.; García-Macía, M.; Suárez, F.M.; Rodríguez-Colunga, M.J.; Solano, J.J.; Coto-Montes, A. Differential inflammatory responses in aging and disease: TNF-α and IL-6 as possible biomarkers. *Free Radic. Biol. Med.* **2010**, *49*, 733–737. [CrossRef] [PubMed]

36. Li, A.; Zhang, X.X.; Shu, M.; Wu, M.J.; Wang, J.; Zhang, J.Y.; Wang, R.; Li, P.; Wang, Y. Arctigenin suppresses renal interstitial fibrosis in a rat model of obstructive nephropathy. *Phytomedicine* **2017**, *30*, 28–41. [CrossRef] [PubMed]
37. Karin, M.; Greten, F.R. NF-κB: Linking inflammation and immunity to cancer development and progression. *Nat. Rev. Immunol.* **2005**, *5*, 749–759. [CrossRef] [PubMed]
38. Viatour, P.; Merville, M.P.; Bours, V.; Chariot, A. Phosphorylation of NF-κB and IκB proteins: Implications in cancer and inflammation. *Trends Biochem. Sci.* **2005**, *30*, 43–52. [CrossRef] [PubMed]
39. Johnson, G.L.; Lapadat, R. Mitogen-activated protein kinase pathways mediated by ERK, JNK, and p38 protein kinases. *Science* **2002**, *298*, 1911–1912. [CrossRef] [PubMed]
40. Arthur, J.S.C.; Ley, S.C. Mitogen-activated protein kinases in innate immunity. *Nat. Rev. Immunol.* **2013**, *13*, 679–692. [CrossRef] [PubMed]
41. Qiu, J.; Chi, G.; Wu, Q.; Ren, Y.; Chen, C.; Feng, H. Pretreatment with the compound asperuloside decreases acute lung injury via inhibiting MAPK and NF-κB signaling in a murine model. *Int. Immunopharmacol.* **2016**, *31*, 109–115. [CrossRef] [PubMed]
42. Viljoen, A.; Mncwangi, N.; Vermaak, I. Anti-inflammatory iridoids of botanical origin. *Curr. Med. Chem.* **2012**, *19*, 2104–2127. [CrossRef] [PubMed]
43. Mantovani, A.; Allavena, P.; Sica, A.; Balkwill, F. Cancer-related inflammation. *Nature* **2008**, *454*, 436–444. [CrossRef] [PubMed]

International Journal of
Molecular Sciences

Article

In Vitro Model of Neuroinflammation: Efficacy of Cannabigerol, a Non-Psychoactive Cannabinoid

Agnese Gugliandolo [1], Federica Pollastro [2], Gianpaolo Grassi [3], Placido Bramanti [1] and Emanuela Mazzon [1,*]

1 IRCCS Centro Neurolesi "Bonino Pulejo", 98124 Messina, Italy; agnesegugli@hotmail.it (A.G.); placido.bramanti@irccsme.it (P.B.)
2 Department of Pharmaceutical Sciences, University of Eastern Piedmont "Amedeo Avogadro", 28100 Novara, Italy; federica.pollastro@uniupo.it
3 Research Centre for Industrial Crops, Council for Agricultural Research and Economics (CREA-CIN), 45100 Rovigo, Italy; giampaolo.grassi@gmail.com
* Correspondence: emazzon.irccs@gmail.com; Tel.: +39-090-60128172

Received: 6 June 2018; Accepted: 6 July 2018; Published: 8 July 2018

Abstract: Inflammation and oxidative stress play main roles in neurodegeneration. Interestingly, different natural compounds may be able to exert neuroprotective actions against inflammation and oxidative stress, protecting from neuronal cell loss. Among these natural sources, *Cannabis sativa* represents a reservoir of compounds exerting beneficial properties, including cannabigerol (CBG), whose antioxidant properties have already been demonstrated in macrophages. Here, we aimed to evaluate the ability of CBG to protect NSC-34 motor neurons against the toxicity induced from the medium of LPS-stimulated RAW 264.7 macrophages. Using MTT assay, we observed that CBG pre-treatment was able to reduce the loss of cell viability induced by the medium of LPS-stimulated macrophages in NSC-34 cells. Indeed, CBG pre-treatment inhibited apoptosis, as shown by the reduction of caspase 3 activation and Bax expression, while Bcl-2 levels increased. Furthermore, CBG pre-treatment counteracted not only inflammation, as demonstrated by the reduction of IL-1β, TNF-α, IFN-γ and PPARγ protein levels assessed by immunocytochemistry, but also oxidative stress in NSC-34 cells treated with the medium of LPS-stimulated RAW 264.7. Indeed, immunocytochemistry showed that CBG pre-treatment reduced nitrotyrosine, SOD1 and iNOS protein levels and restored Nrf-2 levels. All together, these results indicated the neuroprotective effects of CBG, that may be a potential treatment against neuroinflammation and oxidative stress.

Keywords: cannabigerol; *Cannabis sativa*; neuroinflammation; oxidative stress; phytocannabinoid

1. Introduction

Since ancient times, *Cannabis sativa* has been known for its medicinal and psychotropic effects. This plant was discovered to be a reservoir of compounds exerting beneficial properties. Until now about 120 cannabinoids have been isolated from *Cannabis sativa*, including Δ9-tetrahydrocannabinol (Δ9-THC), responsible for the psychotropic effect associated with Cannabis consumption, cannabidiol (CBD) and cannabigerol (CBG) [1]. Other than their psychotropic effects, cannabinoids showed anti-oxidant and anti-inflammatory properties leading to neuroprotection [2–4].

Among cannabinoids, CBD is one of the most studied, and its protective effects on different aspects of human health, including in neurodegenerative disorders, are well known [5,6]. On the contrary, our knowledge about CBG, another non-psychoactive phytocannabinoid, is limited, even if the few studies published on CBG showed promising results and encourage the deepening of its effects on human health. We have already demonstrated the CBG antioxidant properties in RAW 264.7 macrophages stimulated with hydrogen peroxide (H_2O_2) [7]. Also anti-inflammatory and neuroprotective effects were reported for CBG and its derivatives in vitro and in vivo in neurodegenerative disease models [8–12].

The anti-oxidant and anti-inflammatory actions of CBG are particularly interesting taking into account that both inflammation and oxidative stress play pivotal roles in neurodegeneration [13–15]. Indeed, both these processes lead to neuronal cell death, then triggering and amplifying degeneration [16,17]. It is important to consider that the two pathophysiological processes are tightly correlated and influence each other. It is more relevant for the brain that is particularly sensitive to oxidative stress [18]. Indeed, inflammatory cells can produce reactive species at the site of inflammation causing oxidative stress, while reactive oxygen/nitrogen species may initiate an intracellular signaling cascade that induces the expression of pro-inflammatory genes [15,19]. Given the interdependence of these processes, a compound able to act against both inflammation and oxidative stress may be a promising strategy in the treatment of neurodegenerative disorders.

Different cell types participate in the inflammatory process, including macrophages. They act in order to maintain homeostasis and are directly involved in neuroinflammation, when also circulating monocytes are recruited from the periphery and enter into the central nervous system, contributing to the inflammatory process. For these reasons these cells play a pivotal role in central nervous system diseases, such as autoimmune and neurodegenerative diseases [20].

We have already shown the anti-oxidant capacity of CBG in macrophages and in this work, we aimed to deepen our knowledge on CBG properties analyzing its beneficial effects in an in vitro model of neuroinflammation. Specifically, we evaluated whether CBG was able to counteract the toxicity induced in NSC-34 motor neurons by the cell culture medium of (lipopolysaccharide) LPS-stimulated RAW 264.7 macrophages, focusing our attention on the evaluation of CBG anti-inflammatory and anti-oxidant capacities.

2. Results

2.1. CBG Increased Cell Viability in NSC-34 Motor Neurons

In order to evaluate the effects on cell viability of different concentrations of CBG, NSC-34 motor neurons were incubated 24 h with the following CBG doses: 1, 2.5, 5, 7.5, 10, 12.5, 15 and 20 μM. We observed with all doses an increase in cell viability compared to the control, even if the difference was not statistically significant. In particular, for doses from 2.5 to 7.5 μM we observed about a 20% increase in cell viability compared to the control. For higher concentrations, cell proliferation decreased even if it was still higher compared to the control (Figure 1A). We included in our analysis also NSC-34 cells incubated with similar concentrations of dimethyl sulfoxide (DMSO) and no cytotoxicity was observed. On the bases of these results, we decided to perform the other experiments with CBG 7.5 μM, because with this concentration we observed the highest increase in cell viability, even if not significant.

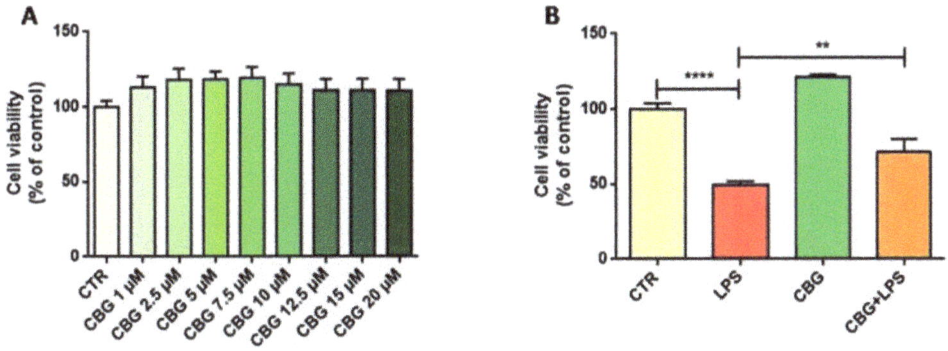

Figure 1. (**A**) Cell viability in NSC-34 motor neurons exposed to different CBG concentrations. All CBG doses increased cell viability compared to the control (CTR). (**B**) Cell viability in NSC-34 exposed to the medium of LPS-stimulated macrophages and in cells pre-treated with CBG. The exposure to the cell culture medium of LPS-stimulated macrophages reduced cell viability, but the pre-treatment with CBG partially restored it. The experiments were performed in triplicate. ** $p < 0.01$ NSC-34 cells treated with the medium of LPS stimulated macrophages vs. NSC-34 cells pre-treated with CBG and then exposed to the medium of LPS stimulated macrophages; **** $p < 0.0001$ NSC-34 treated with the medium of LPS stimulated macrophages vs. control.

2.2. CBG Counteracted the Loss of Cell Viability and Inhibited Apoptosis in NSC-34 Cells Treated with the Medium of LPS-Stimulated Macrophages

The incubation with the medium of LPS-stimulated RAW 264.7 macrophages caused a significant loss of cell viability compared to control cells. Indeed, cell viability decreased of about 50% compared to control NSC-34 cells. Interestingly, the pre-treatment with CBG 7.5 µM was able to reduce the loss of cell viability (Figure 1B).

Accordingly, we observed the induction of apoptosis in NSC-34 motor neurons exposed to the medium of LPS-treated macrophages, as demonstrated by the significant increase of the protein levels of cleaved caspase 3 and Bax, while Bcl-2 expression was reduced (Figure 2). On the contrary the pre-treatment with CBG inhibited apoptosis, abolishing the increase in Bax level and reducing cleaved caspase 3, while Bcl-2 expression increased (Figure 2). Control cells and NSC-34 treated with CBG alone expressed Bcl-2, but neither Bax nor cleaved caspase 3.

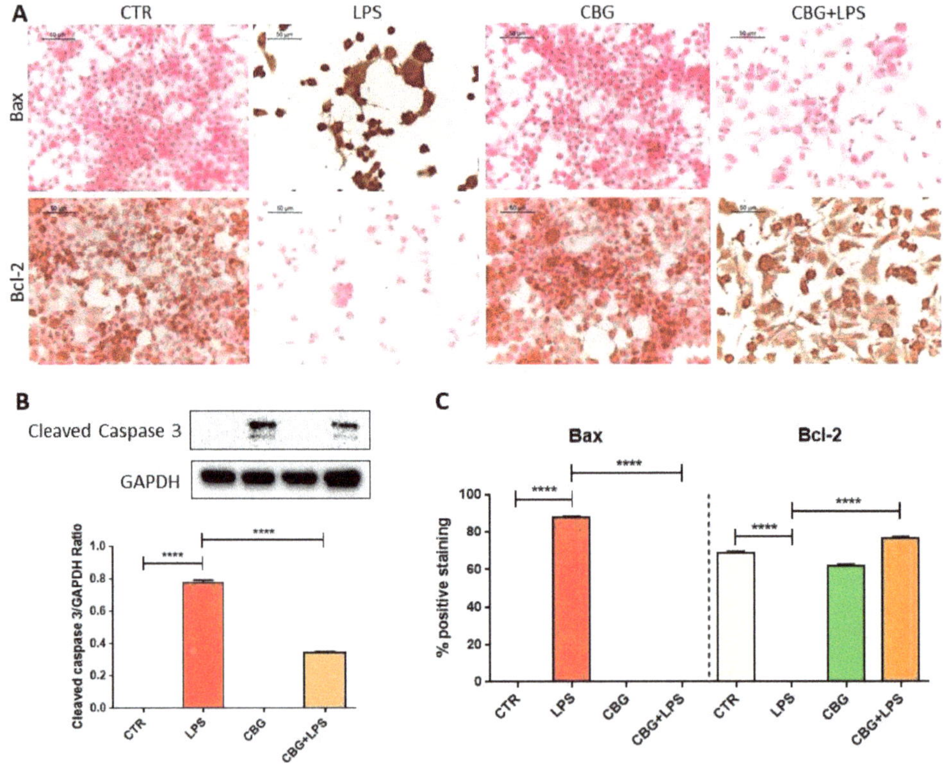

Figure 2. CBG pre-treatment was able to inhibit apoptosis induced by the medium of LPS-stimulated macrophages in NSC-34 motor neurons. (**A**) Immunocytochemistry showed that NSC-34 cells treated with the medium of LPS-stimulated macrophages expressed Bax but not Bcl-2. CBG pre-treatment abolished Bax expression and restored those of Bcl-2. (**B**) The treatment with the medium of LPS-stimulated macrophages induced caspase 3 activation in NSC-34 cells, but CBG pre-treatment reduced its expression. (**C**) Quantitative analysis of positive staining. The experiments were repeated three times. **** $p < 0.0001$, NSC-34 cells treated with the medium of LPS stimulated macrophages vs. NSC-34 pre-treated with CBG and then exposed to the medium of LPS stimulated macrophages, NSC-34 treated with the medium of LPS stimulated macrophages vs. control; Scale bar: 50 µm.

2.3. CBG Reduced the Expression of Pro-Inflammatory Cytokines and Proliferator-Activated Receptor γ (PPARγ)

The treatment of NSC-34 motor neurons with the medium of LPS-stimulated macrophages induced inflammation as demonstrated by the increased protein levels of the pro-inflammatory cytokines interleukin-1β (IL-1β), tumor necrosis factor α (TNF-α) and interferon-γ (IFN-γ) evaluated by immunocytochemical assay (Figure 3). Interestingly, the pre-treatment with CBG was able to reduce IL-1β, TNF-α and IFN-γ protein levels (Figure 3). Control and CBG treated NSC-34 motor neurons did not express pro-inflammatory cytokines.

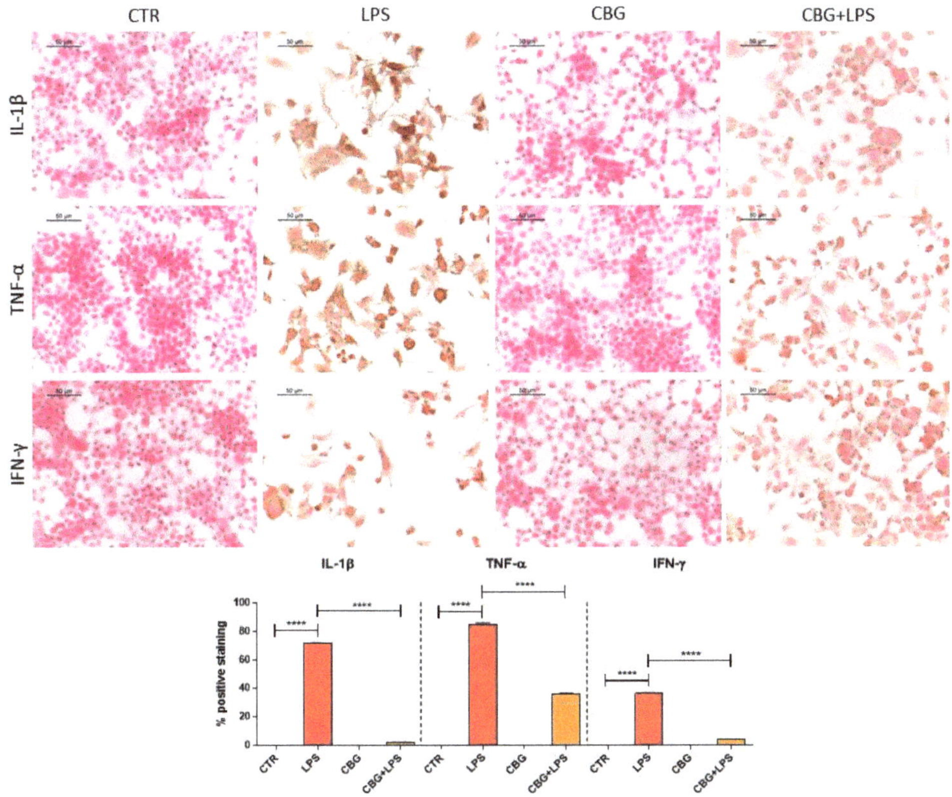

Figure 3. CBG pre-treatment was able to reduce the levels of pro-inflammatory cytokines in NSC-34 cells treated with the medium of LPS-stimulated RAW 264.7 macrophages. Immunocytochemistry with the quantitative analysis of positive staining showed that the treatment with the medium of LPS-stimulated RAW 264.7 macrophages induced the expression of the pro-inflammatory cytokines IL-1β, TNF-α and IFN-γ. CBG pre-treatment reduced the protein levels of the pro-inflammatory cytokines. The immunocytochemical assays were repeated three times. **** $p < 0.0001$, NSC-34 cells treated with the medium of LPS stimulated macrophages vs. NSC-34 pre-treated with CBG and then exposed to the medium of LPS stimulated macrophages, NSC-34 treated with the medium of LPS stimulated macrophages vs. control; Scale bar: 50 μm.

In addition, in NSC-34 motor neurons treated with the medium of LPS-stimulated RAW 264.7 cells, we observed the expression of PPARγ assessed by immunocytochemistry. However, the pre-treatment with CBG reduced PPARγ protein levels (Figure 4).

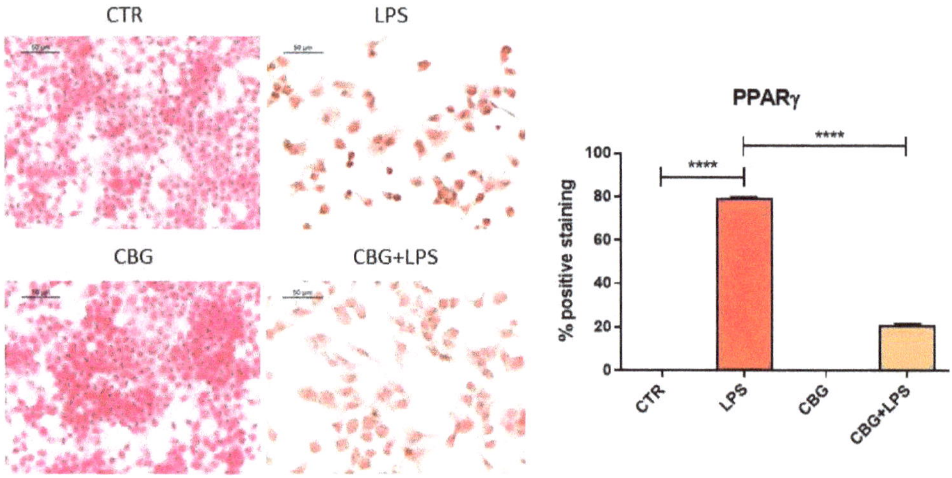

Figure 4. CBG pre-treatment was able to reduce the levels of PPARγ in NSC-34 cells treated with the medium of LPS-stimulated RAW 264.7 macrophages. The treatment with the medium of LPS-stimulated RAW 264.7 macrophages induced the expression of PPARγ, but CBG pre-treatment reduced its levels. The immunocytochemical assays were repeated three times. **** $p < 0.0001$, NSC-34 cells treated with the medium of LPS stimulated macrophages vs. NSC-34 cells pre-treated with CBG and then exposed to the medium of LPS stimulated macrophages, NSC-34 cells treated with the medium of LPS stimulated macrophages vs. control; Scale bar: 50 μm.

2.4. CBG Exerted an Antioxidant Action in NSC-34 Cells Treated with Medium of LPS-Stimulated Macrophages

As we said above, inflammation and oxidative stress are two correlated processes, indeed the treatment of NSC-34 motor neurons with the medium of LPS-stimulated RAW 264.7 induced oxidative stress, as demonstrated by the increase in nitrotyrosine levels evaluated by immunocytochemical assay. However, CBG pre-treatment was able to reduce nitrotyrosine expression (Figure 5). In addition, CBG pre-treatment was able to counteract the increase of superoxide dismutase 1 (SOD1) and inducible nitric oxide synthase (iNOS) expression induced by the treatment with the medium of LPS-stimulated RAW 264.7, reducing their levels (Figure 5) as evidenced by immunocytochemistry. Control NSC-34 motor neurons and cells treated with CBG alone evidenced the absence of oxidative marker expression.

Controls and NSC-34 motor neurons exposed to CBG expressed nuclear factor erythroid 2–related factor 2 (Nrf-2). The exposure of NSC-34 motor neurons to the medium of LPS-stimulated macrophages reduced the levels of Nrf-2 (Figure 6). However, CBG pre-treatment restored Nrf-2 levels.

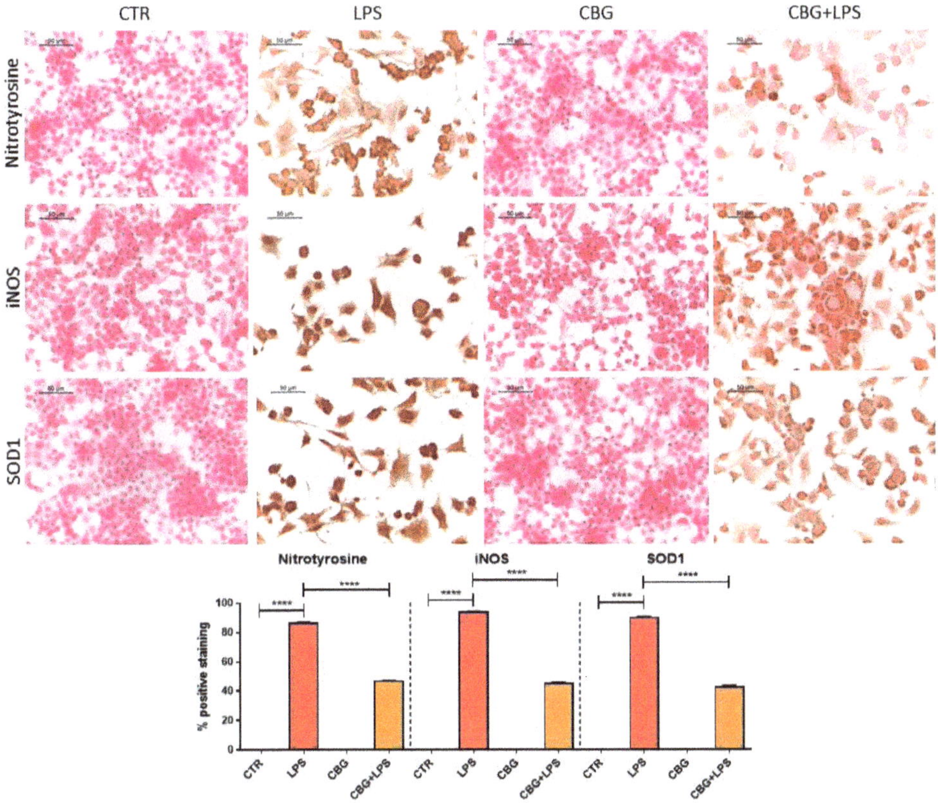

Figure 5. CBG pre-treatment was able to reduce the levels of oxidative stress markers nitrotyrosine, iNOS and SOD1 in NSC-34 cells treated with the medium of LPS-stimulated RAW 264.7 macrophages. The treatment with the medium of LPS-stimulated RAW 264.7 macrophages induced the expression of nitrotyrosine, iNOS and SOD1, but CBG pre-treatment reduced their levels. The immunocytochemical assays were repeated three times. **** $p < 0.0001$, NSC-34 cells treated with the medium of LPS stimulated macrophages vs. NSC-34 cells pre-treated with CBG and then exposed to the medium of LPS stimulated macrophages, NSC-34 cells treated with the medium of LPS stimulated macrophages vs. control; Scale bar: 50 μm.

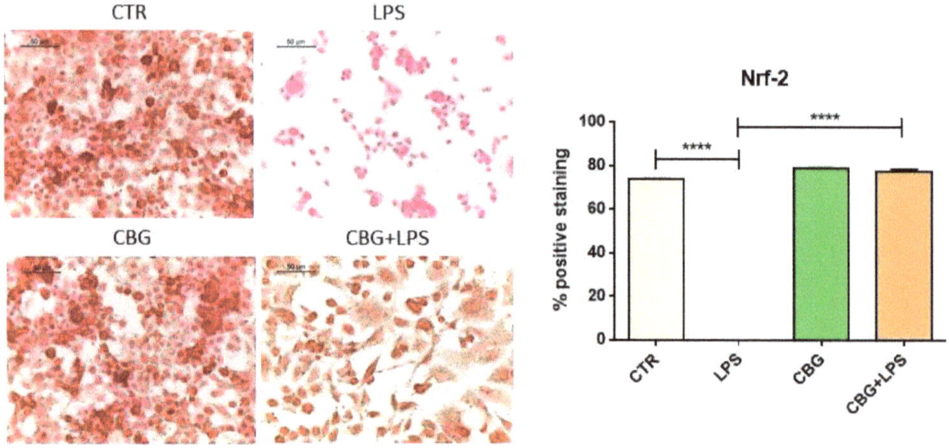

Figure 6. CBG pre-treatment was able to restore Nrf-2 expression in NSC-34 cells treated with the medium of LPS-stimulated RAW 264.7 macrophages. Control cells and NSC-34 cells treated with CBG alone expressed Nrf-2. On the contrary, the treatment with the medium of LPS-stimulated RAW 264.7 macrophages abolished its expression, but CBG pre-treatment restored its levels. The immunocytochemical assays were repeated three times. **** $p < 0.0001$, NSC-34 cells treated with the medium of LPS stimulated macrophages vs. NSC-34 cells pre-treated with CBG and then exposed to the medium of LPS stimulated macrophages, NSC-34 cells treated with the medium of LPS stimulated macrophages vs. control; Scale bar: 50 μm.

3. Discussion

Both oxidative stress and inflammation play a main role in neurodegenerative disorders, including Alzheimer's disease, Parkinson's disease and multiple sclerosis [13,14]. Neurodegeneration represents a major problem for human health, being one of the major causes of mortality and disability. Given that a cure against neurodegenerative disorders is not available, the research is focused on the discovery of new compounds able to exert a beneficial action against neurodegeneration, protecting neuronal cells, and able to stop or delay the progression of this kind of diseases. In particular, compounds with both anti-inflammatory and anti-oxidative actions may represent a successful strategy. Different phytochemicals were shown to exert a protective action, and, among these ones, some cannabinoids extracted from *Cannabis sativa* were studied for their beneficial properties. Even if CBD is one of the most studied non-psychoactive phytocannabinoids, CBG was reported to be able to exert different beneficial actions.

In a previous work we showed that CBG reduced oxidative markers, such as iNOS, nitrotyrosine and Poly (ADP-ribose) polymerase 1 (PARP-1) and increase cell anti-oxidant defense through the modulation of SOD1. We reported that CBG anti-oxidant action depends on the CB2 receptors. Moreover, CBG treatment prevented IκB-α phosphorylation and translocation of the nuclear factor-κB (NF-κB) and modulated the mitogen-activated protein (MAP) kinases pathway. All these actions resulted in an inhibition of cell death [7].

Other than the anti-oxidant action, CBG showed neuroprotective effects in experimental models of Huntington's disease [12] and beneficial actions in a model of inflammatory bowel disease [8]. Furthermore, CBG derivatives showed also neuroprotective effects in models of Parkinson's disease [11], Huntington's disease [21] and multiple sclerosis [9,10].

In this work, we evaluated the beneficial properties exerted by CBG in an in vitro model of neuroinflammation. With this aim, we exposed NSC-34 motor neurons to the cell culture medium of LPS-stimulated RAW 264.7 macrophages.

We observed that CBG increased the number of viable cells compared to the control at all concentrations tested. The highest cell viability was observed at the dose of CBG 7.5 μM, and this concentration was used for further evaluations.

Incubation with the medium of LPS-stimulated RAW 264.7 macrophages caused a 50% loss of cell viability in NSC-34 motor neurons. This result is in line with a study reporting that LPS treatment induced in PC12 rat pheochromocytoma cells, an in vitro model used for neurological and neurochemical studies, loss of cell viability [22]. Interestingly, CBG was able to decrease neuronal cell loss. These results are in line with those obtained with a CBG derivative in M-213 neuronal cells exposed to the conditioned medium of LPS stimulated BV2 cells, in which it was able to reduce M-213 cell death [11]. In addition, the capacity of CBG and of its quinone derivatives to counteract the loss of cell viability induced by neurotoxic stimuli, was also reported in HT22 mouse hippocampal cells and Neuro-2a neuroblastoma cells treated with glutamate [9,21].

Accordingly to the loss of cell viability, the medium of LPS-stimulated macrophages induced apoptosis in NSC-34 motor neurons, as demonstrated by the expression of cleaved caspase 3 and Bax, while Bcl-2 was not expressed. We evaluated cleaved caspase 3 protein level by western blot analysis because this assay better evidenced the presence of the cleaved bands. However, CBG pre-treatment decreased the protein levels of active caspase 3 and Bax was not expressed, instead Bcl-2 levels increased. Similar results were obtained in RAW 264.7 treated with H_2O_2, where it was shown that CBG inhibited apoptosis [7].

The treatment of NSC-34 motor neurons with the medium of LPS-stimulated RAW 264.7 increased the expression of the pro-inflammatory cytokines as already reported by previous works [23,24] and in line with the pro-inflammatory role of LPS. CBG pre-treatment was able to reduce inflammation, decreasing the expression of the pro-inflammatory cytokines IL-1β, TNF-α and IFN-γ. CBG capacity to counteract the release of cytokines was reported in other models. Indeed, in an experimental model of inflammatory bowel disease, CBG reduced IL-1β and IFN-γ levels in inflamed colons [8], while in a model of Huntington's disease, CBG was able to decrease the expression of TNF-α and interleukin 6 (IL-6) [12]. Furthermore, CBG derivatives showed anti-inflammatory properties, such as CBG quinone derivatives that reduced the release of TNF-α and IL-1β in the medium of LPS-treated BV2 cells [11] and the expression of TNF-α and IFN-γ in the spinal cord of a murine model of Experimental Autoimmune Encephalomyelitis (EAE) [10]. Both CBG and its quinone derivative were able to inhibit IL-1β, TNF-α and IL-6 in microglia stimulated with LPS [9]. In our experimental condition, we found that the treatment of NSC-34 motor neurons with the medium of LPS-stimulated RAW 264.7 increased the expression of PPARγ, but CBG pre-treatment reduced its level. PPARγ plays a crucial role in the regulation of proliferation, metabolism, differentiation and inflammatory response in the nervous system. PPARγ agonist can exert anti-inflammatory and anti-oxidant responses [25]. PPARγ was reported to increase in vivo after LPS injection [26,27]. It is known that some cannabinoids can activate PPARγ, that mediates at least in part the analgesic, neuroprotective and anti-inflammatory effects [28]. CBG derivatives exerted neuroprotective, pro-survival and anti-inflammatory actions, at least in part, activating PPARγ [10,11,21].

The incubation with the medium of LPS-stimulated RAW 276.7 increased oxidative stress in NSC-34 cells as demonstrated by the increase in nitrotyrosine levels, a well-known marker of oxidative stress involved also in neurodegenerative disease [29,30]. In parallel, we observed increased levels of iNOS in NSC-34 cells treated with the medium of LPS-stimulated RAW 264.7 macrophages. NOS enzymes mediate the synthesis of nitric oxide (NO) from the conversion of the amino acid L-arginine to L-citrulline. NO can interact with superoxide anion to form peroxynitrite, a potent oxidant agent. It is known that iNOS expression may be induced by both LPS and cytokines [31], such as in our study. However, the pre-treatment with CBG reduced both nitrotyrosine and iNOS expression in NSC-34 motor neurons treated with the medium of LPS-stimulated RAW 264.7 macrophages. CBG ability to reduce the levels of these pro-oxidant markers was demonstrated in vitro in macrophages stimulated with H_2O_2 [7]. However, also in in vivo models of Huntington's disease and experimental inflammatory bowel disease CBG attenuated the expression of iNOS [8,12]. CBG derivatives were reported to decrease iNOS expression in vivo and in vitro [11]. We observed increased SOD1 levels in NSC-34 motor neurons treated with the medium of LPS-stimulated RAW 264.7 macrophages. SOD1 protects cells from harmful amounts of superoxide anions, converting two superoxide anions into oxygen and H_2O_2. The pre-treatment with CBG reduced SOD1 levels.

Decreased levels of the transcription factor Nrf-2 in NSC-34 motor neurons exposed to the medium of LPS-stimulated RAW 276.7 macrophages were found. Nrf-2 takes part in the cell anti-oxidant defense system, being a regulator of the expression of genes involved in the protection against oxidative stress and inflammation in order to maintain mitochondrial function, cellular redox, and protein homeostasis [32]. Indeed, among Nrf-2 target genes there are those encoding for proteins involved in detoxification, antioxidant and anti-inflammatory actions [33]. Interestingly, we observed that the pre-treatment with CBG restored Nrf-2 nuclear protein expression reducing oxidative stress. The antioxidant action of CBG is particularly important taking into account that the brain is particularly sensitive to changes in cellular redox status, making the maintenance of redox homeostasis in the brain a critical point for the prevention of oxidative stress induced cellular damage [34,35]. However, Nrf-2 showed also an anti-inflammatory action, given that evidence showed a mechanism of transcriptional repression of pro-inflammatory cytokines, such as TNF-α, IL-1β, IL-6, interleukin 8 in microglia, macrophages, monocytes, and astrocytes following Nrf-2 activation [36,37]. Interestingly, in our in vitro model of neuroinflammation we observed in parallel to the increased Nrf-2 levels, a reduction of pro-inflammatory cytokines.

Our results are in line with previous studies that showed the beneficial effects and anti-inflammatory activity of CBG and its derivatives. In a model of colitis induced in mice by intracolonic administration of dinitrobenzene sulphonic acid (DNBS), CBG was able to reduce colon weight/colon length ratio, myeloperoxidase activity and exerts an anti-inflammatory activity associated to DNBS administration. In addition, CBG reduced NO production and iNOS protein expression in macrophages [8]. CBG showed neuroprotective effects in a Huntington's disease model, improving motor deficits and reducing microgliosis and inflammatory markers [12]. A derivative of CBG, the CBG quinone VCE-003 showed neuroprotective actions in experimental models of multiple sclerosis [9,10]. Indeed, VCE-003 mitigated disease symptoms, decreased microglia reactivity and modulated the expression of genes involved in multiple sclerosis pathology. In addition, VCE-003 showed anti-inflammatory properties, protecting neurons from excitotoxicity and inhibiting the release of pro-inflammatory mediators in LPS stimulated microglial cells. Another CBG derivative, VCE-003.2 prevented neuronal degeneration in an experimental model of Parkinson's disease, through an anti-inflammatory action [11].

It would be interesting also to perform gene expression analysis, in order to evaluate the transcriptional regulation exerted by CBG. However, we only evaluated protein levels, and then this may be considered a limitation of this study. In addition, it is an in vitro study, then these results have to be confirmed in vivo in a neuroinflammation model, but also in different neurodegenerative disorder models.

4. Materials and Methods

4.1. Plant Material

Cannabis sativa var. Carma was obtained from a greenhouse cultivation at CREA-CIN (Rovigo, Italy), where a voucher specimen is kept. The plant material was harvested in November 2010 and was supplied by Dr. Gianpaolo Grassi (CREA, Rovigo, Italy). The manipulation of the plant was done in accordance with its legal status (Authorization SP/101 of the "Ministerodella Salute", Rome, Italy).

4.2. General Experimental Procedures

^{1}H NMR spectra were measured using JEOL ECP 300—300 MHz spectrometer (JEOL, Pleasanton, CA, USA). Chemical shifts were referenced to the residual solvent signal ($CDCl_3$: δH 7.26). Reverse phase (RP) C-18 (POLYGOPREP60-30 C18) was used to remove waxes and pigments. Silica gel 60 (70–230 mesh) was used for gravity column chromatography. CBG purification was monitored using TLC on Merck 60 F254 (0.25 mm) plates, that were visualized by UV inspection and/or spraying with 5% H_2SO_4 in ethanol and heating.

4.3. Extraction and CBG Isolation

One Kg of dried, powdered flowered aerial parts were heated at 120°C for 2.5 h in order to decarboxylate precannabinoids and then extracted exhaustively with acetone (2 × 9 L) using a shaker. The elimination of the solvent left a black resinous residue (74 g, 7.4%), that was dissolved in MeOH (30 mL/g of extract) and filtered using RP C-18 silica gel to remove waxes and pigments.

The evaporation of methanol afforded 36 g of a dark-green extract that was further purified by gravity column chromatography on silica gel (75 g, petroleum ether-EtOAc, 8:2, as eluent) to afford 5 g of a yellow oil then crystallized with petroleum ether to give 3 g of pure CBG (0.3%). Pure CBG was stored at −8 °C.

4.4. RAW 264.7 Macrophage Cell Culture and LPS Treatment

The murine macrophage RAW 264.7 cell line, obtained from InvivoGen (San Diego, CA, USA), were cultured in monolayer at 37 °C in a moisturized atmosphere of 5% CO_2 and 95% air using DMEM-high glucose medium (Sigma-Aldrich,St. Louis, MO, USA supplemented with 10% fetal bovine serum (FBS) (Sigma-Aldrich). With the aim to induce inflammation, cells were grown until 70–80% confluence was reached, and after they were incubated with 10 ng/mL LPS from Escherichia coli 0111:B4 (Sigma-Aldrich) for 24 h [38]. Untreated cells were used as control. At the end of the treatment the culture medium was collected to carry out experiments with NSC-34 cells.

4.5. NSC-34 Motor Neurons Treatment with the Medium of LPS-Stimulated RAW 264.7

The aim of this work was the evaluation of the anti-inflammatory and anti-oxidative stress properties of CBG in a neuroinflammation model in vitro. In order to reproduce neuroinflammation in vitro, we treated the murine motor neuron cell line NSC-34 with the cell culture medium of LPS-stimulated RAW macrophages. NSC-34 cells, acquired from Cellutions Biosystems Inc., Cedarlane (Burlington, ON, Canada), were cultured in DMEM-high glucose medium (Sigma-Aldrich) with the addition of 10% FBS (Sigma-Aldrich), at 37 °C in a moisturized atmosphere of 5% CO_2 and 95% air. To examine anti-inflammatory effects of CBG against LPS-induced inflammation, NSC-34 cells were pre-treated for 24 h with 7.5 μM CBG. At the end of pre-treatment, medium was replaced with cell-free conditioned medium from LPS-stimulated RAW 264.7 macrophages, and incubated for 24 h. As controls, NSC-34 cells were incubated with the medium of unstimulated RAW 264.7 macrophages. Cells treated with vehicle (<0.1% DMSO) or with the CBG alone were also included as controls. Then, motor neuronal cells were fixed for immunocytochemistry analysis or harvested for western blot. All the experiments were done in triplicate and repeated for three independent times.

4.6. Thiazolyl Blue Tetrazolium Bromide (MTT) Assay

In order to evaluate the effects of CBG and LPS on cell viability the MTT assay was performed. To evaluate the effects of CBG, NSC-34 cells were cultured in 96-well plates and incubated for 24 h with different CBG doses (1, 2.5, 5, 7.5, 10, 12.5, 15 and 20 μM). With the aim to evaluate cell death induced by LPS and whether CBG could counteract the loss of cell viability, NSC-34 motor neurons were cultured in 96-well plates, and after pre-treatment with 7.5 μM CBG for 24 h, cells were incubated with the medium of LPS-stimulated macrophages for 24 h. At the end of the treatments, cells were washed and incubated with fresh medium containing MTT (0.5 mg/mL; Sigma-Aldrich) at 37°C for 4 h. After, formazan crystals were dissolved in acidic isopropanol at 37°C for 1 h and the optical density was evaluated by spectrophotometric measurement of absorbance. All the experiments were done in triplicate and repeated for three independent times.

4.7. Protein Extraction and Western Blot Analysis

At the end of the treatment, NSC-34 motor neurons were collected and lysed using buffer A [320 mM sucrose, 10 mM, 1 mM EGTA, 2 mM EDTA, 5 mM NaN3, 50 mM NaF, β-mercaptoethanol, and protease/phosphatase inhibitor cocktail (Roche Molecular Diagnostics, Branchburg, NJ, USA)] in ice for 15 min, and centrifuged at 1000×*g* for 10 min at 4 °C. The supernatant was collected as cytosolic extract. The obtained pellet was lysed with buffer B [150 mM NaCl, 10 mM Tris-HCl (pH 7.4), 1 mM EGTA, 1 mM EDTA, Triton X-100, and protease/phosphatase inhibitor cocktail (Roche Molecular Diagnostics, Pleasanton, CA, USA)] in ice for 15 min and centrifuged at 15,000×*g* for 30 min at 4 °C. The supernatant was collected as nuclear extract. Protein concentrations were measured through Bradford assay (Bio-Rad Laboratories, Inc., Hercules, CA, USA). Twenty-five µg of proteins were heated for 5 min at 95 °C and resolved by SDS-polyacrylamide gel electrophoresis (SDS-PAGE) and after transferred onto a PVDF membrane (Amersham Hybond, GE Healthcare Life Sciences, Milan, Italy).

Membranes were blocked with 5% skim milk in Phosphate Buffered Saline (PBS) for 1 h at room temperature and incubated overnight at 4 °C with the primary antibody against cleaved caspase 3 (1:1000; Cell Signaling Technology, Danvers, MA, USA). Membranes were washed with PBS 1X and incubated with horse radish peroxidase (HRP)-conjugated anti-rabbit IgG secondary antibody (1:2000; Santa Cruz Biotechnology,Dallas, TX, USA) for 1 h at room temperature. With the aim to analyze if blots were loaded with equal amounts of proteins, membranes were incubated with antibody for glyceraldehyde 3-phosphate dehydrogenase (GAPDH) HRP Conjugated (1:1000; Cell Signaling Technology). The relative expression of protein bands was analyzed through an enhanced chemiluminescence system (Luminata Western HRP Substrates; Millipore, Burlington, MA, USA). Protein bands were acquired using ChemiDoc™ MP System (Bio-Rad Laboratories, Inc.) and quantified through the computer program ImageJ software (developed at the National Institutes of Health, USA, http://rsb.info.nih.gov/ij). All blots are representative of three independent experiments.

4.8. ImmunocytoChemistry

NSC-34 motor neurons were grown on coverslips (12 mm; Thermo Fisher Scientific, Waltham, MA, USA) and, at the end of the treatments, they were fixed with 4% paraformaldehyde at room temperature for 30 min and after washed with PBS (pH 7.5). Afterwards, cells were incubated with 3% H_2O_2 at room temperature for 15 min in order to suppress the endogenous peroxidase activity. After three washes with PBS, cells were blocked with horse serum +0.1% Triton X-100 for 20 min and incubated overnight at 4°C with the following primary antibodies:

- anti Bax (1:50; Santa Cruz Biotechnology);
- anti Bcl-2 (1:50; Santa Cruz Biotechnology);
- anti IL-1β (1:250; Cell Signaling Technology);
- anti IFN-γ (1:50; Santa Cruz Biotechnology);
- anti TNF-α (1:250; Cell Signaling Technology);
- anti SOD1 (1:100; Abcam, Cambridge, UK);
- anti iNOS (1:50; Santa Cruz Biotechnology);
- anti nitrotyrosine (1:1000; Millipore);
- anti Nrf-2 (1:50; Santa Cruz Biotechnology);
- anti PPARγ (1:50; Santa Cruz Biotechnology).

After, cells were washed with PBS and incubated with biotinylated secondary antibody (1:200; Vector Laboratories, Inc., Burlingame, CA, USA) and streptavidin AB Complex-HRP (ABC-kit from

Dako, Glostrup, Denmark). The immunostaining was developed with the DAB peroxidase substrate kit (Vector Laboratories, DBA Italia S.r.l., Milan, Italy; brown color; positive staining) and counterstaining with nuclear fast red (Vector Laboratories, DBA Italia S.r.l.; pink background; negative staining).

The immunocytochemical assays were repeated three times and each experimental group was plated in duplicate, for a total of 6 coverslips for each antibody. With the aim of calculating the percentage of positive cells stained, the images were captured using a light microscopy (LEICA DM 2000 combined with LEICA ICC50 HD camera) with an objective ×40 and the densitometric analysis was carried out using the software LEICA Application Suite ver. 4.2.0 (LEICA, Wetzlar, Germany). Quantitative analysis was performed on 6 coverslips by covering approximately 90% of the total area.

4.9. Statistical Data Analysis

Statistical analysis was carried out using GraphPad Prism version 6.0 software (GraphPad Software, La Jolla, CA, USA). The data were statistically analyzed by one-way ANOVA test and Bonferroni post-hoc test for multiple comparisons. A P value less than or equal to 0.05 was considered statistically significant. Results are reported as mean ± SEM of N experiments.

5. Conclusions

In conclusion, our results indicated that CBG exerted a protective action in an in vitro neuroinflammation model. CBG reduced neuronal death in NSC-34 cells treated with the medium of LPS stimulated macrophages, reducing inflammation and oxidative stress. In particular, CBG restored cell anti-oxidant defense, increasing the expression of Nrf-2, reduced oxidative stress and inflammatory markers. On the bases of these results, thanks to its neuroprotective effects, we encourage the use of CBG against neurodegeneration and in those pathological conditions where neuroinflammation and oxidative stress play a main role.

Author Contributions: A.G. performed in vitro experiments and wrote the manuscript; F.P. and G.G. provided Cannabigerol; P.B. revised the manuscript and acquired funding; E.M. conceived the experiments, performed immunocytochemical analysis and critically revised the manuscript.

Funding: This study was supported by current research funds 2018 of IRCCS "Centro Neurolesi Bonino-Pulejo", Messina, Italy.

Acknowledgments: This study was supported by current research funds 2018 of IRCCS "Centro Neurolesi Bonino-Pulejo", Messina, Italy. The authors would like to thank Prof. Appendino Giovanni (University of Eastern Piedmont "Amedeo Avogadro", Novara, Italy), for his technical assistance and precious contribution during manuscript drafting.

Conflicts of Interest: The authors declare no conflict of interest.

Abbreviations

Δ9-THC	Δ9-tetrahydrocannabinol
CBD	Cannabidiol
CBG	Cannabigerol
H_2O_2	Hydrogen peroxide
LPS	Lipopolysaccharide
DMSO	Dimethyl sulfoxide
PPARγ	Proliferator-activated receptor γ
IL-β	Interleukin-1β
IFN-γ	Interferon-γ
TNF-α	Tumor necrosis factor α
iNOS	Inducible nitric oxide synthase
SOD1	Superoxide dismutase1
Nrf-2	Nuclear factor erythroid 2–related factor 2

PARP-1	Poly [ADP-ribose] polymerase 1
NF-κB	Nuclear factor-κB
MAP	Mitogen-activated protein
IL-6	Interleukin 6
EAE	Experimental Autoimmune Encephalomyelitis
NO	Nitric oxide
DNBS	Dinitrobenzene sulphonic acid
FBS	Fetal bovine serum
MTT	Thiazolyl Blue Tetrazolium Bromide
HRP	Horse radish peroxidase
GAPDH	Glyceraldehyde 3 phosphate dehydrogenase
PBS	Phosphate Buffered Saline

References

1. Morales, P.; Hurst, D.P.; Reggio, P.H. Molecular targets of the phytocannabinoids: A complex picture. *Prog. Chem. Org. Nat. Prod.* **2017**, *103*, 103–131. [PubMed]
2. Jackson, S.J.; Diemel, L.T.; Pryce, G.; Baker, D. Cannabinoids and neuroprotection in cns inflammatory disease. *J. Neurol. Sci.* **2005**, *233*, 21–25. [CrossRef] [PubMed]
3. Cabral, G.A.; Griffin-Thomas, L. Cannabinoids as therapeutic agents for ablating neuroinflammatory disease. *Endocr. Metab. Immune Disord. Drug Targets* **2008**, *8*, 159–172. [CrossRef] [PubMed]
4. Gowran, A.; Noonan, J.; Campbell, V.A. The multiplicity of action of cannabinoids: Implications for treating neurodegeneration. *CNS Neurosci. Ther.* **2011**, *17*, 637–644. [CrossRef] [PubMed]
5. Pisanti, S.; Malfitano, A.M.; Ciaglia, E.; Lamberti, A.; Ranieri, R.; Cuomo, G.; Abate, M.; Faggiana, G.; Proto, M.C.; Fiore, D.; et al. Cannabidiol: State of the art and new challenges for therapeutic applications. *Pharmacol. Ther.* **2017**, *175*, 133–150. [CrossRef] [PubMed]
6. Burstein, S. Cannabidiol (cbd) and its analogs: A review of their effects on inflammation. *Bioorg. Med. Chem.* **2015**, *23*, 1377–1385. [CrossRef] [PubMed]
7. Giacoppo, S.; Gugliandolo, A.; Trubiani, O.; Pollastro, F.; Grassi, G.; Bramanti, P.; Mazzon, E. Cannabinoid cb2 receptors are involved in the protection of raw264.7 macrophages against the oxidative stress: An in vitro study. *Eur. J. Histochem. EJH* **2017**, *61*, 2749. [CrossRef] [PubMed]
8. Borrelli, F.; Fasolino, I.; Romano, B.; Capasso, R.; Maiello, F.; Coppola, D.; Orlando, P.; Battista, G.; Pagano, E.; Di Marzo, V.; et al. Beneficial effect of the non-psychotropic plant cannabinoid cannabigerol on experimental inflammatory bowel disease. *Biochem. Pharmacol.* **2013**, *85*, 1306–1316. [CrossRef] [PubMed]
9. Granja, A.G.; Carrillo-Salinas, F.; Pagani, A.; Gomez-Canas, M.; Negri, R.; Navarrete, C.; Mecha, M.; Mestre, L.; Fiebich, B.L.; Cantarero, I.; et al. A cannabigerol quinone alleviates neuroinflammation in a chronic model of multiple sclerosis. *J. Neuroimmune Pharmacol.* **2012**, *7*, 1002–1016. [CrossRef] [PubMed]
10. Carrillo-Salinas, F.J.; Navarrete, C.; Mecha, M.; Feliu, A.; Collado, J.A.; Cantarero, I.; Bellido, M.L.; Munoz, E.; Guaza, C. A cannabigerol derivative suppresses immune responses and protects mice from experimental autoimmune encephalomyelitis. *PLoS ONE* **2014**, *9*, e94733. [CrossRef] [PubMed]
11. Garcia, C.; Gomez-Canas, M.; Burgaz, S.; Palomares, B.; Gomez-Galvez, Y.; Palomo-Garo, C.; Campo, S.; Ferrer-Hernandez, J.; Pavicic, C.; Navarrete, C.; et al. Benefits of vce-003.2, a cannabigerol quinone derivative, against inflammation-driven neuronal deterioration in experimental parkinson's disease: Possible involvement of different binding sites at the ppargamma receptor. *J. Neuroinflamm.* **2018**, *15*, 19. [CrossRef] [PubMed]
12. Valdeolivas, S.; Navarrete, C.; Cantarero, I.; Bellido, M.L.; Munoz, E.; Sagredo, O. Neuroprotective properties of cannabigerol in huntington's disease: Studies in r6/2 mice and 3-nitropropionate-lesioned mice. *Neurotherapeutics* **2015**, *12*, 185–199. [CrossRef] [PubMed]
13. Liu, Z.; Zhou, T.; Ziegler, A.C.; Dimitrion, P.; Zuo, L. Oxidative stress in neurodegenerative diseases: From molecular mechanisms to clinical applications. *Oxid. Med. Cell. Longev.* **2017**, *2017*, 2525967. [CrossRef] [PubMed]
14. Chen, W.W.; Zhang, X.; Huang, W.J. Role of neuroinflammation in neurodegenerative diseases (review). *Mol. Med. Rep.* **2016**, *13*, 3391–3396. [CrossRef] [PubMed]

15. Leszek, J.; Barreto, G.E.; Gasiorowski, K.; Koutsouraki, E.; Avila-Rodrigues, M.; Aliev, G. Inflammatory mechanisms and oxidative stress as key factors responsible for progression of neurodegeneration: Role of brain innate immune system. *CNS Neurol. Disord. Drug Targets* **2016**, *15*, 329–336. [CrossRef] [PubMed]
16. Chitnis, T.; Weiner, H.L. Cns inflammation and neurodegeneration. *J. Clin. Investig.* **2017**, *127*, 3577–3587. [CrossRef] [PubMed]
17. Angelova, P.R.; Abramov, A.Y. Role of mitochondrial ros in the brain: From physiology to neurodegeneration. *FEBS Lett.* **2018**, *592*, 692–702. [CrossRef] [PubMed]
18. Cobley, J.N.; Fiorello, M.L.; Bailey, D.M. 13 reasons why the brain is susceptible to oxidative stress. *Redox Biol.* **2018**, *15*, 490–503. [CrossRef] [PubMed]
19. Biswas, S.K. Does the interdependence between oxidative stress and inflammation explain the antioxidant paradox? *Oxid. Med. Cell. Longev.* **2016**, *2016*, 5698931. [CrossRef] [PubMed]
20. Mammana, S.; Fagone, P.; Cavalli, E.; Basile, M.S.; Petralia, M.C.; Nicoletti, F.; Bramanti, P.; Mazzon, E. The role of macrophages in neuroinflammatory and neurodegenerative pathways of alzheimer's disease, amyotrophic lateral sclerosis, and multiple sclerosis: Pathogenetic cellular effectors and potential therapeutic targets. *Int. J. Mol. Sci.* **2018**, *19*, 831. [CrossRef] [PubMed]
21. Diaz-Alonso, J.; Paraiso-Luna, J.; Navarrete, C.; Del Rio, C.; Cantarero, I.; Palomares, B.; Aguareles, J.; Fernandez-Ruiz, J.; Bellido, M.L.; Pollastro, F.; et al. Vce-003.2, a novel cannabigerol derivative, enhances neuronal progenitor cell survival and alleviates symptomatology in murine models of huntington's disease. *Sci. Rep.* **2016**, *6*, 29789. [CrossRef] [PubMed]
22. Wang, H.; Xu, Y.S.; Wang, M.L.; Cheng, C.; Bian, R.; Yuan, H.; Wang, Y.; Guo, T.; Zhu, L.L.; Zhou, H. Protective effect of naringin against the lps-induced apoptosis of pc12 cells: Implications for the treatment of neurodegenerative disorders. *Int. J. Mol. Med.* **2017**, *39*, 819–830. [CrossRef] [PubMed]
23. Gugliandolo, A.; Giacoppo, S.; Ficicchia, M.; Aliquo, A.; Bramanti, P.; Mazzon, E. Eruca sativa seed extract: A novel natural product able to counteract neuroinflammation. *Mol. Med. Rep.* **2018**, *17*, 6235–6244. [CrossRef] [PubMed]
24. Rajan, T.S.; Giacoppo, S.; Trubiani, O.; Diomede, F.; Piattelli, A.; Bramanti, P.; Mazzon, E. Conditioned medium of periodontal ligament mesenchymal stem cells exert anti-inflammatory effects in lipopolysaccharide-activated mouse motoneurons. *Exp. Cell Res.* **2016**, *349*, 152–161. [CrossRef] [PubMed]
25. Villapol, S. Roles of peroxisome proliferator-activated receptor gamma on brain and peripheral inflammation. *Cell. Mol. Neurobiol.* **2018**, *38*, 121–132. [CrossRef] [PubMed]
26. Liu, Y.; Lu, J.; Shi, J.; Hou, Y.; Zhu, H.; Zhao, S.; Liu, H.; Ding, B.; Yin, Y.; Yi, G. Increased expression of the peroxisome proliferator-activated receptor gamma in the immune system of weaned pigs after escherichia coli lipopolysaccharide injection. *Vet. Immunol. Immunopathol.* **2008**, *124*, 82–92. [CrossRef] [PubMed]
27. Liu, Y.L.; Shi, J.X.; Lu, J.; Che, Z.Q.; Zhu, H.L.; Hou, Y.Q.; Yin, Y.L.; Zhao, S.J.; Ding, B.Y.; Liu, H.M. Up-regulated expression of peroxisome proliferator-activated receptor gamma in the hypothalamic-pituitary-adrenal axis of weaned pigs after escherichia coli lipopolysaccharide challenge. *Vet. J.* **2010**, *184*, 230–235. [CrossRef] [PubMed]
28. O'Sullivan, S.E. An update on ppar activation by cannabinoids. *Br. J. Pharmacol.* **2016**, *173*, 1899–1910. [CrossRef] [PubMed]
29. Naoi, M.; Maruyama, W.; Shamoto-Nagai, M.; Yi, H.; Akao, Y.; Tanaka, M. Oxidative stress in mitochondria: Decision to survival and death of neurons in neurodegenerative disorders. *Mol. Neurobiol.* **2005**, *31*, 81–93. [CrossRef]
30. Beal, M.F. Oxidatively modified proteins in aging and disease. *Free Radic. Biol. Med.* **2002**, *32*, 797–803. [CrossRef]
31. Forstermann, U.; Sessa, W.C. Nitric oxide synthases: Regulation and function. *Eur. Heart J.* **2012**, *33*, 829–837. [CrossRef] [PubMed]
32. Hayes, J.D.; Dinkova-Kostova, A.T. The nrf2 regulatory network provides an interface between redox and intermediary metabolism. *Trends Biochem. Sci.* **2014**, *39*, 199–218. [CrossRef] [PubMed]
33. Dinkova-Kostova, A.T.; Kostov, R.V.; Kazantsev, A.G. The role of nrf2 signaling in counteracting neurodegenerative diseases. *FEBS J.* **2018**. [CrossRef] [PubMed]
34. Johnson, D.A.; Johnson, J.A. Nrf2–a therapeutic target for the treatment of neurodegenerative diseases. *Free Radic. Biol. Med.* **2015**, *88*, 253–267. [CrossRef] [PubMed]

35. Yamazaki, H.; Tanji, K.; Wakabayashi, K.; Matsuura, S.; Itoh, K. Role of the keap1/nrf2 pathway in neurodegenerative diseases. *Pathol. Int.* **2015**, *65*, 210–219. [CrossRef] [PubMed]
36. Kobayashi, E.H.; Suzuki, T.; Funayama, R.; Nagashima, T.; Hayashi, M.; Sekine, H.; Tanaka, N.; Moriguchi, T.; Motohashi, H.; Nakayama, K.; et al. Nrf2 suppresses macrophage inflammatory response by blocking proinflammatory cytokine transcription. *Nat. Commun.* **2016**, *7*, 11624. [CrossRef] [PubMed]
37. Quinti, L.; Dayalan Naidu, S.; Trager, U.; Chen, X.; Kegel-Gleason, K.; Lleres, D.; Connolly, C.; Chopra, V.; Low, C.; Moniot, S.; et al. Keap1-modifying small molecule reveals muted nrf2 signaling responses in neural stem cells from huntington's disease patients. *Proc. Natl. Acad. Sci. USA* **2017**, *114*, E4676–E4685. [CrossRef] [PubMed]
38. Xagorari, A.; Roussos, C.; Papapetropoulos, A. Inhibition of lps-stimulated pathways in macrophages by the flavonoid luteolin. *Br. J. Pharmacol.* **2002**, *136*, 1058–1064. [CrossRef] [PubMed]

International Journal of
Molecular Sciences

MDPI

Article

The Extracts and Major Compounds Derived from Astragali Radix Alter Mitochondrial Bioenergetics in Cultured Cardiomyocytes: Comparison of Various Polar Solvents and Compounds

Yun Huang [1,2], Kenneth Kin Leung Kwan [2], Ka Wing Leung [1,2], Huaiyou Wang [1], Xiang Peng Kong [1], Tina Ting Xia Dong [1,2] and Karl Wah Keung Tsim [1,2,*]

[1] Shenzhen Key Laboratory of Edible and Medicinal Bioresources, Shenzhen Research Institute, Hi-Tech Park, Nanshan, Shenzhen 518000, China; yhuangbr@connect.ust.hk (Y.H.); lkwing@ust.hk (K.W.L.); hyw@ust.hk (H.W.); xpkong@ust.hk (X.P.K.); botina@ust.hk (T.T.X.D.)

[2] Division of Life Science and Center for Chinese Medicine, The Hong Kong University of Science and Technology, Clear Water Bay, Hong Kong, China; klkwan@connect.ust.hk

* Correspondence: botsim@ust.hk; Tel.: +86-852-2358-7332

Received: 29 March 2018; Accepted: 18 April 2018; Published: 25 May 2018

Abstract: Astragali Radix (AR) is a widely used "Qi-invigorating" herb in China for its tonic effects in strengthening biological tissues. The extract of AR contains abundant antioxidants, including astragalosides and isoflavonoids. However, very few reports have systematically measured the effects of the major components of AR on cell mitochondrial bioenergetics. Here, a systemic approach employing an extracellular flux analyzer was developed to evaluate mitochondrial respiration in cultured cardiomyocyte cells H9C2. The effects of different polar extractives, as well as of the major compounds of AR, were compared. The contents of astragaloside IV, calycosin, formononetin, and genistein in the AR extracts obtained by using water, 50% ethanol, and 90% ethanol were measured by liquid chromatograph-mass spectrometer (LC–MS). The antioxidant activities of the AR extracts, as well as of their major compounds, were determined by measuring the free radical scavenging activity and protective effects in *tert*-butyl hydroperoxide (tBHP)-treated H9C2 cells. By monitoring the real-time oxygen consumption rate (OCR) in tBHP-treated cardiomyocytes with a Seahorse extracellular flux analyzer, the tonic effects of the AR extracts and of their main compounds on mitochondrial bioenergetics were evaluated. AR water extracts possessed the strongest antioxidant activity and protective effects in cardiomyocytes exposed to oxidative stress. The protection was proposed to be mediated via increasing the spare respiratory capacity and mitochondrial ATP production in the stressed cells. The major compounds of AR, astragaloside IV and genistein, showed opposite effects in regulating mitochondrial bioenergetics. These results demonstrate that highly polar extracts of AR, especially astragaloside-enriched extracts, possess better tonic effects on mitochondrial bioenergetics of cultured cardiomyocytes than extracts with a lower polarity.

Keywords: Astragali Radix; astragaloside IV; genistein; mitochondrial bioenergetics; oxygen consumption rate

1. Introduction

Astragali Radix (AR), derived from the dry roots of *Astragalus membranaceus* (Fisch.) Bge. var. *mongholicus* (Bge.) Hsiao and *Astragalus membranaceus* (Fisch.) Bge, is one of the most widely used traditional folk medicines in Asia because of its beneficial effects in invigorating "Qi" and strengthening tissues [1]. According to traditional Chinese medicine (TCM) theory, the interaction between "Yin and Yang" produces "Qi". AR acts mainly by tonifying defensive Qi, which protects the body against disease-causing factors [2]. Hence, multiple pharmacological effects of AR have been reported, e.g., immuno-modulation [3], anti-aging [4], anti-oxidation [5], and enhancement of cardiovascular function [6].

Being considered as a powerful exogenous source of antioxidants, AR provides obvious protective effects to organs in various models of oxidative stress-related diseases [7–9]. Astragaloside and isoflavonoid were proposed to be the major antioxidants of AR [10]. Astragalosides, especially astragaloside IV, have been proved to exert remarkable antioxidant activity and protective effects on mitochondria [11]. Astragaloside IV suppressed heat-induced apoptosis in bronchial epithelial cells by inhibiting the activation of mitochondrial Ca^{2+} uniporter, mitochondrial depolarization, and reactive oxygen species (ROS) production [12]. Other strong antioxidant components of AR are isoflavonoids, e.g., calycosin, formononetin, and genistein. Calycosin showed anti-apoptotic effects by enhancing Akt phosphorylation and activating ERα/β in cardiomyocytes exposed to oxidative stress [13], while formononetin was observed to attenuate apoptosis by regulating ROS formation in various cancer models [14,15]. Genistein was reported to be an anti-cancer agent [16], which could induce the disruption of mitochondrial membrane potential, the release of cytochrome c, and the activation of the apoptosome [17]. Chemical analysis has shown that AR contains different active ingredients, which therefore could account for the aforementioned biological activities [18].

Mitochondria are responsible for the production of ROS in the process of generating ATP. Defects in mitochondria are proposed to be the primary cause of energy decline, as well as of the onset of the aging process [19]. The profile of mitochondrial bioenergetics could be an indicative measurement of a cell energy status. The profile, e.g., the oxygen consumption rate (OCR) and the spare respiratory capacity (SRC), corresponds to the ability of mitochondria to increase ATP. In addition to the spare respiratory capacity, the maximal respiration of cells could be affected by the basal respiration consisting in proton leak and conventional mitochondrial ATP production. Proton leak from the mitochondrial inner membrane results in the uncoupling of oxidative phosphorylation, which is cytoprotective [20]. In addition, this leakage could downregulate ROS generation [21]. However, the proton leak also represents basal respiration not coupled to mitochondrial ATP production, and this could be considered as a sign of mitochondrial damage [22].

AR is considered a "Qi"-invigorating herb, which suggests its beneficial effect resulting in the production of ATP. The possible functions of AR in mitochondrial protection and elimination of ROS formation have been reported [23,24]. However, the real-time effect of AR in mitochondrial bioenergetics of living cells has rarely been studied. Here, a systematic approach to evaluate mitochondrial bioenergetics of intact cultured cardiomyocytes was adopted by using an extracellular flux analyzer. The major compounds of AR, e.g., astragaloside IV, calycosin, formononetin, and genistein, were also analyzed, and their functions in mitochondria were compared.

2. Results

2.1. Quantification of Chemicals and Total Phenolic Compounds in Different Extracts

The contents of calycosin, astragaloside IV, genistein, and formononetin in a water extract of AR (AR_{water}), a 50% ethanol extract of AR (AR_{EtOH50}), and a 90% ethanol extract of AR (AR_{EtOH90}) of three different batches of AR were quantified by LC–MS in multiple reaction monitoring (MRM) detection mode (Table 1 and Figure 1A). The analytical method was optimized on the basis of previous reports [25]. As summarized in Table S1, the fragmentor energy, collision energy, and ion pairs were optimized to attain the highest abundance of detected chemicals. In MS/MS analysis, the calibration curves of the four markers were linear over a concentration range of 1–1000 ng/mL, and the r^2 values of these calibration curves were higher than 0.990 in the analysis (Table S2). The investigation of precision, repeatability, and recovery of those four chemicals in AR extracts proved that the established method was robust enough for simultaneous quantification of various chemicals in AR, as summarized in Table S3.

Table 1. Quantitative assessment of four chemical standards in different AR extracts.

Standards	AR-1 [1]			AR-2			AR-3		
	W [2]	E50	E90	W	E50	E90	W	E50	E90
Calycosin	522.3 ± 6.32 [3]	491.56 ± 6.12	468.26 ± 2.92	467.23 ± 5.86	399.45 ± 7.42	333.22 ± 1.32	498.22 ± 5.89	387.22 ± 5.49	318.98 ± 8.19
Astragaloside IV	686.67 ± 4.23	579.23 ± 3.12	543.98 ± 2.39	537.28 ± 2.89	469.02 ± 2.19	450.22 ± 1.29	543.33 ± 5.67	582.11 ± 5.92	512.45 ± 4.89
Genistein	6.58 ± 0.13	9.14 ± 0.21	7.03 ± 0.22	5.43 ± 0.11	8.99 ± 0.32	7.93 ± 0.12	4.89 ± 0.21	5.89 ± 0.11	5.83 ± 0.12
Formononetin	139.34 ± 7.23	192.29 ± 1.91	179.34 ± 1.21	169.18 ± 5.38	187.29 ± 2.99	166.98 ± 1.11	169.29 ± 4.89	188.27 ± 3.22	138.39 ± 8.29

[1] Three batches of AR, purchased from Shanxi province of China, were used in the present study. [2] W, water extracts of AR; E50, 50% ethanol extracts of AR; E90, 90% ethanol extracts of RA. [3] The values are expressed in mg/g of dried powder of RA, mean ± SD, n = 3.

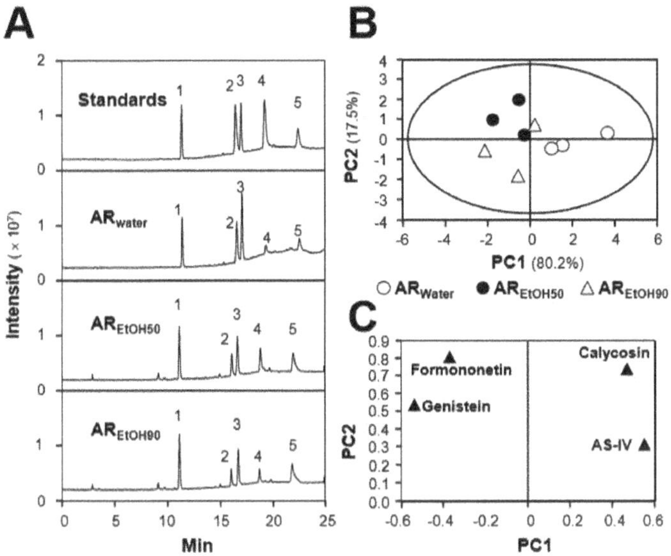

Figure 1. Principal component analysis (PCA) of major compunds in different Astragali Radix (AR) extracts. (**A**) The identification of ginsenoside Rg1 (1; internal control marker), calycosin (2), astragaloside IV (3), genistein (4), and formononetin (5) was made by an MS detector. Representative chromatograms of chemical markers (Standards), water extract of AR (AR_{water}), 50% ethanol extract of AR (AR_{EtOH50}), and 90% ethanol extract of AR (AR_{EtOH90}) under MRM mode are shown. (**B**) The scoring plot of different AR extracts is presented by comparing the contents of chosen major compounds. PC1 and PC2 described ~80.2% and ~17.5% of total variability, respectively. (**C**) The loading plot of PC1 versus PC2 for four compounds is shown. n = 3.

Representative chromatograms of standard markers (Standards), AR_{water}, AR_{EtOH50}, and AR_{EtOH90} under MRM mode are shown (Figure 1A). The chemical markers of ginsenoside Rg1 (internal control), calycosin, astragaloside IV, genistein, and formononetin are indicated. After determination of the contents of selected markers in three batches of AR, a principal component analysis (PCA) analysis was conducted to differentiate the samples extracted with water from those extracted with different ethanol aqueous solutions. As shown in Figure 1B, the two ranking PCs (PC1 and PC2) accounted for 97.7% of total variance, and AR extracts could be obviously distinguished into three distinct groups, according to the extracting solvents. The role of each variable (calycosin, astragaloside IV, genistein, and formononetin) in discriminating the extracts is shown in the loading plot (Figure 1C). Combined with the contents of selected markers recorded in Table 1, the contents of calycosin and astragaloside IV in AR_{water} extract were generally higher than those in AR_{EtOH50} and AR_{EtOH90}, while the for other two compounds the results appeared reversed. The contents of these markers could serve as quality control parameters.

Apart from the quantification of bioactive markers, the antioxidant effects of the AR extracts, i.e., AR_{water}, AR_{EtOH50} and AR_{EtOH90}, were evaluated by measuring their total phenolic content and free radical scavenging activity. Different extracts of AR from batch 1 were used for the subsequent analyses. The total phenolic contents of AR_{water}, AR_{EtOH50}, and AR_{EtOH90} were determined in reference to gallic acid (Figure 2A). Among the three extracts, AR_{EtOH50} exhibited a significant higher content of phenolic compounds, equivalent to ~11.7 mg gallic acid/g of sample, while AR_{water} and AR_{EtOH90} showed ~9.4 mg gallic acid/g and ~9.1 mg gallic acid/g, respectively. Inconsistent with this result, AR_{water} showed a significant higher free radical scavenging activity than the ethanol extracts (Figure 2B), indicating that the phenolic compounds might not be the only antioxidant present in AR.

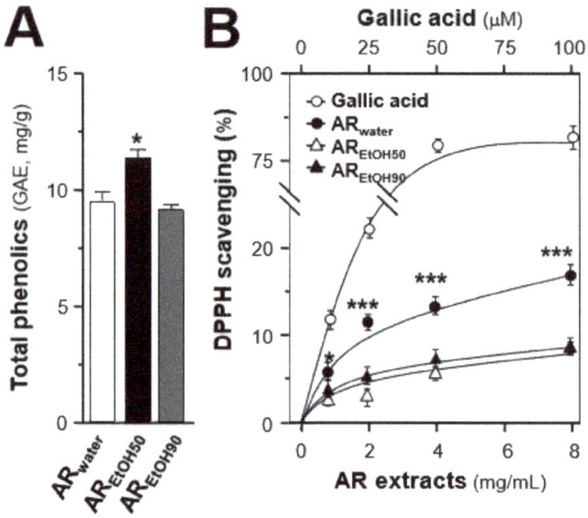

Figure 2. Comparison of total phenolic contents and 1,1-Diphenyl-2-picrylhydrazyl radical 2,2-Diphenyl-1-(2,4,6-trinitrophenyl)hydrazyl (DPPH) radical scavenging activity of different AR extracts. (**A**) The total phenolic contents of the AR extracts was determined using the Folin–Ciocalteu assay. Gallic acid was used as a reference compound, and the total phenolic content of each extract was expressed as the value of gallic acid equivalent (i.e., GAE in mg/g). (**B**) The antioxidant effects of the AR extracts were determined using the DPPH radical scavenging assay. Gallic acid was used as a positive control. All data are expressed as mean ± SD, $n = 5$. Statistical comparison was made with the sample with the lowest value of the corresponding concentration, * $p < 0.05$, *** $p < 0.001$.

2.2. Protection Effects of the AR Extracts in H9C2 Cells Subjected to Oxidative Stressed

H9C2 cell, an embryonic cardiomyocyte cell line, was selected here because of its robust and fast reaction to various stimuli. By treating with different concentrations of tBHP, a stress inducer, cell death of H9C2 cells and intracellular ROS level were induced in a dose-dependent manner. tBHP at 150 μM caused the maximal induction of ROS (Figure S1), and this concentration was used for the subsequent experiments [26]. By using a cell viability assay, the concentration range of the tested extracts and markers was also optimized (Figure S2). The results revealed that all AR extracts could dose-dependently protect the cells against oxidative insult (Figure 3A). Among the three extracts, AR_{water} possessed the best protective effects up to over 60% as compared with the control, while AR_{EtOH50} and AR_{EtOH90} showed almost identical effects corresponding to ~40% compared to the control. Consistent with the protection effects, the AR extracts could dose-dependently decrease tBHP-induced ROS formation: AR_{water} showed the greatest inhibitory effect corresponding to ~42%, as compared with those of the control and of the other extracts (Figure 3B).

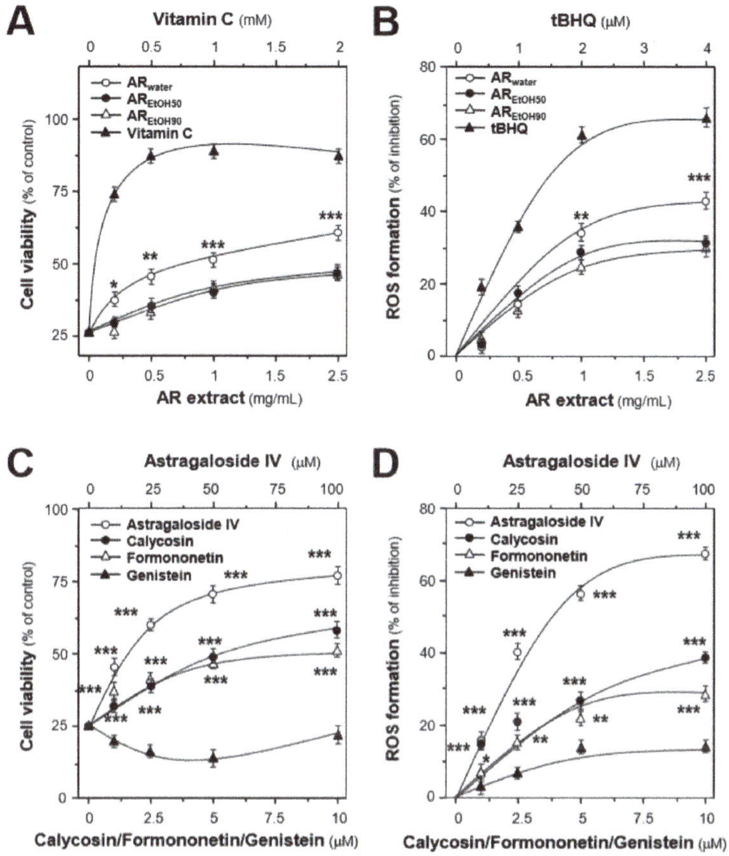

Figure 3. Protection effects of the AR extracts and major compounds in H9C2 cells against oxidative stress. (**A**) The dose-dependent response was determined by pre-treating the cultures with AR extracts (batch AR-1), i.e., water extract of AR (AR_{water}), 50% ethanol extract of AR (AR_{EtOH50}), and 90% ethanol extract of AR (AR_{EtOH90}) for 24 h before the addition of tBHP (150 μM). Vitamin C at various concentrations served as a positive control. (**B**) Cultured H9C2 cells were pre-treated with the AR extracts or *tert*-butyl hydroquinone (tBHQ) for 24 h and then exposed to tBHP (150 μM) for 1 h. The result is in percentage of ROS formation relative to the tBHP-treated control. (**C**) Cultured H9C2 cells were treated with the AR major compounds for 24 h before the addition of tBHP (150 μM). Then, the cell viability was recorded. (**D**) The effects of the chosen markers on ROS formation were compared in tBHP-treated cardiomyocytes. All data are expressed as mean ± SD, $n = 5$, each with triplicate samples. Statistical comparison was made with the sample with the lowest value of the corresponding concentration, * $p < 0.05$, ** $p < 0.01$, *** $p < 0.001$.

The protective effects of the four chemical markers in stressed cells were also evaluated. Apart from genistein, the three compounds could dose-dependently increase cell survival (Figure 3C). Astragaloside IV showed the best protective effects of ~76%, compared with calycosin (~58%) and formononetin (~51%). Genistein showed slight inhibitory effects on tBHP-induced ROS formation.

Among the tested markers, astragaloside IV possessed the best inhibitory effect of ~68%, which was consistent with the enhancement of cell viability (Figure 3D).

To further investigate the effects of AR chemicals on mitochondrial integrity, the mitochondrial membrane potential was measured. As shown in Figure 4, H9C2 cells incubated with astragaloside IV showed a significant slower fluorescence decay rate, as compared with the control during the first 20 min, resulting in a mitochondrial membrane potential ~1.3-fold higher at the end of the recording. Similar to astragaloside IV, calycosin also showed a higher mitochondrial membrane potential throughout the observation process. However, formononetin and genistein both gradually and significantly decreased the mitochondrial membrane potential in H9C2 cells. Furthermore, the concentration-dependent effects of these compounds on the mitochondrial membrane potential were also revealed (Figure 4). By comparing with the mitochondrial membrane potential of the control at 60 min, astragaloside IV and calycosin could dose-dependently increase the mitochondrial membrane potential in cultured H9C2 cells, while formononetin and genistein showed a downward trend.

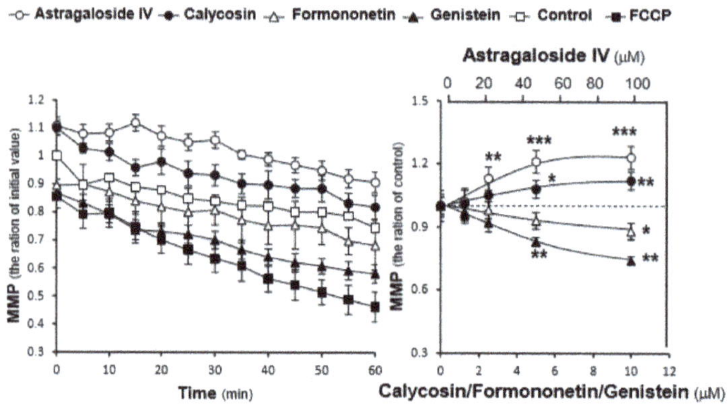

Figure 4. AR compounds regulate the mitochondrial membrane potential of H9C2 cells. Pretreated in 96-well black multi-well plates with a clear bottom for 24 h, H9C2 cells were stained with JC-1 and then washed with PBS-A twice. After adding the indicated concentration of compounds in the wells, the fluorescence of JC-1 aggregates in each sample was measured every 5 min for 60 min at 37 °C. Here, carbonyl cyanide-p trifluoromethoxyphenylhydrazone (FCCP, 100 μM) was used as the positive control. Time course of markers-induced changes in the mitochondrial membrane potential in H9C2 cells (**left panel**). The data are expressed as the ratio of fluorescence intensity of JC-1 aggregates to the respective initial (i.e., 0 min) value. The values given are mean ± SD, with $n = 3$. The dose-dependent effects of the chosen markers on the mitochondrial membrane potential were recorded (**right panel**). The data are expressed as the ratio of fluorescence intensity of JC-1 aggregates to the corresponding value of the control at 60 min. The values given are mean ± SD, with $n = 3$. Statistical comparison was made with the control, * $p < 0.05$, ** $p < 0.01$, *** $p < 0.001$.

2.3. *Effects of the AR Extracts and Compounds on Mitochondrial Bioenergetics*

By using a Seahorse extracellular flux analyzer, the effects of the AR extracts, i.e., AR_{water}, AR_{EtOH50} and AR_{EtOH90}, on the OCR of tBHP-treated H9C2 cells were plotted against time. The profile of the OCR in tBHP-treated H9C2 cells was obtained and appeared to be altered by treatments with the various AR extracts (Figure 5). According to the conversion relationship (Figure S3) [26], various parameters of mitochondrial bioenergetics, i.e., basal respiration, proton leak, mitochondrial ATP production, spare respiratory capacity, maximal respiration, and non-mitochondrial respiration, were evaluated (Figure 6). All AR extracts could dose-dependently increase basal respiration, proton leak, maximal respiration, and non-mitochondrial respiration to different degrees (Figure 6).

Among these responses, AR_{EtOH50} induced the greatest increase in basal respiration, proton leak, and non-mitochondrial respiration; the increase was from 1.6 to 2 folds at the maximum concentration. AR_{water} only increased basal respiration, proton leak, and non-mitochondrial respiration from 1.2 to 1.3 folds, which was significantly lower than compared to AR_{EtOH50}. Similarly, the effects of AR_{water} were totally different from those of AR_{EtOH50} and AR_{EtOH90} with respect to mitochondrial ATP production and spare respiratory capacity. AR_{water} could dose-dependently increase mitochondrial ATP production and spare respiratory capacity up to ~1.5 folds, while AR_{EtOH50} and AR_{EtOH90} showed no difference. Although AR_{water} and AR_{EtOH50} showed opposite effects on mitochondrial ATP production, spare respiratory capacity, and proton leak, both extracts showed a considerable induction of maximal respiration, which was significantly higher than that observed for AR_{EtOH90}.

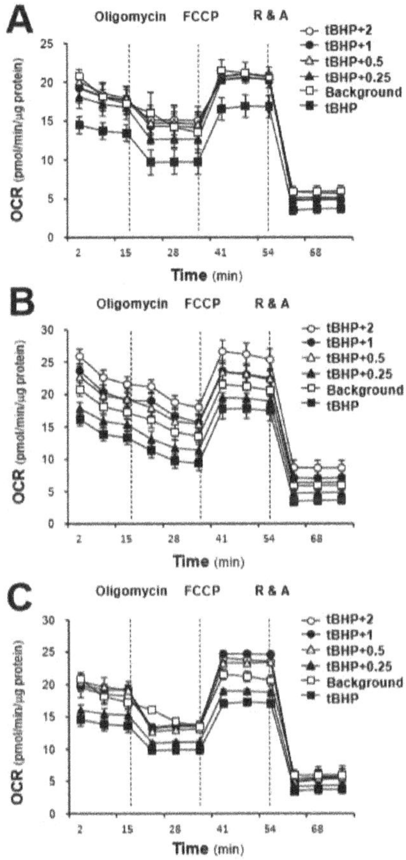

Figure 5. The AR extracts modulate the mitochondrial bioenergetics of H9C2 cells. Cultured H9C2 cells were treated with the AR extracts (from 0.25 to 2 mg/mL as indicated) for 24 h before measuring the oxygen consumption rate (OCR) with the XFp Cell Mito Stress Test. The responses of H9C2 cells after oligomycin (1 μM), FCCP (3 μM), and rotenone/antimycin A (R&A at 1 μM) treatments were recorded. The dotted lines denote the times at which the three inhibitors were applied. Effects of various extracts of AR: (**A**) water extract of AR, (**B**) 50% ethanol extract of AR, (**C**) 90% ethanol extract of AR, at various concentrations on the OCR for four respiration states of H9C2 cells are shown. The OCR values were normalized with respect to the cellular protein content/well. The background are the untreated cell. The data are expressed as mean ± SD, $n = 3$; each experiment was performed with triplicate samples.

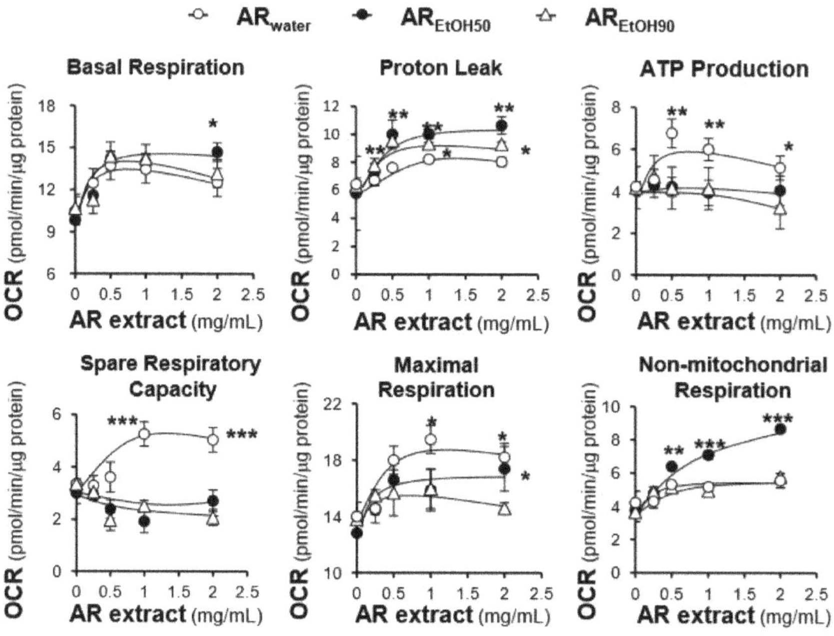

Figure 6. Various parameters of mitochondrial respiration in AR-treated H9C2 cells are compared. Cultured H9C2 cells were treated as in Figure 5. The effects of increasing concentration of AR extracts on basal respiration, proton leak, mitochondrial ATP production, spare respiratory capacity, maximal respiration, non-mitochondrial respiration were measured and compared amongst the three AR extracts. The OCR values were normalized with respect to the cellular protein content. The data are expressed as mean ± SD, $n = 3$, each with triplicate samples. Statistical comparison was made with the sample with the lowest value of the corresponding concentration, * $p < 0.05$, ** $p < 0.01$, *** $p < 0.001$.

Furthermore, the effects of the major compounds of AR on the stressed cells were also determined. On the basis of their effects on the mitochondrial membrane potential, astragaloside IV and genistein, representing two different responses, were selected for the determination of their effects on mitochondrial bioenergetics. Compared with the AR extracts, astragaloside IV and genistein altered the OCR profile of tBHP-treated H9C2 cells dose-dependently and more robustly than the AR extracts (Figure 7). However, their effects on these specific parameters were totally different. Pre-treatment with astragaloside IV at 100 μM of tBHP-treated H9C2 cells increased mitochondrial ATP production of ~1.5 folds and the spare respiratory capacity of ~2 folds, compared with the control, while it showed a negligible impact on proton leak, resulting in a slight increase in basal respiration and a significant increase in maximal respiration (Figure 8). In contrast, genistein at 10 μM increased the proton leak up to ~1.7 folds and decreased mitochondrial ATP production to ~50% and the spare respiratory capacity to ~60%, as compared with the control, which resulted in a slight increase in basal respiration and maximal respiration (Figure 8). Moreover, both compounds could dose-dependently increase the non-mitochondrial respiration to different degrees.

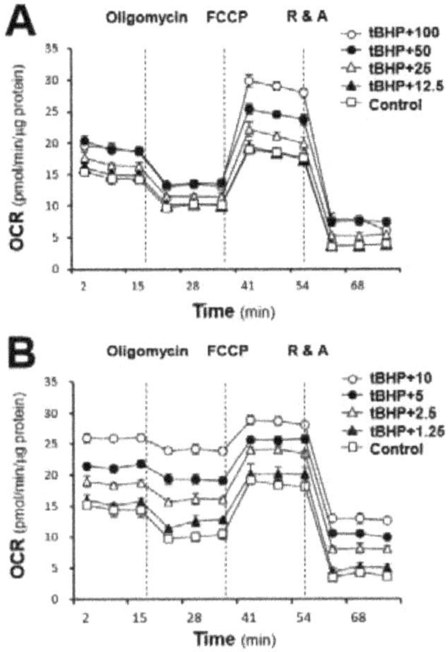

Figure 7. Effects of the major compounds of AR, i.e., (**A**) astragaloside IV and (**B**) genistein, on tBHP-treated H9C2 cells against oxidative stress. Cultured H9C2 cells were pre-treated with astragaloside IV (0–100 µM) and genistein (0–10 µM) for 24 h before being exposed to tBHP (30 µM) for 1 h. The OCR values were normalized with respect to the cellular protein content. The control was tBHP-treated cultures. The data are expressed as mean ± SD, $n = 3$, each with triplicate samples.

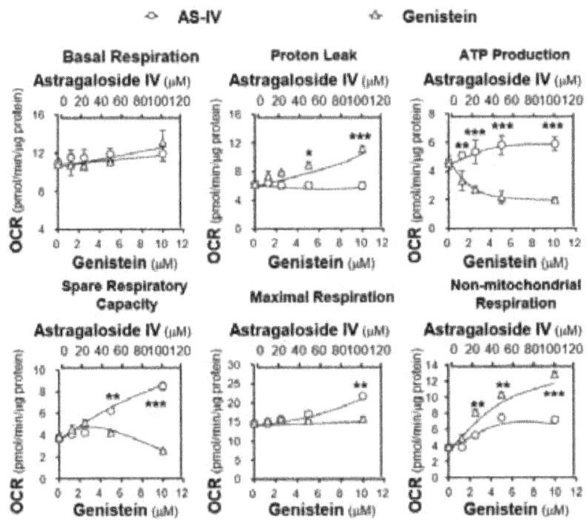

Figure 8. Mitochondrial respiration in tBHP-treated H9C2 cells after pre-treatment with astragaloside IV and genistein. Cultured H9C2 cells were treated as in Figure 7. The basal respiration, proton leak, mitochondrial ATP production, spare respiratory capacity, maximal respiration, non-mitochondrial respiration were measured. The OCR values were normalized with respect to the cellular protein content/well by the Bradford's method. The data are expressed as mean ± SD, $n = 3$, each with triplicate samples. Statistical comparison was made with the sample with the lowest value of the corresponding concentration, * $p < 0.05$, ** $p < 0.01$, *** $p < 0.001$.

3. Discussion

AR is well known for its "Qi-invigorating" action in Chinse medicine and is classified as a top-grade herb in *Shen Nong Ben Cao Jing* [10]. Being the major active compounds of AR, astragalosides and isoflavonoids are generally used as standard chemicals for quality control of AR. Here, simultaneous quantification of four major compounds, i.e., calycosin, astragaloside IV, formononetin, and genistein, in three different polar extracts of AR were performed with LC–MS. The contents of astragaloside IV and calycosin in a water extract of AR were higher than in ethanol extracts, which might be due to the highly polar structures of these compounds [27]. Oppositely, formononetin and genistein were present in higher amounts in the ethanol extracts, especially in the 50% ethanol extract [28]. On the basis of the different content of these compounds, different polar extracts could be obviously classified by PCA, and the distribution of the extracts in the PCA scoring plot was highly consistent with the amounts of the major compounds in the loading plot. These results revealed that the chemical composition of AR extracts might differ a lot when different polar solvents are used for AR extraction.

The total phenolic compound content and free radical scavenging activity of the extracts were determined, to have a rough estimation of the extracts' antioxidant activity. However, the extracts with the most abundant phenolic compounds did not show the best free radical scavenging activity, suggesting that different phenolic compounds might have greatly different antioxidant activity. Thus, the protective effects of the AR extracts and major compounds in cultured H9C2 cells against tBHP-induced oxidative stress were determined. Consistent with their free radical scavenging activity, the water extract showed the best protection in cells exposed to oxidative stress as a result of its inhibitory effects on tBHP-induced ROS. Among the selected AR compounds, astragaloside IV possessed the best protective effects in cultured cells against ROS formation. Interestingly, although genistein showed no influence on cell viability, it could slightly decrease the amount of intracellular ROS. Thus, genistein effect was proposed to be closely related to its effects on mitochondrial permeability transition pore and uncoupling proteins [29]. These results were further confirmed by the analysis of the mitochondrial membrane potential, which was established by determining the different proton concentrations inside and outside the mitochondrial inner membrane [30].

Because of its central role in energy homeostasis, metabolism, signaling, and apoptosis, research on mitochondria is enduring [31]. However, the previous experimental approaches to study mitochondria bioenergetics mainly considered isolated mitochondria, which could result in increased ROS, or other lesions, due to different infiltration environments [32]. Here, the extracellular flux analyzers enabled us to monitor the real-time mitochondrial respiration in live cells, greatly enhancing the credibility of our results [33]. The application of this technology to the AR extracts or to their components is still very limited. Here, only the water extracts of AR showed a dose-dependent enhancement of the spare respiratory capacity and mitochondrial ATP production, which might be due to the high content of tonic compounds in these extracts. This hypothesis was supported by measuring the effects of astragaloside IV and genistein on mitochondrial bioenergetics. In 2015, Lu et al. (2015) found that astragaloside IV could significantly increase mitochondrial OCR and ATP production in vascular smooth muscle cells [34]. Later on, Dong et al. (2017) revealed that the enhancement by astragaloside IV of ATP production was triggered by the stimulation of fatty acid α-oxidation and the inhibition of excessive activation of mitochondrial Ca^{2+} uniporter [35]. Consistent with these studies, the current results showed that astragaloside IV could effectively restore the spare respiratory capacity and ATP production in tBHP-treated cardiomyocytes. Different from astragaloside IV, the effects of genistein on ATP production is still difficult to interpret. According to Rasbach et al. (2008), the treatment of genistein upregulated the expression of PGC-1α and ATP synthase β, which resulted in an increase in O_2 consumption and ATP production in renal proximal tubule cells [36]. However, Zheng et al. (2000) reported a non-competitive inhibitory action of genistein on mitochondrial proton F0F1-ATPase/ATP synthase in rat brain and liver preparations, and, as such, ATP production was reduced [37]. Genistein has been proposed for the treatment of cancer, neurodegeneration, and cardiovascular and endocrine diseases; however, a detail study of genistein-mediated regulation of redox biology and mitochondrial biogenesis is still missing [17]. Here, we showed that genistein possessed small or even negative effects on the spare respiratory capacity and mitochondrial ATP production, while it could dose-dependently increase proton leak. This explained the reduction of intracellular ROS after treatment with genistein. All in all, the opposite effects of compounds like astragaloside IV and genistein on mitochondrial bioenergetics could be the reason for the different effects of the various AR extracts.

In summary, the present research provides a comprehensive investigation of the antioxidant activity of AR extracts and of their effects on mitochondrial bioenergetics. To explain the difference of the tonic effects between water extracts and ethanol extracts, a further study of the major components, i.e., astragaloside IV and genistein, was conducted. The results revealed that astragaloside IV showed significant tonic effects in cells exposed to oxidative stress by dose-dependently increasing the spare respiratory capacity and mitochondrial ATP production, while genistein mainly induced proton leak.

4. Materials and Methods

4.1. Chemicals and Preparation of the RA Extracts

High performance liquid chromatography (HPLC)-grade acetonitrile and ethanol were bought from Merck (Darmstadt, Germany). Ultra-pure water was obtained from a Milli-Q purification system (Millipore, Molsheim, France). Formic acid was purchased from Riedel-de Haen International (Honeywell, Hanover, Germany). The chemical standards of calycosin, astragaloside IV, genistein, and formononetin were purchased from National Institute for the Control of Pharmaceutical and Biological Products (Beijing, China). The purity of these chemical markers was over 98%. Three batches of dried raw materials of *Astragali Radix* (AR; root of *A. membranaceus* var. *mongholicus*) were bought from Shanxi Province of China and then authenticated by Tina Dong at The Hong Kong University of Science and Technology (HKUST), according to the established morphological characteristics. The voucher specimens were stored in the Centre for Chinese Medicine R&D at HKUST. The water extracts (AR_{water}), 50% ethanol extracts (AR_{EtOH50}), and 90% ethanol extracts (AR_{EtOH90}) of RA were prepared using a standardized extraction method. Briefly, 4 grams of the powdered sample were refluxed in 100 mL of solvent for two times (each time for 2 h); the supernatants were combined and then dried under vacuum.

4.2. Standardization of Herbal Extracts

The measurement of chemicals in AR_{water}, AR_{EtOH50}, and AR_{EtOH90} was performed in an Agilent HPLC 1200 series system (Agilent, Waldbronn, Germany), which was equipped with a degasser, a binary pump, an auto sampler, a thermostated column compartment, and a diode array detector (DAD). The samples were separated on an Agilent ZORBAX Eclipse XDB-C18 column (1.8 μm i.d., 50 mm × 4.6 mm; Agilent, Waldbronn, Germany) after filtration with a guard column. The mobile phase was composed of 0.1% formic acid in acetonitrile (A) and 0.1% formic acid in water (B), according to the pre-set gradient program: 0–3 min, linear gradient 20.0–30.0% (A); 3–8 min, linear gradient 30.0–50.0% (A); 8–10 min, isocratic gradient 50.0–50.0% (A); 10–18 min, linear gradient 50.0–58.0% (A), 18–25 min, linear gradient 58.0–80.0% (A). A pre-balance period of 5 min was used between each run. The injection volume was 5 μL, and the flow rate was set at 0.4 mL/min. To get the fingerprints of the AR extracts, the wavelength of a ultraviolet (UV) detector was set to 254 nm with full spectral scanning from 190 to 400 nm. For the MS/MS analysis, an Agilent triple quadrupole tandem mass spectrometry (QQQ-MS/MS, 6410A) equipped with an electron spray ionization (ESI) ion source was operated in negative ion mode. The temperature and the flow of drying gas were set to 325 °C and 10 L/min, respectively. The delta electro multiplier voltage was set to 400 V, and the capillary voltage was set to 4000 V. Two transition pairs were chosen for acquisition in MRM mode for the chemical standards and the internal standard ginsenoside Rg1. The collision energy value and fragmentor voltage were optimized in advance to obtain the highest abundance.

4.3. Cell Culture

H9C2 cell, a cardiomyocyte cell line, was obtained from American Type Culture Collection (ATCC, Manassas, VA, USA). H9C2 cells were grown in high-glucose Dulbecco's modified Eagle's medium (DMEM), supplemented with 10% fetal bovine serum (FBS) and 100 units/mL penicillin/streptomycin in a humidified CO_2 (5%) incubator at 37 °C. The culture reagents were purchased from Invitrogen Technologies (Carlsbad, CA, USA). The culture medium was replaced every 2–3 days, and the cells were grown to 80–90% confluence for experimental use.

4.4. Cell Viability

Cell viability was measured by the 3-(4,5-dimethylthiazol-2-yl)-2,5-diphenyltetra-zolium bromide (MTT; Sigma-Aldrich, St Louis, MO, USA) assay. The cells were seeded in 96-well plates at a density of 1×10^4 cells per well. After 24 h of drug treatment, the cells in each well were incubated with 10 μL MTT (5 mg/mL, Invitrogen) at a final concentration of 0.5 mg/mL for 2 h at 37 °C. After the solution was removed, DMSO was used to re-suspend the purple precipitate inside the cells, and the absorbance was detected at 570 nm. The cell viability was calculated as percentage of the absorbance value of the control (without drug treatment), while the value of the control was 100%.

4.5. Folin–Ciocalteu Assay

The total phenolic content of the AR extracts was measured with the Folin–Ciocalteu assay. To be specific, 20 μL of each extract together with 40 μL 10% (*v*/*v*) of Folin–Ciocalteu reagent (Sigma-Aldrich) was added into each well of a 96-well microplate. Then, 160 μL Na_2CO_3 (700 mM) was added into each well. The assay plates were incubated at room temperature in the dark for 2 h, and then the absorbance at 765 nm was recorded. Here, gallic acid (Sigma-Aldrich, >98%) was used as the reference compound, and the total phenolic content of each extract was expressed in comparison to gallic acid.

4.6. DPPH Radical Scavenging Assay

The free radical scavenging activity of the herbal extracts was measured with the DPPH radical scavenging assay. Briefly, 50 μL of each extract at different concentrations (0–8 mg/mL) was mixed with 150 μL of DPPH solution in each well of a 96-well microplate. After standing for 10 min, the absorbance at 517 nm was recorded. The DPPH free radical scavenging activity was calculated as an inhibition percentage based on the following equation: Inhibition (%) = $100 \times (A_0 - A_1)/A_0$, where A_0 is the absorbance of the control, and A_1 is the absorbance of the AR sample aliquot. Here, gallic acid (0–100 μM) was used as a positive control.

4.7. tBHP-Induced Oxidative Stress Assay

The doses of tBHP (150 μM; Sigma-Aldrich, St. Louis, MO, USA) and of the positive control (vitamin C, 1 mM; Sigma-Aldrich, St. Louis, MO, USA) were optimized with the MTT assay. Similar to the cell viability assay, the cells were cultured in a 96-well plate first. After drug treatment for 24 h, tBHP (150 μM) was added into the wells for 3 h, before MTT, at a final concentration of 0.5 mg/mL, was added. After the solution was removed, the purple precipitate inside the cells was resuspended in DMSO and then measured at 570 nm wavelength.

4.8. ROS Formation Assay

The measurement of ROS content in the cell cultures was performed by using 2′,7′-dichlorofluorescin diacetate (DCFH-DA), an oxidation-sensitive dye. Cultured H9C2 cells (1×10^4 cells/well) in a 96-well plate were pre-treated with the herbal extracts or the standard compounds for 24 h, and the cells were labeled with 100 μM DCFH-DA (Sigma-Aldrich, St. Louis, MO, USA) in HBSS (Hank's Balanced Salt Solution, Sigma-Aldrich, St. Louis, MO, USA) for 1 h at 37 °C. After washing three times with HBSS, the cells were treated with 150 μM tBHP for 1 h at 37 °C. Then, the amount of intracellular tBHP-induced ROS formation was detected by a fluorometric measurement with excitation at 485 nm and emission at 530 nm.

4.9. Measurement of the Mitochondrial Membrane Potential

The mitochondrial membrane potential of tBHP-treated H9C2 cells was determined using JC-1 (5,5′,6,6′-tetrachloro-1,1′,3,3′-tetraethylbenzimidazolyl-carbocyanine iodide; Sigma-Aldrich, St. Louis, MO, USA), a fluorescent probe. H9C2 cells were cultured on a 96-well black multiwell plate with a clear bottom for 24 h. After staining with JC-1, the cells were washed twice with PBS-A and incubated with the examined compounds. The fluorescence of JC-1 aggregates in each sample was measured at an excitation wavelength of 527 nm and an emission wavelength of 590 nm every 5 min for 60 min at 37 °C. Carbonyl cyanide-p trifluoromethoxyphenylhydrazone (FCCP, 100 μM; Sigma-Aldrich, St. Louis, MO, USA), a chemical uncoupler, was used as the positive control. The data were expressed as the ratio of fluorescence intensity of JC-1 aggregates at different time points relative to the initial (i.e., 0 min) value.

4.10. Mitochondrial Bioenergetic Analysis

The mitochondrial bioenergetics of H9C2 cells was measured using a Seahorse Bioscience XFp extracellular flux analyzer (Agilent, Santa Clara, CA, USA), which could measure the real-time oxygen consumption by mitochondria in live cells. According to previous research, the seeding density of H9C2 cell was optimized at 5000 cells per well, and mitochondrial agents (Seahorse Bioscience Cell Mito Stress Test Kit #103010-100; North Billerica, MA, USA) were pre-optimized to elicit the maximal effects on mitochondrial respiration as follows: 1 μM oligomycin (complex V inhibitor), 3 μM FCCP (a respiratory uncoupler), and 1 μM rotenone/antimycin A (inhibitors of complex I and complex III). Background correction wells were used to normalize the data to the background noise. Cultured H9C2 cells were seeded on the XFp cell culture mini-plates and treated with the AR extracts and compounds for 24 h. After the drug treatment, the sensor cartridge of the XFp analyzer was hydrated in a non-CO_2 incubator at 37 °C. Before sensor calibration, the cells were treated with 30 μM tBHP for 1 h and then incubated at 37 °C in a non-CO_2 incubator in XF Base Medium (10 mM glucose, 1 mM pyruvate and 2 mM L-glutamine, pH 7.4) for another 1 h. After calibrating the sensor, the plate was placed onto the XFp extracellular flux analyzer for Mito Stress Test. The OCR was recorded over time and normalized to cellular protein content/well and corrected for extra mitochondrial O_2 consumption. All experiments were repeated four times. Eventually, six parameters of mitochondrial function were calculated from the bioenergetics profile: basal respiration, ATP production, proton leak, maximal respiration, spare respiration capacity, and non-mitochondrial respiration.

4.11. Statistical Analysis

Quantitative data acquisition and processing were conducted using Agilent Mass Hunter workstation software version B.01.00 (Agilent Technologies Inc., Santa Clara, CA, USA). Principal component analysis (PCA) of the peak areas of the standard compounds was performed using SIMCA-P version 12.0 (Umetrics, Umeå, Sweden). The resultant bioenergetics profiles were analyzed with Wave Desktop 2.3.0 (Seahorse Bioscience, North Billerica, MA, USA). All data were expressed as the mean ± SEM for n = 3 to 5, unless otherwise specified. Statistical tests were performed by one-way ANOVA with multiple comparisons using Dunnett's test. Differences were considered significant at $p < 0.05$.

Supplementary Materials: Supplementary materials can be found at http://www.mdpi.com/1422-0067/19/6/1574/s1.

Acknowledgments: This work was supported by Hong Kong Research Grants Council Theme-based Research Scheme (T13-607/12R), General Research Funding (663012, 662713, M-HKUST604/13), TUYF15SC01, Shenzhen Science and Technology Committee Research Grant (CKFW2016082916015476, JCYJ20170413173747440, ZDSYS201707281432317, JCYJ20160229205726699, JCYJ20160229205812004, JCYJ20160229210027564 and 20170326).

Author Contributions: Karl Wah Keung Tsim and Tina Ting Xia Dong conceived and designed the experiments; Yun Huang performed the experiments, analyzed the results, and made figures and tables;

Kenneth Kin Leung Kwan performed the experiments; Ka Wing Leung, Huaiyou Wang, and Xiang Peng Kong contributed to designing the experiments; Karl Wah Keung Tsim and Yun Huang wrote the paper.

Conflicts of Interest: The authors declare no conflict of interest.

References

1. Lin, H.Q.; Gong, A.G.W.; Wang, H.Y.; Duan, R.; Dong, T.T.X.; Zhao, K.J.; Tsim, K.W.K. Danggui Buxue Tang (Astragali Radix and Angelicae Sinensis Radix) for menopausal symptoms: A review. *J. Ethnopharmacol.* **2017**, *199*, 205–210. [CrossRef] [PubMed]
2. Leong, P.K.; Wong, H.S.; Chen, J.H.; Ko, K.M. Yang/Qi invigoration: An herbal therapy for chronic fatigue syndrome with Yang deficiency? *Evid. Based Complement. Altern.* **2015**, *2015*, 945901. [CrossRef] [PubMed]
3. Zhang, R.P.; Zhang, X.P.; Ruan, Y.F.; Ye, S.Y.; Zhao, H.C.; Cheng, Q.H.; Wu, D.J. Protective effect of Radix Astragali injection on immune organs of rats with obstructive jaundice and its mechanism. *World J. Gastroenterol.* **2009**, *15*, 2862–2869. [CrossRef] [PubMed]
4. Wang, P.; Zhang, Z.; Ma, X.; Huang, Y.; Liu, X.; Tu, P.; Tong, T. HDTIC-1 and HDTIC-2, two compounds extracted from Astragali Radix, delay replicative senescence of human diploid fibroblasts. *Mech. Ageing Dev.* **2003**, *124*, 1025–1034. [CrossRef] [PubMed]
5. Chu, C.; Qi, L.W.; Liu, E.H.; Li, B.; Gao, W.; Li, P. Radix Astragali (Astragalus): Latest advancements and trends in chemistry, analysis, pharmacology and pharmacokinetics. *Curr. Org. Chem.* **2010**, *14*, 1792–1807. [CrossRef]
6. Luo, Z.; Zhong, L.; Han, X.; Wang, H.; Zhong, J.; Xuan, Z. *Astragalus membranaceus* prevents daunorubicin-induced apoptosis of cultured neonatal cardiomyocytes: Role of free radical effect of *Astragalus membranaceus* on daunorubicin cardiotoxicity. *Phytother. Res.* **2009**, *23*, 761–767. [CrossRef] [PubMed]
7. Huang, X.; Liu, Y.; Song, F.; Liu, Z.; Liu, S. Studies on principal components and antioxidant activity of different Radix Astragali samples using high-performance liquid chromatography/electrospray ionization multiple-stage tandem mass spectrometry. *Talanta* **2009**, *78*, 1090–1101. [CrossRef] [PubMed]
8. Hasan, A.; Sadiq, A.; Abbas, A.; Mughal, E.; Khan, K.M.; Ali, M. Isolation and synthesis of flavonols and comparison of their antioxidant activity. *Nat. Prod. Res.* **2010**, *24*, 995–1003. [CrossRef] [PubMed]
9. Zhang, L.J.; Liu, H.K.; Hsiao, P.C.; Yang Kuo, L.M.; Lee, I.J.; Wu, T.S.; Chiou, W.F.; Kuo, Y.H. New isoflavonoid glycosides and related constituents from Astragali Radix (*Astragalus membranaceus*) and their inhibitory activity on nitric oxide production. *J. Agric. Food Chem.* **2011**, *59*, 1131–1137. [CrossRef] [PubMed]
10. Fu, J.; Wang, Z.H.; Huang, L.F.; Zheng, S.H.; Wang, D.M.; Chen, S.L.; Zhang, H.T.; Yang, S.H. Review of the botanical characteristics, phytochemistry, and pharmacology of *Astragalus membranaceus* (Huangqi). *Phytother. Res.* **2014**, *28*, 1275–1283. [CrossRef] [PubMed]
11. Zhou, Y.; Hirotani, M.; Lui, K.H.; Furuya, T. Two triglycosidic triterpene astragalosides from hairy root cultures of *Astragalus membranaceus*. *Phytochemistry* **1994**, *38*, 1407–1410. [CrossRef]
12. Dong, Z.W.; Zhang, C.; Chen, Y.J.; Chen, Y.; Yuan, Z.Q.; Peng, Y.Z.; Cao, T.T. Astragaloside-IV protects against heat-induced apoptosis by inhibiting excessive activation of mitochondrial Ca^{2+} uniporter. *Cell. Physiol. Biochem.* **2017**, *42*, 480–494. [CrossRef] [PubMed]
13. Liu, B.; Zhang, J.Z.; Liu, W.H.; Liu, N.N.; Fu, X.Q.; Kwan, H.Y.; Liu, S.J.; Liu, B.R.; Zhang, S.W.; Yu, Z.L.; et al. Calycosin inhibits oxidative stress-induced cardiomyocyte apoptosis via activating estrogen receptor-α/β. *Bioorg. Med. Chem. Lett.* **2016**, *26*, 181–185. [CrossRef] [PubMed]
14. Cheng, Y.Y.; Xia, Z.Y.; Han, Y.F.; Rong, J.H. Plant natural product formononetin protects rat cardiomyocyte H9c2 cells against oxygen glucose deprivation and reoxygenation via inhibiting ROS formation and promoting GSK-3β phosphorylation. *Oxid. Med. Cell. Longev.* **2016**, *2016*, 2060874. [CrossRef] [PubMed]
15. Huang, W.J.; Bi, L.Y.; Li, Z.Z.; Zhang, X.; Ye, Y. Formononetin induces the mitochondrial apoptosis pathway in prostate cancer cells via downregulation of the IGF-1/IGF-1R signaling pathway. *Pharm. Biol.* **2014**, *52*, 466–470. [CrossRef] [PubMed]
16. Russo, M.; Russo, G.L.; Daglia, M.; Kasi, P.D.; Ravi, S.; Nabavi, S.F.; Nabavi, S.M. Understanding genistein in cancer: The "good" and the "bad" effects: A review. *Food Chem.* **2016**, *196*, 589–600. [CrossRef] [PubMed]
17. De Oliveira, M.R. Evidence for genistein as a mitochondriotropic molecule. *Mitochondrion* **2016**, *29*, 35–44. [CrossRef] [PubMed]
18. Kang, D.G.; Yun, C.K.; Lee, H.S. Screening and comparison of antioxidant activity of solvent extracts of herbal medicines used in Korea. *J. Ethnopharmacol.* **2003**, *87*, 231–236. [CrossRef]

19. Navarro, A.; Boveris, A. The mitochondrial energy transduction system and the aging process. *Am. J. Physiol. Cell Physiol.* **2007**, *292*, 670–686. [CrossRef] [PubMed]
20. Brookes, P.S. Mitochondrial H^+ leak and ROS generation: An odd couple. *Free Radic. Biol. Med.* **2005**, *38*, 12–23. [CrossRef] [PubMed]
21. Dott, W.; Mistry, P.; Wright, J.; Cain, K.; Herbert, K.E. Modulation of mitochondrial bioenergetics in a skeletal muscle cell line model of mitochondrial toxicity. *Redox Biol.* **2014**, *2*, 224–233. [CrossRef] [PubMed]
22. Wu, M.; Neilson, A.; Swift, A.L.; Moran, R.; Tamagnine, J.; Parslow, D.; Armistead, S.; Lemire, K.; Orrell, J.; Teich, J.; et al. Multiparameter metabolic analysis reveals a close link between attenuated mitochondrial bioenergetic function and enhanced glycolysis dependency in human tumor cells. *Am. J. Physiol. Cell Physiol.* **2007**, *292*, 125–136. [CrossRef] [PubMed]
23. Li, H.X.; Han, S.Y.; Ma, X.; Zhang, K.; Wang, L.; Ma, Z.Z.; Tu, P.F. The saponin of red ginseng protects the cardiacmyocytes against ischemic injury in vitro and in vivo. *Phytomedicine* **2012**, *19*, 477–483. [CrossRef] [PubMed]
24. Wu, H.W.; Fang, J.; Tang, L.Y.; Lu, P.; Xu, H.Y.; Zhao, Y.; Li, D.F.; Zhang, Y.; Fu, M.H.; Yang, H.J. Quality evaluation of Astragali Radix based on DPPH radical scavenging activity and chemical analysis. *Chin. Herb. Med.* **2014**, *6*, 282–289. [CrossRef]
25. Zheng, K.Y.Z.; Choi, R.C.Y.; Guo, A.J.Y.; Bi, C.W.C.; Zhu, K.Y.; Du, C.Y.Q.; Zhang, Z.X.; Lau, D.T.W.; Dong, T.T.X.; Tsim, K.W.K. The membrane permeability of Astragali Radix-derived formononetin and calycosin is increased by Angelicae Sinensis Radix in Caco-2 cells: A synergistic action of an ancient herbal decoction Danggui Buxue Tang. *J. Pharm. Biomed.* **2012**, *70*, 671–679. [CrossRef] [PubMed]
26. Huang, Y.; Kwan, K.K.L.; Leung, K.W.; Yao, P.; Wang, H.Y.; Dong, T.T.X.; Tsim, K.W.K. Ginseng extracts modulate mitochondrial bioenergetics of live cardiomyoblasts: A functional comparison of different extraction solvents. *J. Ginseng Res.* **2018**. [CrossRef]
27. Chen, C.Y.; Zu, Y.G.; Fu, Y.J.; Luo, M.; Zhao, C.J.; Wang, W.; Zhao, B.S.; Li, J.; Efferth, T. Preparation and antioxidant activity of Radix Astragali residues extracts rich in calycosin and formononetin. *Biochem. Eng. J.* **2011**, *56*, 84–93. [CrossRef]
28. Sun, J.; Jiang, Z.Z.; Yan, R.Q.; Olaleye, O.; Zhang, X.L.; Chai, X.; Wang, Y.F. Quality evaluation of Astragali Radix products by quantitative analysis of multi-components by single marker. *Chin. Herb. Med.* **2013**, *5*, 272–279. [CrossRef]
29. Yoon, H.S.; Moon, S.C.; Kim, N.D.; Park, B.S.; Jeong, M.H.; Yoo, Y.H. Genistein induces apoptosis of RPE-J cells by opening mitochondrial PTP. *Biochem. Biophys. Res. Commun.* **2000**, *276*, 151–156. [CrossRef] [PubMed]
30. Perry, S.W.; Norman, J.P.; Barbieri, J.; Brown, E.B.; Gelbard, H.A. Mitochondrial membrane potential probes and the proton gradient: A practical usage guide. *Biotechniques* **2011**, *50*, 98–115. [CrossRef] [PubMed]
31. Peterson, C.M.; Johannsen, D.L.; Ravussin, E. Skeletal muscle mitochondria and aging: A review. *J. Aging Res.* **2012**, *2012*, 194821. [CrossRef] [PubMed]
32. Li, A.E.; Ito, H.; Rovira, I.I.; Kim, K.S.; Takeda, K.; Yu, Z.Y.; Ferrans, V.J.; Finkel, T. A role for reactive oxygen species in endothelial cell anoikis. *Circ. Res.* **1999**, *85*, 304–310. [CrossRef] [PubMed]
33. Salabei, J.K.; Gibb, A.A.; Hill, B.G. Comprehensive measurement of respiratory activity in permeabilized cells using extracellular flux analysis. *Nat. Protoc.* **2014**, *9*, 421–438. [CrossRef] [PubMed]
34. Lu, Y.; Li, S.; Wu, H.F.; Bian, Z.P.; Xu, J.D.; Gu, C.R.; Chen, X.J.; Yang, D. Beneficial effects of astragaloside IV against angiotensin II-induced mitochondrial dysfunction in rat vascular smooth muscle cells. *Int. J. Mol. Med.* **2015**, *36*, 1223–1232. [CrossRef] [PubMed]
35. Dong, Z.W.; Zhao, P.; Xu, M.; Zhang, C.; Guo, W.; Chen, H.H.; Tian, J.; Wei, H.C.; Iu, R.; Cao, T.T. Astragaloside IV alleviates heart failure via activating PPARα to switch glycolysis to fatty acid β-oxidation. *Sci. Rep.* **2017**, *7*, 2691. [CrossRef] [PubMed]
36. Rasbach, K.A.; Schnellmann, R.G. Isoflavones promote mitochondrial biogenesis. *J. Pharmacol. Exp. Ther.* **2008**, *325*, 536–543. [CrossRef] [PubMed]
37. Zheng, J.; Ramirez, V.D. Inhibition of mitochondrial proton F0F1-ATPase/ATP synthase by polyphenolic phytochemicals. *Br. J. Pharmacol.* **2000**, *130*, 1115–1123. [CrossRef] [PubMed]

International Journal of
Molecular Sciences

MDPI

Article

Neuroprotective Effects of Four Phenylethanoid Glycosides on H_2O_2-Induced Apoptosis on PC12 Cells via the Nrf2/ARE Pathway

Maiquan Li [1], Tao Xu [1], Fei Zhou [1], Mengmeng Wang [1], Huaxin Song [1], Xing Xiao [2] and Baiyi Lu [1,*]

1 National Engineering Laboratory of Intelligent Food Technology and Equipment, Key Laboratory for Agro-Products Postharvest Handling of Ministry of Agriculture and Rural Affairs, Key Laboratory for Agro-Products Nutritional Evaluation of Ministry of Agriculture and Rural Affairs, Zhejiang Key Laboratory for Agro-Food Processing, Fuli Institute of Food Science, College of Biosystems Engineering and Food Science, Zhejiang University, Hangzhou 310058, China; 11413040@zju.edu.cn (M.L.); txu@zju.edu.cn (T.X.); feizhou@zju.edu.cn (F.Z.); 11613027@zju.edu.cn (M.W.); 21713034@zju.edu.cn (H.S.)

2 College of The First Clinical Medical, Guangzhou University of Chinese Medicine, Guangzhou 510006, China; fushengmengxx@gmail.com

* Correspondence: bylu@zju.edu.cn; Tel./Fax: +86-571-8988-2665

Received: 12 March 2018; Accepted: 7 April 2018; Published: 10 April 2018

Abstract: Nuclear factor erythroid 2-related factor 2 (Nrf2) is a key transcription factor against oxidative stress and neurodegenerative disorders. Phenylethanoid glycosides (PhGs; salidroside, acteoside, isoacteoside, and echinacoside) exhibit antioxidant and neuroprotective bioactivities. This study was performed to investigate the neuroprotective effect and molecular mechanism of PhGs. PhGs pretreatment significantly suppressed H_2O_2-induced cytotoxicity in PC12 cells by triggering the nuclear translocation of Nrf2 and reversing the downregulated protein expression of heme oxygenase 1 (HO-1), NAD(P)H quinone oxidoreductase 1 (NQO1), glutamate cysteine ligase-catalytic subunit (GCLC), and glutamate-cysteine ligase modifier subunit (GCLM). Nrf2 siRNA or HO-1 inhibitor zinc protoporphyrin (ZnPP) reduced the neuroprotective effect. PhGs showed potential interaction with the Nrf2 binding site in Kelch-like ECH-association protein 1 (Keap1). This result may support the hypothesis that PhGs are activators of Nrf2. We demonstrated the potential binding between PhGs and the Keap1-activated Nrf2/ARE pathway, and that PhGs with more glycosides had enhanced effects.

Keywords: Keap1; Nrf2; Neuroprotective; PC12 cells; PhGs

1. Introduction

Oxidative stress, which is an imbalance of antioxidant homeostasis, induces lipid peroxidation, injury to protein and DNA, cell aging, and cell death. This process likely contributes to several neurodegenerative disorders, such as Alzheimer's disease (AD), Parkinson's disease (PD), and ischemia/reperfusion [1]. Hydrogen peroxide (H_2O_2), which is one of the main reactive oxygen species (ROS), is known to cause lipid peroxidation and DNA damage [2]. Moreover, H_2O_2 is an endogenous source of hydroxyl free radicals that contributes to the background level of cellular oxidative stress [3,4]. Therefore, therapeutic strategies for preventing oxidative stress-induced apoptosis may have the potential in neurodegenerative diseases treatment.

Nuclear factor erythroid 2-related factor 2 (Nrf2), is a transcription factor that is strongly associated with oxidative stress. Activation of Nrf2 induces the transcription of numerous antioxidant and detoxification genes, including heme oxygenase-1 (HO-1), NAD(P)H quinine oxidoreductase 1 (NQO1), among others [5–7]. This process represents a key step in protecting cells from oxidative stress and is emerging as a promising therapeutic target for neuroprotection [8]. Gaia reported that Nrf2 mitigates LRRK2- and α-synuclein-induced neurodegeneration by potently promoting neuronal protein homeostasis in a cell autonomous and time-dependent manner [9].

Phenylethanoid glycosides (PhGs) are characterized by cinnamic acid and hydroxylphenylethyl moieties attached to a β-glucopyranose through ester and glycosidic linkages, respectively. These molecules are members of a group of water-soluble natural products widely distributed in the plant kingdom [10]. In vitro and in vivo studies have shown that these compounds possess antioxidant [11], neuroprotective [12], antibacterial, anti-inflammatory [13], and immunomodulatory [14] bioactivities. *Osmanthus fragrans* is a common ingredient in several Asian foods and has long been consumed. We previously showed that *O. fragrans* flower extracts enhanced spatial learning and memory, inhibited oxidative damage, and exhibited neuroprotective activities in a d-galactose-induced aging in an ICR mouse model [15]. Salidroside, acteoside, and isoacteoside are the major PhGs response for the antioxidant activities of *O. fragrans* flowers extracts [16].

Studies on the neuroprotective effect of PhGs have obtained desirable results. Salidroside significantly reduced cell apoptosis of PC12 cells that was exposed in MPP^+ [17,18]. Acteoside also alleviated MPP^+-induced apoptosis and oxidative stress in PC12 cells [19] and Aβ25-35-induced SH-SY5Y cell injury [20]. Echinacoside was investigated on tumor necrosis factor-α (TNFα)-induced apoptosis in SH-SY5Y cells [21], MPTP-induced dopaminergic toxicity in mice [22], glutamate-injured primary cultures of rat cortical cells [23], and 6-OHDA-induced damage in PC12 cells [24]. The results indicated that PhGs exhibited cytoprotective effect and are potential agents to treat neurodegenerative diseases. Studies have shown the antioxidant properties of PhGs underly many other bioactivities for these compounds [25]. However, few studies have investigated the molecular mechanism of PhGs against oxidative toxicity.

In our study, we selected four typical PhGs as follows: salidroside (phenylethanoid monosaccharides), acteoside (phenylethanoid disaccharides), isoacteoside (phenylethanoid disaccharides), and echinacoside (phenylethanoid trisaccharides). We employed a model of neuronal death using differentiated PC12 cells [26] to investigate the protective effect and molecular mechanism of PhGs on H_2O_2-induced PC12 cell model. We demonstrated that PhGs activated the Nrf2/ARE pathway by binding to Kelch-like ECH-associated protein 1 (Keap1). This process upregulated the antioxidant enzymes and increased the resistance of PC12 cells to oxidative stress.

2. Results

2.1. PhGs Suppressed H_2O_2-Induced Cytotoxicity in PC12 Cells

Cytotoxic effects of H_2O_2 and PhGs (0.1, 1, 5, and 10 μg/mL) on PC12 cells were tested. The results showed that H_2O_2 induced loss of PC12 cell viability in concentration-dependent and time-dependent manners (Figure 1A). Exposure of PC12 cells to 200 μM H_2O_2 for 2 h resulted in cell viability of 57.4%. Pretreatment of cells with PhGs at 0.1, 1, 5, and 10 μg/mL had no effect on cell viability (Figure 1B) and markedly protected PC12 cells from H_2O_2-induced damage by improving the cell viability as 9.549–22.141%, 12.092–25.289%, 1.470–9.289%, and 3.411–11.441%, respectively (Figure 1C). However, salidroside (0.1 μg/mL), isoacteoside (0.1, 1, 5, and 10 μg/mL), echinacoside (0.1, 1, and 5 μg/mL) pretreatment showed no significant difference on H_2O_2-induced cell injury. Pretreatment of cells with PhGs also ameliorated the morphological characteristic induced by H_2O_2 (Figure 1D).

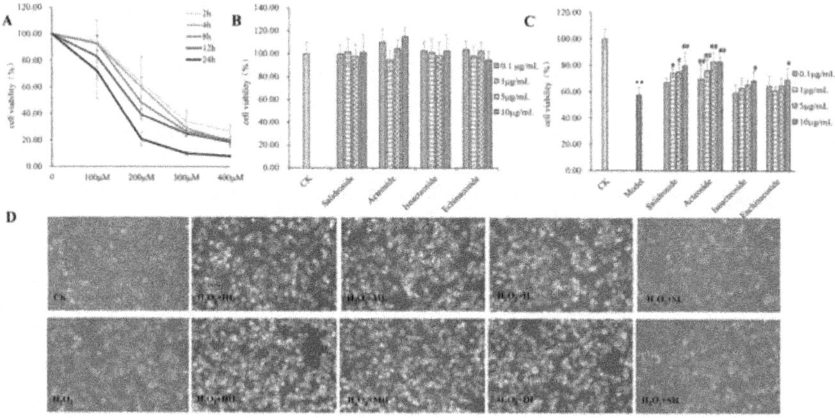

Figure 1. PhGs suppressed H_2O_2-induced cytotoxicity in PC12 cells. Cell viability was detected by MTT assay. Cytotoxic effect of H_2O_2 (**A**) and PhGs (**B**) at different concentrations on PC12 cells. (**C**) PhGs attenuated H_2O_2-induced decrease in cell viability. PC12 cells were incubated with PhGs (0.1, and 10 µg/mL) for 24 h, and then incubated with 200 µM H_2O_2 for another 2 h after the PhGs were removed. (**D**) Morphological observation. Cells after treatment were observed by a phase contrast microscope (×100), CK: normal group, H_2O_2: H_2O_2 treated group, HL: salidroside low dosage treated group, HH: salidroside high dosage treated group, ML: acteoside low dosage treated group, MH: acteoside high dosage treated group, IL: isoacteoside low dosage treated group, IH: isoacteoside high dosage treated group, SL: echinacoside low dosage treated group, SH: echinacoside high dosage treated group. ** $p < 0.01$ versus untreated group; # $p < 0.05$, versus H_2O_2 treated group; ## $p < 0.01$, versus H_2O_2 treated group.

2.2. PhGs Suppressed H_2O_2-Induced Intracellular Accumulation of ROS, Lipid Peroxidation (MDA), and Increased Superoxide Dismutase (SOD) Activities in PC12 Cells

Exposure of PC12 cells to 200 µM H_2O_2 for 2 h increased ROS levels, MDA content and decreased SOD activity (Figure 2). PhGs pretreatment attenuated ROS level, salidroside, and acteoside, and the high dosage of isoacteoside and echinacoside pretreatment significantly attenuated ROS level ($p < 0.01$). Salidroside pretreatment showed no effect on MDA content, but acteoside pretreatment significantly attenuated MDA content ($p < 0.05$). Isoacteoside and echinacoside pretreatment significantly attenuated MDA content to a greater extent ($p < 0.01$). All PhGs significantly increased SOD activity ($p < 0.01$).

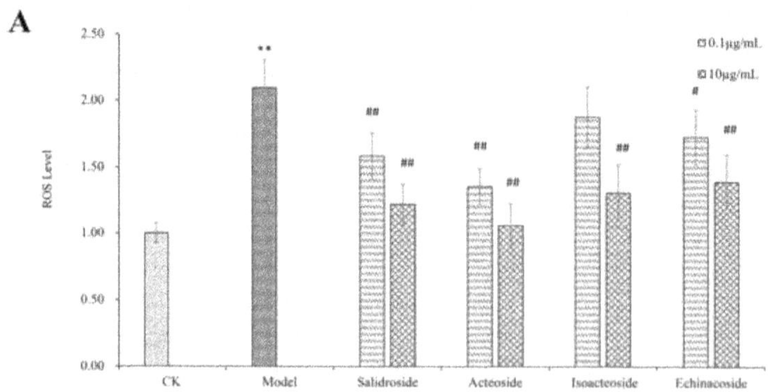

Figure 2. *Cont.*

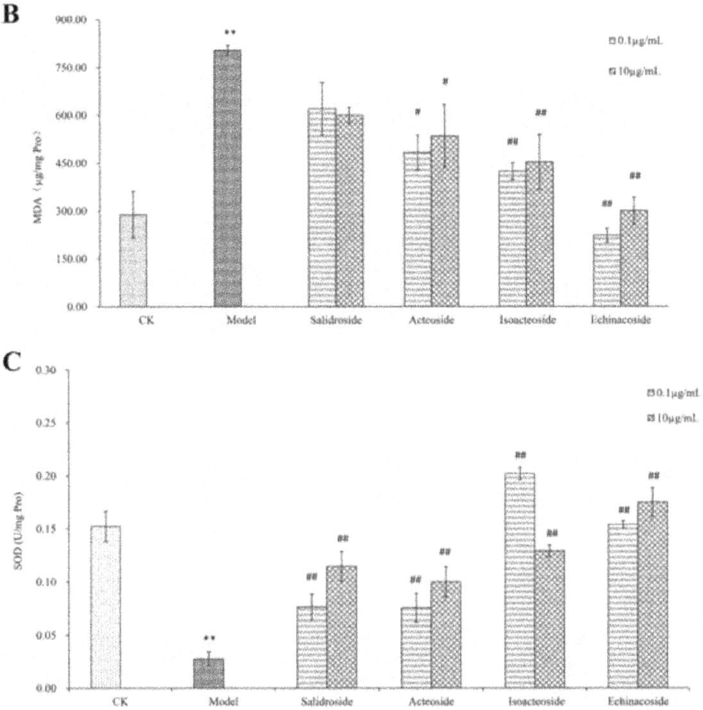

Figure 2. PhGs blocked ROS and MDA accumulation and increased the activities of SOD in PC12 cells. PC12 cells were incubated with PhGs (0.1, and 10 μg/mL) for 24 h, and then incubated with 200 μM H_2O_2 for another 2 h after the PhGs were removed. (**A**) PhGs blocked ROS and MDA accumulation. (**B**) PhGs blocked MDA accumulation. (**C**) PhGs increased the activities of SOD. CK: normal group, Model: H_2O_2 treated group, Salidroside: salidroside treated group, Acteoside: acteoside treated group, Isoacteoside: isoacteoside treated group, Echinacoside: echinacoside treated group. ** $p < 0.01$ versus untreated group; # $p < 0.05$, versus H_2O_2 treated group, ## $p < 0.01$, versus H_2O_2 treated group.

2.3. *PhGs Reversed H_2O_2-Induced Apoptosis in PC12 Cells*

H_2O_2 treatment (200 μM) for 2 h significantly increased apoptosis in PC12 cells, with total apoptotic rate up to 16.02% (Figure 3). However, pretreatment with PhGs (0.1 and 10 μg/mL) for 24 h decreased the apoptosis rate in a concentration-dependent manner ($p < 0.01$). Salidroside, acteoside, isoacteoside, and echinacoside markedly decreased the percentage of cell apoptosis by 4.750–6.627%, 4.413–5.800%, 6.593–10.047%, and 1.530–7.510%, respectively.

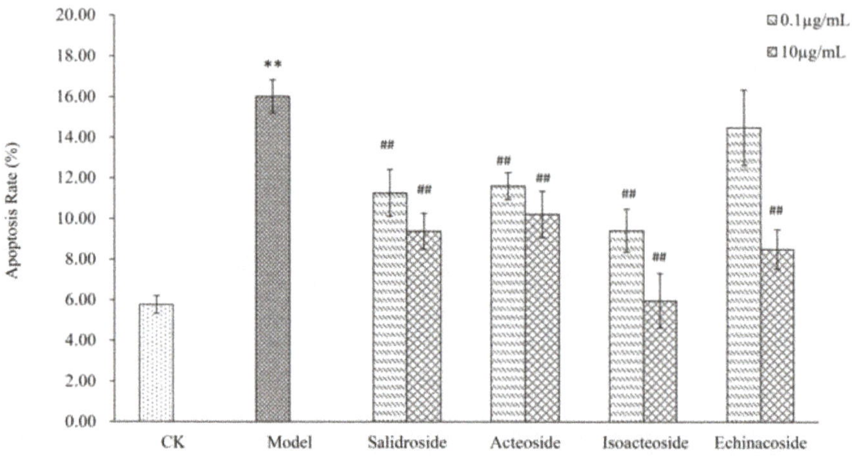

Figure 3. PhGs reversed H_2O_2-induced apoptosis in PC12 cells. PC12 cells were incubated with PhGs (0.1, and 10 μg/mL) for 24 h, and then incubated with 200 μM H_2O_2 for another 2 h after the PhGs were removed. Then, apoptosis was measured by a flow cytometry using PI/FITC fluorescent probe. CK: normal group, Model: H_2O_2 treated group, Salidroside: salidroside treated group, Acteoside: acteoside treated group, Isoacteoside: isoacteoside treated group, Echinacoside: echinacoside treated group. ** $p < 0.01$ versus untreated group; ## $p < 0.01$, versus H_2O_2 treated group.

2.4. *PhGs Alleviated H_2O_2-Induced Dysregulation of the Nrf2-ARE Pathways in PC12 Cells*

The Nrf2-ARE pathway, as one of the major antioxidant pathways in most cell type, is important in regulating cell growth and cell death. Therefore, we investigated whether the Nrf2-ARE pathway is involved in H_2O_2-induced apoptosis by immunofluorescence and Western blot analysis using specific antibodies. The immunofluorescence assay showed that PhGs (0.1 and 10 μg/mL) induced the nuclear translocation of Nrf2 (Figure 4). After treatment of PhGs, isoacteoside, and echinacoside resulted in the partial recovery of the cell normal morphology. The results from Western blotting and gray density analyses showed that PhGs (0.1 and 10 μg/mL) had no significant influence on the expression of Nrf2 in cytoplasm (Figure 5A,B) ($p > 0.05$) but upregulated Nrf2 expression in the nucleus (Figure 5C,D) ($p < 0.01$). Then, we studied the role of Nrf2 in H_2O_2-induced apoptosis by importing the Nrf2 siRNA. The protein and mRNA expression of Nrf2 was significantly downregulated in all Nrf2 siRNA-treated groups (Figure 5E–H). PhGs (0.1 and 10 μg/mL) prevented H_2O_2-induced cytotoxicity in groups without Nrf2 siRNA treatment ($p < 0.01$), but such protection was reversed by Nrf2 siRNA. After Nrf2 siRNA treatment, the cell viability decreased significantly even with PhGs treatment (Figure 5I).

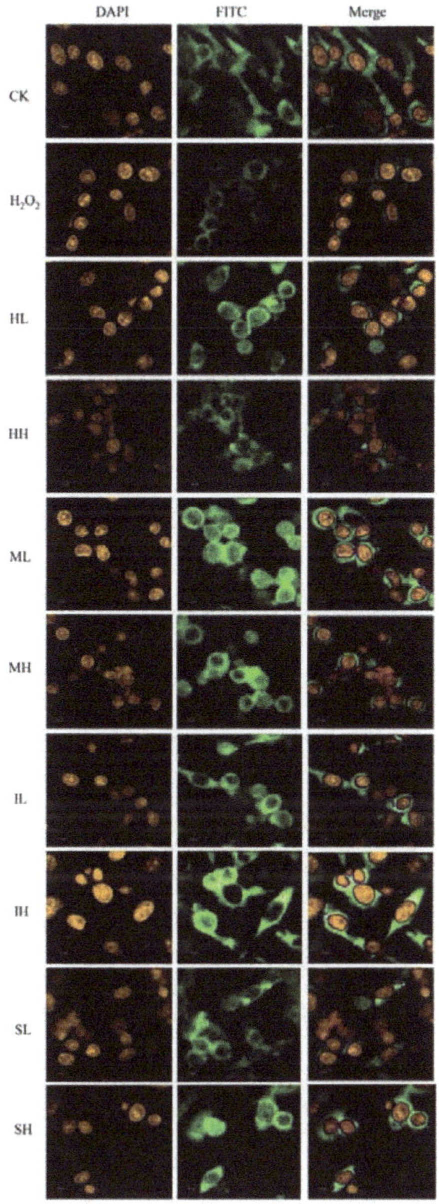

Figure 4. The immunofluorescence assay of Nrf2 in different groups. (×400) PC12 cells were incubated with PhGs (0.1 and 10 μg/mL) for 24 h, and then incubated with 200 μM H_2O_2 for another 2 h after the PhGs were removed. Nrf2 localization was observed under an inverted fluorescence microscope. CK: normal group, H_2O_2:H_2O_2 treated group, HL: 0.1 μg/mL salidroside treated group, HH: 10 μg/mL salidroside treated group, ML: 0.1 μg/mL acteoside treated group, MH 10 μg/mL acteoside treated group, IL: 0.1 μg/mL isoacteoside treated group, IH: 10 μg/mL isoacteoside treated group, SL: 0.1 μg/mL echinacoside treated group, SH: 10 μg/mL echinacoside treated group.

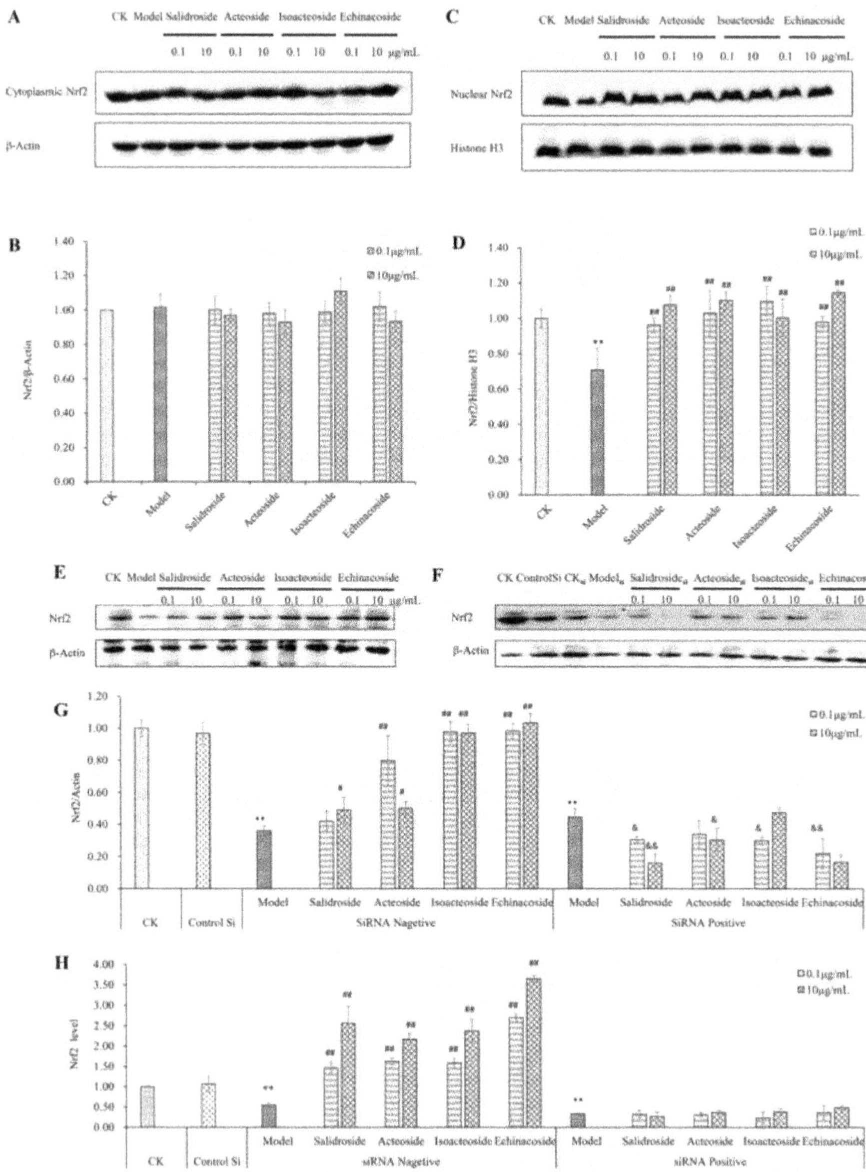

Figure 5. *Cont.*

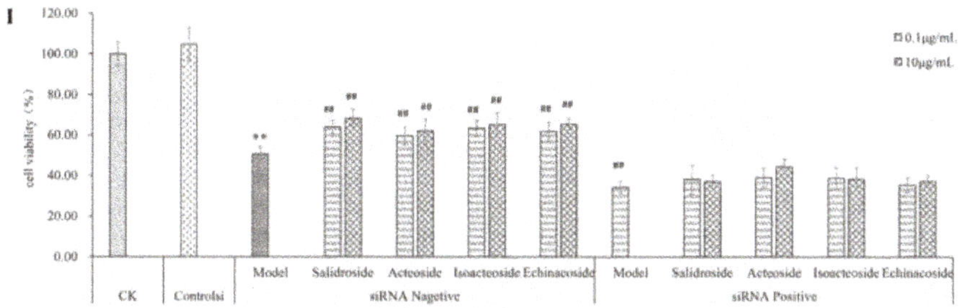

Figure 5. Protective effect of PhGs on Nrf2 in H_2O_2-treated PC12 cells. (**A**) The expression of Nrf2 protein in cytoplasm was detected by immunoblotting using specific antibody. β-Actin was used as loading control. (**B**) The quantitative densitometric analysis of Nrf2 protein in cytoplasm. (**C**) The expression of Nrf2 protein in the nucleus was detected by immunoblotting using specific antibody. Histones H3 was used as loading control. (**D**) The quantitative densitometric analysis of Nrf2 protein in the nucleus. (**E**,**F**) PC12 cells were preincubated without (**E**) or with (**F**) Nrf2 siRNA for 24 h, then incubated with or without PhGs (0.1, and 10 μg/mL) for 24 h, and incubated with H_2O_2 for another 2 h after the PhGs were removed. Total Nrf2 protein expression was detected by immunoblotting using specific antibody, and β-actin was used as loading control. (**G**) The quantitative densitometric analysis of total Nrf2 protein. (**H**) The quantitative analysis of Nrf2 mRNA. (**I**) PC12 cells were preincubated with or without siRNA for 24 h, then incubated with or without PhGs (0.1 and 10 μg/mL) for 24 h, and incubated with H_2O_2 for another 2 h after the PhGs were removed. After treatment, the survival cells were determined by MTT assay. CK: normal group, Model: H_2O_2 treated group, ControlSi: control siRNA treated group, SiRNA Negative: without SiRNA treated group, SiRNA Positive: SiRNA treated group, Salidroside: salidroside treated group, Acteoside: acteoside treated group, Isoacteoside: isoacteoside treated group, Echinacoside: echinacoside treated group. ** $p < 0.01$ versus untreated group; # $p < 0.05$, versus H_2O_2 treated group (without Nrf2 siRNA treated), ## $p < 0.01$, versus H_2O_2 treated group (without Nrf2 siRNA treated); & $p < 0.05$ versus H_2O_2 treated group (with Nrf2 siRNA treated), && $p < 0.01$, versus H_2O_2 treated group (with Nrf2 siRNA treated).

2.5. PhGs Reversed H_2O_2-Induced Downregulation of Protein Expression of HO-1, NQO1, GCLC, and GCLM

HO-1, NQO1, and glutamate-cysteine ligase (GCL) are important cellular antioxidant enzymes, and HO-1, NQO1, and catalytic or modify subunits of GCL (GCLC or GCLM) are Nrf2-regulated downstream genes [27]. Protein expression of HO-1, NQO1, GCLC, and GCLM was observed after treatment. An obvious difference was found between the protein expression of HO-1 and NQO1 with or without H_2O_2 (Figure 6A–C) ($p < 0.01$). PhGs (0.1 and 10 μg/mL) reversed the H_2O_2-induced downregulation of protein expression of HO-1 (except salidroside at 0.1 μg/mL), NQO1 (except acteoside at 0.1 μg/mL) ($p < 0.01$). H_2O_2 also downregulated GCLC and GCLM protein expression ($p < 0.05$) (Figure 6A,D,E). PhGs (0.1 and 10 μg/mL) reversed H_2O_2-induced downregulation of protein expression of GCLC (except echinacoside at 0.1 μg/mL) ($p < 0.01$) and GCLM (except salidroside at 0.1 μg/mL) ($p < 0.01$). Then, the chemical inhibitors for HO-1 were used to further evaluate the roles of the antioxidant enzymes in regulating the protection of PhGs against H_2O_2-induced cytotoxicity. PhGs (0.1 and 10 μg/mL) prevented H_2O_2-induced cytotoxicity, but such protective effect was reversed by HO-1 inhibitor ZnPP ($p < 0.01$) at 20 μM (Figure 6F, $p < 0.01$).

2.6. Keap1 Expression and Molecular Docking Analysis

Under physiological conditions, Keap1 acts as a repressor protein of Nrf2 by binding to the Neh2 domain of Nrf2 and targeting Nrf2 to a Cul3-based E3 ubiquitin ligase for ubiquitination and subsequent degradation by the 26S proteasome [28]. Binding capacity to Keap1 of PhGs was evaluated by molecular docking analysis to investigate the mechanism under their antioxidant effect.

The expression of Keap1 protein did not change before and after PhGs treatment (Figure 7A,B). Molecular docking results showed that the Keap1 protein domain had a relatively active binding pocket (Figure 7D), and PhGs could bind to Keap1 (Figure 7E–H). Analytical results showed that salidroside exhibited relatively weaker binding capacity. C score ≥ 4 and Total-score > 6 of echinacoside, isoacteoside, and acteoside indicated their better binding capacity with Keap1 (Table 1).

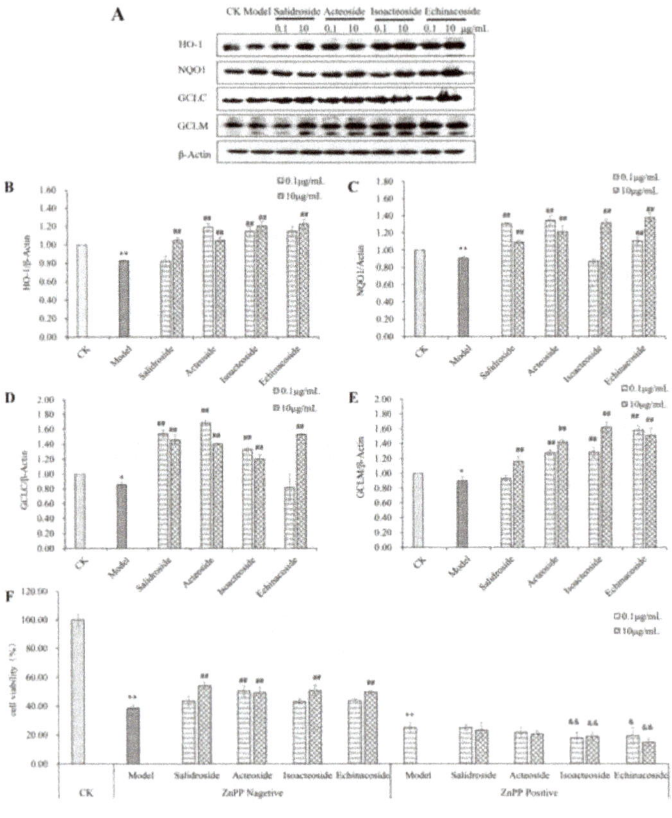

Figure 6. PhGs increased the expression of HO-1, NQO1, GCLC, and GCLM. (**A**) PC12 cells were incubated with PhGs (0.1, and 10 μg/mL) for 24 h, and then incubated with 200 μM H_2O_2 for another 2 h after the PhGs were removed. HO-1, NQO1, GCLC, and GCLM protein expression was detected by immunoblotting using specific antibody, and β-actin was used as loading control. (**B**) The quantitative densitometric analysis of HO-1 protein (**C**) The quantitative densitometric analysis of NQO1 protein. (**D**) The quantitative densitometric analysis of GCLC protein. (**E**) The quantitative densitometric analysis of GCLM protein. (**F**) PC12 cells were preincubated with or without ZnPP (20 mM) for 15 min, then incubated with or without PhGs (0.1, and 10 μg/mL) for 24 h, and incubated with H_2O_2 for another 2 h after the PhGs were removed. After treatment, the survival cells were determined by MTT assay. CK: normal group, Model: H_2O_2 treated group, ZnPP Negative: without ZnPP treated group, ZnPP Positive: ZnPP treated group, Salidroside: salidroside treated group, Acteoside: acteoside treated group, Isoacteoside: isoacteoside treated group, Echinacoside: echinacoside treated group. * $p < 0.05$ versus untreated group, ** $p < 0.01$ versus untreated group; ## $p < 0.01$, versus H_2O_2 treated group (without ZnPP treated); & $p < 0.05$, versus H_2O_2 treated group (with ZnPP treated), && $p < 0.01$, versus H_2O_2 treated group (with ZnPP treated).

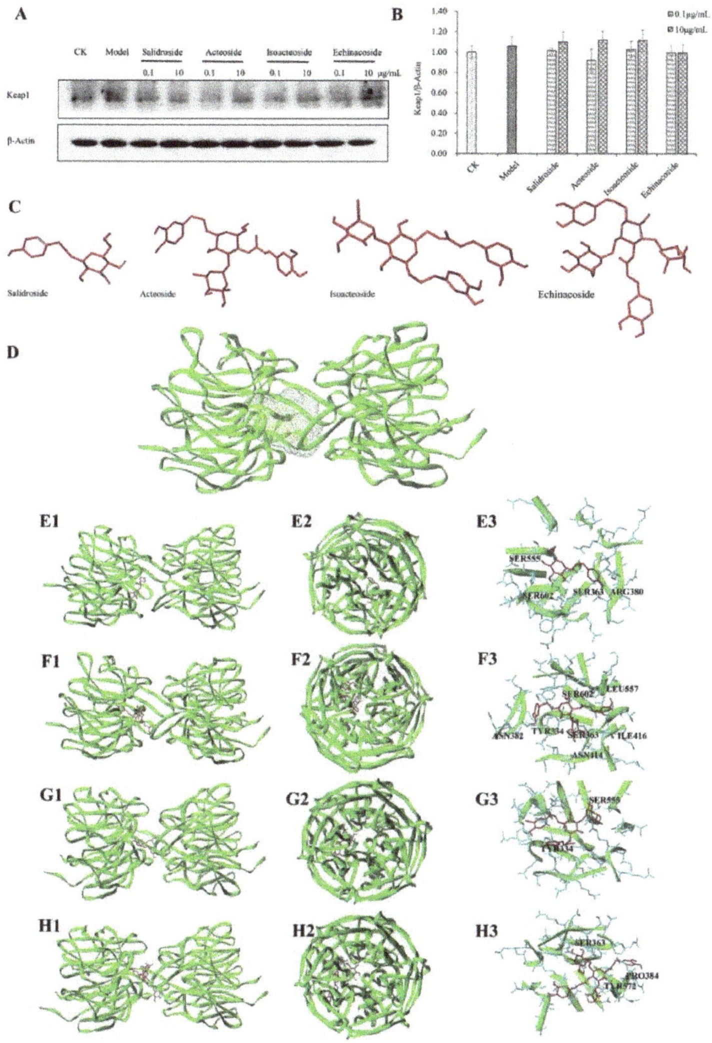

Figure 7. Effect of PhGs on Keap1 expression and molecular docking results. (**A**) PC12 cells were incubated with PhGs (0.1, and 10 μg/mL) for 24 h, and then incubated with 200 μM H_2O_2 for another 2 h after the PhGs were removed. Keap1 protein expression was detected by Western blotting using specific antibody, and β-actin was used as loading control. (**B**) The quantitative densitometric analysis of Keap1 protein. (**C**) 3D structure of salidroside, acteoside, isoacteoside, and echinacoside (**D**) The binding pocket of Keap1. (**E1–E3**) Representative amino acid residues surrounding salidroside (red) in the binding pocket of Keap1 (**E1** front view, **E2** side view, **E3** binding sites). (**F1–F3**) Representative amino acid residues surrounding acteoside (red) in the binding pocket of Keap1 (**F1** front view, **F2** side view, **F3** binding sites). (**G1–G3**) Representative amino acid residues surrounding isoacteoside (red) in the binding pocket of Keap1 (**G1** front view, **G2** side view, **G3** binding sites). (**H1–H3**) Representative amino acid residues surrounding echinacoside (red) in the binding pocket of Keap1 (**H1** front view, **H2** side view, **H3** binding sites). The dotted line (yellow) indicate potential interactions between amino acid residues and PhGs.

Table 1. Molecular docking analysis of PhGs.

Compounds Name	Total-Score	Crash	Polar	D-Score	PMF-Score	G-Score	Chem-Score	C-Score
Salidroside	5.0951	−1.0622	5.1831	−561.448	−30.2413	−115.923	−22.6459	4
Acteoside	7.4971	−2.3674	7.8899	−1562.04	−67.978	-192.18	−33.947	5
Isoacteoside	8.1776	−1.4	6.4762	−1439.24	−88.9989	−155.055	−26.1735	4
Echinacoside	9.3402	−2.6794	9.6386	−1756.32	−82.9345	−187.808	−32.4387	4

Crash: The inadequate penetration between the protein and the ligand. Polar: The hydrogen bonding and electrostatic interactions between the protein and the ligand. D-score: The charge and van der Waals interactions between the protein and the ligand. PMF-score: The helmholtz free energy between the protein and the ligand. G-score: The hydrogen bonding, complex (ligand-protein), and internal (ligand-ligand) energies between the protein and the ligand. Chem-score: The hydrogen bonding, metal-ligand interaction, lipophilic contact, and rotational entropy, along with an intercept term between the protein and the ligand. C-score: The concensus score between the protein and the ligand, comprehensive reflecting the D-score, PMF-score, G-score, and Chem-score.

3. Discussion

We investigated the neuroprotection of PhGs on H_2O_2 induced-cytotoxicity in PC12 cells. The results show that PhGs pretreatment significantly suppressed H_2O_2-induced cytotoxicity, attenuated the intracellular ROS level, improved the level of intracellular antioxidant enzymes, and ultimately reversed H_2O_2-induced cytotoxicity in PC12 cells. Moreover, PhGs increased the transcriptional activation of Nrf2, reversed the H_2O_2-induced downregulation of the protein expression of HO-1, NQO1, GCLC, and GCLM. In addition, PhGs showed potential interaction with Nrf2 binding site in the Keap1 protein.

In the H_2O_2-induced PC12 cell injury, lipid peroxidation, which refers to oxidative degradation of lipid, increased the permeability of membranes, leading to cell damage [29]. MDA formation is widely used as the index of lipid peroxidation [30]. H_2O_2 enhanced ROS production and exhausted antioxidant defense enzymes, such as SOD, catalase, and GPx. This process leads to oxidative stress [31], which plays a key role in the causation and progression of the majority of neurodegenerative disorders. Consistent with previous studies, we observed an increased level of ROS, reduced intracellular antioxidant enzymes, and enhanced apoptosis of PC12 cells after H_2O_2 treatment. PhGs pretreatment significantly attenuated H_2O_2-induced increase in intracellular ROS, improved intracellular antioxidant enzymes, and ultimately reversed H_2O_2-induced cytotoxicity in PC12 cells.

Kuang et al. [32] reported that echinacoside showed significant neuroprotective effect on H_2O_2-induced cytotoxicity in PC12 cells through the mitochondrial apoptotic pathway. In this study, we found that echinacoside, salidroside, acteoside, and isoacteoside showed neuroprotective effect by enhancing the antioxidant activity of PC12 cells because they increased the transcriptional activation of Nrf2 and upregulated the downstream protein expression of HO-1, NQO1, GCLC, and GCLM. Numerous studies have clearly demonstrated that activation of Nrf2 target genes, in particular HO-1, in astrocytes and neurons strongly protect against inflammation, oxidative damage, and cell death. The HO-1 system has been reported to be very active in the central nervous system, and its modulation apparently plays a crucial role in the pathogenesis of neurodegenerative disorders [33]. Recent studies also clarified the role of Nrf2 in the progression and risk of PD [9] and Keap1 as an efficient target for the reactivation of Nrf2 in AD [34]. The results support new evidence for Nrf2 as a therapeutic target in neurodegenerative diseases.

Molecular docking analysis showed that PhGs could bind to Keap1, with the following binding capacities: echinacoside > isoacteoside > acteoside > salidroside. Consistent with these results, PhGs pretreatment led to the Nrf2 nuclear translocation, with the following Nrf2 expression in the nucleus: echinacoside > isoacteoside ≈ acteoside > salidroside. We assumed that the number of glycosides affected the possible binding mode of PhGs and Keap1, and the binding mode further caused the release of Nrf2 from Keap1. This process resulted in the activation of Nrf2 and the downstream genes and ultimately protect PC12 cells from H_2O_2-induced oxidative stress.

In summary, PhGs with more glycosides showed an enhanced effect on Nrf2 activation. PhGs induced Nrf2 activation by blocking the binding between Nrf2 and Keap1. This process activated the Nrf2/ARE pathway and protected PC12 from H_2O_2-induced cytotoxicity.

4. Materials and Methods

4.1. Chemical Compounds and Reagents

Salidroside (CAS No. 10338-51-9), acteoside (CAS No. 61276-17-3), isoacteoside (CAS No. 61303-13-7), and echinacoside (CAS No. 82854-37-3) were purchased from Yuanye Biotechnology Company (Shanghai, China). The PhGs were dissolved in PBS to produce a 10 mg/mL stock solution, which was stored at −20 °C. H_2O_2 was purchased from Aladdin® (Shanghai, China). RPMI-1640 medium and fetal bovine serum were purchased from Hyclone (Logan, UT, USA), and 0.5% trypsin EDTA, penicillin, and streptomycin were purchased from Keyi (Hangzhou, China). MDA, SOD diagnostic kits, MTT, and DCFH-DA were purchased from Beyotime Institute of Biotechnology (Nanjing, Jiangsu, China). Annexin V-FITC/PI double staining Kit was purchased from Solarbio Life Sciences (Beijing, China). Antibodies to Nrf2, Histone H3, Keap1, HO-1, NQO1, GCLC, GCLM, and β-actin, anti-mouse-horseradish peroxide (HRP) IgG, and anti-rabbit-HRP-IgG were purchased from Abcam (London, UK). Inhibitors of HO-1 and ZnPP were purchased from Sigma Chemical Co. (St. Louis, MO, USA). RNAiso Plus, PrimeScript™RT reagent Kit with gDNA Eraser, and SYBR® Premix Ex Taq™ II were bought from Takara (Shiga, Japan). Lipofectamine® RNAiMAX Transfection Reagent was purchased from Thermo Fisher Scientific (Waltham, UK). The Nrf2 siRNA sequences were as follows: forward, CCGAAUUACAGUGUCUUAA; and reverse, UUAAGACACUGUAAUUCGG. Meanwhile, control siRNA sequences were as follows: forward, UUCUCCGAACGUGUCACGU; and reverse, ACGUGACACGUUCGGAGAA.

4.2. Cell Culture

Mouse adrenal pheochromocytoma line (PC12 cells) was obtained from the Institute of Biochemistry and Cell Biology, SIBS, (CAS, Shanghai, China). The cells were maintained in RPMI-1640 (Hyclone) containing 10% fetal bovine serum (Hyclone), 100 U/mL penicillin, and 0.1 mg/mL streptomycin at 37 °C with 5% CO_2. The medium was changed every other day.

4.3. Cell Viability Assay

PC12 cells were seeded in 96-well plates at 2×10^4 cells/well. After attachment, cells were preincubated with or without inhibitor for 20 min, incubated with or without PhGs for 24 h, and then incubated with H_2O_2 for another 2 h after the PhGs were removed. After incubation, the cells were treated with 5 mg/mL MTT for 4 h at 37 °C, and the media were carefully removed. The formazan crystals that had formed by surviving cells were dissolved in 150 μL of DMSO to generate a blue color [35], and the absorbance was measured at 570 nm on a plate reader. Controls utilized the same concentration of medium with DMSO alone. Cell viability was normalized as the percentage of control.

The concentrations of PhGs (0.1, 1, 5, and 10 μg/mL) was chosen depending on the cytotoxicity analysis of PhGs and the reported cytoprotective effect of echinacoside [32]. According to the report there was no cytotoxicity effect shown below 10 μg/mL, and echinacoside was reported to show cytoprotective effect in H_2O_2-injured cell model.

4.4. Apoptosis Assay

Apoptosis was detected with an Annexin V-FITC/PI double staining Kit (Solarbio). PC12 cells were seeded in 6-well plates at 2×10^5 cells/well. After attachment, cells were treated with PhGs (0.1 and 10 μg/mL) for 24 h and incubated with H_2O_2 for another 2 h after the PhGs were removed. After incubation, the cells were washed in cold PBS, centrifuged twice at 1500 rpm for 10 min, and resuspended in 500 μL of binding buffer. FITC-labeled Annexin V (5 μL) and propidium iodide

(PI, 5 μL) were then added to cells. Then, the cells were incubated in the dark at room temperature for 20 min according to the manufacturer's instruction. Cell apoptosis was measured using a Gallios™ flow cytometer (Beckman Coulter, Brea, CA, USA). Annexin V-positive and PI-negative cells were scored as early apoptotic cells, while cells double-stained with both Annexin V and PI were considered as late apoptotic cells. Control cells were negative for both stains.

4.5. Measurement of Intracellular ROS, MDA Production, and SOD

The intracellular ROS level was determined using a ROS-sensitive fluorescent probe, namely, 2,7-dichlorodihydro fluorescent diacetate (DCFH-DA). PC12 cells were seeded in 6-well plates at 2×10^5 cells/well. After attachment, cells were treated with PhGs (0.1 and 10 μg/mL) for 24 h and incubated with H_2O_2 for another 2 h after the PhGs were removed. After incubation, the cells were washed with PBS thrice and subsequently incubated with 10 μM DCFH-DA. After incubation at 37 °C for 20 min, the cells were washed with PBS and collected by gentle centrifugation. Intracellular ROS was measured using a Gallios™ flow cytometer (Beckman Coulter, Brea, CA, USA).

MDA and SOD were measured by assay kits (Beyotime Biotechnology, Nanjing, Jiangsu, China). All procedures completely complied with the manufacturers' instructions. The contents of MDA and SOD were normalized with the corresponding total protein content.

4.6. Nrf2 Nuclear Translocation Immunofluorescence

The PC12 cells were seeded in 6-well glass slides at a density of 2×10^5 per well. After attachment, the cells were treated with PhGs (0.1 and 10 μg/mL) for 24 h and incubated with H_2O_2 for another 2 h after the PhGs were removed. After incubation, the cells were washed in cold PBS and fixed in 4% paraformaldehyde for 15 min at room temperature, followed by membrane permeabilization using 0.5% Triton X-100 in PBS for 5 min. The cells were incubated with anti-Nrf2 Rabbit IgG (Abcam) with 5% FBS overnight at 4 °C. Then, the secondary anti-rabbit antibodies conjugated with FITC were applied to the cells for 20 min at room temperature. The nuclei were stained with 4′,6-diamidino-2-phenylindole (DAPI) at the final preparation step. The slides were rinsed briefly with PBS, air-dried, and mounted in an anti-fluorescence in fading medium. The slides were visualized under a laser confocal microscope (LMS780, Zeiss, Germany).

4.7. Protein Extraction

The PC12 cells were seeded in 100 mm dishes at 1×10^7 cells/dish. After attachment, the cells were treated with PhGs (0.1 and 10 μg/mL) for 24 h and then incubated with H_2O_2 for another 2 h with PhGs removal. After incubation, the cells were washed twice with cold PBS and scraped from the dishes with 1000 μL of PBS. Cell homogenates were centrifuged at 1500 rpm for 10 min. After treatment, cellular proteins were extracted using a Beyotime RIPA cell lysis buffer with 1 mM PMSF according to the manufacturer's instructions. In addition, cytoplasmic and nuclear proteins were isolated as described in the Beyotime nuclear and cytoplasmic extraction kit. Protein concentration of the samples was detected by a Beyotime BCA protein assay kit, and all samples were stored at −80 °C for Western blot analysis.

4.8. Western Blot Analysis

Western blot analysis was performed using standard methods. Briefly, protein samples (20 or 30 μg) were separated by SDS-PAGE and transferred to PVDF membranes. Membranes were blocked in 5% milk-TBST and incubated overnight at 4 °C in primary antibody. Antibodies used included Nrf2 (Abcam), Keap1 (Abcam), HO-1 (Abcam), NQO-1 (Abcam), GCLC (Abcam), GCLM (Abcam), Histone H3 (Abcam), and β-actin (Abcam). Peroxidase-conjugated anti-mouse IgG (Abcam) or anti-rabbit IgG (Abcam) was used as the secondary antibody. The protein bands were visualized using ChemiScope series (Clinx Science Instruments, Shanghai, China). Gray value of protein bands was quantified using ImageJ (National Institutes of Health, Bethesda, MD, USA).

4.9. Quantitative Real-Time PCR

Total RNA was extracted using the RNAiso Plus (Takara, Shiga, Japan), following the manufacturer's instructions. Total RNA samples were reverse transcribed with PrimeScript™RT reagent Kit with gDNA Eraser (Takara, Shiga, Japan) according to the manufacturer's instruction. Quantitative real-time PCR was performed using SYBR® Premix Ex Taq™ II (Takara, Shiga, Japan) in Applied Biosystems ViiA™ 7 Real-Time PCR System. Relative expression of target genes was normalized to β-Actin and analyzed by $2^{-\Delta\Delta Ct}$ method. Primer sequences for Nrf2 were as follows: forward, ACAGTGCTCCTATGCGTGAA and reverse, TCTGGGCGGCGACTTTAT. Primer sequences for β-Actin were as follows: forward, GCTGTCCCTGTATGCCTCT; and reverse, TTGATGTCACGCACGATTT.

4.10. siRNA Transfection

PC12 cells were cultured in 6-well glass slides at a density of 2×10^5 per well (for Western blot analysis) or in 96-well glass slides at a density of 2×10^4 per well (for cell viability analysis). Control siRNA and Nrf2 siRNA were transfected into cells using Lipofectamine RNAiMAX (Thermo Fisher Scientific, Waltham, MA, USA) according to the manufacturer's instructions. After 24 h of incubation, the cells were treated with or without PhGs and H_2O_2 for the indicated times and then used in Western blot analysis, qRT-PCR, or cell viability analysis as described above.

4.11. Molecular Docking Analysis

Molecular docking analysis was performed to investigate the possible binding mode of PhGs to Keap1. The 3D structure of ligands was obtained from NCBI. The crystalized structure of Keap1 (PDB Code: 4L7B) was prepared using correcting structure issues (such as break bond and miss loop) using SYBYL-X 2.0. In this software simulation, crash represents the inadequate penetration between the protein and the ligand. Polar represents the hydrogen bonding and electrostatic interactions between the protein and the ligand. G-score [36] represents the hydrogen bonding, complex (ligand–protein), and internal (ligand–ligand) energies between the protein and the ligand. PMF-score [37] represents the Helmholtz free energy between the protein and the ligand. D-score [38] represents the charge and van der Waals interactions between the protein and the ligand. Chem-score [39] represents the hydrogen bonding, metal-ligand interaction, lipophilic contact, and rotational entropy, along with an intercept term between the protein and the ligand. C score represents the consensus score between the protein and the ligand, comprehensively reflecting the G, PMF, D, and Chem-scores. Tota-score reflects the binding capacity of ligand to protein. The best modes were generated and evaluated using the Total-score (>6) and C-score ($\geq$4).

4.12. Statistical Analysis

Data were analyzed using one-way ANOVA with LSD analyses using SPSS. All results were confirmed from three independent experiments. Data were expressed as means ± SD. Statistically significant differences were considered at $p < 0.05$.

Acknowledgments: This study was supported by the National Major R & D Program of China (No. 2017YFD0400200), the Zhejiang Provincial Natural Science Foundation of China (No. R15C200002) and the Special Project of Agricultural Product Quality Safety Risk Assessment (No. GJFP2018015), Ministry of Agriculture and Rural affairs of China.

Author Contributions: Baiyi Lu and Maiquan Li designed the study. Maiquan Li performed the laboratory work, data analysis and wrote the paper. Maiquan Li, Tao Xu, Fei Zhou, Mengmeng Wang, Huaxin Song, Xing Xiao and Baiyi Lu revised the manuscript.

Conflicts of Interest: The authors declare no conflict of interest.

Abbreviations

GCLC	glutamate cysteine ligase-catalytic subunit
GCLM	glutamate cysteine ligase-catalytic modifier subunit
H_2O_2	hydrogen peroxide
HO-1	heme oxygenase 1
Keap1	Kelch ECH association protein 1
NQO1	NAD(P)H quinone oxidoreductase 1
Nrf2	nuclear factor erythroid 2-related factor 2
PhGs	salidroside, acteoside, isoacteoside, and echinacoside
ROS	reactive oxygen species
ZnPP	zinc protoporphyrin

References

1. Sun, A.Y.; Chen, Y.M. Oxidative stress and neurodegenerative disorders. *J. Biomed. Sci.* **1998**, *5*, 401–414. [CrossRef] [PubMed]
2. Maheshwari, A.; Misro, M.M.; Aggarwal, A.; Sharma, R.K.; Nandan, D. Pathways involved in testicular germ cell apoptosis induced by H_2O_2 in vitro. *FEBS J.* **2009**, *276*, 870–881. [CrossRef] [PubMed]
3. Halliwell, B. Reactive oxygen species and the central nervous system. *J. Neurochem.* **1992**, *59*, 1609–1623. [CrossRef] [PubMed]
4. Richardson, J.S.; Subbarao, K.V.; Ang, L.C. On the possible role of iron-induced free radical peroxidation in neural degeneration in Alzheimer's disease. *Ann. N. Y. Acad. Sci.* **1992**, *648*, 326–327. [CrossRef] [PubMed]
5. Zhang, D.D. Mechanistic studies of the Nrf2-Keap1 signaling pathway. *Drug Metab. Rev.* **2006**, *38*, 769–789. [CrossRef] [PubMed]
6. Itoh, K.; Tong, K.I.; Yamamoto, M. Molecular mechanism activating Nrf2-Keap1 pathway in regulation of adaptive response to electrophiles. *Free Radic. Biol. Med.* **2004**, *36*, 1208–1213. [CrossRef] [PubMed]
7. Kong, A.N.; Owuor, E.; Yu, R.; Hebbar, V.; Chen, C.; Hu, R.; Mandlekar, S. Induction of xenobiotic enzymes by the map kinase pathway and the antioxidant or electrophile response element (ARE/EpRE). *Drug Metab. Rev.* **2001**, *33*, 255–271. [CrossRef] [PubMed]
8. Buendia, I.; Michalska, P.; Navarro, E.; Gameiro, I.; Egea, J.; León, R. Nrf2-ARE pathway: An emerging target against oxidative stress and neuroinflammation in neurodegenerative diseases. *Pharmacol. Ther.* **2016**, *157*, 84–104. [CrossRef] [PubMed]
9. Skibinski, G.; Hwang, V.; Ando, D.M.; Daub, A.; Lee, A.K.; Ravisankar, A.; Modan, S.; Finucane, M.M.; Shaby, B.A.; Finkbeiner, S. Nrf2 mitigates LRRK2- and α-synuclein-induced neurodegeneration by modulating proteostasis. *Proc. Natl. Acad. Sci. USA* **2016**, *114*, 1165–1170. [CrossRef] [PubMed]
10. Jiménez, C.; Riguera, R. Phenylethanoid glycosides in plants: Structure and biological activity. *Nat. Prod. Rep.* **1994**, *11*, 591–606. [CrossRef] [PubMed]
11. Georgiev, M.; Alipieva, K.; Orhan, I.; Abrashev, R.; Denev, P.; Angelova, M. Antioxidant and cholinesterases inhibitory activities of *Verbascum xanthophoeniceum* Griseb. and its phenylethanoid glycosides. *Food Chem.* **2011**, *128*, 100–105. [CrossRef] [PubMed]
12. Li, N.; Wang, J.; Ma, J.; Gu, Z.; Jiang, C.; Yu, L.; Fu, X. Neuroprotective Effects of Cistanches Herba Therapy on Patients with Moderate Alzheimer's Disease. *Evid.-Based Complement. Altern. Med.* **2015**, *2015*, 103985. [CrossRef] [PubMed]
13. Liu, Y.L.; He, W.J.; Mo, L.; Shi, M.F.; Zhu, Y.Y.; Pan, S.; Li, X.R.; Xu, Q.M.; Yang, S.L. Antimicrobial, anti-inflammatory activities and toxicology of phenylethanoid glycosides from *Monochasma savatieri* Franch. ex Maxim. *J. Ethnopharmacol.* **2013**, *149*, 431–437. [CrossRef] [PubMed]
14. Dong, Q.; Yao, J.; Fang, J.N.; Ding, K. Structural characterization and immunological activity of two cold-water extractable polysaccharides from *Cistanche deserticola* Y. C. Ma. *Carbohydr. Res.* **2007**, *342*, 1343–1349. [CrossRef] [PubMed]
15. Xiong, L.; Mao, S.; Lu, B.; Yang, J.; Zhou, F.; Hu, Y.; Jiang, Y.; Shen, C.; Zhao, Y. *Osmanthus fragrans* Flower Extract and Acteoside Protect Against d-Galactose-Induced Aging in an ICR Mouse Model. *J. Med. Food* **2016**, *19*, 54–61. [CrossRef] [PubMed]

16. Jiang, Y.; Mao, S.; Huang, W.; Lu, B.; Cai, Z.; Zhou, F.; Li, M.; Lou, T.; Zhao, Y. Phenylethanoid Glycoside Profiles and Antioxidant Activities of *Osmanthus fragrans* Lour. Flowers by UPLC/PDA/MS and Simulated Digestion Model. *J. Agric. Food Chem.* **2016**, *64*, 2459–2466. [CrossRef] [PubMed]
17. Li, X.; Ye, X.; Li, X.; Sun, X.; Liang, Q.; Tao, L.; Kang, X.; Chen, J. Salidroside protects against MPP^+-induced apoptosis in PC12 cells by inhibiting the NO pathway. *Brain Res.* **2011**, *1382*, 9–18. [CrossRef] [PubMed]
18. Zhang, L.; Ding, W.; Sun, H.; Zhou, Q.; Huang, J.; Li, X.; Xie, Y.; Chen, J. Salidroside protects PC12 cells from MPP^+-induced apoptosis via activation of the PI3K/Akt pathway. *Food Chem. Toxicol.* **2012**, *50*, 2591–2597. [CrossRef] [PubMed]
19. Sheng, G.Q.; Zhang, J.R.; Pu, X.P.; Ma, J.; Li, C.L. Protective effect of verbascoside on 1-methyl-4-phenylpyridinium ion-induced neurotoxicity in PC12 cells. *Eur. J. Pharmacol.* **2002**, *451*, 119–124. [CrossRef]
20. Wang, H.; Xu, Y.; Yan, J.; Zhao, X.; Sun, X.; Zhang, Y.; Guo, J.; Zhu, C. Acteoside protects human neuroblastoma SH-SY5Y cells against beta-amyloid-induced cell injury. *Brain Res.* **2009**, *1283*, 139–147. [CrossRef] [PubMed]
21. Min, D.; Jin, Y.Z.; Yong, J.; Zheng, B.L.; Yao, H.W. Echinacoside rescues the SHSY5Y neuronal cells from TNFα-induced apoptosis. *Chin. Pharmacol. Bull.* **2005**, *505*, 11–18.
22. Zhao, Q.; Gao, J.P.; Li, W.W.; Cai, D.F. Neurotrophic and neurorescue effects of Echinacoside in the subacute MPTP mouse model of Parkinson's disease. *Brain Res.* **2010**, *1346*, 224–236. [CrossRef] [PubMed]
23. Koo, K.A.; Sung, S.H.; Park, J.H.; Kim, S.H.; Lee, K.Y.; Kim, Y.C. In vitro neuroprotective activities of phenylethanoid glycosides from *Callicarpa dichotoma*. *Planta Med.* **2005**, *71*, 778–780. [CrossRef] [PubMed]
24. Liu, Y.G.; Li, X.; Xiong, C.; Yu, B.; Pu, X.; Ye, X.S. Synthetic phenylethanoid glycoside derivatives as potent neuroprotective agents. *Eur. J. Med. Chem.* **2015**, *95*, 313–323. [CrossRef] [PubMed]
25. Fu, G.; Pang, H.; Wong, Y.H. Naturally occurring phenylethanoid glycosides: Potential leads for new therapeutics. *Curr. Med. Chem.* **2008**, *15*, 2592–2613. [CrossRef] [PubMed]
26. Greene, L.A.; Tischler, A.S. Establishment of a noradrenergic clonal line of rat adrenal pheochromocytoma cells which respond to nerve growth factor. *Proc. Natl. Acad. Sci. USA* **1976**, *73*, 2424–2428. [CrossRef] [PubMed]
27. Liang, Q.N.; Sheng, Y.C.; Jiang, P.; Ji, L.L.; Xia, Y.Y.; Min, Y.; Wang, Z.T. The difference of glutathione antioxidant system in newly weaned and young mice liver and its involvement in isoline-induced hepatotoxicity. *Arch. Toxicol.* **2011**, *85*, 1267–1279. [CrossRef] [PubMed]
28. Kobayashi, A.; Kang, M.; Okawa, H.; Ohtsuji, M.; Zenke, Y.; Chiba, T.; Igarashi, K.; Yamamoto, M. Oxidative Stress Sensor Keap1 Functions as an Adaptor for Cul3-Based E3 Ligase To Regulate Proteasomal Degradation of Nrf2. *Mol. Cell. Biol.* **2004**, *24*, 7130–7139. [CrossRef] [PubMed]
29. Cornelius, C.; Crupi, R.; Calabrese, V.; Graziano, A.; Milone, P.; Pennisi, G.; Radak, Z.; Calabrese, E.J.; Cuzzocrea, S. Traumatic brain injury: Oxidative stress and neuroprotection. *Antioxid. Redox Signal.* **2013**, *19*, 836–853. [CrossRef] [PubMed]
30. Hou, Z.; Luo, W.; Sun, X.; Hao, S.; Zhang, Y.; Xu, F.; Wang, Z.; Liu, B. Hydrogen-rich saline protects against oxidative damage and cognitive deficits after mild traumatic brain injury. *Brain Res. Bull.* **2012**, *88*, 560–565. [CrossRef] [PubMed]
31. Ansari, M.A.; Roberts, K.N.; Scheff, S.W. A time course of contusion-induced oxidative stress and synaptic proteins in cortex in a rat model of TBI. *J. Neurotrauma* **2008**, *25*, 513–526. [CrossRef] [PubMed]
32. Kuang, R.; Sun, Y.; Yuan, W.; Lei, L.; Zheng, X. Protective effects of echinacoside, one of the phenylethanoid glycosides, on H_2O_2-induced cytotoxicity in PC12 cells. *Planta Med.* **2009**, *75*, 1499–1504. [CrossRef] [PubMed]
33. Scapagnini, G.; Vasto, S.; Abraham, N.G.; Caruso, C.; Zella, D.; Fabio, G. Modulation of Nrf2/ARE pathway by food polyphenols: A nutritional neuroprotective strategy for cognitive and neurodegenerative disorders. *Mol. Neurobiol.* **2011**, *44*, 192–201. [CrossRef] [PubMed]
34. Kerr, F.; Sofolaadesakin, O.; Ivanov, D.K.; Gatliff, J.; Gomez, P.B.; Bertrand, H.C.; Martinez, P.; Callard, R.; Snoeren, I.; Cochemé, H.M. Direct Keap1-Nrf2 disruption as a potential therapeutic target for Alzheimer's disease. *PLoS Genet.* **2017**, *13*, e1006593. [CrossRef] [PubMed]
35. Hansen, M.B.; Nielsen, S.E.; Berg, K. Re-examination and further development of a precise and rapid dye method for measuring cell growth/cell kill. *J. Immunol. Methods* **1989**, *119*, 203–210. [CrossRef]
36. Press, C. *Virtual Screening in Drug Discovery*; Crc Press: Boca Raton, FL, USA, 2005.

37. Muegge, I.; Martin, Y.C.; Hajduk, P.J.; Fesik, S.W. Evaluation of PMF scoring in docking weak ligands to the FK506 binding protein. *J. Med. Chem.* **1999**, *42*, 2498–2503. [CrossRef] [PubMed]
38. Kuntz, I.D.; Blaney, J.M.; Oatley, S.J.; Langridge, R.; Ferrin, T.E. A geometric approach to macromolecule-ligand interactions. *J. Mol. Biol.* **1982**, *161*, 269–288. [CrossRef]
39. MD, E.; Murray, C.W.; Auton, T.R.; Paolini, G.V.; Mee, R.P. Empirical scoring functions: I. The development of a fast empirical scoring function to estimate the binding affinity of ligands in receptor complexes. *J. Comput.-Aided Mol. Des.* **1997**, *11*, 425–445.

International Journal of
Molecular Sciences

MDPI

Article

Aged (Black) versus Raw Garlic against Ischemia/Reperfusion-Induced Cardiac Complications

Attila Czompa [1], Kitti Szoke [1], Jozsef Prokisch [2], Alexandra Gyongyosi [1], Istvan Bak [1], Gyorgy Balla [3,4], Arpad Tosaki [1] and Istvan Lekli [1,*]

1 Department of Pharmacology, Faculty of Pharmacy, University of Debrecen, 4012 Debrecen, Hungary; czompa.attila@pharm.unideb.hu (A.C.); szoke.kitti@pharm.unideb.hu (K.S.); gyongyosi.alexandra@pharm.unideb.hu (A.G.); bak.istvan@pharm.unideb.hu (I.B.); tosaki.arpad@pharm.unideb.hu (A.T.)

2 Department of Animal Husbandry, Institute of Animal Science, Biotechnology and Nature Conservation, Faculty of Agriculture, Food Science and Environmental Management, University of Debrecen, 4012 Debrecen, Hungary; jprokisch@agr.unideb.hu

3 Department of Pediatrics, Medical and Health Science Center, University of Debrecen, 4012 Debrecen, Hungary; balla@med.unideb.hu

4 Hemostasis, Thrombosis and Vascular Biology Research Group, Hungarian Academy of Sciences, 4012 Debrecen, Hungary

* Correspondence: lekli.istvan@pharm.unideb.hu; Tel.: +36-52-255568

Received: 5 February 2018; Accepted: 22 March 2018; Published: 28 March 2018

Abstract: Recent evidence from studies suggests that aged black garlic also has an effect on health. The major aim of the present study is to compare the effect of raw and aged black garlic on postischemic cardiac recovery. Male Sprague Dawley rats were randomly divided into three groups. Animals of the first group were fed with raw garlic, animals of the second group received aged black garlic, while the third group served as vehicle-treated controls. Upon conclusion of the treatment, isolated hearts were undertaken to ischemia/reperfusion. Heart function and infarct size were measured and the level of HO-1 and iNOS were studied. Superior postischemic cardiac function and reduced infarct size in both garlic treated groups compared to the drug-free control group, indicated cardioprotective effects. However, no significant differences between the garlic treated groups were observed. Western blot analysis revealed that raw garlic enhanced the level of HO-1 before ischemia, while in ischemic samples, we found elevated HO-1 expression in both garlic treated groups. The level of iNOS was the same before ischemia in all groups, however, a markedly reduced iNOS level in ischemic/reperfused hearts originating from control and raw garlic treated animals was observed. Samples from aged black garlic treated animals demonstrated that the level of iNOS was not significantly reduced after ischemia/reperfusion. Taken together these results indicate that not only raw but also aged black garlic possess a cardioprotective effect.

Keywords: garlic; ischemia; heme oxygenase; reperfusion; heart

1. Introduction

Raw garlic (RG) has a long history as a spice and as a medical plant. It is mentioned in ancient literature from different parts of the Word including Egypt, India and Greece. Moreover, different cultures without any connection were associated with similar beneficial effects on for garlic, as summarized by Rivlin [1]. An example is ancient athletes during Olympic Games used garlic to enhance their endurance. Furthermore, garlic bulbs were found in the pyramid of Tutankhamen [2]. Many health-related effects were later confirmed by modern evidence-based medicine. Recent evidence suggests that a processed form of garlic called "Aged black garlic" (ABG) also possesses beneficial to health properties including antidiabetic and antiatherogenic effects [3].

According to the Framingham Heart Study, both diabetes and perturbed lipid homeostasis might contribute to the pathogenesis of ischemic heart diseases [4,5]. Indeed, consequences of atherosclerosis and micro- and macrovascular complications of diabetes often lead to an impaired medical state. Different studies have shown that the consumption of medicinal plants can help to normalize glucose and fat homeostasis. Through normalization of metabolic homeostasis, these plants can indirectly protect the heart from ischemia, for example decreasing the blood sugar level or normalizing the lipid homeostasis, which can reduce the risk of ischemic heart diseases [6], or directly possessing a cardioprotective effect acting on cardiomyocytes or endothelial cells in cardiac vessels. The direct cardioprotective effect might relate to the antioxidant properties of plants, or a direct effect on ion channels or induction of different stress related proteins such as hemoxygenase-1 (HO-1). Indeed, lower levels of HO-1 mRNA and endogen CO production are found to be related to increased risks of reperfusion induced ventricular fibrillation [7]. Furthermore, upregulation of HO-1 by plants or their extracts play a critical role in the prevention of I/R-injury in different organs [8,9]. Recently, ABG was shown to induce HO-1 in an epithelial cell model, which might indicate a tissue protective property of ABG [10]. The major objective of the present study was to compare the effect of ABG and raw garlic (RG) on the pre- and postischemic cardiac function and investigate the underlying molecular mechanisms.

2. Results

2.1. Analysis of the Composition of Raw and Aged Black Garlic

Figure 1 and Table 1 depict the different sulfur-containing molecules in both garlic preparations. It must be noted that amounts and numbers of different sulfur-containing compounds are higher in ABG. The study failed to detect any allicin in ABG (Table 1). During the aging process, the Maillard reaction occurred, which was evidenced by the presence of the 2-acetyl-1-pyrroline in ABG and its absence in raw garlic.

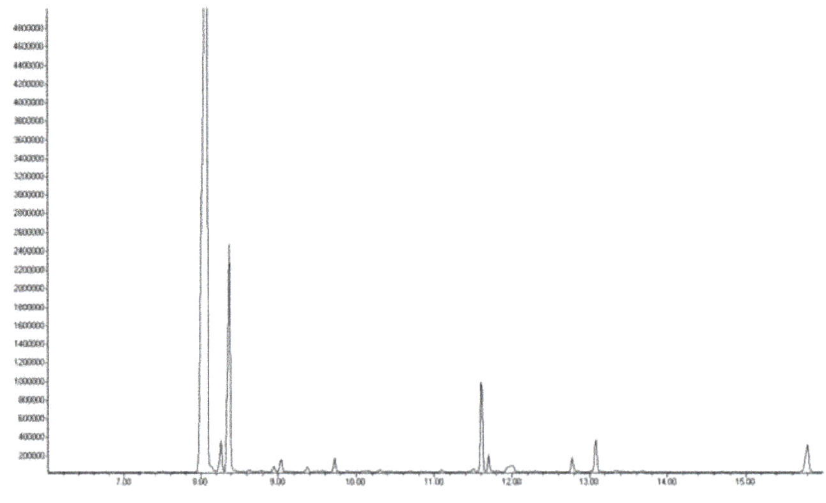

Figure 1. *Cont.*

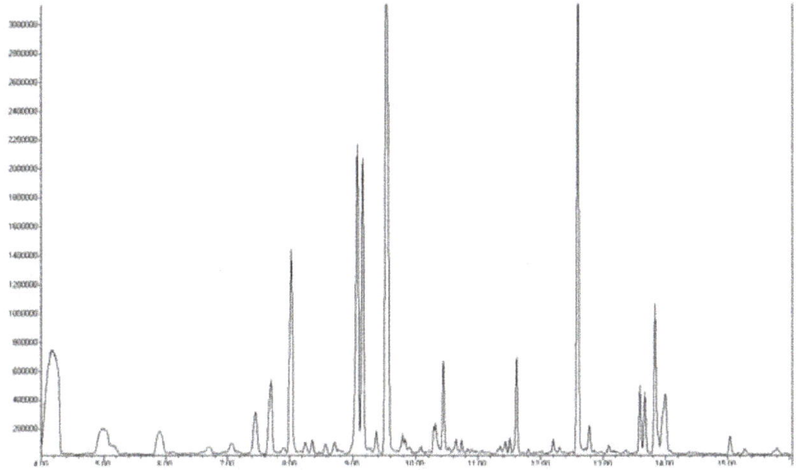

Figure 1. Representative chromatograms of raw garlic (**upper panel**) and black garlic (**lower panel**) Headspace-SPME technique was used to obtained samples followed by GC-MS analysis.

Table 1. Main compounds of raw and black garlic in the gas phase.

Compounds	Retention Time (min)	Raw Garlic	Aged Black Garlic	Structures
2-acetyl-1-pyrroline	7.6	−	+	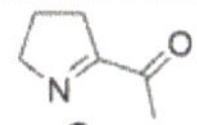
diallyl disulfide	8.0	+	+	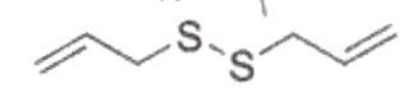
diallyl trisulfide	9.1	+	+	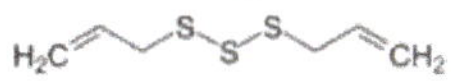
dipropil trisulfide	11.6	+	+	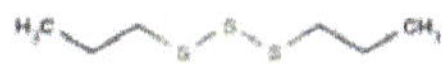
allicin	11.7	+	−	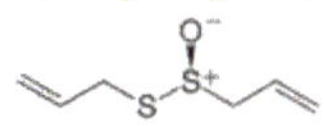

"+" -detectable; "−" non-detectable or just in a very low concentration.

2.2. *Effect of Raw and Aged Garlic on Body Weight and Blood Enzymes*

No significant differences in body weight were seen after 4 weeks of RG- and ABG-treated groups compared to the vehicle-treated group (Figure 2). Following the treatment period with different garlic preparations, peripheral blood was collected, and various blood enzymes were measured. Table 2 shows that the levels of the investigated blood markers remained in the normal range in all groups.

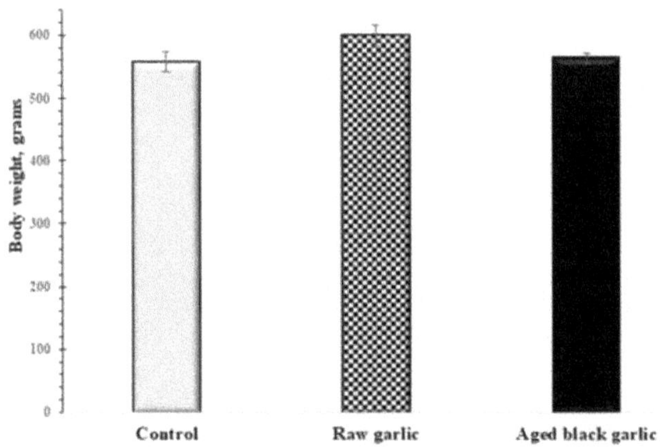

Figure 2. The effects of raw and aged black garlic on bodyweight. Upon conclusion of the treatment with raw (RG) and aged black garlic (ABG) bodyweight was measured. Results are expressed as mean ± SEM. n = 9 in each group.

Table 2. Blood parameters measured from vehicle-, raw- and aged black-treated animals.

Blood Parameters	Control n = 8	Raw Garlic n = 10	Aged Black Garlic n = 9
ALT (U/L)	45.0 ± 3.3	47.1 ± 1.9	44.1 ± 1.4
ALP (U/L)	91.3 ± 9.2	90.2 ± 1.3	84.8 ± 4.4
ASTL (U/L)	89.1 ± 9.1	89.6 ± 3.8	87.9 ± 4.3
CHO (mmol/L)	1.30 ± 0.12	1.41 ± 0.07	1.58 ± 0.05 *
LDL (mmol/L)	0.224 ± 0.020	0.294 ± 0.019 *	0.350 ± 0.021 *
TRIG (mmol/L)	1.35 ± 0.23	1.07 ± 0.12	1.32 ± 0.10
HDL (mmol/L)	1.09 ± 0.11	1.19 ± 0.04	1.25 ± 0.06
LDH (U/L)	811 ± 173	772 ± 88	801 ± 82
CRP (mg/L)	1.35 ± 0.23	1.07 ± 0.12	1.32 ± 0.10
CK–MB (U/L)	765 ± 154	656 ± 66	746 ± 89

* $p < 0.05$ in comparison with the control group.

2.3. Raw and Aged Garlic Treatment Protect the Heart from Ischemia/Reperfusion Injury

To compare the beneficial to health effects of RG and ABG garlic, isolated hearts originating from treated animals were taken to 30 min of global ischemia and 120 min of reperfusion. No significant differences were seen in preischemic values of the studied cardiac functions including CF, AF, AOP, AOdP/dt, CO, and SV alteration. However, Figure 3 shows significantly increased postischemic cardiac function in the presence of raw and aged garlic, respectively, was detected. Thus, after 30 min of ischemia and 120 min of reperfusion, AF was significantly enhanced in the treated groups compared to their control value of 4.3 ± 2.0 mL to 24.1 ± 4.6 mL for raw garlic, and 22.7 ± 3.8 mL for aged garlic. Interestingly, in comparison with the control values of 13.6 ± 1.2 mL superior CF values in the treated groups was observed, in the raw garlic group a value of 19.3 ± 2.8 mL and for aged garlic a value of 19.9 ± 1.4 mL, respectively.

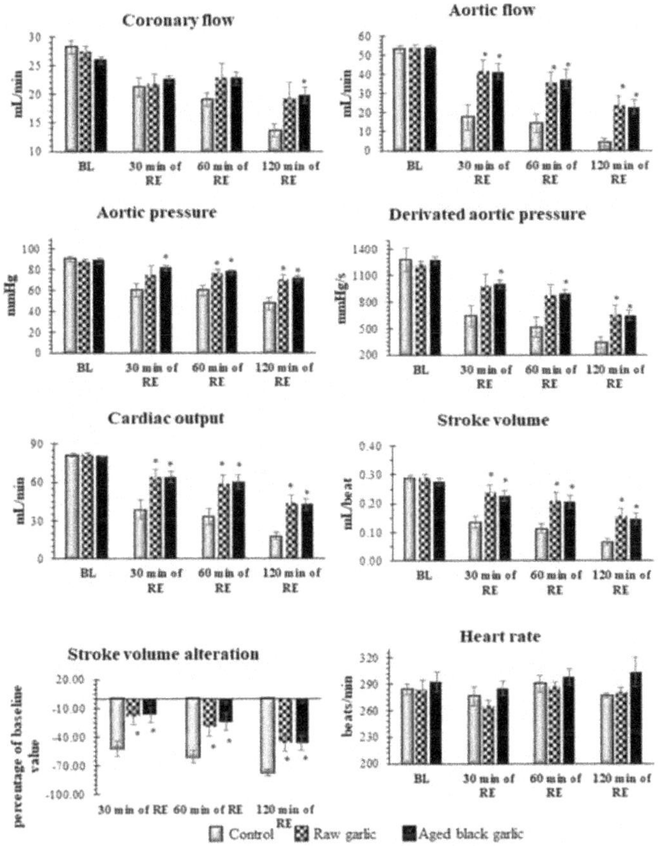

Figure 3. Effects of raw and aged black garlic on pre and postischemic cardiac functions. Following the end of the treatments, isolated hearts were subjected to 30 min of ischemia and 120 min of reperfusion. Pre- and postischemic left ventricular functions including heart rate (HR), coronary flow (CF), aortic flow (AF), aortic pressure (AOP), the first derivative of aortic pressure (AOdP/dt), stroke volume (SV), alteration in stroke volume were studied. Results are expressed as mean ± SEM $n = 9$ in each group. Raw garlic (RG); aged black garlic (ABG). * $p < 0.05$ in comparison with the control parameters within the same period.

2.4. *Infarct Size Reduction by Raw and Aged Black Garlic Treatment in Ischemic Reperfused Myocardium*

To further confirm the cardioprotective effect of the RG and ABG at the end of I/R TTC, staining was carried out to monitor the size of infarcted tissue. It is depicted in Figure 4 that the 27.5 ± 8.4% infarcted volume was in the control group, and both raw and aged garlic were able to significantly reduce the infarct volume to 5.9 ± 2.0% and 6.2 ± 1.2%, respectively. There were no statistically significant differences between the two garlic treated groups.

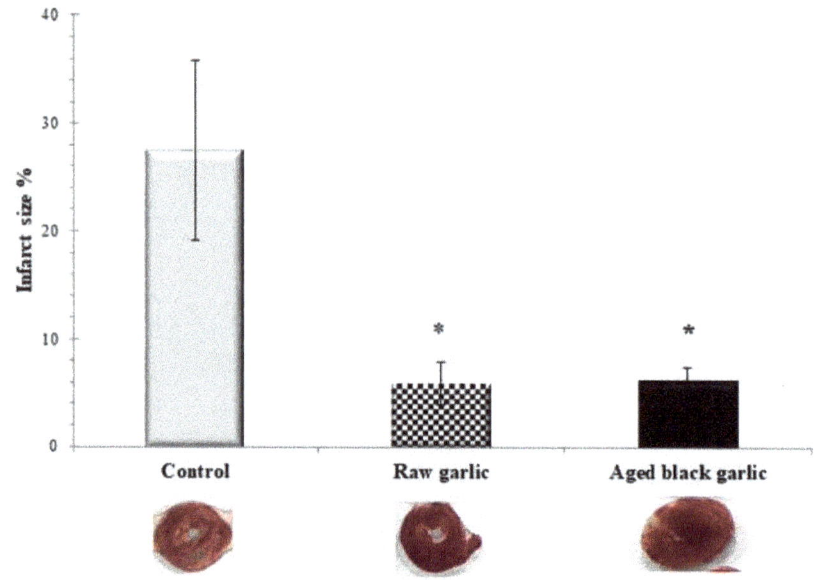

Figure 4. Effects of raw and aged black garlic on infarct size. Following ischemia/reperfusion, hearts were perfused with TTC solution via aortic cannula to assess the infarcted size (infarcted area in white, and non-ischemic region stained in red. Results are expressed as mean ± SEM. $n = 4$ in each group. Raw garlic (RG); Aged black garlic (ABG). * $p < 0.05$ in comparison with the control group.

2.5. Induction of HO-1 and iNOS by Garlic

To explore the molecular mechanisms by which RG and ABG protected the heart against I/R injury, the levels of HO-1 and iNOS were measured by Western blot. Figure 5A illustrates that the study detected the enhanced level of HO-1 for RG preparation before I/R. However, after I/R, in both garlic treated groups, a significantly elevated level of HO-1 was observed. The evaluation of iNOS is depicted in Figure 5B and no significant differences were seen before I/R between the groups. However, after I/R a significantly reduced protein level of iNOS was seen in the control and RG treated hearts, but AGB was able to prevent the reduction of iNOS after I/R. Representative blots are provided as supplementary Figure S1.

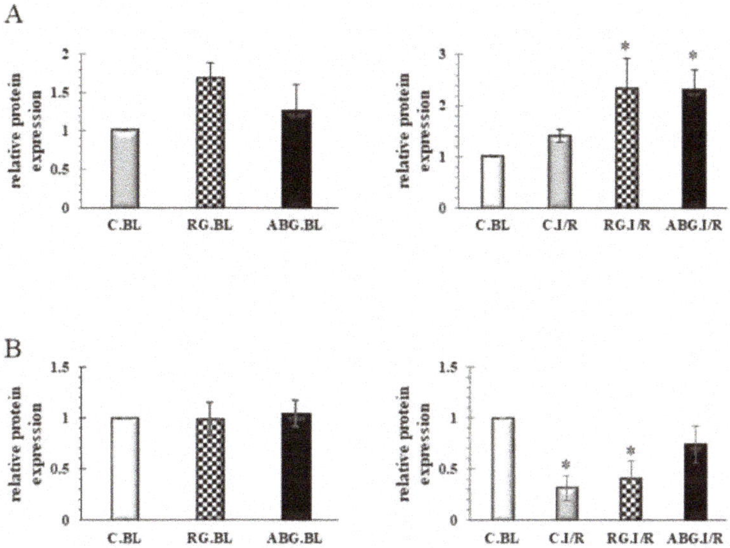

Figure 5. Effect of raw and aged black garlic on HO-1 and iNOS expression. Panel (**A**): Protein samples from hearts originating from animals treated with RG, ABG or vehicle were separated, blotted and probed with the HO-1 antibody. Panel (**B**): Protein samples from hearts originating from animals treated with RG, ABG or vehicle were separated, blotted and probed with iNOS antibody. Results are expressed as mean ± SEM n = 5–7. Raw garlic (RG); aged black garlic (ABG). BL: baseline samples; I/R: ischemia/reperfused samples. * $p < 0.05$ in comparison with the control baseline parameters (CBL).

3. Discussion

A healthy diet is being considered as a keystone of different stages of primary, secondary or tertiary prevention. Nowadays, the so-called functional food is gaining importance in different stages of prevention or might be used as complementary treatment next to medicines. Garlic is being considered as a very healthy spice or medical plant, however, consumption of RG is limited by the intense taste, the foul breath, and the body odor. Even consumption of garlic extracts might have the same effect on body odor. The taste and effect on breath by ABG are very moderate compared to RG. Furthermore, there are preparations of ABG with honey or chocolate, which are very tasty. Intact garlic is abundant in γ-glutamyl cysteine, which can be transformed to alliin. During culinary preparations like cutting, crushing etcetera, alliin is converted to the odiferous allicin by alliinase [11]. During the aging process, when garlic is exposed to a relatively high temperature (70 °C) and high humidity, the major sulfur-containing compound γ-glutamyl cysteine is converted to *S*-allylmercaptocysteine (SAC), which is a major water-soluble antioxidant compound of ABG [12]. These results also verify that during aging, the alliin is being converted to other sulfur-containing compounds and even the level of allicin in ABG remains under the limit of detection. Furthermore, under such conditions, the Maillard reaction also occurs when sugars react with amino acids leading to brownish colors. The compound 2-acetyl-1-pyrroline is present in some plants in raw form; however, it has been shown that during cooking, it forms as a product of the Maillard reaction [13,14]. This study failed to find 2-acetyl-1-pyrroline in RG, however, we were able to detect it in ABG samples, indicating that under this study's conditions, the Maillard reaction also contributes to the "aging and transformation" of RG to ABG. Figure 1 shows that the authors identified different sulphur-containing molecules in both garlic preparations, which might play a role in cardioprotection and possess beneficial to health effects as suggested earlier [15,16]. However, based on these results the authors cannot pick up only one single compound.

The major aim of the present study was to compare the cardiovascular effect of raw and aged black garlic in an experimental model. Consistent with earlier studies [17–19], these results clearly demonstrate that both RG and ABG possess similar very significant cardioprotective effects in I/R-ed myocardium, as evidenced by superior postischemic cardiac functions and smaller infarct size. The study failed to find any significant differences between the two treated groups, indicating that the aging process of garlic does not alter the cardioprotective ability of the preparation. Indeed, different studies have compared the antioxidant and anti-inflammatory effects of RG and ABG under certain conditions [20,21]. Lee and colleagues have shown superior antioxidant properties for ABG over RG in diabetic animals [21]. Earlier, a long term garlic administration was shown to enhance the level of endogen antioxidants such as catalase, SOD in the myocardium in a dose dependent manner [19]. The authors have suggested the contribution of the enhanced antioxidant defense mechanism to the cardioprotective ability of garlic. Consistently, enhanced antioxidant activity was found in ABG by Jeong and co-workers, however, the antioxidant capability was not directly proportional to the anti-inflammatory property of the different garlic preparations in an LPS-stimulated inflammatory model [20]. The authors found that pyruvate and other polyphenols, flavonoids and organosulfur compounds, enriched during the aging process, act synergistically as antioxidants in ABG. Furthermore, the anti-inflammatory effects of pyruvate found in ABG might be perturbed by the sugar component in ABG.

The study did not find any analyzed biomarkers out of the physiological range; since all remained under the physiological level any effect on metabolism cannot be concluded. However, it must be noted that the possibility is quite reasonable since rats were also symptom-free during the treatment period. The same reasoning might explain the unaltered body weight during the experiments. Thus, the metabolic effect of the garlic preparations should be studied in a diabetic or atherosclerotic animal model.

To explore the molecular mechanisms by which the different garlic preparations protect the heart, the levels of HO-1 and iNOS were studied. The study found that treatment with RG can enhance the level of HO-1 before ischemia. Following ischemia in both garlic-treated groups, the level of HO-1 is significantly enhanced. Induction of HO-1 leads to the production of Fe^{2+}, endogen CO and biliverdin/bilirubin as a byproduct of heme metabolism. Enhanced activity of the HO-1/CO system by different natural products has been shown to induce cardioprotection [8,22]. Upregulation of HO-1 might be an adaptive response to different harmful stimuli such as ischemia, or even excess heme levels. Recently, it has been suggested that under special conditions, an excess level of HO-1 and its by-products might fail to protect against I/R. Not long ago, the authors reported that cardioprotection induced by a low dose beta-carotene treatment is absent at a high dose beta-carotene treatment; although in both cases, an enhanced level of HO-1 was observed. The authors have speculated that, probably, the high level of Fe^{2+} in the presence of a high amount of beta-carotene might behave as a pro-oxidant [23]. However, in that circumstance, the authors assumed that mild HO-1 induction was a contributing factor to the cardioprotective effect of HO-1. Earlier, sour cherry seed extract was found to protect the heart via upregulation of HO-1 protein [8]. Ginseng derived ginsenoside was proven to activate the Nrf2/HO-1 pathway and protect H9c2 cells against hypoxia/reoxygenation in a recent study [24]. Furthermore, Issan and colleagues have demonstrated that pharmacological induction of HO-1 by CoPP protects H9c2 cells against hypoxia and also diabetic hearts from ischemia via the modulation of the AKT/GSK3β pathway [25]. However, it must be noted that from this study's results, the authors cannot conclude which component is the major HO-1-inducer since the composition of the two garlic preparations is not the same.

NOSs, possessing three isoforms including eNOS, nNOS, and iNOS, are a group of enzymes producing NO, which is a gaseous transmitter playing a role in different physiological and pathophysiological processes. During the authors' experiments, the level of iNOS was significantly reduced after I/R in the vehicle-treated control and RG-treated groups. A slight decrement was observed in the ABG group, however, it was not at a significant level indicating the ability of ABG to prevent iNOS loss after I/R. Recently, an extract of ABG was shown to possess dose-dependent cardioprotective effects and similarly, an enhanced iNOS expression was found in ABG-treated hearts [15]. Similarly, in a recent study, a reduced level of iNOS mRNA expression was found in hearts obtained from saline-treated animals after infarction. However, fish oil treatment prevented the decreased expression of iNOS after infarction [26]. Furthermore, enhanced expression of iNOS accompanied by smaller infarct size were found in eNOS KO animals in response to I/R-injury in an "ex vivo" model, indicating that NO plays a role in cardioprotection [27]. It must be noted that the authors did not observe any alteration of iNOS expression in WT animals after I/R. Quite the reverse, as "in vivo" studies showed earlier, overexpression of iNOS might contribute to myocardial injury [28,29]. Thus, cardioprotection afforded by Propofol and Sabiporide (Na^+/H^+ exchanger-1 inhibitor) was found to be mediated via the suppression of iNOS. Furthermore, slightly enhanced expression of iNOS was detected in hearts obtained from overfed animals [30]. Moreover, enhanced iNOS activity was found to play a role in cardiomyocyte dysfunction in a regional ischemia in vivo [31]. Interestingly, in another study, enhanced expression of iNOS was observed in the ischemic region of the heart after a "sub-lethal ischemic" insult suggesting a regulatory role of iNOS during the late preconditioning [32]. Based on the above-mentioned outcomes, the role of NO and NOSs in ischemic tissue could be both beneficial and harmful, depending on the environment or tissue damage [33,34]. However, it must be noted that the difference in iNOS expression also might arise from the different experimental models since, in the current study, "ex vivo" 30 min ischemia and 120 min of reperfusion was used to mimic I/R, while in other studies "in vivo" 6–24 h of reperfusion were allowed. Under "in vivo" conditions, the authors cannot rule out the influence of the immune system and platelets on the expression of different proteins [27].

Taken together, this study's results clearly demonstrate that the components of garlic during the aging process are altered, but ABG still possesses beneficial health effects. The outcome of the present study demonstrates that consumption of ABG is also healthy and could reduce I/R-induced cardiac complications. However, further studies need to be carried out to study the cardiovascular effect of different garlic preparations in diseased, diabetic, and atherosclerotic models.

4. Materials and Methods

4.1. Animals

Male Sprague Dawley (SD) rats with an average weight of 575 ± 45 g (n = 9, in each groups) were used. Animals were nutrified with standard rodent chow pellets (R/M-Z+H, ssniff Spezialdiäten GmbH, Soest, Germany) ad libitum with free access to water and kept at an ambient temperature of 25 ± 2 °C, with a relative humidity of 55 ± 5%, and a 12-h light-dark cycle. All animals were treated according to the "Principles of Laboratory Animal Care" formulated by the National Society for Medical Research, and the "Guide for the Care and Use of Laboratory Animals" prepared by the National Academy of Sciences and published by the National Institutes of Health (NIH Publication number 86–23, revised in 1996). Breeding and handling of the animals was approved by the Institutional Animal Care and Use Committee of the University of Debrecen, Debrecen, Hungary (May 2012; 12 March 2012).

4.2. Treatment Protocol

Rats were randomly segregated into three treatment groups as described: GROUP I: control rats, gavage-treated with the mucin-water vehicle (2% hydroxyethylcellulose solution). GROUP II: RG-treated rats, gavaged with mucin-water, supplemented with 300 mg/kg/day dose of RG. GROUP III: ABG-treated rats, gavaged with mucin-water, supplemented with 300 mg/kg/day dose of ABG. The dose of 300 mg/kg is approximately equal with 15–20 cloves of garlic. Hence, it is rather comparable to 2–3 commercially available garlic capsules or tablets.

All animals were treated every day for a period of 4 weeks. Body mass was measured at the end of treatments.

4.3. Preparation of Aged Garlic

Separated and peeled RG cloves were vacuum sealed in heat-resistant plastic bags. After 3 weeks incubation at 75 °C, conversion was completed and the ABG cloves were used for the treatment and GC-MS analyses.

4.4. GC-MS Analyses

Ground raw garlic and aged black garlic cloves were placed into head space vials and were thermostated at 50 °C for 1 h. Solid phase micro-extraction was carried out by using a Supelco fiber assembly with 85 μm polyacrylate-fused silica fiber.

Chromatograms of RG and ABG were taken by a Hewlett-Packard 5890 Series II gas chromatograph-5971A mass spectrometer. Samples were injected into HP-5 stationary phase containing capillary column (25 m × 0.25 mm × 0.25 μm) where the eluent gas was 40 °C helium with 1 mL/min constant flow. Temperatures during analyses were the following: 55 °C for 2 min followed by the scan period to 200 °C with 20 °C/min heating. The overall time of one analysis was 27 min. The temperature of the injector was 200 °C and contained an unpacked liner. Transfer line temperature was 280 °C. Ionization was reached at 70 eV and 10–500 AMU weighed particles were analyzed. Operation of the GC-MS setup, data collecting, and evaluation process was carried out with Hewlett-Packard GC-MS Chemstation rev.3 software (Hewlett-Packard Company, Wilmington, DE, USA. Regarding the mass spectra, components were identified by databases of Nist98 and Wiley.

4.5. Isolated Working Heart Preparation and Cardiac Function Assessments

Following a 4-week treatment period, 24 h after the last treatment, rats were anesthetized with an intraperitoneal pentobarbital sodium injection (60 mg/kg), with heparin as an anticoagulant (1000 U/kg). Following the induction of deep anesthesia, chest cavities were opened, hearts were excised and placed in ice-cold modified Krebs-Henseleit bicarbonate (KHB) buffer (containing 118 mM NaCl, 5.8 mM KCl, 1.8 mM $CaCl_2$, 25 mM $NaHCO_3$, 0.36 mM KH_2PO_4, 1.2 mM $MgSO_4$, and 5.0 mM Glucose) to prevent damage of cardiac tissue. Subsequent to excision, aortas were cannulated, and each heart was perfused with modified KHB buffer at a filling pressure of 100 cm of water, using the non-working (Langendorff) mode of the isolated working heart apparatus for 5 min to flush blood out from the hearts. During the washout period, pulmonary veins were cannulated and heart functions were assessed in working mode at a filling pressure of 17 cm of water with KHB buffer. A total of 10 min of working mode activity was sustained to stabilize the cardiac activity. Upon conclusion of 10 min of working mode perfusion, baseline cardiac parameters were registered, including heart rate (HR), aortic flow (AF), and coronary flow (CF); cardiac output (CO) and stroke volume (SV) were calculated. Next, 30 min of ischemia was induced by closing off atrial inflow and aortic outflow. Upon completion of the ischemic period, reperfusion was initiated by opening the aortic cannula. The first 10 min of reperfusions were conducted in the non-working mode to prevent the development of fatal ventricular arrhythmias. The heart was defibrillated with a square wave impulse if ventricular fibrillation was observed at the onset of the reperfusion. Following the first 10 min of Langendorff reperfusion, hearts were switched to working mode for an additional 110 min. Cardiac parameters were recorded at 30, 60 and 120 min of the reperfusion period to monitor the postischemic recovery of the myocardium. A continuous pressure signal was recorded during the whole experiment with the help of a pressure transducer (ADInstruments, PowerLab, Castle Hill, Australia). HR and AOdP/dt were calculated from the continuously recorded pressure signal. AF was measured by a calibrated flow meter, while CF was assessed by time-collecting the coronary effluent. Cardiac output (CO) was calculated as the sum of AF and CF, while stroke volume (SV) was the ratio of CO and HR. Stroke volume alteration was calculated as a ratio of SV and the baseline of SV [8].

4.6. Infarct Size Measurements

To monitor the degree of infarction, triphenyl tetrazolium chloride (TTC) (Sigma-Aldrich, Inc., St. Louis, MO, USA) staining was carried out. Hearts were perfused with 35 mL of 1% TTC solution via the aortic cannula at the end of the reperfusion. Following 10 min, hearts were stored at −20 °C for 24 h, to allow each heart to solidify. A total of 2–3 mm thick sections were made from the stained frozen hearts. Sections were subsequently scanned on an Epson J232D flat-bed scanner, blotted dry and weighed. The infarcted area (unstained tissue remained white) and the risk area (entire scanned section) were measured using planimetry software (Image J, National Institutes of Health, Bethesda, MD, USA). Estimates of infarcted zone magnitude were subsequently obtained by multiplying infarcted areas by the weight of each section. The resulting numbers represented the weight of the risk zone and the infarcted zone. Infarct size was expressed as a ratio of the weight of infarcted tissue and the weight of risk zone (whole heart). The entire area of each section was considered to be an infarcted risk zone, while the numerical extent of each infarcted area was planimetrically calculated and multiplied by the weight of the section. Outcomes were expressed as the ratio of the total infarcted tissue volume to volume of at-risk tissue.

4.7. Blood Enzymes

Following 4 weeks of treatment with different garlic preparations or mucin-water vehicle prior to sacrifice, peripheral blood was collected from a left external jugular vein of each animal. Analyses of selected serum analytes was conducted using the Cobas 8000 modular analyzer series (Roche Diagnostics GmbH, Mannheim, Germany). The samples were assayed for content of alanine aminotransferase (ALT), alkaline phosphatase (ALP), aspartate aminotransferase (ASTL) total cholesterol (CHO), low-density lipoprotein cholesterol (LDL), triglycerides (TRIG), high-density lipoprotein cholesterol (HDL), lactate dehydrogenase (LDH), C-reactive protein (CRP), and creatine-kinase-myoglobin (CK-MB). Testing was conducted in the Department of Laboratory Medicine, University of Debrecen, Hungary.

4.8. Western Blot Analyses

Approximately 300 mg of heart tissue was lysed in 1 mL isolating buffer (25 mM Tris-HCl, 25 mM NaCl, 1 mM orthovanadate, 10 mM NaF, 10 mM pyrophosphate, 10 mM okadaic acid, 0.5 mM EDTA, 1 mM PMSF, and 1× protease inhibitor cocktail) using a polytron homogenizer. Homogenates were centrifuged at 2000 rpm at 4 °C for 10 min. The supernatant was transferred to a new tube and further centrifuged at 10,000 rpm at 4 °C for 20 min; the resultant supernatant was used as a cytosolic extract. The protein concentration was determined by a BCA Protein Assay Kit (Thermo Scientific, Rockford, IL, USA) using bovine serum albumin (BSA) as the standard. Samples were mixed with Laemmli buffer and boiled for 10 min. A total of 100 µg of protein in each sample was loaded and separated on 12% SDS–PAGE gels (Sigma Aldrich, Schnelldorf, Germany) and then transferred to polyvinylidene difluoride (PVDF) membranes (Bio-Rad Laboratories, Hercules, CA, USA). Following blocking the membranes with 5% of nonfat dry milk powder dissolved in tris-buffered saline buffer with 0.1% Tween 20 (TBST) for 1 h, membranes were incubated with primary antibody solution at 4 °C overnight (HO–1 1/500, Abcam, Cambridge, UK; iNOS, Cell Signaling Technology, Boston, MA, USA). The membranes were washed with TBST 3 times and incubated with horseradish peroxidase (HRP)-conjugated secondary antibody solution (1/2000, Cell Signaling Technology, Boston, MA, USA) for 1 h at room temperature. Subsequent to washing, the membranes were developed using Luminate Forte Western HRP substrate (Millipore, Billerica, MA, USA). Chemiluminescence was detected as well as band intensities were measured by ChemiDoc™ Touch Imaging System and Image Lab software (Bio-Rad Inc., Hercules, CA, USA) [8] and normalized against total protein.

4.9. Statistical Analyses

All data are presented as the average magnitudes of each outcome in a group ± standard error of the mean (SEM). Statistical analysis was performed using one-way analysis of variance (ANOVA), followed by Kruskal–Wallis or Dunnett's multiple comparison tests with GraphPad Prism software for Windows (GraphPad Software Inc., La Jolla, CA, USA). Probability values (p) less than 0.05 were considered statistically significant.

Supplementary Materials: Supplementary materials can be found at http://www.mdpi.com/1422-0067/19/4/1017/s1. Figure S1. Representative Western blots. Upper blot represents protein samples from hearts originating from animals treated with RG, ABG or vehicle were separated, blotted and probed with the HO-1 antibody. Lower blot represents protein samples from hearts originating from animals treated with RG, ABG or vehicle were separated, blotted and probed with the iNOS antibody. Raw garlic (RG); aged black garlic (ABG). BL: baseline samples; I/R: ischemia/reperfused samples.

Acknowledgments: Sources of support: This study was supported by grants from OTKA-PD-111794 (I.L.); NKFI-124719 (A.T.). This research was also supported by the European Union and the State of Hungary, co-financed by the European Social Fund in the framework of TÁMOP 4.2.4. A/2-11-1-2012-0001 (Attila Czompa; Alexandra Gyongyosi; Arpad Tosaki; Istvan Lekli) "National Excellence Program"; GINOP-2.3.2-15-2016-00043; EFOP-3.6.1-16-2016-00022. Supported by the ÚNKP-17-4-III-DE-219 New National Excellence Program of the Ministry of Human Capacities.

Author Contributions: Attila Czompa, Istvan Bak, Gyorgy Balla, Arpad Tosaki, and Istvan Lekli designed research; Attila Czompa, Kitti Szoke, Jozsef Prokisch, and Alexandra Gyongyosi conducted research; Attila Czompa, Arpad Tosaki, and Istvan Lekli wrote the paper. Attila Czompa and Istvan Lekli had primary responsibility for final content. All authors read and approved the final manuscript.

Conflicts of Interest: The authors declare no conflict of interest.

References

1. Rivlin, R.S. Historical perspective on the use of garlic. *J. Nutr.* **2001**, *131*, 951S–954S. [CrossRef] [PubMed]
2. Petrovska, B.B.; Cekovska, S. Extracts from the history and medical properties of garlic. *Pharmacogn. Rev.* **2010**, *4*, 106–110. [CrossRef] [PubMed]
3. Kim, J.H.; Yu, S.H.; Cho, Y.J.; Pan, J.H.; Cho, H.T.; Kim, J.H.; Bong, H.; Lee, Y.; Chang, M.H.; Jeong, Y.J.; et al. Preparation of S-Allylcysteine-Enriched Black Garlic Juice and Its Antidiabetic Effects in Streptozotocin-Induced Insulin-Deficient Mice. *J. Agric. Food Chem.* **2017**, *65*, 358–363. [CrossRef] [PubMed]
4. Kannel, W.B.; Hjortland, M.; Castelli, W.P. Role of diabetes in congestive heart failure: The Framingham study. *Am. J. Cardiol.* **1974**, *34*, 29–34. [CrossRef]
5. Kannel, W.B.; Castelli, W.P.; McNamara, P.M.; McKee, P.A.; Feinleib, M. Role of blood pressure in the development of congestive heart failure. The Framingham study. *N. Engl. J. Med.* **1972**, *287*, 781–787. [CrossRef] [PubMed]
6. Dwivedi, S.; Aggarwal, A. Indigenous drugs in ischemic heart disease in patients with diabetes. *J. Altern. Complement. Med.* **2009**, *15*, 1215–1221. [CrossRef] [PubMed]
7. Bak, I.; Papp, G.; Turoczi, T.; Varga, E.; Szendrei, L.; Vecsernyes, M.; Joo, F.; Tosaki, A. The role of heme oxygenase-related carbon monoxide and ventricular fibrillation in ischemic/reperfused hearts. *Free Radic. Biol. Med.* **2002**, *33*, 639–648. [CrossRef]
8. Czompa, A.; Gyongyosi, A.; Czegledi, A.; Csepanyi, E.; Bak, I.; Haines, D.D.; Tosaki, A.; Lekli, I. Cardioprotection afforded by sour cherry seed kernel: The role of heme oxygenase-1. *J. Cardiovasc. Pharmacol.* **2014**, *64*, 412–419. [CrossRef] [PubMed]
9. Kakuta, Y.; Okumi, M.; Isaka, Y.; Tsutahara, K.; Abe, T.; Yazawa, K.; Ichimaru, N.; Matsumura, K.; Hyon, S.H.; Takahara, S.; et al. Epigallocatechin-3-gallate protects kidneys from ischemia reperfusion injury by HO-1 upregulation and inhibition of macrophage infiltration. *Transpl. Int.* **2011**, *24*, 514–522. [CrossRef] [PubMed]
10. Li, T.; Ito, K.; Sumi, S.I.; Fuwa, T.; Horie, T. Antiapoptosis action of aged garlic extract (AGE) protects epithelial cells from methotrexate induced injury. *Gut* **2005**, *54*, 1819–1820. [CrossRef] [PubMed]
11. Amagase, H.; Petesch, B.L.; Matsuura, H.; Kasuga, S.; Itakura, Y. Intake of garlic and its bioactive components. *J. Nutr.* **2001**, *131*, 955S–962S. [CrossRef] [PubMed]
12. Imai, J.; Ide, N.; Nagae, S.; Moriguchi, T.; Matsuura, H.; Itakura, Y. Antioxidant and radical scavenging effects of aged garlic extract and its constituents. *Planta Medica* **1994**, *60*, 417–420. [CrossRef] [PubMed]
13. Wongpornchai, S.; Sriseadka, T.; Choonvisase, S. Identification and quantitation of the rice aroma compound, 2-acetyl-1-pyrroline, in bread flowers (*Vallaris glabra* Ktze). *J. Agric. Food Chem.* **2003**, *51*, 457–462. [CrossRef] [PubMed]

14. Wei, X.; Handoko, D.D.; Pather, L.; Methven, L.; Elmore, J.S. Evaluation of 2-acetyl-1-pyrroline in foods, with an emphasis on rice flavour. *Food Chem.* **2017**, *232*, 531–544. [CrossRef] [PubMed]
15. García-Villalón, A.L.; Amor, S.; Monge, L.; Fernández, N.; Prodanov, M.; Muñoz, M.; Inarejos-García, A.M.; Granado, M. In vitro studies of an aged black garlic extract enriched in S-allylcysteine and polyphenols with cardioprotective effects. *J. Funct. Foods* **2016**, *27*, 189–200. [CrossRef]
16. Wu, C.C.; Sheen, L.Y.; Chen, H.W.; Kuo, W.W.; Tsai, S.J.; Lii, C.K. Differential effects of garlic oil and its three major organosulfur components on the hepatic detoxification system in rats. *J. Agric. Food Chem.* **2002**, *50*, 378–383. [CrossRef] [PubMed]
17. Rietz, B.; Isensee, H.; Strobach, H.; Makdessi, S.; Jacob, R. Cardioprotective actions of wild garlic (*Allium ursinum*) in ischemia and reperfusion. *Mol. Cell. Biochem.* **1993**, *119*, 143–150. [CrossRef] [PubMed]
18. Banerjee, S.K.; Dinda, A.K.; Manchanda, S.C.; Maulik, S.K. Chronic garlic administration protects rat heart against oxidative stress induced by ischemic reperfusion injury. *BMC Pharmacol.* **2002**, *2*, 16. [CrossRef]
19. Banerjee, S.K.; Maulik, M.; Mancahanda, S.C.; Dinda, A.K.; Gupta, S.K.; Maulik, S.K. Dose-dependent induction of endogenous antioxidants in rat heart by chronic administration of garlic. *Life Sci.* **2002**, *70*, 1509–1518. [CrossRef]
20. Jeong, Y.Y.; Ryu, J.H.; Shin, J.H.; Kang, M.J.; Kang, J.R.; Han, J.; Kang, D. Comparison of Anti-Oxidant and Anti-Inflammatory Effects between Fresh and Aged Black Garlic Extracts. *Molecules* **2016**, *21*, 430. [CrossRef] [PubMed]
21. Lee, Y.M.; Gweon, O.C.; Seo, Y.J.; Im, J.; Kang, M.J.; Kim, M.J.; Kim, J.I. Antioxidant effect of garlic and aged black garlic in animal model of type 2 diabetes mellitus. *Nutr. Res. Pract.* **2009**, *3*, 156–161. [CrossRef] [PubMed]
22. Jayachandran, K.S.; Vasanthi, A.H.; Gurusamy, N. Steroidal Saponin Diosgenin from Dioscorea bulbifera Protects Cardiac Cells from Hypoxia-reoxygenation Injury Through Modulation of Pro-survival and Pro-death Molecules. *Pharmacogn. Mag.* **2016**, *12* (Suppl. 1), S14–S20. [PubMed]
23. Csepanyi, E.; Czompa, A.; Haines, D.; Lekli, I.; Bakondi, E.; Balla, G.; Tosaki, A.; Bak, I. Cardiovascular effects of low versus high-dose beta-carotene in a rat model. *Pharmacol. Res.* **2015**, *100*, 148–156. [CrossRef] [PubMed]
24. Li, Q.; Xiang, Y.; Chen, Y.; Tang, Y.; Zhang, Y. Ginsenoside Rg1 Protects Cardiomyocytes Against Hypoxia/Reoxygenation Injury via Activation of Nrf2/HO-1 Signaling and Inhibition of JNK. *Cell. Physiol. Biochem.* **2017**, *44*, 21–37. [CrossRef] [PubMed]
25. Issan, Y.; Kornowski, R.; Aravot, D.; Shainberg, A.; Laniado-Schwartzman, M.; Sodhi, K.; Abraham, N.G.; Hochhauser, E. Heme oxygenase-1 induction improves cardiac function following myocardial ischemia by reducing oxidative stress. *PLoS ONE* **2014**, *9*, e92246. [CrossRef] [PubMed]
26. Lescano de Souza Junior, A.; Mancini Filho, J.; Pavan Torres, R.; Irigoyen, M.C.; Curi, R. Pretreatment with fish oil attenuates heart ischaemia consequences in rats. *Exp. Physiol.* **2017**, *102*, 1459–1473. [CrossRef] [PubMed]
27. Kanno, S.; Lee, P.C.; Zhang, Y.; Ho, C.; Griffith, B.P.; Shears, L.L., 2nd; Billiar, T.R. Attenuation of myocardial ischemia/reperfusion injury by superinduction of inducible nitric oxide synthase. *Circulation* **2000**, *101*, 2742–2748. [CrossRef] [PubMed]
28. Doods, H.; Wu, D. Sabiporide reduces ischemia-induced arrhythmias and myocardial infarction and attenuates ERK phosphorylation and iNOS induction in rats. *BioMed Res. Int.* **2013**, *2013*, 504320. [CrossRef] [PubMed]
29. Hu, Q.; Zhou, D.; Li, X.; Yang, N.; Guo, P.; Xu, D.; Li, X. Renoprotective effects of propofol on the expression of iNOS protein in rats with ischemia reperfusion injury. *Int. J. Clin. Exp. Med.* **2015**, *8*, 776–780. [PubMed]
30. Granado, M.; Fernandez, N.; Monge, L.; Figueras, J.C.; Carreno-Tarragona, G.; Amor, S.; Garcia-Villalon, A.L. Effects of coronary ischemia-reperfusion in a rat model of early overnutrition. Role of angiotensin receptors. *PLoS ONE* **2013**, *8*, e54984. [CrossRef] [PubMed]
31. Heinzel, F.R.; Gres, P.; Boengler, K.; Duschin, A.; Konietzka, I.; Rassaf, T.; Snedovskaya, J.; Meyer, S.; Skyschally, A.; Kelm, M.; et al. Inducible nitric oxide synthase expression and cardiomyocyte dysfunction during sustained moderate ischemia in pigs. *Circ. Res.* **2008**, *103*, 1120–1127. [CrossRef] [PubMed]
32. Kim, S.J.; Kim, Y.K.; Takagi, G.; Huang, C.H.; Geng, Y.J.; Vatner, S.F. Enhanced iNOS function in myocytes one day after brief ischemic episode. *Am. J. Physiol. Heart Circ. Physiol.* **2002**, *282*, H423–H428. [CrossRef] [PubMed]

33. Lee, J.; Bae, E.H.; Ma, S.K.; Kim, S.W. Altered Nitric Oxide System in Cardiovascular and Renal Diseases. *Chonnam Med. J.* **2016**, *52*, 81–90. [CrossRef] [PubMed]
34. Toda, N.; Toda, H. Coronary hemodynamic regulation by nitric oxide in experimental animals: Recent advances. *Eur. J. Pharmacol.* **2011**, *667*, 41–49. [CrossRef] [PubMed]

International Journal of
Molecular Sciences

MDPI

Article

Protective Effects of Gomisin N against Hepatic Cannabinoid Type 1 Receptor-Induced Insulin Resistance and Gluconeogenesis

Arulkumar Nagappan [1,2], Dae Young Jung [1,2], Ji-Hyun Kim [1,2] and Myeong Ho Jung [1,2,*]

[1] Division of Longevity and Biofunctional Medicine, School of Korean Medicine, Pusan National University, Yangsan 50612, Korea; arulbiotechtnau@gmail.com (A.N.); dyjung999@naver.com (D.Y.J.); kimji77@pusan.ac.kr (J.-H.K.)

[2] Healthy Aging Korean Medical Research Center, School of Korean Medicine, Pusan National University, Yangsan 50612, Korea

* Correspondence: jung0603@pusan.ac.kr; Tel.: +82-051-510-8468

Received: 16 February 2018; Accepted: 21 March 2018; Published: 23 March 2018

Abstract: Activation of the hepatic cannabinoid type 1 receptor (CB1R) induces insulin resistance and gluconeogenesis via endoplasmic reticulum (ER) stress, thereby contributing to hyperglycemia. Gomisin N (GN) is a phytochemical derived from *Schisandra chinensis*. In the current study, we investigated the inhibitory effects of GN on hepatic CB1R-mediated insulin resistance and gluconeogenesis in 2-arachidonoylglycerol (AG; an agonist of CB1R)-treated HepG2 cells and in high-fat diet (HFD)-induced obese mice. Treatment with 2-AG induced the expression of ER stress markers, serine/threonine phosphatase *PHLPP1*, *Lipin1*, and ceramide synthesis genes, but reduced the expression of ceramide degradation genes in HepG2 cells. However, GN reversed 2-AG-mediated effects and improved the 2-AG-mediated impairment of insulin signaling. Furthermore, GN inhibited 2-AG-induced intracellular triglyceride accumulation and glucose production in HepG2 cells by downregulation of lipogenesis and gluconeogenesis genes, respectively. In vivo, GN administration to HFD obese mice reduced the HFD-induced increase in fasting blood glucose and insulin levels, which was accompanied with downregulation of HFD-induced expression of CB1R, ER stress markers, ceramide synthesis gene, and gluconeogenesis genes in the livers of HFD obese mice. These findings demonstrate that GN protects against hepatic CB1-mediated impairment of insulin signaling and gluconeogenesis, thereby contributing to the amelioration of hyperglycemia.

Keywords: cannabinoid type 1 receptor; endoplasmic reticulum stress; gluconeogenesis; gomisin N; lipogenesis; insulin resistance

1. Introduction

The liver plays a major role in maintaining normal blood glucose levels by regulating de novo glucose production and glycogen breakdown. Hepatic glucose production (gluconeogenesis) is essential for the supply of glucose as an energy source to other tissues. However, excessive hepatic gluconeogenesis causes hyperglycemia. Insulin resistance is defined as the disability of insulin to regulate glucose and lipid metabolism in peripheral tissues even at elevated insulin levels in the blood. Hepatic insulin resistance results in the elevation of hepatic glucose production and triglyceride (TG) accumulation by impairing insulin-mediated inhibition of gluconeogenesis and regulating insulin-mediated TG metabolism, respectively, which contributes to hyperglycemia and dyslipidemia [1]. Therefore, the control of hepatic insulin resistance is an attractive therapeutic target for treating type 2 diabetes and hepatic steatosis.

Endogenous cannabinoids, such as arachidonoyl ethanolamide (AEA) and 2-arachidonoylglycerol (2-AG), are bioactive lipid mediators that interact with the cannabinoid type 1 receptor (CB1R) and cannabinoid type 2 receptor (CB2R), and regulate numerous biochemical responses [2]. CB1R is predominantly present in the brain and controls food behavior and energy expenditure [2]. The activation of CB1R in the central nervous system facilitates food intake by modulating the release of orexigenic and anorexigenic neuropeptides in hypothalamic neurons. CB1R is also found in peripheral tissues and controls glucose and lipid metabolism [2]. Activation of hepatic CB1R induces insulin resistance through several mechanisms in the endoplasmic reticulum (ER) stress-dependent manner [3–5]. Activation of CB1R inhibits insulin signaling by elevating inhibitory serine-307 phosphorylation of insulin receptor substrate 1 (IRS1) and by stimulating the dephosphorylation of insulin-activated protein kinase B (PKB/AKT) through upregulation of the S/T phosphatase PH domain and leucine-rich repeats protein phosphatase 1 (*PHLPP1*) [3]. Furthermore, it stimulates the expression of *Lipin1*, a phosphatidic acid phosphatase, via ER stress-inducible transcription factor, cAMP-responsive element-binding protein H (CREBH) [4]. This subsequently leads to accumulation of diacylglycerol (DAG), resulting in the phosphorylation of protein kinase C with inhibition of insulin receptor signaling [4]. In addition, CB1R-mediated ER stress increases the production of ceramide by upregulation of de novo ceramide synthesis and downregulation of ceramide degradation, which inhibits insulin signaling [5]. Moreover, hepatic CB1R activation stimulates the lipogenesis transcription factor, sterol regulatory element-binding transcription factor 1c (SREBP1c), and results in increased TG accumulation by upregulating the expression of its downstream lipogenesis genes, including fatty acid synthase (*FAS*), stearoyl-Coenzyme A desaturase 1 (*SCD1*), and acetyl-CoA carboxylase (*ACC*), which contributes to insulin resistance and steatosis [6]. Furthermore, CB1R also increases the expression of gluconeogenesis genes via CREBH and results in the elevated glucose production [7]. Thus, activation of hepatic CB1R plays a role in the development of insulin resistance, type 2 diabetes, and hepatic steatosis [8]. In this regard, selective inhibition of hepatic CB1R signaling could be a potential molecular target for the treatment of type 2 diabetes and hepatic steatosis.

Schisandra chinensis has been used as a traditional herbal medicine in Asian countries, such as China, Korea, Japan, and Russia. It has diverse pharmacological activities, including anti-oxidant, anti-tumor, anti-obesity, anti-inflammatory, cardioprotective, and hepatoprotective effects [9]. Recently, we reported that *S. chinensis* has a protective effect against ER stress-induced hepatic steatosis [10]. Gomisin N (GN), a lignan derived from *S. chinensis*, possesses hepatoprotective, anti-cancer, and anti-inflammatory effects [11]. Recently, we reported that GN exerts protective effects against obesity-induced hepatic steatosis and hyperglycemia through inhibition of ER stress and AMP-activated protein kinase (AMPK) activation, respectively [12,13]. As activation of hepatic CB1R signaling has been implicated in the development of insulin resistance, hyperglycemia, and hepatic steatosis, targeted inhibition of hepatic CB1R signaling might provide therapeutic approaches to restore insulin receptor signaling and improve hyperglycemia and hepatic steatosis.

Therefore, in the current study, we investigated the inhibitory effect of GN on hepatic CB1R and CB1R-mediated insulin resistance and gluconeogenesis in 2-arachidonoylglycerol (AG; an agonist of CB1R)-treated HepG2 cells and in high-fat diet (HFD)-induced obese mice.

2. Results

2.1. GN Inhibited 2-AG-Induced ER Stress in HepG2 Cells

The 3-(4,5-dimethylthiazol-2-yl)-2,5-diphenyltetrazolium bromide assay revealed that GN had no cytotoxic effect on HepG2 cells at a concentration of 100 μM. Activation of hepatic CB1R induces ER stress, which contributes to insulin resistance and gluconeogenesis [3–5]. Therefore, we first investigated whether GN inhibited CB1R-induced ER stress in HepG2 cells. HepG2 cells were incubated with 2-AG in the absence or presence of different concentrations of GN for 12 h. Treatment with 2-AG increased mRNA level of ER stress markers, including glucose-regulated protein 78 (*GRP78*),

C/EBP homologous protein (*CHOP*), and X box-binding protein 1c (*XBP1c*) (Figure 1A), as well as *CB1R* mRNA level (Figure 1B). However, GN treatment suppressed this increase in mRNA levels in a dose-dependent manner. Western blot analysis also showed that 2-AG treatment increased the protein levels of GRP78, CHOP, and XBP1c, but GN treatment reduced the 2-AG-induced increased in ER stress marker levels (Figure 1C), which was consistent with decrease in mRNA levels. Furthermore, to confirm the inhibitory effect of GN on ER stress, we examined the expression of ER stress markers in HepG2 cells treated with tunicamycin, a chemical ER stress inducer, in the absence or presence of GN for 12 h. As shown in Figure 1D, GN treatment significantly reduced tunicamycin-induced mRNA levels of ER stress markers. Taken together, these results indicate that GN inhibits CB1R-induced ER stress in HepG2 cells.

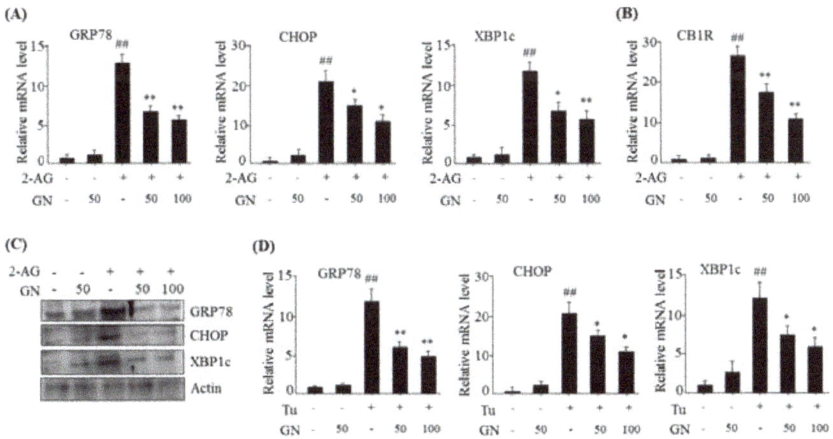

Figure 1. Gomisin N (GN) inhibited 2-AG-induced endoplasmic reticulum (ER) stress in HepG2 cells. HepG2 cells were incubated with 2-AG in the absence or presence of GN (50 or 100 μM) for 12 h. (**A**) qPCR analysis of *GRP78*, *CHOP*, and *XBP1c*; (**B**) qPCR analysis of *CB1R*; (**C**) Western blot analysis of GRP78, CHOP, and XBP1c; (**D**) HepG2 cells were incubated with tunicamycin (Tu) in the absence or presence of GN (50 or 100 μM) for 12 h. qPCR analysis of *GRP78*, *CHOP*, and *XBP1c*. Values are expressed as mean ± SEM (n = 3 independent experiments). ## $p < 0.01$ vs. untreated control. * $p < 0.05$, ** $p < 0.01$ vs. 2-AG or tunicamycin-treated control.

2.2. GN Improved CB1R-Mediated Inhibition of Insulin Signaling in HepG2 Cells

Hepatic CB1R-induced ER stress contributes to insulin resistance by inhibiting insulin signaling via several ER stress-dependent mechanisms [3–5]. CB1R-induced ER stress stimulates the expression of serine/threonine phosphatase *PHLPP1* and CREBH-dependent *Lpin1*, which contribute to inhibit insulin signaling. Therefore, we investigated whether GN suppresses CB1R-induced expression of *PHLPP1*, *CREBH*, and *Lipin1* in 2-AG-treated HepG2 cells. Results of qPCR revealed that 2-AG treatment increased mRNA levels of *PHLPP1* (Figure 2A), *CREBH* (Figure 2B), and *Lipin1* (Figure 2C). However, GN treatment significantly reversed 2-AG-induced effects. Furthermore, it has been reported that CB1R suppresses insulin signaling via regulation of ceramide production, which involves the balance of de novo ceramide synthesis and degradation of ceramides [5]. Therefore, we examined whether GN reverses the effect of CB1R on the expression of de novo ceramide synthesis-associated genes and ceramide degradation-associated genes in HepG2 cells. Treatment with 2-AG increased the mRNA levels of de novo ceramide synthesis-associated genes such as ceramide synthase 6 (*CerS6*) and serine-palmitoyl transferase LC3 (*SPTLC3*) (Figure 2D), whereas reduced the mRNA levels of ceramide degradation-associated genes such as *N*-acylsphingosine amidohydrolase 1 (*Asah1*) and sphingosine kinase 1 (*SPK1*) (Figure 2E). However, GN treatment reversed 2-AG-mediated effects, suggesting that GN suppresses CB1R-induced ceramide production, which might contribute to improve insulin resistance.

Then, we investigated the effects of GN on insulin signaling in 2AG-treated HepG2 cells. As shown in Figure 3A, 2-AG treatment increased the serine-307 phosphorylation of IRS1 at three different times, which inhibits insulin signaling; however, GN treatment reduced serine-307 phosphorylation of IRS1. Next, we investigated the effects of GN on insulin-activated phosphorylation of IRS1 at tyrosine 893 and AKT at serine 473 in 2-AG-treated HpG2 cells. As shown in Figure 3B, incubation with insulin resulted in increased phosphorylation of IRS1 (tyrosine-895) and AKT (serine-473), but 2-AG treatment reduced the expressions of p-IRS1 and p-AKT. However, GN treatment reversed the 2-AG-mediated reduction of insulin-induced phosphorylation of IRS1 and AKT (Figure 3B). These results indicate that GN improves hepatic CB1R-mediated inhibition of insulin signaling.

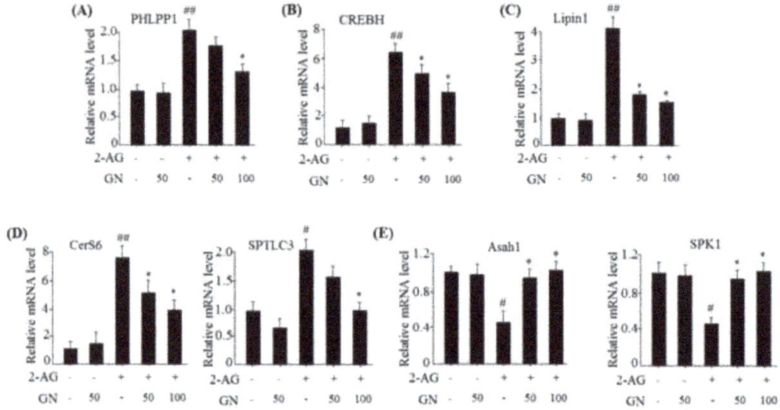

Figure 2. GN reversed 2-AG-mediated expression of insulin resistance-associated genes in HepG2 cells. HepG2 cells were incubated with 2-AG in the absence or presence of GN (50 or 100 μM) for 12 h. qPCR analysis of *PHLPP1* (**A**), *CREBH* (**B**), *Lipin1* (**C**), *Cer6* and *SPTLC3* (**D**), and *Asah1* and *SPK1* (**E**). Values are expressed as mean ± SEM (n = 3 independent experiments). # $p < 0.05$, ## $p < 0.01$ vs. untreated control. * $p < 0.05$ vs. 2-AG-treated control.

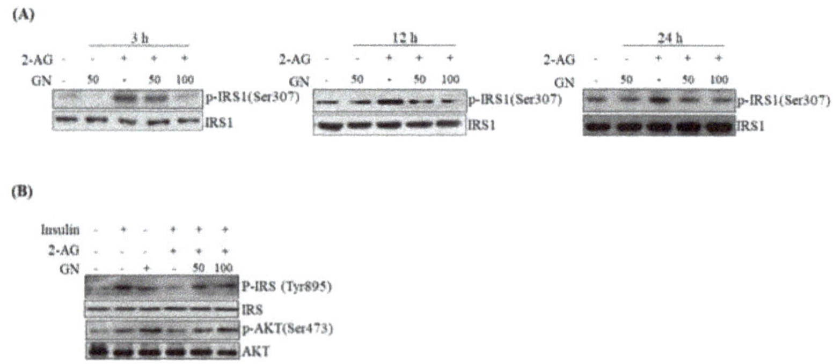

Figure 3. GN improved 2-AG-mediated inhibition of insulin signaling in HepG2 cells. (**A**) HepG2 cells were incubated with 2-AG in the absence or presence of GN (50 or 100 μM) for 3, 12 and 24 h. Serine-307 phosphorylation of IRS1 was detected by western blot analysis; (**B**) HepG2 cells were incubated with 2-AG in the absence or presence of GN (50 or 100 μM) for 12 h, and then incubated with insulin (10 nM) for 30 min. The phosphorylation of IRS1 (tyrosine-895) and AKT (serine-473) was detected by western blot analysis.

2.3. GN Inhibited CB1R-Induced Lipogenesis in HepG2 Cells

Activation of hepatic CB1R induces intracellular TG accumulation through upregulation of lipogenesis, which contributes to dysregulation of insulin signaling [6]. Therefore, we evaluated the inhibitory effects of GN on CB1R-induced lipogenesis in HepG2 cells. The expression of a key lipogenesis transcription factor SREBP1c and its downstream lipogenesis genes was measured in HepG2 cells after incubated with 2-AG in the absence or presence of different concentrations of GN for 24 h. As shown in Figure 4A, qPCR and western blot analyses showed that 2-AG treatment increased mRNA and protein levels of SREBP1c; however, GN reversed these changes. GN also reduced 2-AG-induced SREBP1c protein level even at longer incubation time (48 h). The mRNA levels of SREBP1c downstream lipogenesis genes including *FAS*, *SCD1*, and *ACC* were enhanced by 2-AG treatment, which were efficiently reversed by GN treatment (Figure 4B). In accordance with downregulation of lipogenesis genes, GN suppressed 2-AG-induced intracellular TG accumulation, as shown by TG measurement and ORO staining (Figure 4C).

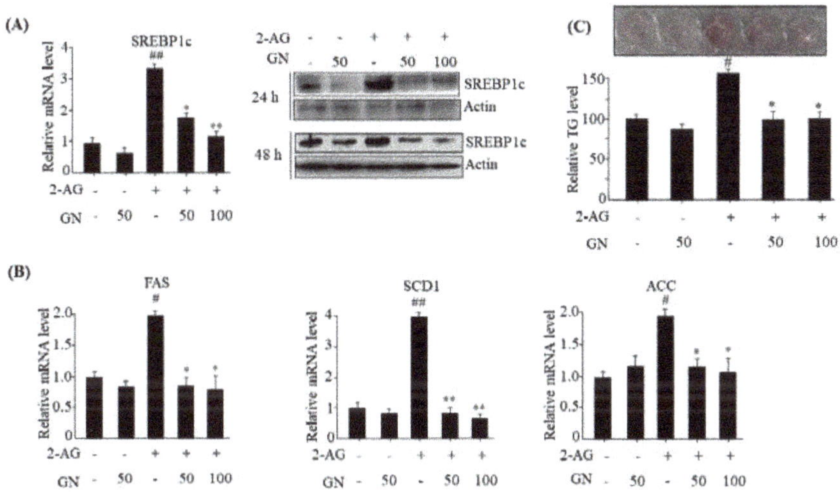

Figure 4. GN inhibited 2-AG-induced lipogenesis in HepG2 cells. HepG2 cells were incubated with 2-AG in the absence or presence of GN (50 or 100 μM) for 24 or 48 h. (**A**) qPCR and western blot analysis of SREBP1c; (**B**) qPCR analysis of *FSA*, *SCD1*, and *ACC*; (**C**) Intracellular TG levels were measured by TG measurement and ORO staining. Values are expressed as mean ± SEM (n = 3 independent experiments). # $p < 0.05$, ## $p < 0.01$ vs. untreated control. * $p < 0.05$, ** $p < 0.01$ vs. 2-AG-treated control.

2.4. GN Inhibited CB1R-Induced Gluconeogenesis in HepG2 Cells

The hepatic CB1R induces gluconeogenesis via upregulation of gluconeogenesis genes [7]. Therefore, we investigated inhibitory effects of GN on hepatic CB1R-induced gluconeogenesis in HepG2 cells. HepG2 cells were incubated with 2-AG in the absence or presence of different concentrations of GN for 12 h, and the expression of gluconeogenesis genes was measured by qPCR. As shown in Figure 5A, 2-AG treatment increased mRNA levels of gluconeogenesis genes such as phosphoenolpyruvate carboxykinase (*PEPCK*) and glucose 6-phosphatase (*G6Pase*); however, GN treatment reversed these changes. Then, we measured glucose production in 2-AG-treated HepG2 cells. Consistent with increased mRNA levels of gluconeogenesis genes, 2-AG treatment resulted in increased glucose production in HepG2 cells (Figure 5B). However, GN treatment markedly suppressed 2-AG-induced glucose production, indicating that GN inhibited CB1R-induced gluconeogenesis. To confirm whether GN-mediated inhibition of gluconeogenesis occurs via the suppression of ER stress, we investigated the inhibitory effects of GN on the expression of gluconeogenesis genes in HepG2 cells. HepG2 cells were incubated with tunicamycin, an ER stress inducer, in the absence or presence of different concentrations of GN for 12 h, and the expression of gluconeogenesis genes was measured by qPCR. As shown in Figure 5C, tunicamycin treatment increased the mRNA levels of *CREBH*, *PEPCK*, and *G6Pase*; however, GN reversed these changes. Taken together, these results suggest that GN might inhibit hepatic CB1R-induced gluconeogenesis via inhibition of ER stress in HepG2 cells.

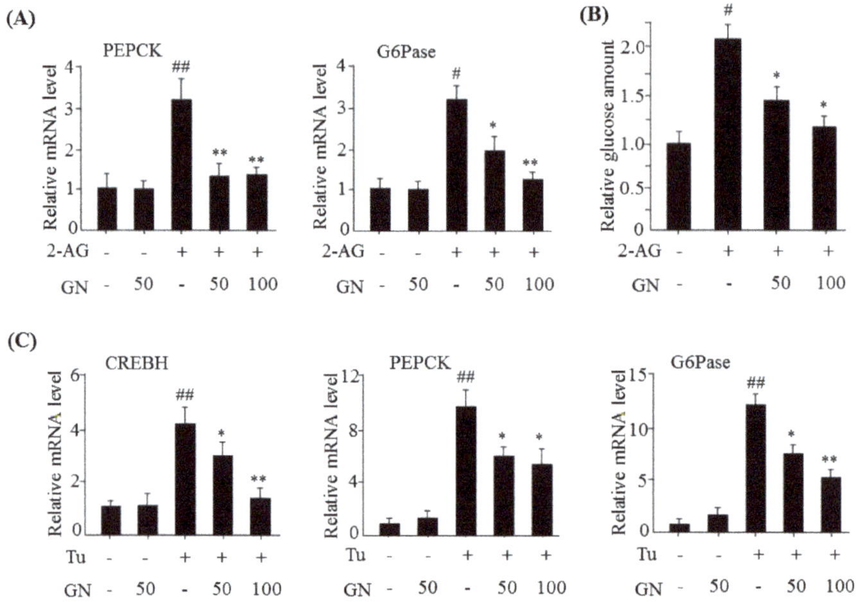

Figure 5. GN inhibited 2-AG-induced gluconeogenesis in HepG2 cells. (**A**) HepG2 cells were incubated with 2-AG in the absence or presence of GN (50 or 100 μM) for 12 h. qPCR analysis of *PEPCK* and *G6Pase*; (**B**) Measurement of glucose production; (**C**) HepG2 cells were incubated with tunicamycin (Tu) in the absence or presence of GN (50 or 100 μM) for 12 h. qPCR analysis of *CREBH*, *PEPCK*, and *G6Pase*. Values are expressed as mean ± SEM (n = 3 independent experiments). $^{\#} p < 0.05$, $^{\#\#} p < 0.01$ vs. untreated control. $^{*} p < 0.05$, $^{**} p < 0.01$ vs. 2-AG or Tu-treated control.

2.5. GN Ameliorated HFD-Induced Hyperglycemia through Inhibition of Hepatic CB1R-Dependent Insulin Resistance and Gluconeogenesis

It has been demonstrated that HFD impairs hepatic insulin signaling via CB1R activation, which contributes to insulin resistance and gluconeogenesis, resulting in hyperglycemia [3]. Thus, pharmacological inhibition of CB1R improves HFD-induced hyperglycemia and glucose tolerance. Previously, we demonstrated that GN reduced the HFD-induced hyperglycemia and improved the glucose tolerance in HFD obese mice [13]. In the current study, we examined whether GN-mediated improvement of hyperglycemia and glucose tolerance is through the inhibition of hepatic CB1R-mediated insulin resistance and gluconeogenesis. HFD induced obesity (Supplementary Figure S1). Consistent with previous results, we observed that GN reduced HFD-induced increase in the serum levels of glucose and insulin in HFD obese mice (Figure 6A). Subsequently, we evaluated the expression of CB1R, ER stress markers, insulin resistance-associated genes, and gluconeogenesis genes in the liver of HFD-induced obese mice. As shown in Figure 6, GN reversed the HFD-induced mRNA levels of *CB1R* (Figure 6B), ER stress markers such as *GRP78*, *CHOP*, and *XBP1c* (Figure 6C),

PHLPP1 (Figure 6D), *Lipin1* (Figure 6E), *CerS6* (Figure 6F), and gluconeogenesis genes such as *PEPCK* and *G6Pase* (Figure 6G). However, GN administration significantly reversed these HFD-induced effects.

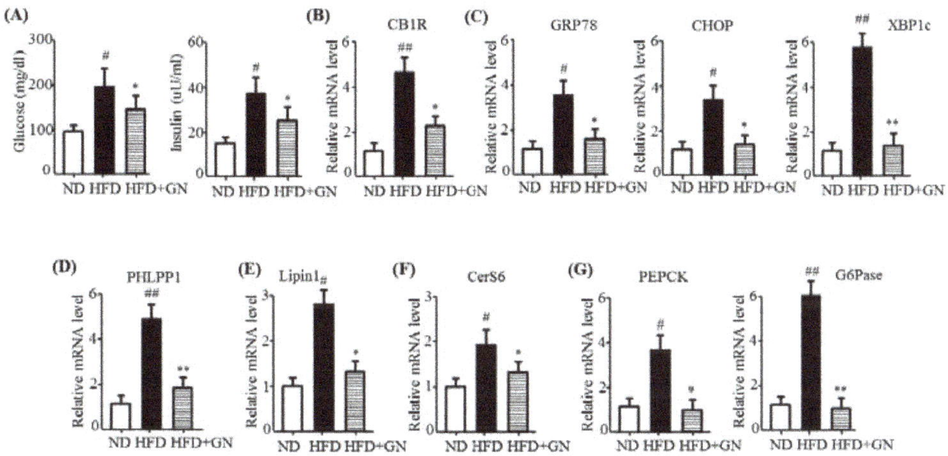

Figure 6. GN ameliorated high-fat diet (HFD)-induced hyperglycemia through inhibition of hepatic CB1R signaling. C57BL6 mice were fed HFD for 12 weeks and orally administered GN for 6 weeks. (**A**) Fasting levels of glucose and insulin. qPCR analysis of *CB1R* (**B**), *GRP78*, *CHOP*, and *XBP1c* (**C**), *PHLPP1* (**D**), *Lipin1* (**E**), *CerS6* (**F**), and *PEPCK* and *G6Pase* (**G**). The values are expressed as mean ± SEM (n = 5 mice per group). # $p < 0.05$, ## $p < 0.01$ vs. ND mice. * $p < 0.05$, ** $p < 0.01$ vs. HFD-induced obese mice control. ND; normal diet.

Finally, we investigated whether GN improved HFD-mediated inhibition of insulin signaling in the liver of HFD-induced obese mice. HFD feeding reduced both phosphorylation of IRS1 at tyrosine 895 and AKT at serine 473 (Figure 7); however, GN administration to HFD obese mice reversed HFD-mediated effects, suggesting that GN reversed the HFD-induced inhibition of insulin signaling in mice. Taken together, these results indicate that GN ameliorates HFD-induced insulin resistance and gluconeogenesis, which may play an important role in GN-mediated improvement of hyperglycemia.

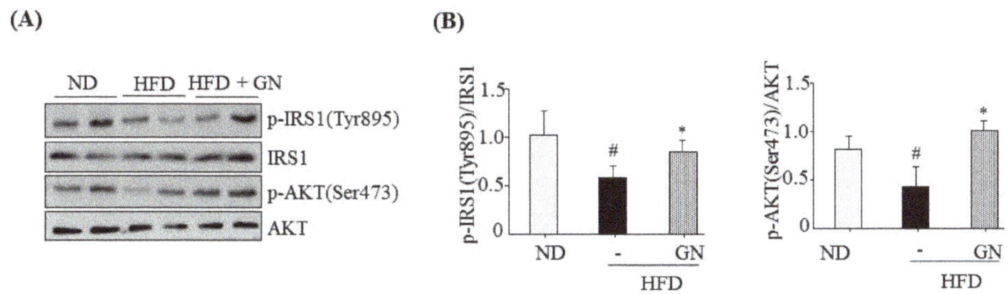

Figure 7. GN reversed HFD-mediated inhibition of insulin signaling in the liver of HFD obese mice. C57BL6 mice were fed HFD for 12 weeks and orally administered GN for 6 weeks. The liver homogenates were subjected to western blot using indicated antibody. (**A**) Representative western blotting. (**B**) Densitometric results. The values are expressed as mean ± SEM (n = 5 mice per group). # $p < 0.05$ vs. ND mice. * $p < 0.05$ vs. HFD-induced obese mice control. ND; normal diet.

3. Discussion

The activation of peripheral CB1Rs has been increasingly recognized as an important regulator of metabolic disorders due to deleterious effects on lipid and glucose metabolism [2]. Among peripheral CB1Rs, activation of the hepatic CB1R induces ER stress-dependent hepatic insulin resistance and gluconeogenesis, resulting in hyperglycemia [3,7]. In addition, hepatic CB1R causes lipid accumulation by upregulation of lipogenesis genes, resulting in hepatic steatosis [6]. Therefore, the inhibition of hepatic CB1R signaling is a promising target for treating type 2 diabetes and hepatic steatosis. GN is a phytochemical derived from *S. chinensis*, a traditional medicinal herb [11]. Previously, we demonstrated that GN exerts protective effects against HFD-induced hyperglycemia and hepatic steatosis in HFD obese mice [12–14]. In the present study, we investigated whether GN-mediated improvement of hyperglycemia and hepatic steatosis is through inhibition of the hepatic CB1R signaling. We examined the inhibitory effect of GN on CB1R-induced insulin resistance and gluconeogenesis in vitro and in vivo.

Recent studies have demonstrated that obesity leads to activation of the hepatic CB1R signaling, which contributes to insulin resistance and gluconeogenesis in the ER stress dependent manner, resulting in hyperglycemia [3–7]. Therefore, hepatic CB1R-mediated ER stress can be a potential target for HFD-induced hyperglycemia. Previously, we demonstrated that GN inhibited fatty acid-induced ER stress and prevented HFD-induced hepatic steatosis and hyperglycemia [12,13]. In the current study, we investigated whether GN also inhibited CB1R-induced ER stress and subsequently improved CB1R-mediated insulin resistance and gluconeogenesis in HepG2 cells. Our data showed that treatment with 2-AG, a CB1R activator, promoted the expression of ER stress markers such as *GRP78*, *CHOP*, and *XBP1c* in HepG2 cells, but GN significantly prevented 2-AG-induced expression of these genes, indicating that GN inhibits CB1R-induced ER stress in HepG2 cells.

It has been reported that CB1R-induced ER stress causes insulin resistance via several mechanisms [3–6]. As described previously, hepatic CB1R-induced ER stress leads to insulin resistance by upregulation of serine phosphatase PHLPP1, Lipin1, and ceramide production. PHLPP1 reverses insulin-activated AKT phosphorylation and inhibits insulin signaling. Lipin1 generates DAG, which subsequently suppresses insulin signaling via PKC activation. Therefore, we examined the inhibitory effects of GN on the expression of *PHLPP1* and *Lipin1* in 2-AG-treated HepG2 cells. Our data revealed that GN treatment significantly reversed 2-AG-induced mRNA levels of both *PHLPP1* and *Lipin1*. CB1R-induced ceramide production, which is regulated by de novo synthesis and degradation of ceramide, also leads to inhibition of insulin signaling. To investigate whether GN affects CB1R-induced ceramide production, we examined the expression of de novo ceramide synthesis genes and ceramide degradation genes in 2-AG-treated HepG2 cells. GN reduced the 2-AG-induced mRNA expression of *CerS6* and *SPTLC3* involved in *de novo* ceramide synthesis, but increased the expression of mRNA levels of *Asah1* and *SPK1* involved in ceramide degradation, which were decreased by 2-AG treatment, indicating that GN suppresses CB1R-induced ceramide production. Taken together, these results suggest that GN might contribute to improvement of hepatic insulin resistance by inhibition of CB1R-induced PHLPP1, Lipin1, and ceramide production. To confirm the ameliorative effect of GN on insulin resistance, we examined insulin signaling in 2-AG-treated HepG2 cells. Treatment with 2-AG increased serine-307 phosphorylation of IRS1, which inhibits AKT phosphorylation, and resulted in reduced insulin-stimulated phosphorylation of IRS1 (tyrosine-895) and AKT (serine-473); however, GN reduced the phosphorylation of IRS1 (serine-307), whereas increased the insulin-stimulated phosphorylation of IRS1 (tyrosine-895) and AKT (serine-473). These results demonstrated that GN reverses the hepatic CB1R-mediated inhibition of insulin signaling.

The hepatic CB1R has been reported to induce TG accumulation via upregulation of lipogenesis genes expression, which leads to dysregulation of insulin signaling [6]. Thus, we tested whether GN inhibits CB1R-induced lipogenesis in 2-AG-treated HepG2 cells. We found that GN inhibited 2-AG-induced expression of lipogenesis genes including *SREBP1c*, *FAS*, *SCD1*, *ACC*, and subsequent intracellular TG accumulation in HepG2 cells. These results suggest that prevention of TG accumulation might also play an important role in GN-mediated improvement of insulin resistance and hepatic steatosis.

The hepatic CB1R stimulates gluconeogenesis via induction of ER stress, which plays a role in HFD-induced hyperglycemia [7]. CB1R-induced ER stress stimulates the expression of gluconeogenesis genes via CREBH. Thus, we investigated the inhibitory effect of GN on gluconeogenesis in 2-AG-treated HepG2 cells. Treatment with 2-AG promoted the expression of *CREBH*, *PEPCK*, and *G6Pase*, and resulted in increased glucose production. However, GN inhibited 2-AG-induced expression of gluconeogenesis genes and subsequent glucose production in HepG2 cells. To confirm whether GN-mediated inhibition of gluconeogenesis is through suppression of ER stress, we assessed the inhibitory effects of GN on the expression of gluconeogenesis genes in tunicamycin-treated HepG2 cells. Consistent with the results in 2-AG-treated HepG2 cells, GN treatment reversed tunicamycin-induced expression of gluconeogenesis genes including *CREBH*, *PEPCK*, and *G6Pase*. Taken together, these results indicate that GN inhibits CB1R-induced gluconeogenesis via suppression of ER stress, which might contribute to improvement of hyperglycemia.

HFD activates hepatic CB1R signaling and results in insulin resistance and hyperglycemia [3]. Our previous study revealed that GN administration to HFD obese mice efficiently reduced HFD-induced hyperglycemia, and improved glucose tolerance in mice [13]. Thus, in the current study, we investigated whether the inhibition of hepatic CB1R signaling plays a role in GN-mediated improvement of hyperglycemia and glucose tolerance. We assessed the inhibitory effects of GN on CB1R-mediated insulin resistance and gluconeogenesis in the liver of HFD obese mice. Results showed that GN administration to HFD obese mice reversed HFD-induced expression of *CB1R*, ER stress markers, *PHLPP1*, ceramide synthase *CerS6*, and recovered reduced phosphorylation of IRS-1 at tyrosine 895 and AKT at serine 473 in the livers of HFD obese mice. Furthermore, GN efficiently reduced HFD-induced expression of gluconeogenesis genes, *PEPCK* and *G6Pase*. These results indicate that GN can ameliorate HFD-induced hyperglycemia through inhibition of CB1R-induced insulin resistance and gluconeogenesis.

Activation of CB1R signaling in the CNS increases food intake and induces obesity [15]. Rimonabant, an inverse agonist of central CB1R, was used as an anti-obesity drug [16]. However, it was withdrawn from the market because of its psychiatric side effects. Since the withdrawal of rimonabant, many investigators have studied peripheral CB1R inhibitors with lesser side effects. Natural products derived from medicinal herbs are usually considered less toxic with fewer side effects. GN is active component of *S. chinensis* that has been used as a traditional herbal medicine and has diverse pharmacological activities [9]. Our results suggest that GN is an attractive and potent compound that inhibits peripheral CB1R signaling and can be useful in the treatment of metabolic disorders including type 2 diabetes.

In conclusion, GN inhibits CB1R-induced ER stress and results in improvement of insulin resistance and gluconeogenesis, which might contribute to the amelioration of hyperglycemia.

4. Materials and Methods

4.1. Reagents

GN (≥98% purity) was obtained from ChemFaces (Wuhan, China). Tunicamycin and 2-AG were purchased from Sigma-Aldrich (St. Louis, MO, USA). Dulbecco's modified Eagle's medium (DMEM), penicillin–streptomycin, and fetal bovine serum (FBS) were obtained from Gibco BRL (Grand Island, NY, USA). Antibodies against GRP78, CHOP, and XBP1c were purchased from Santa Cruz Biotechnology (Santa Cruz, CA, USA). Antibodies against p-IRS1 (serine-307), p-IRS1 (tyrosine-895), p-AKT (serine-473), IRS1, and AKT were purchased from Cellular Signaling Technology (Danvers, MA, USA).

4.2. Cell Culture

The human hepatocellular carcinoma cell line HepG2 was obtained from the American Type Culture Collection (Manassas, VA, USA). HepG2 cells were cultured in DMEM supplemented with 10% heat-inactivated fetal bovine serum, 20 U/mL penicillin, and 20 μg/mL streptomycin.

4.3. Quantitative Polymerase Chain Reaction (qPCR)

Total RNA was isolated from HepG2 cells and mouse livers using TRIzol^{TM} (Invitrogen, Darmstadt, Germany), as per manufacturer's instructions. One microgram of the isolated RNA was reverse-transcribed by using TOPScript RT DryMix (Enzynomics, Daejeon, Korea). Quantitative real-time PCR was performed using a SYBR Green premixed Taq reaction mixture with gene-specific primers. The gene-specific primers used in this study are listed in Supplementary Table S1.

4.4. Western Blots

Proteins (40 μg per well) were separated from HepG2 cells using SDS-PAGE on 8% gels and transferred to polyvinylidene fluoride membranes. The membranes were incubated with primary antibodies, followed by incubation with anti-rabbit or anti-mouse secondary antibodies (Santa Cruz Biotechnology, Dallas, TX, USA) and protein bands were visualized using an enhanced chemiluminescence system (ECL Advance, GE Healthcare, Hatfield, UK).

4.5. Triglyceride (TG) Measurement

HepG2 cell suspensions were mixed with 750 μL of chloroform/methanol/H2O (8:4:3, *v*/*v*/*v*) to extract TG. The cell suspensions were incubated at room temperature for 1 h and centrifuged at 800× *g* for 10 min. The bottom layer (organic phage) obtained was dried overnight and then dissolved in ethanol, followed by measurement of TG concentrations using an AM 157S-K TG kit (Asan Pharmaceutical, Seoul, Korea), which was normalized to the protein concentration.

4.6. Oil Red O Staining

HepG2 were washed twice with phosphate-buffered saline (PBS) and fixed with 10% formalin for 60 min. And then, the cells were then stained with an Oil Red O (ORO) working solution (1.5 mg/mL ORO/60% isopropanol) for 60 min at room temperature. After staining, the cells were washed with distilled water and photographed under a light microscope.

4.7. Glucose Production

Glucose production from HepG2 cells was measured using a colorimetric glucose oxidase assay according to the manufacturer's protocol (Sigma-Aldrich). Briefly, cells were washed three times with PBS and incubated in glucose production buffer (glucose-free DMEM (pH 7.4), 20 mM sodium lactate, 1 mM sodium pyruvate, and 15 mM HEPES) for 3 h at 37 °C in 5% CO_2. Glucose concentration was normalized to cellular protein concentration.

4.8. Animal Study

C57BL/6 mice (male, 6-week-old) were purchased from Jung-Ang Lab Animal, Inc. (Seoul, Korea). The animals were housed in standard conditions of temperature (21–23 °C), humidity (40–60%), and a 12-h light/dark cycle, and were given free access to food and water. The mice were fed a normal diet (ND) or an HFD for 12 weeks. Subsequently, the HFD-fed mice were divided into the following two groups (n = 6 per group): HFD (distilled water-treated) group or HFD + GN (20 mg/kg of body weight) group. The experimental diets were TD.06414, a high-fat in which 60% calories are from fats, and the control diet in which 10% calories are from fat. GN was administered orally every day for 6 weeks. The animal protocol used in this study was reviewed and approved by the Pusan National University's Institutional Animal Care and Use Committee in accordance with established ethical and scientific care procedures (approval number: PNU-2017–1456; 7 February 2017).

4.9. Biochemical Analysis

After starvation for 12 h, the mice were sacrificed. The blood samples were collected and centrifuged at 1000× *g* for 15 min at 4 °C to obtain serum, which was stored at −80°C until analysis.

The concentrations of blood glucose and insulin were determined by using commercial analysis kits (Asan Pharmaceutical, Seoul, Korea).

4.10. Statistical Analysis

All data are presented as the mean ± standard error of the mean (SEM). The statistical differences between various groups were examined by one-way analysis of variance (ANOVA) followed by Tukey's test. Values with $p < 0.05$ were considered statistically significant.

Supplementary Materials: Supplementary materials can be found at http://www.mdpi.com/1422-0067/19/4/968/s1.

Acknowledgments: This study was supported by the National Research Foundation of Korea (NRF) grant funded by the Korean government (MSIP) (No. 2014R1A5A2009936).

Author Contributions: Arulkumar Nagappan performed experiment and analyzed the data; Ji-Hyun Kim performed experiment; Dae Young Jung performed experiment; Myeong Ho Jung designed research and wrote the manuscript.

Conflicts of Interest: We declare that there is no conflict of interest.

Abbreviations

2-AG	2-arachidonoylglycerol
Asah1	*N*-acylsphingosine amidohydrolase1
CB1R	cannabinoid type 1 receptor
CerS6	ceramide synthase 6
CREBH	cAMP-responsive element-binding protein H
CHOP	C/EBP homologous protein
ER	endoplasmic reticulum
G6Pase	glucose 6-phosphatase
GN	gomisin N
GRP78	glucose-regulated protein 78
HFD	high fat diet
PEPCK	phosphoenolpyruvate carboxykinase
PHLPP1	PH domain leucine-rich repeats protein phosphatase 1
SPK1	sphingosine kinase 1
SPTLC3	serine-palmitonyl transferase LC3
XBP1c	X box-binding protein 1, C-terminal

References

1. Biddinger, S.B.; Hernandez-Ono, A.; Rask-Madsen, C.; Haas, J.T.; Alemán, J.Q.; Suzuki, R.; Scapa, E.F.; Agarwal, C.; Carey, M.C.; Stephanopoulos, G.; et al. Hepatic insulin resistance is sufficient to produce dyslipidemia and susceptibility to atherosclerosis. *Cell Metab.* **2008**, *7*, 125–134. [CrossRef] [PubMed]
2. Simon, V.; Cota, D. MECHANISMS IN ENDOCRINOLOGY: Endocannabinoids and metabolism: Past, present and future. *Eur. J. Endocrinol.* **2017**, *176*, R309–R324. [CrossRef] [PubMed]
3. Liu, J.; Zhou, L.; Xiong, K.; Godlewski, G.; Mukhopadhya, B.; Tam, J.; Yin, S.; Gao, P.; Shan, X.; Pickel, J. Hepatic cannabinoid receptor-1 mediates diet-induced insulin resistance via inhibition of insulin signaling and clearance in mice. *Gastroenterology* **2012**, *142*, 1218–1228. [CrossRef] [PubMed]
4. Chanda, D.; Kim, Y.H.; Kim, D.K.; Lee, M.W.; Lee, S.Y.; Park, T.S.; Koo, S.H.; Lee, C.H.; Choi, H.S. Activation of cannabinoid receptor type 1 (Cb1r) disrupts hepatic insulin receptor signaling via cyclic AMP-response element-binding protein H (Crebh)-mediated induction of Lipin1 gene. *J. Biol. Chem.* **2012**, *287*, 38041–38049. [CrossRef] [PubMed]
5. Cinar, R.; Godlewski, G.; Liu, J.; Tam, J.; Jourdan, T.; Mukhopadhyay, B.; Harvey-White, J.; Kunos, G. Hepatic cannabinoid-1 receptors mediate diet-induced insulin resistance by increasing de novo synthesis of long-chain ceramides. *Hepatology* **2014**, *59*, 143–153. [CrossRef] [PubMed]

6. Osei-Hyiaman, D.; DePetrillo, M.; Pacher, P.; Liu, J.; Radaeva, S.; Batkai, S.; Harvey-White, J.; Mackie, K.; Offertaler, L.; Wang, L. Endocannabinoid activation at hepatic CB1 receptors stimulates fatty acid synthesis and contributes to diet-induced obesity. *J. Clin. Investig.* **2005**, *115*, 1298–1305. [CrossRef] [PubMed]
7. Chanda, D.; Kim, D.K.; Li, T.; Kim, Y.H.; Koo, S.H.; Lee, C.H.; Chiang, J.Y.; Choi, H.S. Cannabinoid receptor type 1 (CB1R) signaling regulates hepatic gluconeogenesis via induction of endoplasmic reticulum-bound transcription factor cAMP-responsive element-binding protein H (CREBH) in primary hepatocytes. *J. Biol. Chem.* **2011**, *286*, 27971–27979. [CrossRef] [PubMed]
8. Silvestri, C.; Di Marzo, V. The endocannabinoid system in energy homeostasis and the etiopathology of metabolic disorders. *Cell Metab.* **2013**, *17*, 475–490. [CrossRef] [PubMed]
9. Panossian, A.; Wikman, G. Pharmacology of *Schisandra chinensis* Bail.: An overview of Russian research and uses in medicine. *J. Ethnopharmacol.* **2008**, *118*, 183–212. [CrossRef] [PubMed]
10. Jang, M.K.; Nam, J.S.; Kim, J.H.; Yun, Y.R.; Han, C.W.; Kim, B.J.; Jeong, H.S.; Ha, K.T.; Jung, M.H. *Schisandra chinensis* extract ameliorates nonalcoholic fatty liver via inhibition of endoplasmic reticulum stress. *J. Ethnopharmacol.* **2016**, *185*, 96–104. [CrossRef] [PubMed]
11. Ikeya, H.; Taguchi, I.; Yosioka, H. The constituents of *Schizandra chinensis* Baill. I. Isolation and structure determination of five new lignans, Gomisin A, B, C, F and G, and the absolute structure of schizandrin. *Chem. Pharm. Bull.* **1979**, *27*, 1383–1394. [CrossRef] [PubMed]
12. Jang, M.K.; Yun, Y.R.; Kim, S.H.; Kim, J.H.; Jung, M.H. Protective effect of gomisin N against endoplasmic reticulum stress-induced hepatic steatosis. *Biol. Pharm. Bull.* **2016**, *39*, 832–838. [CrossRef] [PubMed]
13. Jung, D.Y.; Kim, J.H.; Lee, H.; Jung, M.H. Antidiabetic effect of gomisin N via activation of AMP-activated protein kinase. *Biochem. Biophys. Res. Commun.* **2017**, *494*, 587–593. [CrossRef] [PubMed]
14. Yun, Y.R.; Kim, J.H.; Jung, M.H. Protective effects of gomisin N against hepatic steatosis through AMPK activation. *Biochem. Biophys. Res. Commun.* **2017**, *482*, 1095–1101. [CrossRef] [PubMed]
15. Maccarrone, M.; Bab, I.; Bíró, T.; Kunos, G.; Mechoulam, R.; Pacher, P.; Sharkey, K.A.; Zimmer, A. Endocannabinoid signaling at the periphery: 50 years after THC. *Trends Pharmacol. Sci.* **2015**, *36*, 277–296. [CrossRef] [PubMed]
16. Marzo, V.; Di, J.P.; Després, J.P. CB1 antagonists for obesity—What lessons have we learned from rimonabant? *Nat. Rev. Endocrinol.* **2009**, *5*, 633–638. [CrossRef] [PubMed]

International Journal of
Molecular Sciences

MDPI

Article

Hinokitiol Inhibits Migration of A549 Lung Cancer Cells via Suppression of MMPs and Induction of Antioxidant Enzymes and Apoptosis

Thanasekaran Jayakumar [1,†], Chao-Hong Liu [1,2,†], Guan-Yi Wu [1], Tzu-Yin Lee [1], Manjunath Manubolu [3], Cheng-Ying Hsieh [4], Chih-Hao Yang [4,*] and Joen-Rong Sheu [1,4,*]

1. Graduate Institute of Medical Sciences, College of Medicine, Taipei Medical University, Taipei 110, Taiwan; tjaya_2002@yahoo.co.in (T.J.); y4509@yuanhosp.com.tw (C.-H.L.); m120101037@tmu.edu.tw (G.-Y.W.); d119103001@tmu.edu.tw (T.-Y.L.)
2. Department of Dermatology, Yuan's General Hospital, Kaohsiung 249, Taiwan
3. Department of Evolution, Ecology and Organismal Biology, Ohio State University, Columbus, OH 43212, USA; manubolu.1@osu.edu
4. Department of Pharmacology, School of Medicine, College of Medicine, Taipei Medical University, Taipei 110, Taiwan; hsiehcy@tmu.edu.tw

* Correspondence: chyang@tmu.edu.tw (C.-H.Y.); sheujr@tmu.edu.tw (J.-R.S.); Tel.: +886-2-2736-1661 (ext. 3197) (C.-H.Y.); +886-2-2736-1661 (ext. 3199) (J.-R.S.); Fax: +886-2-2739-0450 (J.-R.S.)

† These authors contributed equally to this work.

Received: 23 February 2018; Accepted: 21 March 2018; Published: 22 March 2018

Abstract: Hinokitiol, a natural monoterpenoid from the heartwood of *Calocedrus formosana*, has been reported to have anticancer effects against various cancer cell lines. However, the detailed molecular mechanisms and the inhibiting roles of hinokitiol on adenocarcinoma A549 cells remain to be fully elucidated. Thus, the current study was designed to evaluate the effect of hinokitiol on the migration of human lung adenocarcinoma A549 cells in vitro. The data demonstrates that hinokitiol does not effectively inhibit the viability of A549 cells at up to a 10 μM concentration. When treated with non-toxic doses (1–5 μM) of hinokitiol, the cell migration is markedly suppressed at 5 μM. Hinokitiol significantly reduced p53 expression, followed by attenuation of Bax in A549 cells. A dose-dependent inhibition of activated caspase-9 and -3 was observed in the presence of hinokitiol. An observed increase in protein expression of matrix metalloproteinases (MMPs) -2/-9 in A549 cells was significantly inhibited by hinokitiol. Remarkably, when A549 cells were subjected to hinokitiol (1–5 μM), there was an increase in the activities of antioxidant enzymes catalase (CAT) and superoxide dismutase (SOD) from the reduction in cells. In addition, the incubation of A549 cells with hinokitiol significantly activated the cytochrome c expression, which may be triggered by activation of caspase-9 followed by caspase-3. These observations indicate that hinokitiol inhibited the migration of lung cancer A549 cells through several mechanisms, including the activation of caspases-9 and -3, induction of p53/Bax and antioxidant CAT and SOD, and reduction of MMP-2 and -9 activities. It also induces cytochrome c expression. These findings demonstrate a new therapeutic potential for hinokitiol in lung cancer chemoprevention.

Keywords: A549 cells; hinokitiol; MMPs; p53/Bax; antioxidant enzymes; caspases; migration

1. Introduction

Lung adenocarcinoma is one of the most severe cancers related to deaths globally, and it is becoming more common in numerous countries. Almost 40% of lung cancers are adenocarcinomas, which are non-small cell lung cancers with a normally poor diagnosis and extremely high rate of latent metastasis [1]. Lung adenocarcinomas are identified in most patients when in an advanced stage, and the malignant cells have already extended into distant organs. These patients are not acceptable for invasive resection. In order to advance the treatment of patients detected with lung cancer, evolving innovative therapies is needed for the treatment of lung cancer. As matured lung cancer cells are very aggressive and lead to high death rates, the inhibition of their invasion and metastasis may be effective in the treatment of lung cancer.

Apoptosis is a serious physiological process responsible for the homeostatic mechanisms to maintain cell populations in tissues [2]. There is extensive research on apoptotic cell death, because of the close relationship between the mechanism of apoptosis and the effect of anticancer agents [3]. Natural products have been reported to induce apoptosis in cancer cells via activating reactive oxygen species (ROS) [4]. ROS induce oxidative DNA damage followed by a leakage of cytochrome c, and subsequently activate the caspase cascade [5]. Besides, the agitation in the expression level of Bax and Blc-2 proteins is a vital factor in regulating the vulnerability of tumor cells to anticancer agents [6]. Cancer metastasis, a highly organized and sequential progression, is characterized by separation of cells from the primary tumor, proteolysis of the extracellular matrix (ECM), intravasation, and then invasion into new tissue and growth [6,7].

Matrix metalloproteinases (MMPs) are the major proteases that contribute to tumor cell migration, tissue invasion, and metastasis [8]. Of these, MMP-2 and -9 play crucial roles in the process of metastasis [9]. Activation of these enzymes is associated with increased tumor metastasis, which proposes a crucial functional role for these proteases in the metastatic process [10]. Previous studies found a reduction in the activities of the antioxidant enzymes glutathione peroxidase (GPx), superoxide dismutase (SOD), and catalase (CAT) in lymphoma cell induced tumors in mice [11], and these enzymes are considered as markers of malignant transformation [12]. Therefore, anticancer agents with the ability to activate apoptosis and antioxidants and suppress MMPs are effective in cancer therapy.

The potential of natural products in cancer prevention and therapy were well described in the special issue titled "Bioactive natural products in cancer prevention and therapy: progress and promise" [13]. A detailed review analytically summarized the role of various natural compounds for cancer prevention and therapy via modulation of different transcription factors, multiple signal transduction, and apoptotic cascades [14,15]. Hinokitiol, a natural compound found in *Chamaecyparis taiwanensis* and scrapped from the wood of cupressaceous plants, has miscellaneous biological and pharmacological properties. Antiviral, antibacterial, antifungal, antitumor, and insecticidal tendencies are the noted biological properties of hinokitiol [16,17]. This natural compound accomplished noteworthy anti-inflammatory activity in a variety of cells, achieved by a range of mechanisms [18]. Hinokitiol is reported to have lung tumor suppressing abilities without changing the body weight and inducing toxicity in the host [17]. Our previous study showed that hinokitiol inhibits cell migration via reducing MMP-1 expression followed by the suppression of nuclear factor κ B (NF-κB)/mitogen-activated protein kinase (MAPKs) signaling pathways and in vivo tumor nodule formation in melanoma cells [19]. Despite hinokitiol being found to inhibit the growth of cancer cells, its role on the inhibition of lung cancer is still unclear. Therefore, this study aimed to investigate the inhibitory effect and the molecular mechanisms of hinokitiol on A549 cells in vitro. This study may provide evidence that hinokitiol can inhibit the migration of A549 cells, which suggests that this natural compound inhibits adenocarcinoma.

2. Results

2.1. Cytotoxic Effect of Hinokitiol in A549 Cells

The chemical structure of hinokitiol is shown in Figure 1A. The cytotoxic effect of hinokitiol on human lung adenocarcinoma A549 cells is demonstrated in Figure 1B. The figure demonstrates that the treatment of more than 20 μM hinokitiol (20–100 μM) for 24 h considerably decreased the viability of A549 cells. The data indicate that treatment with hinokitiol at doses of less than 20 μM (i.e., 1–10 μM) for 24 h does not cause cytotoxicity of A549 cells. Thus, we chose the concentration of 1–5 μM for the current study.

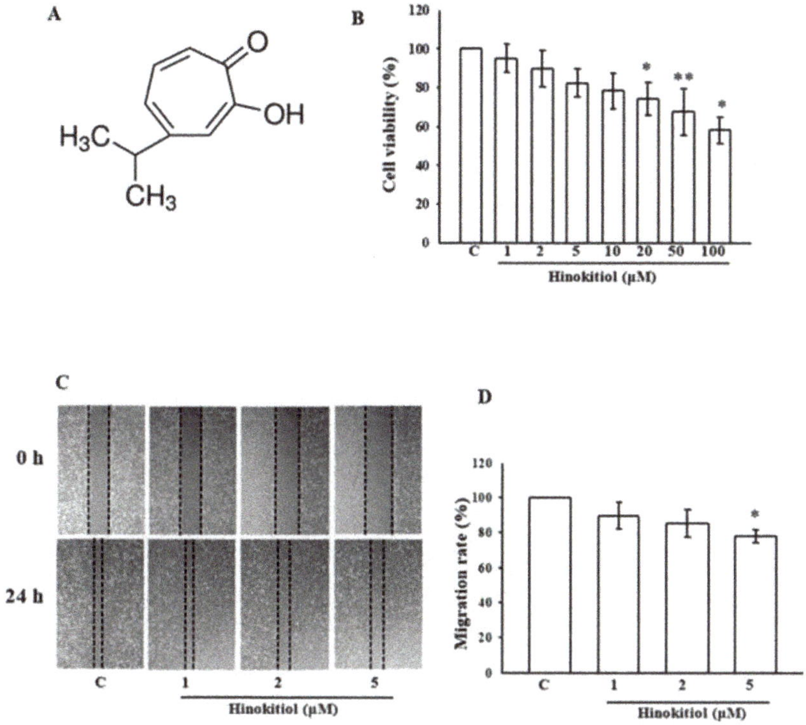

Figure 1. Effects of hinokitiol on the cell viability of the A549 cell line: (**A**) the structure of hinokitiol; (**B**) the viability of A549 cell line during treatment with various concentrations (1~100 μM) of hinokitiol; (**C**,**D**) effects of hinokitiol on A549 cell migration after 24 h of exposure. The figures are representative examples of three independent experiments. * $p < 0.05$ and ** $p < 0.01$ compared with untreated A549 cells.

2.2. Hinokitiol Inhibits the Migration of A549 Cells

Since the higher concentration of hinokitiol seems toxic, it is obligatory to investigate the inhibitory effect of non-toxic doses of hinokitiol on the migration of A549 cells. After incubation with different concentrations (1–5 μM) of hinokitiol for 24 h, we found the high dose of 5 μM suppresses the migration of A549 cells to the denuded zone (Figure 1C). These results demonstrate that hinokitiol inhibited the migration of A549 cells (Figure 1D).

2.3. Effects of Hinokitiol on Caspase Signaling Pathway Activation

To investigate the molecular mechanisms of hinokitiol-mediated apoptosis in A549 cells, activated caspases-9 and -3 were analyzed by Western blot assay. Studies have proposed that caspases are the main enzymes that regulate apoptosis in tissues or cells. Any stimulatory agents that induce apoptosis were found to activate the effector caspases including caspase-9, caspase-3, and caspase-7 [20]. Similarly, treatment of A549 cells with hinokitiol prominently increases the p53 and Bax protein level (Figure 2A,B). Next, the activated caspase-9 and -3 were enhanced upon hinokitiol administration in a dose-dependent manner (Figure 3A,B). Subsequently, cytochrome c (Cyto-c) was up-regulated, inducing apoptosis in A549 cancer cells (Figure 3C).

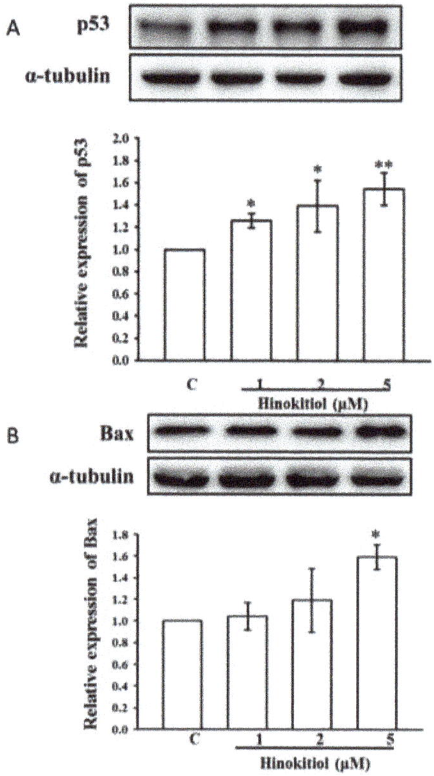

Figure 2. Effects of hinokitiol on phosphorylation of p53 and Bax in A549 cells. A549 adenocarcinoma (5×10^4 cells/well) cells were treated with different concentrations (1–5 μM) of hinokitiol for 30 min. The phosphorylated p53 and Bax proteins in the cell lysate were assayed by Western blotting. Effects of hinokitiol on phosphorylation of p53 (**A**) and Bax (**B**) in A549 adenocarcinoma cells. α-tubulin was used as an internal control. The figures are representative examples of three independent experiments. Data are shown as the mean ± standard errors of the means (SEM) of three independent experiments. * $p < 0.05$, and ** $p < 0.01$ compared with untreated A549 cells.

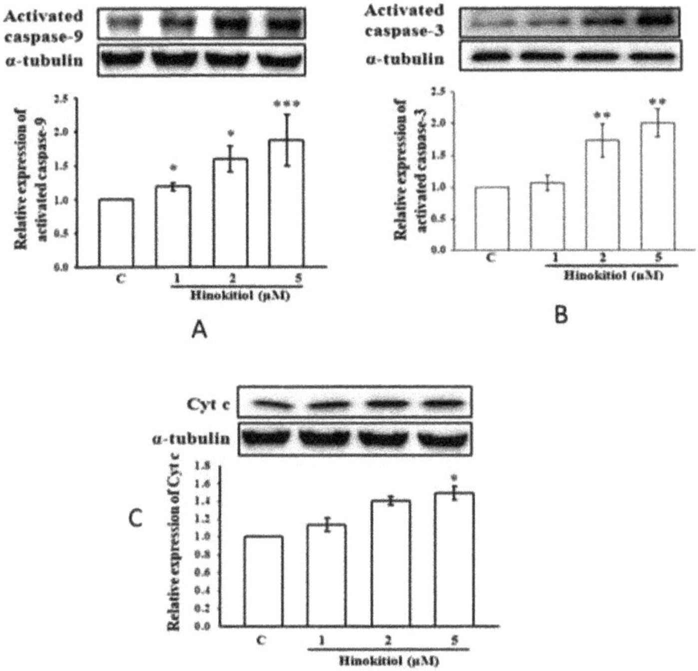

Figure 3. Effect of hinokitiol on caspases activation and cytochrome c release. (**A**,**B**) Relative concentration-dependent activation of activated caspase-9 and -3 in A549 cells treated with various concentrations of hinokitil. Caspase-9 (**A**) was activated in a concentration (1–5 μM) dependent manner, whereas caspase-3 (**B**) was induced significantly only at 2 and 5 μM. (**C**) Meanwhile, cytochrome c was released at the higher concentration (5 μM) of hinokitiol treatment. The data represent the means ± SEM of three independent experiments. * $p < 0.05$, ** $p < 0.01$, and *** $p < 0.001$ compared with untreated A549 cells.

2.4. Hinokitiol Inhibits MMP-9 and MMP-2 Expression

MMP-9 and MMP-2 are recognized as playing a vital role in cancer cell invasion and metastasis among the MMP family. Figure 4A,B exemplifies the expression of MMP-9 and MMP-2 in untreated and hinokitiol treated A549 cells. The results displayed a marked increase in MMP-9 and MMP-2 in untreated A549 cells; this may be due to ROS elevation that triggers MMPs during the rigorous angiogenesis to interrupt the extracellular matrix (ECM). Nevertheless, when cells were treated with hinokitiol, the intracellular protein levels of MMP-9 and MMP-2 were significantly reduced at concentrations of 2 and 5 μM.

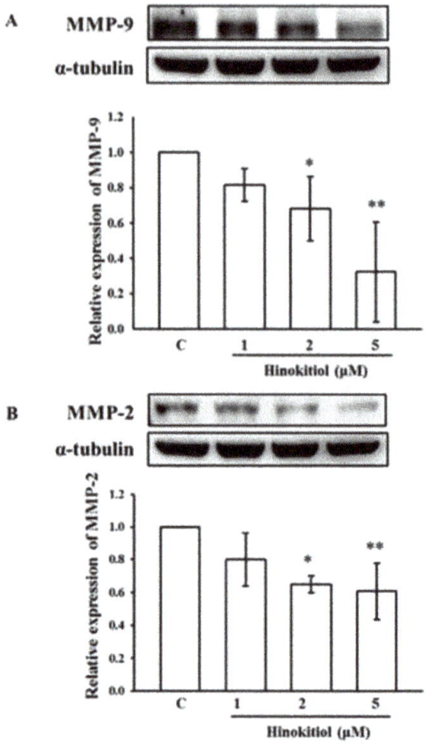

Figure 4. Effects of hinokitiol on matrix metalloproteinases (MMP)-9 and MMP-2 expression in A549 cell line. A549 cells were treated with different concentrations of hinokitiol (1–5 μM) in serum-free media for 24 h. After the treatment periods, cell lysates were collected to detect the expression of MMP-9 (**A**) and MMP-2 (**B**) by using Western blotting. The figures are representative examples of three independent experiments. * $p < 0.05$ and ** $p < 0.01$ compared with untreated A549 cells.

2.5. Hinokitiol Enhances Antioxidants Enzymes in A549 Cells

Some studies have shown decreased antioxidant activities in tumors [21,22]. Changes in antioxidant enzymes are associated with the metastatic progression of cancer [23]. In this study, Figure 5A,B reveal the substrate gel activities of catalase (CAT) and superoxide dismutase (SOD) in untreated and hinokitiol treated A549 cells. The activities of CAT and SOD were decreased in untreated A549 cells. Conversely, a concentration-dependent elevation of CAT was observed in hinokitiol treated cells; the highest increase was noticed in 5 μM hinokitiol treated cells (Figure 5A). Likewise, a significant increase in the activity of SOD was also found in 2 and 5 μM hinokitiol-treated cells (Figure 5B). These results propose that hinokitiol can abolish cancer cells through the up-regulation of antioxidant enzymes CAT and SOD.

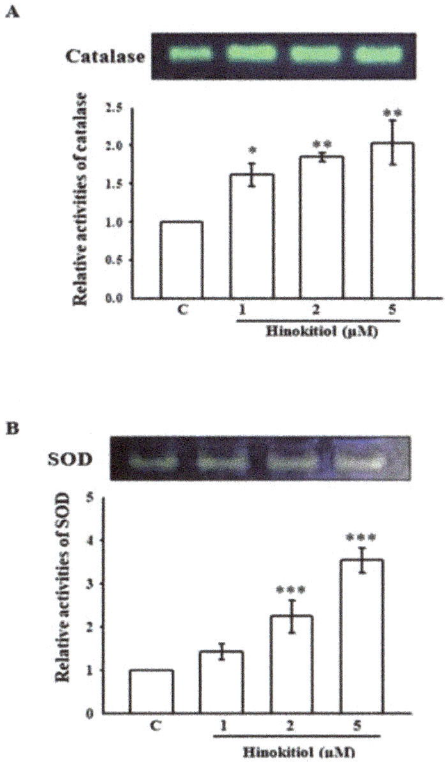

Figure 5. Effects of hinokitiol on catalase (CAT) and superoxide dismutase (SOD) activity in A549 cell line. A549 cells were treated with different concentrations of hinokitiol (1–5 μM) in serum-free media for 24 h. Cell lysates were obtained for the assay of CAT (**A**) and SOD (**B**) activities by using native-PAGE. The figures are representative examples of three independent experiments. * $p < 0.05$, ** $p < 0.01$, and *** $p < 0.001$ compared with untreated A549 cells.

3. Discussion

Chemotherapy with anticancer drugs is more valuable for treating different tumors, mostly in end-stage cancer patients. Nevertheless, the therapeutic methods may encounter drug resistance, as cancer cells can have a diversity of molecular mechanisms to attempt to stay alive by fighting the therapeutic drugs. Hinokitiol is a natural monoterpenoid originally extracted from Taiwanese hinoki, and this compound induces apoptosis in cancer cells via a caspase 3-dependent pathway or through cell cycle arrest [24]. Previous studies indicated that hinokitiol could work as a novel anti-cancer compound. The results of the present study reveal that hinokitiol holds anticancer effects against adenocarcinoma A549 cells via induction of tumor suppressor proteins p53 and Bax and apoptotic markers (activated caspase-9 and -3, cytochrome c), down regulation of MMPs-9 and MMP-2, and up regulation of antioxidants enzymes catalase (CAT) and superoxide dismutase (SOD). This study shows treatment with hinokitiol at doses of less than 20 μM (i.e., 1–10 μM) for 24 h does not cause cytotoxicity in A549 cells. Our previous study found that hinokitiol at the concentrations of 1, 2, and 5 μM did not affect the viability of lymphocytes after treatment for 24 h [25]. Another study from our group also established that hinokitiol (1, 2, 10, and 50 μM) incubated with platelets for 20 min did not significantly increase lactate dehydrogenase (LDH) activity; the study indicated that hinokitiol did not affect platelet permeability or induce platelet cytolysis [26]. These findings clearly show that hinokitiol has no acute cytotoxic effects, as well, it does not induce cytotoxicity in normal cells.

Apoptosis is an important physiological process that arises in cells during growth and normal cellular development [27]. Several cellular signals induce apoptosis and change mitochondrial permeability, resulting in a cascade of actions, such as the release of apoptosis activators from mitochondria [28]. Bax, a pro-apoptotic protein, has been shown to be involved in the cytochrome c release from mitochondria to cytosol via dimerization and translocation to the outer mitochondrial membrane [29]. Moreover, the tumor suppressor p53 induces the cell cycle and apoptosis, which supports genome stability and integrity by responding to cellular stress and DNA damage [30]. The increased levels of p53 inhibit the cyclin expression that is vital for transitioning from G1 into S phase. In this study, p53 and Bax were found to be activated upon hinokitiol administration; this may induce apoptosis. Caspase activation is involved in an energy-dependent cascade of molecular events towards apoptosis. Two major groups of caspases have been recognized to be associated in apoptosis pathways, including executioner caspases-3, -6, -7 and initiator caspases-2, -8, -9, -10 [31]. Initiator caspases-9 and -8 trigger intrinsic and extrinsic pathways, respectively. A previous study reported that activation of these caspases consequently induces executioner caspase-3 [32]. In the present study, we investigated whether hinokitiol triggers the caspases in A549 cells when treated with different concentrations. The expression of caspase-9 and -3 were significantly elevated in hinokitiol treated cells. Our results indicated that induced apoptosis of A549 cells by hinokitiol was mediated through caspase-9 and -3 activation.

Pericellular proteolysis of the extracellular matrix (ECM) is essential for cell projection during cell invasion. The proteolytic degradation of ECM is facilitated by extracellular proteases, such as MMPs, and is required for cancer cell invasion. Among these, MMP-9 and MMP-2 play a critical role in the progression of lung cancer [33]. The inhibition of expression of these MMPs is a potential target for the prevention of the metastasis of cancer [34]. Numerous earlier studies have also established that natural compounds such as quercetin [35], baicalein [36], and gallic acid [37] suppress MMPs to exert their anticancer activity. Consistent with these reports, our study demonstrated that anticancer effects of hinokitiol are associated with a decline in MMP-9 and MMP-2 expression in A549 cells.

Antioxidant systems, which includes SOD, CAT, and glutathione-dependent enzymes are well recognized in lung tissues [38]. SOD enzymes comprise intracellular manganese (Mn)-SOD, copper-zinc (CuZn)-SOD, and an extracellular SOD that occurs in epithelial lining fluid and blood vessels [39]. SOD enzymes convert superoxide anions to H_2O_2, and H_2O_2 is further converted to water and oxygen by CAT [40]. Previous studies have found reduced antioxidant activity in lung cancers [20,41]. Another study showed reduced catalase activity in lung cancer due to its protein and mitochondrial RNA (mRNA) reduction in tumor cells [42]. Though studies have shown increased antioxidant activities in tumor cells or in individuals with lung cancer [43], others have found the reduction of antioxidant activities in lung tumors [20]. In this study, the antioxidant enzymes CAT and SOD were increased in hinokitiol treated A549 cells.

4. Materials and Methods

4.1. Materials

Hinikitiol with more than 90% purity was purchased from Sigma (St. Louis, MO, USA). Sodium dodecylsulfate (SDS), phenylmethylsulfonyl fluoride (PMSF), leupeptin, aprotinin, sodium fluoride, sodium orthovanadate, sodium pyrophosphate, diethyl pyrocarbonate (DEPC), bovine serum albumin (BSA), potassium ferricyanide, ferric chloride, nitroblue tetrazolium (NBT), and riboflavin were all purchased from Sigma-Aldrich (St. Louis, MO, USA). An antibody against MMP-9 was purchased from LabVision/NeoMarkers (Fremont, CA, USA). Antibodies against MMP-2 and active caspase-9 and -3 were purchased from BioVision (Mountain View, CA, USA). Anti-mouse and anti-rabbit immunoglobulin G-conjugated horseradish peroxidase (HRP) was purchased from Amersham

Biosciences (Sunnyvale, CA, USA) and/or Jackson-Immuno Research (West Grove, PA, USA). The Hybond-P polyvinylidene difluoride (PVDF) membrane, and enhanced chemiluminescence (ECL) Western blotting detection reagents and analysis systems were obtained from Amersham (Buckinghamshire, UK).

4.2. Cell Cultivation and Hinokitiol Treatment

Human adenocarcinoma A549 cells were obtained from American Type Culture Collection (Manassas, VA, USA). A549 cells were cultured in RPMI1640 medium contained with 3.65 mM L-glutamine, 90 units/mL penicillin, 90 μg/mL streptomycin, 18 mM HEPES, 23.57 mM $NaHCO_3$, and 10% heat-inactivated fetal bovine serum (FBS) at 37 °C in humidified air with 5% CO_2. In this study, A549 cells were seeded at 5×10^4 per well and cultured until 90% confluent. After 24 h, cells were transferred into serum-free media. Twenty-four hours after changing to serum-free media, cells were treated with hinokitiol (1–5 μM) for another 24 h. At the end of the incubation period, cell supernatants were collected and stored at −80 °C for the Western blot assay.

4.3. Cell Viability

The 3-(4,5-dimethylthiazol-2-yl)-2,5-diphenyltetrazolium bromide (MTT) method was used to detect the cell viability. Briefly, 5×10^4 cells were seeded in a 96-well plate containing RPMI1640 medium with 10% fetal bovine serum. After the required confluence was reached, cells were treated with various concentrations of hinokitiol (1–100 μM) for 24 h in a 5% CO_2 incubator at 37 °C. At 22 h, the medium was changed to fresh medium having 0.5 mg/mL MTT. After 2 h incubation, the dark blue MTT formazan crystals formed in intact cells were solubilized in dimethyl sulfoxide (DMSO), and the absorbance was measured at 550 nm in a spectrophotometer. The percent cell viability was calculated using the following formula:

Percentage cell viability = (absorbance of the experiment samples/absorbance of the control) × 100%

4.4. Wound Healing Migration Assay

According to a previously described study, the wound healing migration assay was executed [44]. In brief, A549 cells were seeded in 12-well plates to achieve the required growth. The monolayer culture was then scrape-wounded with a sterile micropipette tip to create a denuded zone with constant width. After removing the cellular debris using PBS, cells were treated with various concentrations (1–5 μM) of hinokitiol for 24 h. A549 cell migration to the wounded region was monitored by photographing at 0 and 24 h using an Image pro Express, version 6.0.0.319 for Windows XP/Professional (Media Cybernetics Inc., Bethesda, MD, USA). To quantify cell migration, images of the initial wounded monolayers were equated to the corresponding pictures of cells at later time points. Migrated cells in each of five random fields were counted.

4.5. Western Blotting

Cells with required confluence were pre-incubated with 1–5 μM hinokitiol for 24 h for MMPs-9 and MMP-2, activated caspases-9 and -3, and cytochrome c and 30 min for p53 and Bax. After the experimental periods, the proteins were extracted with 60 μL lysis buffer. Samples containing 50 μg of protein were separated by 10% SDS–PAGE, and the proteins were electrotransferred to the PVDF membranes using a Bio-Rad semi dry transfer unit (Hercules, CA, USA). The membranes were blocked with 5% (*w*/*v*) non-fat milk in TBST (10 mM Tris-base, 100 mM NaCl, and 0.01% Tween 20) for 40 min, and blotted with the various primary antibodies. Subsequently, the membranes were incubated with an appropriate secondary antibody (horseradish peroxidase-conjugated goat anti-mouse or anti-rabbit IgG). The immunoreactive bands were visualized with enhanced chemiluminescent reagents (ECL, Amersham, UK).

4.6. Non-Denaturing Polyacrylamide Gel Electrophoresis (Native PAGE)

The activity of the antioxidant enzymes CAT and SOD was detected by using native PAGE. For this, the buffers and samples were not heated in the absence of SDS before electrophoresis. The PAGE was run based on the equal amounts of 50 μg protein in an 8% gel for CAT and 10% gel for SOD. The electrophoretic gel was run at 4 °C with a constant power supply of 80 V for stacking gel and 100 V for separating gel.

4.6.1. CAT Activity Staining

The activity of the CAT enzyme was identified according to the method described by Woodbury et al. [45]. In this, the gel was incubated in 5 mM H_2O_2 solution for 10 min, washed with deionized water, and stained with a reaction mixture containing 1% potassium ferricyanide (*w*/*v*) and 1% ferric chloride. The appearance of a yellow band on a dark green background is considered to be indicative of the CAT enzyme. The reaction was ended by adding water, and the gel was photographed.

4.6.2. SOD Activity Staining

SOD activity was identified according to the method described by Beauchamp and Fridovich [46]. The gel was incubated in 50 mM Tris-HCl buffer (pH 8) containing 10 mg nitroblue tetrazolium (NBT), 1 mg ethylene diamine tetra acetic acid (EDTA), and 2 mg riboflavin (50 mL final volume) and reserved in a dark place for 30 min. The gel was then taken to an illuminated light box to detect the area of SOD activity, which looked like a clear zone on a bluish-violet background.

4.7. Statistical Analysis

The results are expressed as the mean ± standard errors of the means (SEM) and are accompanied by the number of observations. For analysis of the data, a one-way analysis of variance (ANOVA) test was performed using the Sigma Stat v3.5 software (SAS Inc., Cary, NC, USA). When group comparisons displayed a significant difference, the Student-Newman-Keuls test was applied. p-value < 0.05 was considered statistically significant.

5. Conclusions

This study shows the inhibitory effect of hinokitiol on the migration of human adenocarcinoma A549 cells. The anticancer potential of hinokitiol is supported by the evidence provided in the present study, including, upregulation of Bax/p53, increase in the level of cytochrome c, and activation of caspases-9/-3 and antioxidant enzymes CAT and SOD. Moreover, we found the inhibitory effect of hinokitiol on the A549 cell migration was accompanied by downregulation of MMPs-9 and MMP-2. These results may illustrate a new therapeutic value of hinokitiol in anticancer therapy.

Acknowledgments: This work was supported by grants from the Ministry of Science and Technology of Taiwan (MOST 104-2622-B-038-003, MOST 104-2320-B-038-045-MY2, MOST 106-2320-B-038-012) and Yuan's General Hospital-Taipei Medical University (104-YGH-TMU-01-2).

Author Contributions: Joen-Rong Sheu and Thanasekaran Jayakumar conceived and designed the experiments. Thanasekaran Jayakumar, Chao-Hong Liu, and Guan-Yi Wu performed most of the experiments. Thanasekaran Jayakumar and Joen-Rong Sheu wrote the paper. Tzu-Yin Lee, Manjunath Manubolu, Cheng-Ying Hsieh, and Chih-Hao Yang contributed interpretations and assistance on the manuscript. All authors contributed clarifications and guidance on the manuscript. All authors were involved in editing the manuscript. All authors read and approved the final manuscript.

Conflicts of Interest: The authors declare no conflict of interest.

References

1. Shivapurkar, N.; Reddy, J.; Chaudhary, P.M.; Gazdar, A.F. Apoptosis and lung cancer: A review. *J Cell. Biochem.* **2003**, *88*, 885–898. [CrossRef] [PubMed]

2. Kim, S.S.; Cho, H.J.; Kang, J.Y.; Kang, H.K.; Yoo, T.K. Inhibition of androgen receptor expression with small interfering RNA enhances cancer cell apoptosis by suppressing survival factors in androgen insensitive, late stage LNCaP cells. *Sci. World J.* **2013**, *2013*. [CrossRef] [PubMed]
3. Ocker, M.; Höpfner, M. Apoptosis-modulating drugs for improved cancer therapy. *Eur. Surg. Res.* **2012**, *48*, 111–120. [CrossRef] [PubMed]
4. Moghadamtousi, S.Z.; Goh, B.H.; Chan, C.K.; Shabab, T.; Kadir, H.A. Biological activities and phytochemicals of *Swietenia macrophylla* king. *Molecules* **2013**, *18*, 10465–10483. [CrossRef] [PubMed]
5. Simon, H.U.; Haj-Yehia, A.; Levi-Schaffer, F. Role of reactive oxygen species (ROS) in apoptosis induction. *Apoptosis* **2000**, *5*, 415–418. [CrossRef] [PubMed]
6. Martinou, J.C.; Youle, R.J. Mitochondria in apoptosis: Bcl-2 family members and mitochondrial dynamics. *Dev. Cell* **2011**, *21*, 92–101. [CrossRef] [PubMed]
7. Yang, F.; Jove, V.; Chang, S.; Hedvat, M.; Liu, L.; Buettner, R.; Tian, Y.; Scuto, A.; Wen, W.; Yip, M.L.R.; et al. Bortezomib induces apoptosis and growth suppression in human medulloblastoma cells, associated with inhibition of AKT and NF-kB signaling, and synergizes with an ERK inhibitor. *Cancer Biol. Ther.* **2012**, *13*, 349–357. [CrossRef] [PubMed]
8. Itoh, Y.; Nagase, H. Matrix metalloproteinases in cancer. *Essays Biochem.* **2002**, *38*, 21–36. [CrossRef] [PubMed]
9. Bernhard, E.J.; Gruber, S.B.; Muschel, R.J. Direct evidence linking expression of matrix metalloproteinase 9 (92-kDa gelatinase/collagenase) to the metastatic phenotype in transformed rat embryo cells. *Proc. Natl. Acad. Sci. USA* **1994**, *91*, 4293–4297. [CrossRef] [PubMed]
10. Mook, O.R.; Frederiks, W.M.; Van Noorden, C.J. The role of gelatinases in colorectal cancer progression and metastasis. *Biochim. Biophys. Acta* **2004**, *1705*, 69–89. [CrossRef] [PubMed]
11. Loganayaki, M.; Manian, S. Antitumor activity of the methanolic extract of *Ammannia baccifera* L. against Dalton's ascites lymphoma induced ascetic and solid tumors in mice. *J. Ethnopharmacol.* **2012**, *142*, 305–309. [CrossRef] [PubMed]
12. Kavitha, K.; Manoharan, S. Anticarcinogenic and antilipidperoxidative effects of *Tephrosia purpurea* (Linn) pers. In 7, 12-dimethyl benz (a) anthracene (DMBA) induced hamster buccal pouch carcinoma. *Ind. J. Pharmacol.* **2006**, *38*, 185–189.
13. Bishayee, A.; Sethi, G. Bioactive natural products in cancer prevention and therapy: Progress and promise. *Semin. Cancer Biol.* **2016**, *40–41*, 1–3. [CrossRef] [PubMed]
14. Shanmugam, M.K.; Lee, J.H.; Chai, E.Z.; Kanchi, M.M.; Kar, S.; Arfuso, F.; Dharmarajan, A.; Kumar, A.P.; Ramar, P.S.; Looi, C.Y.; et al. Cancer prevention and therapy through the modulation of transcription factors by bioactive natural compounds. *Semin. Cancer Biol.* **2016**, *40–41*, 35–47. [CrossRef] [PubMed]
15. Shanmugam, M.K.; Kannaiyan, R.; Sethi, G. Targeting cell signaling and apoptotic pathways by dietary agents: Role in the prevention and treatment of cancer. *Nutr. Cancer* **2011**, *63*, 161–173. [CrossRef] [PubMed]
16. Baba, T.; Nakano, H.; Tamai, K.; Sawamura, D.; Hanada, K.; Hashimoto, I.; Arima, Y. Inhibitory effect of beta-thujaplicin on ultraviolet B-induced apoptosis in mouse keratinocytes. *J. Investig. Dermatol.* **1998**, *110*, 24–28. [CrossRef] [PubMed]
17. Li, L.H.; Wu, P.; Lee, J.Y.; Li, P.R.; Hsieh, W.Y.; Ho, C.C.; Ho, C.L.; Chen, W.J.; Wang, C.C.; Yen, M.Y.; et al. Hinokitiol induces DNA damage and autophagy followed by cell cycle arrest and senescence in gefitinib-resistant lung adenocarcinoma cells. *PLoS ONE* **2014**, *9*, e104203. [CrossRef] [PubMed]
18. Shih, Y.H.; Lin, D.J.; Chang, K.H.; Hsia, S.M.; Ko, S.Y.; Lee, S.Y.; Hsue, S.S.; Wang, T.H.; Chen, Y.L.; Shieh, T.M. Evaluation physical characteristics and comparison antimicrobial and anti-inflammation potentials of dental root canal sealers containing hinokitiol in vitro. *PLoS ONE* **2014**, *9*, e94941. [CrossRef] [PubMed]
19. Huang, C.H.; Lu, S.H.; Chang, C.C.; Thomas, P.A.; Jayakumar, T.; Sheu, J.R. Hinokitiol, a tropolone derivative, inhibits mouse melanoma (B16-F10) cell migration and in vivo tumor formation. *Eur. J. Pharmacol.* **2015**, *746*, 148–157. [CrossRef] [PubMed]
20. Lavrik, I.N.; Golks, A.; Krammer, P.H. Caspases: Pharmacological manipulation of cell death. *J. Clin. Investg.* **2005**, *115*, 2665–2672. [CrossRef] [PubMed]
21. Guner, G.; Islekel, H.; Oto, O.; Hazan, E.; Acikel, U. Evaluation of some antioxidant enzymes in lung carcinoma tissue. *Cancer Lett.* **1996**, *103*, 233–239. [CrossRef]
22. Coursin, D.B.; Cihla, H.P.; Sempf, J.; Oberley, T.D.; Oberley, L.W. An immunohistochemical analysis of antioxidant and glutathione s-transferase enzyme levels in normal and neoplastic human lung. *Histol. Histopathol.* **1996**, *11*, 851–860. [PubMed]

23. Lewis, A.; Du, J.; Liu, J.; Ritchie, J.M.; Oberley, L.W.; Cullen, J.J. Metastatic progression of pancreatic cancer: Changes in antioxidant enzymes and cell growth. *Clin. Exp. Metast.* **2005**, *22*, 523–532. [CrossRef] [PubMed]
24. Lee, Y.S.; Choi, K.M.; Kim, W.; Jeon, Y.S.; Lee, Y.M.; Hong, J.T.; Yun, Y.P.; Yoo, H.S. Hinokitiol inhibits cell growth through induction of S-phase arrest and apoptosis in human colon cancer cells and suppresses tumor growth in a mouse xenograft experiment. *J. Nat. Prod.* **2013**, *76*, 2195–2202. [CrossRef] [PubMed]
25. Chung, C.L.; Leung, K.W.; Lu, W.J.; Yen, T.L.; He, C.F.; Sheu, J.R.; Lin, K.H.; Lien, L.M. Hinokitiol negatively regulates immune responses through cell cycle arrest in concanavalin A-activated lymphocytes. *Evid. Based Complement. Altern. Med.* **2015**, *2015*, 595824. [CrossRef] [PubMed]
26. Lin, K.H.; Kuo, J.R.; Lu, W.J.; Chung, C.L.; Chou, D.S.; Huang, S.Y.; Lee, H.C.; Sheu, J.R. Hinokitiol inhibits platelet activation ex vivo and thrombus formation in vivo. *Biochem. Pharmacol.* **2013**, *85*, 1478–1485. [CrossRef] [PubMed]
27. Abedin, M.J.; Wang, D.; McDonnell, M.A.; Lehmann, U.; Kelekar, A. Autophagy delays apoptotic death in breast cancer cells following DNA damage. *Cell Death Differ.* **2007**, *14*, 500–510. [CrossRef] [PubMed]
28. Xiong, X.; Wu, M.; Zhang, H.; Li, J.; Lu, B.; Guo, Y.; Zhou, T.; Guo, H.; Peng, R.; Li, X.; et al. Atg5 siRNA inhibits autophagy and enhances norcantharidin-induced apoptosis in hepatocellular carcinoma. *Int. J. Oncol.* **2015**, *47*, 1321–1328. [CrossRef] [PubMed]
29. Zamzami, N.; Kroemer, G. The mitochondrion in apoptosis: How Pandora's box opens. *Nat. Rev. Mol. Cell Biol.* **2001**, *2*, 67–71. [CrossRef] [PubMed]
30. Baldwin, A.S. Control of oncogenesis and cancer therapy resistance by the transcription factor NF-κB. *J. Clin. Investg.* **2001**, *107*, 241–246. [CrossRef] [PubMed]
31. Hill, M.M.; Adrain, C.; Duriez, P.J.; Creagh, E.M.; Martin, S.J. Analysis of the composition, assembly kinetics and activity of native Apaf-1 apoptosomes. *EMBO J.* **2004**, *23*, 2134–2145. [CrossRef] [PubMed]
32. Elmore, S. Apoptosis: A review of programmed cell death. *Toxicol. Pathol.* **2007**, *35*, 495–516. [CrossRef] [PubMed]
33. Bodey, B.; Bodey, B., Jr.; Groger, A.M.; Siegel, S.E.; Kaiser, H.E. Invasion and metastasis: The expression and significance of matrix metalloproteinases in carcinomas of the lung. *In Vivo* **2001**, *15*, 175–180. [PubMed]
34. Hrabec, E.; Strek, M.; Nowak, D.; Greger, J.; Suwalski, M.; Hrabec, Z. Activity of type IV collagenases (MMP-2 and MMP-9) in primary pulmonary carcinomas: A quantitative analysis. *J. Cancer Res. Clin. Oncol.* **2002**, *128*, 197–204. [CrossRef] [PubMed]
35. Lai, W.W.; Hsu, S.C.; Chueh, F.S.; Chen, Y.Y.; Yang, J.S.; Lin, J.P.; Lien, J.C.; Tsai, C.H.; Chung, J.G. Quercetin inhibits migration and invasion of SAS human oral cancer cells through inhibition of NF-κB and matrix metalloproteinase-2/-9 signaling pathways. *Anticancer Res.* **2013**, *33*, 1941–1950. [PubMed]
36. Chandrashekar, N.; Selvamani, A.; Subramanian, R.; Pandi, A.; Thiruvengadam, D. Baicalein inhibits pulmonary carcinogenesis-associated inflammation and interferes with COX-2, MMP-2 and MMP-9 expressions in-vivo. *Toxicol. Appl. Pharmacol.* **2012**, *261*, 10–21. [CrossRef] [PubMed]
37. Subramanian, V.; Venkatesan, B.; Tumala, A.; Vellaichamy, E. Topical application of Gallic acid suppresses the 7, 12-DMBA/Croton oil induced two-step skin carcinogenesis by modulating anti-oxidants and MMP-2/MMP-9 in Swiss albino mice. *Food Chem. Toxicol.* **2014**, *66*, 44–55. [CrossRef] [PubMed]
38. Seidman, M.D.; Quirk, W.S.; Shirwany, N.A. Reactive oxygen metabolites, antioxidants and head and neck cancer. *Head Neck* **1999**, *21*, 467–479. [CrossRef]
39. Erzurum, S.C.; Danel, C.; Gillissen, A.; Chu, C.S.; Trapnell, B.C.; Crystal, R.G. In vivo antioxidant gene expression in human airway epithelium of normal individuals exposed to 100% O_2. *J. Appl. Physiol.* **1993**, *75*, 1256–1262. [CrossRef] [PubMed]
40. Putnam, C.D.; Arvai, A.S.; Bourne, Y.; Tainer, J.A. Active and inhibited human catalase structures: Ligand and NADPH binding and catalytic mechanism. *J. Mol. Biol.* **2000**, *296*, 295–309. [CrossRef] [PubMed]
41. Crawford, E.L.; Khuder, S.A.; Durham, S.J.; Frampton, M.; Utell, M.; Thilly, W.G.; Weaver, D.A.; Ferencak, W.J.; Jennings, C.A.; Hammersley, J.R.; et al. Normal bronchial epithelial cell expression of glutathione transferase P1, glutathione transferase M3, and glutathione peroxidase is low in subjects with bronchogenic carcinoma. *Cancer Res.* **2000**, *60*, 1609–1618. [PubMed]
42. Ho, C.J.; Zheng, S.; Comhair, S.A.A.; Farver, C.; Erzurum, S.C. Differential expression of manganese superoxide dismutase and catalase in lung cancer. *Cancer Res.* **2001**, *61*, 8578–8585.

43. Melloni, B.; Lefebvre, M.; Bonnaud, F.; Vergnenegre, A.; Grossin, L.; Rigaud, M.; Cantin, A. Antioxidant activity in bronchoalveolar lavage fluid from individuals with lung cancer. *Am. J. Respir. Crit. Care Med.* **1996**, *154*, 1706–1711. [CrossRef] [PubMed]
44. Lu, M.K.; Shih, Y.W.; Chang, T.T.; Fang, L.H.; Huang, H.C.; Chen, P.S. α-Solanine inhibits human melanoma cell migration and invasion by reducing matrix metalloproteinase-2/9 activities. *Biol. Pharm. Bull.* **2010**, *33*, 1685–1691. [CrossRef] [PubMed]
45. Woodbury, W.; Speacer, A.K.; Stahman, M.A. An improved procedure using ferricyanide for detecting catalase isozymes. *Anal. Biochem.* **1971**, *44*, 301–305. [CrossRef]
46. Beauchamp, C.; Fridovich, I. Superoxide dismutase: Improved assays and an assay applicable to acrylamide gels. *Anal. Biochem.* **1971**, *44*, 276–287. [CrossRef]

International Journal of
Molecular Sciences

MDPI

Article

Calorie Restriction Effect of Heat-Processed Onion Extract (ONI) Using In Vitro and In Vivo Animal Models

Yu-Ri Kang [1], Hwang-Yong Choi [1], Jung-Yun Lee [1], Soo In Jang [1], Hanna Kang [1], Jung-Bae Oh [2], Hae-Dong Jang [1,*] and Young-In Kwon [1,*]

[1] Department of Food and Nutrition, Hannam University, Daejeon 34054, Korea; djsdnd12@nate.com (Y.-R.K.); kelolo123@naver.com (H.-Y.C.); seembeeks@hanmail.net (J.-Y.L.); sooin8042@nate.com (S.I.J.); hanna9506@daum.net (H.K.)

[2] Institute of Functional Foods, KunpoongBio Co. Ltd., Jeju 63010, Korea; denisoh89@naver.com

* Correspondence: headong@hnu.kr (H.-D.J.); youngk@hnu.kr (Y.-I.K.); Tel.: +82-42-629-8795 (H.-D.J.); +82-10-2238-7228 (Y.-I.K.)

Received: 16 January 2018; Accepted: 9 March 2018; Published: 15 March 2018

Abstract: Onion (*Allium cepa* L.) is widely consumed as food or medicinal plant due to its well-defined health benefits. The antioxidant and antihyperlipidemic effects of onion and its extracts have been reported well. However, very limited information on anti-hyperglycemic effect is available in processed onion extracts. In our previous study, we reported that Amadori rearrangement compounds (ARCs) produced by heat-processing in Korean ginseng can reduce carbohydrate absorption by inhibiting intestinal carbohydrate hydrolyzing enzymes in both in vitro and in vivo animal models. To prove the enhancement of anti-hyperglycemic effect and ARCs content by heat-processing in onion extract, a correlation between the anti-hyperglycemic activity and the total content of ARCs of heat-processed onion extract (ONI) was investigated. ONI has a high content of ARCs and had high rat small intestinal sucrase inhibitory activity (0.34 ± 0.03 mg/mL, IC_{50}) relevant for the potential management of postprandial hyperglycemia. The effect of ONI on the postprandial blood glucose increase was investigated in Sprague Dawley (SD) rats fed on sucrose or starch meals. The maximum blood glucose levels (C*max*) of heat-processed onion extract were significantly decreased by about 8.7% (from 188.60 ± 5.37 to 172.27 ± 3.96, $p < 0.001$) and 14.2% (from 204.04 ± 8.73 to 175.13 ± 14.09, $p < 0.01$) in sucrose and starch loading tests, respectively. These results indicate that ARCs in onion extract produced by heat-processing have anti-diabetic effect by suppressing carbohydrate absorption via inhibition of intestinal sucrase, thereby reducing the postprandial increase of blood glucose. Therefore, enhancement of ARCs in onion by heat-processing might be a good strategy for the development of the new product on the management of hyperglycemia.

Keywords: heat-process; onion; calorie restriction; Amadori rearrangement compounds; hyperglycemia

1. Introduction

Hyperglycemia is a common symptom of diabetes with blood sugar levels higher than normal and is a condition in which an excessive amount of glucose circulates in the blood plasma. Chronic hyperglycemia causes various complications such as nephropathy, retinopathy, neuropathy, stroke, and cardiovascular diseases in type 2 diabetes mellitus (T2DM) patients [1]. Therefore, regulation of postprandial hyperglycemia is an important strategy used for treatment in T2DM patients. Dietary carbohydrates are broken down into monosaccharides by carbohydrate hydrolyzing enzymes such as α-amylase and α-glucosidases (sucrase, maltase, and glucoamylase) before their absorption [2]. Inhibition of these enzymes can suppress or retard the absorption of monosaccharides such as glucose, fructose, and galactose. Modulation of activities of these enzymes can prevent postprandial hyperglycemia and maintain normal blood glucose levels [3].

Recent studies report that intestinal α-glucosidase inhibitors from medicinal plants could be as effective as commercial drugs with lower side effect [4]. Phytochemicals present in medicinal plants have various health-promoting activities and have been shown to exert intestinal α-glucosidase inhibitory effects in vitro [5].

Herbs, onions, and beans that are important and traditional nutritive components have elevated polyphenol contents [1]. Plants belonging to the *Allium* species, such as onions and garlic, are used as foodstuffs, condiments, flavorings, and folk medicines [2]. Onion is rich in flavonoids such as quercetin and organosulfur compounds such as allyl propyl disulfide and S-methyl cysteine sulfoxide. It was reported that quercetin has antioxidant, anti-inflammatory, and antidiabetic effect [6–8]. Moreover, S-methyl cysteine sulfoxide has a lipid-lowering, antidiabetic, and antioxidant effects in alloxan diabetic rats [9,10]. The degree to which phytochemicals change during processing depends on the sensitivity of the phytochemical to modification or degradation, and length of exposure to a processing technique [11,12]. The content of quercetin in processed vegetables is dramatically decreased in the alkaline conditions, especially during heat-processing [10]. These results indicate that food processing conditions play an important role for food quality and functionality.

In addition, specific compounds, such as Amadori rearrangement compounds (ARCs) and Maillard reaction produts (MRPs), are produced by the heat-treatment of onions. It is reported that the production of MRPs and ARCs such as arginyl-fructose (AF) and fructosyl-lysine due to heat-treatment of onion results to the increase of antioxidant activity of onions [13–15].

During steaming and drying processes that are necessary for the production of Korean red ginseng or onion, certain components undergo non-enzymatic browning reaction, otherwise known as a Maillard reaction [16]. In the early stage of Maillard reaction, AF and arginyl-fructosyl-glucose (AFG) are formed through Amadori rearrangement of arginine with glucose or maltose in ginseng or onion, respectively [17]. In our previous study, we reported that arginyl-fructose (AF) and arginyl-fructosyl-glucose (AFG) produced by heat-processing in Korean ginseng can reduce carbohydrate absorption by inhibiting intestinal carbohydrate hydrolyzing enzymes in both in vitro and in vivo animal models [16,17]. The postprandial anti-hyperglycemia effect of AF from heat-processed Korean ginseng in db/db animal model and human clinical trials was also reported by our previous study [18,19].

However, very limited information is available about the enhancement of ARCs content in plant foods, except for red ginseng and subsequent enhanced antidiabetic activity. Therefore, to investigate the benefit of the heat-processing of onions for improving the antidiabetic activity and maximizing the production of ARCs, it is essential to measure the effect of heat-processing. Consequently, the purpose of this study was (i) to identify how heat processing affects ARC production in onion extracts and (ii) to evaluate the anti-hyperglycemic effect of heat-processed onion extracts such as heat-treated onion extract containing high ARCs (ONI_H) and heat-treated onion extract containing low ARCs (ONI_L) using in vitro alpha-glucosidase and sucrase inhibition assays as well as an in vivo animal model.

2. Results

2.1. Sample Preparation

As seen in Table 1 and Figure 1, two sample powders—which have a different contents of total ARCs, arginyl-fructose, glucose, fructose, and quercetin due to the different processing condition were prepared. Each sample was named by the content of ARCs, ONI_H (13.3% of AF and 33% of total ARCs), and ONI_L (5.55% of AF and 18% of total ARCs), respectively. In regards to ARC contents ONI_H and ONI_L treatments resulted to significantly higher contents of ARC when compared to quercetin (Table 1). These results indicate that reaction time for heating onions is an important factor for producing ARCs. Furthermore, we observed that ONI_H had higher ARC and quercetin contents, when compared to ONI_L (Table 1). Although both ARC and quercetin contents increased with heat treatment, since ARCs account for 38.02% of the total weight of the tested extract, we suspect that the observed bioactivities are due to ARCS, but we cannot exclude the possible synergistic effect of quercetin, which has a well-defined anti-hyperglycaemic effect.

Table 1. The composition of two different onion extracts (ONI_H and ONI_L).

Samples	pH	Brix	AF (%)	Arg (%)	Glu (%)	Fru (%)	Que (ug/g)	Total [1] (%)
ONI_H	6.97	30.1	13.3	8.56	6.08	10.08	200	38.02
ONI_L	7.59	28.3	5.55	9.46	6.86	6.99	103	28.90

[1] Total: AF + Arg + Glu + Fru; AF: arginyl-fructose, Arg: arginine, Glu: glucose, Fru: fructose, Que: quercetin.

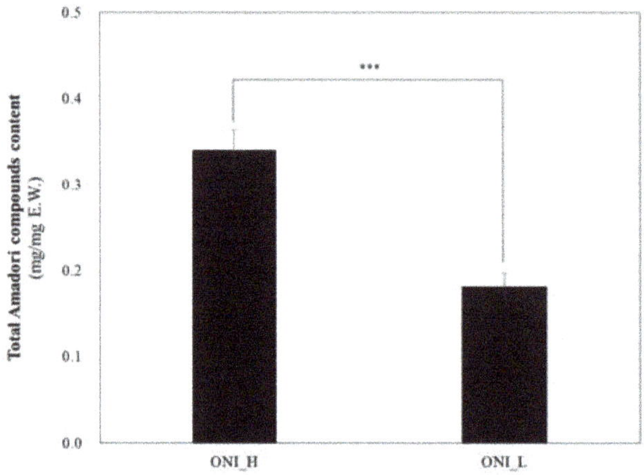

Figure 1. Total ARCs content of two different onion extracts (ONI_H and ONI_L). The results were expressed as mean ± S.D. Statistical significances were determined by Student's *t*-test (*** $p < 0.001$).

2.2. α-Glucosidase Inhibitory Activity

The α-glucosidase inhibitors, which interfere with enzymatic action in the brush-border of the small intestine, could inhibit the liberation of D-glucose from oligosaccharides and disaccharides, resulting in reduced postprandial plasma glucose levels.

α-Glucosidase inhibitory activities of ONI_H and ONI_L are shown in Figure 2. As expected, ONI_H (high ARCs content sample), showed higher α-glucosidase inhibitory activity (5.87 mg/mL of IC_{50}) (Table 2) than that of ONI_L (>12.59 mg/mL of IC_{50}) (Table 2). In terms of sucrase inhibition, ONI_H inhibits sucrase activity in a dose-dependent manner, but ONI_L showed almost no inhibition at all tested doses (Figure 3). The half-maximal inhibitory concentration (IC_{50}) of ONI_H was 0.34 mg/mL.

Table 2. The half-maximal inhibitory concentration (IC_{50}) values for rat intestinal α-glucosidase and sucrase by two different onion extracts (ONI_H and ONI_L).

	IC_{50} (mg/mL)	
Enzymes	ONI_H	ONI_L
Sucrase	0.34 ± 0.03	ND [1]
α-glucosidase	5.87 ± 0.60	>12.59 ± 0.27

[1] ND—Not determined.

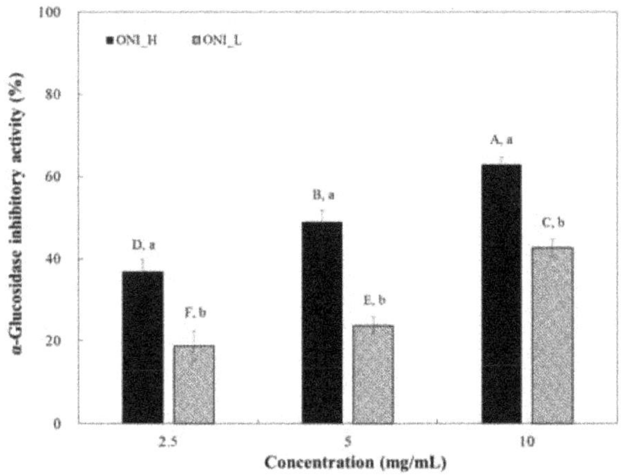

Figure 2. Dose dependent changes in rat small intestinal α-glucosidase inhibitory activities (% inhibition) of two different onion extracts (ONI_H and ONI_L). The results were expressed as mean ± S.D. with three independent experiments in triplicate. Different corresponding letters indicate significant differences at $p < 0.05$ by Duncan's test. A–F The first letters in uppercase indicate significant differences among all samples and a–b the second letters in lowercase are different between ONI_H and ONI_L within the same concentration.

As seen in Figures 2 and 3, ONI_H which has a higher content of AF and ARC than ONI_L showed high α-glucosidase and sucrase inhibitory activities. Interestingly, inhibitory activity of both ONI_H and ONI_L against sucrase was higher than that of α-glucosidase. This result may due to the enzyme inhibition specificity of AF, a major ingredient in both extracts. According to a previous report by Ha et al. (2011), AF yielded to superior inhibitory effect against sucrase (IC_{50}, 6.40 mM) [17] suggesting possible bioactive components were present in the heat-processed onions.

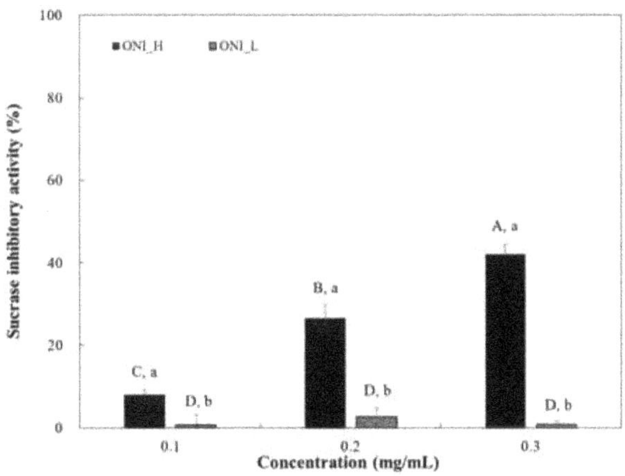

Figure 3. Dose dependent changes in rat small intestinal sucrase inhibitory activities (% inhibition) of two different onion extracts (ONI_H and ONI_L). The results were expressed as mean ± S.D. with three independent experiments in triplicate. Different corresponding letters indicate significant differences at $p < 0.05$ by Duncan's test. A–D The first letters in uppercase indicate significant differences among all samples and a–b the second letters in lowercase are different between ONI_H and ONI_L within same concentration.

Our observations suggest that the increased content of AF or ARCs is critical for enzyme inhibitory activity of heat-processed onion extract. These results indicate that ARCs produced by heat treatment plays an important role in the enhancement of functionality of onion-based products.

2.3. Blood Glucose Lowering Effect of Onion Extracts In Vivo

ONI_H and ONI_L showed significant inhibition against α-glucosidases especially for sucrase, which is a membrane-bound enzyme at the epithelia of the small intestine and a key enzyme of sucrose digestion (Table 2). Inhibition of sucrase may lead to a delayed and reduced rise in postprandial blood glucose levels. To confirm the in vitro sucrase inhibitory activity of samples, the in vivo blood glucose reducing effects of ONI_H and ONI_L were evaluated with SD rats and the results are illustrated in Figure 4.

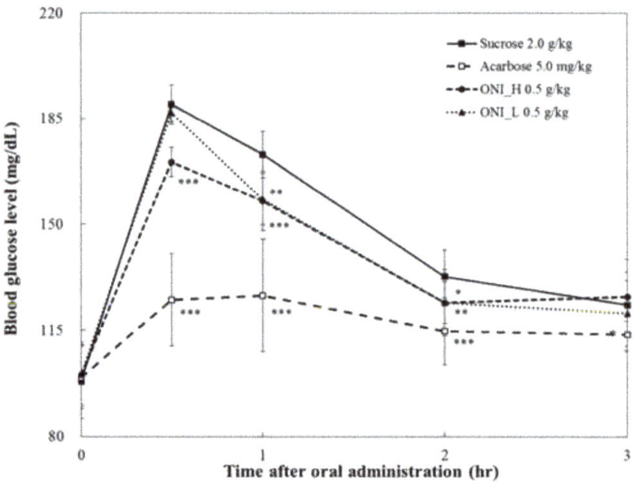

Figure 4. Comparison of postprandial blood glucose-lowering effects of ONI_H and ONI_L in sucrose loading test. After fasting for 24 h, five-week-old, male SD rats were orally administered sucrose solution (2.0 g/kg) with or without samples (onion extracts). The results were expressed as mean ± S.D. Statistical significances were determined by Student's t-test (* $p < 0.05$; ** $p < 0.01$; and *** $p < 0.001$).

In the ONI_L-treated group with sucrose, the blood glucose level was 186.90 ± 2.92 mg/dL at 30 min after administration and not significantly different to the sucrose control group (189.67 ± 6.50 mg/dL) (Figure 4). On the other hand, ONI_H-treated group (170.63 ± 4.87 mg/dL, $p < 0.001$) suppresses the rising of plasma glucose level by 19.04 mg/dL compared to the sucrose control group at 30 min after administration.

In terms of starch loading test, blood glucose level in the ONI_H-treated group was 173.33 ± 16.41 mg/dL ($p < 0.01$) at 30 min after administration (Figure 5). This is lower than the ONI_L-treated group (191.60 ± 12.08 mg/dL) and the starch group (197.50 ± 12.42 mg/dL) by 18.27 mg/dL and 24.17 mg/dL respectively. At 1 h after administration, the blood glucose level of ONI_H-treated group (153.82 ± 11.44 mg/dL, $p < 0.001$) was lower than both the ONI_L-treated group (164.62 ± 13.43 mg/dL) and starch group (187.67 ± 3.51 mg/dL).

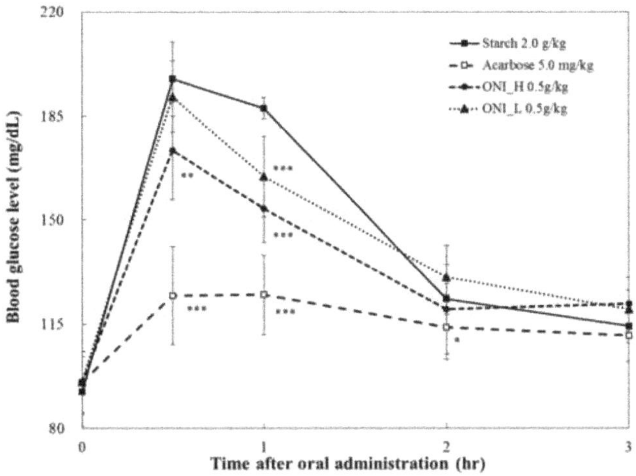

Figure 5. Comparison of postprandial blood glucose-lowering effects of pyridoxine, pyridoxal, and pyridoxamine in starch loading test. After fasting for 24 h, five-week-old, male SD rats were orally administered starch solution (2.0 g/kg) with or without samples (onion extracts). The results were expressed as mean ± S.D. Statistical significances were determined by Student's *t*-test (* $p < 0.05$; ** $p < 0.01$; and *** $p < 0.001$).

2.4. Pharmacodynamics Parameters

Pharmacodynamic (PD) parameters of the sucrose and starch loading tests are shown in Table 3. In terms of T*max*, there is no significant difference among sucrose and both ONI_H and ONI_L-treated groups. In contrast, ONI_H-treated groups resulted significantly reduced C*max* and AUC*t*, however this reduction was less effective than the acarbose-treated group. Specifically for C*max*, the maximum blood glucose levels (C*max*) of ONI_H administration group decreased by about 8.6% (from 188.60 ± 5.37 to 172.27 ± 3.96) and 14.3% (from 204.04 ± 8.73 to 175.13 ± 14.09) in sucrose and starch loading tests, respectively, when compared to control in pharmacodynamics study.

Our findings suggest health beneficial effect of ONI_H against high blood glucose levels, following sucrose and starch administration. Based on the above observations, it is expected that the resulting reduction of glucose levels could be due to the inhibitory effect of ONI_H against carbohydrate hydrolyzing enzymes.

Table 3. Changes in pharmacodynamic (PD) parameters of control and after administration of ONI_H, ONI_L, and acarbose with sucrose or starch ingestions

Groups	PD Parameters		
	C*max* (mg/dL)	T*max* (h)	AUC*t* (h·mg/dL)
Sucrose 2.0 g/kg	188.60 ± 5.37 [a]	0.50 ± 0.00 [b]	442.22 ± 18.45 [a]
Acarbose 5.0 mg/kg	129.47 ± 15.84 [c]	1.10 ± 0.55 [a]	353.65 ± 34.41 [b]
ONI_H 0.5 g/kg	172.27 ± 3.96 [b]	0.50 ± 0.00 [b]	418.11 ± 13.83 [a]
ONI_L 0.5 g/kg	187.00 ± 1.90 [a]	0.50 ± 0.00 [b]	422.33 ± 14.38 [a]
Starch 2.0 g/kg	204.04 ± 8.73 [a]	0.75 ± 0.29 [a]	451.90 ± 3.94 [a]
Acarbose 5.0 mg/kg	133.43 ± 10.28 [c]	1.00 ± 0.61 [a]	350.48 ± 19.40 [c]
ONI_H 0.5 g/kg	175.13 ± 14.09 [b]	0.50 ± 0.00 [a]	406.69 ± 22.62 [b]
ONI_L 0.5 g/kg	193.77 ± 11.48 [a]	0.50 ± 0.00 [a]	434.95 ± 19.47 [a]

The results were expressed as mean ± S.D. [a–c] Different letters indicate statistically significant differences between groups one-way ANOVA followed by Duncan's test of $p < 0.05$.

3. Discussion

It is reported that the production of Maillard reaction products (MRPs) and Amodori rearrangement compounds (ARCs) such as arginyl-fructose and fructosyl-lysine due to heat-treatment of onion positively affects the antioxidant activity of onion [11–13]. ARCs such as arginyl-fructose (AF) and arginyl-fructosyl-glucose (AFG) in red ginseng possess antioxidant and antidiabetic activity [14,15]. However, very limited information is available about the enhancement of ARCs content in various plant foods extracts, except for red ginseng [20–22].

In this study, the optimum condition for improving the antidiabetic activity and maximizing the production of ARCs in onion extract was investigated. ARCs production was positively proportional to the reaction temperature and controlled by the amount of arginine and food-grade acid additions. ARCs content was also correlated with inhibitory activity against α-glucosidase and sucrase, which are membrane-bound enzymes at the epithelia of the small intestine and key enzymes of carbohydrate digestion.

Furthermore, to confirm the in vitro α-glucosidase and sucrase inhibitory activities of samples, the in vivo blood glucose reducing effects of onion extract with high ARCs content (ONI_H) and low ARCs content (ONI_L) were evaluated with SD rats and the results were similar with in vitro data. The postprandial blood glucose levels of the ONI_H-treated group were decreased more effectively than the ONI_L-treated group in sucrose and starch loading tests.

These results suggest that ARCs—such as AF—in heat-processed onions could be the reason for the resulting reduction in postprandial blood glucose levels, as previously described by Ha et al. [15]. Also, it is reported that ARCs from ginseng could be great antioxidant compounds [14]. Even though the quercetin contents were significantly lower when compared to ARC contents, we cannot exclude the possible synergistic effect of ARCs and quercetin, since the anti-diabetic effect of quercetin is well-defined. Our findings suggest that the observed postprandial glucose reduction effect of ONI_H correlate to ARCs and quercetin contents and therefore can have an additional health-benefits, such as the reduction of oxidation-induced complication of diabetes.

These results indicate that heat-processing of onion supplemented with arginine resulted in the formation of ARCs which could be effectively designed as complementary therapies for postprandial hyperglycemia linked to type 2 diabetes prevention.

4. Materials and Methods

4.1. Materials

Korean onion (*Allium cepa* L.) was purchased from a local market in Jeju, Korea. Rat intestinal acetone powders of α-glucosidase (EC 3.2.1.20) and nitro blue tetrazolium (NBT) were purchased from Sigma-Aldrich Co. (St. Louis, MO, USA). Sodium carbonate was purchased from DUKSAN Pure Chemicals Co. (Ansan, Kyounggi-Do, Korea). Unless noted, all chemicals were purchased from Sigma-Aldrich Co. (St. Louis, MO, USA).

4.2. Sample Preparation

In order to produce a high mass of heat-processed onion extract, the scale-up process with 500 kg onions was performed, using the facilities in KunpoongBio Co., Ltd. (Jeju city, Jeju-Do, Korea). The onions, whole without peeling, were crushed and enzymatically digested with 0.5% Celluclast + Pectinex (Novozyme Korea Ltd., Seoul, Korea) mix for 2 h at 50 °C, and then the enzyme was inactivated for 20 min at 100 °C and the filtered using a sieve (10 mesh). The filtrate sieved (10 mesh) was concentrated at 60 °C using vacuum evaporator. Citric acid and arginine were used as a pH regulator. It was then heated for 3 or 5 h at 90 °C. Finally, the two reactants such as 3 h (ONI_L) and 5 h (ONI_H) reactants were spray-dried, respectively. After all this process, total ARCs, arginyl-fructose, residue glucose, fructose, and quercetin contents of the two samples were measured. Finally, dextrin—an extender—was added and spray dried. Samples were stored at −20 °C until analysis.

4.3. Total Amadori Compounds Analysis

Fructosamine measurement method was modified and used as an experimental method [23]. Sodium carbonate was prepared as 0.1 M, pH 10.3 and 0.57 mM of NBT dissolved in 0.1 M sodium carbonate was prepared. The sample solution (50 µL) and NBT solution (150 µL) was added to each well and incubated at 37 °C. The absorbance was measured at 540 nm at 10 and 20 min time points. The concentration of total ARCs was calculated compared to fructosyl-arginine as a standard.

4.4. α-Glucosidase Inhibition Assay

Rat intestinal α-glucosidase assay referred to the method of Kwon et al. [3] with a slight modification. A total of 1 g of rat-intestinal acetone powder was suspended in 3 mL of 0.1 M sodium phosphate buffer (pH 6.9), and the suspension was sonicated 12 times for 30 s at 4 °C. After centrifugation (10,000× g, 30 min, 4 °C), the resulting supernatant was used for the assay. Sample solution (50 µL) and 0.1 M sodium phosphate buffer (pH 6.9, 100 µL) containing glucosidase solution (1.0 U/mL) was incubated at 37 °C for 10 min. After pre-incubation, 5 mM p-nitrophenyl-α-D-glucopyranoside solution (50 µL) in 0.1 M sodium phosphate buffer (pH 6.9) was added to each well at timed intervals. The reaction mixtures were incubated at 37 °C for 30 min. After incubation, absorbance was read at 405 nm and compared to a control which had 50 µL of buffer solution in place of the extract by micro-plate reader (SUNRISE; Tecan Trading AG, Salzburg, Austria). The α-glucosidase inhibitory activity was expressed as inhibition % and was calculated as follows:

$$\text{Inhibition (\%)} = \left(\left[\frac{\Delta A_{405}^{\text{Control}} - \Delta A_{405}^{\text{Extract}}}{\left[\Delta A_{405}^{\text{Control}}\right]} \right] \right) \times 100$$

4.5. Sugar Loading Test

Effect on hyperglycemia induced by carbohydrate loads in Sprague Dawley (SD) rats was determined by the inhibitory action of processed onion extract and acarbose on postprandial hyperglycemia [17]. All animal procedures were approved by Institutional Animal Care and Use Committee (IACUC) of the Hannam University (Approval number: HNU2017-003, 14/03/2017). Five-week-old male SD rats were purchased from Raon Bio Co. (Yongin, Kyounggi-Do, Korea) and fed a solid diet (Samyang Diet Co., Seoul, Korea) for one week. The rats were housed in a ventilated room at 25 ± 2 °C with 50 ± 7% relative humidity and under an alternating 12 h light/dark cycle. After 6 groups of 5 male SD rats (180–200 g) fasted for 24 h, 2.0 g/kg of sucrose were orally administrated concurrently with 0–500 mg/kg or onion extracts or acarbose. The blood samples were then taken from the tail after administration and blood glucose levels were measured at 0, 0.5, 1, 2, and 3 h. The glucose level in blood was determined by glucose oxidase method and compared with that of the control group, which had not taken the inhibitors. The parameters for blood glucose levels were calculated using PKsolver. Maximum observed peak blood glucose level (C_{max}) and the time at which it is observed (T_{max}) were determined based on the observed data. The area under the blood glucose–time curve up to the last sampled time-point (AUC_t) was estimated by the trapezoidal rule.

4.6. Statistical Analysis

All data are presented as mean ± S.D. Statistical analyses were carried out using the statistical package SPSS 11 (Statistical Package for Social Science 11, SPSS Inc., Chicago, IL, USA) program and significance of each group was verified with the analysis of one-way ANOVA followed by Duncan's test of $p < 0.05$. In addition, statistical significances in animal study were determined by Student's t-test (* $p < 0.05$; ** $p < 0.01$; and *** $p < 0.001$).

5. Conclusions

Hyperglycemia has been identified as a major risk factor for cardiovascular complications linked to T2DM, and thereby known as an effective therapeutic target in the treatment of T2DM. Our data presented in this study strongly suggest that heat-processed onion extract can be a significant source of AF, a major bioactive ARCs in ONI, and phenolic compounds that exert postprandial blood glucose-lowering and antioxidant effects, respectively. Taking into consideration that AF is present in a wide variety of heat-processed food products, knowledge of this additional health benefit of heat-processed foods can assist in the development of efficacious anti-hyperglycemia supplements and give rationale for further clinical study.

Although further work is still needed to optimize the condition for production of anti-hyperglycemic components in the ONI and evaluate pharmacological effect in human clinical trial, our in vitro and in vivo data offer a biochemical rationale to support further clinical studies. These results also provide the basis for developing valuable alternatives to synthetic drugs to manage glycemic control from heat-processed food products in food industry.

Acknowledgments: This research was financially supported by the Ministry of Trade, Industry, and Energy (MOTIE), Korea, under the "Regional Specialized Industry Development Program" supervised by the Korea Institute for Advancement of Technology (KIAT).

Author Contributions: Young-In Kwon and Hae-Dong Jang designed the experiment and directed its process, including data analysis. Yu-Ri Kang and Hwang-Yong Choi prepared introduction and the Methods and the Discussion sections of the text. Jung-Yun Lee, and Soo In Jang performed the animal study and statistically analyzed the data. Jung-Bae Oh and Hanna Kang manufactured samples and conducted all scale-up processes. All the authors read and approved the final manuscript.

Conflicts of Interest: The authors declare no conflict of interest.

Abbreviations

ARCs	Amadori rearrangement compounds
SD rat	Sprague Dawley rat
MRPs	Maillard reaction products
AF	Arginyl-fructose
AFG	Arginyl-fructosyl-glucose
ONI_H	Heat-treated onion extract containing high ARCs
ONI_L	Heat-treated onion extract containing low ARCs

References

1. Kim, S.H.; Jo, S.H.; Kwon, Y.I.; Hwang, J.K. Effects of onion (*Allium cepa* L.) extract administration on intestinal α-glucosidases activities and spikes in postprandial blood glucose levels in SD rats model. *Int. J. Mol. Sci.* **2011**, *12*, 3757–3769. [CrossRef] [PubMed]
2. Singh, U.; Singh, S.; Kochhar, A. Therapeutic potential of antidiabetic neutraceuticals. *Phytopharmacol* **2012**, *2*, 144–169.
3. Kwon, Y.I.; Apostolidis, E.; Kim, Y.C.; Shetty, K. Health benefits of traditional corn, beans, and pumpkin: In vitro studies for hyperglycemia and hypertension management. *J. Med. Food* **2007**, *10*, 266–275. [CrossRef] [PubMed]
4. Kwon, Y.I.; Vattem, D.A.; Shetty, K. Evaluation of clonal herbs of Lamiaceae species for management of diabetes and hypertension. *Asia Pac. J. Clin. Nutr.* **2006**, *15*, 107–118. [PubMed]
5. Rasheed, D.; Porzel, A.; Frolov, A.; El Saedi, H.R.; Wessjohann, L.A.; Farag, M.A. Comparative analysis of Hibiscus sabdariffa (roselle) hot and cold extracts in respect to their potential for α-glucosidase inhibition. *Food Chem.* **2018**, *250*, 236–244. [CrossRef] [PubMed]
6. Guardia, T.; Rotelli, A.E.; Juarez, A.O.; Pelzer, L.E. Anti-inflammatory properties of plant flavonoids. Effects of rutin, quercetin and hesperidin on adjuvant arthritis in rat. *Farmaco* **2001**, *56*, 683–687. [CrossRef]
7. Vessal, M.; Hemmati, M.; Vasei, M. Antidiabetic effects of quercetin in streptozocin-induced diabetic rats. *Comp. Biochem. Physiol. Part C Toxicol. Pharmacol.* **2003**, *135*, 357–364. [CrossRef]

8. Coskun, O.; Kanter, M.; Korkmaz, A.; Oter, S. Quercetin, a flavonoid antioxidant, prevents and protects streptozotocin-induced oxidative stress and β-cell damage in rat pancreas. *Pharmacol. Res.* **2005**, *51*, 117–123. [CrossRef] [PubMed]
9. Kumari, K.; Augusti, K.T. Antidiabetic and antioxidant effects of S-methyl cysteine sulfoxide isolated from onions (*Allium cepa* Linn) as compared to standard drugs in alloxan diabetic rats. *Indian J. Exp. Biol.* **2002**, *40*, 1005–1009. [PubMed]
10. Kumari, K.; Augusti, K.T. Lipid lowering effect of S-methyl cysteine sulfoxide from Allium cepa Linn in high cholesterol diet fed rats. *J. Ethnopharmacol.* **2007**, *109*, 367–371. [CrossRef] [PubMed]
11. Breene, W.M. Healthfulness and nutritional quality of fresh versus processed fruits and vegetables: A review. *J. Foodserv.* **1994**, *8*, 1–45. [CrossRef]
12. Lombard, K.; Peffley, E.; Geoffriau, E.; Thompson, L.; Herring, A. Quercetin in onion (*Allium cepa* L.) after heat-treatment simulating home preparation. *J. Food Compost. Anal.* **2005**, *18*, 571–581. [CrossRef]
13. Moreno, F.J.; Corzo-Martı, M.; Del Castillo, M.D.; Villamiel, M. Changes in antioxidant activity of dehydrated onion and garlic during storage. *Food Res. Int.* **2006**, *39*, 891–897. [CrossRef]
14. Woo, K.S.; Hwang, I.G.; Kim, T.M.; Kim, D.J.; Hong, J.T.; Jeong, H.S. Changes in the antioxidant activity of onion (*Allium cepa*) extracts with heat treatment. *Food Sci. Biotechnol.* **2007**, *16*, 828–831.
15. Hwang, I.G.; Kim, H.Y.; Lee, S.H.; Hwang, C.R.; Oh, S.H.; Woo, K.S.; Kim, D.J.; Lee, J.S.; Jeong, H.S. Isolation and identification of an antioxidant substance from heated onion (*Allium cepa* L.). *J. Korean Soc. Food Sci. Nutr.* **2011**, *40*, 470–474. [CrossRef]
16. Lee, J.S.; Kim, G.N.; Lee, S.H.; Kim, E.S.; Ha, K.S.; Kwon, Y.I.; Jeong, H.S.; Jang, H.D. In vitro and cellular antioxidant activity of arginyl-fructose and arginyl-fructosyl-glucose. *Food Sci. Biotechnol.* **2009**, *18*, 1505–1510.
17. Ha, K.S.; Jo, S.H.; Kang, B.H.; Apostolidis, E.; Lee, M.S.; Jang, H.D.; Kwon, Y.I. In Vitro and In Vivo Antihyperglycemic Effect of 2 Amadori Rearrangement Compounds, Arginyl-Fructose and Arginyl-Fructosyl-Glucose. *J. Food Sci.* **2011**, *76*, H188–H193. [CrossRef] [PubMed]
18. Lee, K.-H.; Ha, K.S.; Jo, S.H.; Lee, C.-M.; Kim, Y.-C.; Chung, K.-H.; Kwon, Y.-I. Effect of long-term dietary arginyl-fructose (AF) on hyperglycemia and HbA1c in diabetic db/db mice. *Int. J. Mol. Sci.* **2014**, *15*, 8352–8359. [CrossRef] [PubMed]
19. Park, S.E.; Kin, O.-H.; Kwak, J.H.; Lee, K.H.; Kwon, Y.-I.; Chung, K.H.; Lee, J.H. Antihyperglycemic effect of short-term arginyl-fructose supplementation in subjects with prediabetes and newly diagnosed type 2 diabetes: Randomized, double-blinded, placebo-controlled trial. *Trials* **2015**, *16*, 521–528. [CrossRef] [PubMed]
20. Yukinaga, M.; Yinan, Z.; Takeshi, T.; Kenji, K.; Hiromichi, O. Isolation and Physiological Activites of a New Amino Acid Derivative from Korean Red Ginseng. *J. Ginseng Res.* **1994**, *18*, 204–211.
21. Takaku, T.; Han, L.K.; Kameda, K.; Ninomiya, H.; Okuda, H. Production of arginyl-fructosyl-glucose during processing of red ginseng. *J. Tradit. Med.* **1996**, *13*, 118–123.
22. Suzuki, Y.; Choi, K.J.; Uchida, K.; Ko, S.R.; Sohn, H.J.; Park, J.D. Arginyl-fructosyl-glucose and arginyl-fructose, compounds related to browning reaction in the model system of steaming and heat-drying processes for the preparation of red ginseng. *J. Ginseng Res.* **2004**, *28*, 143–148.
23. Jariyapamornkoon, N.; Yibchok-anun, S.; Adisakwattana, S. Inhibition of advanced glycation end products by red grape skin extract and its antioxidant activity. *BMC Complement. Altern. Med.* **2013**, *13*, 171. [CrossRef] [PubMed]

International Journal of
Molecular Sciences

MDPI

Review

Therapeutic Potential of Plants and Plant Derived Phytochemicals against Acetaminophen-Induced Liver Injury

Sandeep B. Subramanya [1], Balaji Venkataraman [1], Mohamed Fizur Nagoor Meeran [2], Sameer N. Goyal [3,4], Chandragouda R. Patil [4] and Shreesh Ojha [2,*]

1 Department of Physiology, College of Medicine and Health Sciences, PO Box # 17666, United Arab Emirates University, Al Ain 17666, UAE; sandeep.bs@uaeu.ac.ae (S.B.S.); balajiv@uaeu.ac.ae (B.V.)
2 Department of Pharmacology and Therapeutics, College of Medicine and Health Sciences, PO Box # 17666, United Arab Emirates University, Al Ain 17666, UAE; nagoormeeran1985@uaeu.ac.ae
3 Department of Pharmacology, SVKM's Institute of Pharmacy, Dhule, Maharashtra 424 001, India; goyal.aiims@gmail.com
4 Department of Pharmacology, R. C. Patel Institute of Pharmaceutical Education and Research, Shirpur, Dhule, Maharashtra 425 405, India; pchandragouda@yahoo.com
* Correspondence: shreeshojha@uaeu.ac.ae; Tel.: +971-3-7137524

Received: 14 July 2018; Accepted: 15 September 2018; Published: 28 November 2018

Abstract: Acetaminophen (APAP), which is also known as paracetamol or *N*-acetyl-*p*-aminophenol is a safe and potent drug for fever, pain and inflammation when used at its normal therapeutic doses. It is available as over-the-counter drug and used by all the age groups. The overdose results in acute liver failure that often requires liver transplantation. Current clinical therapy for APAP-induced liver toxicity is the administration of *N*-acetyl-cysteine (NAC), a sulphydryl compound an approved drug which acts by replenishing cellular glutathione (GSH) stores in the liver. Over the past five decades, several studies indicate that the safety and efficacy of herbal extracts or plant derived compounds that are used either as monotherapy or as an adjunct therapy along with conventional medicines for hepatotoxicity have shown favorable responses. Phytochemicals mitigate necrotic cell death and protect against APAP-induced liver toxicityby restoring cellular antioxidant defense system, limiting oxidative stress and subsequently protecting mitochondrial dysfunction and inflammation. Recent experimental evidences indicat that these phytochemicals also regulate differential gene expression to modulate various cellular pathways that are implicated in cellular protection. Therefore, in this review, we highlight the role of the phytochemicals, which are shown to be efficacious in clinically relevant APAP-induced hepatotoxicity experimental models. In this review, we have made comprehensive attempt to delineate the molecular mechanism and the cellular targets that are modulated by the phytochemicals to mediate the cytoprotective effect against APAP-induced hepatotoxicity. In this review, we have also defined the challenges and scope of phytochemicals to be developed as drugs to target APAP-induced hepatotoxicity.

Keywords: APAP; acetaminophen; hepatotoxicity; hpatoprotection; paracetamol; animals; preclinical studies; natural products; small molecules; phytochemicals; plants

---

1. Introduction

Acetaminophen (APAP), which is also known as paracetamol or *N*-acetyl-*p*-aminophenol appears as a safe and potent drug for fever, pain and inflammation at its normal therapeutic doses. It is indicated for all age groups and is often available as over-the-counter medicine. However, the overdoses of APAP whether intentional or unintentional may cause dose-dependent acute liver failure, a potentially fatal liver necrosis that has limited treatment options except liver transplantation [1]. APAP is metabolized by sulfation and glucuronidation in liver with less than 5–10% being metabolized by the hepatic cytochrome P450 (CYP450) system. Simultaneously, glutathione redox system also plays an important role for inactivating the formed metabolite by glutathione conjugation that leads to the consumption of GSH in the liver. The rapid conversion of APAP in to the reactive metabolite *N*-acetyl-*p*-benzoquinone imine (NAPQI) by CYP450 enzymes, mainly CYP2E1 results in the generation of free radicals and which binds covalently with the cellular nucleophiles such as DNA, RNA and proteins that leads cell death [2,3]. Although, NAPQI is detoxified by GSH which results in depletion of the cellular GSH stores and formation of protein adducts. Oxidative stress in the mitochondria further leads to the activation of the enzymes of signaling cascade such as redox-sensitive MAP kinases and the phosphorylation of c-jun-*N*-terminal kinase (JNK) [4–9]. This mitochondrial oxidative and nitrosative stress initiates the overt activation of mitochondrial permeability transition (MPT) and it causes interruption and destabilizes the membrane potential which leads mitochondrial swelling and rupture of the membranes [10,11]. Following the rupture of the membrane, there is a massive release of apoptosis-inducing factor (AIF), endonuclease G and caspases activators into the cytoplasm and concomitant tranlocation into the nucleus to initiate nuclear DNA fragmentation [5,12]. Together, mitochondrial impairment along with DNA fragmentation are the prime cause of hepatocyte necrosis observed in APAP-induced liver toxicity [13].

Biochemically, CYP450, the heme-containing monoxygenases that are predominantly present in liver is believed to play a regulatory and catalytic activity in the metbolism of APAP and represent an important therapeutic target for metabolic modulation [14]. Among the various isoforms of CYP450 (CYP1A1, CYP1A2, CYP1B1, CYP2A6, CYP2E1 and CYP3A), CYP2E1 is the major mediator of APAP-induced bioactivation [15]. It appears critical to NAPQI formation and have shown to contribute to 30–78% of APAP metabolism [16]. Furthermore, CYP2E1 mediates NADPH oxidase activity resulting in the generation of free radicals that leads to hepatic injury. Therefore, inhibiting CYP2E1 activity can affect APAP metabolism and represent a plausible pharmacological mechanism for therapeutic interventions for APAP-induced liver injury [17–19].

Excessive metabolites formation depletes GSH from liver, therefore the treatment of APAP toxicity is based on replenishing GSH stores in the liver by the use of glutathione precursor; *N*-acetylcysteine (NAC), a sulphydryl compound [20]. NAC is the only drug approved and available as an antidote for APAP-induced hepatotoxicity, that seems to be effective only when it is administered either orally or intravenously within 10h of APAP overdose [21]. Therefore, it is reasonable to conceive that the inhibitors of glutathione synthesis will exacerbate APAP-induced hepatotoxicity and the precursor of GSH formation will be hepatoprotective against APAP. The graphical representation relevant to the hepatic injury that is caused by APAP metabolism as well as the efficaciousness of the phytochemicals or plant extracts/formulations is depicted in Figure 1.

Over the past five decades, the safety and efficacy of several herbal extracts and plant derived compounds either as monotherapy or as an adjunct to conventional medicines for APAP-induced hepatotoxicity appears to be favorable due to their ability to limit APAP-induced hepatotoxicity. Since the recognition of APAP associated liver toxicity in 1960s, experimental models including both in vivo (animal models) and in vitro (cell lines) have been employed for screening hepatoprotective properties [22,23] either of synthetic origin or plant derived natural extracts. Many experimental studies carried out using natural products have shown heptoprotective properties in clinically relevant APAP-induced liver toxicity model [24]. Therefore, this review renders an account of all the plant derived natural compounds, namely, phytochemicals that have been shown efficacious in APAP-induced hepatotoxicity.

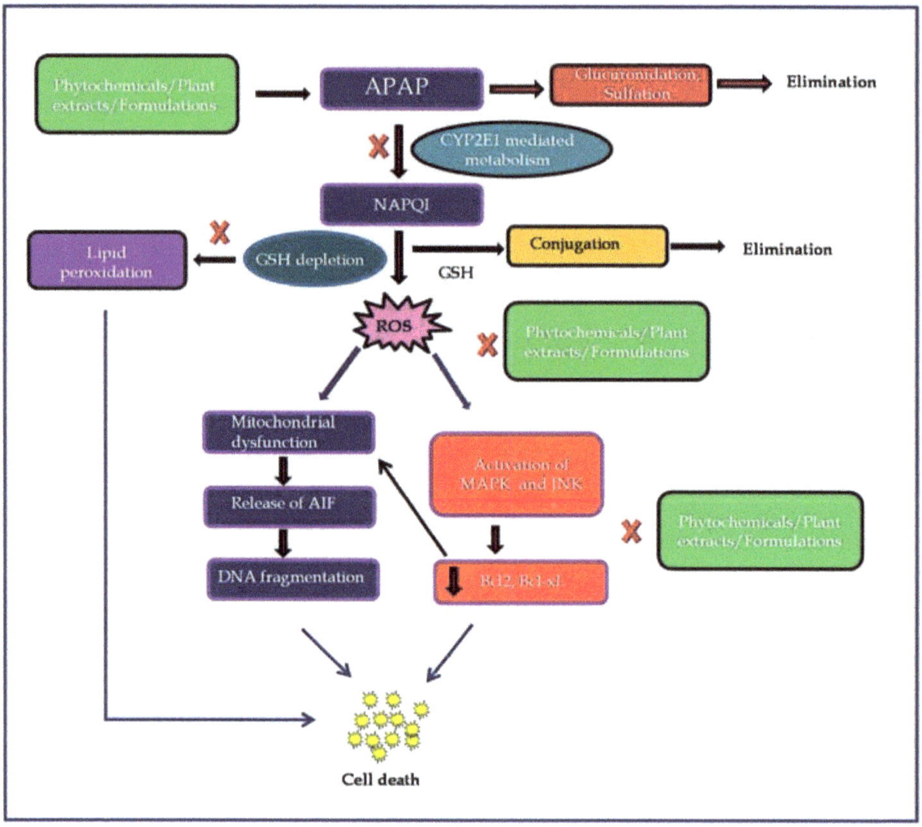

Figure 1. Schematic representation of phytochemical attenuate acetaminophen-induced liver toxicity.

This review summarized the current literature and comprehensively discussed the hepatoprotective properties of all the phytochemicals that were investigated in APAP-induced hepatotoxicity. This review also assessed the challenges and scope of the phytochemicals that can be developed as potential new hepatoprotective drugs for APAP-induced hepatotoxicity. The details of each phytochemical showed hepatoprotective are represented in the individual paragraphs. The dose of the phytochemicals investigated, the regimen of APAP used to induce liver toxicity in the in vivo or in vitro models and the parameters assessed are presented in the synoptic Tables 1–3 respectively. The electronic databases including Pub Med, Scopus, Google, and Google scholar were searched with the keywords "hepatoprotective", "hepatotoxicity", "liver toxicity" or "liver injury" with "plant", "extract", "herb", or "phytochemical", "natural product", "small molecules" with "acetaminophen", and "paracetamol". Table 4 in this review enlists all of the plants extract that showed hepatoprotective in experimental models of APAP-induced liver toxicity. The name of the medicinal plants has been arranged following the data retrieved from PubMed/Medline, Google Scholar, Science direct, and Scopus. We did not elaborate the detailed investigations performed with all these plant extracts herein as we focus mainly on phytochemicals which could be stepping stone for the drug discovery. Nearly all of the plant extracts have been reported hepatoprotective based on the biochemical and histopathological assessments of liver injury and protection. Briefly, these natural drugs appear hepatoprotective by restoring the antioxidant defense, preventing the occurrence of oxidative stress and subsequently curbing mitochondrial dysfunction and inflammation, as well as limiting the resultant necrotic cell death [25,26]. The phytochemicals that are enumerated in this review have shown to attenuate liver injury either in the in vitro; cell-based assays (microsomes or cell lines) or in vivo; in rats and mice models of liver toxicity in preclinical studies. In next paragraphs, each phytochemical has been discussed emphasizing their source, chemical name and their effect as well as underlying mechanism in countering APAP-induced liver toxicity.

1.1. Acanthoic Acid

Acanthoic acid, which is a pimarane-type diterpene, chemically known as [(1R,4aR,7S)-7-ethenyl-1,4a,7-trimethyl-3,4,6,8,8a,9,10,10a-octahydro-2H-phenanthrene-1-carboxylic-acid] or (−)-primara-9(11),15-dien-19-oic acid is obtained from the bark of *Acanthopanax koreanum* Nakai roots and *Croton oblongifolius* stems. Wu et al. (2010) have shown that pretreatment with acanthoic acid restored liver enzymes, improved antioxidants and inhibited lipid peroxidation in addition to histological salvage [27]. Further, it inhibited apoptosis, as shown by amelioration of hypoxia inducible factor-1α (HIF-1α) and caspase-3 in liver tissues [28].

1.2. Ajoene

Ajoene, an allylsulfur compound, chemically known as [(E)-1-(prop-2-enyldisulfanyl)-3-prop-2-enylsulfinylprop-1-ene)], is isolated from processed garlic in an *E*/*Z*-mixture [29]. Ajoene dose dependently inhibited depletion of thiol content and GSH from liver and restored the liver enzymes in mice model of APAP-induced hepatotoxicity [30].

1.3. Alpha Hederin

α-Hederin, an oleanane-type saponin is present in many plants including *Nigella sativa* and *Hedera helix*, is reputed for its benefits in respiratory diseases. α-Hederin was found to attenuate hepatotoxicity in mice induced by several liver toxicants including APAP, by dose dependently suppressing CYP450, CYPB5, CYP1A, CYP2A and CYP3A enzymes as well as NADPH-cytchrome-C-reductase activity in liver microsomes. α-Hederin also reduced activities of 7-ethoxyresorufin-*O*-dealkylation, 7-pentoxyresorufin-*O*-dealkylation, coumarin-7-hydroxylation, 7-ethoxycoumarin-*O*-deethylation, caffeine-N3-demethylation, chlorzoxazone-6-hydroxylation and the oxidation of testosterone to 2α-,6α-,15α-,15β-,16α-,16β-, and 18/12 α-hydroxyltestosterone, androstenedione, and 6-dehydroxytestosterone [31].

1.4. Amyrin

Amyrin, a triterpene exists as anisomeric mixture of α and β-amyrin in the resin exudate of *Protium heptaphyllum*. Amyrin isomers showed to ameliorate liver toxicity by the restoration of liver enzymes and GSH levels in the liver, along with histopathological salvage and reduced mortality. The effects were found to be comparable to NAC [32].

1.5. Andrographolide

Andrographolide, which is a diterpene lactone chemically known as (3E,4S)-3-[2-[(1R,4aS,5R,6R,8aS)-6-hydroxy-5-(hydroxymethyl)-5,8a-dimethyl-2-methylidene-3,4,4a,6,7,8-hexahydro-1H-naphthalen-1-yl]ethylidene]-4-hydroxyoxolan-2-one is isolated from *Andrographis paniculata*, a reputed natural remedy in traditional Chinese and Indian medicine. Handa and Sharma (1990) have reported its hepatoprotective activity against APAP and galactosamine-induced hepatotoxicity for the first time in rats [33]. Visen et al. (1993) further showed the protective effects in rat hepatocytes and found to be more efficacious than silymarin [34]. Roy et al. (2013) had developed nanoparticles of andrographolide incorporated in PLGA along with heparin. These nanoparticles found to be more bioavailable inliver tissues and protected mouse liver against APAP by rapid restoration of antioxidants and GSH content [35].

1.6. Anthocyanins

Anthocyanins belong to a group of natural pigments that were isolated from the dried calyx of *Hibiscus sabdariffa* L. was found protective against APAP-induced hepatotoxicity in rats by improving liver enzymes but failed to improve the liver histology [36]. The anthocyanin isolated from purple-fleshed sweet potato was also reported to attenuate hepatotoxicity in mice. It restored liver enzymes, improved antioxidant enzymes, inhibited lipid peroxidation and diminished the depletion of GSH from liver. The improved histology and dose-dependent reduction of CYP2E1, as well as CYP2E1-dependent aniline hydroxylation further showed the hepatoprotective effect. It also showed free radical scavenging activity and antioxidant action against ferric chloride and ascorbate-induced lipid peroxidation in mouse liver [37]. In another study, anthocyanin fraction exhibited antioxidant and free radical scavenging activity and improved histology, along with favourable modulation of numerous signaling pathways in hepatoprotection [38].

1.7. Apigenin

Apigenin, which is a flavone chemically known as 4′,5,7-trihydroxyflavone is abundantly found in numerous edible plants, such as parsley, oranges, grapefruit, celery, onions, thyme, lemon balm, chamomile, and wheat sprouts. It is reputed for its organoprotective properties and also found hepatoprotective in mice model of APAP-induced toxicity by salvaging liver tissues, restoring antioxidants, liver enzymes and GSH content along with the inhibition of lipid peroxidation [39].

1.8. Arjunolic Acid

Arjunolic acid, which is a triterpene chemically known as 2,3,23-Trihydroxyolean-12-en-28-oic acid is obtained from the bark of *Terminalia arjuna* and is present in the plants of the Combretaceae family. Arjunolic acid reported hepatoprotective in chemical induced hepatotoxicity and hepatocarcinogenesis models [40]. Ghosh et al. (2010) have reported that it prevented GSH depletion from liver and APAP metabolite formation by inhibiting the specific forms of CYP450 that aid in the metabolic activation of APAP to *N*-acetyl-*p*-benzoquinone-imine [41]. Further, it prevented the dissipation of mitochondrial membrane potential, release of cytochrome-C along with decreased activation of JNK and mitochondrial permeabilization as well as downstream Bcl-2 and Bcl-xL phosphorylation.

1.9. Berberine

Berberine, which is an alkaloid chemically known as 5,6-dihydro-9,10-dimethoxybenzo(g)-1,3-benzodioxolo(5,6-a) quinolizinium sulfate is obtained from several dietary plants, including *Berberis aristata* and it is widely studied for its pharmacological properties, including hepatoprotective. For the first time, Janbaz and Gilani (2009) showed its hepatoprotective effects against APAP-induced hepatotoxicity [42]. It also increased pentobarbital-induced sleeping time and strychnine-induced toxicity that indicated its inhibitory effect on microsomal drug metabolizing enzymes, CYPs [42]. Recently, Vivoli et al. (2016) have demonstrated its effect in various experimental models like APAP-induced liver toxicity, methionine, and choline deficient diet induced steatohepatitis and in cultured murine macrophages [43]. Berberine also reduced mortality, restored liver enzymes, and inhibited the inflammasomes components, the major mediator of inflammation which requires activation of the cytokines IL-1β and IL-18 that are generated upon caspase-1 activation. The activation of inflammasomes in APAP-induced hepatotoxicity seems to be a major mediator in hepatocyte injury, immune cell activation and amplification of inflammation and cell death. Thus, inhibiting activation of $P2X_7$, the purinergic receptors that mediates inflammasome activation by berberine appears a novel approach [43].

1.10. Bixin

Bixin, a group of carotenoids extracted from the seeds of *Bixa orellana* (Annatto) is a FDA approved popular food additive and colorant in cosmetics. It showed potent antioxidant and anti-inflammatory properties and protection against DNA damage and lipid peroxidation in liver. Rao et al. (2014) showed that solid lipid nanoparticle formulation of bixin exhibit sustained release following the first order diffusion kinetics and non-Fickian type of release mechanism. The in vivo studies revealed that the hepatoprotective property followed by the localization of bixin nanoparticals in liver tissues of rats [44].

1.11. Boswellic Acid

Boswellic acid, which is a mixture of triterpenic acids is chemically known as [(3R,4R,4aR,6aR, 6bS,8aR,11R,12S,12aR,14aR,14bR)-3-hydroxy-4,6a,6b,8a,11,12,14b-heptamethyl-2,3,4a,5,6,7,8,9,10,11,12, 12a,14,14a-tetradecahydro-1H-picene-4-carboxylic acid)]. It is principal constituent in the oleo gum resin of *Boswellia* species such as *B carteri, B serrata* and *B sacra*. Boswellic acid was found bioavailable in liver tissues following the oral ingestion. It protected against APAP-induced hepatotoxicity in mice by improving glutathione redox, inhibiting oxidative stress and attenuating pro-inflammatory cytokines and chemokines along with histopathologic salvage. It produced restoration of glutathione reductase (GR) and heme oxygenase-1 (HO-1) activities and inhibited CYP2E1 concomitant with reduced expression of toll-like receptors; TLR-3 and -4, MyD88, NF-κBp50, NF-κB p65 and JNK in liver tissues [45].

1.12. Brusatol

Brusatol, which is a natural quassinoid terpenoid, chemically known as methyl 13,20-epoxy-3, 11,12-trihydroxy-15-((3-methyl-1-oxo-2-butenyl) oxy)-2,16-dioxopicras has been isolated from the fruit of *Brucea javanica*. Recently, Olayanju et al. (2015) found that brusatol treatment attenuated nuclear factor-like 2 (Nrf2) signaling following post-transcriptional mechanism in mouse hepatoma Hepa-1c1c7 cells [46]. Italso sensitized these cells to the chemical insult induced by the hepatotoxic metabolites of APAP including 2,4-dinitrochlorobenzene, iodoacetamide and *N*-acetyl-*p*-benzoquinone imine. The inhibitory effects were found to be independent of its repressor kelch-like ECH-associated protein-1 (Keap1), the proteasomal and autophagic protein degradation system and protein kinase signaling pathways that reveal the novel roles of Nrf2 regulation.

1.13. Caffeic Acid

Caffeic acid, which is a polyphenolic compound chemically known as trans-3,4-dihydroxycinnamic acid is abundantly found in edible plants including many fruits, coffee, and honey. For the first time, caffeic acid was showed to attenuate liver toxicity by restoring liver enzymes in rats [47]. In another study, caffeic acid showed to attenuate APAP-induced liver injury by restoring GSH and liver enzymes as well as reducing myeloperoxidase (MPO) activity, ROS levels and histopathologic salvage. It was also improved cell viability and suppressed ROS formation in L-02 cells from normal human liver and HepG2 cells. Further, it enhanced expression of endogenous antioxidants such as Nrf2, HO-1 and NAD(P)H:quinone oxidoreductase 1 (NQO1) and reduced expression of Keap1 there by prevented the binding of Keap1 to Nrf2 and thus activating Nrf2 in hepatocytes. The in silico data showed the interaction of Nrf2 binding site in the Keap1 protein and the in vitro study showed minimal effect on the enzymatic activity of CYP3A4 and CYP2E1 [48]. In another in vitro and in vivo study, authors showed the hepatoprotective mechanism of caffeic acid by down-regulating mRNA expression and transcriptional activation of early growth response-1. Caffeic acid also reduced the expression of growth arrest and DNA-damage-inducible protein (Gadd45) α and inhibited activation of extracellular-regulated protein kinase (ERK1/2) signaling cascade. Altogether, the studies reveal the inhibitory effect of caffeic acid on ERK1/2-mediated Egr1 transcriptional activation that is attributed to the detoxification of APAP-induced liver injury [49].

1.14. Calamusins

Calamusins compounds are isolated from the ethanol extract of rhizomes of *Acorus calamus*. Calmusins A to H are the sesquiterpenes, while calamusin-I is a norsesquiterpene. Calamusin C, D, F and I (10 μM) have been reported to exert hepatoprotective activity against APAP-induced toxicity in HepG2 cells [50].

1.15. Carnosic Acid

Carnosic acid, which is a phenolic diterpene chemically known as (4aR,10aS)-5,6-dihydroxy-1,1-dimethyl-7-propan-2-yl-2,3,4,9,10,10a-hexahydrophenanthrene-4a-carboxylic acid) is isolated from the leaves of *Rrosmarinus officinalis* (Rosemary) and Sage. Guo et al. (2016) have shown that carnosic acid exert hepatoprotective effects by restoring liver enzymes and reducing liver necrosis [51]. Further, it was found to inhibit lipid peroxidation, pro-inflammatory cytokines and chemokines and phosphorylated IκBα and p65 proteins in the liver and suppressed cleaved caspase-3, Bax and phosphorylated JNK protein expression. It also facilitated Nrf2 translocation into nucleus through blocking interaction between Nrf2 and Keap1 that resulted in the up-regulation of antioxidant genes. However, in another study, Dickmann et al. (2012) showed that carnosic acid did not exhibit significant time dependent inhibition for any of the cytochrome P450 enzymes in primary human hepatocytes and human liver microsomes [52]. It dose dependently induced CYP2B6 and CYP3A4 and inhibited CYP2C9 and CYP3A4 enzymes catalyzed reactions. The increase in the activities of CYP2B6 and CYP3A enzymes were found to be comparable to phenobarbital and rifampicin, respectively. Though, the safety needs to be confirmed further.

1.16. Chlorogenic Acid

Chlorogenic acid, the esters of caffeic and quinic acid are abundantly found in numerous plants and consumed through diet or beverages. Zheng et al. (2015) showed its hepatoprotective effect by the inhibition of pro-inflammatory cytokines, MPO expression and activity, restoration of liver enzymes and salvage of liver tissues along with diminution of raised expression of TLR-3, TLR-4 and MyD88 and the increased phosphorylation of inhibitor of kappa B (IκB) and p65 subunit of NF-κB in liver [53]. Further, it also improved cell viability in L-02 cells and showed the inhibition of activities of CYP2E1 and CYP1A2 in addition to improved antioxidant signals against APAP-induced cytotoxicity [54].

1.17. Chrysin

Chrysin, which is a flavone chemically known as 5,7-dihydroxy-2-phenylchromen-4-one is abundantly found in many plants, including fruits, vegetables and mushrooms. Chrysin was found an inhibitor of sulfo-conjugation of APAP by human liver cytosol with IC_{50} values < 1 μM. The inhibitory actions were attributed to the presence of 7-hydroxyl group in structure [55]. In another study, Morimitsu et al. (2004) have shown that chrysin elicit inhibitory effects on sulfo- and glucurono conjugation of APAP in rat cultured hepatocytes and liver subcellular preparations [56]. Recently, chrysin was reported as modulator of intestinal *P*-glycoprotein (*P*-gp) and drug-metabolizing enzymes that plays an important role in the first-pass-metabolism and pharmacokinetics of APAP in the in vitro non-everted gut sacs preparation and rats [57]. It was observed that chrysin increases the systemic exposure of APAP which needs to be studied in detail for clear conclusive remarks.

1.18. Corynoline, Acetylcorynoline and Protopine

Corynoline, acetylcorynoline or protopine were found to ameliorate liver injury in mice and liver microsomes with a pronounced efficacy of acetylcorynoline than corynoline and protopine.

These compounds also showed biphasic response (inhibition followed by induction) on P450 in mice liver [58]. In another study, protopine was found to attenuate APAP-induced hepatotoxicity and suppress microsomal enzymes in rats. Protopine restored the liver enzymes mediating the inhibition of microsomal drug metabolizing enzymes [59].

1.19. Curcumin

Curcumin, a yellow polyphenol pigment chemically known as (1E,6E)-1,7-bis(4-hydroxy-3-methoxyphenyl) hepta-1,6-diene-3,5-dione is the main bioactive constituent in the rhizomes of *Curcuma longa*, popularly known as turmeric and reputed for its use in dietary, culinary, and cosmetic purposes. Several in vitro and in vivo studies have demonstrated that the protective effects of curcumin against liver injury mediating attenuation of oxidative stress, inflammation, and cell death. The cytoprotective effect against APAP was demonstrated in rat hepatocytes by attenuating lipid peroxidation, but no effect was found on depletion of lactae dehydrogenase (LDH) and GSH and in time dependent action at low concentrations. However, higher doses have shown the protective effects [60]. The effects were confirmed in vivo in rats, wherein it dose-dependently attenuated liver and renal toxicity by improving antioxidants, restoring liver enzymes and salvage histology. It potentiated the protective effects of NAC and also reduced the therapeutic dose of NAC [61,62]. In another study, curcumin provided protection against genomic instability, cell death, and oxidative stress in the liver. It was found to restore liver enzymes, inhibit lipid peroxidation, modulate APAP-induced alterations in genes expression of antioxidant and inflammatory cytokines, matrix metalloproteinase, DNA fragmentation and apoptosis [63]. The hepatoprotective effects were further reconfirmed in mice models [64–66].

1.20. Diallyl Sulfide

Diallyl sulfide, which is chemically known as 3-prop-2-enylsulfanylprop-1-ene is isolated from garlic known to impart flavor to garlic. It has been demonstrated to protect against APAP-induced liver toxicity as evidenced by restoration of liver enzymes and reduction in mortality in a time- and dose-dependent manner. In liver microsomes, it showed the hepatoprotective effect by the inhibition of APAP metabolism [67]. In another study, diallyl sulfone, a metabolite of diallyl sulfide was shown to protect against APAP-induced liver toxicity in mice by improving histopathology, liver enzymes and restoration of hepatic GSH levels. It also suppressed oxidative APAP metabolites in the plasma with no effect on non-oxidative metabolites of APAP. It repressed the rate of APAP oxidation to *N*-acetyl-*p*-benzoquinone imine, a glutathione conjugate by inhibiting CYP2E1 activity in liver microsomes [18]. Further, the organosulfur compounds of garlic were reported to protect against hepatotoxicity by inhibiting P450-mediated APAP bioactivation. The presence of *S*-allyl pharmacophore seems to confer the CYP2E1 inhibitory property to the sulfide compounds of garlic [68]. Diallyl sulfide gets converted into diallyl sulfoxide and diallyl sulfone by CYP2E1 and all of these are competitive inhibitors of CYP2E1. They also believed to induce other CYPs and phase II enzymes as well as augments enzymatic and non-enzymatic hepatic antioxidants [69].

1.21. Dioscin

Dioscin, a steroid saponin chemically known as 3-*O*-[α-L-Rha-(1->4)-[α-L-Rha-(1->2)]-β-D-Glc]-diosgenin is abundantly found in dietary plants *Dioscorea pseudojaponica*. Zhao et al. (2012) reported that dioscin in HepG2 cells attenuates mitochondrial impairment and cell death and improves cell viability [70]. The in vivo study showed similar effects and proteomic analysis revealed that *Suox*, *Krt18*, *Rgn*, *Prdx1*, *MDH* and *PNP* proteins were involved in the hepatoprotection. Additionally, it decreased expression of ATP2A2 and mitochondrial cardiolipin and regulated Ca^{2+} levels in mitochondria by attenuating and CYP2E1 activation. Further, it also modulated apoptotic proteins Bcl-2, Bid, Bax, Bak and p53 and activated aryl hydrocarbon receptor (AhR).

1.22. Diosmin

Diosmin, a flavanoid chemically known as 3′,5,7-Trihydroxy-4′-methoxyflavone 7-rutinoside is abundantly found in citrus fruits and available clinically for the management of venous insufficiency. Diosmin was found to attenuate APAP-induced liver toxicity by inhibiting GSH depletion from liver and improving the enzymes activating glutathion-*s*-transferases permitting the captation of the reactive metabolites of the APAP and other liver toxicants [71].

1.23. (−)-Epigallocatechin-3-gallate

(−)-Epigallocatechin-3-gallate, a polyphenolic compound is one of the most abundant catechin in tea with numerous pharmacological properties and therapeutic benefits. EGCG was found to curb metabolism and toxicity of APAP in rats by restoring liver enzymes, suppressing the activities of hepatic CYP3A, CYP2E1, uridine diphosphate glucuronosyltransferase and sulfotransferase. It also reduced APAP-glucuronate and -glutathione contents in plasma and liver [72].

1.24. Esculetin

Esculetin, which is a coumarin class of polyphenolic compound is chemically known as 6,7-dihydroxycoumarin and abundantly found in many medicinal plants, including *Artemisia capillaries, Artemisia scoparia, Citrus limonia, Ceratostigma willmottianum, Cichorium intybus* and *Bougainvllra spectabillis*. Gilani et al. (1998) have reported that esculetin restored the liver enzymes and reduce mortality in mice [73]. The inhibition of lipoxygenase pathway is believed to account for hepatoprotective action of esculetin.

1.25. Ferulic Acid

Ferulic acid, which is a polyphenolic compound with structural resemblance to curcumin is abundantly found in leaves and seeds of many vegetables, fruits and cereals such as brown rice, whole wheat, and oats. Wand and Penf (1994) for the first time demonstrated the hepatoprotective activity of sodium ferulate, an active ingredient of *Angelica sinensis* Diels [74]. Sodium ferulate restored the liver enzymes and improved glutathione redox cycles and antioxidants, along with inhibition of lipid peroxidation in mice. Recently, ferulic acid dose-dependently restored liver enzymes, improved antioxidants, inhibited pro-inflammatory cytokines, *TLR4* expression and p38 mitogen-activated (MAPK), and activation of *NF-κB* in mice. The hepatoprotective effects involve inhibition of TLR4-mediated inflammatory responses and the expression of CYP2E1 [75].

1.26. Fulvotomentosides

Fulvotomentosides are the total saponins that were obtained from the flower extracts of *Lonicera fulvotomentosa*. Fulvotomentosides were found to ameliorate APAP-induced hepatotoxicity in mice by restoration of liver enzymes and reduced hepatic CYP450, CYPB5, and NADPH-cytochrome-C reductase. They exhibited reduced APAP-glutathione level, increased hepatic glucuronyltransferase activity and increased urinary elimination of APAP-glucuronide, with no effect on liver UDP-glucuronic acid in mice microsomes. This indicated that detoxification involves CYP450 and glucuronidation of APAP [76]. In another study, fulvomentosides showed similar hepatoprotective effects against hepatotoxicity induced by APAP [77]. Another derivative of fulvotomentoside known as sapindoside B ameliorated APAP-induced hepatotoxicity in mice by salvaging liver tissues and preventing GSH depletion and restoring liver enzymes along with reduction in mortality. It also promoted urinary excretion of APAP that is attributed to the suppression of hepatic CYP450 [78].

1.27. Galangin

Galangin, a flavonoid that is chemically known as 3,5,7-trihydroxyflavone is widely found in many plants including *Alpinia officinarum* and *Helichrysum aureonitens*. Galangin showed hepatoprotective effect in mice against propacetamol, a water soluble derivative of APAP. Galangin attenuated oxidative stress, increased GSH levels and inhibited microsomal CYP2E1 levels in the liver and found more potent than silymarin and NAC. However, galangin did not reduce mortality significantly [79].

1.28. Gallic Acid

Gallic acidand its derivatives are polyphenolic compounds that were widely distributed in different parts of plants and fruits, thus being often consumed directly or indirectly by humans as food stuffs and preservatives etc. Rasool et al. (2010) reported its hepatoprotective effects against hepatotoxicity in mice by restoring liver enzymes, inhibiting lipid peroxidation and pro-inflammatory cytokines and enhancing antioxidant defense by improving glutathione redox cycle [80].

1.29. Genistein

Genistein, a phytoestrogen and isoflavone that is chemically known as 4′,5,7-trihydroxyisoflavone is abundantly found in numerous edible plants including soybeans and mainly varieties of pulses. Genistein was found bioavailable in liver and amelioratedlipid peroxidation and restored liver enzymes by modulating APAP biotransformation. It also accelerated and promoted APAP glucuronidation by activating UGTs and glutathione peroxidase and inhibiting CYP2E1 [81]. Genistein get metabolized by CYP1A2 and CYP2E1 and CYP1A2 was predominantly responsible for 3′-OH-genistein formation; primary metabolite of genistein since its formation was inhibited [82]. Genistein was showed to reduce the formation of sulphate derivative of APAP and its raised excretion into bile arises from the inhibition of sinusoidal efflux transport [83]. Recently, genistein showed to inhibit APAP-induced cytotoxicity in fetal hepatocyte cell line (L-02), HepG2 and Hep3b cells, as evidenced by improved antioxidants, cell viability, hepatic enzymes and GSH redox in a dose-dependent manner. It also enhanced the metabolic transformation of APAP to glucuronic acid inL-02, HepG2, and Hep3b cells via the Nrf2/Keap1 pathway [84].

1.30. Geranylgeranylacetone

Geranylgeranylacetone, which is an acyclic polyisoprenoid chemically known as 6,10,14,18-tetramethyl-5,9,13,17-nonadecatetraen-2-one is reputed as an anti-ulcer agent with minimal adverse effects. It has been shown to ameliorate liver necrosis by inhibiting lipid peroxidation and myeloperoxidase activity as well as restoring liver enzymes. However, it did not suppress hepatic CYP2E1 activity nor prevent depletion of GSH contents from liver [85].

1.31. Gingerol

6-Gingerol, which is chemically known as (5S)-5-hydroxy-1-(4-hydroxy-3-methoxyphenyl) decan-3-one is one of the major bioactive component of a widely used plant; *Zingiber officinalis*. It was reported to restore the liver enzymes, correct total bilirubin, inhibits lipid peroxidation and normalizes antioxidant status in liver in mice model of hepatotoxicity and found to be comparable to the standard drug, silymarin [86].

1.32. Ginkgolide

Ginkgolide A, a terpenic lactone that is chemically known as 9H-1,7a-(Epoxymethano)-1H,6aH-cyclopenta(c)furo(2,3-b) is abundantly present in the leaves of *Ginkgo biloba* that is widely-used herbal dietary supplement for its effects on health promoting and therapeutic benefits. The extract contains bilobalide and Ginkgolide A which played different roles in the modulation of CYP2B1 and CYP3A23 gene expression and enzyme activities. Ginkgolide A showed its protective effects on APAP toxicity in hepatocytes isolated from adult male Long-Evans rats. Ginkgolide A was found to increase CYP3A23 mRNA levels and CYP3A mediated enzyme activity that in part account to the potentiating effect on APAP toxicity. Whereas, other derivatives, such as ginkgolide B, ginkgolide C, ginkgolide J, quercetin, kaempferol, isorhamnetin and isorhamnetin-3-O-rutinoside failed to affect LDH leakage that is caused by APAP [87].

1.33. Glycyrrhetinic Acid

Glycyrrhetinic acid isomers are pentacyclic triterpenoid isolated from the roots of licorice plant; *Glycyrrhiza glabra* and possess various pharmacological properties such as antioxidant, antitumor and anti-inflammatory activities. Liu et al. (1994) for the first time reported that glycyrrhizin, 18 α-glycyrrhetinic acid and 18 β-glycyrrhetinic acid treatment were found to protect mice against APAP and other liver toxicants. In addition to histopathological salvage, these compounds restored serum activities of liver enzymes and sorbitol dehydrogenase [31]. Glycyrrhizin was also found to affect glucuronidation in the liver by increasing the activities of *p*-nitrophenol UDP-glucuronosyltransferase (UGT), known as UGT1A, which is indicative of its detoxificating property of xenobiotics [88]. Lin et al. (1997) have reported that hepatoprotective effect of *Scutellaria rivularis* Benth fractions known as Ban-zhi-lian against APAP and other toxicant models of liver toxicity while using glycyrrhizin as standard reference medicine [89]. In an in vivo study using metabolomics, glycyrrhetinic acid showed to protect against APAP by histological salvage and restoration of liver enzymes [90].

1.34. Glycyrrhizin

Glycyrrhizin or glycyrrhizic acid, a pentacyclic triterpenoid glycoside, chemically known as 29-Hydroxy-11,29-dioxoolean-12-en-3-yl 2-O-hexopyranuronosylhexopyranosiduronic is one of the bioactive constituent in roots of *Glycyrrhiza glabra*, popularly known as licorice. It is one of the highly consumed herbs and is widely studied for its therapeutic benefits in experimental and human studies. For the first time, Liu et al. (1994) in a preliminary study reported its hepatoprotective activity against APAP [31]. It has been suggested to detoxify xenobiotics by activating glucuronidation via increasing UGT and intracellular concentrations of hepatic UDP-glucuronic acid in rat liver [88]. In another study, Wan et al. (2009) reported that glycyrrhizin in combination with matrin that is extracted from *Sophora flavescens* [91]. It reduced mortality in APAP-induced hepatotoxicity in mice through immunosuppressive properties and inhibiting inflammation that was further supported by improved liver function and histology.

1.35. Gomisin A

Gomisin A, which is a lignan compound chemically known as 5,6,7,8-tetrahydro-1,2,3,12-tetramethoxy-6,7-dimethyl-10,11-methylenedioxy-6-dibenzo(a,c)cyclooctenol is isolated from *Shizandra* fruits. GomisinA was found to restore the liver enzymes, inhibit lipid peroxidation and reduce the necrotic changes in liver, as examined in histological and biochemical analysis [92]. In addition, similar results were observed in another study wherein it reported to suppress lipid peroxidation and induce hepatocyte growth factor [93].

1.36. Guajavadimer A

Guajavadimer A, a dimeric monoterpenoid of sesquiterpene origin consisting of two caryophyllenes, a benzylphlorogulcinol and a flavonone-fused structure is isolated from the leaves of *Psidium guajava* L. Guajavadimer A in a preliminary study in HepG2 cells showed to attenuate APAP-induced liver toxicity [94].

1.37. Hesperidin

Hesperidin, a biflavonoid and flavanone glycoside consisting of the flavone hesperitin bound to the disaccharide rutinose, which is chemically known as 3′,5′-ihydroxy-4′-methoxy-7-rutinosyloxyflavan-4-on, is found in highly nutritious foods such as oranges, tangelos, tangerines, grapefruits, and other citrus fruits. Hesperidin showed hepatoprotective property in many experimental models, including APAP-induced hepatotoxicity [95]. It has been found to restore the levels of antioxidant enzymes and serum levels of liver enzymes and it prevents apoptotic death and inflammatory cytokines.

1.38. Homopterocarpin

Homopterocarpin, which is an isoflavonoid chemically known as (6aS,11aS)-3,9-dimethoxy-6a, 11a-dihydro-6H-[1]benzofuro[3,2-c]chromene is obtained from the ethanolic extract of stem bark of *Pterocarpus erinaceus* Poir. It was found to restore liver enzymes, inhibit lipid peroxidation and restore antioxidants in liver and corrected altered liver function [96].

1.39. Hyperoside

Hyperoside, which is a flavonol glycoside chemically known as (2-(3,4-dihydroxyphenyl)-5,7-dihydroxy-3-[(2S,3R,4S,5R,6R)-3,4,5-trihydroxy-6-(hydroxymethyl)oxan-2-yl]oxychromen-4-one) is obtained from *Hypericum perforatum*, *Crataegus oxycantha*, and *Apocynum venetum* L. Xie et al. (2016) showed that hyperoside dose dependently ameliorated lipid peroxidation, oxidative and nitrosative stress and increased activities and expression of uridine diphoshate glucuronosyltransferases and sulfotransferases [97]. It was also found to inhibit CYP2E1 activities that attrbute to the APAP detoxification.

1.40. Isoquercitrin

Isoquercitin or hirsutrin, a naturally occurring glycoside of quercetin is chemically known as (2-(3,4-dihydroxyphenyl)-5,7-dihydroxy-3-[(2S,3R,4S,5S,6R)-3,4,5-trihydroxy-6-(hydroxymethyl) oxan-2-yl]oxychromen-4-one). Xie et al. (2016) demonstrated the hepatoprotective effect of isoquercitrin, as evidenced by the amelioration of oxidative/nitrosative stress and inflammation by blocking the NF-κB and MAPK pathways [98]. It was also found to restore the liver enzymes and diminish centrilobular necrosis by regulating the activities of sulfotransferases and CYP2E1 that enhances hepatic detoxification of APAP. In a recent study, a microbiota-derived metabolite of quercetin; 3,4-dihydroxyphenylacetic acid has also been found to restore liver enzymes, attenuate lipid peroxidation, augment antioxidants and salvage the histology. It was found to promote Nrf2 translocation to the nucleus and enhance the expression of phase II enzymes and antioxidant enzymes that promotes APAP detoxification [99].

1.41. Isorhamnetin

Isorhamnetin, a polyphenolic metabolite of quercetin that is chemically known as quercetin-3-methyl-ether is isolated from the leaves of *Cistus laurifolius Linn.* In a preliminary study, it has been reported to restore liver enzymes, improve GSH content in liver and inhibit lipid peroxidation in plasma and liver in mice model of hepatotoxicity [100].

1.42. Kaempferol Derivatives

Kaempferol8-C-β-galactoside, a congener of kaempferol is isolated from extract of *Solanum elaeagnifolium*. It was shown to protect against APAP-hepatotoxicity by improving liver enzymes and salvaging liver tissues, comparable to silymarin [101]. Another kaempferol derivative known as kaempferol-3,7-dimethyl-ether is isolated from the extracts of leaves of *Cistus laurifolius* L. It was also found to improve cellular GSH levels, inhibit lipid peroxidation in plasma and liver and restore liver enzymes in mice model [100].

1.43. Lophirones

Lophirones are chalcone dimers that are isolated from stem bark of *Lophira alata* and reported to exhibit antioxidant, chemopreventive, antimutagenic, anticarcinogenic and hepatoprotective activity.

Recently, Ajiboye (2016) demonstrated the hepatoprotective effect of lophirone B and C in mice by restoration of liver enzymes, enzymatic and non-enzymatic antioxidants along with attenuation of oxidative stress, pro-inflammatory cytokines, lipid peroxidation and reduced formation of conjugated dienes, protein carbonyl, lipid hydroperoxides, and fragmented DNA [102].

1.44. Lupeol

Lupeol, a pentacyclic triterpenoid that is chemically known as (1R,3aR,5aR,5bR,7aR,9S,11aR, 11bR,13aR,13bR)-3a,5a,5b,8,8,11a-hexamethyl-1-prop-1-en-2-yl-1,2,3,4,5,6,7,7a,9,10,11,11b,12,13,13a, 13b-hexadecahydrocyclopenta[a]chrysen-9-ol) is abundantly found in several dietary plants such as Crataeva, Mango, andOlive etc. Kumari and Kakkar (2012) have demonstrated its hepatoprotective activity against APAP-induced hepatotoxicity in rat hepatocytes [102]. It inhibited lipid peroxidation, ROS generation, and mitochondrial depolarization and restored liver enzymes as well as antioxidants and has shown the improved viability of hepatocytes. It also inhibited DNA damage and cell death by preventing downregulation of Bcl-2, upregulation of Bax, release of cytochrome-C, and the activation of caspase 9/3. The protective effects were further confirmed in vivo based on the attenuation of oxidative stress and histological salvage [103].

1.45. Luteolin

Luteolin, a flavone that is chemically known as 2-(3,4-dihydroxyphenyl)-5,7-dihydroxychromen-4-one is predominantly found in many plants, fruits and flowers and are reputed for its health benefits including liver diseases. Luteolin was found to inhibit sulfation in isolated liver cytosolic and microsomal preparations [56]. Recently, Tai et al. (2015) showed its antioxidant and anti-inflammatory activities against APAP in mice [104]. Luteolin restored liver enzymes, augmented the endogenous antioxidant defense, and inhibited lipid peroxidation and endoplasmic reticulum stress and GSH depletion from liver. It also inhibited pro-inflammatory cytokines and inflammatory mediators including iNOS, TNF-α, NF-κB, and nitrotyrosine. The inhibition of conjugation depends on both C5 and 7 hydroxyl substitutions on the A-ring of the flavone structure. Another derivative, luteolin 7-*O*-β-galacturonyl-(2–>1)-*O*-β-galacturonide, a new digalacturonide flavone is isolated from extract of flowers of *Lantana camara*, elicited potent hepatoprotective activity against APAP. It exerted free radical scavenging and antioxidant activity and restored the liver enzymes, along with histological salvage of liver tissues [105]. Luteolin-7-glucoside that was also isolated from the plant, *Glossogyne tenuifolia* Cassini was found to elicit hepatoprotection against APAP in BALB/c mice mediating antioxidant activity [106].

1.46. Magnolol

Magnolol, a biphenolic compound which is chemically known as (2-(2-hydroxy-5-prop-2-enylphenyl)-4-prop-2-enylphenol), is isolated from the bark of *Magnolia officinalis* is widely used in traditional Chinese and Japanese medicines. It has been shown to inhibit CYP1A and 2C in rats with no effect on CYP3A and play a role in the metabolic balance of lipids through liver X receptor α. Chen et al. (2009) have demonstrated the hepatoprotective activity of magnolol on APAP-induced hepatotoxicity in the rats by improving antioxidants, liver enzymes and ameliorating of lipid peroxidation along with liver tissues salvage [107].

1.47. Meso-Zeaxanthin

Meso-zeaxanthin, a xanthophyll carotenoid, is not a constituent of a normal human diet but comprises one-third of the primate macular pigment rarely found in diet and is believed to be formed at the macula by metabolic transformations of ingested carotenoids. Meso-zeaxanthin along with lutein and zeaxanthin known as macular pigment is believed to protect against age-related macular degeneration and is reputed nutrient for eye health. Lutein and zeaxanthin are obtained from dietary sources such as green leafy vegetables and orange and yellow fruits and vegetables. It was found to augment antioxidants, normalize GSH levels and restore liver enzymes along with histologic salvage against APAP and other liver toxicants in rats [108].

1.48. Methoxypsoralen

5-Methoxypsoralen, a naturally occurring linear furocoumarin chemically known as 4-Methoxy-7H-furo[3,2-g]chromen-7-one is obtained from the essential oils of bergamot, and citrus fruits, including grapefruits. It has been reputed in therapeutics for its use in combination with ultraviolet A irradiation to manage psoriasis and vitiligo. It was found to ameliorate liver necrosis by reducing the infiltration of inflammatory cells and dose dependent inhibition of lipid peroxidation, restoration of liver enzymes, and normalization of glutathione ratio [109].

1.49. Methyl Sulfonylmethane

Methyl sulfonylmethane, a sulfur rich compound that is commonly present in many dietary plants consumed as grains, fruits, vegetables and beverages. Bohlooli et al. (2013) have reported that it prevented APAP-induced liver toxicity in rats due to its antioxidant and sulfur donating properties. It also prevented lipid peroxidation, MPO formation and GSH depletion from liver and restored liver enzymes along with improving antioxidants [110].

1.50. Morin

Morin, a flavonoid that is chemically known as (2-(2,4-dihydroxyphenyl)-3,5,7-trihydroxychromen-4-one), is isolated from many fruits including *Maclura pomifera* (Osage orange), *Maclura tinctoria* (old fustic), and from the leaves of *Psidium guajava* (guava). Morin treatment ameliorated liver necrosis by reducing release of HMGB1, NALP3 and caspase-1 along with histological salvage and restoration of liver enzymes [111]. It also strengthened cellular defense by the attenuation of oxidative stress induced deactivation of Akt (Ser473) causes suppression in GSK3β and Fyn kinase activation. It regulated PHLPP2 activity by suppressing Nrf2 ubiquitination and enhanced nuclear Nrf2 retention as well as ARE-Nrf2 binding affinity.

1.51. Naphthoflavone

β-naphthaflavone, a synthetic derivative of a naturally occurring flavonoid is a ligand of the aryl hydrocarbon receptor, which mediates the potent activation of CYP1A. It caused a potentiation of APAP toxicity and/or death of both obese and lean Zucker rats. APAP overdose produced reduction of hepatic cytochrome P450 enzyme-substrate activities in lean Zucker rats. However, obese Zucker rats are less affected by the hepatotoxic effects of APAP overdoses [112].

1.52. Naringenin

Naringenin, a flavonoid aglycone of naringin that is chemically known as 5,7-dihydroxy-2-(4-hydroxyphenyl) chroman-4-one is commonly found in citrus fruits. Recently, it was found hepatoprotective against APAP in metallothionein null mice. Naringenin inhibited lipid peroxidation, normalized gluathione redox and restored liver enzymes along with improved histopathology [113]. It did not inhibit DNA and protein synthesis [114]. However, it has been reported to cause a weak inhibition of APAP oxidation [115].

1.53. Oleanolic Acid

Oleanolic acid (OA), a pentacyclic triterpene chemically known as 3-β-3-Hydroxyolean-12-en-28-oic acidis abundantly found in medicinal plants used in traditional Chinese medicine. It has been found to exhibit potent anticancer, anti-osteoporosis, antiobesity, antidiabetic, antihyperlipidemic, anti-inflammatory, antioxidant, and immunoregulatory and hepatoprotective effects. Liu et al. (1993) for the first time demonstrated its hepatoprotective property against APAP in mice as evidenced by improved antioxidant defense and restoration of liver enzymes in liver [116]. It did not affect liver UDP-glucuronic acid concentration, but it increased hepatic glucuronosyl transferase activity toward APAP. Further, it was found to increase hepatic metallothionein levels in Cd/hemoglobin assay and appears protective against hepatotoxicants, such as D-galactosamine plus endotoxin, thioacetamide, furosemide, colchicine, carbon tetrachloride, APAP, cadmium and bromobenzene [31]. In another study, OA was showed to ameliorate hepatotoxicity induced by chemical toxicants, including APAP [77]. The authors showed that OA decreased mouse liver CYP1A and CYP2A enzymes with minimal effect on CYP3A enzymes. It also increased GSH content in liver without affecting GSH peroxidase and GSH reductases [117]. The hepatoprotective activities were further confirmed as OA prevented APAP-induced the overproduction of NO and decline in GSH levels in liver along with reduced mortality [118]. Mechanistically, OA enhanced the expression of metallothionein, *Nrf2*, NQO1, HO-1, and glutamate-cysteine ligases (Gclc and Gclm) in liver and induced genes that were involved in proliferation with the suppression of P450 genes against hepatotoxicants [119]. Reisman et al. (2009) reconfirmed that OA protect liver by Nrf2-dependent and Nrf2-independent mechanism following the nuclear accumulation of Nrf2 that leads to the induction of Nrf2-dependent genes and contributes in hepatoprotection [120]. Recently, 2-cyano-3,12 dioxooleana-1,9-diene-28-imidazolide (CDDO-Im) a more efficacious and potent triterpenoid derivative from OA was synthesized [121]. It has been shown as a potent antioxidant and anti-inflammatory agent by diminishing iNOS production and activating the Nrf2-Keap1 pathway.

1.54. Paenol

Paenol, chemically known as 2′-hydroxy-4′-methoxyacetophenone is isolated from the root bark of *Paeonia spp.* and popular as *Moutan cortex* root in traditional Chinese medicine. Paeonol treatment attenuated lipid peroxidation, liver necrosis, and restored the liver enzymes, as well as antioxidants in liver along with inhibition of APAP-induced phosphorylated JNK protein expression without affecting p38 and Erk1/2 [122]. Moreover, it also prevented against APAP-induced cytotoxicity in primary mouse hepatocytes evidenced by the attenuation of pro-inflammatory cytokines and ROS formation along with suppression of IKKα/β, IκBα, and p65 phosphorylation. All of these mechanisms were attributed to the hepatoprotective effect of paenol.

1.55. Panaxatriol

Panaxatriols are the saponin constituents mainly isolated from *Panax notoginseng* which is major source of ginsenosides consists of two groups based on the types of the panaxadiol group (e.g., ginsenoside-Rb1 and -Rc) and the panaxatriol group (e.g., ginsenoside-Rg1 and -Re). The ginsenosides are widely studied for their therapeutic potential mediating multiple pharmacological properties. It has been shown that the ginsenoside-Rg1 and -Re had no CYP3A inhibitory effect [123], thus it may be devoid of ginseng-drug interaction. Wang et al. (2014) reported that panaxatriol inhibited pro-inflammatory cytokines, restored the thioredoxin-1 expression, an important redox regulator that play an important role in countering oxidative stress and subsequent inflammation [124]. Panaxatriol also inhibited apoptosis by regulating pro-caspase-12 expression. Also, ginsenoside-Rg3 enhanced the GSH content and multidrug resistance-associated protein expression in NAPQI induced rat hepatocytes [125].

1.56. Procyanidins

Procyanidins are the polymeric flavan-3-ols isolated from skin of *Prunus amygdalus* popularly known as almond, a dietary nut that has shown to exhibit antioxidant, anti-inflammatory, antiatherosclerotic and anticancer properties. It has been shown to enhance the expression of *Nrf2* and antioxidant respons element (ARE) reporter gene activity in HepG2 cells and induce the expression of phase II enzymes includingNQO1, catalase, glutathione peroxidase, and superoxide dismutase.

In APAP-induced hepatotoxicity in mice, it attenuated hepatotoxicity through the activation of Nrf2/ARE-mediated phase II detoxifying/antioxidant enzymes [126].

1.57. Pterostilbene

Pterostilbene, a dimethylated resveratrol derivative that is chemically known as 4'-Hydroxy-3,5-dimethoxy-trans-stilbene, is mainly found in blueberries and are found to show potent pharmacological actions, including antioxidant, anti-inflammatory, and anti-apoptotic and therapeutic benefits in liver diseases. El-Sayed et al. (2015) have shown that pterostilbene exerted hepatoprotective effect against APAP-induced hepatotoxicity by restoring liver enzymes, inhibiting pro-inflammatory cytokines and lipid peroxidation and augmenting antioxidant activity along with the suppression of cell death [127]. Further, the hepatoprotective effects were affirmed by histopathological preservation and they were found to be comparable to silymarin.

1.58. Punicalagin and Punicalin

Punicalagin, an ellagitannin polyphenolic compound is abundantly found in fruit, husk and juice of pomegranate. Punicalagin and punicalin were also extracted from the leaves of a Combretaceous plant, *Terminalia catappa*. They exhibited multiple pharmacological properties such as neuroprotective, cardioprotective and hepatoprotective due to potent antioxidant and anti-inflammatory properties. Lin et al. (2001) have shown that hepatoprotective property of punicalagin and punicalin were exhibited through restoration of the liver enzymes and the inhibition of lipid peroxidation, along with improved antioxidant defense against APAP-induced hepatotoxicity in rats [128]. The histopathological salvage further confirmed the protective effects, though at high doses they appear hepatotoxic.

1.59. Quercetin

Quercetin is one of the most popular polyphenolic flavonol type compound reported to contain many phenol structural units. It predominantly found in glycosides form in large number of dietary plants including fruits, vegetables, beverages, spices and ornamental plants. Till date, it is extensively studied for its health and therapeutic benefits in experimental and clinical studies and it is considered as one of the highly consumed dietary flavonoid in day to day life across the world. Gilani et al. (1997) first reported the hepatoprotective activity of quercetin [129]. It was shown to reduce APAP-induced liver toxicity by promoting the repletion of GSH and the enzymes activating glutathione-s-transferases permitting the captation of the reactive metabolites of the APAP and other liver toxicants [71,130]. Quercetin was found to attenuate liver toxicity by restoring liver enzymes in rats [49]. Another derivative, quercetin-3,7-dimethyl-ether which was isolated from leaves of *Cistus laurifolius* L. has been shown to protect APAP-induced liver toxicity by antioxidant action [102]. Quercetin was found to ameliorate APAP-induced liver injury by restoring liver enzymes and antioxidants, inhibiting lipid peroxidation concomitant to histological salvage and correcting alter liver function tests similar to the standard drug, NAC [62]. It was also shown to ameliorate hepatorenal toxicity in rats by attenuating oxidative and nitrosative stress in liver and kidney and improving mitochondrial energy production [131]. However, recently, quercetinand chrysin have been shown to enhance the systemic exposure of APAP by inhibiting intestinal *P*-glycoprotein and metabolism of APAP [57]. In an approach to improve the drug delivery of quercetin, quercetin loaded self-nanoemulsifying drug delivery system was developed, which protected the liver injury. The optimized quercetin formulation was shown to enhance solubility and dissolution and it displayed potent protection by biochemical and histopathological improvement against APAP-induced hepatotoxicity in the form of free radical scavenging, antioxidant augmenting, and antilipiperoxidative activity [132]. In another recent study, quercetin inhibited APAP-induced cytotoxicity in human liver cells mediating *Nrf2* antioxidative signaling pathway inducing *p62* expression, inhibiting the binding of *Keap1* to *Nrf2* in L-02 cells. It enhanced the nuclear translocation of Nrf2 and induced the expression of the ARE-dependent genes like catalytic or modify subunit of glutamate-cysteine ligase (Gclc/Gclm), and HO-1. Docking studies indicated that the interaction of quercetin with the Nrf2-binding site in Keap1 protein, but it did not affect Keap1 expression. It also enhanced the expression of p62 and p62 siRNA and activated JNK in hepatocytes [133].

1.60. Resveratrol

Resveratrol, a polyphenol compound of stilbene group that is chemically known as 3,4,5-trihydroxystilbene, is abundantly present in grapes, berries, nuts and beverages. It is one of the comprehensively studied compounds for health benefits and pharmaceutical development. A convincing number of experimental studies [134–138] along with some detailed reviews [139,140] in the past few years reported the benefits of resveratrol in liver diseases. Sener et al. (2006) for the first time demonstrated its hepatoprotective property against APAP-induced liver toxicity in mice [138]. Resveratrol was found to attenuate hepatotoxicity by inhibiting the activation of pro-inflammatory cytokines, oxidative stress, lipid peroxidation and myeloperoxidase activity. The restoration of liver enzymes and histological preservation of liver tissues further confirmed the hepatoprotective effects of resveratrol due to its potent antioxidant and anti-inflammatory properties [138]. In another study, resveratrol treatment was found to be protective against APAP-induced liver injury in CD-1 mice with an observation that Th1-dominant response in Th1/Th2 cytokine balance and TNF-play an important role in APAP-induced liver injury [137]. Du et al. (2015) investigated the hepatoprotective mechanism and showed that resveratrol did not affect the formation of reactive metabolites, protein bindings and JNK pathway. It was found to inhibit downstream nuclear DNA fragmentation and release of apoptosis-inducing factor and endonuclease G from mitochondria independent of Bax pore formation along with reduction in protein nitration following APAP challenge due to scavenging of peroxynitrite [136]. In another study, resveratrol was found to inhibit bioactivation of APAP by suppressing activation of CYP2E1, CYP3A11, and CYP1A2 activities and inducing Sirtuin 1 activation; an important player in energy metabolism and regulates cell cycle, apoptosis, and inflammation. Further, sirtuin activation negatively regulated p53 signaling to induce cell proliferation-associated proteins including cyclin D1, cyclin dependent kinase 4, and proliferating cell nuclear antigenand facilitated hepatocyte proliferation. It also inhibited the activation of JNK pathway and protected against mitochondrial injury [135]. The sirtuins mediated hepatoprotective effects were further confirmed in vivo and in vitro models of APAP-induced hepatotoxicity. Resveratrol was found to increase APAP-reduced SIRT1 activity comparable to the selective synthetic sirtuins activators [134]. Taken together, the studies are suggestive of hepatoprotective properties of resveratrol in APAP-induced liver toxicity and the activation of sirtuins appear to be a novel mechanism of hepatoprotection.

1.61. Rhein

Rhein, an anthraquinone glycoside, which is chemically known as 4,5-dihydroxy-9,10-dioxoanthracene-2-carboxylic acid, is abundantly found in many plants including *Rheum palmatum* L., *Aloe barbadensis* Miller, *Cassia angustifolia* Vahl, and *Polygonum multiflorum* Thunb. Rhein has been shown potent antioxidant, anti-inflammatory, antitumor, neuroprotective, and hepatoprotective properties. It has been reported to confer protection dose dependently against APAP-induced liver and renal toxicity in rats, by normalizing antioxidants, restoring liver enzymes and GSH levels along with suppressed lipid peroxidation and histological salvage due to potent antioxidant action [141].

1.62. Rutin

Rutin or vitamin P or quercetin-3-*O*-rutinoside is a polyphenolic bioflavonoid that is chemically known as 3,3′,4′,5,7-pentahydroxyflavone-3-rhamnoglucoside and abundantly found in vegetables, beverages, and dietary plants, including *Artemisia scoparia*. Its cytoprotective effect, such as gastroprotective, hepatoprotective, and anti-diabetic has been shown via antioxidant, anti-inflammatory, and organoprotection in several studies. It has been showed to reduce mortality and restore liver enzymes [142].

1.63. Saikosaponin D

Saikosaponin D, which is chemically known as β-D-Galactopyranoside, (3β,4α,16α)-13,28-epoxy-16,23-dihydroxyolean-11-en is a major constituent isolated from *Bupleurum falcatum* that is popularly used for liver diseases in eastern Asian countries. Liu et al. (2014) reported that Saikosaponin D protected against APAP-induced hepatotoxicity by down-regulating *NF-κB* and STAT3-mediated inflammatory signaling as evidenced by decreased phosphorylation of *NF-κB* and signal transducer and STAT3 and suppressed *NF-κB* target genes such as pro-inflammatory cytokine *IL-6* and *Ccl2*, and *STAT3* genes such as suppressor of cytokine signaling 3 (*Socs3*) and fibrinogen gene analysis (*Fga*, *Fgb* and *Fgg*). Also, it increased the expression of anti-inflammatory cytokine IL-10 mRNA [143].

1.64. Salidroside

Salidroside or p-tyrosol, a phenylethanoid glycoside is chemically known as (2R,3S,4S,5R,6R)-2-(hydroxymethyl)-6-[2-(4-hydroxyphenyl) ethoxy]oxane-3,4,5-triol) is a major constituent of perennial flowering plant *Rhodiola* species mainly *Rhodiolarosea* and *Rhodiola imbricata*, *Rhodiola algida* and *Rhodiola crenulata*. In traditional medicine, it is used for the management of many chronic degenerative diseases and has shown numerous pharmacological properties including adaptogenic, neuroprotective, anti-tumor, cardioprotective, antidepressant, antioxidant, anti-inflammatory and hepatoprotective. Wu et al. (2008) have demonstrated that salidroside protects against APAP-induced hepatotoxicity by inhibiting lipid peroxidation, pro-inflammatory cytokines and restoring liver enzymes along with antioxidants [144]. It was also displayed histopathological salvage and suppression of caspase-3 and hypoxia inducible factor-1α (HIF-1α) expression in liver. The protective effects of salidroside were found to be comparable to that of NAC. In another study, Guo et al. (2014) developed and validated a simple and specific LC-MS/MS method for the determination of salidroside and its metabolite p-tyrosol in rat liver tissues that suggested its bioavailability in the liver tissues and its hepatoprotective effect [145].

1.65. Salvianolic Acids

Salvianolic acid B, a polyphenolic compound, is isolated from the aqueous factions of extracts of *Salvia miltiorrhiza* Bunge, popularly used in traditional Chinese medicine and represents one of the highly used medications with application from oral to intravenous. It is one of the most potent antioxidant, anti-inflammatory agent and reported to protect various organs, such as brain, heart, kidney, and liver from oxidative stress [146]. Salvianolic acid B was found to confer hepatoprotective effects against APAP by inducing Nrf2 expression [147]. Salvianolic acid B treatment restored liver enzymes, enhanced the expression of Nrf2, HO-1 and glutamate-l-cysteine ligase catalytic subunit (Gclc). Furthermore, it also activated the phosphatidylinositol-3-kinase (PI3K) and protein kinase C (PKC) signaling pathways. In another study, salvianolic acid B showed to maintain redox status and mitochondrial metabolic activity in rat hepatocytes, but fail to inhibit CYP2E1 [146]. Altogether, it appears that salvianolic B protects against liver toxicity via the activation of the PI3K and PKC pathways.

1.66. Saponarin

Saponarin, a favone glycoside that is chemically known as (5-hydroxy-2-(4-hydroxyphenyl)-6-[(2S,3R,4R,5S,6R)-3,4,5-trihydroxy-6-(hydroxymethyl)oxan-2-yl]-7-[(2S,3R,4R,5S,6R)-3,4,5-trihydroxy-6-(hydroxymethyl)oxan-2-yl] oxychromen-4-one) is naturally occurring apigenin-6-C-glucosyl-7-*O*-glucoside isolated from *Gypsophila trichotoma*. It has been reported to possess antihyperglycemic, antimicrobial, antioxidant, anti-inflammatory and hepatoprotective properties. Simeonova et al. (2013) reported hepatoprotective effects in the in vitro/in vivo studies. In isolated rat hepatocytes, saponarin dose dependently improved cell viability and antioxidant defense and inhibited lipid peroxidation as well as LDH leakage [148]. Similar results were replicated in vivo in addition to the histological salvage of liver tissues. However, no changes in phase I enzyme activities of Aniline 4-Hydroxylase (AH) and Ethylmorphine-N-Demethylase (EMND) and cytochrome P450 quantity were detected. The protective effects were comparable to silymarin.

1.67. Sauchinone

Sauchinone, a polyphenolic lignin isolated from *Saururus chinensis* exhibits potent antioxidant and anti-inflammatory activity and protects hepatocytes against iron-induced toxicity [149]. Kay et al. (2011), have shown that sauchinone attenuated APAP-induced liver injury and its protective mechanism as activating *Nrf2* through the *PKCδ-GSK3β* pathway [150]. In hepatocytes, sauchinone activated Nrf2, leads to increased nuclear accumulation of *Nrf2*, activation of *NQO1*- ARE reporter gene and glutamate-cysteine ligase and NQO1 protein that imparts the restoration of hepatic GSH content. Sauchinone also activated protein kinase C-δ (PKCδ) that enhanced Nrf2 phosphorylation with a reciprocal decrease in its interaction with Keap1 and activated Nrf2 phosphorylation. Further, it was also found to enhance the inhibitory phosphorylation of glycogen synthase kinase-3β (GSK3β), suppressing Nrf2 activity dependent on PKCδ activation.

1.68. Schisandrol Derivatives

Schisandrin A, schisandrin B, schisandrin C, schisandrol A, schisandrol B and schisantherin A are the lignan compounds isolated from *Schisandra sphenanthera*, a reputed herb in traditional Chinese medicine for the treatment of many diseases including liver. These derivatives have been shown hepatoprotective against APAP-induced liver toxicity in mice [151]. The protective effects of these compounds were evidenced by restoration of GSH in liver, inhibition of lipid peroxidation, and restoration of liver enzymes in a dose-dependent manner. They were also found to attenuate the enzymatic activities of CYP450 isoforms viz. CYP2E1, CYP1A2 and CYP3A11 and alter APAP bioactivation mechanism [151]. This results in the reduced formation of toxic intermediate N-acetyl-p-benzoquinone imine NAPQI-GSH in vivo and in vitro both. Among these derivatives, schisandrol B was studied extensively and showed to attenuate activation of p53 and p21 and promote liver regeneration along with enhancement in antiapoptotic proteins such as cyclin D1, PCNA and BCL-2. Further, in silico studies also demonstrated that schisandrol B interferes with CYP2E1 and CYP3A4 active sites [152]. Schisandrol B exhibited a significant protective effect toward APAP-induced liver toxicity, potentially through inhibition of CYP-mediated APAP bioactivation and regulation of the p53, p21, CCND1, PCNA, and BCL-2 to promote liver regeneration [153]. In a recent study, schisandrol B further showed to attenuate APAP-induced hepatotoxicity in mice by the activation of Nrf2/ARE pathway and the regulation of *Nrf2* target genes *Nrf2/ARE* signaling pathway [153]. Schisandrol B treatment ameliorated liver toxicity and increased the nuclear accumulation of Nrf2 as well as expression of Nrf2 downstream proteins, including Gclc, GSR, NQO1, GSTs, MRP2, MRP3 and MRP4 in APAP-treated mice. The mechanism was further confirmed in HepG2 cells. Based on these studies, all of the lignans appear promising with better potential of schisandrol B in reducing hepatotoxicity by improving antioxidant defense and inhibiting the CYP mediated bioactivation of APAP.

1.69. Sesamol

Sesamol, a flavonoid lignin that is chemically known as 1,3-benzodioxol-5-ol is obtained fromthe oil that was extracted from seeds of *Sesamum indicum*. Chandrasekaran et al. (2009) demonstrated the ameliorative effect of sesamol pretreatment against APAP by improved liver enzymes and the inhibition of free radicals generation and subsequent lipid peroxidation and centrilobular necrosis [154]. In another report, authors reconfirmed the findings and showed that hepatoprotective effects were comparable to NAC at the equimolar doses post-treatment [155].

1.70. Silybin

Silybin dihemisuccinate, which is a soluble form of the flavonoid silymarin, was found to prevent GSH depletion and inhibit lipid peroxidation in liver along with restoration of liver enzymes altered by APAP [156,157]. In another study, silybin inhibited lipid peroxidation in isolated rat hepatocytes [158]. Conti et al. (1992) demonstrated the hepatoprotective properties of silipide, a silybin-phosphatidylcholine complex abbreviated as IdB 1016. Silipide dose dependently ameliorated APAP-induced liver toxicity due to its antioxidant action and bolstering of RNA and resultant protein synthesis [159].

1.71. Sweroside

Sweroside, an iridoid glycoside that is chemically known as (3S,4R,4aS)-4-ethenyl-3-[(2S,3R,4S, 5S,6R)-3,4,5-trihydroxy-6-(hydroxymethyl)oxan-2-yl]oxy-4,4a,5,6-tetrahydro-3H-pyrano[3,4-*c*]pyran-8-one, is isolated from the flower buds of *Lonicera japonica* Thunb and *Swertia pseudochinensis* Hara. It has been traditionally used in treatment of liver diseases and showed hepatoprotective in chemical models of liver injury. Its high bioavailability in liver tissues is attributed to its liver regenerating and hepatoprotective activity [160]. The metabolic profile revealed the presence of several phase I, phase II and aglycone-related metabolites in rat urine [161]. Though, in one preliminary study, Liu et al. (1994) did not find protective of sweroside against APAP [77].

1.72. Syringic Acid

Syringic acid, a naturally occurring phenolic compound that is chemically known as *O*-methylated trihydroxybenzoic acid, is abundantly found in many edible mushrooms and vegetable, food and beverages plants. Syringic acid possesses high proteasome inhibitory activity and showed to alleviate APAP-induced liver injury by improving enzymatic and non-enzymatic antioxidant defense and restoration of liver enzymes along with histopathological preservation of liver tissues [162].

1.73. Tannic Acid

Tannic acid, a polyphenolic compound is naturally occurring tannins and abundantly found in edible plants, including fruits, vegetables, tea, strawberries, beans, grapes, coffee, persimmons, cocoa, and nuts. Recently, tannic acid has been shown to be protective against APAP-induced hepatotoxicity [163]. It restored activities of antioxidant and liver enzymes and inhibited endothelin-1, nitric oxide and malondialdehyde formation. It also suppressed the activation of pro-inflammatory cytokines, and apoptotic mediators, such as *c-Fos*, *c-Jun*, *NF-κB (p65)* and caspase-3 and increased Bax along with decreased Bcl-2 and increased Nrf2 and HO-1. The histologic salvage of liver tissues reconfirmed the protective effects and anti-oxidant, anti-inflammatory, and anti-apoptotic effects were attributed to confer hepatoprotective effects [163].

1.74. Thymoquinone

Thymoquinone, a quinone compound that is chemically known as 2-methyl-5-propan-2-ylcyclohexa-2,5-diene-1,4-dione, is found abundantly in the oil from the seeds of *Nigella sativa* and represent one of the widely studied molecule. In a study, Nagi et al. (2010) first showed that thymoquinone dose-dependently protect against hepatotoxicity in mice by reversing rise in liver enzymes in serum, total nitrate/nitrite, lipid peroxide, and a fall in GSH and ATP in APAP-induced hepatotoxicity. Though, it did not affect the metabolic activation of APAP [164].

1.75. Withferin A

Withaferin A, a withanolide alkaloid that is chemically known as (4β,5β,6β,22*R*)-4,27-dihydroxy-5,6-22,26-diepoxyergosta-2,24-diene-1,26-di), is isolated from the leaves of *Withania somnifera* popularly known as 'Indian ginseng'. Withaferin A showed protection against liver necrosis by decreasing the activities of liver marker enzymes and prevents lipid peroxidation by improving antioxidant statusin mice model of hepatotoxicity [165]. It also suppressed JNK activation, mitochondrial Bax translocation, nitrotyrosine production, and upregulated *Nrf2*, *Gclc* and *NQO1* expression as well as down-regulated pro-inflammatory cytokines. In AML12 hepatocytes, it also reduced H_2O_2-induced oxidative stress and necrosis.

1.76. Miscellaneous

The lignans, 2,4′-epoxy-8,5′-neolignans and 7,9′;7′,9-diepoxylignans isolated from extract of *Penthorum chinese* was shown its hepatoprotective activity in hepatocytes [166]. The isoflavonoid compounds, such as 7-hydroxy-4′,5,6-trimethoxyisoflavone, 7-hydroxy-5,6-dimethoxy-2′,3′-methylenedioxyisoflavone, and 5,6-dimethoxy-2′,3′-methylenedioxy-7-C-β-*d*-gluco-pyranosyl isoflavone isolated from the seeds of *Lepidium sativum* L., displayed the amelioration of APAP-induced hepatotoxicity in rats by augmenting the endogenous antioxidants, improving the liver enzymes along with salvage of liver tissues [167]. Myricetin was found to inhibit microsomal CYP2E1 and CYP3A activities, but others, such as tangeretin, quercetin, naringenin and nobiletin does not inhibit [115]. Thymol and carvacrol found to enhance antioxidant and free radical scavenging activity and reduce activation of pro-inflammatory cytokines that are comparable to NAC in HepG2 cells [168]. Oxymatrine does not confer protective effects against AP-induced hepatotoxicity [77]. In a preliminary study, several triterpenoids, such as oleanolic acid, ursolicacid, uvaol, alpha-hederin, hederagenin, glycyrrhizin, 18-α-glycyrrhetinic acid, 18-β-glycyrrhetinic acid, 19-α-hydroxylasiatic acid, 28-*O*-β-D-glucoside, and 19-α-hydroxyl Asiatic acid were evaluated against APAP-induced hepatotoxicity. Uvaol, hederagenin, 19 alpha-hydroxyl Asiatic acid, 28-*O*-β-D-glucoside and 19-α-hydroxyl asiatic acid had no effect on APAP-hepatotoxicity whereas, glycyrrhizin, 18-α-glycyrrhetinic acid, 18-β-glycyrrhetinic acid, alpha-hederin, ursolic acid and oleanolic acid has reduced APAP-induced hepatotoxicity [31]. Girish et al. (2009) reported the hepatoprotective activity of ellagic acid against APAP-induced acute hepatotoxicity in a preliminary study and found the effects were comparable to silymarin.The protective effects were mediated by antioxidant activity and the restoration of liver cytochrome P450 enzymes [169].

Table 1. Phytochemicals showed hepatoprotective effect in the mice model of acetaminophen-induced liver toxicity.

Phytochemical	Dose of Phytochemical	Dose of APAP and Route	Efficacy and Major Mechanisms	CYP2E1 Inhibition	References
Acanthoic acid	50, 100 mg/kg, *p. o.* 2h before APAP	300 mg/kg, *i. p.*	LFT, antioxidants, anti-inflammatory, antiapoptotic and antinecrotic	No	[27]
Ajoene	20,50,100 mg/kg, *p. o.*, 2 & 24 h before APAP	300 mg/kg, *p. o.*	LFT, GSH	No	[30]
Apigenin	100, 200 mg/kg	350 mg/kg, *i. p.*	LFT, antioxidants, H&E	No	[39]
Astaxanthin	30, 60 mg/kg, *p. o.* × 14 days	300 mg/kg, *i. p.*	LFT, antioxidants, pro-inflammatory cytokines, inhibition of JNK signal pathway and phosphorylation of ERK and P38	No	[170]
Baicalin	15, 30, 60 mg/kg, *p. o.*	300 mg/kg, *i. p.*	LFT, cytokines, H&E, decrease hepatic phosphorylated extracellular signal-regulated kinase expression	No	[171,172]
Berberine	1 or 5 mg/kg, *i. p*	500 mg/kg, *i. p.*	LFT, mortality, NLRP3 inflammasome pathway	No	[43]
Boswellic acid	0.05, 0.1% in diet × 4 weeks	400 mg/kg, *i. p.*	LFT, antioxidants, cytokines and chemokines, toll-like receptor signaling and H&E	Yes	[45]
Carnosic acid	100 mg/kg × 3 days	400 mg/kg, *i. p.*	LFT, antioxidants, Nrf2/Keap pathway, H&E	No	[51]
Chlorogenic acid	5, 10, 20 or 40 mg/kg × 7days	300 mg/kg, *i. g*	LFT, antioxidants, antiapoptotic, ERK1/2, JNK, p38 kinases mediated MAPK pathway	No	[173]
Chlorogenic acid	10, 20, 40 mg/kg at 1h after given AP	400 mg/kg, and another 3h later	LFT, MPO, H&E, pro-inflamatory cytokines, chemokines, TLR3/4 and NFκB signaling	No	[53]
Corynoline, acetylcorynoline and protopine	50, 100 mg/kg, 8 to 24 h before APAP	-	LFT, antioxidants	Yes	[58]
Esculentoside A	2.5 mg/kg, *i. p.* twice in a day	400, 900 mg/kg, *i. p.*	LFT, antioxidants, H&E, increases Nrf2 expression and phosphorylation of AMPK, Akt and GSK3β	No	[174]
Ferulic acid	30, 100 mg/kg, *p. o.*, t.d. × 3 days	350 mg/kg, *i. p.*	LFT, antioxidants, H&E, MAPK and TLR4 pathway	Yes	[75]
Gallic acid	100 mg/kg, *i. p.* 30 min after APAP	900 mg/kg, *i. p.*	LFT, pro-inflammatory cytokines, antioxidants	No	[80]
6-Gingerol	30 mg/kg, 30 min after APAP	900 mg/kg	LFT, antioxidants, comparable to the standard drug silymarin	No	[86]
Glycyrrhetinic acid	500 mg/kg × 20 days before APAP	400 mg/kg, *i. p.*	LFT, metabolism pathway of fatty acids, palmtioylcarnitine and oleoylcarnitine	No	[90]

Table 1. *Cont.*

Phytochemical	Dose of Phytochemical	Dose of APAP and Route	Efficacy and Major Mechanisms	CYP2E1 Inhibition	References
Glycyrrhizin	Oral, *i. p.* and *i. v.*	200-600 mg/kg, *i. p.*	LFT, antioxidants, pro-inflammatory cytokines, antiapptotic, H & E, only *i. p.*, *i. v.* effective	Yes	[175]
Hyperoside	10, 50, 100 mg/kg, *p. o.* for 3 days before APAP	300 mg/kg, *i. p.*	LFT, antioxidants, Nrf2/Keap pathway, Phase II enzymes	Yes	[97]
Isoquercitrin	10, 20, or 50 mg/kg, *p. o.* for 3 days before APAP	300 mg/kg, *i. p.*	LFT, Pro-inflammatory cytokines, antioxidants, NF-κB/MAPK pathway	Yes	[98]
Kaempferoll8-C-β-galactoside and C-glycoside	25, 50, 75 mg/kg	500 mg/kg	LFT, H&E, comparable to silymarin	No	[101]
Luteolin and quercetin 3-β-d-glucoside	200, 400 mg/kg, *p. o.* for 14 days	2 g/kg, *p. o.* × 14 days	LFT, antioxidants, H&E	No	[176]
Lycopene	10, 100mg/kg, *p. o.*	500 mg/kg, *p. o.*	LFT, antioxidants, MMP-2, H&E, morphometry	No	[177,178]
Naringenin	200, 400, and 800 mg/kg, *p. o.*	250 mg/kg, *s. c.*	LFT, antioxidants, H&E	No	[113]
Paeonol	25, 50, 100 mg/kg, *p. o.*, 6 and 24 h before APAP	400 mg/kg, *i. p.*	LFT, antioxidants, chemokines and cytokines, JNK pathways	No	[122]
Fulvotomentosides, oleanolic acid, total saponins of *Panax japonicus* & *Panax* notoginseng, sweroside, oxymatrine, dimethyl dicarboxylate biphenyl,	-	-	LFT, H&E, Fulvomentosides found most potent, oleanic acid, total saponins of *Panax japonicus* and *Panax notoginseng* had moderate hepatoprotective effects, sweroside, oxymatrine and dimethyl dicarboxylate biphenyl had no effect on APAP toxicity	No	[77]
α-Hederin and sapindoside B	20 mg/kg, *s. c.* twice	-	LFT, H&E, mortality	No	[78]
Procyanidins	1 or 10 mg/kg, *p. o.*	300 mg/kg, *i. p.*	LFT, enhanced Nrf2/ARE activity and phase II detoxifying/antioxidant enzymes	Yes	[126]
Rutin	20 mg/kg, *p. o.*	640 mg/kg, *p. o.*	LFT, antioxidants	No	[142]
Sodium ferulate	100 mg/kg, *p. o.*, q.d. × 10 days	130 mg/kg, *i. p.*	LFT, antioxidants	No	[74]
Salidroside	50, 100 mg/kg 2 h before APAP	300 mg/kg, *i. p.*	LFT, pro-inflammatory cytokines, antioxidants, antiapoptotic, H&E, parallel with NAC	No	[144]
Salvianolic acid B	25 and 50 mg/kg, *i. g.* × 3 days	300 mg/kg, *i. g.*	LFT, antioxidants, Nrf2, HO-1 and Gclc activation of the PI3K and PKC pathways	Yes	[147]
Sauchinone	6 h after APAP	500 mg/kg, *i. p.*	LFT, antioxidants, H&E, Keap1/Nrf2 and GSK3β-PKCδ pathway	No	[150]

Table 1. *Cont.*

Phytochemical	Dose of Phytochemical	Dose of APAP and Route	Efficacy and Major Mechanisms	CYP2E1 Inhibition	References
Schisandrol B	200 mg/kg, *p. o.* for 3 days before APAP	400 mg/kg, *i. p.*	LFT, H&E, antioxidants, Nrf2/ARE signaling pathway	No	[153]
Schisandrol B	6.25, 25 and 100 mg/kg for 7 days before APAP	400 mg/kg, *i. p.*	LFT, antioxidants, antiapoptotic (p53, p21, CCND1, PCNA, and BCL-2)	Yes	[152]
Schisandrin derivatives	200 mg/kg/day, *p. o.*	400 mg/kg, *i. p.*	LFT, antioxidants, H&E	Yes	[151]
Silipide	400 mg/kg, *p. o.*	-	LFT, antioxidant activities	No	[159]
Quercitrin	10, 50 mg/kg, *p. o.* × 7 days	300 mg/kg, *i. p.*	LFT, antioxidants and Nrf2/ARE, anti-inflammatory, MAPK pathways including ERK, JNK, and p38 MAPK, comparable to silymarin	No	[179]
Tannic acid	25, 50 mg/kg, *p. o.* × 3 days	400 mg/kg, *p. o.*	LFT, antioxidants, pro-inflammatory cytokines, H&E, suppressed c-Fos, c-Jun, NF-κB (p65) and caspase-3, regulated Bax/Bcl-2, Nrf2 and HO-1	No	[163]
Trans-anethole	62.5, 125, 250 mg/kg, *p. o.*	250 mg/kg, *p. o.* in mice	LFT, antioxidants, pro-inflammatory cytokines, morphometrics, H&E	No	[180]
Withaferin A	7 mg/kg, *p. o.* in Nrf2 KO mice	250 mg/kg, *i. p.*	LFT, Keap1-independent & Pten/PI_3K/Akt-dependent	No	[181]

Table 2. Phytochemicals showed hepatoprotective effect in the rat model of acetaminophen-induced liver injury.

Phytochemical	Dose of Phytochemical	Route and Dose of APAP	Efficacy and Major Mechanisms	CYP2E1 Inhibition	References
Andrographolide	200 mg/kg, *i. p.*, 1, 4 & 7 h after APAP	3 g/kg, *p. o.*	LFT, H&E, antioxidants	No	[33]
Berberine	4 mg/kg; *p. o.* twice × 2 days or 4 mg/kg every 6 h	-	LFT, antioxidants	Yes	[42]
Chlorogenic acid	40 mg/kg *p. o.* × 7 days	300 mg/kg, intragastric	LFT, antioxidants LFT, antioxidants	Yes	[54]
Esculetin	6 mg/kg	640 mg/kg, *p. o.*	LFT, antioxidants	No	[73]
Gomisin A	50 mg/kg	750 mg/kg *i. p.*	LFT, antioxidants, antiapoptotic, H&E	No	[92]
Hesperidin	100, 200 mg/kg × 14 days	750 mg/kg, *p. o.*	LFT, antioxidants, antioapoptotic, H&E	No	[95]
Liquiritigenin & Schisandrin C derivative	*p. o.* or *i. v.*, 2–4 days		LFT, H & E, liquiritigenin and combination showed protection while schisandrin C derivative failed	No	[182]
Lupeol	150 mg/kg, *p. o.* × 30 days	1 g/kg	LFT, antioxidants, antiapoptotic, H&E	No	[183]
Magnolol	0.01, 0.1, 1 µg/kg 0.5 h after APAP	500 mg/kg, *i. p.* × 8 and 24 h	LFT, H&E, antioxidants	No	[107]
Pterostilbene	50, 100 mg/kg, *p. o.* × 15 days before APAP	800 mg/kg, *i. p.*	LFT, lipid profiles, pro-inflammatory cytokines, antioxidants, antiapoptotitic, antifibrotic, comparable to silymarin	No	[127]
Punicalagin and Punicalin	1,5,12.5 or 25 mg/kg, *i. p.*	500 mg/kg, *i. p.*	LFT, antioxidants, H&E	No	[128]
Rutin	20 mg/kg, *p. o.* × 11 days	500 mg/kg *p. o.* from day 1–3 in rats	LFT, H&E, TEM, antioxidants, comparable to silymarin	No	[184]
Saponarin	80 mg/kg, *p. o.* × 7 days	600 mg/kg, *i. p.*	LFT, antioxidants, H&E	Yes	[148]
Silybin	-	-	LFT, GSH and lipid peroxidation	No	[157]
Syringic acid	25, 50 and 100 mg/kg *p. o.*	750 mg/kg *i. p.*	LFT, H&E, comparable to silymarin	No	[162]

Table 3. Phytochemicals showed hepatoprotective effect in the in vitro model of acetaminophen-induced liver injury.

Phytochemicals	Dose of Phytochemical	Cells and Dose of APAP	Efficacy and Major Mechanisms	CYP2E1 Inhibition	References
Andrographolide	0.75–12 mg/kg *p. o.* × 7 days	Rat hepatocytes	LFT, viability, more potent than silymarin	No	[34]
Lupeol	10 μM	Rat hepatocytes, APAP (675 μM)	Maintaining redox and preventing mitochondria-mediated apoptosis	No	[103]
Paeonol	20, 40, 80 μM	Mouse hepatocytes H_2O_2 or APAP	LDH, ROS and pro-inflammatory genes and reduced IKKα/β, IκBα and p65 phosphorylation	No	[122]
Silibin	25 μM	Rat hepatocytes, APAP (25–30 mM)	Inhibited APAP toxicity, prevented DNA strand breaks formation	No	[185]
CalamusinsA-I	10 μM	HepG2 cells	Weak hepatoprotective activities against APAP	No	[50]
α-Hederin	10, 30 μM/kg, *s. c.* × 3 days	Rat liver microsomes	Dose-dependent suppression of liver cytochrome P450 enzymes	Yes	[186]
Saponarin	60-0.006 μg/mL	Rat hepatocytes, APAP (100 μM)	Cell viability, LDH, GSH, MDA	Yes	[148]
Chlorogenic acid	1, 10, 25, 50 and 100 μM/L	L-02 cells	LFT, cell viability	Yes	[54]
Procyanidins	10, 25 and 50 μg/L	HepG2 cells	Enhanced phase II detoxifying and antioxidant enzymes and Nrf2/ARE activity	Yes	[126]
Thymol and carvacrol	25, 50 and 100 μM	HepG2 cells	Antioxidants, pro-inflammatory cytokines, comparable to NAC	No	[168]

Table 4. The medicinal plants showed to ameliorate the acetaminophen-induced hepatotoxicity in different models.

Plant Names	Plant Names	Plant Names	Plant Names	Plant Names
Abelmoschus moschatus	*Boswellia ovalifoliolata*	*Eugenia jambolana*	*Mucuna capitataRoxb.*	*Sargassum tenerrimum*
Abutilon indicum	*Boswellia serrata*	*Fagonia olivieri*	*Mucuna pruriens*	*Sargassum variegatum*
Acacia auriculiformis	*Brassica juncea Linn.*	*Fermented ginseng*	*Muntingia calabura*	*Schisandra chinensis*
Acacia indica	*Bridelia micrantha*	*Fermented red ginseng*	*Musa paradisiaca*	*Schoenoplectus grossus*
Acathopanax senticosus	*Bryophylum pinnatum*	*Ficus exasperate*	*Musanga cecropioides*	*Scutia myrtina*
Achillea wilhelmsii C.	*Bupleurus spp.*	*Ficus hispida Linn*	*Mussaenda erythrophylla*	*Senecio scandens*
Acronychia laurifolia	*Caesalpinia bonduc Linn.*	*Ficus microcarpa Linn.*	*Myrica rubra Sieb.*	*Sesamum indicum*
Adansonia digitata Linn.	*Caesalpinia gilliesii*	*Ficus mollis*	*Nasturtium officinale*	*Sida acuta Burm. f.*
Adhatoda vasica	*Cajanus cajan*	*Ficus religisoa Linn.*	*Nauclea latifolia*	*Silene aprica*

Table 4. *Cont.*

Plant Names	Plant Names	Plant Names	Plant Names	Plant Names
Aegle marmelos	*Cajanus indicus*	*Flos lonicerae*	*Nigella sativa*	*Silybum marianum*
Agaricus blazei	*Calotropis procera*	*Foeniculum vulgare*	*Ocimum gratissimum*	*Smilax zeylanica Linn.*
Ageratum conyzoides	*Camelia sinesis*	*Fumaria indica*	*Opuntia robusta*	*Solanum alatum*
Alcea rosea	*Capparis sepiaria L.*	*Fumaria officinalis*	*Opuntia streptacantha*	*Solanum fastigiatum*
Alchornea cordifolia	*Caralluma umbellate*	*Fumaria parviflora*	*Ornithogalum saundersiae*	*Solanum indicum*
Allium cepa	*Cardiospermum halicacabum*	*Ganoderma amboinense*	*Oroxylum indicum*	*Solanum nigrum*
Allium sativum	*Carica papaya*	*Garcinia indica*	*Osbeckia octandra*	*Sophora flavescens*
Alnus japonica	*Carissa carandas Linn.*	*Garcinia kola*	*Oxalis corniculata*	*Sphaeranthus indicus*
Aloe barbadensis	*Carum copticum*	*Genista quadriflora*	*Oxalis strictalinn*	*Swertia chirata*
Aloe vera	*Cassia fistula*	*Gentiana manshurica*	*Paederia foetida*	*Swertia longifolia Boiss*
Alpinia galanga	*Cassia occidentalis L*	*Glossogyne tenuifolia*	*Paeonia anomala*	*Swertia punicea*
Alstonia scholaris R. Br.	*Ceiba pentandra Linn.*	*Glycosmis arborea*	*Pandanus odoratissimus*	*Swietenia mahagoni L.*
Amaranthus caudatus	*Centaurium erythraea*	*Glycosmis pentaphylla*	*Parinari curatellifolia*	*Syzygium aromaticum*
Ambrosia maritima	*Chelidonium majus*	*Gongronema latifolium*	*Pavonia zeylanica*	*Taraxacum officinale*
Amorphophallus paeoniifolius	*Cichorium endivia*	*Gossypium herbacium*	*Penthorum chinese*	*Taraxacum syriacum*
Andrographis paniculata	*Cichorium glandulosum*	*Gymnaster koraiensis*	*Pergularia daemia*	*Telfairia occidentalis*
Anisochilus carnosus	*Cinnamomum tamala*	*Gymnosporia montana*	*Phyllanthus acidus*	*Tephrosia purprea*
Annona muricata	*Cinnamomum zeylanicum*	*Gynostemma pentaphyllum*	*Phyllanthus amarus*	*Terminalia chebula*
Anoectochilus formosanus	*Cistus laurifolius Linn.*	*Gypsophila trichotoma*	*Phyllanthus emblica*	*Terminalia paniculata*
Apium graveolens Linn.	*Citrullus colocynthis*	*Haplophylum tuberculatum*	*Phyllanthus maderaspatensis*	*Tetracera loureiri*
Apocynum venetum Linn.	*Citrus hystrix*	*Harungana madagascariensis*	*Phyllanthus niruri Linn.*	*Teucrium poliumgeyrii*
Aquilegia vulgaris	*Citrus maxima*	*Hedyotis corymbosa*	*Phyllanthus polyphyllus*	*Teucrium stocksianum*
Arctium lappa Linn	*Citrus microcarpa*	*Hemodiscus indicus*	*Phyllanthus urinariae*	*Thymus vulgaris*
Argania spinosa	*Clausena dentata*	*Hibiscus hispidissimus*	*Piper methysticum*	*Tinospora cordifolia*
Artemisia absinthium	*Cleome chelidonii*	*Hibiscus sabdariffa L*	*Piper puberulum*	*Tournefortia sarmentosa*
Artemisia capillaris	*Clerodendron Inerme*	*Hippocratea africana*	*Pisonia aculeate*	*Trianthema portulacastrum*
Artemisia maritima	*Clitoria ternatea Linn.*	*Hippophae rhamnoides*	*Pittosporum neilgherrense*	*Tribulus terrestris Linn.*
Artemisia pallens Walls	*Cnidoscolus aconitifolius*	*Holostemma ada Kodien*	*Plantago major*	*Trichopus zeylanicus*
Artemisia sacrorumLedeb.	*Coldenia procumbens*	*Hordeum vulgare Linn.*	*Platycodon grandiflorum*	*Trichosanthes dioica*
Artemisia scoparia	*Conyza bonariensis*	*Hypericum perforatum*	*Pleurotus ostreatus*	*Trichosanthes lobata*
Artichoke	*Copaiba oil*	*Indigofera tinctoria Linn.*	*Pluchea arguta*	*Tridax procumbens Linn*

Table 4. *Cont.*

Plant Names	Plant Names	Plant Names	Plant Names	Plant Names
Asparagus falcatus	*Cornus officinalisSieb.*	*Iris spuria*	*Plumbago zeylanica*	*Trifolium alexandrinum*
Asparagus racemosus	*Corylus avellana*	*Ixeris chinensis*	*Polyalthia longifolia*	*Ulva reticulata*
Asteracantha longifolia	*Costus igneus*	*Khaya gradifoliola*	*Polygonum odoratum*	*Urtica dioica*
Astragalus corniculatus	*Crataegus songarica*	*Khaya senegalensis*	*Pongamia pinnata*	*Uvaria afzelli*
Astragalus persicus	*Croton zehntneri*	*Kigelia africana*	*Porphyra yezoensis*	*Vernonia amygdalina*
Astragalus tournefortii	*Cucurbita pepo*	*Kohautia grandiflora*	*Pouteria campechiana*	*Vigna angularis*
Atropa acuminata	*Cuscuta australis*	*Kombucha tea*	*Premna tomentosa*	*Vitellaria paradoxa*
Auricularia polytricha	*Cuscuta chinensis*	*Lawsonia inermis*	*Prosopis africana*	*Vitex doniana*
Averrhoa bilimbi	*Cyathea gigantea*	*Leea asiatica*	*Prosopis farcta*	*Wedelia calendulacea*
Averrhoa carambola	*Cynanchum atratum*	*Leonotis nepetifolia*	*Psidium guajava*	*Wedelia paludosa*
Azadirachta indica	*Cynara scolymus*	*Lepidium sativum Linn.*	*Pterocarpus osun Craib*	*Woodfordia fruticosa*
Azolla microphylla	*Cyperus scariosus*	*Lopatherum gracile*	*Pueraria lobata*	*Ximenia americana Linn.*
Baccharis dracunculifolia	*Cyperus segetum*	*Lophira lanceolata*	*Pyropia yezoensis*	*Xylopia aethiopica*
Baccharis trimera	*Dalbergia paniculata*	*Lycopersicum esculentum*	*Raphanus sativus*	*Zea mays Linn.*
Balanites aegyptiaca	*Desmodium adscendens*	*Lycopodium clavatum*	*Rhazya stricta*	*Zingiber officinale*
Barleria prionitis Linn.	*Dicranopteris linearis*	*Malva sylvestris Linn.*	*Rhodiola imbricata*	*Zingiber zerumbet*
Basella alba	*Dioscorea alata Linn.*	*Mangifera india*	*Rosa damascena*	*Zizyphus jujube*
Bauhinia purpurea	*Ecballium elaterium*	*Markhamia platycalyx*	*Rosa laevigataMichx*	*Zizyphus spina*
Berberis aristata	*Echinophora platyloba*	*Maytenus emerginata*	*Rosmarinus officinalis*	
Beta vulgaris	*Eclipta alba Hassk.*	*Melastoma malabathricum*	*Rubia cordifolia*	
Bidens pilosa Linn.	*Embelia ribes*	*Mesona palustris BL*	*Salacia oblonga*	
Bixa orellana Linn.	*Enantia chlorantha*	*Momordica charantia*	*Salvia miltiorrhiza*	
Blumea mollis	*Entada africana*	*Monochoria vaginalis*	*Santallum album*	
Boehmeria nivea	*Epaltes divaricate*	*Moringa oleifera Lam.*	*Sargassum binderi*	
Boerhaavia diffusa	*Eucalyptus maculata*	*Moutan cortex*	*Sargassum polycystum*	

2. Discussions

As represented in the tables, a large number of phytochemicals (Tables 1–3), plant extracts (Table 4), and herbal formulations (Table 5) have been shown to ameliorate APAP-induced liver injury. The available experimental studies reveal that phytochemicals and plant extracts exert hepatoprotective effects against APAP-induced liver toxicity due to their multiple pharmacological properties, including anti-inflammatory, antioxidant and antiapoptotic. Among them, the majority of them are linked to cascades that are involved in oxidative stress, inflammatory cytokine signaling, and cell death [187,188]. Mechanistically, phytochemicals and plant extracts showed to restore antioxidant defense by preventing glutathione depletion, improving antioxidants enzymes along with attenuation of lipid peroxidation and subsequently limiting inflammation and cell death.

Many plant extracts have been shown to improve the endogenous enzymatic and non-enzymatic antioxidants to inhibit lipid peroxidation and the activation and release of pro-inflammatory cytokines concomitant with prevention of depletion of GSH from the liver. The cardinal characteristic of APAP-induced liver injury is massive retrograde degeneration of the liver tissues resulting in the loss of liver enzymes followed by depletion of GSH and lipid peroxidation and inflammation. The dramatic depletion of glutathione is known to be responsible for the clinical manifestation of hepatotoxicity. In majority of the studies, the hepatoprotective effects of plant extracts against APAP-induced liver injury were confirmed by liver function tests, as evidenced by the restoration of the liver enzymes and attenuation of the rise of liver enzymes in the serum concomitant improvement in cellular architecture and reduced liver necrosis. The whole plant extract known to have various phytoconstituents that act synergistically to enhance efficacy and prevent toxicity when it is used as an adjuvant along with the modern medicine [189]. Therefore, the synergy of phytoconstituents could be beneficial to enhance their efficacy.

Several formulations containing plant extracts of a single plant or many plants known as polyherbal formulation are often available in the market for treating liver disorders [190–196]. The polyherbal or single herb or herbomineral formulations showed hepatoprotective effects are represented in Table 5. One such example for single herb formulation that is quite popular from traditional to modern medicine is silymarin, a reputed hepatoprotective herbal drug preparation containing a single herb, known as Milk thistle [197]. Whereas, Liv 52® represents a popular polyherbal preparation for liver diseases. Though, the management of liver disorders by a simple and precise herbal drug is still an intriguing problem. Silymarin is an extract from the seeds of milk thistle mainly contains flavonolignan isomers such as silybin, isosilybin, silydianin and silychristin with silybin is the most potent constituent [198]. On oral administration, silymarin absorbs quickly and eliminates mainly through bile as sulphates and conjugates. Silymarin has been shown to protect numerous preclinical models of liver diseases due to its antioxidative, anti-lipid peroxidative, antifibrotic, anti-inflammatory, membrane stabilizing, immunomodulatory, and liver regenerating properties [199]. Clinically, silymarin is found to be useful in alcoholic liver disease, liver cirrhosis, Amanita mushroom poisoning, viral hepatitis, toxic and drug induced liver diseases and in also diabetic patients [200–205]. The safety and efficacy of herbal medicines either as monotherapy or as an adjunct to conventional therapy for hepatotoxicity appears to be favorable, as indicated by many studies [206–209], thus the plant extract are believed to hold a promise in the management of APAP-associated hepatotoxicity. However, it is important to note that, very few of these plant extracts have been showed to attenuate necrotic or apoptotic cell death cascades but favorably modulate the antioxidant signaling pathways that are mediated by *Nrf2* and *Keap1*, along with modulation of different kinases viz. *JNK* and *MAPK*. Further, very few of them demonstrated the prevention of the metabolic activation of APAP by suppressing CYP2E1, a plausible mechanism believed to alter the bioactivation of APAP. In studies employing phytochemicals/plant extracts to investigate APAP-induced hepatotoxicity, very few studies have been compared with silymarin as a positive reference phytochemical for the comparative evaluation of hepatoprotective effects [205,210–212].

This may be attributed to the huge variation observed in the dose (25–200 mg/kg) and the dosing regimen (1–15 days) of silymarin treatment.

The model systems adapted to evaluate hapatoprotective agents whether it is in vitro or in vivo have its own merits and demerits; however the choice of model system selection mainly depends on the goals of the particular experimental paradigm. Several in vitro assays invovling cell lines and in vivo animal models have been developed to understand the pathogenesis of APAP-induced liver toxicity and to investigate the hepatoprotective agents. Recently, Kuo et al. (2016) have suggested that the natural antioxidants tested in non-suitable animal models may prove efficacious but it will impose ambiguity when these preclinical data are used as a baseline to design clinical studies. Thus, careful selection of suitable animal model is imperative to carry out well-defined preclinical studies. One such example is using rat as a model animal to evaluate APAP-induced hapatotoxicity, which is relatively resistant to APAP toxicity [26]; therefore, any data generated using this model system will impose inherent experimental bias. Many in vitro studies using phytochemicals/plant extracts to investigate the hapatoprotective effects have employed human hepatoma cell lines (e.g., HepG2, Hep3B, Huh7). These cell lines lack CYP enzymes, which are involved in the formation of hepatotoxic metabolites of APAP [213] therefore, such studies lose the clinical relevance due to the inherent variation of cellular physiologic and biochemical system. The CYP enzyme isoforms, mainly CYP2E1 is responsible for the bioactivation of AAP in humans and animals, which may represent a therapeutic target for APAP-induced hepatotoxicity.

Among the in vivo models, APAP-induced hepatotoxicity in mice is considered to be one of the best physiologically and clinically relevant model systems that represent the most of the pathophysiological features of APAP toxicity in humans. Whereas, among the in vitro models screening agents in primary mouse hepatocytes is considered to be closest to in vivo settings [214,215]. Additionally, the HepaRG cells also mimic the pathological changes similar to humans with APAP toxicity (except the requirement for JNK) [216,217]. Freshly isolated primary human hepatocytes are considered as gold standard for drug toxicity studies, including APAP-induced hepatotoxicity [218]. Jeschke and colleagues comprehensively reviewed the pathogenesis of APAP-induced toxicity and suggested that it is vital to choose a right animal species/in vitro system, timing/doses of APAP, as well as the assessments of signaling events, metabolic activation and protein adduct formation, the role of lipid peroxidation, and the apoptotic/necrotic cell death to elucidate hepatoprotective mechanisms and provide correct conclusion by avoiding the potential bias and pitfalls in the evaluation of hepatoprotectants [12,219].

The available literature reviewed herein reveal that a large number of plants and phytochemicals mediating antioxidant and anti-inflammatory properties appear hepatoprotective in preclinical models of APAP-induced liver injury. About five hundred plant extracts and fifty phytochemicals have shown to be hepatoprotective in preclinical studies with negligible clinical data. A vast majority of them have been shown to be hepatoprotective based on the biochemical, morphological, and histopathological assessments. All of them were shown to restore the liver enzymes and also protect liver cellular architecture. These plants and phytochemicals may provide novel chemical entities for future drug discovery and development against APAP-induced liver toxicity. Among many phytochemicals showed hepatoprotective against APAP few of them found to inhibit CYP2E1 that could be promising for further evaluation in APAP-induced liver toxicity. Despite a large number of plant extracts being demonstrated as hepatoprotective, the use of medicinal plants may have many issues, such as lack of standardization, quality control, heavy metal contamination, and presence of bacterial toxins.

Though, a large number of plant extracts and phytochemicals have been demonstrated hepatoprotective against APAP-induced liver toxicity, but those that shown hepatoprotective in numerous model systems and their effect on APAP bioactivation by inhibiting CYP2E1 has been demonstrated that could be promising to investigate further in detail. Although, the present preclinical data are markedly speculative for clinical usage, but it could be substantial for further evaluation of these plants and phytochemicals in clinical settings provided their human safety.

Table 5. The polyherbal or single herb formulations showed protective against APAP-induced liver toxicity.

S. No.	Polyherbal/Single HerbFormulation
1	999 Ganmaoling®
2	A formulation of *Andrographis paniculata, Tinospora cordifolia* and *Solanum nigrum*
3	A polyherbal formulation containing eight herbs; Vasaguduchyadi Kwatha®
4	A polyherbal formulation containing a mixture of leaves of *Gongronema latifolia, Ocimum gratissimum* and *Vernonia amygdalina*
5	A polyherbal formulation containing aqueous extracts of *Ocinnim larrilifolium, Crassocephaluin vitellitiurn, Guizotia scabra* and *Vernonia lasiopus*
6	A polyherbal formulation containing extracts of *Butea monosperma, Bauhinia variegata* and *Ocimum gratissimum*
7	A polyherbal formulation containing *Hydrocotyle asiatica, Tephrosia purpurea, Solanum nigrum, Citrullus colocynthis, Momordica charantia*
8	A polyherbal formulation HP-4® is a combination of 80% alcoholic extract of leaves of *Aloe vera, Bacopa monniera, Moringa oleifera* and rhizome of *Zingiber officinale*
9	A polyherbal formulation, HD-03®
10	A polyherbal formulations containing five bioactive fractionated extracts of *Butea monosperma, Bauhinia variegata* and *Ocimum gratissimum*
11	A polyherbal formulation containing extracts of *Andrographis paniculata* Nees., *Phyllanthus niruri* Linn., *Phyllanthus emblica* Linn.
12	A polyherbal mixture of *Tinospora cordifolia, Boerhavia diffusa, Phyllanthus amaraus, Euphorbia hirta, Wedelia chinensis*
13	A polyherbal Siddha formulation, Karisalai Karpam®
14	A polyherbal Siddha medicine, Amukkara chooranam®
15	Ban-zhi-lian
16	Bazhen decoction
17	Biherbal formulations of *Aerva lanata* and *Achyranthes aspera*
18	Chai-Hu-Ching-Kan-Tang®
19	D-003®
20	DA-9601®, a quality-controlled extract of *Artemisia asiatica*
21	Fengxiang Yigankang®
22	Fourteen vitex honeys
23	Gn-3®, a stilbene polymer isolated from *Gnetum parvifolium*
24	Habb-e-Asgand®, polyherbal Unani formulation
25	Hepax®, a polyherbal formulation
26	Himoliv®, a polyherbal formulation
27	Huanglian-Jie-Du-Tang®
28	Hwang-hua-mih-tsay (*Wedelia chinensis*)
29	IH636 grape seed extract
30	Karisalai Karpam tablet®
31	Kava herbal dietary supplements
32	Liu weiwuling Tablets®
33	Livartho®, a polyherbal formulations consist of 10 active constituents of medicinal plants viz, *Andrographis paniculata, Cichorium intybus, Tephrosia purpurea, Solanum nigrum, Phyllanthus amarus, Tinospora cordifolia, Eclipta alba, Berberis aristata, Piper longum* and *Emblica officinalis*
34	Livina®, a polyherbal formulation
35	Majoon -e-Dabeed-ul-Ward
36	MAP, a Standardized Herbal Composition, Blend Comprising *Myristica fragrans, Astragalus membranaceus* and *Poriacocos*
37	Picroliv®
38	Polyherbal ayurvedic formulations, Liv 52®, Livergen®, Livokin®, Octogen®, Stimuliv®, Triphala® and Tefroliv®, Tritone® (Livosone)
39	Shekwasha®
40	Somanathitamrabhasma®, a tamra bhasma preparation containing shudhatamra, parada, gandhaka, haritala and manashila
41	'Teng-khia-u'
42	Yang-Gan-Wan

Funding: The research work in the authors laboratory are supported by intramural grants from College of Medicine and Health Sciences, United Arab Emirates University, United Arab Emirates.

Conflicts of Interest: The other authors declare no conflict of interest.

References

1. Thomas, S.H. Paracetamol (acetaminophen) poisoning. *Pharmacol. Ther.* **1993**, *60*, 91–120. [CrossRef]
2. Nelson, S.D. Molecular mechanisms of the hepatotoxicity caused by acetaminophen. *Semin. Liver Dis.* **1990**, *10*, 267–278. [CrossRef] [PubMed]
3. Bessems, J.G.; Vermeulen, N.P. Paracetamol (acetaminophen)-induced toxicity: Molecular and biochemical mechanisms, analogues and protective approaches. *Crit. Rev. Toxicol.* **2001**, *31*, 55–138. [CrossRef] [PubMed]
4. Cohen, S.D.; Khairallah, E.A. Selective protein arylation and acetaminophen-induced hepatotoxicity. *Drug Metab. Rev.* **1997**, *29*, 59–77. [CrossRef] [PubMed]
5. Jaeschke, H.; McGill, M.R.; Ramachandran, A. Oxidant stress, mitochondria, and cell death mechanisms in drug-induced liver injury: Lessons learned from acetaminophen hepatotoxicity. *Drug Metab. Rev.* **2012**, *44*, 88–106. [CrossRef] [PubMed]
6. McGill, M.R.; Jaeschke, H. Metabolism and disposition of acetaminophen: Recent advances in relation to hepatotoxicity and diagnosis. *Pharm. Res.* **2013**, *30*, 2174–2187. [CrossRef] [PubMed]
7. Han, D.; Dara, L.; Win, S.; Than, T.A.; Yuan, L.; Abbasi, S.Q.; Liu, Z.X.; Kaplowitz, N. Regulation of drug-induced liver injury by signal transduction pathways: Critical role of mitochondria. *Trends Pharmacol. Sci.* **2013**, *34*, 243–253. [CrossRef] [PubMed]
8. Hanawa, N.; Shinohara, M.; Saberi, B.; Gaarde, W.A.; Han, D.; Kaplowitz, N. Role of JNK translocation to mitochondria leading to inhibition of mitochondria bioenergetics in acetaminophen-induced liver injury. *J. Biol. Chem.* **2008**, *283*, 13565–13577. [CrossRef] [PubMed]
9. Saito, C.; Lemasters, J.J.; Jaeschke, H. c-Jun N-terminal kinase modulates oxidant stress and peroxynitrite formation independent of inducible nitric oxide synthase in acetaminophen hepatotoxicity. *Toxicol. Appl. Pharmacol.* **2010**, *246*, 8–17. [CrossRef] [PubMed]
10. Kon, K.; Kim, J.S.; Jaeschke, H.; Lemasters, J.J. Mitochondrial permeability transition in acetaminophen-induced necrosis and apoptosis of cultured mouse hepatocytes. *Hepatology* **2004**, *40*, 1170–1179. [CrossRef] [PubMed]
11. Cover, C.; Mansouri, A.; Knight, T.R.; Bajt, M.L.; Lemasters, J.J.; Pessayre, D.; Jaeschke, H. Peroxynitrite-induced mitochondrial and endonuclease-mediated nuclear DNA damage in acetaminophen hepatotoxicity. *J. Pharmacol. Exp. Ther.* **2005**, *315*, 879–887. [CrossRef] [PubMed]
12. Bajt, M.L.; Cover, C.; Lemasters, J.J.; Jaeschke, H. Nuclear translocation of endonuclease G and apoptosis-inducing factor during acetaminophen-induced liver cell injury. *Toxicol. Sci.* **2006**, *94*, 217–225. [CrossRef] [PubMed]
13. Gujral, J.S.; Knight, T.R.; Farhood, A.; Bajt, M.L.; Jaeschke, H. Mode of cell death after acetaminophen overdose in mice: Apoptosis or oncotic necrosis? *Toxicol. Sci.* **2002**, *67*, 322–328. [CrossRef] [PubMed]
14. Gonzalez, F.J. Role of cytochromes P450 in chemical toxicity and oxidative stress: Studies with CYP2E1. *Mutat. Res.* **2005**, *569*, 101–110. [CrossRef] [PubMed]
15. Jollow, D.J.; Mitchell, J.R.; Potter, W.Z.; Davis, D.C.; Gillette, J.R.; Brodie, B.B. Acetaminophen-induced hepatic necrosis. II. Role of covalent binding in vivo. *J. Pharmacol. Exp. Ther.* **1973**, *187*, 195–202. [PubMed]
16. Raucy, J.L.; Lasker, J.M.; Lieber, C.S.; Black, M. Acetaminophen activation by human liver cytochromes P450IIE1 and P450IA2. *Arch. Biochem. Biophys.* **1989**, *271*, 270–283. [CrossRef]
17. Laine, J.E.; Auriola, S.; Pasanen, M.; Juvonen, R.O. Acetaminophen bioactivation by human cytochrome P450 enzymes and animal microsomes. *Xenobiotica* **2009**, *39*, 11–21. [CrossRef] [PubMed]
18. Lin, M.C.; Wang, E.J.; Patten, C.; Lee, M.J.; Xiao, F.; Reuhl, K.R.; Yang, C.S. Protective effect of diallyl sulfone against acetaminophen-induced hepatotoxicity in mice. *J. Biochem. Toxicol.* **1996**, *11*, 11–20. [CrossRef]
19. Das, J.; Ghosh, J.; Manna, P.; Sil, P.C. Taurine protects acetaminophen-induced oxidative damage in mice kidney through APAP urinary excretion and CYP2E1 inactivation. *Toxicology* **2010**, *269*, 24–34. [CrossRef] [PubMed]
20. Polson, J.; Lee, W.M. AASLD position paper: The management of acute liver failure. *Hepatology* **2005**, *41*, 1179–1197. [CrossRef] [PubMed]

21. Smilkstein, M.J.; Knapp, G.L.; Kulig, K.W.; Rumack, B.H. Efficacy of oral N-acetylcysteine in the treatment of acetaminophen overdose. Analysis of the national multicenter study (1976 to 1985). *N. Engl. J. Med.* **1988**, *319*, 1557–1562. [CrossRef] [PubMed]
22. Casas-Grajales, S.; Muriel, P. Antioxidants in liver health. *World J. Gastrointest. Pharmacol. Ther.* **2015**, *6*, 59–72. [CrossRef] [PubMed]
23. Madrigal-Santillan, E.; Madrigal-Bujaidar, E.; Alvarez-Gonzalez, I.; Sumaya-Martinez, M.T.; Gutierrez-Salinas, J.; Bautista, M.; Morales-Gonzalez, A.; Garcia-Luna y Gonzalez-Rubio, M.; Aguilar-Faisal, J.L.; Morales-Gonzalez, J.A. Review of natural products with hepatoprotective effects. *World J. Gastroenterol.* **2014**, *20*, 14787–14804. [CrossRef] [PubMed]
24. Thomson, J.S.; Prescott, L.F. Liver damage and impaired glucose tolerance after paracetamol overdosage. *Br. Med. J.* **1966**, *2*, 506–507. [CrossRef] [PubMed]
25. Mitchell, J.R.; Jollow, D.J.; Potter, W.Z.; Davis, D.C.; Gillette, J.R.; Brodie, B.B. Acetaminophen-induced hepatic necrosis. I. Role of drug metabolism. *J. Pharmacol. Exp. Ther.* **1973**, *187*, 185–194. [PubMed]
26. Du, K.; Ramachandran, A.; Jaeschke, H. Oxidative stress during acetaminophen hepatotoxicity: Sources, pathophysiological role and therapeutic potential. *Redox Biol.* **2016**, *10*, 148–156. [CrossRef] [PubMed]
27. Wu, Y.L.; Jiang, Y.Z.; Jin, X.J.; Lian, L.H.; Piao, J.Y.; Wan, Y.; Jin, H.R.; Joon Lee, J.; Nan, J.X. Acanthoic acid, a diterpene in Acanthopanax koreanum, protects acetaminophen-induced hepatic toxicity in mice. *Phytomedicine* **2010**, *17*, 475–479. [CrossRef] [PubMed]
28. Nan, J.X.; Jin, X.J.; Lian, L.H.; Cai, X.F.; Jiang, Y.Z.; Jin, H.R.; Lee, J.J. A diterpenoid acanthoic acid from Acanthopanax koreanum protects against D-galactosamine/lipopolysaccharide-induced fulminant hepatic failure in mice. *Biol. Pharm. Bull.* **2008**, *31*, 738–742. [CrossRef] [PubMed]
29. Kaschula, C.H.; Hunter, R.; Stellenboom, N.; Caira, M.R.; Winks, S.; Ogunleye, T.; Richards, P.; Cotton, J.; Zilbeyaz, K.; Wang, Y.; et al. Structure-activity studies on the anti-proliferation activity of ajoene analogues in WHCO1 oesophageal cancer cells. *Eur. J. Med. Chem.* **2012**, *50*, 236–254. [CrossRef] [PubMed]
30. Hattori, A.; Yamada, N.; Nishikawa, T.; Fukuda, H.; Fujino, T. Protective effect of ajoene on acetaminophen-induced hepatic injury in mice. *Biosci. Biotechnol. Biochem.* **2001**, *65*, 2555–2557. [CrossRef] [PubMed]
31. Liu, J.; Liu, Y.; Mao, Q.; Klaassen, C.D. The effects of 10 triterpenoid compounds on experimental liver injury in mice. *Toxicol. Sci.* **1994**, *22*, 34–40. [CrossRef]
32. Oliveira, F.A.; Chaves, M.H.; Almeida, F.R.; Lima, R.C., Jr.; Silva, R.M.; Maia, J.L.; Brito, G.A.; Santos, F.A.; Rao, V.S. Protective effect of alpha- and beta-amyrin, a triterpene mixture from Protium heptaphyllum (Aubl.) March. trunk wood resin, against acetaminophen-induced liver injury in mice. *J. Ethnopharmacol.* **2005**, *98*, 103–108. [CrossRef] [PubMed]
33. Handa, S.S.; Sharma, A. Hepatoprotective activity of andrographolide against galactosamine & paracetamol intoxication in rats. *Indian J. Med. Res.* **1990**, *92*, 284–292. [PubMed]
34. Visen, P.K.; Shukla, B.; Patnaik, G.K.; Dhawan, B.N. Andrographolide protects rat hepatocytes against paracetamol-induced damage. *J. Ethnopharmacol.* **1993**, *40*, 131–136. [CrossRef]
35. Roy, P.; Das, S.; Auddy, R.G.; Saha, A.; Mukherjee, A. Engineered andrographolide nanoparticles mitigate paracetamol hepatotoxicity in mice. *Pharm. Res.* **2013**, *30*, 1252–1262. [CrossRef] [PubMed]
36. Ali, B.H.; Mousa, H.M.; El-Mougy, S. The effect of a water extract and anthocyanins of hibiscus sabdariffa L on paracetamol-induced hepatoxicity in rats. *Phytother. Res.* **2003**, *17*, 56–59. [CrossRef] [PubMed]
37. Choi, J.H.; Choi, C.Y.; Lee, K.J.; Hwang, Y.P.; Chung, Y.C.; Jeong, H.G. Hepatoprotective effects of an anthocyanin fraction from purple-fleshed sweet potato against acetaminophen-induced liver damage in mice. *J. Med. Food* **2009**, *12*, 320–326. [CrossRef] [PubMed]
38. Wang, W.; Li, J.; Wang, Z.; Gao, H.; Su, L.; Xie, J.; Chen, X.; Liang, H.; Wang, C.; Han, Y. Oral hepatoprotective ability evaluation of purple sweet potato anthocyanins on acute and chronic chemical liver injuries. *Cell. Biochem. Biophys.* **2014**, *69*, 539–548. [CrossRef] [PubMed]
39. Yang, J.; Wang, X.Y.; Xue, J.; Gu, Z.L.; Xie, M.L. Protective effect of apigenin on mouse acute liver injury induced by acetaminophen is associated with increment of hepatic glutathione reductase activity. *Food Funct.* **2013**, *4*, 939–943. [CrossRef] [PubMed]
40. Manna, P.; Sinha, M.; Pal, P.; Sil, P.C. Arjunolic acid, a triterpenoid saponin, ameliorates arsenic-induced cyto-toxicity in hepatocytes. *Chem. Biol. Interact.* **2007**, *170*, 187–200. [CrossRef] [PubMed]

41. Ghosh, J.; Das, J.; Manna, P.; Sil, P.C. Arjunolic acid, a triterpenoid saponin, prevents acetaminophen (APAP)-induced liver and hepatocyte injury via the inhibition of APAP bioactivation and JNK-mediated mitochondrial protection. *Free Radic. Biol. Med.* **2010**, *48*, 535–553. [CrossRef] [PubMed]
42. Janbaz, K.H.; Gilani, A.H. Studies on preventive and curative effects of berberine on chemical-induced hepatotoxicity in rodents. *Fitoterapia* **2000**, *71*, 25–33. [CrossRef]
43. Vivoli, E.; Cappon, A.; Milani, S.; Piombanti, B.; Provenzano, A.; Novo, E.; Masi, A.; Navari, N.; Narducci, R.; Mannaioni, G.; et al. NLRP3 inflammasome as a target of berberine in experimental murine liver injury: Interference with $P2X_7$ signalling. *Clin. Sci.* **2016**, *130*, 1793–1806. [CrossRef] [PubMed]
44. Rao, M.P.; Manjunath, K.; Bhagawati, S.T.; Thippeswamy, B.S. Bixin loaded solid lipid nanoparticles for enhanced hepatoprotection—Preparation, characterisation and in vivo evaluation. *Int. J. Pharm.* **2014**, *473*, 485–492. [CrossRef] [PubMed]
45. Chen, L.C.; Hu, L.H.; Yin, M.C. Alleviative effects from boswellic acid on acetaminophen-induced hepatic injury. *Biomedicine* **2016**, *6*, 9. [CrossRef] [PubMed]
46. Olayanju, A.; Copple, I.M.; Bryan, H.K.; Edge, G.T.; Sison, R.L.; Wong, M.W.; Lai, Z.Q.; Lin, Z.X.; Dunn, K.; Sanderson, C.M.; et al. Brusatol provokes a rapid and transient inhibition of Nrf2 signaling and sensitizes mammalian cells to chemical toxicity-implications for therapeutic targeting of Nrf2. *Free Radic. Biol. Med.* **2015**, *78*, 202–212. [CrossRef] [PubMed]
47. Janbaz, K.H.; Saeed, S.A.; Gilani, A.H. Studies on the protective effects of caffeic acid and quercetin on chemical-induced hepatotoxicity in rodents. *Phytomedicine* **2004**, *11*, 424–430. [CrossRef] [PubMed]
48. Pang, C.; Zheng, Z.; Shi, L.; Sheng, Y.; Wei, H.; Wang, Z.; Ji, L. Caffeic acid prevents acetaminophen-induced liver injury by activating the Keap1-Nrf2 antioxidative defense system. *Free Radic. Biol. Med.* **2016**, *91*, 236–246. [CrossRef] [PubMed]
49. Pang, C.; Shi, L.; Sheng, Y.; Zheng, Z.; Wei, H.; Wang, Z.; Ji, L. Caffeic acid attenuated acetaminophen-induced hepatotoxicity by inhibiting ERK1/2-mediated early growth response-1 transcriptional activation. *Chem. Biol. Interact.* **2016**, *260*, 186–195. [CrossRef] [PubMed]
50. Hao, Z.Y.; Liang, D.; Luo, H.; Liu, Y.F.; Ni, G.; Zhang, Q.J.; Li, L.; Si, Y.K.; Sun, H.; Chen, R.Y.; et al. Bioactive sesquiterpenoids from the rhizomes of Acorus calamus. *J. Nat. Prod.* **2012**, *75*, 1083–1089. [CrossRef] [PubMed]
51. Guo, Q.; Shen, Z.; Yu, H.; Lu, G.; Yu, Y.; Liu, X.; Zheng, P. Carnosic acid protects against acetaminophen-induced hepatotoxicity by potentiating Nrf2-mediated antioxidant capacity in mice. *Korean J. Physiol. Pharmacol.* **2016**, *20*, 15–23. [CrossRef] [PubMed]
52. Dickmann, L.J.; VandenBrink, B.M.; Lin, Y.S. In vitro hepatotoxicity and cytochrome P450 induction and inhibition characteristics of carnosic acid, a dietary supplement with antiadipogenic properties. *Drug Metab. Dispos.* **2012**, *40*, 1263–1267. [CrossRef] [PubMed]
53. Zheng, Z.; Sheng, Y.; Lu, B.; Ji, L. The therapeutic detoxification of chlorogenic acid against acetaminophen-induced liver injury by ameliorating hepatic inflammation. *Chem. Biol. Interact.* **2015**, *238*, 93–101. [CrossRef] [PubMed]
54. Pang, C.; Sheng, Y.C.; Jiang, P.; Wei, H.; Ji, L.L. Chlorogenic acid prevents acetaminophen-induced liver injury: The involvement of CYP450 metabolic enzymes and some antioxidant signals. *J. Zhejiang Univ. Sci. B* **2015**, *16*, 602–610. [CrossRef] [PubMed]
55. Eaton, E.A.; Walle, U.K.; Lewis, A.J.; Hudson, T.; Wilson, A.A.; Walle, T. Flavonoids, potent inhibitors of the human P-form phenolsulfotransferase. Potential role in drug metabolism and chemoprevention. *Drug Metab. Dispos.* **1996**, *24*, 232–237. [PubMed]
56. Morimitsu, Y.; Sugihara, N.; Furuno, K. Inhibitory effect of flavonoids on sulfo- and glucurono-conjugation of acetaminophen in rat cultured hepatocytes and liver subcellular preparations. *Biol. Pharm. Bull.* **2004**, *27*, 714–717. [CrossRef] [PubMed]
57. Pingili, R.B.; Pawar, A.K.; Challa, S.R. Systemic exposure of Paracetamol (acetaminophen) was enhanced by quercetin and chrysin co-administration in Wistar rats and in vitro model: Risk of liver toxicity. *Drug Dev. Ind. Pharm.* **2015**, *41*, 1793–1800. [CrossRef] [PubMed]
58. Wei, H.L.; Liu, G.T. Protective action of corynoline, acetylcorynoline and protopine against experimental liver injury in mice. *Yao Xue Xue Bao* **1997**, *32*, 331–336. [PubMed]

59. Janbaz, K.H.; Saeed, S.A.; Gilani, A.H. An assessment of the potential of protopine to inhibit microsomal drug metabolising enzymes and prevent chemical-induced hepatotoxicity in rodents. *Pharmacol. Res.* **1998**, *38*, 215–219. [CrossRef] [PubMed]
60. Donatus, I.A.; Sardjoko; Vermeulen, N.P. Cytotoxic and cytoprotective activities of curcumin. Effects on paracetamol-induced cytotoxicity, lipid peroxidation and glutathione depletion in rat hepatocytes. *Biochem. Pharmacol.* **1990**, *39*, 1869–1875. [CrossRef]
61. Kheradpezhouh, E.; Panjehshahin, M.R.; Miri, R.; Javidnia, K.; Noorafshan, A.; Monabati, A.; Dehpour, A.R. Curcumin protects rats against acetaminophen-induced hepatorenal damages and shows synergistic activity with N.-acetyl cysteine. *Eur. J. Pharmacol.* **2010**, *628*, 274–281. [CrossRef] [PubMed]
62. Yousef, M.I.; Omar, S.A.; El-Guendi, M.I.; Abdelmegid, L.A. Potential protective effects of quercetin and curcumin on paracetamol-induced histological changes, oxidative stress, impaired liver and kidney functions and haematotoxicity in rat. *Food Chem. Toxicol.* **2010**, *48*, 3246–3261. [CrossRef] [PubMed]
63. Bulku, E.; Stohs, S.J.; Cicero, L.; Brooks, T.; Halley, H.; Ray, S.D. Curcumin exposure modulates multiple pro-apoptotic and anti-apoptotic signaling pathways to antagonize acetaminophen-induced toxicity. *Curr. Neurovasc. Res.* **2012**, *9*, 58–71. [CrossRef] [PubMed]
64. Somanawat, K.; Thong-Ngam, D.; Klaikeaw, N. Curcumin attenuated paracetamol overdose induced hepatitis. *World J. Gastroenterol.* **2013**, *19*, 1962–1967. [CrossRef] [PubMed]
65. Li, G.; Chen, J.B.; Wang, C.; Xu, Z.; Nie, H.; Qin, X.Y.; Chen, X.M.; Gong, Q. Curcumin protects against acetaminophen-induced apoptosis in hepatic injury. *World J. Gastroenterol.* **2013**, *19*, 7440–7446. [CrossRef] [PubMed]
66. Soliman, M.M.; Abdo Nassan, M.; Ismail, T.A. Immunohistochemical and molecular study on the protective effect of curcumin against hepatic toxicity induced by paracetamol in Wistar rats. *BMC Complement. Altern. Med.* **2014**, *14*, 457. [CrossRef] [PubMed]
67. Hu, J.J.; Yoo, J.S.; Lin, M.; Wang, E.J.; Yang, C.S. Protective effects of diallyl sulfide on acetaminophen-induced toxicities. *Food Chem. Toxicol.* **1996**, *34*, 963–969. [CrossRef]
68. Wang, E.J.; Li, Y.; Lin, M.; Chen, L.; Stein, A.P.; Reuhl, K.R.; Yang, C.S. Protective effects of garlic and related organosulfur compounds on acetaminophen-induced hepatotoxicity in mice. *Toxicol. Appl. Pharmacol.* **1996**, *136*, 146–154. [CrossRef] [PubMed]
69. Yang, C.S.; Chhabra, S.K.; Hong, J.Y.; Smith, T.J. Mechanisms of inhibition of chemical toxicity and carcinogenesis by diallyl sulfide (DAS) and related compounds from garlic. *J. Nutr.* **2001**, *131*, 1041S–1045S. [CrossRef] [PubMed]
70. Zhao, X.; Cong, X.; Zheng, L.; Xu, L.; Yin, L.; Peng, J. Dioscin, a natural steroid saponin, shows remarkable protective effect against acetaminophen-induced liver damage in vitro and in vivo. *Toxicol. Lett.* **2012**, *214*, 69–80. [CrossRef] [PubMed]
71. Lahouel, M.; Boulkour, S.; Segueni, N.; Fillastre, J.P. The flavonoids effect against vinblastine, cyclophosphamide and paracetamol toxicity by inhibition of lipid-peroxydation and increasing liver glutathione concentration. *Pathol. Biol.* **2004**, *52*, 314–322. [CrossRef] [PubMed]
72. Yao, H.T.; Yang, Y.C.; Chang, C.H.; Yang, H.T.; Yin, M.C. Protective effects of (-)-epigallocatechin-3-gallate against acetaminophen-induced liver injury in rats. *Biomedicine* **2015**, *5*, 15. [CrossRef] [PubMed]
73. Gilani, A.H.; Janbaz, K.H.; Shah, B.H. Esculetin prevents liver damage induced by paracetamol and CCL4. *Pharmacol. Res.* **1998**, *37*, 31–35. [CrossRef] [PubMed]
74. Wang, H.; Peng, R.X. Sodium ferulate alleviated paracetamol-induced liver toxicity in mice. *Zhongguo Yao Li Xue Bao* **1994**, *15*, 81–83. [PubMed]
75. Yuan, J.; Ge, K.; Mu, J.; Rong, J.; Zhang, L.; Wang, B.; Wan, J.; Xia, G. Ferulic acid attenuated acetaminophen-induced hepatotoxicity though down-regulating the cytochrome P 2E1 and inhibiting toll-like receptor 4 signaling-mediated inflammation in mice. *Am. J. Transl. Res.* **2016**, *8*, 4205–4214. [PubMed]
76. Liu, Y.P.; Liu, J.; Jia, X.S.; Mao, Q.; Madhu, C.; Klaassen, C.D. Protective effects of fulvotomentosides on acetaminophen-induced hepatotoxicity. *Zhongguo Yao Li Xue Bao* **1992**, *13*, 209–212. [PubMed]
77. Liu, J.; Liu, Y.; Klaassen, C.D. The effect of Chinese hepatoprotective medicines on experimental liver injury in mice. *J. Ethnopharmacol.* **1994**, *42*, 183–191. [PubMed]
78. Shi, J.Z.; Liu, G.T. Protective effect of the fulvotomentosides on paracetamol-induced hepatotoxicity in mice. *Yao Xue Xue Bao* **1995**, *30*, 311–314. [PubMed]

79. Tsai, M.S.; Chien, C.C.; Lin, T.H.; Liu, C.C.; Liu, R.H.; Su, H.L.; Chiu, Y.T.; Wang, S.H. Galangin Prevents Acute Hepatorenal Toxicity in Novel Propacetamol-Induced Acetaminophen-Overdosed Mice. *J. Med. Food* **2015**, *18*, 1187–1197. [CrossRef] [PubMed]
80. Rasool, M.K.; Sabina, E.P.; Ramya, S.R.; Preety, P.; Patel, S.; Mandal, N.; Mishra, P.P.; Samuel, J. Hepatoprotective and antioxidant effects of gallic acid in paracetamol-induced liver damage in mice. *J. Pharm. Pharmacol.* **2010**, *62*, 638–643. [CrossRef] [PubMed]
81. Fan, Y.J.; Rong, Y.; Li, P.F.; Dong, W.L.; Zhang, D.Y.; Zhang, L.; Cui, M.J. Genistein protection against acetaminophen-induced liver injury via its potential impact on the activation of UDP-glucuronosyltransferase and antioxidant enzymes. *Food Chem. Toxicol.* **2013**, *55*, 172–181. [CrossRef] [PubMed]
82. Hu, M.; Krausz, K.; Chen, J.; Ge, X.; Li, J.; Gelboin, H.L.; Gonzalez, F.J. Identification of CYP1A2 as the main isoform for the phase I hydroxylated metabolism of genistein and a prodrug converting enzyme of methylated isoflavones. *Drug Metab. Dispos.* **2003**, *31*, 924–931. [CrossRef] [PubMed]
83. Lucas, A.N.; Nation, R.L.; Milne, R.W.; Reynolds, G.D.; Evans, A.M. The effects of phytoestrogenic isoflavones on the formation and disposition of paracetamol sulfate in the isolated perfused rat liver. *J. Pharm. Pharmacol.* **2003**, *55*, 639–646. [CrossRef] [PubMed]
84. Fan, Y.; Wei, W.; Luo, J.; Jin, Y.; Dai, Z. Genistein promotes the metabolic transformation of acetaminophen to glucuronic acid in human L-O2, HepG2 and Hep3b cells via the Nrf2/Keap1 pathway. *Food Funct.* **2016**, *7*, 4683–4692.
85. Nishida, T.; Matsura, T.; Nakada, J.; Togawa, A.; Kai, M.; Sumioka, I.; Minami, Y.; Inagaki, Y.; Ishibe, Y.; Ito, H.; et al. Geranylgeranylacetone protects against acetaminophen-induced hepatotoxicity by inducing heat shock protein 70. *Toxicology* **2006**, *219*, 187–196. [CrossRef] [PubMed]
86. Sabina, E.P.; Pragasam, S.J.; Kumar, S.; Rasool, M. 6-gingerol, an active ingredient of ginger, protects acetaminophen-induced hepatotoxicity in mice. *Zhong Xi Yi Jie He Xue Bao* **2011**, *9*, 1264–1269. [CrossRef] [PubMed]
87. Rajaraman, G.; Chen, J.; Chang, T.K. Ginkgolide A contributes to the potentiation of acetaminophen toxicity by Ginkgo biloba extract in primary cultures of rat hepatocytes. *Toxicol. Appl. Pharmacol.* **2006**, *217*, 225–233. [CrossRef] [PubMed]
88. Moon, A.; Kim, S.H. Effect of Glycyrrhiza glabra roots and glycyrrhizin on the glucuronidation in rats. *Planta Med.* **1997**, *63*, 115–119. [CrossRef] [PubMed]
89. Lin, C.C.; Shieh, D.E.; Yen, M.H. Hepatoprotective effect of the fractions of Ban-zhi-lian on experimental liver injuries in rats. *J. Ethnopharmacol.* **1997**, *56*, 193–200. [CrossRef]
90. Yang, H.; Jiang, T.; Li, P.; Mao, Q. The protection of glycyrrhetinic acid (GA) towards acetaminophen (APAP)-induced toxicity partially through fatty acids metabolic pathway. *Afr. Health Sci.* **2015**, *15*, 1023–1027. [CrossRef] [PubMed]
91. Wan, X.Y.; Luo, M.; Li, X.D.; He, P. Hepatoprotective and anti-hepatocarcinogenic effects of glycyrrhizin and matrine. *Chem. Biol. Interact.* **2009**, *181*, 15–19. [CrossRef] [PubMed]
92. Yamada, S.; Murawaki, Y.; Kawasaki, H. Preventive effect of gomisin A, a lignan component of shizandra fruits, on acetaminophen-induced hepatotoxicity in rats. *Biochem. Pharmacol.* **1993**, *46*, 1081–1085. [CrossRef]
93. Shiota, G.; Yamada, S.; Kawasaki, H. Rapid induction of hepatocyte growth factor mRNA after administration of gomisin A, a lignan component of shizandra fruits. *Res. Commun. Mol. Pathol. Pharmacol.* **1996**, *94*, 141–146. [PubMed]
94. Li, C.J.; Ma, J.; Sun, H.; Zhang, D.; Zhang, D.M. Guajavadimer A, a Dimeric Caryophyllene-Derived Meroterpenoid with a New Carbon Skeleton from the Leaves of Psidium guajava. *Org. Lett.* **2016**, *18*, 168–171. [CrossRef] [PubMed]
95. Ahmad, S.T.; Arjumand, W.; Nafees, S.; Seth, A.; Ali, N.; Rashid, S.; Sultana, S. Hesperidin alleviates acetaminophen induced toxicity in Wistar rats by abrogation of oxidative stress, apoptosis and inflammation. *Toxicol. Lett.* **2012**, *208*, 149–161. [CrossRef] [PubMed]
96. Akinmoladun, A.C.; Olaleye, M.T.; Komolafe, K.; Adetuyi, A.O.; Akindahunsi, A.A. Effect of homopterocarpin, an isoflavonoid from Pterocarpus erinaceus, on indices of liver injury and oxidative stress in acetaminophen-provoked hepatotoxicity. *J. Basic Clin. Physiol. Pharmacol.* **2015**, *26*, 555–562. [CrossRef] [PubMed]

97. Xie, W.; Jiang, Z.; Wang, J.; Zhang, X.; Melzig, M.F. Protective effect of hyperoside against acetaminophen (APAP) induced liver injury through enhancement of APAP clearance. *Chem. Biol. Interact.* **2016**, *246*, 11–19. [CrossRef] [PubMed]
98. Xie, W.; Wang, M.; Chen, C.; Zhang, X.; Melzig, M.F. Hepatoprotective effect of isoquercitrin against acetaminophen-induced liver injury. *Life Sci.* **2016**, *152*, 180–189. [CrossRef] [PubMed]
99. Xue, H.; Xie, W.; Jiang, Z.; Wang, M.; Wang, J.; Zhao, H.; Zhang, X. 3,4-Dihydroxyphenylacetic acid, a microbiota-derived metabolite of quercetin, attenuates acetaminophen (APAP)-induced liver injury through activation of Nrf-2. *Xenobiotica* **2016**, *46*, 931–939. [CrossRef] [PubMed]
100. Kupeli, E.; Orhan, D.D.; Yesilada, E. Effect of Cistus laurifolius L. leaf extracts and flavonoids on acetaminophen-induced hepatotoxicity in mice. *J. Ethnopharmacol.* **2006**, *103*, 455–460. [CrossRef] [PubMed]
101. Hawas, U.W.; Soliman, G.M.; Abou El-Kassem, L.T.; Farrag, A.R.; Mahmoud, K.; Leon, F. A new flavonoid C-glycoside from Solanum elaeagnifolium with hepatoprotective and curative activities against paracetamol-induced liver injury in mice. *Z. Naturforsch. C* **2013**, *68*, 19–28. [PubMed]
102. Ajiboye, T.O. Lophirones B and C Attenuate Acetaminophen-Induced Liver Damage in Mice: Studies on Hepatic, Oxidative Stress and Inflammatory Biomarkers. *J. Biochem. Mol. Toxicol.* **2016**, *30*, 497–505. [CrossRef] [PubMed]
103. Kumari, A.; Kakkar, P. Lupeol protects against acetaminophen-induced oxidative stress and cell death in rat primary hepatocytes. *Food Chem. Toxicol.* **2012**, *50*, 1781–1789. [CrossRef] [PubMed]
104. Tai, M.; Zhang, J.; Song, S.; Miao, R.; Liu, S.; Pang, Q.; Wu, Q.; Liu, C. Protective effects of luteolin against acetaminophen-induced acute liver failure in mouse. *Int. Immunopharmacol.* **2015**, *27*, 164–170. [CrossRef] [PubMed]
105. Abou El-Kassem, L.T.; Mohammed, R.S.; El Souda, S.S.; El-Anssary, A.A.; Hawas, U.W.; Mohmoud, K.; Farrag, A.R. Digalacturonide flavones from Egyptian Lantana camara flowers with in vitro antioxidant and in vivo hepatoprotective activities. *Z. Naturforsch. C* **2012**, *67*, 381–390. [CrossRef] [PubMed]
106. Tien, Y.H.; Chen, B.H.; Wang Hsu, G.S.; Lin, W.T.; Huang, J.H.; Lu, Y.F. Hepatoprotective and anti-oxidant activities of Glossogyne tenuifolia against acetaminophen-induced hepatotoxicity in mice. *Am. J. Chin. Med.* **2014**, *42*, 1385–1398. [CrossRef] [PubMed]
107. Chen, Y.H.; Lin, F.Y.; Liu, P.L.; Huang, Y.T.; Chiu, J.H.; Chang, Y.C.; Man, K.M.; Hong, C.Y.; Ho, Y.Y.; Lai, M.T. Antioxidative and hepatoprotective effects of magnolol on acetaminophen-induced liver damage in rats. *Arch. Pharm. Res.* **2009**, *32*, 221–228. [CrossRef] [PubMed]
108. Firdous, A.P.; Sindhu, E.R.; Kuttan, R. Hepato-protective potential of carotenoid meso-zeaxanthin against paracetamol, CCl4 and ethanol induced toxicity. *Indian J. Exp. Biol.* **2011**, *49*, 44–49. [PubMed]
109. Liu, W.X.; Jia, F.L.; He, Y.Y.; Zhang, B.X. Protective effects of 5-methoxypsoralen against acetaminophen-induced hepatotoxicity in mice. *World J. Gastroenterol.* **2012**, *18*, 2197–2202. [CrossRef] [PubMed]
110. Bohlooli, S.; Mohammadi, S.; Amirshahrokhi, K.; Mirzanejad-Asl, H.; Yosefi, M.; Mohammadi-Nei, A.; Chinifroush, M.M. Effect of Methylsulfonylmethane Pretreatment on Aceta-minophen Induced Hepatotoxicity in Rats. *Iran. J. Basic Med. Sci.* **2013**, *16*, 896–900. [PubMed]
111. Rizvi, F.; Mathur, A.; Kakkar, P. Morin mitigates acetaminophen-induced liver injury by potentiating Nrf2 regulated survival mechanism through molecular intervention in PHLPP2-Akt-Gsk3beta axis. *Apoptosis* **2015**, *20*, 1296–1306. [CrossRef] [PubMed]
112. Tuntaterdtum, S.; Chaudhary, I.P.; Cibull, M.; Robertson, L.W.; Blouin, R.A. Acetaminophen hepatotoxicity: Influence of phenobarbital and beta-naphthoflavone treatment in obese and lean Zucker rats. *Toxicol. Appl. Pharmacol.* **1993**, *123*, 219–225. [CrossRef] [PubMed]
113. Lv, Y.; Zhang, B.; Xing, G.; Wang, F.; Hu, Z. Protective effect of naringenin against acetaminophen-induced acute liver injury in metallothionein (MT)-null mice. *Food Funct.* **2013**, *4*, 297–302. [CrossRef] [PubMed]
114. Wong, W.S.; McLean, A.E. Effects of phenolic antioxidants and flavonoids on DNA synthesis in rat liver, spleen, and testis in vitro. *Toxicology* **1999**, *139*, 243–253. [CrossRef]
115. Li, Y.; Wang, E.; Patten, C.J.; Chen, L.; Yang, C.S. Effects of flavonoids on cytochrome P450-dependent acetaminophen metabolism in rats and human liver microsomes. *Drug Metab. Dispos.* **1994**, *22*, 566–571. [PubMed]
116. Liu, J.; Liu, Y.; Madhu, C.; Klaassen, C.D. Protective effects of oleanolic acid on acetaminophen-induced hepatotoxicity in mice. *J. Pharmacol. Exp. Ther.* **1993**, *266*, 1607–1613. [PubMed]

117. Liu, J.; Liu, Y.; Parkinson, A.; Klaassen, C.D. Effect of oleanolic acid on hepatic toxicant-activating and detoxifying systems in mice. *J. Pharmacol. Exp. Ther.* **1995**, *275*, 768–774. [PubMed]
118. Abdel-Zaher, A.O.; Abdel-Rahman, M.M.; Hafez, M.M.; Omran, F.M. Role of nitric oxide and reduced glutathione in the protective effects of aminoguanidine, gadolinium chloride and oleanolic acid against acetaminophen-induced hepatic and renal damage. *Toxicology* **2007**, *234*, 124–134. [CrossRef] [PubMed]
119. Liu, J.; Wu, Q.; Lu, Y.F.; Pi, J. New insights into generalized hepatoprotective effects of oleanolic acid: Key roles of metallothionein and Nrf2 induction. *Biochem. Pharmacol.* **2008**, *76*, 922–928. [CrossRef] [PubMed]
120. Reisman, S.A.; Aleksunes, L.M.; Klaassen, C.D. Oleanolic acid activates Nrf2 and protects from acetaminophen hepatotoxicity via Nrf2-dependent and Nrf2-independent processes. *Biochem. Pharmacol.* **2009**, *77*, 1273–1282. [CrossRef] [PubMed]
121. Honda, T.; Rounds, B.V.; Gribble, G.W.; Suh, N.; Wang, Y.; Sporn, M.B. Design and synthesis of 2-cyano-3,12-dioxoolean-1,9-dien-28-oic acid, a novel and highly active inhibitor of nitric oxide production in mouse macrophages. *Bioorg. Med. Chem. Lett.* **1998**, *8*, 2711–2714. [CrossRef]
122. Ding, Y.; Li, Q.; Xu, Y.; Chen, Y.; Deng, Y.; Zhi, F.; Qian, K. Attenuating Oxidative Stress by Paeonol Protected against Acetaminophen-Induced Hepatotoxicity in Mice. *PLoS ONE* **2016**, *11*, e0154375. [CrossRef] [PubMed]
123. Liu, Y.; Li, W.; Li, P.; Deng, M.C.; Yang, S.L.; Yang, L. The inhibitory effect of intestinal bacterial metabolite of ginsenosides on CYP3A activity. *Biol. Pharm. Bull.* **2004**, *27*, 1555–1560. [CrossRef] [PubMed]
124. Wang, S.; Wang, X.; Luo, F.; Tang, X.; Li, K.; Hu, X.; Bai, J. Panaxatriol saponin ameliorated liver injury by acetaminophen via restoring thioredoxin-1 and pro-caspase-12. *Liver Int.* **2014**, *34*, 1068–1073. [CrossRef] [PubMed]
125. Gum, S.I.; Cho, M.K. The amelioration of N-acetyl-p-benzoquinone imine toxicity by ginsenoside Rg3: The role of Nrf2-mediated detoxification and Mrp1/Mrp3 transports. *Oxid. Med. Cell. Longev.* **2013**, *2013*, 957947. [CrossRef] [PubMed]
126. Truong, V.L.; Bak, M.J.; Jun, M.; Kong, A.N.; Ho, C.T.; Jeong, W.S. Antioxidant defense and hepatoprotection by procyanidins from almond (Prunus amygdalus) skins. *J. Agric. Food Chem.* **2014**, *62*, 8668–8678. [CrossRef] [PubMed]
127. El-Sayed el, S.M.; Mansour, A.M.; Nady, M.E. Protective effects of pterostilbene against acetaminophen-induced hepatotoxicity in rats. *J. Biochem. Mol. Toxicol* **2015**, *29*, 35–42. [CrossRef] [PubMed]
128. Lin, C.C.; Hsu, Y.F.; Lin, T.C.; Hsu, H.Y. Antioxidant and hepatoprotective effects of punicalagin and punicalin on acetaminophen-induced liver damage in rats. *Phytother. Res.* **2001**, *15*, 206–212. [CrossRef] [PubMed]
129. Gilani, A.H.; Janbaz, K.H.; Shah, B.H. Quercetin exhibits hepatoprotective activity in rats. *Biochem. Soc. Trans.* **1997**, *25*, S619. [CrossRef] [PubMed]
130. Bousova, I.; Skalova, L. Inhibition and induction of glutathione S-transferases by flavonoids: Possible pharmacological and toxicological consequences. *Drug Metab. Rev.* **2012**, *44*, 267–286. [CrossRef] [PubMed]
131. El-Shafey, M.M.; Abd-Allah, G.M.; Mohamadin, A.M.; Harisa, G.I.; Mariee, A.D. Quercetin protects against acetaminophen-induced hepatorenal toxicity by reducing reactive oxygen and nitrogen species. *Pathophysiology* **2015**, *22*, 49–55. [CrossRef] [PubMed]
132. Ahmed, O.A.; Badr-Eldin, S.M.; Tawfik, M.K.; Ahmed, T.A.; El-Say, K.M.; Badr, J.M. Design and optimization of self-nanoemulsifying delivery system to enhance quercetin hepatoprotective activity in paracetamol-induced hepatotoxicity. *J. Pharm. Sci.* **2014**, *103*, 602–612. [CrossRef] [PubMed]
133. Ji, L.L.; Sheng, Y.C.; Zheng, Z.Y.; Shi, L.; Wang, Z.T. The involvement of p62-Keap1-Nrf2 antioxidative signaling pathway and JNK in the protection of natural flavonoid quercetin against hepatotoxicity. *Free Radic. Biol. Med.* **2015**, *85*, 12–23. [CrossRef] [PubMed]
134. Wojnarova, L.; Kutinova Canova, N.; Farghali, H.; Kucera, T. Sirtuin 1 modulation in rat model of acetaminophen-induced hepatotoxicity. *Physiol. Res.* **2015**, *64*, S477. [PubMed]
135. Wang, Y.; Jiang, Y.; Fan, X.; Tan, H.; Zeng, H.; Chen, P.; Huang, M.; Bi, H. Hepato-protective effect of resveratrol against acetaminophen-induced liver injury is associated with inhibition of CYP-mediated bioactivation and regulation of SIRT1-p53 signaling pathways. *Toxicol. Lett.* **2015**, *236*, 82–89. [CrossRef] [PubMed]
136. Du, K.; McGill, M.R.; Xie, Y.; Bajt, M.L.; Jaeschke, H. Resveratrol prevents protein nitration and release of endonucleases from mitochondria during acetaminophen hepatotoxicity. *Food Chem. Toxicol.* **2015**, *81*, 62–70. [CrossRef] [PubMed]

137. Masubuchi, Y.; Sugiyama, S.; Horie, T. Th1/Th2 cytokine balance as a determinant of acetaminophen-induced liver injury. *Chem. Biol. Interact.* **2009**, *179*, 273–279. [CrossRef] [PubMed]
138. Sener, G.; Toklu, H.Z.; Sehirli, A.O.; Velioglu-Ogunc, A.; Cetinel, S.; Gedik, N. Protective effects of resveratrol against acetaminophen-induced toxicity in mice. *Hepatol. Res.* **2006**, *35*, 62–68. [CrossRef] [PubMed]
139. McGill, M.R.; Du, K.; Weemhoff, J.L.; Jaeschke, H. Critical review of resveratrol in xenobiotic-induced hepatotoxicity. *Food Chem. Toxicol.* **2015**, *86*, 309–318. [CrossRef] [PubMed]
140. Bishayee, A.; Darvesh, A.S.; Politis, T.; McGory, R. Resveratrol and liver disease: From bench to bedside and community. *Liver Int.* **2010**, *30*, 1103–1114. [CrossRef] [PubMed]
141. Zhao, Y.L.; Zhou, G.D.; Yang, H.B.; Wang, J.B.; Shan, L.M.; Li, R.S.; Xiao, X.H. Rhein protects against acetaminophen-induced hepatic and renal toxicity. *Food Chem. Toxicol.* **2011**, *49*, 1705–1710. [CrossRef] [PubMed]
142. Janbaz, K.H.; Saeed, S.A.; Gilani, A.H. Protective effect of rutin on paracetamol- and CCl4-induced hepatotoxicity in rodents. *Fitoterapia* **2002**, *73*, 557–563. [CrossRef]
143. Liu, A.; Tanaka, N.; Sun, L.; Guo, B.; Kim, J.H.; Krausz, K.W.; Fang, Z.; Jiang, C.; Yang, J.; Gonzalez, F.J. Saikosaponin d protects against acetaminophen-induced hepatotoxicity by inhibiting NF-kappaB and STAT3 signaling. *Chem. Biol. Interact.* **2014**, *223*, 80–86. [CrossRef] [PubMed]
144. Wu, Y.L.; Piao, D.M.; Han, X.H.; Nan, J.X. Protective effects of salidroside against acetaminophen-induced toxicity in mice. *Biol. Pharm. Bull.* **2008**, *31*, 1523–1529. [CrossRef] [PubMed]
145. Guo, N.; Ding, W.; Wang, Y.; Hu, Z.; Wang, Z. An LC-MS/MS method for the determination of salidroside and its metabolite p-tyrosol in rat liver tissues. *Pharm. Biol.* **2014**, *52*, 637–645. [CrossRef] [PubMed]
146. Zhou, X.; Cheung, C.M.; Yang, J.M.; Or, P.M.; Lee, W.Y.; Yeung, J.H. Danshen (Salvia miltiorrhiza) water extract inhibits paracetamol-induced toxicity in primary rat hepatocytes via reducing CYP2E1 activity and oxidative stress. *J. Pharm. Pharmacol.* **2015**, *67*, 980–989. [CrossRef] [PubMed]
147. Lin, M.; Zhai, X.; Wang, G.; Tian, X.; Gao, D.; Shi, L.; Wu, H.; Fan, Q.; Peng, J.; Liu, K.; et al. Salvianolic acid B protects against acetaminophen hepatotoxicity by inducing Nrf2 and phase II detoxification gene expression via activation of the PI3K and PKC signaling pathways. *J. Pharmacol. Sci.* **2015**, *127*, 203–210. [CrossRef] [PubMed]
148. Simeonova, R.; Vitcheva, V.; Kondeva-Burdina, M.; Krasteva, I.; Manov, V.; Mitcheva, M. Hepatoprotective and antioxidant effects of saponarin, isolated from Gypsophila trichotoma Wend. on paracetamol-induced liver damage in rats. *Biomed. Res. Int.* **2013**, *2013*, 757126. [CrossRef] [PubMed]
149. Song, H.; Kim, Y.C.; Moon, A. Sauchinone, a lignan from Saururus chinensis, inhibits staurosporine-induced apoptosis in C6 rat glioma cells. *Biol. Pharm. Bull.* **2003**, *26*, 1428–1430. [CrossRef] [PubMed]
150. Kay, H.Y.; Kim, Y.W.; Ryu, D.H.; Sung, S.H.; Hwang, S.J.; Kim, S.G. Nrf2-mediated liver protection by sauchinone, an antioxidant lignan, from acetaminophen toxicity through the PKCdelta-GSK3beta pathway. *Br. J. Pharmacol.* **2011**, *163*, 1653–1665. [CrossRef] [PubMed]
151. Jiang, Y.; Fan, X.; Wang, Y.; Tan, H.; Chen, P.; Zeng, H.; Huang, M.; Bi, H. Hepato-protective effects of six schisandra lignans on acetaminophen-induced liver injury are partially associated with the inhibition of CYP-mediated bioactivation. *Chem. Biol. Interact.* **2015**, *231*, 83–89. [CrossRef] [PubMed]
152. Jiang, Y.; Fan, X.; Wang, Y.; Chen, P.; Zeng, H.; Tan, H.; Gonzalez, F.J.; Huang, M.; Bi, H. Schisandrol B protects against acetaminophen-induced hepatotoxicity by inhibition of CYP-mediated bioactivation and regulation of liver regeneration. *Toxicol. Sci.* **2015**, *143*, 107–115. [CrossRef] [PubMed]
153. Jiang, Y.M.; Wang, Y.; Tan, H.S.; Yu, T.; Fan, X.M.; Chen, P.; Zeng, H.; Huang, M.; Bi, H.C. Schisandrol B protects against acetaminophen-induced acute hepatotoxicity in mice via activation of the NRF2/ARE signaling pathway. *Acta pharmacol. Sin.* **2016**, *37*, 382–389. [CrossRef] [PubMed]
154. Chandrasekaran, V.R.; Hsu, D.Z.; Liu, M.Y. The protective effect of sesamol against mitochondrial oxidative stress and hepatic injury in acetaminophen-overdosed rats. *Shock* **2009**, *32*, 89–93. [CrossRef] [PubMed]
155. Chandrasekaran, V.R.; Chien, S.P.; Hsu, D.Z.; Liu, M.Y. Anti-hepatotoxic effects of 3,4-methylenedioxyphenol and N-acetylcysteine in acutely acetaminophen-overdosed mice. *Hum. Exp. Toxicol.* **2011**, *30*, 1609–1615. [CrossRef] [PubMed]
156. Campos, R.; Garrido, A.; Guerra, R.; Valenzuela, A. Acetaminophen hepatotoxicity in rats is attenuated by silybin dihemisuccinate. *Prog. Clin. Biol. Res.* **1988**, *280*, 375–378. [PubMed]

157. Campos, R.; Garrido, A.; Guerra, R.; Valenzuela, A. Silybin dihemisuccinate protects against glutathione depletion and lipid peroxidation induced by acetaminophen on rat liver. *Planta Med.* **1989**, *55*, 417–419. [CrossRef] [PubMed]
158. Garrido, A.; Arancibia, C.; Campos, R.; Valenzuela, A. Acetaminophen does not induce oxidative stress in isolated rat hepatocytes: Its probable antioxidant effect is potentiated by the flavonoid silybin. *Pharmacol. Toxicol.* **1991**, *69*, 9–12. [CrossRef] [PubMed]
159. Conti, M.; Malandrino, S.; Magistretti, M.J. Protective activity of silipide on liver damage in rodents. *Jpn. J. Pharmacol.* **1992**, *60*, 315–321. [CrossRef] [PubMed]
160. Luo, Y.D.; Chen, J.; Cao, J.; Wen, X.D.; Li, P. Determination of sweroside in rat plasma and bile for oral bioavailability and hepatobiliary excretion. *Chem. Pharm. Bull.* **2009**, *57*, 79–83. [CrossRef] [PubMed]
161. Han, H.; Zeng, W.; He, C.; Bligh, S.W.; Liu, Q.; Yang, L.; Wang, Z. Characterization of metabolites of sweroside in rat urine using ultra-high-performance liquid chromatography combined with electrospray ionization quadrupole time-of-flight tandem mass spectrometry and NMR spectroscopy. *J. Mass Spectrom.* **2014**, *49*, 1108–1116. [CrossRef] [PubMed]
162. Ramachandran, V.; Raja, B. Protective effects of syringic acid against acetaminophen-induced hepatic damage in albino rats. *J. Basic Clin. Physiol. Pharmacol.* **2010**, *21*, 369–385. [CrossRef] [PubMed]
163. Zhang, J.; Song, Q.; Han, X.; Zhang, Y.; Zhang, X.; Chu, X.; Zhang, F.; Chu, L. Multi-targeted protection of acetaminophen-induced hepatotoxicity in mice by tannic acid. *Int. Immunopharmacol.* **2017**, *47*, 95–105. [CrossRef] [PubMed]
164. Nagi, M.N.; Almakki, H.A.; Sayed-Ahmed, M.M.; Al-Bekairi, A.M. Thymoquinone supplementation reverses acetaminophen-induced oxidative stress, nitric oxide production and energy decline in mice liver. *Food Chem. Toxicol.* **2010**, *48*, 2361–2365. [CrossRef] [PubMed]
165. Jadeja, R.N.; Urrunaga, N.H.; Dash, S.; Khurana, S.; Saxena, N.K. Withaferin-A Reduces Acetaminophen-Induced Liver Injury in Mice. *Biochem. Pharmacol.* **2015**, *97*, 122–132. [CrossRef] [PubMed]
166. He, Y.C.; Zou, Y.; Peng, C.; Liu, J.L.; He, C.J.; Guo, L.; Xie, X.F.; Xiong, L. Penthorin A and B, two unusual 2,4′-epoxy-8,5′-neolignans from Penthorum chinese. *Fitoterapia* **2015**, *100*, 7–10. [CrossRef] [PubMed]
167. Sakran, M.; Selim, Y.; Zidan, N. A new isoflavonoid from seeds of *Lepidium sativum* L. and its protective effect on hepatotoxicity induced by paracetamol in male rats. *Molecules* **2014**, *19*, 15440–15451. [CrossRef] [PubMed]
168. Palabiyik, S.S.; Karakus, E.; Halici, Z.; Cadirci, E.; Bayir, Y.; Ayaz, G.; Cinar, I. The protective effects of carvacrol and thymol against paracetamol-induced toxicity on human hepatocellular carcinoma cell lines (HepG2). *Hum. Exp. Toxicol.* **2016**, *35*, 1252–1263. [CrossRef] [PubMed]
169. Girish, C.; Koner, B.C.; Jayanthi, S.; Ramachandra Rao, K.; Rajesh, B.; Pradhan, S.C. Hepatoprotective activity of picroliv, curcumin and ellagic acid compared to silymarin on paracetamol induced liver toxicity in mice. *Fundam. Clin. Pharmacol.* **2009**, *23*, 735–745. [CrossRef] [PubMed]
170. Zhang, J.; Zhang, S.; Bi, J.; Gu, J.; Deng, Y.; Liu, C. Astaxanthin pretreatment attenuates acetaminophen-induced liver injury in mice. *Int. Immunopharmacol.* **2017**, *45*, 26–33. [CrossRef] [PubMed]
171. Liao, C.C.; Day, Y.J.; Lee, H.C.; Liou, J.T.; Chou, A.H.; Liu, F.C. ERK Signaling Pathway Plays a Key Role in Baicalin Protection Against Acetaminophen-Induced Liver Injury. *Am. J. Chin. Med.* **2017**, *45*, 105–121. [CrossRef] [PubMed]
172. Liao, C.C.; Day, Y.J.; Lee, H.C.; Liou, J.T.; Chou, A.H.; Liu, F.C. Baicalin Attenuates IL-17-Mediated Acetaminophen-Induced Liver Injury in a Mouse Model. *PLoS ONE* **2016**, *11*, e0166856. [CrossRef] [PubMed]
173. Ji, L.; Jiang, P.; Lu, B.; Sheng, Y.; Wang, X.; Wang, Z. Chlorogenic acid, a dietary polyphenol, protects acetaminophen-induced liver injury and its mechanism. *J. Nutr. Biochem.* **2013**, *24*, 1911–1919. [CrossRef] [PubMed]
174. Wang, L.; Zhang, S.; Cheng, H.; Lv, H.; Cheng, G.; Ci, X. Nrf2-mediated liver protection by esculentoside A against acetaminophen toxicity through the AMPK/Akt/GSK3beta pathway. *Free Radic. Biol. Med.* **2016**, *101*, 401–412. [CrossRef] [PubMed]
175. Yan, T.; Wang, H.; Zhao, M.; Yagai, T.; Chai, Y.; Krausz, K.W.; Xie, C.; Cheng, X.; Zhang, J.; Che, Y.; et al. Glycyrrhizin Protects against Acetaminophen-Induced Acute Liver Injury via Alleviating Tumor Necrosis Factor alpha-Mediated Apoptosis. *Drug Metab. Dispos.* **2016**, *44*, 720–731. [CrossRef] [PubMed]

176. Shanmugam, S.; Thangaraj, P.; Lima, B.D.; Chandran, R.; de Souza Araujo, A.A.; Narain, N.; Serafini, M.R.; Junior, L.J. Effects of luteolin and quercetin 3-beta-d-glucoside identified from Passiflora subpeltata leaves against acetaminophen induced hepatotoxicity in rats. *Biomed. Pharmacother.* **2016**, *83*, 1278–1285. [CrossRef] [PubMed]
177. Bandeira, A.C.; da Silva, T.P.; de Araujo, G.R.; Araujo, C.M.; da Silva, R.C.; Lima, W.G.; Bezerra, F.S.; Costa, D.C. Lycopene inhibits reactive oxygen species production in SK-Hep-1 cells and attenuates acetaminophen-induced liver injury in C57BL/6 mice. *Chem. Biol. Interact.* **2017**, *263*, 7–17. [CrossRef] [PubMed]
178. Bandeira, A.C.; da Silva, R.C.; Rossoni, J.V.J.; Figueiredo, V.P.; Talvani, A.; Cangussu, S.D.; Bezerra, F.S.; Costa, D.C. Lycopene pretreatment improves hepatotoxicity induced by acetaminophen in C57BL/6 mice. *Bioorg. Med. Chem.* **2017**, *25*, 1057–1065. [CrossRef] [PubMed]
179. Truong, V.L.; Ko, S.Y.; Jun, M.; Jeong, W.S. Quercitrin from Toona sinensis (Juss.) M.Roem. Attenuates Acetaminophen-Induced Acute Liver Toxicity in HepG2 Cells and Mice through Induction of Antioxidant Machinery and Inhibition of Inflammation. *Nutrients* **2016**, *8*, 431. [CrossRef] [PubMed]
180. da Rocha, B.A.; Ritter, A.M.; Ames, F.Q.; Goncalves, O.H.; Leimann, F.V.; Bracht, L.; Natali, M.R.; Cuman, R.K.; Bersani-Amado, C.A. Acetaminophen-induced hepatotoxicity: Preventive effect of trans anethole. *Biomed. Pharmacother.* **2017**, *86*, 213–220. [CrossRef] [PubMed]
181. Palliyaguru, D.L.; Chartoumpekis, D.V.; Wakabayashi, N.; Skoko, J.J.; Yagishita, Y.; Singh, S.V.; Kensler, T.W. Withaferin A induces Nrf2-dependent protection against liver injury: Role of Keap1-independent mechanisms. *Free Radic. Biol. Med.* **2016**, *101*, 116–128. [CrossRef] [PubMed]
182. Kim, Y.W.; Ki, S.H.; Lee, J.R.; Lee, S.J.; Kim, C.W.; Kim, S.C.; Kim, S.G. Liquiritigenin, an aglycone of liquiritin in Glycyrrhizae radix, prevents acute liver injuries in rats induced by acetaminophen with or without buthionine sulfoximine. *Chem. Biol. Interact.* **2006**, *161*, 12538. [CrossRef] [PubMed]
183. Kumari, A.; Kakkar, P. Lupeol prevents acetaminophen-induced in vivo hepatotoxicity by altering the Bax/Bcl-2 and oxidative stress-mediated mitochondrial signaling cascade. *Life Sci.* **2012**, *90*, 561–570. [CrossRef] [PubMed]
184. Reddy, M.K.; Reddy, A.G.; Kumar, B.K.; Madhuri, D.; Boobalan, G.; Reddy, M.A. Protective effect of rutin in comparison to silymarin against induced hepatotoxicity in rats. *Vet. World* **2017**, *10*, 74–80. [CrossRef] [PubMed]
185. Lewerenz, V.; Hanelt, S.; Nastevska, C.; El-Bahay, C.; Rohrdanz, E.; Kahl, R. Antioxidants protect primary rat hepatocyte cultures against acetaminophen-induced DNA strand breaks but not against acetaminophen-induced cytotoxicity. *Toxicology* **2003**, *191*, 179–187. [CrossRef]
186. Liu, J.; Liu, Y.; Bullock, P.; Klaassen, C.D. Suppression of liver cytochrome P450 by alpha-hederin: Relevance to hepatoprotection. *Toxicol. Appl. Pharmacol.* **1995**, *134*, 124–131. [CrossRef] [PubMed]
187. Iorga, A.; Dara, L.; Kaplowitz, N. Drug-Induced Liver Injury: Cascade of Events Leading to Cell Death, Apoptosis or Necrosis. *Int. J. Mol. Sci.* **2017**, *18*, 1018. [CrossRef] [PubMed]
188. Woolbright, B.L.; Jaeschke, H. Sterile inflammation in acute liver injury: Myth or mystery? *Expert Rev. Gastroenterol. Hepatol.* **2015**, *9*, 1027–1029. [CrossRef] [PubMed]
189. Wagner, H.; Ulrich-Merzenich, G. Synergy research: Approaching a new generation of phytopharmaceuticals. *Phytomedicine* **2009**, *16*, 97–110. [CrossRef] [PubMed]
190. Lahon, K.; Das, S. Hepatoprotective activity of Ocimum sanctum alcoholic leaf extract against paracetamol-induced liver damage in Albino rats. *Pharm. Res.* **2011**, *3*, 13–18. [CrossRef] [PubMed]
191. Chandan, B.K.; Saxena, A.K.; Shukla, S.; Sharma, N.; Gupta, D.K.; Suri, K.A.; Suri, J.; Bhadauria, M.; Singh, B. Hepatoprotective potential of Aloe barbadensis Mill. against carbon tetrachloride induced hepatotoxicity. *J. Ethnopharmacol.* **2007**, *111*, 560–566. [CrossRef] [PubMed]
192. Ranawat, L.; Bhatt, J.; Patel, J. Hepatoprotective activity of ethanolic extracts of bark of Zanthoxylum armatum DC in CCl4 induced hepatic damage in rats. *J. Ethnopharmacol.* **2010**, *127*, 777–780. [CrossRef] [PubMed]
193. Wang, L.; Cheng, D.; Wang, H.; Di, L.; Zhou, X.; Xu, T.; Yang, X.; Liu, Y. The hepatoprotective and antifibrotic effects of Saururus chinensis against carbon tetrachloride induced hepatic fibrosis in rats. *J. Ethnopharmacol.* **2009**, *126*, 487–491. [CrossRef] [PubMed]
194. Shi, Y.; Sun, J.; He, H.; Guo, H.; Zhang, S. Hepatoprotective effects of Ganoderma lucidum peptides against D-galactosamine-induced liver injury in mice. *J. Ethnopharmacol.* **2008**, *117*, 415–419. [CrossRef] [PubMed]

195. Morita, T.; Jinno, K.; Kawagishi, H.; Arimoto, Y.; Suganuma, H.; Inakuma, T.; Sugiyama, K. Hepatoprotective effect of myristicin from nutmeg (Myristica fragrans) on lipopolysaccharide/d-galactosamine-induced liver injury. *J. Agric. Food Chem.* **2003**, *51*, 1560–1565. [CrossRef] [PubMed]
196. Hase, K.; Kasimu, R.; Basnet, P.; Kadota, S.; Namba, T. Preventive effect of lithospermate B from Salvia miltiorhiza on experimental hepatitis induced by carbon tetrachloride or D-galactosamine/lipopolysaccharide. *Planta Med.* **1997**, *63*, 22–26. [CrossRef] [PubMed]
197. Surai, P.F. Silymarin as a Natural Antioxidant: An Overview of the Current Evidence and Perspectives. *Antioxidants* **2015**, *4*, 204–247. [CrossRef] [PubMed]
198. Vargas-Mendoza, N.; Madrigal-Santillan, E.; Morales-Gonzalez, A.; Esquivel-Soto, J.; Esquivel-Chirino, C.; Garcia-Luna, Y.G.-R.M.; Gayosso-de-Lucio, J.A.; Morales-Gonzalez, J.A. Hepatoprotective effect of silymarin. *World J. Hepatol.* **2014**, *6*, 144–149. [CrossRef] [PubMed]
199. Freitag, A.F.; Cardia, G.F.; da Rocha, B.A.; Aguiar, R.P.; Silva-Comar, F.M.; Spironello, R.A.; Grespan, R.; Caparroz-Assef, S.M.; Bersani-Amado, C.A.; Cuman, R.K. Hepatoprotective Effect of Silymarin (Silybum marianum) on Hepatotoxicity Induced by Acetaminophen in Spontaneously Hypertensive Rats. *Evid. Based Complement. Alternat. Med.* **2015**, *2015*, 538317. [CrossRef] [PubMed]
200. Wu, J.W.; Lin, L.C.; Hung, S.C.; Lin, C.H.; Chi, C.W.; Tsai, T.H. Hepatobiliary excretion of silibinin in normal and liver cirrhotic rats. *Drug Metab. Dispos.* **2008**, *36*, 589–596. [CrossRef] [PubMed]
201. Tong, T.C.; Hernandez, M.; Richardson, W.H., 3rd; Betten, D.P.; Favata, M.; Riffenburgh, R.H.; Clark, R.F.; Tanen, D.A. Comparative treatment of alpha-amanitin poisoning with N-acetylcysteine, benzylpenicillin, cimetidine, thioctic acid, and silybin in a murine model. *Ann. Emerg. Med.* **2007**, *50*, 282–288. [CrossRef] [PubMed]
202. Papackova, Z.; Heczkova, M.; Dankova, H.; Sticova, E.; Lodererova, A.; Bartonova, L.; Poruba, M.; Cahova, M. Silymarin prevents acetaminophen-induced hepatotoxicity in mice. *PLoS ONE* **2018**, *13*, e0191353. [CrossRef] [PubMed]
203. Lirussi, F.; Beccarello, A.; Zanette, G.; De Monte, A.; Donadon, V.; Velussi, M.; Crepaldi, G. Silybin-beta-cyclodextrin in the treatment of patients with diabetes mellitus and alcoholic liver disease. Efficacy study of a new preparation of an anti-oxidant agent. *Diabetes Nutr. Metab.* **2002**, *15*, 222–231. [PubMed]
204. Huseini, H.F.; Larijani, B.; Heshmat, R.; Fakhrzadeh, H.; Radjabipour, B.; Toliat, T.; Raza, M. The efficacy of *Silybum marianum* (L.) Gaertn. (silymarin) in the treatment of type II diabetes: A randomized, double-blind, placebo-controlled, clinical trial. *Phytother. Res.* **2006**, *20*, 1036–1039. [CrossRef] [PubMed]
205. Heidarian, E.; Saffari, J.; Jafari-Dehkordi, E. Hepatoprotective action of Echinophora platyloba DC leaves against acute toxicity of acetaminophen in rats. *J. Diet. Suppl.* **2014**, *11*, 53–63. [CrossRef] [PubMed]
206. de Avelar, C.R.; Pereira, E.M.; de Farias Costa, P.R.; de Jesus, R.P.; de Oliveira, L.P.M. Effect of silymarin on biochemical indicators in patients with liver disease: Systematic review with meta-analysis. *World J. Gastroenterol.* **2017**, *23*, 5004–5017. [CrossRef] [PubMed]
207. Darvishi Khezri, H.; Salehifar, E.; Kosaryan, M.; Aliasgharian, A.; Jalali, H.; Hadian Amree, A. Potential Effects of Silymarin and Its Flavonolignan Components in Patients with beta-Thalassemia Major: A Comprehensive Review in 2015. *Adv. Pharmacol. Sci.* **2016**, *2016*, 3046373. [PubMed]
208. Yang, Z.; Zhuang, L.; Lu, Y.; Xu, Q.; Chen, X. Effects and tolerance of silymarin (milk thistle) in chronic hepatitis C virus infection patients: A meta-analysis of randomized controlled trials. *Biomed. Res. Int.* **2014**, *2014*, 941085. [CrossRef] [PubMed]
209. Huseini, H.F.; Alavian, S.M.; Heshmat, R.; Heydari, M.R.; Abolmaali, K. The efficacy of Liv-52 on liver cirrhotic patients: A randomized, double-blind, placebo-controlled first approach. *Phytomedicine* **2005**, *12*, 619–624. [CrossRef] [PubMed]
210. Chaphalkar, R.; Apte, K.G.; Talekar, Y.; Ojha, S.K.; Nandave, M. Antioxidants of *Phyllanthus emblica* L. Bark Extract Provide Hepatoprotection against Ethanol-Induced Hepatic Damage: A Comparison with Silymarin. *Oxid. Med. Cell. Longev.* **2017**, *2017*, 3876040. [CrossRef] [PubMed]
211. Das, S.; Bandyopadhyay, S.; Ramasamy, A.; Mondal, S. Evaluation of hepatoprotective activity of aqueous extracts of leaves of Basella alba in albino rats. *Nat. Prod. Res.* **2015**, *29*, 1059–1064. [CrossRef] [PubMed]

212. Zakaria, Z.A.; Yahya, F.; Mamat, S.S.; Mahmood, N.D.; Mohtarrudin, N.; Taher, M.; Hamid, S.S.; Teh, L.K.; Salleh, M.Z. Hepatoprotective action of various partitions of methanol extract of Bauhinia purpurea leaves against paracetamol-induced liver toxicity: Involvement of the antioxidant mechanisms. *BMC Complement. Altern. Med.* **2016**, *16*, 175. [CrossRef] [PubMed]
213. Qu, Q.; Qu, J.; Han, L.; Zhan, M.; Wu, L.X.; Zhang, Y.W.; Zhang, W.; Zhou, H.H. Inhibitory effects of phytochemicals on metabolic capabilities of CYP2D6(*)1 and CYP2D6(*)10 using cell-based models in vitro. *Acta pharmacol. Sin.* **2014**, *35*, 685–696. [CrossRef] [PubMed]
214. Maes, M.; Vinken, M.; Jaeschke, H. Experimental models of hepatotoxicity related to acute liver failure. *Toxicol. Appl. Pharmacol.* **2016**, *290*, 86–97. [CrossRef] [PubMed]
215. Godoy, P.; Hewitt, N.J.; Albrecht, U.; Andersen, M.E.; Ansari, N.; Bhattacharya, S.; Bode, J.G.; Bolleyn, J.; Borner, C.; Bottger, J.; et al. Recent advances in 2D and 3D in vitro systems using primary hepatocytes, alternative hepatocyte sources and non-parenchymal liver cells and their use in investigating mechanisms of hepatotoxicity, cell signaling and ADME. *Arch. Toxicol.* **2013**, *87*, 1315–1530. [CrossRef] [PubMed]
216. Du, K.; Xie, Y.; McGill, M.R.; Jaeschke, H. Pathophysiological significance of c-jun N-terminal kinase in acetaminophen hepatotoxicity. *Expert Opin. Drug Metab. Toxicol.* **2015**, *11*, 1769–1779. [CrossRef] [PubMed]
217. McGill, M.R.; Yan, H.M.; Ramachandran, A.; Murray, G.J.; Rollins, D.E.; Jaeschke, H. HepaRG cells: A human model to study mechanisms of acetaminophen hepatotoxicity. *Hepatology* **2011**, *53*, 974–982. [CrossRef] [PubMed]
218. Xie, Y.; McGill, M.R.; Dorko, K.; Kumer, S.C.; Schmitt, T.M.; Forster, J.; Jaeschke, H. Mechanisms of acetaminophen-induced cell death in primary human hepatocytes. *Toxicol. Appl. Pharmacol.* **2014**, *279*, 266–274. [CrossRef] [PubMed]
219. Jaeschke, H.; McGill, M.R.; Williams, C.D.; Ramachandran, A. Current issues with acetaminophen hepatotoxicity—A clinically relevant model to test the efficacy of natural products. *Life Sci.* **2011**, *88*, 737–745. [CrossRef] [PubMed]

International Journal of
Molecular Sciences

MDPI

Review

Hair-Growth Potential of Ginseng and Its Major Metabolites: A Review on Its Molecular Mechanisms

Bu Young Choi

Department of Pharmaceutical Science and Engineering, Seowon University, Cheongju 28674, Korea; bychoi@seowon.ac.kr; Tel.: +82-43-299-8411; Fax: +82-43-299-8470

Received: 25 August 2018; Accepted: 8 September 2018; Published: 11 September 2018

Abstract: The functional aspect of scalp hair is not only to protect from solar radiation and heat/cold exposure but also to contribute to one's appearance and personality. Progressive hair loss has a cosmetic and social impact. Hair undergoes three stages of hair cycle: the anagen, catagen, and telogen phases. Through cyclical loss and new-hair growth, the number of hairs remains relatively constant. A variety of factors, such as hormones, nutritional status, and exposure to radiations, environmental toxicants, and medications, may affect hair growth. Androgens are the most important of these factors that cause androgenic alopecia. Other forms of hair loss include immunogenic hair loss, that is, alopecia areata. Although a number of therapies, such as finasteride and minoxidil, are approved medications, and a few others (e.g., tofacitinib) are in progress, a wide variety of structurally diverse classes of phytochemicals, including those present in ginseng, have demonstrated hair growth-promoting effects in a large number of preclinical studies. The purpose of this review is to focus on the potential of ginseng and its metabolites on the prevention of hair loss and its underlying mechanisms.

Keywords: ginseng; human-hair-follicle dermal papilla cells; WNT/β-catenin; Shh/Gli; TGF-β; BMP/Smad; mouse-hair growth

1. Introduction

The hair-growth cycle comprises three distinct phases, the anagen, catagen, and telogen phases of independent hair follicles. Hair continues to grow during the anagen phase, followed by a transitional period of the catagen phase, which enters into the telogen phase, when hair is released from the follicle and falls. The anagen phase can be classified into a propagating anagen phase that involves the activation of new hair follicles, and an autonomous anagen phase, when hair growth and differentiation of hair follicles actively occur [1]. The normal hair-growth cycle is repeated about 20 times; however, it can be modified or shortened by internal or external factors such as hormones, stress, concurrent disease, exposure to environmental pollution, and smoking. Changes in the growth cycle leading to hair loss may be represented with the shortening of the anagen phase, premature ingression of the catagen phase, and the prolongation of the telogen phase. Early hair loss is medically termed as alopecia [2,3]. The number of people suffering from alopecia is increasing and approaching approximately 10 million throughout the world. Considering the pathological background of alopecia and its impact on an individual's health and social value, there is now a growing interest in the development of novel therapeutics for its medical management. To date, the United States Food and Drug Administration (US-FDA) has approved two medications, minoxidil and finasteride, for the treatment of alopecia. Finasteride has been shown to prevent male pattern hair loss through the inhibition of type II 5α-reductase, which affects androgen metabolism. Although the exact mechanism of minoxidil has still not been elucidated, available research findings suggest that the hair-growth promotional effects of minoxidil are mediated through enhanced nutrient supply to hair follicles through vasodilation, opening of the K^+ channel, and the activation of extracellular signal-regulated kinase (ERK) and protein kinase B (AKT/PKB) signaling, resulting in increased cell proliferation and inhibition of apoptosis in dermal papilla cells [4,5]. However, these drugs exhibit certain adverse effects, such as allergic contact dermatitis, erythema, and itching. While discontinuation of minoxidil leads to recurrence of alopecia, prolonged use of finasteride causes male sexual dysfunction and appears as a major cause of infertility and teratogenicity in females [6,7]. Thus, nontoxic chemicals with persistent hair-growth promoting effects have long been sought from the vast resources of natural products [8–10].

Ginseng is an ancient herbal remedy that was recorded in The Herbal Classic of the Divine Plowman, the oldest comprehensive Materia Medica, which was scripted approximately 2000 years ago. Contemporary science has revealed that ginseng contains a wide variety of bioactive constituents, especially a group of saponin compounds collectively known as ginsenosides, which are accredited with diverse biological activities, including the hair-growth potential of ginseng. Depending on the number of hydroxyl groups available for glycosylation via dehydration reactions, ginsenosides can be classified as protopanaxadiol (PPD) and protopanaxatriol (PPT). Common PPD-type ginsenosides include ginsenosides Rb1, Rb2, Rc, Rd, Rg3, F2, Rh2, compound K (cK), and PPD, whereas PPT-type ginsenosides include Re, Rf, Rg1, Rg2, F1, Rh1, and PPT [1]. Ginseng extract or its specific ginsenosides have been tested for their potential to promote hair growth. This review sheds light on the potential of ginseng and ginsenosides in promoting hair growth and delineating the mechanisms by which they function.

2. Biochemical Basis of Hair-Growth Promotion by Ginseng

There has been mounting evidence suggesting that ginseng and its major bioactive constituents, ginsenosides, promote hair growth by enhancing proliferation of dermal papilla and preventing hair loss via modulation of various cell-signaling pathways [11–13]. While the role of 5α-reductase enzyme in the hair-loss process has been well-documented [14,15], the emerging biochemical mechanisms of hair-follicle proliferation and the hair-loss process unravel new targets for designing novel therapeutics for the management of hair loss and alopecia (Figure 1). These targets include, but are not limited to, WNT/Dickkopf homologue 1 (DKK1), sonic hedgehog (Shh), vascular endothelial growth factor (VEGF), transforming growth factor-beta (TGF-β), matrix metalloproteinases (MMPs), extracellular signal-regulated protein kinase (ERK), and Janus-activated kinase (JAK). The following section summarizes the role of ginseng and its metabolites on hair growth.

2.1. Prevention of Radiation-Induced Skin Damage

Photoaging is one of the long-term effects of chronic sun exposure characterized by different inflammatory responses to ultraviolet radiation (UVR). Although exposure to solar UVR induces the synthesis of vitamin D, melanocortins, adrenocorticotropic hormone, and corticotropin- releasing hormone in human skin, and shows a beneficial effect, excessive UV irradiation is known to cause skin photodamage by inducing reactive oxygen species (ROS), precipitating skin inflammation, and promoting keratinocyte cell death. The impact of UVR exposure further leads to skin photoaging and carcinogenesis. However, the influence of UVR on skin appendages such as hair follicles is still in progress in many aspects. Accumulating evidence suggests that UVR exposure not only causes the damage of the hair shaft as an extracellular tissue, but also alters the hair-growth cycle by affecting keratinocyte and dermal papilla growth [16]. UV irradiation causes accumulation of ROS and activates MMPs, a class of tissue-degrading enzymes, thereby compromising dermal and epidermal structural integrity. Irradiation of normal human dermal papilla cells (nHDPC) with ultraviolet B (UVB) ($\geq$50 mJ/cm^2) exhibited ROS-mediated induction of apoptotic cell death [17]. Ginsenosides Rb2 [4] and 20 (S) PPD, but not 20 (R) PPD [4], have been reported to reduce the formation of ROS and MMP-2 secretion in cultured human keratinocytes (HaCaT) cells after exposure to UVB radiation. Likewise, ginsenoside Rg3 20 (S), but not 20 (R), reduced ROS generation in HaCaT cells and human dermal fibroblasts without affecting cell viability. The 20 (S) Rg3 also attenuated UVB-induced MMP-2 levels in HaCaT cells [6]. In another study, ginsenoside Rh2 epimers reduced UVB radiation-induced expression and activity of MMP-2 in HaCaT cells, but UVB-induced ROS formation was only suppressed by 20 (S)-Rh2 [7]. Because the extracellular matrix plays a critical role in hair-follicle function, degradation and matrix remodeling by MMPs affect the hair cycle [18,19]. The inhibitory effect of ginsenosides on UVB-induced activation of MMP2 suggests the potential of these ginseng saponins in hair-growth regulation.

Ginsenosides have also been shown to improve hair growth by attenuating radiation-induced cell death in the skin. Total-root saponins and ginsenoside Rb1 diminished apoptotic cells, as revealed by the accumulation of Ki-67-positive cells and elevated expression of Bcl-2, an antiapoptotic protein, in UVB-exposed human keratinocytes [20]. Ginsenoside F1, an enzymatically modified derivative of ginsenoside Rg1, also protected keratinocytes from radiation-induced apoptosis by maintaining a constant level of Bcl-2 and Brn-3a expression in UVB-irradiated HaCaT cells [21].

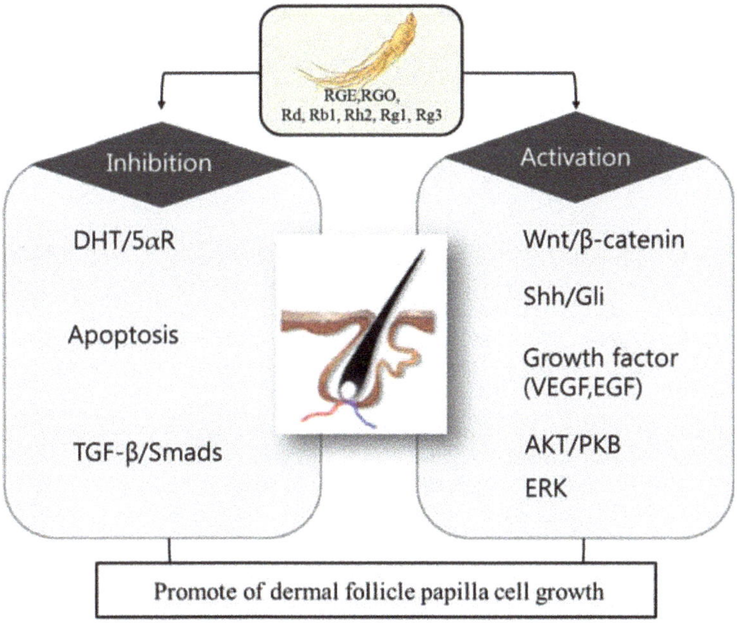

Figure 1. Potential molecular targets of ginseng in hair growth and loss. Ginseng exhibits therapeutic potential for hair growth and preventing hair loss by preventing the apoptosis of dermal follicle papilla cells. Ginseng components: RGE (red ginseng extract), RGO (red ginseng oil), ginsenoside Rd, Rb1, Rh2, Rg1, Rg3. antiandrogenic: DHT (dihydrotestosterone), 5-aR (5α-reductase). Apoptosis inhibition: TGF-β (transforming growth factor beta), Smads (homologues of the Drosophila protein, mothers against decapentaplegic (Mad) and the *Caenorhabditis elegan* sprotein Sma). Proliferation activation: WNT (wingless-type MMTV integration site family member), Shh (Sonic hedgehog), Gli (glioma-associated oncogene homolog), VEGF (vascular endothelial growth factor), EGF (epidermal growth factor), AKT/PKB (protein kinase B), ERK (extracellular-signal-regulated kinases).

2.2. *Antiaging Effects of Ginsenosides*

Several studies have reported on the antiaging effects of various ginsenosides [22,23]. As a general outcome of antiaging effects, ginseng extract and ginsenosides maintain skin structural integrity and regulate hair-growth promotion. For instance, incubation of cultured human dermal fibroblasts with *Panax ginseng* for three days significantly increased cell proliferation and collagen synthesis [24].

The antiaging effects of *P. ginseng* root extract were attributed to the induction of type-1 pro-collagen via phosphorylation of Smad2 and activation of human collagen-A2 promoter in human dermal fibroblast. According to this study, *P. ginseng* root extract did not exhibit any sensitivity reaction to human skin [25]. Another marker of the aging process is wrinkle formation, which is often associated with a reduced level of hyaluronan in the dermis. Topical application of a major ginseng metabolite (compound K) on mouse skin elevated the expression of hyaluronan synthase-2, an enzyme that catalyzes the synthesis of hyaluronan, through Src kinase-dependent activation of ERK and AKT/PKB kinases in the dermis and papillary dermis of mice [26,27]. These antiaging effects result in improved skin health, thereby ensuring hair-follicle health and a regular hair cycle.

2.3. Modulation of TGF-β Signaling

The role of TGF-β in hair loss has been documented through the study revealing that treatment with a TGF-β antagonist can promote hair growth via preventing catagen progression [28]. Since TGF-β1 induces catagen in hair follicles and acts as a pathogenic mediator of androgenic alopecia [28], red ginseng extract can delay the catagen phase and holds the potential to promote hair growth. Administration of red ginseng extract at a dose of 20 or 60 mg/kg twice daily by gavage decreased TGF-β1 levels in UVB-irradiated mouse skin [29]. Likewise, topical administration of ginsenoside Re on to the back skin of nude mice for up to 45 days significantly increased hair-shaft length and hair existent time, and stimulated hair-shaft elongation in the ex vivo cultures of hair follicles isolated from C57BL/6 mouse. The hair-growth-promoting effects of ginsenoside Re were associated with the downregulation of TGF-β-pathway-related genes, which are involved in the control of hair-growth phase-transition-related signaling pathways [30]. It has been reported that brain-derived neurotrophic factor (BDNF) enhances transition from the anagen to the catagen phase through the activation of TGF-β [31]. Protopanaxatriol-type gisenoside Re promotes hair growth through the inhibition of TGF-β signaling pathways [30]. TGF-β-induced hair loss is associated with the hyperactivation of the c-Jun-N-terminal kinase (JNK) pathway [32]. The inhibition of JNK by Korean red ginseng has been attributed to the protective effects of ginseng on radiation-induced apoptosis of HaCaT cells [33].

Moreover, hair-follicle regression is partly regulated by the p75 neurotrophin receptor (p75NTR), which is a classical BDNF [34]. Since neurotrophins elicit their effects by interacting with high-affinity neurotrophin receptors, it would be a rational approach to develop neurotrophin-receptor antagonists as potential therapy for the treatment of hair loss, particularly androgenetic alopecia. A recent study has demonstrated that *P. ginseng* hexane extracts, which largely contain polyacetylenes, strongly inhibited β-nerve growth factor (β-NGF) interaction with p75NTR. Thus *P. ginseng*-derived polyacetylenes would be a potential therapeutic choice for the treatment of hair-growth disorders [35].

2.4. Inhibition of 5α-Reductase Enzyme

Progressive hair loss, also known as alopecia, occurs due to alternations in cell-signaling pathways in hair follicular cells resulting in the induction of apoptosis, changes in usual pattern of hair cycling and thinning, or fracture of the hair shaft. One of the major triggers for hair loss is the exposure to androgens, which in most cases are genetically predetermined among the individuals who have androgenic alopecia. The androgen that mainly plays a role in altering hair cycling is 5α-dihydrotestosterone (DHT), which is a metabolite of testosterone. The conversion of testosterone to DHT is mediated by the 5α-reductase (5αR) enzyme in each follicle [27]. Treatment with 5α-reductase inhibitors, e.g., finasteride, prevents the development of alopecia and increases scalp-hair growth. In several in vivo experiments, topical application of ginseng extract or ginsenosides was reported to enhance hair growth. Rhizomes of *P. ginseng* (red ginseng) containing a considerable amount of ginsenoside Ro inhibited the activity of 5α-reductase. Ginsenoside Rg3 and Rd also exhibited similar inhibitory effects on this enzyme [36]. The inhibition of 5αR enzyme activity was more pronounced with extracts of red-ginseng rhizomes as compared to that of ginseng main-root extract. Ginsenosides Ro derived from rhizome extract and ginsenoside Rg3 obtained from main-root extract attenuated the 5αR enzyme activity with IC_{50} values of 259.4 and 86.1 μm, respectively. Another variety of ginseng, the *Parribacus japonicas* rhizome extract that contains a larger quantity of ginsenoside Ro also inhibited 5αR enzyme activity. Topical administration of red-ginseng rhizome extracts (2 mg/mouse) and ginsenoside Ro (0.2 mg/mouse) onto shaved skin of C57BL/6 mice abrogated testosterone-mediated suppression of hair regrowth [36].

2.5. Modulation of Wnt/Dickkopf Homologue 1 (DKK1) Signaling

Wingless-type integration-site (WNT) signaling plays a key role in hair-follicle development. The blockade of Wnt signaling by overexpression of the WNT inhibitor, DKK1, prevents hair-follicle formation in mice [37]. β-catenin signaling is essential for epithelial stem-cell fate since keratinocytes adopt an epidermal fate in the absence of β-catenin [38]. Treatment with ginsenoside F2 resulted in a 30% increase in the proliferation of HHDPC and HaCaT cells as compared to that of finasteride. Ginsenoside F2 increased the expression of β-catenin and its transcriptional coactivator Lef-1, while it decreased the expression of DKK-1 in HHDPC as well as in the skin of C57BL/6. Administration of ginsenoside F2 promoted hair growth as compared to finasteride, as revealed by an increase in the number of hair follicles, thickness of the epidermis, and follicles of the anagen phase, suggesting that F2 induces the anagen phase and stimulates hair growth through the modulation of the Wnt signal pathway [39]. In another study by Matsuda et al., the hair growth-stimulating activity of the methanol extract of red ginseng in an organ culture of mouse vibrissal follicles was attributable to ginsenosides Rg3 and Rb1 [40]. Treatment of cultured outer root sheath (ORS) keratinocytes with *P. ginseng* extract in the presence or absence of DKK-1 has revealed that *P. ginseng*-extract treatment increased the Bcl-2 to Bax ratio, and the anagen to catagen ratio, and reversed DKK-1-mediated suppression of the Bcl-2/Bax ratio. *P. ginseng* extract antagonizes DKK-1-induced catagen-like changes, in part, through the regulation of apoptosis-related gene expression in hair follicles [41].

2.6. Modulation of Sonic Hedgehog (Shh) Signaling

Shh/Gli (glioma-associated oncogene homolog) regulates hair-follicle development during embryonic life and influences the cycling and growth of hair follicles in adults by promoting telogen-to-anagen transition of follicular cells and epidermal growth [42–44]. Mice harboring the mutant form of Shh have small dermal papillae characterized by the presence of abnormal hair follicular cells that are incapable of maintaining normal hair morphogenesis [44]. Attenuation of Shh activity by a monoclonal antibody targeting Shh diminished hair growth in mice, indicating the importance of Shh signaling in hair-growth promotion [45]. Treatment with red-ginseng oil reversed testosterone-induced suppression of hair regeneration in C57BL/6 mice by increasing the expression of Shh/Gli pathway-related proteins, including Shh, Smoothened (Smo), and Gli1. Additionally, two major compounds in red-ginseng oil, linoleic acid and β-sitosterol, were also found to activate the Shh/Gli signaling pathway in testosterone-treated mice. Topical application of bicycle (10.1.0) tridec-1-ene was unlikely to significantly accelerate protein levels of Shh and Gli1, but likely to increase Smo expression [46].

2.7. Modulation of JAK2-STAT3 Signaling

Cytokines, such as interleukins (ILs) and interferons (IFN), are inflammatory-signaling molecules that, upon overexpression and/or secretion, cause skin inflammation. Hair follicles are usually immune-tolerated areas, where natural killer (NK) cells remain suppressed [47]. Such immune activation is supported by the presence of CD8+ T cells and NKG2D+ cells around the peribulbar area of the affected hair follicles [48] and upregulation of several ILs, such as IL-2, IL-7, IL-15, and IL-21, and IFN-γ [49]. Loss of immune tolerance or immune activation, due to the upregulation of major histocompatibility complex (MHC class I) or UL16-binding protein 3 (ULBP3) molecules, leads to the activation of a cytotoxic cluster of differentiation 8-positive (CD8+) and NK group 2D-positive

(NKG2D+) T cells to the hair follicles [50,51], thereby leading to hair-follicle dystrophy and acceleration of the catagen phase [52]. Since JAK/Signal transducer and activator of transcription-3 (STAT3) pathway plays a critical role in mediating the activation of CD8+ NKG2D+ T cells, the inhibition of JAK appears as a plausible target for developing a therapy for hair loss [49]. In fact, a number of JAK inhibitors, such as tofacitinib and roxulitinib, are in the progress of developing a therapy for alopecia [53]. Ginsenoside Rk1 inhibited the lipopolysaccharide- stimulated phosphorylation of JAK2 and STAT3 in murine macrophage cells [54]. It would be interesting to investigate whether ginsenoside Rk1 or other ginsenosides can target JAK2 signaling in dermal papilla and diminish activation of NKG2D+ T cells. Moreover, the pathogenesis of alopecia areata is believed to involve inflammatory cytokines IL-17A and monoclonal antibodies against IL-17A secukinumab-caused hair regrowth in human volunteers [55]. Treatment of Th17 cells with *Panax notoginseng* saponins diminished the proliferation and differentiation of Th17 cells and decreased IL-17 expression [56]. Topical application of ginsenoside F2 also ameliorated phorbol ester-induced dermal inflammation by inhibiting the production of IL-17 and ROS in $\gamma\delta$T cells and neutrophils, respectively, in mouse-ear skin [57]. These findings suggest that ginsenosides may enhance hair growth in alopecia areata by regulating IL-17 secretion.

2.8. Activation of Dermal Papillary Cell Proliferation

Various intracellular signaling molecules, including kinases and growth factors, play a critical role in stimulating hair growth by promoting dermal papillary-cell proliferation. VEGF, which is released from the epithelium, is a signaling protein that increases the vascular network surrounding the hair follicle [58]. Ginsenoside Rg3 promotes hair growth by upregulating VEGF expression [36]. Shin et al. also demonstrated that Rg3 increased the proliferation of human dermal papillary cells, which was associated with elevating the mRNA level of VEGF. In mouse-hair follicles in vivo, Rg3 not only increased the expression of VEGF but also stimulated stem cells by upregulating factor-activating CD34, and promoted hair growth even more than minoxidil [39].

Signaling pathway ERK, usually activated by mitogens, plays an important role in the proliferation of human hair-follicle dermal papillary cells (HHDPCs) [59]. Both red-ginseng extract (RGE) and ginsenoside-Rb1 activated the ERK signaling pathway. Thus, the proliferation of HHDPCs by red ginseng may be mediated by the ERK signaling pathways [12]. Another intercellular kinase, AKT/PKB, transmits critical signals for cell survival, and also regulates the survival of dermal papillary cells (DPCs) as an antiapoptotic molecule [60]. Therefore, the activation of AKT/PKB by red-ginseng extract and ginsenoside-Rb1 may prolong the survival of HHDPCs [12].

The Bcl-2 family proteins consists of more than a dozen members, which are either antiapoptotic or proapoptotic in nature [61]. During the hair cycle, the DPC is the only region where Bcl-2 is expressed consistently and is considered to resist apoptosis [62]. *Fructus panax ginseng* extract increases the expression of Bcl-2 but decreases Bax expression, a proapoptotic species, in cultured DPCs [63].

3. Evidence from In Vivo Animal Studies

Ginsenosides Rb1 and Rd from *P. ginseng* also exert a stimulating effect on hair follicles, and thus, appear as potential therapeutic agents. One suggested mechanism for this effect of ginsenosides Rb1 and Rd is the induction of p63 [64]. Topical application of *P. ginseng* extract (2.5%) failed to stimulate hair growth as compared to minoxidil in athymic nude mice [8]. The lack of the hair growth-promoting effect of ginseng in this study compared to other herbal products exhibiting hair growth may not be appropriately judged, as the nude mice are basically hairless or have limited fine hairs with poorly defined hair cycles. However, application of *P. ginseng* extract by intraperitoneal or per oral prior to gamma irradiation to adult N:GP mice diminished apoptosis and promoted hair medullary-cell repair [65]. In another study, C57BL/6 mice were subjected to treatment with ginsenoside F2 or finasteride. As compared to the finasteride-treated group, the ginsenoside F2-treated group showed 20% higher hair-growth rates as evidenced by increased number of hair follicles, epidermal thickness, and proportion of follicles in the anagen phase. This hair-growth promoting effect of ginsenoside F2 was mediated, at least in part, through the activation of the Wnt-β-catenin pathway via blockade of Dkk [39]. Truong and colleagues [46] also reported that hair-regenerative capacity was significantly restored by treatment of red-ginseng oil and its major compounds in testosterone-treated mice.

4. Human Clinical Studies

Although individual ginsenosides are yet to be investigated for hair-growth promotion in human clinical trials, there have been few interesting human studies documenting the potential of Korean red ginseng in hair-growth promotion. Oh et al. studied hair-growth efficacy and safety of Korean red ginseng (KRG) in alopecia areata (AA), a model of androgenic alopecia, in human subjects. According to this study, human volunteers were treated with corticosteroid intralesional injection (ILI) with or without treatment with KRG. Hair growth in both the ILI-alone and ILI-plus-KRG patient group was monitored using Folliscope 2.5 for 12 weeks. Average hair density and hair thickness were significantly increased upon addition of KRG with ILI, suggesting that KRG may be considered as a useful complimentary food for gaining efficacy in the treatment for AA [66]. Kim et al. reported the effectiveness of Korean red ginseng in increasing the thickness and density of hair in human volunteers [11]. Moreover, combination treatment with topical minoxidil and oral KRG is more effective than topical minoxidil treatment alone for promoting hair growth. Therefore, KRG is expected to be a helpful supplement in the treatment of hair loss [67]. Keum et al. examined the potential of KRG in preventing premature hair-follicle dystrophy using a human hair-follicle organ-culture model. According to this study, human occipital scalp-skin specimens were obtained from patients undergoing hair-transplantation surgery, and follicular keratinocytes cells (FKC) were cultured in vitro. Treatment of FKCs with 4-hydroxycyclophosphamide (4-HC), a metabolite of chemotherapeutic agent cyclophosphamide, attenuated human hair growth, induced premature catagen development, diminished proliferation, and stimulated apoptosis of hair matrix keratinocytes. Pretreatment with KRG protected against 4-HC-induced hair-growth inhibition and premature catagen development partly by blocking 4-HC-induced p53 and Bax/Bcl2 expression [13].

5. Conclusions

The use of plant products in therapy has long been practiced and has appeared to be generally safe. Ginseng is a multipurpose natural medicine with a long history of medical application throughout the world, particularly in Eastern countries. The medical use of ginseng is not only restricted to the improvement of general wellness, but also extended to the treatment of organ-specific pathological conditions. In the field of dermatology, ginseng and ginsenosides have been shown to regulate the expression and activity of major proteins involved in hair-cycling phases. The promotion of hair growth and prevention of hair loss by ginseng and its metabolites are associated with the induction of anagen and delaying of catagen phases. Although the underlying mechanisms by which ginseng and its metabolites regulate hair cycling have been explored to a limited extent, further studies, especially focusing on extended human trials, are required to establish this natural remedy for hair loss. Alopecia, originating from a variety of causes, including hyperactivation of androgenic signals, exposure to chemotherapeutics, aging, or skin photodamage, is considered as a skin pathology and has great psychosocial impact. Thus, it would be a plausible approach to develop hair growth-stimulating formulations, either as FDA-approved therapeutics or as cosmeceuticals, by using the index component of red ginseng (Table 1).

Table 1. Molecular mechanisms underlying hair-proliferative and antiapoptosis-inducing activity of ginseng.

Type	Study Model	Dosage	Action Mechanism	Target	Reference
Fructus panax ginseng extract (FPG) (95% EtOH)	Human hair dermal papilla cells Male six-week-old C57BL/6 mice	0.8, 4, 20, 100, 500 μg/mL 1 mg/mL	FPG elicited the proliferation of DPC by the upregulation of antiapoptotic Bcl-2 accompanied by the inhibition of apoptotic Bax expression	Apoptosis	[4]
Ginsenoside Re	Male six-week-old C57BL/6 mice Cultured C57BL/6 mouse HFs HeLa cells	1 or 5 mg/d 10 or 50 mg/L 10 mg/L	Ginsenoside Re is the effective constituent in Panax ginseng that promotes hair growth through inhibition of transition related TGF-β signaling pathways.	TGF	[5]
Polyacetylenes isolated from *P. ginseng*	Neurotrophin receptor-binding inhibition assay	sample solution (10, 30, and 100 μM)	Inhibits BDNF-TrkB binding.	Growth	[6]
Ginsenoside F2	Human hair dermal papilla cells Human keratinocyte (HaCaT) cells Male six-week-old C57BL/6 mice	0.01, 0.1, 1, and 10 μM 0. 5 and 2.5 mg/kg	(1) Stimulates proliferation of HHDPC and HaCaT; (2) increases β-catenin and Lef-1 expression and decreases DKK-1 expression in HHDPC; (3) hair anagen induction and acceleration of hair growth in mouse model; (4) increases β-catenin expression and decreases DKK-1 expression in mouse tissue.	WNT	[7]
Root of PG extract (70% EtOH)	Human ORS keratinocytes Anagen HFs from human scalp-skin specimens	20 ppm	PG extract may enhance ORS and hDPC stimulation of hair follicle growth despite the presence of DKK-1, a strong catagen inducer	WNT	[29]
Korean Red Ginseng (KRG)	Human (patients diagnosed with AA)	Treated with corticosteroid ILI while taking KRG	KRG can result in improved hair regrowth in AA patients.		[20]
KRG extract	Follicular keratinocytes (FKCs) Human anagen hair follicles	0~1000 μg/mL 500 μg/mL	KRG may protect against 4-HC-induced premature dystrophy as it occurs in CIA in vivo. Possible mechanisms include the stimulation of hair matrix keratinocyte proliferation and inhibition of hair matrix keratinocyte apoptosis, which are possibly mediated through modulation of p53 and Bax/Bcl-2 expression.	Apotosis	[21]

Table 1. *Cont.*

Type	Study Model	Dosage	Action Mechanism	Target	Reference
Red ginseng extract (RGE) RGE, insenoside-Rb1	Six-week-old female C57BL/6 mice Human hair follicles	3% 100 μg/mL	RGE and its ginsenosides may enhance hDPC proliferation, activate the ERK and AKT/PKB signaling pathways in hDPCs, upregulate hair matrix keratinocyte proliferation, and inhibit DHT-induced androgen receptor transcription.	Growth 5aR	[16]
Red ginseng oil (RGO)	C57BL/6 mice	RGO 10%	Upregulates Wnt/-catenin and Shh/Gli pathways-mediated expression of genes such as β-catenin, Lef-1, Sonic hedgehog, Smoothened, Gli-1, Cyclin D1, and Cyclin E in TES-treated mice. RGO and its major components reduce the protein level of TGF-β but enhance the expression of antiapoptotic protein Bcl-2.	WNT Shh Growth TGF Apoptosis	[25]
KRG	Human (patients with female pattern hair loss)	Oral	Patients about the size of the vertex spot, hair loss on the top of scalp, bitemporal recession, hair shedding, hair quality, and overall satisfaction; group 2 was more satisfied at 24 weeks.		[68]
Ginsenoside Rg3	Human DP cells Female C57BL/6 mice	1, 5, 10 μM 1000 μM	Dose-dependent increases in VEGF, CD8, CD34 Rg3 might increase hair growth through stimulation of hair-follicle stem cells	Growth	[69]
Red ginseng (RGE) White ginseng (WGE) Ginsenoside-Rb1 (G-Rb1), Rg1 (G-Rg1), -Ro (G-Ro)	B6C3F1 mice Mouse vibrissal hair follicles	20, 50 μg/mL 10 μg/mL	Hair growth-promoting assay using mouse vibrissal follicles in organ culture	Growth	[26]
Ginseng rhizome Ginsenoside Ro	C57BL/6 mice	extracts of red ginseng rhizomes (2 mg/mouse) and ginsenoside Ro (0.2 mg/mouse)	Inhibitory activity against 5αR in the androgenetic alopecia model.	5aR	[27]
Ginsenosides Rb1, Re, and Rg1	Cultured hHFs	2, 5, and 10 mg/mL PG extracts and 1 mM of the ginsenosides Rb1, Re and Rg1	PG extract using hHF organ culture, and promoting hair growth through similar mechanisms to those of minoxidil.	5aR	[36]

Funding: This research received no external funding.

Acknowledgments: I wish to thank Joydeb Kumar Kundu for his helpful comments on the manuscript.

Conflicts of Interest: The author declares no conflict of interest.

References

1. Dong Hyun, K. Review: Herbal medicines are activated by intestinal microflora. *Nat. Prod. Sci.* **2002**, *8*, 35–43.
2. Tawab, M.A.; Bahr, U.; Karas, M.; Wurglics, M.; Schubert-Zsilavecz, M. Degradation of ginsenosides in humans after oral administration. *Drug Metab. Dispos.* **2003**, *31*, 1065–1071. [CrossRef] [PubMed]
3. Rees, J.L. The genetics of sun sensitivity in humans. *Am. J. Hum. Genet.* **2004**, *75*, 739–751. [CrossRef] [PubMed]
4. Oh, S.J.; Kim, K.; Lim, C.J. Suppressive properties of ginsenoside Rb2, a protopanaxadiol-type ginseng saponin, on reactive oxygen species and matrix metalloproteinase-2 in UV-B-irradiated human dermal keratinocytes. *Biosci. Biotechnol. Biochem.* **2015**, *79*, 1075–1081. [CrossRef] [PubMed]
5. Oh, S.J.; Lee, S.; Kho, Y.E.; Kim, K.; Jin, C.D.; Lim, C.J. Stereoselective suppressive effects of protopanaxadiol epimers on uv-b-induced reactive oxygen species and matrix metalloproteinase-2 in human dermal keratinocytes. *Can. J. Physiol. Pharmacol.* **2015**, *93*, 91–95. [CrossRef] [PubMed]
6. Lim, C.J.; Choi, W.Y.; Jung, H.J. Stereoselective skin anti-photoaging properties of ginsenoside Rg3 in UV-B-irradiated keratinocytes. *Biol. Pharm. Bull.* **2014**, *37*, 1583–1590. [CrossRef] [PubMed]
7. Oh, S.J.; Lee, S.; Choi, W.Y.; Lim, C.J. Skin anti-photoaging properties of ginsenoside Rh2 epimers in UV-B-irradiated human keratinocyte cells. *J. Biosci.* **2014**, *39*, 673–682. [CrossRef] [PubMed]
8. Begum, S.; Lee, M.R.; Gu, L.J.; Hossain, M.J.; Kim, H.K.; Sung, C.K. Comparative hair restorer efficacy of medicinal herb on nude (foxn1nu) mice. *Biomed Res. Int.* **2014**, *2014*, 319795. [CrossRef] [PubMed]
9. Gottumukkala, V.R.; Annamalai, T.; Mukhopadhyay, T. Phytochemical investigation and hair growth studies on the rhizomes of nardostachys jatamansi dc. *Pharmacogn. Mag.* **2011**, *7*, 146–150. [CrossRef] [PubMed]
10. Tanaka, S.; Saito, M.; Tabata, M. Bioassay of crude drugs for hair growth promoting activity in mice by a new simple method. *Planta Med.* **1980**, *40*, 84–90. [CrossRef] [PubMed]
11. Jae Hwan, K.; Sang Min, Y.; Jae Eun, C.; Sang Wook, S. Study of the efficacy of Korean red ginseng in the treatment of androgenic alopecia. *J. Ginseng Res.* **2009**, *33*, 223–228.
12. Park, G.H.; Park, K.Y.; Cho, H.I.; Lee, S.M.; Han, J.S.; Won, C.H.; Chang, S.E.; Lee, M.W.; Choi, J.H.; Moon, K.C.; et al. Red ginseng extract promotes the hair growth in cultured human hair follicles. *J. Med. Food* **2015**, *18*, 354–362. [CrossRef] [PubMed]
13. Keum, D.I.; Pi, L.Q.; Hwang, S.T.; Lee, W.S. Protective effect of korean red ginseng against chemotherapeutic drug-induced premature catagen development assessed with human hair follicle organ culture model. *J. Ginseng Res.* **2016**, *40*, 169–175. [CrossRef] [PubMed]
14. Inui, S.; Itami, S. Androgen actions on the human hair follicle: Perspectives. *Exp. Dermatol.* **2013**, *22*, 168–171. [CrossRef] [PubMed]
15. Traish, A.M. Negative impact of testosterone deficiency and 5α-reductase inhibitors therapy on metabolic and sexual function in men. *Adv. Exp. Med. Biol.* **2017**, *1043*, 473–526. [PubMed]
16. Rattan, S.I.; Kryzch, V.; Schnebert, S.; Perrier, E.; Nizard, C. Hormesis-based anti-aging products: A case study of a novel cosmetic. *Dose Response* **2013**, *11*, 99–108. [CrossRef] [PubMed]
17. Cha, H.J.; Kim, O.Y.; Lee, G.T.; Lee, K.S.; Lee, J.H.; Park, I.C.; Lee, S.J.; Kim, Y.R.; Ahn, K.J.; An, I.S.; et al. Identification of ultraviolet b radiationinduced micrornas in normal human dermal papilla cells. *Mol. Med. Rep.* **2014**, *10*, 1663–1670. [CrossRef] [PubMed]
18. Chen, W.X.; Qin, Z.H.; Zeng, D.; Han, Z.Z.; Zhan, R.T.; Tan, Y.; Chen, W.W. Comparative study on effects of anti-contusion injury, analgesia and anti-inflammation of root and stem of zanthoxylum nitidum. *Zhong Yao Cai* **2015**, *38*, 2358–2363. [PubMed]
19. Hou, C.; Miao, Y.; Wang, J.; Wang, X.; Chen, C.Y.; Hu, Z.Q. Collagenase iv plays an important role in regulating hair cycle by inducing VEGF, IGF-1, and TGF-β expression. *Drug Des. Dev. Ther.* **2015**, *9*, 5373–5383. [CrossRef] [PubMed]
20. Kim, Y.G.; Sumiyoshi, M.; Sakanaka, M.; Kimura, Y. Effects of ginseng saponins isolated from red ginseng on ultraviolet B-induced skin aging in hairless mice. *Eur. J. Pharmacol.* **2009**, *602*, 148–156. [CrossRef] [PubMed]

21. Lee, E.H.; Cho, S.Y.; Kim, S.J.; Shin, E.S.; Chang, H.K.; Kim, D.H.; Yeom, M.H.; Woe, K.S.; Lee, J.; Sim, Y.C.; et al. Ginsenoside F1 protects human hacat keratinocytes from ultraviolet-B-induced apoptosis by maintaining constant levels of Bcl-2. *J. Investig. Dermatol.* **2003**, *121*, 607–613. [CrossRef] [PubMed]
22. Pham, Q.L.; Jang, H.J.; Kim, K.B. Antiwrinkle effect of fermented black ginseng on human fibroblasts. *Int. J. Mol. Med.* **2017**, *39*, 681–686. [CrossRef] [PubMed]
23. Hwang, E.; Park, S.Y.; Yin, C.S.; Kim, H.T.; Kim, Y.M.; Yi, T.H. Antiaging effects of the mixture of *panax ginseng* and crataegus pinnatifida in human dermal fibroblasts and healthy human skin. *J. Ginseng Res.* **2017**, *41*, 69–77. [CrossRef] [PubMed]
24. Lee, G.Y.; Park, K.G.; Namgoong, S.; Han, S.K.; Jeong, S.H.; Dhong, E.S.; Kim, W.K. Effects of *panax ginseng* extract on human dermal fibroblast proliferation and collagen synthesis. *Int. Wound J.* **2016**, *13*, 42–46. [CrossRef] [PubMed]
25. Lee, J.; Jung, E.; Lee, J.; Huh, S.; Kim, J.; Park, M.; So, J.; Ham, Y.; Jung, K.; Hyun, C.G.; et al. *Panax ginseng* induces human Type I collagen synthesis through activation of smad signaling. *J. Ethnopharmacol.* **2007**, *109*, 29–34. [CrossRef] [PubMed]
26. Li, X.; Lin, Z.; Huang, Y.; Deng, Q.; Xu, H. Study on antiradiation effect of panaxatriol. *Zhong Yao Cai* **2002**, *25*, 805–808. [PubMed]
27. Kaufman, K.D.; Olsen, E.A.; Whiting, D.; Savin, R.; DeVillez, R.; Bergfeld, W.; Price, V.H.; Van Neste, D.; Roberts, J.L.; Hordinsky, M.; et al. Finasteride in the treatment of men with androgenetic alopecia. Finasteride male pattern hair loss study group. *J. Am. Acad. Dermatol.* **1998**, *39*, 578–589. [CrossRef]
28. Foitzik, K.; Lindner, G.; Mueller-Roever, S.; Maurer, M.; Botchkareva, N.; Botchkarev, V.; Handjiski, B.; Metz, M.; Hibino, T.; Soma, T.; et al. Control of murine hair follicle regression (catagen) by TGF-β1 in vivo. *FASEB J.* **2000**, *14*, 752–760. [CrossRef] [PubMed]
29. Kim, Y.G.; Sumiyoshi, M.; Kawahira, K.; Sakanaka, M.; Kimura, Y. Effects of red ginseng extract on ultraviolet b-irradiated skin change in C57BL mice. *Phytother. Res.* **2008**, *22*, 1423–1427. [CrossRef] [PubMed]
30. Li, Z.; Ryu, S.W.; Lee, J.; Choi, K.; Kim, S.; Choi, C. Protopanaxatirol type ginsenoside re promotes cyclic growth of hair follicles via inhibiting transforming growth factor β signaling cascades. *Biochem. Biophys. Res. Commun.* **2016**, *470*, 924–929. [CrossRef] [PubMed]
31. Peters, E.M.; Hansen, M.G.; Overall, R.W.; Nakamura, M.; Pertile, P.; Klapp, B.F.; Arck, P.C.; Paus, R. Control of human hair growth by neurotrophins: Brain-derived neurotrophic factor inhibits hair shaft elongation, induces catagen, and stimulates follicular transforming growth factor β2 expression. *J. Investig. Dermatol.* **2005**, *124*, 675–685. [CrossRef] [PubMed]
32. Hibino, T.; Nishiyama, T. Role of tgf-β2 in the human hair cycle. *J. Dermatol. Sci.* **2004**, *35*, 9–18. [CrossRef] [PubMed]
33. Chang, J.W.; Park, K.H.; Hwang, H.S.; Shin, Y.S.; Oh, Y.T.; Kim, C.H. Protective effects of korean red ginseng against radiation-induced apoptosis in human hacat keratinocytes. *J. Radiat. Res.* **2014**, *55*, 245–256. [CrossRef] [PubMed]
34. Botchkarev, V.A.; Botchkareva, N.V.; Albers, K.M.; Chen, L.H.; Welker, P.; Paus, R. A role for p75 neurotrophin receptor in the control of apoptosis-driven hair follicle regression. *FASEB J.* **2000**, *14*, 1931–1942. [CrossRef] [PubMed]
35. Suzuki, A.; Matsuura, D.; Kanatani, H.; Yano, S.; Tsunakawa, M.; Matsuyama, S.; Shigemori, H. Inhibitory effects of polyacetylene compounds from *panax ginseng* on neurotrophin receptor-mediated hair growth. *Biol. Pharm. Bull.* **2017**, *40*, 1784–1788. [CrossRef] [PubMed]
36. Shin, D.H.; Cha, Y.J.; Yang, K.E.; Jang, I.S.; Son, C.G.; Kim, B.H.; Kim, J.M. Ginsenoside rg3 up-regulates the expression of vascular endothelial growth factor in human dermal papilla cells and mouse hair follicles. *Phytother. Res.* **2014**, *28*, 1088–1095. [CrossRef] [PubMed]
37. Andl, T.; Reddy, S.T.; Gaddapara, T.; Millar, S.E. Wnt signals are required for the initiation of hair follicle development. *Dev. Cell* **2002**, *2*, 643–653. [CrossRef]
38. Kretzschmar, K.; Cottle, D.L.; Schweiger, P.J.; Watt, F.M. The androgen receptor antagonizes Wnt/β-catenin signaling in epidermal stem cells. *J. Investig. Dermatol.* **2015**, *135*, 2753–2763. [CrossRef] [PubMed]
39. Shin, H.S.; Park, S.Y.; Hwang, E.S.; Lee, D.G.; Song, H.G.; Mavlonov, G.T.; Yi, T.H. The inductive effect of ginsenoside F2 on hair growth by altering the Wnt signal pathway in telogen mouse skin. *Eur. J. Pharmacol.* **2014**, *730*, 82–89. [CrossRef] [PubMed]

40. Matsuda, H.; Yamazaki, M.; Asanuma, Y.; Kubo, M. Promotion of hair growth by ginseng radix on cultured mouse vibrissal hair follicles. *Phytother. Res.* **2003**, *17*, 797–800. [CrossRef] [PubMed]
41. Lee, Y.; Kim, S.N.; Hong, Y.D.; Park, B.C.; Na, Y. *Panax ginseng* extract antagonizes the effect of DKK1-induced catagen-like changes of hair follicles. *Int. J. Mol. Med.* **2017**, *40*, 1194–1200. [CrossRef] [PubMed]
42. Kishimoto, J.; Burgeson, R.E.; Morgan, B.A. Wnt signaling maintains the hair-inducing activity of the dermal papilla. *Genes Dev.* **2000**, *14*, 1181–1185. [PubMed]
43. Sato, N.; Leopold, P.L.; Crystal, R.G. Effect of adenovirus-mediated expression of sonic hedgehog gene on hair regrowth in mice with chemotherapy-induced alopecia. *J. Natl. Cancer Inst.* **2001**, *93*, 1858–1864. [CrossRef] [PubMed]
44. St-Jacques, B.; Dassule, H.R.; Karavanova, I.; Botchkarev, V.A.; Li, J.; Danielian, P.S.; McMahon, J.A.; Lewis, P.M.; Paus, R.; McMahon, A.P. Sonic hedgehog signaling is essential for hair development. *Curr. Biol.* **1998**, *8*, 1058–1068. [CrossRef]
45. Wang, L.C.; Liu, Z.Y.; Gambardella, L.; Delacour, A.; Shapiro, R.; Yang, J.; Sizing, I.; Rayhorn, P.; Garber, E.A.; Benjamin, C.D.; et al. Regular articles: Conditional disruption of hedgehog signaling pathway defines its critical role in hair development and regeneration. *J. Investig. Dermatol.* **2000**, *114*, 901–908. [CrossRef] [PubMed]
46. Truong, V.L.; Bak, M.J.; Lee, C.; Jun, M.; Jeong, W.S. Hair regenerative mechanisms of red ginseng oil and its major components in the testosterone-induced delay of anagen entry in C57BL/6 mice. *Molecules* **2017**, *22*, 1505. [CrossRef] [PubMed]
47. Paus, R.; Ito, N.; Takigawa, M.; Ito, T. The hair follicle and immune privilege. *J. Investig. Dermatol. Symp. Proc.* **2003**, *8*, 188–194. [CrossRef] [PubMed]
48. Ito, T.; Ito, N.; Saatoff, M.; Hashizume, H.; Fukamizu, H.; Nickoloff, B.J.; Takigawa, M.; Paus, R. Maintenance of hair follicle immune privilege is linked to prevention of NK cell attack. *J. Investig. Dermatol.* **2008**, *128*, 1196–1206. [CrossRef] [PubMed]
49. Xing, L.; Dai, Z.; Jabbari, A.; Cerise, J.E.; Higgins, C.A.; Gong, W.; de Jong, A.; Harel, S.; DeStefano, G.M.; Rothman, L.; et al. Alopecia areata is driven by cytotoxic t lymphocytes and is reversed by Jak inhibition. *Nat. Med.* **2014**, *20*, 1043–1049. [CrossRef] [PubMed]
50. Petukhova, L.; Duvic, M.; Hordinsky, M.; Norris, D.; Price, V.; Shimomura, Y.; Kim, H.; Singh, P.; Lee, A.; Chen, W.V.; et al. Genome-wide association study in alopecia areata implicates both innate and adaptive immunity. *Nature* **2010**, *466*, 113–117. [CrossRef] [PubMed]
51. Betz, R.C.; Petukhova, L.; Ripke, S.; Huang, H.; Menelaou, A.; Redler, S.; Becker, T.; Heilmann, S.; Yamany, T.; Duvic, M.; et al. Genome-wide meta-analysis in alopecia areata resolves HLA associations and reveals two new susceptibility loci. *Nat. Commun.* **2015**, *6*, 5966. [CrossRef] [PubMed]
52. Ito, T.; Ito, N.; Saathoff, M.; Bettermann, A.; Takigawa, M.; Paus, R. Interferon-gamma is a potent inducer of catagen-like changes in cultured human anagen hair follicles. *Br. J. Dermatol.* **2005**, *152*, 623–631. [CrossRef] [PubMed]
53. Triyangkulsri, K.; Suchonwanit, P. Role of janus kinase inhibitors in the treatment of alopecia areata. *Drug Des. Dev. Ther.* **2018**, *12*, 2323–2335. [CrossRef] [PubMed]
54. Yu, Q.; Zeng, K.W.; Ma, X.L.; Jiang, Y.; Tu, P.F.; Wang, X.M. Ginsenoside Rk1 suppresses pro-inflammatory responses in lipopolysaccharide-stimulated RAW264.7 cells by inhibiting the Jak2/Stat3 pathway. *Chin. J. Nat. Med.* **2017**, *15*, 751–757. [CrossRef]
55. Guttman-Yassky, E.; Nia, J.K.; Hashim, P.W.; Mansouri, Y.; Alia, E.; Taliercio, M.; Desai, P.N.; Lebwohl, M.G. Efficacy and safety of secukinumab treatment in adults with extensive alopecia areata. *Arch. Dermatol. Res.* **2018**. [CrossRef] [PubMed]
56. Wei, Y.; Huyghues-Despointes, B.M.; Tsai, J.; Scholtz, J.M. Nmr study and molecular dynamics simulations of optimized β-hairpin fragments of protein g. *Proteins* **2007**, *69*, 285–296. [CrossRef] [PubMed]
57. Park, S.H.; Seo, W.; Eun, H.S.; Kim, S.Y.; Jo, E.; Kim, M.H.; Choi, W.M.; Lee, J.H.; Shim, Y.R.; Cui, C.H.; et al. Protective effects of ginsenoside F2 on 12-*O*-tetradecanoylphorbol-13-acetate-induced skin inflammation in mice. *Biochem. Biophys. Res. Commun.* **2016**, *478*, 1713–1719. [CrossRef] [PubMed]
58. Mattioli, M.; Barboni, B.; Turriani, M.; Galeati, G.; Zannoni, A.; Castellani, G.; Berardinelli, P.; Scapolo, P.A. Follicle activation involves vascular endothelial growth factor production and increased blood vessel extension. *Biol. Reprod.* **2001**, *65*, 1014–1019. [CrossRef] [PubMed]

59. Li, W.; Man, X.Y.; Li, C.M.; Chen, J.Q.; Zhou, J.; Cai, S.Q.; Lu, Z.F.; Zheng, M. VEGF induces proliferation of human hair follicle dermal papilla cells through VEGFR-2-mediated activation of ERK. *Exp. Cell Res.* **2012**, *318*, 1633–1640. [CrossRef] [PubMed]
60. Han, J.H.; Kwon, O.S.; Chung, J.H.; Cho, K.H.; Eun, H.C.; Kim, K.H. Effect of minoxidil on proliferation and apoptosis in dermal papilla cells of human hair follicle. *J. Dermatol. Sci.* **2004**, *34*, 91–98. [CrossRef] [PubMed]
61. Adams, J.M.; Cory, S. The Bcl-2 protein family: Arbiters of cell survival. *Science* **1998**, *281*, 1322–1326. [CrossRef] [PubMed]
62. Lindner, G.; Botchkarev, V.A.; Botchkareva, N.V.; Ling, G.; van der Veen, C.; Paus, R. Analysis of apoptosis during hair follicle regression (catagen). *Am. J. Pathol.* **1997**, *151*, 1601–1617. [PubMed]
63. Park, S.; Shin, W.S.; Ho, J. *Fructus panax ginseng* extract promotes hair regeneration in C57BL/6 mice. *J. Ethnopharmacol.* **2011**, *138*, 340–344. [CrossRef] [PubMed]
64. Li, Z.; Li, J.J.; Gu, L.J.; Zhang, D.L.; Wang, Y.B.; Sung, C.K. Ginsenosides Rb1 and Rd regulate proliferation of mature keratinocytes through induction of p63 expression in hair follicles. *Phytother. Res.* **2013**, *27*, 1095–1101. [CrossRef] [PubMed]
65. Kim, S.H.; Jeong, K.S.; Ryu, S.Y.; Kim, T.H. *Panax ginseng* prevents apoptosis in hair follicles and accelerates recovery of hair medullary cells in irradiated mice. *In Vivo* **1998**, *12*, 219–222. [PubMed]
66. Oh, G.N.; Son, S.W. Efficacy of korean red ginseng in the treatment of alopecia areata. *J. Ginseng Res.* **2012**, *36*, 391–395. [CrossRef] [PubMed]
67. Ryu, H.J.; Yoo, M.G.; Son, S.W. The efficacy of 3% minoxidil vs. Combined 3% minoxidil and korean red ginseng in treating female pattern alopecia. *Int. J. Dermatol.* **2014**, *53*, e340–e342. [CrossRef] [PubMed]
68. Kim, S.; Kang, B.Y.; Cho, S.Y.; Sung, D.S.; Chang, H.K.; Yeom, M.H.; Kim, D.H.; Sim, Y.C.; Lee, Y.S. Compound k induces expression of hyaluronan synthase 2 gene in transformed human keratinocytes and increases hyaluronan in hairless mouse skin. *Biochem. Biophys. Res. Commun.* **2004**, *316*, 348–355. [CrossRef] [PubMed]
69. Lim, T.G.; Jeon, A.J.; Yoon, J.H.; Song, D.; Kim, J.E.; Kwon, J.Y.; Kim, J.R.; Kang, N.J.; Park, J.S.; Yeom, M.H.; et al. 20-O-β-D-glucopyranosyl-20(S)-protopanaxadiol, a metabolite of ginsenoside Rb1, enhances the production of hyaluronic acid through the activation of ERK and AKT/PKB mediated by Src tyrosin kinase in human keratinocytes. *Int. J. Mol. Med.* **2015**, *35*, 1388–1394. [CrossRef] [PubMed]

International Journal of
Molecular Sciences

MDPI

Review

Natural Products for the Treatment of Autoimmune Arthritis: Their Mechanisms of Action, Targeted Delivery, and Interplay with the Host Microbiome

Steven Dudics [1,2], David Langan [1,2,†], Rakeshchandra R. Meka [1,2,†], Shivaprasad H. Venkatesha [1,2], Brian M. Berman [3,4], Chun-Tao Che [5] and Kamal D. Moudgil [1,2,6,*,‡]

1 Baltimore Veterans Affairs Medical Center, Baltimore, MD 21201, USA; sdudics1@gmail.com (S.D.); david.langan@umaryland.edu (D.L.); Rmeka@som.umaryland.edu (R.R.M.); hvshivaprasad@gmail.com (S.H.V.)
2 Department of Microbiology and Immunology, University of Maryland School of Medicine, Baltimore, MD 21201, USA
3 Family and Community Medicine, University of Maryland School of Medicine, Baltimore, MD 21201, USA; bberman@som.umaryland.edu
4 Center for Integrative Medicine, University of Maryland School of Medicine, Baltimore, MD 21201, USA
5 Medicinal Chemistry and Pharmacognosy, College of Pharmacy, University of Illinois at Chicago, Chicago, IL 60612, USA; chect@uic.edu
6 Division of Rheumatology, Department of Medicine, University of Maryland School of Medicine, Baltimore, MD 21201, USA
* Correspondence: kmoudgil@som.umaryland.edu; Fax: +1-410-706-2129
† These authors contributed equally to this manuscript.
‡ Supv. Research Health Scientist, Veterans Affairs.

Received: 23 July 2018; Accepted: 18 August 2018; Published: 24 August 2018

Abstract: Rheumatoid arthritis (RA) is a chronic, debilitating illness characterized by painful swelling of the joints, inflammation of the synovial lining of the joints, and damage to cartilage and bone. Several anti-inflammatory and disease-modifying drugs are available for RA therapy. However, the prolonged use of these drugs is associated with severe side effects. Furthermore, these drugs are effective only in a proportion of RA patients. Hence, there is a need to search for new therapeutic agents that are effective yet safe. Interestingly, a variety of herbs and other natural products offer a vast resource for such anti-arthritic agents. We discuss here the basic features of RA pathogenesis; the commonly used animal models of RA; the mainstream drugs used for RA; the use of well-characterized natural products possessing anti-arthritic activity; the application of nanoparticles for efficient delivery of such products; and the interplay between dietary products and the host microbiome for maintenance of health and disease induction. We believe that with several advances in the past decade in the characterization and functional studies of natural products, the stage is set for widespread clinical testing and/or use of these products for the treatment of RA and other diseases.

Keywords: adjuvant-induced arthritis; arthritis; celastrol; curcumin; dietary supplements; EGCG; green tea; inflammation; liposomes; microbiome; nanoparticles; natural products; resveratrol; rheumatoid arthritis; targeted delivery; traditional medicine; Tripterygium wilfordii; triptolide

---

1. Introduction

Rheumatoid arthritis (RA) is a multifactorial disease that involves both genetic predisposition and environmental components [1–5]. RA is prevalent worldwide with approximately 1.3 million people affected by RA in the United States alone [6–10]. Moreover, women are more likely to develop RA than men [7]. It is anticipated that with people living longer, the incidence of RA is likely to increase [11–14]. RA is typically characterized by chronic inflammation of the synovial membrane that lines the joints, damage to the cartilage, and erosion of the bone [15–17]. Swelling and redness of the hands and feet is the most common sign of RA along with pain in the afflicted areas [15]. Ulnar deviation [18], Swan neck deformity [19], and subcutaneous nodules [20,21] are among the clinical manifestations of untreated severe RA. The most common serum biomarkers for RA are rheumatoid factor (RF) and anti-citrullinated protein/peptide antibodies (ACPA) [22]. Furthermore, ACPA can also be used as prognostic markers for RA similarly to RF, as they are present a median of 4.5 years prior to clinical onset of the disease [23]. A relatively new potential biomarker for RA is the oncoprotein survivin [24], which is already a known biomarker for cancer. In one study, survivin was detected in 50.7% of RA patients but only 5.6% in controls, which indicates its high specificity [24].

2. The Cellular and Soluble Mediators of Arthritic Inflammation

Under normal conditions, the mature T cells encounter self-antigens in the periphery all the time; however, their activation is kept under control via diverse mechanisms, including unresponsiveness due to lack of adequate interaction between the peptide-MHC (major histocompatibility complex) complex and the T cell receptor (TCR) (ignorance), induction of anergy in the absence of co-stimulation, or suppression by T regulatory (Treg) cells [25,26]. The initiation of RA involves an interplay among components of the innate and adaptive immune responses leading to unintended activation of autoreactive T cells specific for potentially arthritogenic self-antigens in the peripheral lymphoid organs (Figure 1) [15,27]. Antigen-presenting cells (APCs), including dendritic cells, macrophages as well as activated B cells, present arthritogenic autoantigens to T cells that have specific TCRs that can recognize these autoantigens. At the same time, upregulation of co-stimulatory molecules expressed by the APCs under inflammatory conditions facilitates activation of these potentially arthritogenic T cells. Further, the cytokine milieu of the inflammatory environment (such as interleukin-12 (IL-12) and interferon-γ (IFN-γ) for T helper 1 (Th1), and IL6 and IL-1β for Th17) facilitates the differentiation of activated T cells into pathogenic T cell subsets (Th1, Th17), the key drivers of RA pathology [28,29]. This process results in break in tolerance leading to expansion of pathogenic T cells in the peripheral lymphoid organs.

The development of inflammatory arthritis in the joints involves the migration of activated pathogenic T cells from the peripheral lymphoid tissues into the joint tissue (synovial tissue), which is mediated primarily by a chemotactic process [15,27]. These T cells initiate joint-destructive activities by secreting cytokines and other mediators described below. This creates an inflammatory environment which attracts other cell types such as neutrophils, macrophages and fibroblasts to the local site. Collectively, these cells together with various effector molecules (e.g., cytokines, prostaglandins, proteolytic enzymes and other osteoclastogenic factors) induce joint inflammation and cartilage and bone damage. The B cells contribute to the pathogenesis of RA, not only through antigen presentation to the T cells, but also through the production of cytokines and autoantibodies, such as RF and ACPA, which can further reinforce the inflammation induced by the T cells [15,27,30,31]. Similarly, the Th17 cells produce receptor activator of nuclear factor kappa-B ligand (RANKL), which along with other soluble mediators produced by myeloid cells, facilitates osteoclastogenesis. These osteoclasts can cause bone damage via secreting matrix-degrading enzymes such as matrix metalloproteinases (MMPs) and cathepsin K.

RA is associated with increased production of citrullinated proteins/peptides, which is usually attributed to smoke inhalation. Smoking causes irritation of the lungs and airways, in turn leading to an increase in peptidyl arginine deiminase (PAD) 2 [3], which catalyzes the conversion of arginine to citrulline in certain proteins. This increase in citrullinated proteins/peptides can cause an upregulation of antibodies to citrullinated protein/peptide antigens (ACPA), and individuals with certain human leukocyte antigen (HLA) alleles (e.g., HLA-DRB1) are more prone to mount an immune response to these modified antigens than others [4,5].

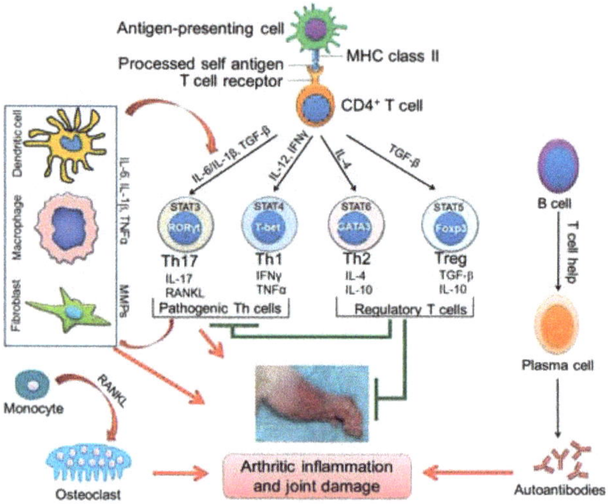

Figure 1. Immunopathogenesis of experimental autoimmune arthritis. Schematic representation of the key pathways is shown: The presentation of an autoantigen to autoreactive T cells and their differentiation into major T helper (Th) cell subsets under the influence of various cytokines; the activation and secretion of pro-inflammatory cytokines by myeloid cells; the T-B cell collaboration leading to autoantibody production by plasma cells; and the osteoimmune cross-talk leading to osteoclast differentiation. These intricate pathways regulate autoimmune inflammation of the synovial joint as shown by arrows (leading to activation/induction) and blunt ends (leading to suppression/inhibition).

3. Animal Models of RA for Studying Disease Pathogenesis and Testing Therapeutic Agents

There are several different animal models used to study the disease process and test novel therapeutics for RA. One of the most well-known models is the collagen-induced arthritis (CIA) model. Here, DBA/1 mice are immunized with type II collagen (CII) emulsified in complete Freund's adjuvant (CFA). This initiates both a B and T cell response to CII, leading to arthritis induction [32,33]. Another commonly used model is the adjuvant-induced arthritis (AA) model [34,35]. In AA, Lewis rats are immunized with heat-killed *Mycobacterium tuberculosis* $H_{37}R_a$ (Mtb) emulsified in mineral oil. This immunization activates a T cell response to mycobacterial heat-shock protein 65 (Bhsp65), which in turn leads to destruction of the joints [33,36–38]. A relatively newer transgenic mouse model to study RA is the K/BxN mouse [39], which were generated by crossing the TCR-transgenic KRN mice with non-obese diabetic (NOD) mice expressing the MHC class II molecule I-A^{g7}. The K/BxN mice develop a severe and destructive form of arthritis, which is associated with high titers of antibodies recognizing glucose-6-phosphate isomerase (GPI), making it a valuable serum transfer model of arthritis [33,40]. Several researchers also use the proteoglycan-induced arthritis (PGIA) model in BALB/c mice, which is a T cell–dependent and autoantibody/B cell–driven disease [41]. Humanized mice are also used to study arthritis [2,33,42]. These mice express the human form of RA-susceptible MHC, HLA-DR4 and/or HLA-DQ8. This allows the researchers to study arthritis in mice but correlate the pathology to humans due to the human genetic background [2,33,42].

4. Currently Used Drugs for Arthritis Therapy and Their Limitations

There are multiple drugs currently being utilized to treat RA patients. The most widely used class of drugs is the non-steroidal anti-inflammatory drugs (NSAIDs) [43]. There are several different drugs under this category, including Ibuprofen, Aspirin, and Naproxone. A majority of them target and suppress prostaglandins (PGs) through inhibition of the cyclooxygenase (COX) enzymes [43]. Patients taking NSAIDs may experience a wide variety of symptoms including renal, hepatic, and cardiovascular toxicity [43]. Certain COX-2-selective agents can cause myocardial infarction (heart attack) and stroke [43]. The second major class of antirheumatic drugs is the disease-modifying antirheumatic drugs (DMARDs), and they belong to two categories, chemical and biologic [44]. Methotrexate (MTX) is one of the gold standards of therapy for RA, and it is a chemical DMARD. There is some evidence that MTX can suppress the production of proinflammatory cytokines [45,46] as well as modulate the levels of specific MMPs [47,48]. Another proposition that has been corroborated in animal models and humans is the augmentation of adenosine levels through the reduction of adenosine deaminase in lymphocytes [49]. Adenosine exerts its anti-inflammatory properties via inhibiting proinflammatroy cytokine production, attenuating neutrophil trafficking to sites of inflammation, and suppressing Th17 cell differentiation, while stimulating Treg differentiation [50]. Adenosine binds to the A_{2A} receptor, which is increased on the surface of lymphocytes in RA patients, and exert its immunosuppressive properties [50]. While the MTX response rate in RA patients is approximately 50% [51], the long-term use of this drug can lead to liver fibrosis, which in some cases may require a liver transplant for its management [52–54].

The biologic DMARDs include monoclonal antibodies targeting tumor necrosis factor (TNF)-α (anti-TNF-α) and IL-6 receptor (anti-IL6R), thereby inhibiting these two cytokines that are major players in promoting RA pathogenesis. Anti-TNF-α is currently the standard of care for RA patients, and it is widely used either alone or in combination with other drugs such as MTX [55,56]. Approximately 10–30% of patients do not respond to initial treatment with anti-TNF-α, and another 23–46% lose responsiveness over time [57]. Moreover, due to the immunosuppressive effect of blocking TNF-α, RA patients are at an increased risk of recurrent infections [58]. Anti-IL6R has been shown to be efficacious in suppressing RA [59,60], and it can be useful in patients not responding to other forms of treatment [61]. However, anti-IL6R has similar side-effects as anti-TNF-α [62].

Corticosteroids are another group of biologic DMARDs, which has been used for RA therapy for the past several decades [63]. Corticosteroids suppress inflammation by binding to the glucocorticoid receptor (GR), also known as NR3C1 (nuclear receptor subfamily 3 group C member 1), in turn leading to the transcription of multiple genes that inhibit several inflammatory pathways. These genes include glucocorticoid-induced leucine zipper protein (GILZ) and MAP kinase phosphatase-1 (MKP-1), which suppress the nuclear factor kappa light chain enhancer of activated B cells (NF-κB) (and Activator protein 1 (AP-1)) and p38 MAP kinase, respectively [64]. Moreover, corticosteroids can lead to an epigenetic modification of histones, subsequently resulting in reduction in inflammation [64]. Corticosteroids have unwanted side effects, including osteoporosis, peptic ulcer, and increased rate of infections [65,66].

5. The Use of Plant Natural Products for Arthritis Therapy

While the above-mentioned mainstream drugs are widely prescribed to patients, they have unwanted side effects. Moreover, some of these drugs are quite expensive. Owing to these limitations, an increasing number of patients have started to turn to natural products to relieve symptoms of RA and related ailments [67], with over 36% of adults in the USA using complementary and alternative (CAM) therapies [68]. Natural products have been studied extensively in multiple different ailments such as cancer [69], infectious diseases [70], and autoimmunity [71–75]. However, difficulties in evaluating the efficacy of these products as well as inadequate information about their mechanism of action are among the reasons for skepticism from both the public and professional communities [76,77]. Therefore, defining the mechanism of action of natural products is a high priority, as also emphasized by National Center for Complementary and Integrative Health (NCCIH)/National Institutes of Health (NIH), USA. A summary of significant validation of some of the common natural products in arthritis therapy is given below.

Natural products can control arthritic inflammation through multiple pathways, for example, inhibition of effector molecules (e.g., pro-inflammatory cytokines and chemokines), induction of anti-inflammatory mediators (e.g., IL-4, IL-10), regulation of the Th17/Treg balance, and modulation of the osteo-immune cross-talk [34,78–81]. These effects are in turn the outcome of the control of molecular mediators of inflammation such as NF-κB (nuclear factor kappa-light-chain-enhancer of activated B cells), MAPK (mitogen-activated protein kinase), and STAT3 (signal transducer and activator of transcription 3) by the bioactive components of plant-derived or other natural products. Furthermore, natural products can modulate the Th17/Treg balance by controlling the relative levels of key cytokines (e.g., IL-1β, IL-6, and TGF-β (transforming growth factor-β)) and certain transcription factors such as STAT3, RORγt (RAR-related orphan receptor gamma), IRF-4 (interferon Regulatory Factor 4), and Foxp3 (forkhead box P3) [34,82]. Similarly, acting via certain cytokines (e.g., IL-17) and other mediators such as RANKL, natural products can influence not only the T cell response, but also the osteo-immune cross-talk and bone health [80,83–85]. In this regard, natural products possessing the above properties can serve as potential therapeutic agents to treat RA either alone or in combination with certain mainstream anti-arthritic drugs. However, such combination therapies need to be fully assessed for their compatibility in regard to any unexpected drug interactions that might affect efficacy and side effects of these therapeutic agents.

We have discussed below in more detail some of the well-studied natural products for arthritis therapy. Most of the information is derived from testing in animal models, but where applicable, results of clinical testing in patients are also summarized.

5.1. *Tripterygium wilfordii Hook F*

5.1.1. Tripterygium wilfordii Hook F (TwHF)

One of the most well-studied natural products for its therapeutic properties in RA, TwHF has the capabilities to suppress numerous pro-inflammatory mediators. For example, TwHF extract reduces in vitro production of prostaglandin E2 (PGE2) through the suppression of COX-2 [86,87]. In addition, TwHF inhibits the production of nitric oxide (NO) by targeting and attenuating the transcription of the inducible nitric oxide synthase (iNOS) gene [86,88]. Moreover, in human synovial fibroblasts, TwHF reduces the expression of MMP1 and MMP3, while augmenting tissue inhibitors of metalloproteinases (TIMPs) that inhibit MMP1 and MMP2 [86,89]. Furthermore, TwHF blocks the transcription of MMP3 and MMP13, thereby reducing their levels [86,90]. The transcription of iNOS and COX2 is under the control of NF-κB, and TwHF has been shown to prevent NF-κB from binding to DNA, inhibiting its activation [86,90]. In turn, this leads to reduced levels of NO and COX2. Furthermore, TwHF can suppress the production of numerous proinflammatory cytokines (e.g., TNF-α, IL-1β, IL-6, IL-8, and IFN-γ) from T cells and macrophages. The balance of the T cell subsets and their differentiation is crucial for the development and propagation of RA [91]. It has been shown that TwHF can suppress T/B cell proliferation and synovial fibroblast growth [92–94] as well as induce T cell apoptosis [95].

Finally, the testing of TwHF in RA patients showed that it is an efficacious form of therapy for RA both alone and in combination with conventional (mainstream) therapies such as MTX, sulfasalazine (a chemical DMARD), or other DMARDs [96–103]. These included randomized, placebo controlled trials as well. One study used local application of TwHF formulation, but the rest used oral administration of TwHF. Different treatment regimen used in these studies can be summarized as follows: (a) RA patients treated with TwHF alone compared with control group that received placebo, or not [97]; (b) RA patients treated with TwHF compared with those treated with a DMARD (either MTX or sulfasalazine) [96,99,100,103]; and (c) RA patients treated with a combination of TwHF and MTX compared with control group that received MTX alone [98,101,102]. Taken together, the results of these studies, which also included meta-analysis, showed that TwHF alone was just as effective as either MTX or sulfasalazine alone. However, the most efficacious outcome was with a combination of TwHF with MTX. The safety profile of TwHF alone or in combination with a DMARD was comparable to that of DMARD alone. While TwHF is generally safe for human consumption, patients in these trials reported some side effects, the most common being gastrointestinal distress [103].

5.1.2. Triptolide

A bioactive component of TwHF, triptolide can induce T cell apoptosis and inhibit the phosphorylation of STAT3 [104,105]. In addition, triptolide can attenuate the NF-κB activity and several other pathways induced by TNF and TLR4 in RA [106–108]. Also, in CIA, triptolide can protect against bone damage by targeting RANKL-mediated ERK/Akt signaling [106,108]. Triptolide can also target and suppress the IL-6/STAT3/SOCS3 pathway in lamina propria mononuclear cells and promote their apoptosis [106,109], as well as attenuate angiogenesis [110].

5.1.3. Celastrol

Another bioactive component of TwHF, celastrus, and some other members of celastraceae family, celastrol has multiple anti-arthritic properties. Studies from our laboratory [34,79,80,84,111] and others [78,111] have demonstrated that celastrol can reduce arthritis severity in the AA model in Lewis rats [84]. Moreover, celastrol can suppress proinflammatory cytokine production as well as skew the T cell balance to a regulatory phenotype in the target organ, the joints [34,79,84]. In addition, celastrol can protect against bone erosion by targeting the RANKL pathway and deviating the RANKL/osteoprotegerin ratio that aids in the inhibition of osteoclastic activity. In turn, this reduces the osteoclast numbers and subsequent bone damage [80].

5.2. Green Tea

Green tea (*Camellia sinensis*) has several anti-inflammatory properties [112,113]. It has been demonstrated that feeding green tea polyphenols to CIA mice prevented the onset and progression of arthritis [114]. This was associated with marked reduction of COX-2, IFN-γ and TNF-α in the joints, and of antibodies to CII in serum and arthritic joints. Similarly, feeding the green tea polyphenols to AA rats significantly reduced arthritic scores [112]. Moreover, these rats had reduced IL-17 levels and increased IL-10 levels in the draining lymph node cells (LNCs). Also, serum analysis showed a significant reduction in anti-Bhsp65 antibodies compared to controls [112]. Another study in the same model revealed that green tea had superior anti-arthritic capabilities compared to black tea. Here, rats treated with green tea had reduced arthritic scores compared to both black tea-treated and non-treated controls [113]. Proinflammatory cytokine (TNF-α and IL-1β) levels in the serum were significantly reduced in the rats given green tea compared to non-treated controls and black tea-treated rats [113]. Also, protein levels of C–C chemokine receptor type 5 (CCR5) in the joint were decreased in rats given green tea [113].

One of the main bioactive molecules of green tea is epigallocatechin-3-gallate (EGCG) [115], and it has been shown to target multiple inflammatory pathways. Using the rat AA model, it was shown that EGCG can inhibit arthritis, which was associated with inhibition of IL-6 synthesis as well as trans-signaling [116]. The latter effect was attributable to increased synthesis of soluble gp130. EGCG and other catechins in green tea can interfere with IL-1β signaling and reduce the levels of pro-inflammatory mediators IL-8 and IL-1β in synovial fibroblasts [117,118]. Further analysis revealed that EGCG was able to effectively target and inhibit transforming growth factor beta-activated kinase 1 (TAK-1) activity, subsequently reducing IL-8, IL-1β as well as MMP2 and COX2 levels [117,118]. Moreover, EGCG was able to suppress p38 and NF-κB activity more effectively than the other catechins [117]. Also, EGCG was shown to increase Nrf2 (nuclear factor, erythroid 2-like 2) and HO-1 (heme oxygenase-1) activities, subsequently upregulating the production of indoleamine-2,3-dioxygenase (IDO). IDO is able to suppress the differentiation of pathogenic T cell subsets, while inducing Treg differentiation [119]. Another study demonstrated that EGCG can also regulate and suppress Th17 cell production and inhibit osteoclastogenesis by inhibiting STAT3 signaling [120]. Moreover, MMP2 and MMP9 levels were reduced in osteoclasts that were treated with EGCG compared to non-treated controls [121], which further shows the ability of EGCG to inhibit bone erosion. Finally, there have been multiple studies detailing the effects of green tea consumption in RA patients and reduction in disease activity score-28 (DAS28) as well as better pain management. Moreover, green tea was shown to prevent RA more effectively when compared with high fat beverages [122].

5.3. Curcumin

Curcumin possesses a wide variety of anti-inflammatory properties which make it a potent anti-arthritic bioactive molecule. Curcumin is derived from turmeric (*Curcuma longa*), a plant product that has been shown to attenuate inflammation [123–125]. A recent study using the AA model in Lewis rats demonstrated that curcumin was as effective at treating arthritis as MTX [126]. Rats treated with curcumin showed attenuated disease and histopathology scores, as well as reduced levels of pro-inflammatory cytokines (TNF-α and IL-1β) in the serum and synovial fluid compared to controls [126]. Curcumin inhibits NF-κB activity, which, in turn, leads to the reduction in proinflammatory cytokines as well as prevents TNF-α-induced adhesion of monocytes to endothelial cells [73,127,128]. Curcumin also regulates the cyclooxygenase (COX) and lipoxygenase (LOX) enzymes, leading to the suppression of various proinflammatory mediators, including MMP9 and MMP13 [73,129–132], and subsequent inflammation [73,133]. Furthermore, curcumin has been shown to suppress IL-1β signaling in articular chondrocytes [134] through the downregulation of mitogen-activated protein kinase (MAPK), activator protein 1 (AP-1), and NF-κB pathways. In turn, this leads to the reduction of MMP9 and MMP13 production [134]. Finally, curcumin can reduce the osteoclastogenic potential of peripheral blood mononuclear cells (PBMCs) of RA patients [135]. This was evident from the inhibition of expression of receptor activator of nuclear factor κB (RANK), c-Fos and nuclear factor of activated T cells (NFATc1) following curcumin treatment [135]. Also suppressed were extracellular signal-regulated kinases 1 (ERK1) and ERK2, p38 and c-Jun N-terminal kinase (JNK) [135].

5.4. Resveratrol

Resveratrol, a polyphenol, is found in red grape and other plant sources [136]. Resveratrol can suppress arthritis in CIA mice [137,138]. The T cell profile of these mice showed a reduction in the number of Th17 cells in the draining lymph node as well as decreased levels of circulating pro-inflammatory cytokines, such as IL-17, and CII-specific antibodies [137,138]. Resveratrol also has osteoprotective properties [139,140]. CIA mice treated with resveratrol showed a reduction in bone erosion as well as cartilage damage as evidenced by Safranin-O and tartrate-resistant acid phosphatase (TRAP) staining, in addition to radiographic imaging of the paws [140]. Moreover, resveratrol treatment leads to the suppression of wingless-related integration site (Wnt) signaling, an important pathway for bone remodeling and synovial inflammation [141], by targeting Wnt5a and inhibiting its expression [139]. Intra-articular injection of resveratrol suppressed signs of inflammatory arthritis in rabbits as evidenced by reduced histological scores [142]. Resveratrol is able to modulate the MEK-ERK1/2, MAPK, AP-1 and NF-κB pathways in various tissues [143]. Furthermore, resveratrol plays a role in regulating the aryl hydrocarbon receptor (AhR), which is known to affect several immune-mediate pathways in RA [143–146]. A previous study has indicated that resveratrol can ameliorate arthritis and synovial hyperplasia by inhibiting angiogenesis [147]. Resveratrol-treated rats showed significantly attenuated articular cartilage degradation, and higher caspase-3 levels in inflammatory cells compared to non-treated controls [147].

5.5. Other Natural Products

There are several other natural products besides those described above that possess anti-inflammatory activities and are reported to be beneficial in the treatment of arthritis and some other musculoskeletal disorders in patients and experimental models [75]. Some of these are summarized in Table 1.

Table 1. Natural products with anti-inflammatory/anti-arthritic activity.

Plant Name	Bioactive Compounds	Mediators of Inflammation Targeted by the Natural Product	References
Boswellia serrata	Boswellic acids	Proinflammatory cytokines, 5-LOX	[148,149]
Harpagophytum procumbens	Harpagoside, Harpagide	COX-2, MAPK, NF-κB, NO	[150,151]
Rosa canina	Carotenoids, organic acids	COX-1, COX-2	[152,153]
Uncaria tomentosa	Mitraphylline	Pro-inflammatory cytokines, anti-oxidant, NF-κB	[154,155]
Urtica dioica	Flavonoid glycosides, terpenoids	NF-κB, PLA2	[156,157]
Zingiber officinale	Zingerone, Gingerol	COX-2, NF-κB	[158,159]
Several grains, vegetables, fruits	Quercetin	MAPK, NF-κB, PI3K/Akt, JAK3	[160,161]

LOX, lipoxygenase; NF-κB, nuclear factor-kappa B; PLA2, phospholipase A2; COX; cyclooxygenase; MAPK, mitogen-activated protein kinase; NO, nitric oxide; PI3K, phosphatidylinositol-3-kinase; Akt, also known as PKB, protein kinase B; JAK, janus kinase.

6. Nanoparticle-Based Delivery of Plant Natural Products and Other Drugs for Arthritis Therapy

A major challenge in the treatment of diseases using natural products is their poor absorption. This results in loss of bioavailability and efficacy, and it requires consumption of a large amount of the natural product to achieve the required therapeutic effects. This increase in dosage can lead to unwanted toxicity [162–164]. Therefore, novel methods for delivering natural products are needed to improve therapeutic efficacy as well as reduce toxicity. Nanotechnology is an attractive approach in this regard [165,166]. Currently, there are many types of nanoparticles that have been approved for clinical use, and these nanoparticles are being used for therapeutic and diagnostic purposes (Figure 2) [167,168]. Encapsulating the bioactive natural products into nanoparticles can increase their in vivo stability, extend their circulation time, and allow for their controlled and sustained release [169,170]. Furthermore, with suitable modifications, nanoparticles can deliver drugs to a particular target site, including inflamed tissues [171–174]. For this purpose the surface of the nanoparticles can be modified with a peptide, an antibody, a protein, or a small molecule [172] to direct them to the desired inflamed tissue or organ [170,175,176]. The most common types of nanoparticles used for drug delivery for therapeutic purpose are micelles, lipid nanoparticles, liposomes, polymeric nanoparticles and emulsions [177].

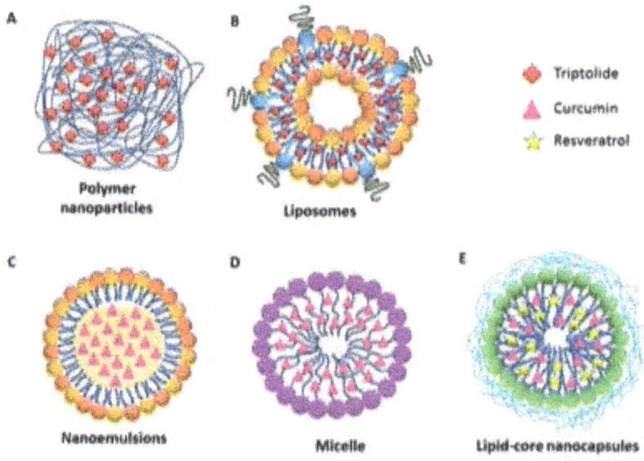

Figure 2. Schematic representation of different types of nanoparticles for the delivery of natural products. (**A**) Polymer nanoparticles encapsulating triptolide; (**B**) Liposomes loaded with triptolide; (**C**) Nanoemulsions entrapping curcumin; (**D**) Micelles encapsulating curcumin; and (**E**) Lipid core nanocapsules co-encapsulating resveratrol and curcumin.

6.1. Polymer Nanoparticles

Polymer Nanoparticles are biodegradable, biocompatible, minimally immunogenic, and suitable for targeted delivery of therapeutic drugs [178]. For example, triptolide-loaded PGA (poly-γ-glutamic acid) polymer nanoparticles (Figure 2A) were found to be more safe and efficacious compared to free triptolide, when tested at similar dosage [179]. In that study, mice treated intravenously (i.v.) with nanoparticle -triptolide showed increased survival rates and significantly reduced liver and kidney toxicity, when compared with free triptolide-treated mice [179]. In another study, TNF-α transgenic mice treated with nanoparticle-triptolide had a survival rate of 100% and no body weight changes compared to the survival rate of 70% and 20% body weight loss, respectively in mice treated with free triptolide [180]. However, the difference between the two groups in the bone volume of astragalus (ankle bone) was not significant [180].

6.2. Liposomes

Liposomes are spherical-shaped nanovesicles that are extensively used as carriers for the delivery of therapeutic drugs [181]. Liposomes can encapsulate both hydrophobic and hydrophilic drugs and can release the entrapped drug at designated targets [182,183]. A study using triptolide-entrapped liposomes (Figure 2B) in a rat model of CIA [184] showed slower release and a longer half-life in plasma as well as decreased hepatic and digestive tract toxicity when compared to free triptolide. Furthermore, there was a decrease in IL-1β and IL-6 levels in serum as well as reduced expression of Flk-1, Flt-4, and HIF-1α in synovium of liposome-triptolide group when compared to arthritic control group [184]. In a recent study, we have shown that liposomes encapsulating an immunomodulatory cytokine IL-27 and displaying a joint-homing peptide [185] on their surface are more effective in suppressing AA in rats compared with liposomes containing IL-27 but lacking the peptide on the cell surface as well as free IL-27 [186]. We propose that IL-27 combined with a natural product such as celastrol [186] might have an additive or synergistic protective effect against AA, and we plan to test this in the near future.

6.3. Nanoemulsions

Nanoemulsions result from the dispersion of two immiscible liquids, typically water and oil, and are stabilized using an appropriate surfactant [187]. In a study on AA [126], free curcumin was administrated i.v., whereas the curcumin-nanoemulsion formulation (Figure 2C) was administrated orally. The plasma concentration of curcumin was increased three-fold, whereas the levels of TNF-α and

IL-1β in both synovial fluid and serum were reduced two-fold in the curcumin-nanoemulsion-treated group compared to free curcumin-treated group [126].

6.4. Nanomicelles

Nanomicelles are self-assembling colloidal constructs composed of amphiphilic monomers (Figure 2D). Their hydrophobic core can encapsulate hydrophobic drugs/natural products, whereas the hydrophilic shell helps enhance the solubility of the drug. The surface of the nanomicelles is suitable for conjugation with cell/tissue-targeting ligands [188,189]. Nanomicelles were shown to improve the therapeutic efficacy of curcumin in CIA [190]. Curcumin-nanomicelles caused a significant reduction in paw edema, whereas free curcumin failed to reduce the paw swelling. Moreover, serum levels of IL-1β and vascular endothelial growth factor (VEGF) were significantly decreased in curcumin-nanomicelles-treated rats compared to free curcumin-treated rats [190].

6.5. Lipid-Core Nanocapsules

Lipid-Core Nanocapsules are composed of triglycerides/grape seed oil and sorbitan monostearate surrounded by a polymeric wall, which protects both the nanoparticle as well as the drug from degradation, and it also helps control drug release (Figure 2E) [191,192]. In one study, resveratrol and curcumin were co-encapsulated in lipid-core nanocapsules [137], and then administered intraperitoneally (i.p.) to arthritic rats, followed by monitoring of arthritis severity. These nanocapsules improved the edema-reducing activity of resveratrol and curcumin compared to their free counterparts, and no toxic side-effects were reported.

7. Interplay between Dietary Products and the Host Microbiome for Maintenance of Health and Disease Modulation

The human microbiota is composed of bacteria, fungi, and viruses, whose total population exceeds that of the host cells, and whose metabolic contribution to our state of health is essential [193–195]. From here on, the prefix 'micro' will be used to refer exclusively to prokaryotic organisms. The microbiome is an untapped source for identification of novel natural products for the treatment and prevention of disease such as RA. The associations between certain taxa of microbes and RA have been reported [196,197]. In addition, a variety of bioactive molecules produced by the human microbiome can have significant effects on the immune system [198]. There are three general approaches to harnessing the microbiome for RA prevention and treatment, namely the use of prebiotics, probiotics, and microbial-derived xenobiotics. Prebiotics are certain dietary ingredients metabolized by the microbiome to facilitate growth of beneficial bacteria in the gut, which in turn produce substances that are optimal for the local microenvironment and health of the intestines. Probiotics consist of living strains of beneficial bacteria. Microbial-derived xenobiotics are the molecules produced by the action of the microbiome action, for example, metabolic degradation/alteration of the dietary products consumed by the host and/or of the products released from the host's cellular processes.

The best known examples of prebiotics are plant-derived fibers inulin and oligofructose. These are present in several grains (e.g., wheat), fruits (e.g., bananas), and vegetables (e.g., onion and garlic). These prebiotic fibers serve as a fuel for microbiota, which then produce substances that contribute to the optimal health and function of intestinal cells. Another way for microbiota to influence immune system is via production of xenobiotic metabolites. For example, *Bifidobacterium* spp., including *B. bifidum*, convert dietary carbohydrates into butyrate. In addition to propionate and acetate, these essential short-chain fatty acids (SCFAs) affect host cells by inhibiting histone-deacetylase to promote anti-inflammatory responses [198]. Oral administration of SCFAs prior to induction of CIA has been shown to reduce arthritis severity [199]. SCFAs were shown to inhibit osteoclastogenesis in vitro, and to prevent bone loss in the CIA and K/BxN models of arthritis when administered orally [200]. These studies illustrate the potential benefits of xenobiotic supplementation. It also enforces the importance of a complex carbohydrate rich diet. In addition to SCFAs, unexplored microbial-derived ligands for the AhR could prove efficacious for RA treatment, as other ligands of the AhR are either currently licensed for RA treatment or have been shown to alter disease in animal models [145,201]. In the dairy-derived *P. freudenreichii*, beneficial metabolites produced could include SCFAs as well as the metabolite 1,4-Dihydroxy-2-naphthoic acid (DHNA), a known AhR ligand.

8. Concluding Remarks

While current therapies are effective at mitigating RA, their prolonged use is associated with unwanted side effects. It is clear that natural products can be effective forms of therapy for RA. We described in detail four such natural products and their bioactive components, but there are many more that have been shown to possess anti-inflammatory and anti-arthritic properties. One of the major hurdles of using natural products for therapy is their poor bioavailability. In order to combat this issue, researchers are turning to nanoparticle delivery of such products, and have reported successful application of these approaches. Nanoparticles are designed for the delivery of drugs/biologics to improve their pharmacological and therapeutic properties. They can protect the drug against degradation and deliver the drug to a specific target. In consequence, lower dose of the drug is required to achieve the desired efficacy. Thus, nanoparticles can ensure controlled release of drugs and reduce their toxicity. Furthermore, natural products might also contain prebiotic components, whose interaction with the host microbiome can have a significant impact on health and disease. This is a new area of research that would further help optimize the selection of natural products for therapy and define their mechanisms of action. Taken together, in the past couple decades, there has been a gradual increase in the use of natural products for the maintenance of health and treatment of arthritis and other diseases all over the world. It is hoped that in the near future, with additional research efforts and controlled clinical testing, natural products will be more widely accepted and used as therapeutics, either alone or as adjuncts to mainstream allopathic (Western) drugs, for RA and other diseases.

Acknowledgments: This work was supported in part by R01 AT004321 (K.D.M.), F31 AT009421 (S.D.), R24 AT001293 (B.M.B.), and P01 AT002605 (B.M.B., P.I.; K.D.M., Sub-project # 3) grants from the National Institutes of Health, Bethesda, MD, USA; and Merit Review Award # 5 I01 BX002424 (K.D.M.) from the United States (U.S.) Department of Veterans Affairs (Biomedical Laboratory Research and Development Service).

Conflicts of Interest: The authors declare no conflicts of interest.

Declaration: The contents do not represent the views of the U.S. Department of Veterans Affairs or the United States Government.

References

1. Du Montcel, S.T.; Michou, L.; Petit-Teixeira, E.; Osorio, J.; Lemaire, I.; Lasbleiz, S.; Pierlot, C.; Quillet, P.; Bardin, T.; Prum, B.; et al. New classification of HLA-DRB1 alleles supports the shared epitope hypothesis of rheumatoid arthritis susceptibility. *Arthritis Rheumatol.* **2005**, *52*, 1063–1068. [CrossRef] [PubMed]
2. Fugger, L.; Svejgaard, A. Association of MHC and rheumatoid arthritis. HLA-DR4 and rheumatoid arthritis: Studies in mice and men. *Arthritis Res.* **2000**, *2*, 208–211. [CrossRef] [PubMed]
3. Makrygiannakis, D.; Hermansson, M.; Ulfgren, A.K.; Nicholas, A.P.; Zendman, A.J.; Eklund, A.; Grunewald, J.; Skold, C.M.; Klareskog, L.; Catrina, A.I. Smoking increases peptidylarginine deiminase 2 enzyme expression in human lungs and increases citrullination in BAL cells. *Ann. Rheum. Dis.* **2008**, *67*, 1488–1492. [CrossRef] [PubMed]
4. Snir, O.; Widhe, M.; von Spee, C.; Lindberg, J.; Padyukov, L.; Lundberg, K.; Engstrom, A.; Venables, P.J.; Lundeberg, J.; Holmdahl, R.; et al. Multiple antibody reactivities to citrullinated antigens in sera from patients with rheumatoid arthritis: Association with HLA-DRB1 alleles. *Ann. Rheum. Dis.* **2009**, *68*, 736–743. [CrossRef] [PubMed]

5. Van der Helm-van Mil, A.H.; Verpoort, K.N.; Breedveld, F.C.; Huizinga, T.W.; Toes, R.E.; de Vries, R.R. The HLA-DRB1 shared epitope alleles are primarily a risk factor for anti-cyclic citrullinated peptide antibodies and are not an independent risk factor for development of rheumatoid arthritis. *Arthritis Rheumatol.* **2006**, *54*, 1117–1121. [CrossRef] [PubMed]
6. Alamanos, Y.; Drosos, A.A. Epidemiology of adult rheumatoid arthritis. *Autoimmun. Rev.* **2005**, *4*, 130–136. [CrossRef] [PubMed]
7. Crowson, C.S.; Matteson, E.L.; Myasoedova, E.; Michet, C.J.; Ernste, F.C.; Warrington, K.J.; Davis, J.M., III; Hunder, G.G.; Therneau, T.M.; Gabriel, S.E. The lifetime risk of adult-onset rheumatoid arthritis and other inflammatory autoimmune rheumatic diseases. *Arthritis Rheumatol.* **2011**, *63*, 633–639. [CrossRef] [PubMed]
8. Helmick, C.G.; Felson, D.T.; Lawrence, R.C.; Gabriel, S.; Hirsch, R.; Kwoh, C.K.; Liang, M.H.; Kremers, H.M.; Mayes, M.D.; Merkel, P.A.; et al. Estimates of the prevalence of arthritis and other rheumatic conditions in the United States. Part I. *Arthritis Rheumatol.* **2008**, *58*, 15–25. [CrossRef] [PubMed]
9. Silman, A.J.; Pearson, J.E. Epidemiology and genetics of rheumatoid arthritis. *Arthritis Res.* **2002**, *4*, S265–S272. [CrossRef] [PubMed]
10. Symmons, D.; Turner, G.; Webb, R.; Asten, P.; Barrett, E.; Lunt, M.; Scott, D.; Silman, A. The prevalence of rheumatoid arthritis in the United Kingdom: New estimates for a new century. *Rheumatology* **2002**, *41*, 793–800. [CrossRef] [PubMed]
11. Hootman, J.M.; Helmick, C.G.; Barbour, K.E.; Theis, K.A.; Boring, M.A. Updated projected prevalence of self-reported doctor-diagnosed arthritis and arthritis-attributable activity limitation among US adults, 2015–2040. *Arthritis Rheumatol.* **2016**, *68*, 1582–1587. [CrossRef] [PubMed]
12. Horiuchi, A.C.; Pereira, L.H.C.; Kahlow, B.S.; Silva, M.B.; Skare, T.L. Rheumatoid arthritis in elderly and young patients. *Rev. Bras. Reumatol.* **2017**, *57*, 491–494. [CrossRef] [PubMed]
13. Kato, E.; Sawada, T.; Tahara, K.; Hayashi, H.; Tago, M.; Mori, H.; Nishino, J.; Matsui, T.; Tohma, S. The age at onset of rheumatoid arthritis is increasing in Japan: A nationwide database study. *Int. J. Rheum. Dis.* **2017**, *20*, 839–845. [CrossRef] [PubMed]
14. Kobak, S.; Bes, C. An autumn tale: Geriatric rheumatoid arthritis. *Ther. Adv. Musculoskelet. Dis.* **2018**, *10*, 3–11. [CrossRef] [PubMed]
15. Harris, E.D., Jr. Rheumatoid arthritis. Pathophysiology and implications for therapy. *N. Engl. J. Med.* **1990**, *322*, 1277–1289. [PubMed]
16. McInnes, I.B.; Schett, G. The pathogenesis of rheumatoid arthritis. *N. Engl. J. Med.* **2011**, *365*, 2205–2219. [CrossRef] [PubMed]
17. Yanni, G.; Whelan, A.; Feighery, C.; Bresnihan, B. Synovial tissue macrophages and joint erosion in rheumatoid arthritis. *Ann. Rheum. Dis.* **1994**, *53*, 39–44. [CrossRef] [PubMed]
18. Morco, S.; Bowden, A. Ulnar drift in rheumatoid arthritis: A review of biomechanical etiology. *J. Biomech.* **2015**, *48*, 725–728. [CrossRef] [PubMed]
19. Eberhardt, K.; Johnson, P.M.; Rydgren, L. The occurrence and significance of hand deformities in early rheumatoid arthritis. *Br. J. Rheumatol.* **1991**, *30*, 211–213. [CrossRef] [PubMed]
20. Palmer, D.G.; Hogg, N.; Highton, J.; Hessian, P.A.; Denholm, I. Macrophage migration and maturation within rheumatoid nodules. *Arthritis Rheumatol.* **1987**, *30*, 728–736. [CrossRef]
21. Sayah, A.; English, J.C., III. Rheumatoid arthritis: A review of the cutaneous manifestations. *J. Am. Acad. Dermatol.* **2005**, *53*, 191–209. [CrossRef] [PubMed]
22. Gavrila, B.I.; Ciofu, C.; Stoica, V. Biomarkers in Rheumatoid Arthritis, what is new? *J. Med. Life* **2016**, *9*, 144–148. [PubMed]
23. Deane, K.D.; Norris, J.M.; Holers, V.M. Preclinical rheumatoid arthritis: Identification, evaluation, and future directions for investigation. *Rheum. Dis. Clin. N. Am.* **2010**, *36*, 213–241. [CrossRef] [PubMed]
24. Chun-Lai, T.; Murad, S.; Erlandsson, M.C.; Hussein, H.; Sulaiman, W.; Dhaliwal, J.S.; Bokarewa, M.I. Recognizing rheumatoid arthritis: Oncoprotein survivin opens new possibilities: A population-based case-control study. *Medicine* **2015**, *94*, e468. [CrossRef] [PubMed]
25. Lohr, J.; Knoechel, B.; Nagabhushanam, V.; Abbas, A.K. T-cell tolerance and autoimmunity to systemic and tissue-restricted self-antigens. *Immunol. Rev.* **2005**, *204*, 116–127. [CrossRef] [PubMed]
26. Ring, G.H.; Lakkis, F.G. Breakdown of self-tolerance and the pathogenesis of autoimmunity. *Semin. Nephrol.* **1999**, *19*, 25–33. [PubMed]

27. Veale, D.J.; Orr, C.; Fearon, U. Cellular and molecular perspectives in rheumatoid arthritis. *Semin. Immunopathol.* **2017**, *39*, 343–354. [CrossRef] [PubMed]
28. Bluestone, J.A.; Mackay, C.R.; O'Shea, J.J.; Stockinger, B. The functional plasticity of T cell subsets. *Nat. Rev. Immunol.* **2009**, *9*, 811–816. [CrossRef] [PubMed]
29. Mucida, D.; Cheroutre, H. The many face-lifts of CD4 T helper cells. *Adv. Immunol.* **2010**, *107*, 139–152. [PubMed]
30. Calabresi, E.; Petrelli, F.; Bonifacio, A.F.; Puxeddu, I.; Alunno, A. One year in review 2018: Pathogenesis of rheumatoid arthritis. *Clin. Exp. Rheumatol.* **2018**, *36*, 175–184. [PubMed]
31. Guo, Q.; Wang, Y.; Xu, D.; Nossent, J.; Pavlos, N.J.; Xu, J. Rheumatoid arthritis: Pathological mechanisms and modern pharmacologic therapies. *Bone Res.* **2018**, *6*, 1–14. [CrossRef] [PubMed]
32. Brand, D.D.; Latham, K.A.; Rosloniec, E.F. Collagen-induced arthritis. *Nat. Protoc.* **2007**, *2*, 1269–1275. [CrossRef] [PubMed]
33. Choudhary, N.; Bhatt, L.K.; Prabhavalkar, K.S. Experimental animal models for rheumatoid arthritis. *Immunopharmacol. Immunotoxicol.* **2018**, *40*, 193–200. [CrossRef] [PubMed]
34. Astry, B.; Venkatesha, S.H.; Laurence, A.; Christensen-Quick, A.; Garzino-Demo, A.; Frieman, M.B.; O'Shea, J.J.; Moudgil, K.D. Celastrol, a Chinese herbal compound, controls autoimmune inflammation by altering the balance of pathogenic and regulatory T cells in the target organ. *Clin. Immunol.* **2015**, *157*, 228–238. [CrossRef] [PubMed]
35. Dudics, S.; Venkatesha, S.H.; Moudgil, K.D. The micro-RNA expression profiles of autoimmune arthritis reveal novel biomarkers of the disease and therapeutic response. *Int. J. Mol. Sci.* **2018**, *19*, 2293. [CrossRef] [PubMed]
36. De Castro Costa, M.; De Sutter, P.; Gybels, J.; Van Hees, J. Adjuvant-induced arthritis in rats: A possible animal model of chronic pain. *Pain* **1981**, *10*, 173–185. [CrossRef]
37. Whitehouse, M.W. Adjuvant arthritis 50 years on: The impact of the 1956 article by CM Pearson, 'Development of arthritis, periarthritis and periostitis in rats given adjuvants'. *Inflamm. Res.* **2007**, *56*, 133–138. [CrossRef] [PubMed]
38. Whiteley, P.E.; Dalrymple, S.A. Models of inflammation: Adjuvant-induced arthritis in the rat. *Curr. Protoc. Pharmacol.* **2001**. [CrossRef]
39. Kouskoff, V.; Korganow, A.S.; Duchatelle, V.; Degott, C.; Benoist, C.; Mathis, D. Organ-specific disease provoked by systemic autoimmunity. *Cell* **1996**, *87*, 811–822. [CrossRef]
40. Christensen, A.D.; Haase, C.; Cook, A.D.; Hamilton, J.A. K/BxN serum-transfer arthritis as a model for human inflammatory arthritis. *Front. Immunol.* **2016**, *7*, 213. [CrossRef] [PubMed]
41. Glant, T.T.; Radacs, M.; Nagyeri, G.; Olasz, K.; Laszlo, A.; Boldizsar, F.; Hegyi, A.; Finnegan, A.; Mikecz, K. Proteoglycan-induced arthritis and recombinant human proteoglycan aggrecan G1 domain-induced arthritis in BALB/c mice resembling two subtypes of rheumatoid arthritis. *Arthritis Rheumatol.* **2011**, *63*, 1312–1321. [CrossRef] [PubMed]
42. Nabozny, G.H.; Baisch, J.M.; Cheng, S.; Cosgrove, D.; Griffiths, M.M.; Luthra, H.S.; David, C.S. HLA-DQ8 transgenic mice are highly susceptible to collagen-induced arthritis: A novel model for human polyarthritis. *J. Exp. Med.* **1996**, *183*, 27–37. [CrossRef] [PubMed]
43. Crofford, L.J. Use of NSAIDs in treating patients with arthritis. *Arthritis Res. Ther.* **2013**, *15* (Suppl. 3), S2. [CrossRef] [PubMed]
44. Schett, G.; Emery, P.; Tanaka, Y.; Burmester, G.; Pisetsky, D.S.; Naredo, E.; Fautrel, B.; van Vollenhoven, R. Tapering biologic and conventional DMARD therapy in rheumatoid arthritis: Current evidence and future directions. *Ann. Rheum. Dis.* **2016**, *75*, 1428–1437. [CrossRef] [PubMed]
45. Gerards, A.H.; de Lathouder, S.; de Groot, E.R.; Dijkmans, B.A.; Aarden, L.A. Inhibition of cytokine production by methotrexate. Studies in healthy volunteers and patients with rheumatoid arthritis. *Rheumatology* **2003**, *42*, 1189–1196. [CrossRef] [PubMed]
46. Rudwaleit, M.; Yin, Z.; Siegert, S.; Grolms, M.; Radbruch, A.; Braun, J.; Sieper, J. Response to methotrexate in early rheumatoid arthritis is associated with a decrease of T cell derived tumour necrosis factor alpha, increase of interleukin 10, and predicted by the initial concentration of interleukin 4. *Ann. Rheum. Dis.* **2000**, *59*, 311–314. [CrossRef] [PubMed]
47. Brown, P.M.; Pratt, A.G.; Isaacs, J.D. Mechanism of action of methotrexate in rheumatoid arthritis, and the search for biomarkers. *Nat. Rev. Rheumatol.* **2016**, *12*, 731–742. [CrossRef] [PubMed]

48. Tchetverikov, I.; Kraan, M.C.; van El, B.; Hanemaaijer, R.; DeGroot, J.; Huizinga, T.W. Leflunomide and methotrexate reduce levels of activated matrix metalloproteinases in complexes with α2 macroglobulin in serum of rheumatoid arthritis patients. *Ann. Rheum. Dis.* **2008**, *67*, 128–130. [CrossRef] [PubMed]
49. Cronstein, B.N. Going with the flow: Methotrexate, adenosine, and blood flow. *Ann. Rheum. Dis.* **2006**, *65*, 421–422. [CrossRef] [PubMed]
50. Hasko, G.; Cronstein, B. Regulation of inflammation by adenosine. *Front. Immunol.* **2013**, *4*, 85. [CrossRef] [PubMed]
51. Lopez-Olivo, M.A.; Siddhanamatha, H.R.; Shea, B.; Tugwell, P.; Wells, G.A.; Suarez-Almazor, M.E. Methotrexate for treating rheumatoid arthritis. *Cochrane Database Syst. Rev.* **2014**. [CrossRef] [PubMed]
52. Carneiro, S.C.; Cassia, F.F.; Lamy, F.; Chagas, V.L.; Ramos-e-Silva, M. Methotrexate and liver function: A study of 13 psoriasis cases treated with different cumulative dosages. *J. Eur. Acad. Dermatol. Venereol.* **2008**, *22*, 25–29. [CrossRef] [PubMed]
53. Cheng, H.S.; Rademaker, M. Monitoring methotrexate-induced liver fibrosis in patients with psoriasis: Utility of transient elastography. *Psoriasis* **2018**, *8*, 21–29. [CrossRef] [PubMed]
54. Conway, R.; Carey, J.J. Risk of liver disease in methotrexate treated patients. *World J. Hepatol.* **2017**, *9*, 1092–1100. [CrossRef] [PubMed]
55. Monaco, C.; Nanchahal, J.; Taylor, P.; Feldmann, M. Anti-TNF therapy: Past, present and future. *Int. Immunol.* **2015**, *27*, 55–62. [CrossRef] [PubMed]
56. Weinblatt, M.E.; Keystone, E.C.; Furst, D.E.; Moreland, L.W.; Weisman, M.H.; Birbara, C.A.; Teoh, L.A.; Fischkoff, S.A.; Chartash, E.K. Adalimumab, a fully human anti-tumor necrosis factor alpha monoclonal antibody, for the treatment of rheumatoid arthritis in patients taking concomitant methotrexate: The ARMADA trial. *Arthritis Rheumatol.* **2003**, *48*, 35–45. [CrossRef] [PubMed]
57. Roda, G.; Jharap, B.; Neeraj, N.; Colombel, J.F. Loss of Response to Anti-TNFs: Definition, Epidemiology, and Management. *Clin. Transl. Gastroenterol.* **2016**, *7*, e135. [CrossRef] [PubMed]
58. Goh, L.; Jewell, T.; Laversuch, C.; Samanta, A. A systematic review of the influence of anti-TNF on infection rates in patients with rheumatoid arthritis. *Rev. Bras. Reumatol.* **2013**, *53*, 501–515. [CrossRef] [PubMed]
59. Kim, G.W.; Lee, N.R.; Pi, R.H.; Lim, Y.S.; Lee, Y.M.; Lee, J.M.; Jeong, H.S.; Chung, S.H. IL-6 inhibitors for treatment of rheumatoid arthritis: Past, present, and future. *Arch. Pharm. Res.* **2015**, *38*, 575–584. [CrossRef] [PubMed]
60. Oldfield, V.; Dhillon, S.; Plosker, G.L. Tocilizumab: A review of its use in the management of rheumatoid arthritis. *Drugs* **2009**, *69*, 609–632. [CrossRef] [PubMed]
61. Navarro-Millan, I.; Singh, J.A.; Curtis, J.R. Systematic review of tocilizumab for rheumatoid arthritis: A new biologic agent targeting the interleukin-6 receptor. *Clin. Ther.* **2012**, *34*, 788–802. [CrossRef] [PubMed]
62. Smolen, J.S.; Schoels, M.M.; Nishimoto, N.; Breedveld, F.C.; Burmester, G.R.; Dougados, M.; Emery, P.; Ferraccioli, G.; Gabay, C.; Gibofsky, A.; et al. Consensus statement on blocking the effects of interleukin-6 and in particular by interleukin-6 receptor inhibition in rheumatoid arthritis and other inflammatory conditions. *Ann. Rheum. Dis.* **2013**, *72*, 482–492. [CrossRef] [PubMed]
63. Hench, P.S.; Kendall, E.C.; Slocumb, C.H.; Polley, H.F. Effects of cortisone acetate and pituitary ACTH on rheumatoid arthritis, rheumatic fever and certain other conditions. *Arch. Intern. Med.* **1950**, *85*, 545–666. [CrossRef]
64. Barnes, P.J. How corticosteroids control inflammation: Quintiles Prize Lecture 2005. *Br. J. Pharmacol.* **2006**, *148*, 245–254. [CrossRef] [PubMed]
65. Mundell, L.; Lindemann, R.; Douglas, J. Monitoring long-term oral corticosteroids. *BMJ Open Qual.* **2017**, *6*, e000209. [CrossRef] [PubMed]
66. Youssef, J.; Novosad, S.A.; Winthrop, K.L. Infection risk and safety of corticosteroid use. *Rheum. Dis. Clin. N. Am.* **2016**, *42*, 157–176. [CrossRef] [PubMed]
67. Clarke, T.C.; Black, L.I.; Stussman, B.J.; Barnes, P.M.; Nahin, R.L. *Trends in the Use of Complementary Health Approaches Among Adults: United States, 2002–2012*; U.S. Department of Health and Human Services, Centers for Disease Control and Prevention, National Center for Health Statistics: Hyattsville, MD, USA, 2013.
68. Barnes, P.M.; Bloom, B.; Nahin, R.L. *Complementary and Alternative Medicine Use Among Adults and Children: United States, 2007*; National Health Statistics Reports; U.S. Department of Health and Human Services, Centers for Disease Control and Prevention, National Center for Health Statistics: Hyattsville, MD, USA, 2008; pp. 1–23.

69. Rajesh, E.; Sankari, L.S.; Malathi, L.; Krupaa, J.R. Naturally occurring products in cancer therapy. *J. Pharm. Bioallied Sci.* **2015**, *7*, S181–S183. [CrossRef] [PubMed]
70. Kim, K.J.; Liu, X.; Komabayashi, T.; Jeong, S.I.; Selli, S. Natural products for infectious diseases. *Evid.-Based Complement. Altern. Med.* **2016**, *2016*, 9459047. [CrossRef] [PubMed]
71. Shamsizadeh, A.; Roohbakhsh, A.; Ayoobi, F.; Moghaddamahmadi, A. The role of natural products in the prevention and treatment of multiple sclerosis. In *Nutrition and Lifestyle in Neurological Autoimmune Diseases*; Academic Press/Elsevier: Cambridge, MA, USA, 2017; pp. 249–260. ISBN 978-240-212-805298-805293.
72. Chang, C.L.; Chen, Y.C.; Chen, H.M.; Yang, N.S.; Yang, W.C. Natural cures for type 1 diabetes: A review of phytochemicals, biological actions, and clinical potential. *Curr. Med. Chem.* **2013**, *20*, 899–907. [PubMed]
73. Kapoor, B.; Gupta, R.; Gupta, M. Natural products in treatment of rheumatoid arthritis. *Int. J. Green Pharm.* **2017**, *11*, S356–S363.
74. Venkatesha, S.H.; Rajaiah, R.; Berman, B.M.; Moudgil, K.D. Immunomodulation of autoimmune arthritis by herbal CAM. *Evid.-Based Complement. Altern. Med.* **2011**, *2011*, 986797. [CrossRef] [PubMed]
75. Venkatesha, S.; Acharya, B.; Moudgil, K. Natural products as source of anti-inflammatory drugs. In *Inflammation: From Molecular and Cellular Mechanisms to the Clinic*; Cavaillo, J.-M., Singer, M., Eds.; Wiley-VCH Verlag GmbH & Co. KGaA: Weinheim, Germany, 2018; Chapter 64; pp. 1607–1635.
76. Ben-Arye, E.; Frenkel, M.; Klein, A.; Scharf, M. Attitudes toward integration of complementary and alternative medicine in primary care: Perspectives of patients, physicians and complementary practitioners. *Patient Educ. Couns.* **2008**, *70*, 395–402. [CrossRef] [PubMed]
77. Ekor, M. The growing use of herbal medicines: Issues relating to adverse reactions and challenges in monitoring safety. *Front. Pharmacol.* **2014**, *4*, 177. [CrossRef] [PubMed]
78. Cascao, R.; Vidal, B.; Raquel, H.; Neves-Costa, A.; Figueiredo, N.; Gupta, V.; Fonseca, J.E.; Moita, L.F. Effective treatment of rat adjuvant-induced arthritis by celastrol. *Autoimmun. Rev.* **2012**, *11*, 856–862. [CrossRef] [PubMed]
79. Venkatesha, S.H.; Dudics, S.; Astry, B.; Moudgil, K.D. Control of autoimmune inflammation by celastrol, a natural triterpenoid. *Pathog. Dis.* **2016**, *74*, ftw059. [CrossRef] [PubMed]
80. Nanjundaiah, S.M.; Venkatesha, S.H.; Yu, H.; Tong, L.; Stains, J.P.; Moudgil, K.D. Celastrus and its bioactive celastrol protect against bone damage in autoimmune arthritis by modulating osteoimmune cross-talk. *J. Biol. Chem.* **2012**, *287*, 22216–22226. [CrossRef] [PubMed]
81. Zhang, R.X.; Fan, A.Y.; Zhou, A.N.; Moudgil, K.D.; Ma, Z.Z.; Lee, D.Y.; Fong, H.H.; Berman, B.M.; Lao, L. Extract of the Chinese herbal formula Huo Luo Xiao Ling Dan inhibited adjuvant arthritis in rats. *J. Ethnopharmacol.* **2009**, *121*, 366–371. [CrossRef] [PubMed]
82. Busbee, P.B.; Rouse, M.; Nagarkatti, M.; Nagarkatti, P.S. Use of natural AhR ligands as potential therapeutic modalities against inflammatory disorders. *Nutr. Rev.* **2013**, *71*, 353–369. [CrossRef] [PubMed]
83. Che, C.T.; Wong, M.S.; Lam, C.W. Natural products from chinese medicines with potential benefits to bone health. *Molecules* **2016**, *21*, 239. [CrossRef] [PubMed]
84. Venkatesha, S.H.; Yu, H.; Rajaiah, R.; Tong, L.; Moudgil, K.D. Celastrus-derived celastrol suppresses autoimmune arthritis by modulating antigen-induced cellular and humoral effector responses. *J. Biol. Chem.* **2011**, *286*, 15138–15146. [CrossRef] [PubMed]
85. Che, C.T.; Wong, M.S. Ligustrum lucidum and its Constituents: A mini-review on the anti-osteoporosis potential. *Nat. Prod. Commun.* **2015**, *10*, 2189–2194. [PubMed]
86. Bao, J.; Dai, S.M. A Chinese herb Tripterygium wilfordii Hook F in the treatment of rheumatoid arthritis: Mechanism, efficacy, and safety. *Rheumatol. Int* **2011**, *31*, 1123–1129. [CrossRef] [PubMed]
87. Tao, X.; Schulze-Koops, H.; Ma, L.; Cai, J.; Mao, Y.; Lipsky, P.E. Effects of Tripterygium wilfordii Hook F extracts on induction of cyclooxygenase 2 activity and prostaglandin E2 production. *Arthritis Rheumatol.* **1998**, *41*, 130–138. [CrossRef]
88. Guo, W.; Ma, L.; Tao, X. In vitro inhibitive effects of Tripterygium wilforii on NO production, iNOS activity, and iNOS-mRNA expression in chondrocyrtes of patients with rheumatoid arthritis. *Zhonghua Yi Xue Za Zhi* **2001**, *81*, 1035–1037. [PubMed]
89. Lin, N.; Sato, T.; Ito, A. Triptolide, a novel diterpenoid triepoxide from Tripterygium wilfordii Hook F, suppresses the production and gene expression of pro-matrix metalloproteinases 1 and 3 and augments those of tissue inhibitors of metalloproteinases 1 and 2 in human synovial fibroblasts. *Arthritis Rheumatol.* **2001**, *44*, 2193–2200.

90. Sylvester, J.; Liacini, A.; Li, W.Q.; Dehnade, F.; Zafarullah, M. Tripterygium wilfordii Hook F extract suppresses proinflammatory cytokine-induced expression of matrix metalloproteinase genes in articular chondrocytes by inhibiting activating protein-1 and nuclear factor-κB activities. *Mol. Pharmacol.* **2001**, *59*, 1196–1205. [CrossRef] [PubMed]
91. Pandya, J.M.; Lundell, A.C.; Hallstrom, M.; Andersson, K.; Nordstrom, I.; Rudin, A. Circulating T helper and T regulatory subsets in untreated early rheumatoid arthritis and healthy control subjects. *J. Leukoc. Biol.* **2016**, *100*, 823–833. [CrossRef] [PubMed]
92. Chan, M.A.; Kohlmeier, J.E.; Branden, M.; Jung, M.; Benedict, S.H. Triptolide is more effective in preventing T cell proliferation and interferon-γ production than is FK506. *Phytother. Res.* **1999**, *13*, 464–467. [CrossRef]
93. Tong, K.K.; Yang, D.; Chan, E.Y.; Chiu, P.K.; Yau, K.S.; Lau, C.S. Downregulation of lymphocyte activity and human synovial fibroblast growth in rheumatoid arthritis by triptolide. *Drug Dev. Res.* **1999**, *47*, 144–153. [CrossRef]
94. Li, X.W.; Weir, M.R. Radix Tripterygium wilfordii—A Chinese herbal medicine with potent immunosuppressive properties. *Transplantation* **1990**, *50*, 82–86. [CrossRef] [PubMed]
95. Ho, L.J.; Chang, D.M.; Chang, M.L.; Kuo, S.Y.; Lai, J.H. Mechanism of immunosuppression of the antirheumatic herb TWHf in human T cells. *J. Rheumatol.* **1999**, *26*, 14–24. [PubMed]
96. Jiang, M.; Zha, Q.; Zhang, C.; Lu, C.; Yan, X.; Zhu, W.; Liu, W.; Tu, S.; Hou, L.; Wang, C.; et al. Predicting and verifying outcome of Tripterygium wilfordii Hook F based therapy in rheumatoid arthritis: From open to double-blinded randomized trial. *Sci. Rep.* **2015**, *5*, 9700. [CrossRef] [PubMed]
97. Jiao, J.; Tang, X.P.; Yuan, J.; Liu, X.; Liu, H.; Zhang, C.Y.; Wang, L.Y.; Jiang, Q. Effect of external applying compound Tripterygium wilfordii Hook F on joint pain of rheumatoid arthritis patients. *Zhongguo Zhong Xi Yi Jie He Za Zhi* **2016**, *36*, 29–34. [PubMed]
98. Lv, Q.W.; Zhang, W.; Shi, Q.; Zheng, W.J.; Li, X.; Chen, H.; Wu, Q.J.; Jiang, W.L.; Li, H.B.; Gong, L.; et al. Comparison of Tripterygium wilfordii Hook F with methotrexate in the treatment of active rheumatoid arthritis (TRIFRA): A randomised, controlled clinical trial. *Ann. Rheum. Dis.* **2015**, *74*, 1078–1086. [CrossRef] [PubMed]
99. Wang, H.L.; Jiang, Q.; Feng, X.H.; Zhang, H.D.; Ge, L.; Luo, C.G.; Gong, X.; Li, B. Tripterygium wilfordii Hook F versus conventional synthetic disease-modifying anti-rheumatic drugs as monotherapy for rheumatoid arthritis: A systematic review and network meta-analysis. *BMC Complement. Altern. Med.* **2016**, *16*, 215. [CrossRef] [PubMed]
100. Wang, J.; Chen, N.; Fang, L.; Feng, Z.; Li, G.; Mucelli, A.; Zhang, X.; Zhou, X. A systematic review about the efficacy and safety of Tripterygium wilfordii Hook F preparations used for the management of rheumatoid arthritis. *Evid.-Based Complement. Altern. Med.* **2018**, *2018*, 1567463.
101. Wang, X.; Zu, Y.; Huang, L.; Yu, J.; Zhao, H.; Wen, C.; Chen, Z.; Xu, Z. Treatment of rheumatoid arthritis with combination of methotrexate and Tripterygium wilfordii: A meta-analysis. *Life Sci.* **2017**, *171*, 45–50. [CrossRef] [PubMed]
102. Zhou, Y.Y.; Xia, X.; Peng, W.K.; Wang, Q.H.; Peng, J.H.; Li, Y.L.; Wu, J.X.; Zhang, J.Y.; Zhao, Y.; Chen, X.M.; et al. The Effectiveness and Safety of Tripterygium wilfordii Hook F Extracts in Rheumatoid Arthritis: A Systematic Review and Meta-Analysis. *Front. Pharmacol.* **2018**, *9*, 356. [CrossRef] [PubMed]
103. Goldbach-Mansky, R.; Wilson, M.; Fleischmann, R.; Olsen, N.; Silverfield, J.; Kempf, P.; Kivitz, A.; Sherrer, Y.; Pucino, F.; Csako, G.; et al. Comparison of Tripterygium wilfordii Hook F versus sulfasalazine in the treatment of rheumatoid arthritis: A randomized trial. *Ann. Intern. Med.* **2009**, *151*, 229–240. [CrossRef] [PubMed]
104. Liu, Q.; Chen, T.; Chen, G.; Li, N.; Wang, J.; Ma, P.; Cao, X. Immunosuppressant triptolide inhibits dendritic cell-mediated chemoattraction of neutrophils and T cells through inhibiting Stat3 phosphorylation and NF-κB activation. *Biochem. Biophys. Res. Commun.* **2006**, *345*, 1122–1130. [CrossRef] [PubMed]
105. Yang, Y.; Liu, Z.; Tolosa, E.; Yang, J.; Li, L. Triptolide induces apoptotic death of T lymphocyte. *Immunopharmacology* **1998**, *40*, 139–149. [CrossRef]
106. Chen, S.R.; Dai, Y.; Zhao, J.; Lin, L.; Wang, Y.; Wang, Y. A mechanistic overview of triptolide and celastrol, natural products from Tripterygium wilfordii Hook F. *Front. Pharmacol.* **2018**, *9*, 104. [CrossRef] [PubMed]
107. Huang, J.; Zhou, L.; Wu, H.; Pavlos, N.; Chim, S.M.; Liu, Q.; Zhao, J.; Xue, W.; Tan, R.X.; Ye, J.; et al. Triptolide inhibits osteoclast formation, bone resorption, RANKL-mediated NF-κB activation and titanium particle-induced osteolysis in a mouse model. *Mol. Cell. Endocrinol.* **2015**, *399*, 346–353. [CrossRef] [PubMed]

108. Gong, Y.; Huang, X.; Wang, D.; Li, M.; Liu, Z. Triptolide protects bone against destruction by targeting RANKL-mediated ERK/AKT signalling pathway in the collagen-induced rheumatoid arthritis. *Biomed. Res.* **2017**, *28*, 4111–4116.
109. Li, Y.; Tian, Y.; Zhu, W.; Gong, J.; Zhang, W.; Yu, C.; Gu, L.; Li, N.; Li, J. Triptolide induces suppressor of cytokine signaling-3 expression and promotes lamina propria mononuclear cells apoptosis in Crohn's colitis. *Int. Immunopharmacol.* **2013**, *16*, 268–274. [CrossRef] [PubMed]
110. Zhang, W.; Li, F.; Gao, W. Tripterygium wilfordii Inhibiting Angiogenesis for Rheumatoid Arthritis Treatment. *J. Natl. Med. Assoc.* **2017**, *109*, 142–148. [CrossRef] [PubMed]
111. Cascao, R.; Vidal, B.; Lopes, I.P.; Paisana, E.; Rino, J.; Moita, L.F.; Fonseca, J.E. Decrease of CD68 Synovial Macrophages in Celastrol Treated Arthritic Rats. *PLoS ONE* **2015**, *10*, e0142448. [CrossRef] [PubMed]
112. Kim, H.R.; Rajaiah, R.; Wu, Q.L.; Satpute, S.R.; Tan, M.T.; Simon, J.E.; Berman, B.M.; Moudgil, K.D. Green tea protects rats against autoimmune arthritis by modulating disease-related immune events. *J. Nutr.* **2008**, *138*, 2111–2116. [CrossRef] [PubMed]
113. Ramadan, G.; El-Beih, N.M.; Talaat, R.M.; Abd El-Ghffar, E.A. Anti-inflammatory activity of green versus black tea aqueous extract in a rat model of human rheumatoid arthritis. *Int. J. Rheum. Dis.* **2017**, *20*, 203–213. [CrossRef] [PubMed]
114. Haqqi, T.M.; Anthony, D.D.; Gupta, S.; Ahmad, N.; Lee, M.S.; Kumar, G.K.; Mukhtar, H. Prevention of collagen-induced arthritis in mice by a polyphenolic fraction from green tea. *Proc. Natl. Acad. Sci. USA* **1999**, *96*, 4524–4529. [CrossRef] [PubMed]
115. Bhutia Pemba, H.; Sharangi, A.B.; Lepcha, R.; Tamang, D. Bioactive Compounds and Antioxidant Properties of Tea: Status, Global Research and Potentialities. *J. Tea Sci. Res.* **2015**, *5*, 1–13.
116. Ahmed, S.; Marotte, H.; Kwan, K.; Ruth, J.H.; Campbell, P.L.; Rabquer, B.J.; Pakozdi, A.; Koch, A.E. Epigallocatechin-3-gallate inhibits IL-6 synthesis and suppresses transsignaling by enhancing soluble gp130 production. *Proc. Natl. Acad. Sci. USA* **2008**, *105*, 14692–14697. [CrossRef] [PubMed]
117. Fechtner, S.; Singh, A.; Chourasia, M.; Ahmed, S. Molecular insights into the differences in anti-inflammatory activities of green tea catechins on IL-1β signaling in rheumatoid arthritis synovial fibroblasts. *Toxicol. Appl. Pharmacol.* **2017**, *329*, 112–120. [CrossRef] [PubMed]
118. Singh, A.K.; Umar, S.; Riegsecker, S.; Chourasia, M.; Ahmed, S. Regulation of transforming growth factor β-activated kinase activation by epigallocatechin-3-gallate in rheumatoid arthritis synovial fibroblasts: suppression of K63-linked Autoubiquitination of tumor necrosis factor receptor-associated factor 6. *Arthritis Rheumatol.* **2016**, *68*, 347–358. [CrossRef] [PubMed]
119. Min, S.Y.; Yan, M.; Kim, S.B.; Ravikumar, S.; Kwon, S.R.; Vanarsa, K.; Kim, H.Y.; Davis, L.S.; Mohan, C. Green tea epigallocatechin-3-gallate suppresses autoimmune arthritis through indoleamine-2,3-dioxygenase expressing dendritic cells and the nuclear factor, erythroid 2-like 2 antioxidant pathway. *J. Inflamm.* **2015**, *12*, 53. [CrossRef] [PubMed]
120. Lee, S.Y.; Jung, Y.O.; Ryu, J.G.; Oh, H.J.; Son, H.J.; Lee, S.H.; Kwon, J.E.; Kim, E.K.; Park, M.K.; Park, S.H.; et al. Epigallocatechin-3-gallate ameliorates autoimmune arthritis by reciprocal regulation of T helper-17 regulatory T cells and inhibition of osteoclastogenesis by inhibiting STAT3 signaling. *J. Leukoc. Biol.* **2016**, *100*, 559–568. [CrossRef] [PubMed]
121. Oka, Y.; Iwai, S.; Amano, H.; Irie, Y.; Yatomi, K.; Ryu, K.; Yamada, S.; Inagaki, K.; Oguchi, K. Tea polyphenols inhibit rat osteoclast formation and differentiation. *J. Pharmacol. Sci.* **2012**, *118*, 55–64. [CrossRef] [PubMed]
122. Rambod, M.; Nazarinia, M.; Raieskarimian, F. The impact of dietary habits on the pathogenesis of rheumatoid arthritis: A case-control study. *Clin. Rheumatol.* **2018**. [CrossRef] [PubMed]
123. Gupta, S.C.; Kismali, G.; Aggarwal, B.B. Curcumin, a component of turmeric: From farm to pharmacy. *Biofactors* **2013**, *39*, 2–13. [CrossRef] [PubMed]
124. Srivastava, S.; Saksena, A.K.; Khattri, S.; Kumar, S.; Dagur, R.S. Curcuma longa extract reduces inflammatory and oxidative stress biomarkers in osteoarthritis of knee: A four-month, double-blind, randomized, placebo-controlled trial. *Inflammopharmacology* **2016**, *24*, 377–388. [CrossRef] [PubMed]
125. Zdrojewicz, Z.; Szyca, M.; Popowicz, E.; Michalik, T.; Smieszniak, B. Turmeric—Not only spice. *Polski Merkuriusz Lekarski* **2017**, *42*, 227–230. [PubMed]
126. Zheng, Z.; Sun, Y.; Liu, Z.; Zhang, M.; Li, C.; Cai, H. The effect of curcumin and its nanoformulation on adjuvant-induced arthritis in rats. *Drug Des. Dev. Ther.* **2015**, *9*, 4931–4942.

127. Kumar, A.; Dhawan, S.; Hardegen, N.J.; Aggarwal, B.B. Curcumin (*Diferuloylmethane*) inhibition of tumor necrosis factor (TNF)-mediated adhesion of monocytes to endothelial cells by suppression of cell surface expression of adhesion molecules and of nuclear factor-κB activation. *Biochem. Pharmacol.* **1998**, *55*, 775–783. [CrossRef]
128. Yeh, C.H.; Chen, T.P.; Wu, Y.C.; Lin, Y.M.; Jing Lin, P. Inhibition of NF-κB activation with curcumin attenuates plasma inflammatory cytokines surge and cardiomyocytic apoptosis following cardiac ischemia/reperfusion. *J. Surg. Res.* **2005**, *125*, 109–116. [CrossRef] [PubMed]
129. Aggarwal, B.B.; Gupta, S.C.; Sung, B. Curcumin: An orally bioavailable blocker of TNF and other pro-inflammatory biomarkers. *Br. J. Pharmacol.* **2013**, *169*, 1672–1692. [CrossRef] [PubMed]
130. Shakibaei, M.; John, T.; Schulze-Tanzil, G.; Lehmann, I.; Mobasheri, A. Suppression of NF-κB activation by curcumin leads to inhibition of expression of cyclo-oxygenase-2 and matrix metalloproteinase-9 in human articular chondrocytes: Implications for the treatment of osteoarthritis. *Biochem. Pharmacol.* **2007**, *73*, 1434–1445. [CrossRef] [PubMed]
131. Moore, B.A.; Aznavoorian, S.; Engler, J.A.; Windsor, L.J. Induction of collagenase-3 (MMP-13) in rheumatoid arthritis synovial fibroblasts. *Biochim. Biophys. Acta* **2000**, *1502*, 307–318. [CrossRef]
132. Xue, M.; McKelvey, K.; Shen, K.; Minhas, N.; March, L.; Park, S.Y.; Jackson, C.J. Endogenous MMP-9 and not MMP-2 promotes rheumatoid synovial fibroblast survival, inflammation and cartilage degradation. *Rheumatology* **2014**, *53*, 2270–2279. [CrossRef] [PubMed]
133. Rao, C.V. Regulation of COX and LOX by curcumin. *Adv. Exp. Med. Biol.* **2007**, *595*, 213–226. [PubMed]
134. Kapil Kumar, A.K.R. Curcumin: A yellow magical spice of kitchen for treatment of rheumatoid arthritis. *Int. Res. J. Pharm.* **2011**, *2*, 29–31.
135. Shang, W.; Zhao, L.J.; Dong, X.L.; Zhao, Z.M.; Li, J.; Zhang, B.B.; Cai, H. Curcumin inhibits osteoclastogenic potential in PBMCs from rheumatoid arthritis patients via the suppression of MAPK/RANK/c-Fos/NFATc1 signaling pathways. *Mol. Med. Rep.* **2016**, *14*, 3620–3626. [CrossRef] [PubMed]
136. Pandey, K.B.; Rizvi, S.I. Plant polyphenols as dietary antioxidants in human health and disease. *Oxid. Med. Cell. Longev.* **2009**, *2*, 270–278. [CrossRef] [PubMed]
137. Coradini, K.; Friedrich, R.B.; Fonseca, F.N.; Vencato, M.S.; Andrade, D.F.; Oliveira, C.M.; Battistel, A.P.; Guterres, S.S.; da Rocha, M.I.; Pohlmann, A.R.; et al. A novel approach to arthritis treatment based on resveratrol and curcumin co-encapsulated in lipid-core nanocapsules: In vivo studies. *Eur. J. Pharm. Sci.* **2015**, *78*, 163–170. [CrossRef] [PubMed]
138. Xuzhu, G.; Komai-Koma, M.; Leung, B.P.; Howe, H.S.; McSharry, C.; McInnes, I.B.; Xu, D. Resveratrol modulates murine collagen-induced arthritis by inhibiting Th17 and B-cell function. *Ann. Rheum. Dis.* **2012**, *71*, 129–135. [CrossRef] [PubMed]
139. Koca, S.S.; Yolbas, S.; Yildirim, A.; Celik, Z.B.; Onalan, E.E.; Akin, M. AB0108 resveratrol inhibits canonical wnt signaling and ameliorates experimental arthritis. *Ann. Rheum. Dis.* **2016**, *75*, 933. [CrossRef]
140. Cheon, Y.H.; Kim, H.O.; Suh, Y.S.; Hur, J.H.; Jo, W.; Lim, H.S.; Hah, Y.S.; Sung, M.J.; Kwon, D.Y.; Lee, S.I. Inhibitory effects for rheumatoid arthritis of dietary supplementation with resveratrol in collagen-induced arthritis. *J. Rheum. Dis.* **2015**, *22*, 93–101. [CrossRef]
141. Miao, C.G.; Yang, Y.Y.; He, X.; Li, X.F.; Huang, C.; Huang, Y.; Zhang, L.; Lv, X.W.; Jin, Y.; Li, J. Wnt signaling pathway in rheumatoid arthritis, with special emphasis on the different roles in synovial inflammation and bone remodeling. *Cell. Signal.* **2013**, *25*, 2069–2078. [CrossRef] [PubMed]
142. Elmali, N.; Baysal, O.; Harma, A.; Esenkaya, I.; Mizrak, B. Effects of resveratrol in inflammatory arthritis. *Inflammation* **2007**, *30*, 1–6. [CrossRef] [PubMed]
143. Nguyen, C.; Savouret, J.F.; Widerak, M.; Corvol, M.T.; Rannou, F. Resveratrol, potential therapeutic interest in joint disorders: A critical narrative review. *Nutrients* **2017**, *9*, 45. [CrossRef] [PubMed]
144. Nguyen, C.H.; Nakahama, T.; Dang, T.T.; Chu, H.H.; Van Hoang, L.; Kishimoto, T.; Nguyen, N.T. Expression of aryl hydrocarbon receptor, inflammatory cytokines, and incidence of rheumatoid arthritis in Vietnamese dioxin-exposed people. *J. Immunotoxicol.* **2017**, *14*, 196–203. [CrossRef] [PubMed]
145. Nguyen, N.T.; Nakahama, T.; Nguyen, C.H.; Tran, T.T.; Le, V.S.; Chu, H.H.; Kishimoto, T. Aryl hydrocarbon receptor antagonism and its role in rheumatoid arthritis. *J. Exp. Pharmacol.* **2015**, *7*, 29–35. [PubMed]

146. Ogando, J.; Tardáguila, M.; Díaz-Alderete, A.; Usategui, A.; Miranda-Ramos, V.; Martínez-Herrera, D.J.; de la Fuente, L.; García-León, M.J.; Moreno, M.C.; Escudero, S.; et al. Notch-regulated miR-223 targets the aryl hydrocarbon receptor pathway and increases cytokine production in macrophages from rheumatoid arthritis patients. *Sci. Rep.* **2016**, *6*, 20223. [CrossRef] [PubMed]
147. Almonte-Becerril, M.; Fernandez-Rodriguez, J.A.; Ramil-Gómez, O.; Riveiro-Naveira, R.R.; Hermida-Carballo, L.; Blanco, F.J.; Lopez-Armada, M.J. Resveratrol attenuates synovial hyperplasia in an acute antigen-induced arthritis model by augmenting autophagy and decreasing angiogenesis. *Osteoarthr. Cartil.* **2017**, *25*, S90–S91. [CrossRef]
148. Abdel-Tawab, M.; Werz, O.; Schubert-Zsilavecz, M. *Boswellia serrata*: An overall assessment of in vitro, preclinical, pharmacokinetic and clinical data. *Clin. Pharmacokinet.* **2011**, *50*, 349–369. [CrossRef] [PubMed]
149. Ammon, H.P. Modulation of the immune system by *Boswellia serrata* extracts and boswellic acids. *Phytomedicine* **2010**, *17*, 862–867. [CrossRef] [PubMed]
150. Chrubasik, S.; Conradt, C.; Roufogalis, B.D. Effectiveness of Harpagophytum extracts and clinical efficacy. *Phytother. Res.* **2004**, *18*, 187–189. [CrossRef] [PubMed]
151. Grant, L.; McBean, D.E.; Fyfe, L.; Warnock, A.M. A review of the biological and potential therapeutic actions of Harpagophytum procumbens. *Phytother. Res.* **2007**, *21*, 199–209. [CrossRef] [PubMed]
152. Chrubasik, C.; Roufogalis, B.D.; Muller-Ladner, U.; Chrubasik, S. A systematic review on the *Rosa canina* effect and efficacy profiles. *Phytother. Res.* **2008**, *22*, 725–733. [CrossRef] [PubMed]
153. Saaby, L.; Jager, A.K.; Moesby, L.; Hansen, E.W.; Christensen, S.B. Isolation of immunomodulatory triterpene acids from a standardized rose hip powder (*Rosa canina* L.). *Phytother. Res.* **2011**, *25*, 195–201. [CrossRef] [PubMed]
154. Erowele, G.I.; Kalejaiye, A.O. Pharmacology and therapeutic uses of cat's claw. *Am. J. Health Syst. Pharm.* **2009**, *66*, 992–995. [CrossRef] [PubMed]
155. Rosenbaum, C.C.; O'Mathuna, D.P.; Chavez, M.; Shields, K. Antioxidants and antiinflammatory dietary supplements for osteoarthritis and rheumatoid arthritis. *Altern. Ther. Health Med.* **2010**, *16*, 32–40. [PubMed]
156. Di Lorenzo, C.; Dell'Agli, M.; Badea, M.; Dima, L.; Colombo, E.; Sangiovanni, E.; Restani, P.; Bosisio, E. Plant food supplements with anti-inflammatory properties: A systematic review (II). *Crit. Rev. Food Sci. Nutr.* **2013**, *53*, 507–516. [CrossRef] [PubMed]
157. Randall, C.; Randall, H.; Dobbs, F.; Hutton, C.; Sanders, H. Randomized controlled trial of nettle sting for treatment of base-of-thumb pain. *J. R. Soc. Med.* **2000**, *93*, 305–309. [CrossRef] [PubMed]
158. Lakhan, S.E.; Ford, C.T.; Tepper, D. Zingiberaceae extracts for pain: A systematic review and meta-analysis. *Nutr. J.* **2015**, *14*, 50. [CrossRef] [PubMed]
159. Semwal, R.B.; Semwal, D.K.; Combrinck, S.; Viljoen, A.M. Gingerols and shogaols: Important nutraceutical principles from ginger. *Phytochemistry* **2015**, *117*, 554–568. [CrossRef] [PubMed]
160. Ji, J.J.; Lin, Y.; Huang, S.S.; Zhang, H.L.; Diao, Y.P.; Li, K. Quercetin: A potential natural drug for adjuvant treatment of rheumatoid arthritis. *Afr. J. Tradit. Complement. Altern. Med.* **2013**, *10*, 418–421. [PubMed]
161. Russo, M.; Spagnuolo, C.; Tedesco, I.; Bilotto, S.; Russo, G.L. The flavonoid quercetin in disease prevention and therapy: Facts and fancies. *Biochem. Pharmacol.* **2012**, *83*, 6–15. [CrossRef] [PubMed]
162. Efferth, T.; Kaina, B. Toxicities by herbal medicines with emphasis to traditional Chinese medicine. *Curr. Drug Metab.* **2011**, *12*, 989–996. [CrossRef] [PubMed]
163. Byard, R.W. A review of the potential forensic significance of traditional herbal medicines. *J. Forensic. Sci.* **2010**, *55*, 89–92. [CrossRef] [PubMed]
164. Kim, E.J.; Chen, Y.; Huang, J.Q.; Li, K.M.; Razmovski-Naumovski, V.; Poon, J.; Chan, K.; Roufogalis, B.D.; McLachlan, A.J.; Mo, S.L.; et al. Evidence-based toxicity evaluation and scheduling of Chinese herbal medicines. *J. Ethnopharmacol.* **2013**, *146*, 40–61. [CrossRef] [PubMed]
165. Watkins, R.; Wu, L.; Zhang, C.; Davis, R.M.; Xu, B. Natural product-based nanomedicine: Recent advances and issues. *Int. J. Nanomed.* **2015**, *10*, 6055–6074.
166. Shi, J.; Votruba, A.R.; Farokhzad, O.C.; Langer, R. Nanotechnology in drug delivery and tissue engineering: From discovery to applications. *Nano Lett.* **2010**, *10*, 3223–3230. [CrossRef] [PubMed]
167. Anselmo, A.C.; Mitragotri, S. Nanoparticles in the clinic. *Bioeng. Transl. Med.* **2016**, *1*, 10–29. [CrossRef] [PubMed]
168. Parveen, S.; Misra, R.; Sahoo, S.K. Nanoparticles: A boon to drug delivery, therapeutics, diagnostics and imaging. *Nanomedicine* **2012**, *8*, 147–166. [CrossRef] [PubMed]

169. Bonifacio, B.V.; Silva, P.B.; Ramos, M.A.; Negri, K.M.; Bauab, T.M.; Chorilli, M. Nanotechnology-based drug delivery systems and herbal medicines: A review. *Int. J. Nanomed.* **2014**, *9*, 1–15.
170. Obeid, M.A.; Al Qaraghuli, M.M.; Alsaadi, M.; Alzahrani, A.R.; Niwasabutra, K.; Ferro, V.A. Delivering natural products and biotherapeutics to improve drug efficacy. *Ther. Deliv.* **2017**, *8*, 947–956. [CrossRef] [PubMed]
171. Suri, S.S.; Fenniri, H.; Singh, B. Nanotechnology-based drug delivery systems. *J. Occup. Med. Toxicol.* **2007**, *2*, 16. [CrossRef] [PubMed]
172. Singh, R.; Lillard, J.W., Jr. Nanoparticle-based targeted drug delivery. *Exp. Mol. Pathol.* **2009**, *86*, 215–223. [CrossRef] [PubMed]
173. Yu, X.; Trase, I.; Ren, M.; Duval, K.; Guo, X.; Chen, Z. Design of Nanoparticle-Based Carriers for Targeted Drug Delivery. *J. Nanomater.* **2016**, *2016*, 1–15. [CrossRef] [PubMed]
174. Yu, X.; Pishko, M.V. Nanoparticle-based biocompatible and targeted drug delivery: Characterization and in vitro studies. *Biomacromolecules* **2011**, *12*, 3205–3212. [CrossRef] [PubMed]
175. Jain, S.; Heeralal, B.; Swami, R.; Swarnakar, N.K.; Kushwah, V. Improved oral bioavailability, therapeutic efficacy, and reduced toxicity of tamoxifen-loaded liquid crystalline nanoparticles. *AAPS PharmSciTech* **2018**, *19*, 460–469. [CrossRef] [PubMed]
176. Jain, S.; Spandana, G.; Agrawal, A.K.; Kushwah, V.; Thanki, K. Enhanced Antitumor Efficacy and Reduced Toxicity of Docetaxel Loaded Estradiol Functionalized Stealth Polymeric Nanoparticles. *Mol. Pharm.* **2015**, *12*, 3871–3884. [CrossRef] [PubMed]
177. Jahangirian, H.; Lemraski, E.G.; Webster, T.J.; Rafiee-Moghaddam, R.; Abdollahi, Y. A review of drug delivery systems based on nanotechnology and green chemistry: Green nanomedicine. *Int. J. Nanomed.* **2017**, *12*, 2957–2978. [CrossRef] [PubMed]
178. Banik, B.L.; Fattahi, P.; Brown, J.L. Polymeric nanoparticles: The future of nanomedicine. *Wiley Interdiscip. Rev. Nanomed. Nanobiotechnol.* **2016**, *8*, 271–299. [CrossRef] [PubMed]
179. Zhang, L.; Wang, T.; Li, Q.; Huang, J.; Xu, H.; Li, J.; Wang, Y.; Liang, Q. Fabrication of novel vesicles of triptolide for antirheumatoid activity with reduced toxicity in vitro and in vivo. *Int. J. Nanomed.* **2016**, *11*, 2663–2673.
180. Zhang, L.; Chang, J.; Zhao, Y.; Xu, H.; Wang, T.; Li, Q.; Xing, L.; Huang, J.; Wang, Y.; Liang, Q. Fabrication of a triptolide-loaded and poly-γ-glutamic acid-based amphiphilic nanoparticle for the treatment of rheumatoid arthritis. *Int. J. Nanomed.* **2018**, *13*, 2051–2064. [CrossRef] [PubMed]
181. Sercombe, L.; Veerati, T.; Moheimani, F.; Wu, S.Y.; Sood, A.K.; Hua, S. Advances and Challenges of Liposome Assisted Drug Delivery. *Front. Pharmacol.* **2015**, *6*, 286. [CrossRef] [PubMed]
182. Allen, T.M.; Cullis, P.R. Liposomal drug delivery systems: From concept to clinical applications. *Adv. Drug Deliv. Rev.* **2013**, *65*, 36–48. [CrossRef] [PubMed]
183. Akbarzadeh, A.; Rezaei-Sadabady, R.; Davaran, S.; Joo, S.W.; Zarghami, N.; Hanifehpour, Y.; Samiei, M.; Kouhi, M.; Nejati-Koshki, K. Liposome: Classification, preparation, and applications. *Nanoscale Res. Lett.* **2013**, *8*, 102. [CrossRef] [PubMed]
184. Chen, G.; Hao, B.; Ju, D.; Liu, M.; Zhao, H.; Du, Z.; Xia, J. Pharmacokinetic and pharmacodynamic study of triptolide-loaded liposome hydrogel patch under microneedles on rats with collagen-induced arthritis. *Acta Pharm. Sin. B* **2015**, *5*, 569–576. [CrossRef] [PubMed]
185. Yang, Y.H.; Rajaiah, R.; Ruoslahti, E.; Moudgil, K.D. Peptides targeting inflamed synovial vasculature attenuate autoimmune arthritis. *Proc. Natl. Acad. Sci. USA* **2011**, *108*, 12857–12862. [CrossRef] [PubMed]
186. Meka, R.; Venkatesha, S.; Moudgil, K.D. Peptide-directed liposomal delivery improves the therapeutic index of an immunomodulatory cytokine in controlling autoimmune arthritis. *J. Control. Release* **2018**, *286*, 279–288. [CrossRef] [PubMed]
187. Singh, Y.; Meher, J.G.; Raval, K.; Khan, F.A.; Chaurasia, M.; Jain, N.K.; Chourasia, M.K. Nanoemulsion: Concepts, development and applications in drug delivery. *J. Control. Release* **2017**, *252*, 28–49. [CrossRef] [PubMed]
188. Vadlapudi, A.D.; Mitra, A.K. Nanomicelles: An emerging platform for drug delivery to the eye. *Ther. Deliv.* **2013**, *4*, 1–3. [CrossRef] [PubMed]
189. Trivedi, R.; Kompella, U.B. Nanomicellar formulations for sustained drug delivery: Strategies and underlying principles. *Nanomedicine* **2010**, *5*, 485–505. [CrossRef] [PubMed]

190. Fan, Z.; Li, J.; Liu, J.; Jiao, H.; Liu, B. Anti-inflammation and joint lubrication dual effects of a novel hyaluronic acid/curcumin nanomicelle improve the efficacy of rheumatoid arthritis therapy. *ACS Appl. Mater. Interfaces* **2018**. [CrossRef] [PubMed]
191. Venturini, C.G.; Jäger, E.; Oliveira, C.P.; Bernardi, A.; Battastini, A.M.; Guterres, S.S.; Pohlmann, A.R. Formulation of lipid core nanocapsules. *Colloids Surf. A Physicochem. Eng. Asp.* **2011**, *375*, 200–208. [CrossRef]
192. Frank, L.A.; Contri, R.V.; Beck, R.C.; Pohlmann, A.R.; Guterres, S.S. Improving drug biological effects by encapsulation into polymeric nanocapsules. *Wiley Interdiscip. Rev. Nanomed. Nanobiotechnol.* **2015**, *7*, 623–639. [CrossRef] [PubMed]
193. Holmes, E.; Li, J.V.; Athanasiou, T.; Ashrafian, H.; Nicholson, J.K. Understanding the role of gut microbiome-host metabolic signal disruption in health and disease. *Trends Microbiol.* **2011**, *19*, 349–359. [CrossRef] [PubMed]
194. Huang, X.; Fang, S.; Yang, H.; Gao, J.; He, M.; Ke, S.; Zhao, Y.; Chen, C.; Huang, L. Evaluating the contribution of gut microbiome to the variance of porcine serum glucose and lipid concentration. *Sci. Rep.* **2017**, *7*, 14928. [CrossRef] [PubMed]
195. Riedl, R.A.; Atkinson, S.N.; Burnett, C.M.L.; Grobe, J.L.; Kirby, J.R. The Gut Microbiome, Energy Homeostasis, and Implications for Hypertension. *Curr. Hypertens. Rep.* **2017**, *19*, 27. [CrossRef] [PubMed]
196. Chen, J.; Wright, K.; Davis, J.M.; Jeraldo, P.; Marietta, E.V.; Murray, J.; Nelson, H.; Matteson, E.L.; Taneja, V. An expansion of rare lineage intestinal microbes characterizes rheumatoid arthritis. *Genome Med.* **2016**, *8*, 43. [CrossRef] [PubMed]
197. Zhang, X.; Zhang, D.; Jia, H.; Feng, Q.; Wang, D.; Liang, D.; Wu, X.; Li, J.; Tang, L.; Li, Y.; et al. The oral and gut microbiomes are perturbed in rheumatoid arthritis and partly normalized after treatment. *Nat. Med.* **2015**, *21*, 895–905. [CrossRef] [PubMed]
198. Haase, S.; Haghikia, A.; Wilck, N.; Muller, D.N.; Linker, R.A. Impacts of microbiome metabolites on immune regulation and autoimmunity. *Immunology* **2018**, *154*, 230–238. [CrossRef] [PubMed]
199. Mizuno, M.; Noto, D.; Kaga, N.; Chiba, A.; Miyake, S. The dual role of short fatty acid chains in the pathogenesis of autoimmune disease models. *PLoS ONE* **2017**, *12*, e0173032. [CrossRef] [PubMed]
200. Lucas, S.; Omata, Y.; Hofmann, J.; Bottcher, M.; Iljazovic, A.; Sarter, K.; Albrecht, O.; Schulz, O.; Krishnacoumar, B.; Kronke, G.; et al. Short-chain fatty acids regulate systemic bone mass and protect from pathological bone loss. *Nat. Commun.* **2018**, *9*, 55. [CrossRef] [PubMed]
201. Dong, L.; Xia, S.; Gao, F.; Zhang, D.; Chen, J.; Zhang, J. 3,3′-Diindolylmethane attenuates experimental arthritis and osteoclastogenesis. *Biochem. Pharmacol.* **2010**, *79*, 715–721. [CrossRef] [PubMed]

International Journal of
Molecular Sciences

MDPI

Review

Biological Activities and Safety of *Citrus* spp. Essential Oils

Noura S. Dosoky [1] and William N. Setzer [1,2,*]

[1] Aromatic Plant Research Center, 230 N 1200 E, Suite 102, Lehi, UT 84043, USA; ndosoky@aromaticplant.org
[2] Department of Chemistry, University of Alabama in Huntsville, Huntsville, AL 35899, USA
* Correspondence: wsetzer@chemistry.uah.edu; Tel.: +1-256-824-6519

Received: 6 June 2018; Accepted: 3 July 2018; Published: 5 July 2018

Abstract: *Citrus* fruits have been a commercially important crop for thousands of years. In addition, *Citrus* essential oils are valuable in the perfume, food, and beverage industries, and have also enjoyed use as aromatherapy and medicinal agents. This review summarizes the important biological activities and safety considerations of the essential oils of sweet orange (*Citrus sinensis*), bitter orange (*Citrus aurantium*), neroli (*Citrus aurantium*), orange petitgrain (*Citrus aurantium*), mandarin (*Citrus reticulata*), lemon (*Citrus limon*), lime (*Citrus aurantifolia*), grapefruit (*Citrus* × *paradisi*), bergamot (*Citrus bergamia*), Yuzu (*Citrus junos*), and kumquat (*Citrus japonica*).

Keywords: sweet orange; bitter orange; neroli; orange petitgrain; mandarin; lemon; lime; grapefruit; bergamot; yuzu; kumquat

1. Introduction

The genus *Citrus* (Rutaceae) is one of the ancient, most traded, and most popular crops. The earliest records of its cultivation date back to 2100 BC [1]. The origin of *Citrus* is still controversial; however, it is believed to have originated from Southeast Asia [2]. *Citrus* is grown widely all over the world for its numerous health benefits. *Citrus* fruits are consumed as a fresh fruit desert or used for making juice and jam. They are an excellent source of vitamins, especially vitamin C. Processing *Citrus* fruits results in a significant amount of waste (peels, seeds, and pulps), which accounts for 50% of the fruit [3]. *Citrus* waste is a valuable source of *d*-limonene, flavonoids, carotenoids, dietary fibers, soluble sugars, cellulose, hemicellulose, pectin, polyphenols, ascorbic acid, methane, and essential oils [4–6]. Interestingly, the essential oil (EO) is the most vital by-product of *Citrus* processing. *Citrus* EOs are broadly used as natural food additives in several food and beverage products [7] because they have been classified as generally recognized as safe (GRAS) [8]. Furthermore, *Citrus* EOs are used as natural preservatives due to their broad spectrum of biological activities including antimicrobial and antioxidant effects [9]. The presence of terpenes, flavonoids, carotenes, and coumarins is thought to be responsible for the strong anti-oxidative and antimicrobial activities [10–14]. Due to their pleasant refreshing smell and rich aroma, *Citrus* EOs are also used in air-fresheners, household cleaning products, perfumes, cosmetics, and medicines.

Because of their high economic importance, numerous studies have investigated the chemical composition of the peel, leaf, and flower essential oils of different *Citrus* species. It is worth noting that there is a great variation in the chemical composition of *Citrus* oils due to differences in origin, genetic background, season, climate, age, ripening stage, method of extraction, etc. [15–19]. The key volatile components are presented in Figure 1. Sweet orange, bitter orange, mandarin, and grapefruit EOs are rich in monoterpenes with the major component being *d*-limonene (65.3–95.9%) (Table 1) [8]. The main components in the essential oil of bitter orange leaf are linalyl acetate and linalool [16], while the flower EO contained linalool as the major component, followed by *d*-limonene and linalyl acetate [20]. Some of the *Citrus* EOs are prepared by expression, which results in the presence of non-volatile components (Figure 2) that can cause photosensitivity and skin irritation [8]. The percentages of these non-volatile constituents in expressed oils are given in Table 2.

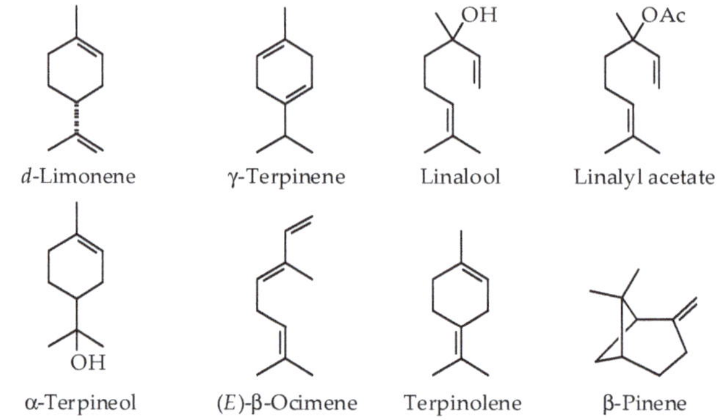

Figure 1. Chemical structures of key volatile components in *Citrus* essential oils.

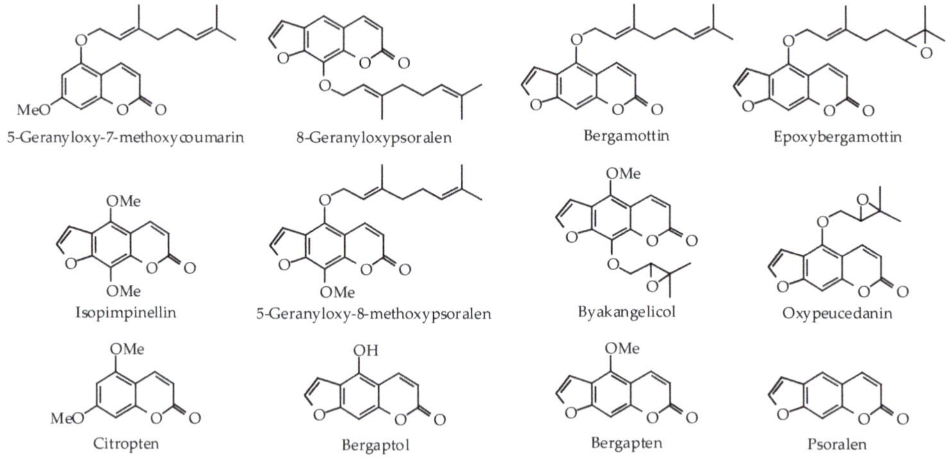

Figure 2. Chemical structures of key non-volatile components in expressed *Citrus* essential oils.

The objective of this review is to summarize the reported biological activities and safety of the essential oils of sweet orange (*Citrus sinensis* L.), bitter orange (*Citrus aurantium* L.), neroli (*Citrus aurantium* L.), orange petitgrain (*Citrus aurantium* L.), mandarin (*Citrus reticulata* Blanco), lemon (*Citrus limon* Osbeck), lime (*Citrus aurantifolia*), grapefruit (*Citrus* × *paradisi* Macfady), bergamot (*Citrus bergamia* Risso & Poit), Yuzu (*Citrus junos* Sieb. ex Tanaka), and kumquat (*Citrus japonica* Thunb).

Table 1. Major volatile components in essential oils of different *Citrus* spp.

	Citrus EO	Sweet Orange [8,21]	Bitter Orange [8]	Neroli (Egyptian) [8]	Petitgrain [8]	Mandarin [8]	Lemon (D) [8]	Lemon (Ex) [8]	Lime (D) [8,22,23]	Lime (Ex) [8,22]	Bergamot (FCF) [8,24]	Bergamot (Ex) [8,24,25]	Grapefruit [8,26]	Yuzu [8,27]
	Plant Part	**Fruit Peel**	**Fruit Peel**	**Flower**	**Leaf**	**Fruit Peel**	**Fruit Peel**	**Fruit Peel**	**Fruit Peel**	**Fruit Peel**	**Fruit Peel**	**Fruit Peel**	**Fruit Peel**	**Fruit Peel**
Essential oil Composition	*d*-Limonene	83.9–95.9%	89.7–94.7%	6.0–10.2%	0.4–8.0%	65.3–74.2%	64.0–70.5%	56.6–76.0%	40.4–49.4%	48.2%	28.0–45.0%	27.4–52.0%	84.8–95.4%	63.1%
	Linalool	0–5.6%	0.1–2.0%	43.7–54.3%	12.3–24.2%						4.0–20.0%	1.7–20.6%		2–8%
	Linalyl acetate			3.5–8.6%	51.0–71.0%						18.0–28.0%	17.1–40.4%		
	β-Pinene			3.5–5.3%	0.3–2.7%	1.4–2.1%	8.2–14.0%	6.0–17.0%	2.0–2.9%	21.1%	4.0–11.0%	4.4–11.0%		1.1%
	γ-Terpinene					16.4–22.7%	8.4–10.7%	3.0–13.3%	9.5–10.7%	8.1%	3.0–12.0%	5.0–11.4%		12.5%
	α-Pinene	0.6–1.0%				2.0–2.7%	1.1–2.1%	1.3–4.4%	1.2–2.1%	2.5%	1.0–1.8%	0.7–2.2%	0.2–1.6%	2.7%
	β-Myrcene	1.3–3.3%	1.6–2.4%	1.4–2.1%	0–2.0%	1.5–1.8%	1.4–1.6%	tr–2.2%	1.3–2.1%	1.3%		0.6–1.8%	1.4–3.6%	3.2%
	α-Terpineol			3.9–5.8%	2.1–5.2%			0.1–8.0%	5.4–12.7%					
	(*E*)-β-Ocimene			4.6–5.8%	0.2–2.2%									
	Sabinene	0.2–1.0%		0.4–1.6%			0.8–1.7%	0.5–2.4%		3.1%			0.4–1.0%	
	Neral	0–1.3%					0.5–1.5%	0.4–2.0%		1.4%				
	Geranial	0–1.8%					0.7–2.2%	0.5–4.3%		2.4%				
	Bicyclogermacrene													2.0%
	(*E*)-β-Farnesene													1.3%
	Geranyl acetate			3.4–4.1%	1.9–3.4%									
	Terpinolene					0.7–1.0%			8.1–8.7%					
	(*E*)-Nerolidol			1.3–4.0%										
	Geraniol			2.8–3.6%	1.4–2.3%									
	Nerol			1.1–1.3%	0.4–1.1%									
	p-Cymene					0.1–1.4%		tr–2.3%	1.6–2.5%					
	(*E,E*)-Farnesol			1.6–3.2%										
	(*E,Z*)-Farnesol													
	Neryl acetate			1.7–2.1%	0–2.6%			0.1–1.5%				0.1–1.2%		
	Terpinen-4-ol							tr–1.9%	0.7–1.9%					
	(*Z*)-β-Ocimene			0.7–1.0%										
	α-Thujene					0.7–1.0%								
	1,4-Cineole								2.0–3.0%					
	Terpinen-1-ol								1.0–2.3%					
	(*Z*)-β-Terpineol								0.5–2.2%					
	α-Terpinene								tr–2.1%					
	β-Bisabolene								1.6–1.8%	1.8%				
	α-Fenchol								0.6–1.4%					
	Borneol								0.5–1.4%					
	Camphene								0.5–1.3%					
	γ-Terpineol								0.8–1.6%					
	(*E*)-α-Bergamotene									1.1%				
	β-Caryophyllene									1.0%				
	(2*E*,6*E*)-α-Farnesene									1.0%				
	β-Phellandrene													5.4%
	Nootkatone												0.1–0.8%	

D = Distilled; Ex = Expressed; FCF = Furanocoumarin-Free.

Table 2. Non-volatile components of some expressed *Citrus* oils.

Non-Volatile Components	Bitter Orange [8,26]	Lemon [8]	Lime [8,26]	Grapefruit [8,26]	Bergamot [8,24,25]	Bergamot (FCF) [8,24]	Mandarin [8]
Bergamottin	-	0.16–0.54%	1.7–3.0%	<0.11%	0.68–2.75%	0–1.625%	0–0.001%
Bergapten	0.035–0.073%	0.0001–0.035%	0.17–0.33%	0.012–0.19%	0.11–0.33%	0–0.0091%	0–0.0003%
Oxypeucedanin	-	0.09–0.82%	0.02–0.3%	-	-	-	-
5-Geranloxy-7-methoxycoumarin	-	0.18–0.28%	1.7–3.2%	-	0.08–0.68%	0–0.19%	-
Citropten	-	0.05–0.17%	0.4–2.2%	-	0.01–0.35%	0–0.0052%	-
Byakangelicol	-	0.006–0.16%	-	-	-	-	-
8-Geranyloxypsoralen	-	0.01–0.045%	0.10–0.14%	-	-	-	-
Isopimpinellin	-	0–0.011%	0.1–1.3%	-	-	-	-
5-Geranoxy-8-methoxypsoralen	-	-	0.2–0.9%	-	-	-	-
Epoxybergamottin	0.082%	-	-	0.1126%	-	-	-
Psoralen	0.007%	-	-	-	0–0.0026%	-	-
Bergaptol	-	-	-	-	0–0.19%	-	-

FCF = Furanocoumarin-Free.

2. Biological Properties

A summary of the biological activities of different *Citrus* essential oils is presented in Table 3.

Table 3. Biological activities of different *Citrus* essential oils.

Essential Oil	Biological Activity	Ref.
Sweet orange	Anticarcinogenic	[28,29]
	Relaxant	[30]
	Anxiolytic	[31–33]
	Pain relief	[34]
	Hepatocarcinogenesis suppressant	[35]
	Anti-tumor	[36]
	Antioxidant	[37]
	Food preservative	[38]
	Acne treatment (with sweet basil oil)	[39]
	Antibacterial	[40–43]
	Antifungal	[10,44,45]
	Anti-aflatoxigenic (at 500 ppm)	[44]
	Larvicidal	[46,47]
	Insecticidal	[48–50]
	Anthelmintic	[51]
	Growth promoter (in Tilapia)	[52]
Bitter orange	Mild sedative, hypnotic, soothing, calming, and motor relaxant	[53]
	Sleep inducer	[54]
	Anxiolytic and antidepressant	[53,55–58]
	Pain relief	[34,59]
	Antiseizure and anticonvulsant agent	[54]
	Anti-spasmodic and sexual desire enhancer	[59]
	Gastroprotective and ulcer healing	[60]
	Digestive disorders treatment	[53]
	Hepatocarcinogenesis suppressant	[35]
	Antioxidant	[53,61]
	Nephroprotective	[62]
	Antibacterial	[53,63–65]
	Pimple and acne treatment	[53]
	Antifungal	[15,53,66]
	Fumigant and anti-cholinesterase	[67]
	Larvicidal	[46]
Neroli	Sedative, soothing, calming, and motor relaxant	[55,68]
	Anxiolytic and antidepressant	[53,57,69,70]
	Antiseizure and anticonvulsant	[71,72]
	Central and peripheral antinociceptive effects	[73]
	Anti-inflammatory	[73]
	Menopausal symptoms relief	[74]
	Premenstrual syndrome (PMS) relief	[75]
	Sexual desire enhancer	[59]
	Endothelium- and smooth muscle-dependent vasodilator	[76]
	Hypotensive	[77]
	Antioxidant	[20,78]
	Anti-amnesic	[72]
	Antibacterial	[53,79]
	Antifungal	[20,53,75,79]
Orange petitgrain	Antioxidant	[78,80]
	Antibacterial	[81]
	Antifungal	[81]

Table 3. *Cont.*

Essential Oil	Biological Activity	Ref.
Mandarin	Anti-proliferative	[82]
	Chemoprotective	[82]
	Antioxidant	[83]
	Antibacterial	[83,84]
	Antifungal	[84–87]
Lemon	Stress relief	[88,89]
	Cytotoxic	[28,90]
	Chemoprotective	[91]
	Anti-obesity	[92]
	Antioxidant	[93]
	Neuroprotective	[94,95]
	Anti-anxiety	[96]
	Creativity and mood enhancer	[97]
	Analgesic	[98]
	Relief of nausea and vomiting of pregnancy	[99]
	Anti-spasmodic	[89]
	Attention level, concentration, cognitive performance, mood, and memory enhancer	[89,100]
	Skin penetration enhancer	[101]
	Antibacterial	[102,103]
	Antifungal	[10]
	Insect repellent	[104]
	Miticidal	[105]
Lime	Anti-obesity	[106]
	Spasmolytic agent	[107,108]
	Selective acetylcholinesterase and buytrylcholinesterase inhibitor	[109]
	Antioxidant	[109]
	Anti-inflammatory	[110]
	Flavoring agent	[111,112]
	Antibacterial	[111,113]
	Antifungal	[111,113]
	Insecticidal	[114]
	Phytotoxic	[113]
Grapefruit	Anti-obesity	[92,115–117]
	Cravings and hunger reducer (mixed with patchouli oil)	[116]
	Body cleansing promoter	[116]
	Cytotoxic	[28,90]
	Antibacterial	[118,119]
	Antifungal	[118–120]
	Larvicidal	[121–124]
Bergamot	Melanogenic component in suntan preparations	[125,126]
	Pain relief	[127–129]
	Peripheral antinociceptive	[129,130]
	Antiallodynic	[127,131]
	Wound healing	[132]
	Cytotoxic	[125,133–135]
	Anti-tumor	[136]
	Neuroprotective	[137,138]
	Sedative, calming, and soothing	[139]
	Anxiolytic	[139,140]
	Mood enhancer	[141]
	Antioxidant	[109]
	Antibacterial	[142–144]
	Antifungal	[142,143,145]
	Anti-dermatophyte	[146,147]
	Antimycoplasmal	[148]

Table 3. *Cont.*

Essential Oil	Biological Activity	Ref.
Yuzu	Anti-carcinogenic	[149]
	Anti-inflammatory	[150]
	Anti-anxiety	[151]
	Mood disturbance, tension-anxiety, anger-hostility, and fatigue reducer	[152,153]
	Mind and body health promoter	[152]
	Odor suppressant	[154]
	Anti-cancer	[155]
	Hypocholesterolemic	[156]
	Anti-diabetic	[157]
	Anti-obesity	[158]
	Platelet aggregation inhibitor	[159]
	Heart failure treatment	[160]
Kumquat	Antiproliferative	[161]
	Antioxidant	[161,162]
	Antibacterial	[163]
	Antifungal	[163]

2.1. *Sweet Orange (Citrus sinensis L.) Essential Oil*

Sweet orange EO showed anticarcinogenic potential via inducing apoptosis in human leukemia (HL-60) cells [28] and human colon cancer cells [29], and inhibiting angiogenesis and metastasis [29]. Olfactory stimulation using orange EO induced physiological and psychological relaxation. Inhalation of orange EO for 90 s caused a significant decrease in oxyhemoglobin concentration in the right prefrontal cortex of the brain which increases comfortable, relaxed, and natural feelings [30]. The odor of sweet orange decreases the symptoms of anxiety and improves the mood [31]. The oil showed strong anxiolytic activity in Wistar rats [32]. When female dental patients were exposed to sweet orange odor diffused in the waiting room prior to a dental procedure, they showed lower levels of state-anxiety compared to control patients who were exposed to air only [33]. Sweet orange EO in combination with ginger and accompanied by a massage was effective in alleviating moderate to severe knee pain among the elderly in Hong Kong [34]. Moreover, sweet orange EO suppressed pre-neoplastic hepatic lesions during *N*-nitrosodiethylamine (DEN)-induced hepatocarcinogenesis in rats by restoring the normal phenotype and upregulating junctional complexes [35]. Injections of orange EO in mice 24 h after subcutaneous injections with dibenzo-[α]-pyrene (DBP) reduced the tumor incidence to less than 50% after 30 weeks [36]. In addition, the oil was reported to have a good radical-scavenging activity [37], mainly due to the high *d*-limonene content [12,13]. It is used in combination with thyme oil to improve the quality traits of marinated chicken meat [38]. Moreover, formulations based on orange and sweet basil oils were effective in treating acne [39]. Improvement of the acne condition was observed with 43–75% clearance of lesions. It should be noted that there were some side effects, such as burning and redness that disappeared within a few minutes of completing the application [39]. Sweet orange EO was reported to inhibit the growth of several bacteria including *Staphylococcus aureus*, *Listeria monocytogenes*, *Vibrio parahaemolyticus*, *Salmonella typhimurium*, *Escherichia coli*, and *Pseudomonas aeruginosa* [40–43], as well as several fungal species, such as *Aspergillus flavus*, *A. fumigatus*, *A. niger*, *A. terreus*, *Alternaria alternata*, *Cladosporium herbarum*, *Curvularia lunata*, *Fusarium oxysporum*, *Helminthosporium oryzae*, *Penicillium chrysogenum*, *P. verrucosum*, and *Trichoderma viride* [10,44,45]. It also showed a good anti-aflatoxigenic effects (inhibited aflatoxin B_1) at 500 ppm [44]. In addition, it has an intense larvicidal activity against the malaria vector, *Anopheles labranchiae* [46], and the vector of yellow and dengue fever, *Aedes aegypti* [47]. Sweet orange EO is a potent fumigant against house flies, cockroaches, and mosquitoes [48,49]. It can be used for controlling subterranean termites [50]. It is also an effective anthelmintic agent against gastrointestinal nematodes; five times more effective on *Haemonchus contortus* eggs than tea tree EO [51]. Moreover, sweet orange EO acted as a growth promoter, increased immunity, and improved disease resistance to *Streptococcus iniae* in Tilapia [52].

2.2. Bitter Orange (Citrus aurantium L.) Essential Oil

Bitter orange EO is used as a mild sedative and hypnotic for its soothing, calming, and motor relaxant effects [53]. It also enhances sleeping time and is used to treat insomnia [54]. Bitter orange odor decreases the symptoms of anxiety, improves mood, and creates a sense of well-being [53]. It showed strong anxiolytic activity in rodents without any motor impairment, even after 15 consecutive days of treatment [55]. It increased social interactions for rats (time spent in active social interaction), and increased exploration time in the open arms of the elevated plus-maze (EPM) [55]. It was also effective in treating the symptoms of anxiety in patients with chronic myeloid leukemia prior to the collection of medullary material [56]. It exerted its antianxiety effects by regulating serotonin (5-HT) receptors in rats [57] and its antidepressant effects through the monoaminergic system in mice [58]. Furthermore, bitter orange EO was effective in reducing the severity of first-stage labor pain and anxiety in primiparous women [59], as well as in alleviating moderate and severe knee pain [34]. Bitter orange EO is used as a natural antiseizure and anticonvulsant agent. It has been used in treating epilepsy and seizures [54]. It has been reported to have anti-spasmodic effect and to enhance sexual desire [59]. Due to the presence of limonene, bitter orange EO possesses its gastroprotective and ulcer healing actions through increasing the gastric production of mucus, which is useful as a secondary intervention in the treatment of chronic inflammatory diseases [60]. It is used as a treatment for digestive disorders such as slow digestion, constipation, flatulence, gastric problems, etc. [53]. Bitter orange EO suppressed preneoplastic hepatic lesions during DEN-induced hepatocarcinogenesis in rats by restoring the normal phenotype and upregulating junctional complexes [35]. Bitter orange EO showed good radical-scavenging activity [53], largely due to the high *d*-limonene content [12,13] and its microencapsulated form, which was effective in reducing oxidative stress in acute otitis media rats [61]. Due to its free radical-scavenging properties, bitter orange extract showed nephroprotective effects against gentamicin-induced renal damage [62]. The antibacterial activity of bitter orange EO was manifested by inhibiting the growth of *Listeria innocua*, *Salmonella enterica*, *Escherichia coli*, *Pseudomonas fluorescens*, and *Aeromonas hydrophila* [53,63,64]. It was also effective in controlling multi-species biofilms [65]. Due to its antimicrobial effects, bitter orange EO is used for treating colds, dull skin, flu, gums and mouth, and chronic bronchitis, as well as a food preservative [53]. The diluted oil is used to treat pimples and acne [53]. In addition, bitter orange EO inhibits the growth of *Penicillium digitatum*, and *P. italicum* [15,53]. The oil was mentioned as a topical treatment for skin fungal infections like ringworm, jock itch, and athlete's foot [66]. Furthermore, bitter orange EO showed potent fumigant and anti-cholinesterase activities against the silverleaf whitefly, *Bemisia tabaci* [67]. It was also effective against the larvae of the malaria vector, *Anopheles labranchiae* [46].

2.3. Neroli (Citrus aurantium L.) Essential Oil

Neroli EO is used as a sedative for its soothing, calming, and motor relaxant effects by healthcare centers in Puerto Rico, Guatemala, Mexico, Italy, Martinique, and Spain [55]. Neroli EO is effective for cardiac palpitations resulting from shock or fear [68]. Similar to the fruit peel oil, the odor of neroli decreases the symptoms of anxiety, improves mood, and creates a sense of well-being [53]. It was proven to be effective in reducing preoperative anxiety before minor operations [69]. Neroli EO reduced the mean anxiety scores in postmenopausal women [70]. It exerted its antianxiety effects by regulating 5-HT receptors in rats [57]. Neroli EO is used as a natural antiseizure and anticonvulsant agent [71]. It has been used in treating insomnia, epilepsy, and seizures [72]. Neroli EO has central and peripheral antinociceptive effects which support the ethnomedicinal claims of its use in the management of pain and inflammation [73]. Neroli EO possesses significant anti-inflammatory activity against acute and chronic inflammation [73]. Neroli EO is effective in reducing stress and improving the endocrine system. Inhalation of neroli EO helps in relieving menopausal symptoms, reducing blood pressure, and increasing sexual desire in postmenopausal women [74]. It also decreased the overall symptoms of premenstrual syndrome (PMS) in university students. It showed positive effects on the mood, blood pressure, pain, inflammation, bloating, and indigestion in addition to its anti-depressant effects [75]. Inhaling neroli odor enhances sexual desire [59]. Neroli EO is an endothelium- and smooth-muscle-dependent vasodilator that can alleviate cardiovascular symptoms. The endothelial component is mediated by the nitric oxide to soluble guanylyl cyclase pathway, while the smooth muscle component involves inhibiting extracellular Ca^{2+} influx and store-operated Ca^{2+} release mediated by the ryanodine receptor (RyR) signaling pathway [76]. Inhaling a mixture of lavender, ylang-ylang, marjoram, and neroli (20:15:10:2) decreased systolic and diastolic blood pressure, as well as the concentration of salivary cortisol in prehypertensive and hypertensive subjects [77]. These positive effects were immediate and continuous [77]. Furthermore, neroli EO is a strong antioxidant. It showed a 100% singlet oxygen scavenging activity at all concentrations between 0.1 and 2% [20,78]. Interestingly, the *C. aurantium* flower extract showed anti-amnesic and repairing effects on memory, learning impairments, and behavioral disorders induced by scopolamine, and has the potential to treat Alzheimer's disease [72]. Neroli EO inhibits the growth of several bacteria including *Bacillus subtilis*, *B. cereus*, *Staphylococcus aureus*, *S. epidermis*, *Enterococcus faecalis*, *Micrococcus luteus*, *Listeria monocytogenes*, *Salmonella enteritidis*, *Escherichia coli*, *Pseudomonas aeruginosa*, and *Klebsiella pneumonia* [53,79], as well as several fungi including *Aspergillus niger*, *A. flavus*, *A. nidulans*, *A. fumigatus*, *Fusarium graminearum*, *F. oxysporum*, *F. culmorum*, and *Alternaria alternata* [20,53,75,79].

2.4. Orange Petitgrain (Citrus aurantium L.) Essential Oil

Orange petitgrain EO showed a remarkable radical-scavenging activity, higher than the flower oil (neroli) and fruit peel oil (bitter orange) from the same plant [78,80]. The potent antioxidant effect could be attributed to the high *d*-limonene content [12,13]. It also inhibited the growth of *Bacillus subtilis*, *Staphylococcus aureus*, *Escherichia coli*, *Saccharomyces cerevisiae*, *Mucor ramannianus*, and *Fusarium culmorum* [81].

2.5. Mandarin (Citrus reticulata Blanco) Essential Oil

Citrus reticulata EO showed an anti-proliferative effect against human embryonic lung fibroblasts (HELFs) and showed protective effects against bleomycin (BLM)-induced pulmonary fibrosis in rats. The mechanism is thought to be through adjusting the unbalance of oxidation and antioxidation, down-regulating the expressions of connective tissue growth factor (CTGF) and mRNA in lung tissues, and reducing collagen deposition and fibrosis [82]. *C. reticulata* EO showed a moderate radical scavenging activity [83] mainly due to the high *d*-limonene content [12]. Mandarin oil is well known for its broad spectrum antibacterial and antifungal actions. It inhibits the growth of several bacteria including *Escherichia coli*, *Bacillus subtilis*, *Pseudomonas aeruginosa*, and *Staphylococcus aureus* [83,84], as well as several fungi including *Penicillium italicum*, *P. digitatum*, *P. chrysogenum*, *Aspergillus niger*, *A. flavus*, *Alternaria alternata*, *Rhizoctonia solani*, *Curvularia lunata*, *Fusarium oxysporum*, and *Helminthosporium oryzae* [84–87].

2.6. Lemon (Citrus limon Osbeck) Essential Oil

Lemon EO is a natural stress reliever. Inhaling lemon EO causes anti-stress effects through modulating the 5-HT and dopamine (DA) activities in mice [88,89]. Lemon EO showed cytotoxic effects against human prostate, lung, and breast cancer cells [90]. It also induced apoptosis in HL-60 cells due to the presence of citral, decanal, and octanal [28]. Oral administration of lemon EO inhibited 4-(methylnitrosamino)-1-(3-pyridyl)-1-butanone (NNK)-induced neoplasia of the lungs and forestomach of female mice [91]. Lemon EO causes activation of the sympathetic nerve activity innervating the white adipose tissue (WAT), which increases lipolysis and results in the suppression of body weight gain [92]. Lemon EO significantly reduces lipid peroxidation levels and nitrile content, but increases reduced glutathione (GSH) levels, as well as superoxide dismutase, catalase, and glutathione peroxidase activities in mouse hippocampus [93]. The neuroprotective effect of lemon EO is attributed to its remarkable radical-scavenging activity [94,95]. Prolonged exposure (for 2 weeks) to lemon EO induces significant changes in neuronal circuits involved in anxiety and pain in rats [96]. Lemon EO improves creativity and mood, and is thought to affect heart rhythm [97]. The analgesic effect of lemon EO is induced by dopamine-related activation of anterior cingulate cortex (ACC) and the descending pain inhibitory system [98]. Inhalation of lemon EO reduces the intensity of nausea and vomiting of pregnancy (NVP) by 33% [99]. It also showed anti-spasmodic activity [89]. Lemon EO significantly enhanced attention level, concentration, cognitive performance, mood, and memory of students during the learning process [100]. Rats exposed to lemon EO were able to find a target point faster than a control group [89]. Lemon EO is a safe and effective penetration enhancer for topical administration of lipid- and water-soluble vitamins which are critical issues for the protection of anti-ageing formulations. It significantly enhances the trans-epidermal release of α-tocopherol (vitamin E), retinyl acetate (vitamin A), pyridoxine (vitamin B_6), and ascorbic acid (vitamin C) from topical emulsions in reconstructed human epidermis [101]. In addition, lemon EO is a potent antibacterial against *Bacillus cereus, Mycobacterium smegmatis, Listeria monocytogenes, Lactobacillus curvatus, L. sakei, Micrococcus luteus, Escherichia coli, Klebsiella pneumoniae, Pseudococcus aeruginosa, Proteus vulgaris, Enterobacter gergoviae, E. ammnigenus, Staphylococcus aureus, S. carnosus,* and *S. xylosus* [102,103], and a strong antifungal against *Aspergillus niger, A. flavus, Penicillium verrucosum, P. chrysogenum, Kluyveromyces fragilis, Rhodotorula rubra, Candida albicans, Hanseniaspora guilliermondii,* and *Debaryomyces hansenii* [10]. Lemon EO has insect repellent effects against the malaria vector, *Anopheles stephensi* [104]. It also showed remarkable miticidal activity against *Sarcoptes scabiei* var. *cuniculi,* both in vitro and in vivo. When lemon EO was tested at 20% and applied topically on the infected parts of rabbits once a week for four successive weeks, the infected rabbits completely recovered after the second week of treatment [105].

2.7. Key Lime (Citrus aurantifolia) Essential Oil

Lime EO has been used to relieve common cold, flu, asthma, arthritis, and bronchitis [111,164]. It could be useful in weight loss and the treatment of drug-induced obesity and related diseases. It displayed a reduction in body weight and food consumption in ketotifen-induced obese mice [106]. It has been reported as a potent spasmolytic agent [107,108]. Lime EO could also be useful in treating Alzheimer's disease since it is a strong selective acetylcholinesterase and buytrylcholinesterase inhibitor [109]. It has a remarkable radical-scavenging activity (IC_{50} = 19.6 μg/mL) [109] due to the high *d*-limonene content [12,13]. Lime EO exhibited anti-inflammatory effects by reducing cell migration, cytokine production, and protein extravasation induced by carrageenan [110]. Lime EO is used as a flavoring agent in syrups and suspensions [111,112]. In addition, it is a potent antibacterial against *Escherichia coli, Listeria monocytogenes, Bacillus subtilis, Enterococcus durans, E. hirae, Staphylococcus epidermidis, S. aureus, Enterobacter cloacae, Pseudomonas aeruginosa, Serratia marcescens, Shigella flexnerii, Streptococcus faecalis, Citrobacter* spp., *Klebsiella pneumoniae, and Salmonella typhi* [111,113]. It also inhibits the growth of many fungi including *Colletotrichum gloeosporioides, Rhizopus stolonifer, Aspergillus niger, A. parasiticus, Rhizoctonia solani, Candida albicans,* and *C. parapsilosis* [111,113]. Lime EO has insecticidal activity (contact, fumigation, and feeding deterrent activities) against the maize weevil, *Sitophilus zeamais* [114]. It showed phytotoxic activities against *Avena fatua* L., *Echinochloa crus-galli* (L.) Beauv, *Allium cepa* L., and *Phalaris minor* Retz [113].

2.8. Grapefruit (Citrus × paradisi Macfady) Essential Oil

Because of its anti-obesity effects, grapefruit EO is called the "dieter's friend" [116]. The fragrance of grapefruit EO causes activation of the sympathetic nerve activity innervating the WAT, which facilitates lipolysis, then results in a suppression of body weight gain [92,115]. It efficiently inhibits adipogenesis via inhibiting the accumulation of triglycerides [117]. When mixed with patchouli oil, grapefruit EO is known to lower cravings and hunger, which makes it a great tool to lose weight in a healthy way [116]. The bright, refreshing scent of grapefruit EO energizes and uplifts the senses. Grapefruit EO promotes body cleansing and removal of toxins and excess fluids [116]. Grapefruit EO was cytotoxic against human prostate and lung cancer cells [90]. It also induced apoptosis in HL-60 cells due to the presence of citral, decanal, and octanal [28]. Moreover, it showed a strong antibacterial activity against *Bacillus cereus, Enterococus faecalis, Escherichia coli, Klebsiella pneumoniae, Pseudococcus* sp., *Salmonella thyphimurium, Shigella flexneri*, and *Staphylococcus aureus* [118,119], and a strong antifungal activity against *Aspergillus niger, Candida albicans, Cladosporium cucumerinum, Penicillium digitatum, P. italicum*, and *P. chrysogenum* [118–120]. Grapefruit EO was 95% lethal to eggs and larvae of *Anastrepha fraterculus* and *Ceratitis capitata* [121]. It completely inhibited the viability of *Aedes aegypti* eggs exposed at 400 ppm, and inhibits its larval development at 100 ppm [122]. Also, grapefruit EO is a potent larvicide against *Anopheles stephensi* at 80 ppm [123]. It caused an 89.6% decrease of *Eimeria*-induced coccidiosis contamination with 5 mg/kg for 30 days [124].

2.9. Bergamot (Citrus bergamia Risso & Poit) Essential Oil

Bergamot EO is widely used in the perfumery, pharmaceutical, cosmetic, and food industries [125]. It is used in suntan preparations due to the presence of bergapten, which is the active melanogenic component [126]. Bergamot EO is used in complementary medicine to treat chronic nociceptive and neuropathic pain via modulating sensitive perception of pain [127–129]. Intraplantar injection of bergamot EO, linalool, and linalyl acetate showed a peripheral antinociception effect in the capsaicin test mediated by a peripheral opioid mechanism [129,130]. A combination of a low dose of morphine with inactive doses of bergamot oil or linalool was sufficient to induce antiallodynic effects in mice via inhibiting spinal extracellular signal-regulated protein kinase (ERK) phosphorylation [127,131]. The oil is used to facilitate wound healing [132]. Bergamot EO was reported to be cytotoxic against SH-SY5Y human neuroblastoma cells, suppressing their growth rate through a mechanism related to both apoptotic and necrotic cell death [133,134]. Bergamottin and 5-geranyloxy-7-methoxycoumarin were identified as the bioactive molecules responsible for the cytotoxic effect of bergamot EO [133]. Bergamot EO inhibited tumor formation by the carcinogen NDMA in vitro by more than 70% [136]. Bergamot oil and its *d*-Limonene were reported to modulate autophagic pathways in SH-SY5Y cells [125]. Liposomal bergamot oil showed improved anticancer activity against SH-SY5Y cells because of its higher stability and higher bioavailability [135]. In addition, it has been shown to reduce neuronal damage caused in vitro by excitotoxic stimuli by preventing an injury-induced decrease of phosphorylated protein kinase B (phospho-Akt) and phosphorylated glycogen synthase kinase 3β (phospho-GSK-3β) levels [137,138]. Bergamot EO is used as a mild sedative that acts by calming and soothing the nervous system [139]. In rodent experiments, the pleasant, refreshing odor of bergamot decreased the symptoms of stress-induced anxiety and minimized behavior-related depressive disorders in chronic stressed rats [139]. Inhalation of bergamot EO was reported to increase the release of amino acid neurotransmitters (glutamate, gamma-aminobutyric acid (GABA), aspartate, glycine, and taurine) in rat hippocampuses, both in vivo and in vitro, which suggested that the oil may interfere with exocytosis [165]. Similar to diazepam, bergamot oil exerted anxiolytic-like behaviors and attenuated hypothalamic-pituitary-adrenal (HPA) axis activity via reducing the corticosterone response to acute stress caused by EPM [140]. A pilot study performed in the waiting room of a mental health treatment center (Utah, USA) revealed that inhalation of bergamot EO for 15 minutes improves positive feelings [141]. Furthermore, bergamot EO showed a good radical scavenging activity evaluated by β-carotene bleaching test (IC_{50} = 42.6 μg/mL) [109] due to the high *d*-limonene content [12,13]. Bergamot EO inhibits the growth of several bacteria including *Escherichia coli, Staphylococcus aureus, Bacillus cereus, Salmonella enterica, S. typhimurium, Pseudomonas putida, Arcobacter butzleri, Enterococcus faecium, E. faecalis*, and *Listeria monocytogenes* [142–144]. Several studies showed a broad spectrum antifungal activity of bergamot EO against *Hanseniaspora guilliermondii, Debaryomyces hansenii, Kluyveromyces fragilis, Rhodotorula rubra, Candida albicans, Aspergillus niger, A. flavus, Penicillium italicum, Fusarium solani, F. sporotrichioides, F. oxysporum, Curvularia lunata, Verticillium dahliae, Phomopsis* sp., *Phoma* sp., and *Myrothechium verrucaria* [142,143,145]. It was also reported to have antifungal effects against dermatophytes of the genera *Trichophyton*, *Microsporum*, and *Epidermophyton* [146]. It could be used in the treatment of dermatophytosis in animals [147]. The mechanism underlying its antimicrobial and antifungal effect is thought to be via increasing reactive oxygen species (ROS) production, relevant to its action in human polymorphonuclear leukocytes [132]. Bergamot EO also showed strong antimycoplasmal activity against *Mycoplasma hominis*, *M. fermentans*, and *M. pneumoniae* [148].

2.10. Yuzu or Yuja (Citrus junos Sieb. ex Tanaka) Essential Oil

Yuzu EO inhibited the formation of the carcinogen *N*-nitrosodimethylamine (NDMA) in vegetables (by 22–59%) and saliva (by 24–62%) [149]. Yuzu EO is useful in treating bronchial asthma due to its anti-inflammatory activities. It inhibits the production of cytokines and ROS, and reduces eosinophil migration [150]. Yuzu odor was reported to decrease maternal anxiety for a sick child receiving an infusion at a pediatric clinic [151]. A 10 min inhalation of the yuzu odor significantly decreased the heart rate and increased the high frequency power of heart rate variability reflecting parasympathetic nervous system activity, regardless of menstrual phase. Inhalation of the yuzu oil decreased total mood disturbance, tension-anxiety, anger-hostility, and fatigue, which are common premenstrual symptoms [152,153]. Yuzu odor promotes mind and body health in Japan [152]. It is also used to suppress the odor of Niboshi soup stock [154]. Yuzu peel ethanol extract is useful in preventing colitis and colorectal cancer through reducing cyclooxygenase-2 (COX-2) expression [155]. This extract also showed hypocholesterolemic effect both in vitro and in vivo by reducing the weight gain, lipid accumulation, liver fat content, liver weight, total cholesterol, and low-density lipoprotein (LDL) cholesterol [156]. Yuzu extract was reported to exert anti-diabetic activity through increasing glucose uptake in C_2C1_2 myotubes by modulating the AMP-activated protein kinase (AMPK) and peroxisome proliferator-activated receptor gamma (PPAR-γ) signaling pathways. It improved insulin resistance (IR) in mice that were fed a high-fat diet [157]. Moreover, yuzu peel extract showed anti-obesity effects in a zebrafish model via activating hepatic PPAR-α and adipocyte PPAR-γ pathways [158]. The methanol extract of yuzu could be beneficial for individuals at high risk of cardiovascular disease because it inhibits platelet aggregation [159]. Yuzu extract could be useful in treating heart failure as it prevents myocardial infarction (MI)-induced ventricular dysfunction and structural remodeling of myocardium [160].

2.11. Kumquat (Citrus japonica Thunb) Essential Oil

Kumquat EO showed antiproliferative action against human prostate cancer (LNCaP) cells via inducing apoptosis and inhibition of inflammation [161]. The oil also showed a considerable radical-scavenging activity evaluated by a 2,2-diphenyl-1-picrylhydrazyl (DPPH) test [161,162] due to the high *d*-limonene content [12,13]. Kumquat EO exhibits potent antibacterial effects against *Escherichia coli*, *Staphylococcus aureus*, *Bacillus cereus*, *Bacillus subtilis*, *Bacillus laterosporus*, *Salmonella typhimurium*, and *Lactobacillus bulgaricus*, as well as antifungal effects against *Candida albicans* [163].

3. Safety of *Citrus* Oils

Generally speaking, *Citrus* EOs are non-toxic, non-mutagenic, and non-carcinogenic [8]. They are not hazardous in pregnancy and do not alter the maternal reproductive outcome [8,166]. Sweet orange, bitter orange, neroli, petitgrain, lemon, lime (both distilled and expressed), bergamot, and grapefruit oils have GRAS status [8]. However, there is a possible skin sensitization issue if old or oxidized oil is used. The distilled oils are not phototoxic, while the expressed oils carry a low to moderate risk of phototoxicity (Table 4) [167] due to the presence of furanocoumarins [168]. In case of applying expressed EOs to the skin in a dose higher than the maximum dermal use level, it is recommended to avoid exposure to sunlight for at least 12 h [8]. Neroli and yuzu oils are neither irritating nor sensitizing [167]. Expressed sweet orange oil was neither irritating nor sensitizing to 25 volunteers when tested at 8 and 100% [167], whereas it caused sensitivity to 0.13% of total dermatitis patients when tested at 2% [169]. Bitter orange EO was neither irritating nor sensitizing to 25 volunteers when tested at 10% [167], while it caused sensitivity to 1.5% of total dermatitis patients when tested at 2% [169]. Lemon oil was neither irritating nor sensitizing to volunteers when tested at 10% [167], and similar results were observed for distilled lime oil when tested at 15 and 100% [167]. No irritation or sensitization data were found for the expressed lime oil. The high citral content of lime EO causes potential toxic and myelotoxic effects [110]. Grapefruit oil was neither irritating nor sensitizing to volunteers when tested at 10 and 100% [167]. Mandarin EO was neither irritating nor sensitizing to 25 volunteers when tested at 5 and 8% [167]. The expressed bergamot oil was neither irritating nor sensitizing to 25 volunteers when tested at 10% [167]. It caused no irritation when tested at 2% on 1200 dermatitis patients, with only two (0.17%) patients showing sensitivity reaction [170], whereas when tested at 10% in 590 eczema patients, 0.5% of the patients had reactions [171]. Expressed bergamot oil caused severe phototoxic effects in hairless mice and pigs using simulated sunlight, and in humans using natural sunlight and may be photocarcinogenic [167]. When applied to mice, then irradiated with UV light, bergamot oil showed a carcinogenic action due to the presence of bergapten [172]. Chronic skin pigmentation (also known as berloque dermatitis, bergapten dermatitis, or photophytodermatitis) can also develop. Increased exposure to UV light can lead to serious burns [8]. In the absence of UV light, bergamot oil is not carcinogenic and even low concentration sunscreens can completely inhibit bergapten-enhanced phototumorigenesis [172]. No hazards found for the furanocoumarin-free (FCF) or rectified bergamot oil. The rectified oil was not sensitizing when tested at 30% on 25 volunteers [173].

Table 4. Phototoxicity risk, irritation of the undiluted oil, acute dermal LD_{50} in rabbits, acute oral LD_{50} in rats, and maximum dermal use level for different essential oils from *Citrus* species.

Acute Toxicity	Phototoxicity Risk [167]	Irritation of Undiluted Oil [8]	Acute Dermal LD_{50} in Rabbits (g/kg) [167]	Acute Oral LD_{50} in Rats (g/kg) [167]	Maximum Dermal Use Level [8]
Sweet orange EO	Low risk	Moderately irritating to rabbits but not irritating to mice	>5	>5	-
Bitter orange EO	low risk	Moderately irritating to rabbits	>10	>5	1.25%
Neroli EO	Not phototoxic	Not irritating	>5	4.55	-
Petitgrain EO	Not phototoxic	Slightly irritating to rabbits, but not irritating to mice or pigs	<2	>5	-
Lemon EO (distilled)	Not phototoxic	Moderately irritating to rabbits and slightly irritating to mice	>5	>5	20%
Lemon EO (expressed)	Low risk	Not irritating	>5	>5	2%
Lime EO (distilled)	Not phototoxic	Slightly irritating to rabbits	>5	>5	-
Lime EO (expressed)	moderate risk	No data available	>5	>5	0.7%
Grapefruit EO	Low risk	Slightly irritating to rabbits, but not irritating to mice or pigs	>5	>5	4%
Bergamot EO (FCF)	Not phototoxic	Mildly irritating to rabbits	>20	>10	0.4%
Bergamot EO (expressed)	Moderate risk	Moderately irritating to rabbits	-	-	-
Yuzu EO	Not phototoxic	Not irritating	-	-	-
Mandarin	Not phototoxic	Moderately irritating (produces slight edema and erythema) to rabbits, mice, and pigs	>5	>5	30%

To avoid oxidation of *d*-limonene, *Citrus* oils should be stored in a dark air-tight container and placed at 4 °C [8]. The use of old or oxidized oils should be avoided. To avoid any possible adverse skin reactions, it is recommended to dilute *Citrus* oils with a carrier oil before topical use [174]. Also, adding an antioxidant to preparations containing *Citrus* oils is recommended [8].

4. Bioactivity and Safety of Individual Key Components

4.1. d-Limonene

d-Limonene has been shown to possess antioxidant, anti-inflammatory [12], and anticarcinogenic [8] effects. It is not acutely toxic, nephrotoxic, or carcinogenic, but the oxidized *d*-limonene may carry some toxicity. Unoxidized *d*-limonene is listed as an allergen by the EU, and moderately allergenic in Germany [8]. Unoxidized *d*-limonene was allergenic in 0.2% of dermatitis patients when tested at 2–3% [8]. No positive skin reactions were observed when testing the 98% pure *d*-limonene at 20% in dermatitis patients [175]. Undiluted *d*-limonene was moderately irritating to rabbits [167]. *d*-Limonene was irritating at concentrations of 70–80%, a weak irritant at 50%, and a non-irritant at concentrations of 20–30%. The acute dermal LD_{50} of *d*-limonene was >5 g/kg in rabbits, while the acute oral LD_{50} was >5 g/kg in rats [167].

4.2. γ-Terpinene

γ-Terpinene is an antioxidant [176]. It is neither irritating nor sensitizing [167]. It possesses minimal toxicity. Depending on concentration, it may be mutagenic or non-mutagenic [8]. The acute dermal LD_{50} of γ-terpinene was >5 g/kg in rabbits, while the acute oral LD_{50} was 3.65 g/kg in rats [167].

4.3. Linalool

Linalool is a sedative, an antidepressant, and an anticancer, antifungal, and pesticidal EO [177–180]. It is neither toxic nor irritable to skin. It presents an extremely low risk of skin sensitization [8]. No positive skin reactions were observed when testing the 97% pure linalool at 20%, or to oxidized linalool tested at 1% in dermatitis and eczema patients [175,181]. Linalool does not cause photo-irritation or photo-allergy because it does not absorb UV light in the range of 290–400 nm [182]. No fetal toxicity was observed [8]. No carcinogenic, mutagenic, or genotoxic activities were found [8]. The acute dermal LD_{50} was 5.61 g/kg in rabbits, while the acute oral LD_{50} was 2.79 g/kg in rats [183] and 2.2–3.92 g/kg in mice [184]. High doses of linalool cause ataxia and narcosis [185].

4.4. Linalyl Acetate

Linalyl acetate has narcotic effects [177]. It is non-toxic, and is very minimally skin reactive [8]. When tested at 5–20%, no skin reaction was observed [186]. Similar to linalool, linalyl acetate does not cause photo-irritation or photo-allergy because it does not absorb UV light in the range of 290–400 nm [182]. It has no carcinogenic activity [8]. The acute dermal LD_{50} was higher than 5 g/kg in rabbits, while the acute oral LD_{50} was 14.5 g/kg in rats and 13.5 g/kg in mice [184].

4.5. α-Terpineol

α-Terpineol has anticarcinogenic activity [187]. It is a non-irritant at 1–15%, and non-phototoxic [188]. It is not mutagenic or genotoxic. The acute dermal LD_{50} of the mixed isomer terpineol was >3 g/kg in rabbits, while the acute oral LD_{50} was 4.3 g/kg in rats [167].

4.6. Geranyl Acetate

Geranyl acetate has anti-inflammatory [189], antifungal [189], and antimicrobial properties [190]. It is a very weak skin sensitizer [167]. It is neither toxic nor carcinogenic [8]. It was not mutagenic in the Ames test [191], and had no genotoxic effect [192]. The acute oral LD_{50} of geranyl acetate is 6.33 g/kg in rats [183].

4.7. Terpinolene

Terpinolene is an antioxidant [193]. It is neither irritating nor sensitizing at 20% [167]. Limited data suggests minimal toxicity. The acute oral LD_{50} was 4.4 mL/kg in rats and mice [167]. Thresholds of terpinolene skin sensitization are not known.

4.8. β-Pinene

β-Pinene showed antiproliferative and cytotoxic effects [19,194]. It is not mutagenic or genotoxic [8]. It is generally a non-irritant and non-sensitizing. Undiluted β-pinene was moderately irritating to rabbits [8]. β-pinene was irritating at concentrations of 70–80%, a weak irritant at 50%, and a non-irritant at concentrations of 25–30% to dermatitis patients [195]. β-Pinene was classified as a category B substance in Germany, meaning it is considered moderately allergenic [196]. The acute dermal LD_{50} of β-pinene was >5 g/kg in rabbits, subcutaneous LD_{50} was 1.42 g/kg in mice, and the acute oral LD_{50} was >5 g/kg in rats [167].

5. Conclusions

Citrus essential oils are well known for their flavor and fragrance properties, as well as numerous aromatherapeutic and medicinal applications. With the exception of some phototoxicity of expressed oils, they are generally safe to use with negligible toxicity to humans. These readily available essential oils will undoubtedly continue to play important roles in the food and beverage industries, as well as for medicinal, cosmetic, and "green" pest-control uses.

Author Contributions: Writing-Original Draft Preparation, N.S.D.; Writing-Review & Editing, N.S.D. & W.N.S.

Funding: This work was carried out as part of the activities of the Aromatic Plant Research Center. (APRC, https://aromaticplant.org/). The authors are grateful to dōTERRA International (https://www.doterra.com/US/en) for financial support of the APRC.

Conflicts of Interest: The authors declare no conflict of interest. dōTERRA International had no role in the writing or the decision to publish this manuscript.

Abbreviations

5-HT	serotonin
ACC	anterior cingulate cortex
AMPK	AMP-activated protein kinase
BLM	bleomycin
COX-2	cyclooxygenase-2
CTGF	connective tissue growth factor
DA	dopamine
DBP	Dibenzo-[α]-pyrene
DENA	*N*-nitrosodiethylamine
DPPH	2,2-diphenyl-1-picrylhydrazyl
EO	essential oil
EPM	elevated plus-maze
ERK	extracellular signal-regulated protein kinase
FCF	furanocoumarin-free
GABA	gamma-aminobutyric acid
GRAS	generally recognized as safe
GSH	glutathione
HELFs	human embryonic lung fibroblasts
HL-60	human leukemia cells
HPA	hypothalamic-pituitary-adrenal
IC_{50}	median inhibitory concentration

IR	insulin resistance
LD_{50}	median lethal dose
LDL	low-density lipoprotein
LNCaP	human prostate acedocarcinoma cells
MI	myocardial infarction
NDMA	*N*-nitrosodimethylamine
NNK	4-(methylnitrosoamine)-1-(3-pyridyl)-1-butanone
NVP	nausea and vomiting of pregnancy
phospho-Akt	phosphorylated protein kinase B
phospho-GSK-3β	phosphorylated glycogen synthase kinase 3 beta
PMS	premenstrual syndrome
PPAR-γ	peroxisome proliferator-activated receptor gamma
ppm	parts per million
ROS	reactive oxygen species
RyR	ryanodine receptor
SH-SY5Y	human neuroblasoma cells
WAT	white adipose tissue

References

1. Moore, G.A. Oranges and lemons: Clues to the taxonomy of *Citrus* from molecular markers. *Trends Genet.* **2001**, *17*, 536–540. [CrossRef]
2. Mabberley, D.J. *Citrus* (Rutaceae): A review of recent advances in etymology, systematics and medical applications. *Blumea* **2004**, *49*, 481–498. [CrossRef]
3. Anwar, F.; Naseer, R.; Bhanger, M.I.; Ashraf, S.; Talpur, F.N.; Aladedunye, F.A. Physico-chemical characteristics of citrus seeds and seed oils from Pakistan. *J. Am. Oil Chem. Soc.* **2008**, *85*, 321–330. [CrossRef]
4. Sharma, K.; Mahato, N.; Cho, M.H.; Lee, Y.R. Converting citrus wastes into value-added products: Economic and environmently friendly approaches. *Nutrition* **2017**, *34*, 29–46. [CrossRef] [PubMed]
5. Martín, M.A.; Siles, J.A.; Chica, A.F.; Martín, A. Biomethanization of orange peel waste. *Bioresour. Technol.* **2010**, *101*, 8993–8999. [CrossRef] [PubMed]
6. Rezzadori, K.; Benedetti, S.; Amante, E.R. Proposals for the residues recovery: Orange waste as raw material for new products. *Food Bioprod. Process.* **2012**, *90*, 606–614. [CrossRef]
7. Ferhat, M.A.; Meklati, B.Y.; Smadja, J.; Chemat, F. An improved microwave Clevenger apparatus for distillation of essential oils from orange peel. *J. Chromatogr. A* **2006**, *1112*, 121–126. [CrossRef] [PubMed]
8. Tisserand, R.; Young, R. *Essential Oil Safety*, 2nd ed.; Elsevier: New York, NY, USA, 2014.
9. Mitropoulou, G.; Fitsiou, E.; Spyridopoulou, K.; Tiptiri-Kourpeti, A.; Bardouki, H.; Vamvakias, M.; Panas, P.; Chlichlia, K.; Pappa, A.; Kourkoutas, Y. *Citrus medica* essential oil exhibits significant antimicrobial and antiproliferative activity. *LWT Food Sci. Technol.* **2017**, *84*, 344–352. [CrossRef]
10. Viuda-Martos, M.; Ruiz-Navajas, Y.; Fernández-López, J.; Perez-Álvarez, J. Antifungal activity of lemon (*Citrus limon* L.), mandarin (*Citrus reticulata* L.), grapefruit (*Citrus paradisi* L.) and orange (*Citrus sinensis* L.) essential oils. *Food Control* **2008**, *19*, 1130–1138. [CrossRef]
11. Ali, N.; Chhetri, B.; Dosoky, N.; Shari, K.; Al-Fahad, A.; Wessjohann, L.; Setzer, W. Antimicrobial, antioxidant, and cytotoxic activities of *Ocimum forskolei* and *Teucrium yemense* (Lamiaceae) essential oils. *Medicines* **2017**, *4*, 17. [CrossRef] [PubMed]
12. Yu, L.; Yan, J.; Sun, Z. D-limonene exhibits anti-inflammatory and antioxidant properties in an ulcerative colitis rat model via regulation of iNOS, COX-2, PGE2 and ERK signaling pathways. *Mol. Med. Rep.* **2017**, *15*, 2339–2346. [CrossRef] [PubMed]
13. Roberto, D.; Micucci, P.; Sebastian, T.; Graciela, F.; Anesini, C. Antioxidant activity of limonene on normal murine lymphocytes: Relation to H_2O_2 modulation and cell proliferation. *Basic Clin. Pharmacol. Toxicol.* **2010**, *106*, 38–44. [CrossRef] [PubMed]
14. Kostova, I.; Bhatia, S.; Grigorov, P.; Balkansky, S.; Parmar, V.S.; Prasad, A.K.; Saso, L. Coumarins as antioxidants. *Curr. Med. Chem.* **2011**, *18*, 3929–3951. [CrossRef] [PubMed]

15. Caccioni, D.R.; Guizzardi, M.; Biondi, D.M.; Renda, A.; Ruberto, G. Relationship between volatile components of citrus fruit essential oils and antimicrobial action on *Penicillium digitatum* and *Penicillium italicum*. *Int. J. Food Microbiol.* **1998**, *43*, 73–79. [CrossRef]
16. De Pasquale, F.; Siragusa, M.; Abbate, L.; Tusa, N.; De Pasquale, C.; Alonzo, G. Characterization of five sour orange clones through molecular markers and leaf essential oils analysis. *Sci. Hortic.* **2006**, *109*, 54–59. [CrossRef]
17. Dosoky, N.S.; Moriarity, D.M.; Setzer, W.N. Phytochemical and biological investigations of *Conradina canescens*. *Nat. Prod. Commun.* **2016**, *11*, 25–28. [PubMed]
18. Dosoky, N.S.; Stewart, C.D.; Setzer, W.N. Identification of essential oil components from *Conradina canescens*. *Am. J. Essent. Oils Nat. Prod.* **2014**, *2*, 24–28.
19. da Silva, J.K.; da Trindade, R.; Moreira, E.C.; Maia, J.G.S.; Dosoky, N.S.; Miller, R.S.; Cseke, L.J.; Setzer, W.N. Chemical diversity, biological activity, and genetic aspects of three *Ocotea* species from the Amazon. *Int. J. Mol. Sci.* **2017**, *18*, 1081. [CrossRef] [PubMed]
20. Ammar, A.H.; Bouajila, J.; Lebrihi, A.; Mathieu, F.; Romdhane, M.; Zagrouba, F. Chemical composition and in vitro antimicrobial and antioxidant activities of *Citrus aurantium* L. flowers essential oil (Neroli oil). *Pak. J. Biol. Sci.* **2012**, *15*, 1034–1040. [CrossRef] [PubMed]
21. Zhu, L.F.; Li, Y.H.; Li, B.L.; Lu, B.Y.; Xia, N.H. *Aromatic Plants and Their Essential Constitutes*; South China Inst. Bot., Chinese Academy of Sciences, Peace Book Co.: Hong Kong, China, 1993.
22. Kubeczka, K.-H. *Essential Oils Analysis by Capillary Gas Chromatography and Carbon-13 NMR Spectroscopy*; Wiley: Chichester, UK, 2002.
23. Pino, J.A.; Rosado, A. Comparative investigation of the distilled lime oils (*Citrus aurantifolia* Swingle and *Citrus latifolia* Tanaka) from Cuba. *J. Essent. Oil Res.* **2001**, *13*, 179–180. [CrossRef]
24. Dugo, P.; Mondello, L.; Proteggente, A.R.; Cavazza, A.; Dugo, G. Oxygen heterocyclic compounds of bergamot essential oils. *Riv. Ital. EPPOS* **1999**, *27*, 31–41.
25. Verzera, A.; Trozzi, A.; Stagno d'Alcontres, I.; Mondello, L.; Dugo, G.; Sebastiani, E. The composition of the volatile fraction of calabrian bergamot essential oil. *Riv. Ital. EPPOS* **1998**, *25*, 17–38.
26. Dugo, P.; Mondello, L.; Sebastiani, E.; Ottanà, R.; Errante, G.; Dugo, G. Identification of minor oxygen heterocyclic compounds of citrus essential oils by liquid chromatography-atmospheric pressure chemical ionisation mass spectrometry. *J. Liq. Chromatogr. Relat. Technol.* **1999**, *22*, 2991–3005. [CrossRef]
27. Sawamura, M.; Hasegawa, K.; Kashiwagi, T.; Nguyen Thi, L.-P.; Wada, M.; Kumagai, C. Determination of bergapten in Japanese citrus essential oils. *Jpn. J. Aromather.* **2009**, *9*, 30–37.
28. Hata, T.; Sakaguchi, I.; Mori, M.; Ikeda, N.; Kato, Y.; Minamino, M.; Watabe, K. Induction of apoptosis by *Citrus paradisi* essential oil in human leukemic (HL-60) cells. *In Vivo* **2003**, *17*, 553–559. [PubMed]
29. Chidambara Murthy, K.N.; Jayaprakasha, G.K.; Patil, B.S. D-limonene rich volatile oil from blood oranges inhibits angiogenesis, metastasis and cell death in human colon cancer cells. *Life Sci.* **2012**, *91*, 429–439. [CrossRef] [PubMed]
30. Igarashi, M.; Ikei, H.; Song, C.; Miyazaki, Y. Effects of olfactory stimulation with rose and orange oil on prefrontal cortex activity. *Complement. Ther. Med.* **2014**, *22*, 1027–1031. [CrossRef] [PubMed]
31. Goes, T.C.; Antunes, F.D.; Alves, P.B.; Teixeira-Silva, F. Effect of sweet orange aroma on experimental anxiety in humans. *J. Altern. Complement. Med.* **2012**, *18*, 798–804. [CrossRef] [PubMed]
32. Faturi, C.B.; Leite, J.R.; Alves, P.B.; Canton, A.C.; Teixeira-Silva, F. Anxiolytic-like effect of sweet orange aroma in Wistar rats. *Prog. Neuro-Psychopharmacol. Biol. Psychiatry* **2010**, *34*, 605–609. [CrossRef] [PubMed]
33. Lehrner, J.; Eckersberger, C.; Walla, P.; Potsch, G.; Deecke, L. Ambient odor of orange in a dental office reduces anxiety and improves mood in female patients. *Physiol. Behav.* **2000**, *71*, 83–86. [CrossRef]
34. Yip, Y.B.; Tam, A.C.Y. An experimental study on the effectiveness of massage with aromatic ginger and orange essential oil for moderate-to-severe knee pain among the elderly in Hong Kong. *Complement. Ther. Med.* **2008**, *16*, 131–138. [CrossRef] [PubMed]
35. Bodake, H.B.; Panicker, K.N.; Kailaje, V.; Rao, K.V. Chemopreventive effect of orange oil on the development of hepatic preneoplastic lesions induced by *N*-nitrosodiethylamine in rats: An ultrastructural study. *Indian J. Exp. Biol.* **2002**, *40*, 245–251. [PubMed]
36. Homburger, F.; Treger, A.; Boger, E. Inhibition of murine subcutaneous and intravenous benzo(rst)pentaphene carcinogenesis by sweet orange oils and d-limonene. *Oncology* **1971**, *25*, 1–10. [CrossRef] [PubMed]

37. Asjad, H.; Akhtar, M.; Bashir, S.; Gulzar, B.; Khalid, R.; Asad, M. Phenol, flavonoid contents and antioxidant activity of six common citrus plants in Pakistan. *J. Pharm. Cosmet. Sci.* **2013**, *1*, 1–5.
38. Rimini, S.; Petracci, M.; Smith, D.P. The use of thyme and orange essential oils blend to improve quality traits of marinated chicken meat. *Poult. Sci.* **2014**, *93*, 2096–2102. [CrossRef] [PubMed]
39. Matiz, G.; Osorio, M.R.; Camacho, F.; Atencia, M.; Herazo, J. Effectiveness of antimicrobial formulations for acne based on orange (*Citrus sinensis*) and sweet basil (*Ocimum basilicum* L.) essential oils. *Biomedica* **2012**, *32*, 125–133. [CrossRef] [PubMed]
40. Franco-Vega, A.; Reyes-Jurado, F.; Cardoso-Ugarte, G.A.; Sosa-Morales, M.E.; Palou, E.; Lopez-Malo, A. *Sweet Orange (Citrus Sinensis) Oils*; Elsevier Inc.: New York, NY, USA, 2015; ISBN 9780124166448.
41. Settani, L.; Palazzolo, E.; Guarrasi, V.; Aleo, A.; Mammina, C.; Moschetti, G.; Germaná, M. Inhibition of foodborne pathogen bacteria by essential oils extracted from citrus fruits cultivated in Sicily. *Food Control* **2012**, *26*, 326–330. [CrossRef]
42. Lin, C.M.; Sheu, S.R.; Hsu, S.C.; Tsai, Y.H. Determination of bactericidal efficacy of essential oil extracted from orange peel on the food contact surfaces. *Food Control* **2010**, *21*, 1710–1715. [CrossRef]
43. Bourgou, S.; Zohra, F.; Ourghemmi, I.; Saidani, M. Changes of peel essential oil composition of four Tunisian citrus during fruit maturation. *Sci. World J.* **2012**, *2012*, 528593. [CrossRef] [PubMed]
44. Singh, P.; Shukla, R.; Prakash, B.; Kumar, A.; Singh, S.; Mishra, P.K.; Dubey, N.K. Chemical profile, antifungal, antiaflatoxigenic and antioxidant activity of *Citrus maxima* Burm. and *Citrus sinensis* (L.) Osbeck essential oils and their cyclic monoterpene, DL-limonene. *Food Chem. Toxicol.* **2010**, *48*, 1734–1740. [CrossRef] [PubMed]
45. Sharma, N.; Tripathi, A. Effects of *Citrus sinensis* (L.) Osbeck epicarp essential oil on growth and morphogenesis of *Aspergillus niger* (L.) Van Tieghem. *Microbiol. Res.* **2008**, *163*, 337–344. [CrossRef] [PubMed]
46. El-Akhal, F.; Lalamia, A.E.O.; Guemmouh, R. Larvicidal activity of essential oils of *Citrus sinensis* and *Citrus aurantium* (Rutaceae) cultivated in Morocco against the malaria vector *Anopheles labranchiae* (Diptera: Culicidae). *Asian Pac. J. Trop. Dis.* **2015**, *5*, 458–462. [CrossRef]
47. Galvão, J.G.; Silva, V.F.; Ferreira, S.G.; França, F.R.M.; Santos, D.A.; Freitas, L.S.; Alves, P.B.; Araújo, A.A.S.; Cavalcanti, S.C.H.; Nunes, R.S. β-Cyclodextrin inclusion complexes containing *Citrus sinensis* (L.) Osbeck essential oil: An alternative to control *Aedes aegypti* larvae. *Thermochim. Acta* **2015**, *608*, 14–19. [CrossRef]
48. Rossi, Y.E.; Palacios, S.M. Fumigant toxicity of *Citrus sinensis* essential oil on *Musca domestica* L. adults in the absence and presence of a P450 inhibitor. *Acta Trop.* **2013**, *127*, 33–37. [CrossRef] [PubMed]
49. Ezeonu, F.C.; Chidume, G.I.; Udedi, S.C. Insecticidal properties of volatile extracts of orange peels. *Bioresour. Technol.* **2001**, *76*, 273–274. [CrossRef]
50. Raina, A.; Bland, J.; Doolittle, M.; Lax, A.; Folkins, M.; Raina, A.; Bland, J.; Doolittle, M.; Lax, A.; Boopathy, R.A.J.; et al. Effect of orange oil extract on the Formosan subterranean termite (Isoptera: Rhinotermitidae). *J. Econ. Entomol.* **2007**, *100*, 880–885. [CrossRef] [PubMed]
51. Gaínza, Y.A.; Domingues, L.F.; Perez, O.P.; Rabelo, M.D.; López, E.R.; de Souza Chagas, A.C. Anthelmintic activity in vitro of *Citrus sinensis* and *Melaleuca quinquenervia* essential oil from Cuba on *Haemonchus contortus*. *Ind. Crop. Prod.* **2015**, *76*, 647–652. [CrossRef]
52. Acar, U.; Kesbiç, O.S.; Yilmaz, S.; Gültepe, N.; Türker, A. Evaluation of the effects of essential oil extracted from sweet orange peel (*Citrus sinensis*) on growth rate of tilapia (*Oreochromis mossambicus*) and possible disease resistance against *Streptococcus iniae*. *Aquaculture* **2015**, *437*, 282–286. [CrossRef]
53. Anwar, S.; Ahmed, N.; Speciale, A.; Cimino, F.; Saija, A. *Bitter Orange (Citrus Aurantium L.) Oils*; Elsevier Inc.: New York, NY, USA, 2015; ISBN 9780124166448.
54. Carvalho-Freitas, M.I.R.; Costa, M. Anxiolytic and sedative effects of extracts and essential oil from *Citrus aurantium* L. *Biol. Pharm. Bull.* **2002**, *25*, 1629–1633. [CrossRef] [PubMed]
55. De Moraes Pultrini, A.; Almeida Galindo, L.; Costa, M. Effects of the essential oil from *Citrus aurantium* L. in experimental anxiety models in mice. *Life Sci.* **2006**, *78*, 1720–1725. [CrossRef] [PubMed]
56. Pimenta, F.C.F.; Alves, M.F.; Pimenta, M.B.F.; Melo, S.A.L.; de Almeida, A.A.F.; Leite, J.R.; Pordeus, L.C.D.M.; Diniz, M.D.F.F.M.; de Almeida, R.N. Anxiolytic effect of *Citrus aurantium* L. on patients with chronic myeloid leukemia. *Phyther. Res.* **2016**, *30*, 613–617. [CrossRef] [PubMed]
57. Costa, C.A.R.A.; Cury, T.C.; Cassettari, B.O.; Takahira, R.K.; Florio, J.C.; Costa, M. *Citrus aurantium* L. essential oil exhibits anxiolytic-like activity mediated by 5-HT1A-receptors and reduces cholesterol after repeated oral treatment. *BMC Complement. Altern. Med.* **2013**, *13*, 42. [CrossRef] [PubMed]

58. Yi, L.-T.; Xu, H.-L.; Feng, J.; Zhan, X.; Zhou, L.-P.; Cui, C.-C. Involvement of monoaminergic systems in the antidepressant like effect of nobiletin. *Physiol. Behav.* **2011**, *102*, 1–6. [CrossRef] [PubMed]
59. Namazi, M.; Ali Akbari, S.A.; Mojab, F.; Talebi, A.; Majd, H.A.; Jannesari, S. Effects of *Citrus aurantium* (bitter orange) on the severity of first-stage labor pain. *Iran. J. Pharm. Res.* **2014**, *13*, 1011–1018. [PubMed]
60. Moraes, T.M.; Kushima, H.; Moleiro, F.C.; Santos, R.C.; Machado Rocha, L.R.; Marques, M.O.; Vilegas, W.; Hiruma-Lima, C.A. Effects of limonene and essential oil from *Citrus aurantium* on gastric mucosa: Role of prostaglandins and gastric mucus secretion. *Chem. Biol. Interact.* **2009**, *180*, 499–505. [CrossRef] [PubMed]
61. Lv, Y.X.; Zhao, S.P.; Zhang, J.Y.; Zhang, H.; Xie, Z.H.; Cai, G.M.; Jiang, W.H. Effect of orange peel essential oil on oxidative stress in AOM animals. *Int. J. Biol. Macromol.* **2012**, *50*, 1144–1150. [CrossRef] [PubMed]
62. Ullah, N.; Khan, M.A.; Khan, T.; Ahmad, W. Nephroprotective potentials of *Citrus aurantium*: A prospective pharmacological study on experimental models. *Pak. J. Pharm. Sci.* **2014**, *27*, 505–510. [PubMed]
63. Friedman, M.; Henika, P.R.; Levin, C.E.; Mandrell, R.E. Antibacterial activities of plant essential oils and their components against *Escherichia coli* O157:H7 and *Salmonella enterica* in apple juice. *J. Agric. Food Chem.* **2004**, *52*, 6042–6048. [CrossRef] [PubMed]
64. Iturriaga, L.; Olabarrieta, I.; de Marañón, I.M. Antimicrobial assays of natural extracts and their inhibitory effect against Listeria innocua and fish spoilage bacteria, after incorporation into biopolymer edible films. *Int. J. Food Microbiol.* **2012**, *158*, 58–64. [CrossRef] [PubMed]
65. Oliveira, S.A.C.; Zambrana, J.R.M.; di Iorio, F.B.R.; Pereira, C.A.; Jorge, A.O.C. The antimicrobial effects of *Citrus limonum* and *Citrus aurantium* essential oils on multi-species biofilms. *Braz. Oral Res.* **2014**, *28*, 22–27. [CrossRef] [PubMed]
66. Ramadan, W.; Mourad, B.; Ibrahim, S.; Sonbol, F. Oil of bitter orange: New topical antifungal agent. *Int. J. Dermatol.* **1996**, *35*, 448–449. [CrossRef] [PubMed]
67. Zarrad, K.; Hamouda, A.B.; Chaieb, I.; Laarif, A.; Jemâa, J.M. Ben Chemical composition, fumigant and anti-acetylcholinesterase activity of the Tunisian *Citrus aurantium* L. essential oils. *Ind. Crop. Prod.* **2015**, *76*, 121–127. [CrossRef]
68. Battaglia, S. *The Complete Guide to Aromatherapy Brisbane*; The International Centre of Holistic Aromatherapy: Brisbane, Australia, 2003.
69. Akhlaghi, M.; Shabanian, G.; Rafieian-Kopaei, M.; Parvin, N.; Saadat, M.; Akhlaghi, M. *Citrus aurantium* blossom and preoperative anxiety. *Rev. Bras. Anestesiol.* **2011**, *61*, 702–712. [CrossRef]
70. Farshbaf-Khalili, A.; Kamalifard, M.; Namadian, M. Comparison of the effect of lavender and bitter orange on anxiety in postmenopausal women: A triple-blind, randomized, controlled clinical trial. *Complement. Ther. Clin. Pract.* **2018**, *31*, 132–138. [CrossRef] [PubMed]
71. Azanchi, T.; Shafaroodi, H.; Asgarpanah, J. Anticonvulsant activity of *Citrus aurantium* blossom essential oil (neroli): Involvment of the GABAergic system. *Nat. Prod. Commun.* **2014**, *9*, 1615–1618. [PubMed]
72. Rahnama, S.; Rabiei, Z.; Alibabaei, Z.; Mokhtari, S.; Rafieian-Kopaei, M.; Deris, F. Antiamnesic activity of *Citrus aurantium* flowers extract against scopolamine-induced memory impairments in rats. *Neurol. Sci.* **2014**, *36*, 553–560. [CrossRef] [PubMed]
73. Khodabakhsh, P.; Shafaroodi, H.; Asgarpanah, J. Analgesic and anti-inflammatory activities of *Citrus aurantium* L. blossoms essential oil (neroli): Involvement of the nitric oxide/cyclic-guanosine monophosphate pathway. *J. Nat. Med.* **2015**, *69*, 324–331. [CrossRef] [PubMed]
74. Choi, S.Y.; Kang, P.; Lee, H.S.; Seol, G.H. Effects of inhalation of essential oil of *Citrus aurantium* L. var. amara on menopausal symptoms, stress, and estrogen in postmenopausal women: A randomized controlled trial. *Evid.-Based Complement. Altern. Med.* **2014**, *2014*. [CrossRef] [PubMed]
75. Heydari, N.; Abootalebi, M.; Jamalimoghadam, N.; Kasraeian, M.; Emamghoreishi, M.; Akbarzade, M. Investigation of the effect of aromatherapy with *Citrus aurantium* blossom essential oil on premenstrual syndrome in university students: A clinical trial study. *Complement. Ther. Clin. Pract.* **2018**, *32*, 1–5. [CrossRef]
76. Kang, P.; Ryu, K.H.; Lee, J.M.; Kim, H.K.; Seol, G.H. Endothelium- and smooth muscle-dependent vasodilator effects of *Citrus aurantium* L. var. *amara*: Focus on Ca^{2+} modulation. *Biomed. Pharmacother.* **2016**, *82*, 467–471. [CrossRef] [PubMed]
77. Kim, I.H.; Kim, C.; Seong, K.; Hur, M.H.; Lim, H.M.; Lee, M.S. Essential oil inhalation on blood pressure and salivary cortisol levels in prehypertensive and hypertensive subjects. *Evid.-Based Complement. Altern. Med.* **2012**, *2012*, 984203. [CrossRef] [PubMed]

78. Ao, Y.; Satoh, K.; Shibano, K.; Kawahito, Y.; Shioda, S. Singlet oxygen scavenging activity and cytotoxicity of essential oils from Rutaceae. *J. Clin. Biochem. Nutr.* **2008**, *43*, 6–12. [CrossRef] [PubMed]
79. Ben Hsouna, A.; Hamdi, N.; Ben Halima, N.; Abdelkafi, S. Characterization of essential oil from *Citrus aurantium* L. flowers: Antimicrobial and antioxidant activities. *J. Oleo Sci.* **2013**, *62*, 763–772. [CrossRef] [PubMed]
80. Sarrou, E.; Chatzopoulou, P.; Dimassi-Theriou, K.; Therios, I. Volatile constituents and antioxidant activity of peel, flowers and leaf oils of *Citrus aurantium* L. growing in Greece. *Molecules* **2013**, *18*, 10639–10647. [CrossRef] [PubMed]
81. Ellouze, I.; Abderrabba, M.; Sabaou, N.; Mathieu, F.; Lebrihi, A.; Bouajila, J. Season's variation impact on *Citrus aurantium* leaves essential oil: Chemical composition and biological activities. *J. Food Sci.* **2012**, *77*, 1–2. [CrossRef] [PubMed]
82. Zhou, X.M.; Zhao, Y.; He, C.C.; Li, J.X. Preventive effects of *Citrus reticulata* essential oil on bleomycin-induced pulmonary fibrosis in rats and the mechanism. *J. Chin. Integr. Med.* **2012**, *10*, 200–209. [CrossRef]
83. Yi, F.; Jin, R.; Sun, J.; Ma, B.; Bao, X. Evaluation of mechanical-pressed essential oil from Nanfeng mandarin (*Citrus reticulata* Blanco cv. Kinokuni) as a food preservative based on antimicrobial and antioxidant activities. *LWT Food Sci. Technol.* **2018**, *95*, 346–353. [CrossRef]
84. Tao, N.; Jia, L.; Zhou, H. Anti-fungal activity of *Citrus reticulata* Blanco essential oil against *Penicillium italicum* and *Penicillium digitatum*. *Food Chem.* **2014**, *153*, 265–271. [CrossRef] [PubMed]
85. Matan, N.; Matan, N. Antifungal activities of anise oil, lime oil, and tangerine oil against molds on rubberwood (*Hevea brasiliensis*). *Int. Biodeterior. Biodegrad.* **2008**, *62*, 75–78. [CrossRef]
86. Wu, T.; Cheng, D.; He, M.; Pan, S.; Yao, X.; Xu, X. Antifungal action and inhibitory mechanism of polymethoxylated flavones from *Citrus reticulata* Blanco peel against *Aspergillus niger*. *Food Control* **2014**, *35*, 354–359. [CrossRef]
87. Chutia, M.; Deka Bhuyan, P.; Pathak, M.G.; Sarma, T.C.; Boruah, P. Antifungal activity and chemical composition of *Citrus reticulata* Blanco essential oil against phytopathogens from North East India. *LWT Food Sci. Technol.* **2009**, *42*, 777–780. [CrossRef]
88. Komiya, M.; Takeuchi, T.; Harada, E. Lemon oil vapor causes an anti-stress effect via modulating the 5-HT and DA activities in mice. *Behav. Brain Res.* **2006**, *172*, 240–249. [CrossRef] [PubMed]
89. Ogeturk, M.; Kose, E.; Sarsilmaz, M.; Akpinar, B.; Kus, I.; Meydan, S. Effects of lemon essential oil aroma on the learning behaviors of rats. *Neurosciences* **2010**, *15*, 292–293. [PubMed]
90. Zu, Y.; Yu, H.; Liang, L.; Fu, Y.; Efferth, T.; Liu, X.; Wu, N. Activities of ten essential oils towards *Propionibacterium acnes* and PC-3, A-549 and MCF-7 cancer cells. *Molecules* **2010**, *15*, 3200–3210. [CrossRef] [PubMed]
91. Wattenberg, L.; Coccia, J.B. Inhibition of 4-(methylnitrosamino)-1-(3-pyridyl)-1-butanone carcinogenesis in mice by D-limonene and citrus fruit oils. *Carcinogenesis* **1991**, *12*, 115–117. [CrossRef] [PubMed]
92. Niijima, A.; Nagai, K. Effect of Olfactory stimulation with flavor of grapefruit oil and lemon oil on the activity of sympathetic branch in the white adipose tissue of the epididymis. *Exp. Biol. Med.* **2003**, *228*, 1190–1192. [CrossRef]
93. Campêlo, L.M.; Moura Gonçalves, F.C.; Feitosa, C.M.; de Freitas, R.M. Antioxidant activity of *Citrus limon* essential oil in mouse hippocampus. *Pharm. Biol.* **2011**, *49*, 709–715. [CrossRef] [PubMed]
94. Choi, H.-S.; Song, H.S.; Ukeda, H.; Sawamura, M. Radical-scavenging activities of citrus essential oils and their components: Detection using 1,1-diphenyl-2-picrylhydrazyl. *J. Agric. Food Chem.* **2000**, *48*, 4156–4161. [CrossRef] [PubMed]
95. De Freitas, R.M.; Campêlo, L.M.L.; de Almeida, A.A.C.; de Freitas, R.L.M.; Cerqueira, G.S.; de Sousa, G.F.; Saldanha, G.B.; Feitosa, C.M. Antioxidant and antinociceptive effects of *Citrus limon* essential oil in mice. *J. Biomed. Biotechnol.* **2011**. [CrossRef]
96. Ceccarelli, I.; Lariviere, W.R.; Fiorenzani, P.; Sacerdote, P.; Aloisi, A.M. Effects of long-term exposure of lemon essential oil odor on behavioral, hormonal and neuronal parameters in male and female rats. *Brain Res.* **2004**, *1001*, 78–86. [CrossRef] [PubMed]
97. Ceccarelli, I.; Masi, F.; Fiorenzani, P.; Aloisi, A.M. Sex differences in the citrus lemon essential oil-induced increase of hippocampal acetylcholine release in rats exposed to a persistent painful stimulation. *Neurosci. Lett.* **2002**, *330*, 25–28. [CrossRef]

98. Ikeda, H.; Takasu, S.; Murase, K. Contribution of anterior cingulate cortex and descending pain inhibitory system to analgesic effect of lemon odor in mice. *Mol. Pain* **2014**, *10*, 14. [CrossRef] [PubMed]
99. Yavari Kia, P.; Safajou, F.; Shahnazi, M.; Nazemiyeh, H. The effect of lemon inhalation aromatherapy on nausea and vomiting of pregnancy: A double-blinded, randomized, controlled clinical trial. *Iran. Red Crescent Med. J.* **2014**, *16*. [CrossRef] [PubMed]
100. Akpinar, B. The effects of olfactory stimuli on scholastic performance. *Ir. J. Educ.* **2005**, *36*, 86–90.
101. Valgimigli, L.; Gabbanini, S.; Berlini, E.; Lucchi, E.; Beltramini, C.; Bertarelli, Y.L. Lemon (*Citrus limon*, Burm.f.) essential oil enhances the trans-epidermal release of lipid-(A, E) and water-(B_6, C) soluble vitamins from topical emulsions in reconstructed human epidermis. *Int. J. Cosmet. Sci.* **2012**, *34*, 347–356. [CrossRef] [PubMed]
102. Viuda-Martos, M.; Ruiz-Navajas, Y.; Fernández-López, J.; Perez-Álvarez, J. Antibacterial activity of lemon (*Citrus limon* L.), mandarin (*Citrus reticulata* L.), grapefruit (*Citrus paradisi* L.) and orange (*Citrus sinensis* L.) essential oils. *J. Food Saf.* **2008**, *28*, 567–576. [CrossRef]
103. Viuda-Martos, M.; Mohamady, M.A.; Fernández-López, J.; Abd ElRazik, K.A.; Omer, E.A.; Pérez-Alvarez, J.A.; Sendra, E. In vitro antioxidant and antibacterial activities of essentials oils obtained from Egyptian aromatic plants. *Food Control* **2011**, *22*, 1715–1722. [CrossRef]
104. Oshaghi, M.A.; Ghalandari, R.; Vatandoost, H.; Shayeghi, M.; Abolhassani, M.; Hashemzadeh, M. Repellent effect of extracts and essential oils of *Citrus limon* (Rutaceae) and *Melissa officinalis* (Labiatae) against main malaria vector, *Anopheles stephensi* (Diptera: Culicidae). *Iran. J. Public Health* **2003**, *32*, 47–52.
105. Aboelhadid, S.M.; Mahrous, L.N.; Hashem, S.A.; Abdel-Kafy, E.-S.M.; Miller, R.J. In vitro and in vivo effect of *Citrus limon* essential oil against sarcoptic mange in rabbits. *Parasitol. Res.* **2016**, *115*, 3013–3020. [CrossRef] [PubMed]
106. Asnaashari, S.; Delazar, A.; Habibi, B.; VasÒ, R.; Nahar, L.; Hamedeyazdan, S.; Sarker, S.D. Essential oil from *Citrus aurantifolia* prevents ketotifen-induced weight-gain in mice. *Phyther. Res.* **2010**, *24*, 1893–1897. [CrossRef] [PubMed]
107. Shafreen, R.B.; Lubinska, M.; Różańska, A.; Dymerski, T.; Namieśnik, J.; Katrich, E.; Gorinstein, S. Human serum interactions with phenolic and aroma substances of Kaffir (*Citrus hystrix*) and Key lime (*Citrus aurantifolia*) juices. *J. Lumin.* **2018**. [CrossRef]
108. Spadaro, F.; Costa, R.; Circosta, C.; Occhiuto, F. Volatile composition and biological activity of key lime *Citrus aurantifolia* essential oil. *Nat. Prod. Commun.* **2012**, *7*, 1523–1526. [PubMed]
109. Tundis, R.; Loizzo, M.R.; Bonesi, M.; Menichini, F.; Mastellone, V.; Colica, C.; Menichini, F. Comparative study on the antioxidant capacity and cholinesterase inhibitory activity of *Citrus aurantifolia* Swingle, *C. aurantium* L., and *C. bergamia* Risso and Poit. peel essential oils. *J. Food Sci.* **2012**, *77*, H40–H46. [CrossRef] [PubMed]
110. Amorim, J.L.; Simas, D.L.R.; Pinheiro, M.M.G.; Moreno, D.S.A.; Alviano, C.S.; Da Silva, A.J.R.; Fernandes, P.D. Anti-inflammatory properties and chemical characterization of the essential oils of four *Citrus* species. *PLoS ONE* **2016**, *11*, e0153643. [CrossRef] [PubMed]
111. Cruz-Valenzuela, M.R.; Tapia-Rodriguez, M.R.; Vazquez-Armenta, F.J.; Silva-Espinoza, B.A.; Ayala-Zavala, J.F. *Lime (Citrus aurantifolia) Oils*; Elsevier Inc.: New York, NY, USA, 2015; ISBN 9780124166448.
112. Ruberto, G. Analysis of Volatile Components of Citrus Fruit Essential Oils. In *Analysis of Taste and Aroma*; Springer: Berlin/Heidelberg, Germany, 2002.
113. Fagodia, S.K.; Singh, H.P.; Batish, D.R.; Kohli, R.K. Phytotoxicity and cytotoxicity of *Citrus aurantiifolia* essential oil and its major constituents: Limonene and citral. *Ind. Crop. Prod.* **2017**, *108*, 708–715. [CrossRef]
114. Fouad, H.A.; da Camara, C.A.G. Chemical composition and bioactivity of peel oils from *Citrus aurantiifolia* and *Citrus reticulata* and enantiomers of their major constituent against *Sitophilus zeamais* (Coleoptera: Curculionidae). *J. Stored Prod. Res.* **2017**, *73*, 30–36. [CrossRef]
115. Nagai, K.; Niijima, A.; Horii, Y.; Shen, J.; Tanida, M. Olfactory stimulatory with grapefruit and lavender oils change autonomic nerve activity and physiological function. *Auton. Neurosci. Basic Clin.* **2014**, *185*, 29–35. [CrossRef] [PubMed]
116. Stiles, K.G. *The Essential Oils Complete Reference Guide: Over 250 Recipes for Natural Wholesome Aromatherapy*; Page Street Publishing: Salem, MA, USA, 2017; ISBN 1624143067.
117. Lim, T.K. *Edible Medicinal and Non-Medicinal Plants*; Springer Science & Business Media: New York, NY, USA, 2012; Volume 4, ISBN 978-94-007-4052-5.

118. Okunowo, W.O.; Oyedeji, O.; Afolabi, L.O.; Matanmi, E. Essential oil of grape fruit (*Citrus paradisi*) peels and its antimicrobial activities. *Am. J. Plant Sci.* **2013**, *4*, 1–9. [CrossRef]
119. Churata-Oroya, D.E.; Ramos-Perfecto, D.; Moromi-Nakata, H.; Martínez-Cadillo, E.; Castro-Luna, A.; Garcia-de-la-Guarda, R. Antifungal effect of *Citrus paradisi* "grapefruit"on strains of *Candida albicans* isolated from patients with denture stomatitis. *Rev. Estomatol. Hered.* **2016**, *26*, 78–84. [CrossRef]
120. Tirillini, B. Grapefruit: The last decade acquisitions. *Fitoterapia* **2000**, *71*. [CrossRef]
121. Ruiz, M.J.; Juaìrez, M.L.; Alzogaray, R.A.; Arrighi, F.; Arroyo, L.; Gastaminza, G.; Willink, E.; del Valle Bardoìn, A.; Vera, T. Toxic effect of citrus peel constituents on *Anastrepha fraterculus* Wiedemann and *Ceratitis capitata* Wiedemann immature stages. *J. Agric. Food Chem.* **2014**, *62*, 10084–10091. [CrossRef] [PubMed]
122. Ivoke, N.; Ogbonna, P.C.; Ekeh, F.N.; Ezenwaji, N.E.; Atama, C.I.; Ejere, V.C.; Onoja, U.S.; Eyo, J.E. Effects of grapefruit (*Citrus paradisi* MACF) (Rutaceae) peel oil against developmental stages of *Aedes aegypti* (Diptera: Culicidae). *Southeast Asian J. Trop. Med. Public Health* **2013**, *44*, 970–978. [PubMed]
123. Sanei-Dehkord, A.; Sedaghat, M.M.; Vatandoost, H.; Abai, M.R. Chemical compositions of the peel essential oil of *Citrus aurantium* and its natural larvicidal activity against the malaria vector *Anopheles stephensi* (Diptera: Culicidae) in comparison with *Citrus paradisi*. *J. Arthropod Borne Dis.* **2016**, *10*, 577–585.
124. Pérez, A.; Alcala, Y.; Salem, A.Z.M.; Alberti, A.B. Anticoccidial efficacy of naringenin and a grapefruit peel extract in growing lambs naturally-infected with *Eimeria* spp. *Vet. Parasitol.* **2016**, *232*, 58–65. [CrossRef] [PubMed]
125. Russo, R.; Cassiano, M.G.V.; Ciociaro, A.; Adornetto, A.; Varano, G.P.; Chiappini, C.; Berliocchi, L.; Tassorelli, C.; Bagetta, G.; Corasaniti, M.T. Role of d-limonene in autophagy induced by bergamot essential oil in SH-SY5Y neuroblastoma cells. *PLoS ONE* **2014**, *9*, e0113682. [CrossRef] [PubMed]
126. Moysan, A.; Morlière, P.; Averbeck, D.; Dubertret, L. Evaluation of phototoxic and photogenotoxic risk associated with the use of photosensitizers in suntan preparations: Application to tanning preparations containing bergamot oil. *Skin Pharmacol. Physiol.* **1993**, *6*, 282–291. [CrossRef]
127. Rombolà, L.; Amantea, D.; Russo, R.; Adornetto, A.; Berliocchi, L.; Tridico, L.; Corasaniti, M.; Sakurada, S.; Sakurada, T.; Bagetta, G.; et al. Rational basis for the use of bergamot essential oil in complementary medicine to treat chronic pain. *Mini-Rev. Med. Chem.* **2016**, *16*, 721–728. [CrossRef] [PubMed]
128. Lauro, F.; Ilari, S.; Giancotti, L.A.; Morabito, C.; Malafoglia, V.; Gliozzi, M.; Palma, E.; Salvemini, D.; Muscoli, C. The protective role of bergamot polyphenolic fraction on several animal models of pain. *PharmaNutrition* **2016**, *4*, S35–S40. [CrossRef]
129. Sakurada, T.; Mizoguchi, H.; Kuwahata, H.; Katsuyama, S.; Komatsu, T.; Morrone, L.A.; Corasaniti, M.T.; Bagetta, G.; Sakurada, S. Intraplantar injection of bergamot essential oil induces peripheral antinociception mediated by opioid mechanism. *Pharmacol. Biochem. Behav.* **2011**, *97*, 436–443. [CrossRef] [PubMed]
130. Katsuyama, S.K.; Towa, A.O.; Amio, S.K.; Ato, K.S.; Agi, T.Y.; Ishikawa, Y.K.; Omatsu, T.K.; Agetta, G.B.; Akurada, T.S.; Akamura, H.N. Effect of plantar subcutaneous administration of bergamot essential oil and linalool on formalin-induced nociceptive behavior in mice. *Biomed. Res.* **2015**, *36*, 47–54. [CrossRef] [PubMed]
131. Kuwahata, H.; Komatsu, T.; Katsuyama, S.; Corasaniti, M.T.; Bagetta, G.; Sakurada, S.; Sakurada, T.; Takahama, K. Peripherally injected linalool and bergamot essential oil attenuate mechanical allodynia via inhibiting spinal ERK phosphorylation. *Pharmacol. Biochem. Behav.* **2013**, *103*, 735–741. [CrossRef] [PubMed]
132. Cosentino, M.; Luini, A.; Bombelli, R.; Corasaniti, M.T.; Bagetta, G.; Marino, F. The essential oil of bergamot stimulates reactive oxygen species production in human polymorphonuclear leukocytes. *Phyther. Res.* **2014**, *28*, 1232–1239. [CrossRef] [PubMed]
133. Navarra, M.; Ferlazzo, N.; Cirmi, S.; Trapasso, E.; Bramanti, P.; Lombardo, G.E.; Minciullo, P.L.; Calapai, G.; Gangemi, S. Effects of bergamot essential oil and its extractive fractions on SH-SY5Y human neuroblastoma cell growth. *J. Pharm. Pharmacol.* **2015**, *67*, 1042–1053. [CrossRef] [PubMed]
134. Berliocchi, L.; Ciociaro, A.; Russo, R.; Cassiano, M.G.V.; Blandini, F.; Rotiroti, D.; Morrone, L.A.; Corasaniti, M.T. Toxic profile of bergamot essential oil on survival and proliferation of SH-SY5Y neuroblastoma cells. *Food Chem. Toxicol.* **2011**, *49*, 2780–2792. [CrossRef] [PubMed]

135. Celia, C.; Trapasso, E.; Locatelli, M.; Navarra, M.; Ventura, C.A.; Wolfram, J.; Carafa, M.; Morittu, V.M.; Britti, D.; Di Marzio, L.; et al. Anticancer activity of liposomal bergamot essential oil (BEO) on human neuroblastoma cells. *Colloids Surf. B Biointerfaces* **2013**, *112*, 548–553. [CrossRef] [PubMed]
136. Sawamura, M. *Citrus Essential Oils: Flavor and Fragrance*; Wiley: Hoboken, NJ, USA, 2010.
137. Bagetta, G.; Morrone, L.A.; Rombolà, L.; Amantea, D.; Russo, R.; Berliocchi, L.; Sakurada, S.; Sakurada, T.; Rotiroti, D.; Corasaniti, M.T. Neuropharmacology of the essential oil of bergamot. *Fitoterapia* **2010**, *81*, 453–461. [CrossRef] [PubMed]
138. Amantea, D.; Fratto, V.; Maida, S.; Rotiroti, D.; Ragusa, S.; Corasaniti, M.T. Prevention of glutamate accumulation and upregulation of phospho-Akt may account for neuroprotection afforded by bergamot essential oil against brain injury induced by focal cerebral ischemia in rat. *Int. Rev. Neurobiol.* **2009**, *85*, 389–405. [PubMed]
139. Saiyudthong, S.; Mekseepralard, C. Effect of Inhaling bergamot oil on depression-related behaviors in chronic stressed rats. *J. Med. Assoc. Thail.* **2015**, *98*, S152–S159.
140. Saiyudthong, S.; Marsden, C.A. Acute effects of bergamot oil on anxiety-related behaviour and corticosterone level in rats. *Phyther. Res.* **2011**, *25*, 858–862. [CrossRef] [PubMed]
141. Han, X.; Gibson, J.; Eggett, D.L.; Parker, T.L. Bergamot (*Citrus bergamia*) essential oil inhalation improves positive feelings in the waiting room of a mental health treatment center: A pilot study. *Phyther. Res.* **2017**, *31*, 812–816. [CrossRef] [PubMed]
142. Avila-Sosa, R.; Navarro-Cruz, A.R.; Sosa-Morales, M.E.; López-Malo, A.; Palou, E. *Bergamot (Citrus Bergamia) Oils*; Elsevier Inc.: New York, NY, USA, 2015; ISBN 9780124166448.
143. Kirbaslar, F.G.; Tavman, A.; Dülger, B.; Türker, G. Antimicrobial activity of Turkish citrus peel oils. *Pak. J. Bot.* **2009**, *41*, 3207–3212.
144. Fisher, K.; Phillips, C.A. The effect of lemon, orange and bergamot essential oils and their components on the survival of *Campylobacter jejuni*, *Escherichia coli* O157, *Listeria monocytogenes*, *Bacillus cereus* and *Staphylococcus aureus* in vitro and in food systems. *J. Appl. Microbiol.* **2006**, *101*, 1232–1240. [CrossRef] [PubMed]
145. Stević, T.; Berić, T.; Šavikin, K.; Soković, M.; Gođevac, D.; Dimkić, I.; Stanković, S. Antifungal activity of selected essential oils against fungi isolated from medicinal plant. *Ind. Crop. Prod.* **2014**, *55*, 116–122. [CrossRef]
146. Sanguinetti, M.; Posteraro, B.; Romano, L.; Battaglia, F.; Lopizzo, T.; De Carolis, E.; Fadda, G. In vitro activity of *Citrus bergamia* (bergamot) oil against clinical isolates of dermatophytes. *J. Antimicrob. Chemother.* **2007**, *59*, 305–308. [CrossRef] [PubMed]
147. El-Ashmawy, W.R.; Elsaeed, M.; Gebely, M. Randomized clinical trial on evaluation of the effect of bergamot oil on treatment of ring worm infection in calves and cats. *Int. J. Infect. Dis.* **2016**, *45*, 312–313. [CrossRef]
148. Furneri, P.M.; Mondello, L.; Mandalari, G.; Paolino, D.; Dugo, P.; Garozzo, A.; Bisignano, G. In vitro antimycoplasmal activity of *Citrus bergamia* essential oil and its major components. *Eur. J. Med. Chem.* **2012**, *52*, 66–69. [CrossRef] [PubMed]
149. Sawamura, M.; Wu, Y.; Fujiwara, C.; Urushibata, M. Inhibitory effect of yuzu essential oil on the formation of *N*-nitrosodimethylamine in vegetables. *J. Agric. Food Chem.* **2005**, *53*, 4281–4287. [CrossRef] [PubMed]
150. Hirota, R.; Roger, N.N.; Nakamura, H.; Song, H.S.; Sawamura, M.; Suganuma, N. Anti-inflammatory effects of limonene from yuzu (*Citrus junos* Tanaka) essential oil on eosinophils. *J. Food Sci.* **2010**, *75*, 20492298. [CrossRef] [PubMed]
151. Ueki, S.; Niinomi, K.; Takashima, Y.; Kimura, R.; Komai, K.; Murakami, K.; Fujiwara, C. Effectiveness of aromatherapy in decreasing maternal anxiety for a sick child undergoing infusion in a paediatric clinic. *Complement. Ther. Med.* **2014**, *22*, 1019–1026. [CrossRef] [PubMed]
152. Matsumoto, T.; Kimura, T.; Hayashi, T. Aromatic effects of a Japanese citrus fruit-yuzu (*Citrus junos* Sieb. ex Tanaka)-on psychoemotional states and autonomic nervous system activity during the menstrual cycle: A single-blind randomized controlled crossover study. *Biopsychosoc. Med.* **2016**, *10*, 11. [CrossRef] [PubMed]
153. Matsumoto, T.; Kimura, T.; Hayashi, T. Does Japanese citrus fruit yuzu (*Citrus junos* Sieb. ex Tanaka) fragrance have lavender-like therapeutic effects that alleviate premenstrual emotional symptoms? A single-blind randomized crossover Study. *J. Altern. Complement. Med.* **2017**, *23*, 461–470. [CrossRef] [PubMed]
154. Kasahara, K.; Takahashi, E.; Nishibori, K. Suppressing effect of yuzu peel on the odor of Niboshi soup stock. *Bull. Jpn. Soc. Sci. Fish.* **1993**, *59*, 673–675. [CrossRef]

155. Kim, S.H.; Shin, E.J.; Hur, H.J.; Park, J.H.; Sung, M.J.; Kwon, D.Y.; Hwang, J.T. *Citrus junos* Tanaka peel extract attenuates experimental colitis and inhibits tumour growth in a mouse xenograft model. *J. Funct. Foods* **2014**, *8*, 301–308. [CrossRef]
156. Hwang, J.T.; Shin, E.J. Ethanol extract of *Citrus junos* Tanaka exerts hypocholesterolemic effect in mice fed a high cholesterol diet. *Atherosclerosis* **2013**, *241*, e195. [CrossRef]
157. Kim, S.H.; Hur, H.J.; Yang, H.J.; Kim, H.J.; Kim, M.J.; Park, J.H.; Sung, M.J.; Kim, M.S.; Kwon, D.Y.; Hwang, J.T. *Citrus junos* Tanaka peel extract exerts antidiabetic effects via AMPK and PPAR-γboth in vitro and in vivo in mice fed a high-fat diet. *Evid.-Based Complement. Altern. Med.* **2013**, *2013*, 921012.
158. Zang, L.; Shimada, Y.; Kawajiri, J.; Tanaka, T.; Nishimura, N. Effects of yuzu (*Citrus junos* Siebold ex Tanaka) peel on the diet-induced obesity in a zebrafish model. *J. Funct. Foods* **2014**, *10*, 499–510. [CrossRef]
159. Yu, H.Y.; Park, S.W.; Chung, I.M.; Jung, Y.S. Anti-platelet effects of yuzu extract and its component. *Food Chem. Toxicol.* **2011**, *49*, 3018–3024. [CrossRef] [PubMed]
160. Yu, H.Y.; Ahn, J.H.; Park, S.W.; Jung, Y.-S. Preventive effect of yuzu and hesperidin on left ventricular remodeling and dysfunction in rat permanent left anterior descending coronary artery occlusion model. *PLoS ONE* **2015**, *10*, e110596. [CrossRef] [PubMed]
161. Jayaprakasha, G.; Murthy, K.C.; Demarais, R.; Patil, B. Inhibition of prostate cancer (LNCaP) cell proliferation by volatile components from Nagami kumquats. *Planta Med.* **2012**, *78*, 974–980. [CrossRef] [PubMed]
162. Nouri, A.; Shafaghatlonbar, A. Chemical constituents and antioxidant activity of essential oil and organic extract from the peel and kernel parts of *Citrus japonica* Thunb. (kumquat) from Iran. *Nat. Prod. Res.* **2016**, *30*, 1093–1097. [CrossRef] [PubMed]
163. Wang, Y.W.; Zeng, W.C.; Xu, P.Y.; Lan, Y.J.; Zhu, R.X.; Zhong, K.; Huang, Y.N.; Gao, H. Chemical composition and antimicrobial activity of the essential oil of kumquat (*Fortunella crassifolia* Swingle) peel. *Int. J. Mol. Sci.* **2012**, *13*, 3382–3393. [CrossRef] [PubMed]
164. Md Othman, S.; Hassan, M.; Nahar, L.; Basar, N.; Jamil, S.; Sarker, S. Essential Oils from the Malaysian *Citrus* (Rutaceae) medicinal plants. *Medicines* **2016**, *3*, 13. [CrossRef] [PubMed]
165. Morrone, L.A.; Rombolà, L.; Pelle, C.; Corasaniti, M.T.; Zappettini, S.; Paudice, P.; Bonanno, G.; Bagetta, G. The essential oil of bergamot enhances the levels of amino acid neurotransmitters in the hippocampus of rat: Implication of monoterpene hydrocarbons. *Pharmacol. Res.* **2007**, *55*, 255–262. [CrossRef] [PubMed]
166. Volpato, G.T.; Francia-Farje, L.A.D.; Damasceno, D.C.; Renata, V.O.; Clélia, A.H.-L.; Wilma, G.K. Effect of essential oil from *Citrus aurantium* in maternal reproductive outcome and fetal anomaly frequency in rats. *An. Acad. Bras. Ciênc.* **2015**, *87*, 407–415. [CrossRef] [PubMed]
167. Opdyke, D.L.J. Monographs on fragrance raw materials. *Food Cosmet. Toxicol.* **1974**, *12*, 807–1016. [CrossRef]
168. Naganuma, M.; Hirose, S.; Nakayama, Y.; Nakajima, K.; Someya, T. A study of the phototoxicity of lemon oil. *Arch. Dermatol. Res.* **1985**, *278*, 31–36. [CrossRef] [PubMed]
169. Rudzki, E.; Grzywa, Z.; Bruo, W.S. Sensitivity to 35 essential oils. *Contact Dermat.* **1976**, *2*, 196–200. [CrossRef]
170. Santucci, B.; Cristaudo, A.; Cannistraci, C.; Picardo, M. Contact dermatitis to fragrances. *Contact Dermat.* **1987**, *16*, 93–95. [CrossRef]
171. Menenghini, C.L.; Rantuccio, F.; Lomuto, M. Additives, vehicles and active drugs of topical medicaments as causes of delayed-type allergic dermatitis. *Dermatologica* **1971**, *143*, 137–147. [CrossRef] [PubMed]
172. Young, A.R.; Walker, S.L.; Kinley, J.S.; Plastow, S.R.; Averbeck, D.; Morlière, P.; Dubertret, L. Phototumorigenesis studies of 5-methoxypsoralen in bergamot oil: Evaluation and modification of risk of human use in an albino mouse skin model. *J. Photochem. Photobiol. B* **1990**, *7*, 231–250. [CrossRef]
173. Opdyke, D.L.S. Fragrance raw materials Monographs. *Food Cosmet. Toxicol.* **1973**, *11*, 873–874. [CrossRef]
174. Bouhlal, K.; Meynadier, J.; Peyron, J.L.; Meynadier, J.; Peyron, L.; Senaux, M.S. The cutaneous effects of the common concretes and absolutes used in the perfume industry. In *The Antimicrobial/Biological Activity of Essential Oils*; Lawrence, B.M., Ed.; Allured: Carol Stream, IL, USA, 2005; pp. 10–23.
175. Christensson, J.B.; Forsstrom, P.; Wennberg, A.M.; Karlberg, A.T. Air oxidation increases skin irritation from fragrance terpenes. *Contact Dermat.* **2009**, *60*, 32–40. [CrossRef] [PubMed]
176. Li, G.X.; Liu, Z.Q. Unusual antioxidant behavior of alpha- and gamma-terpinene in protecting methyl linoleate, DNA, and erythrocyte. *J. Agric. Food Chem.* **2009**, *57*, 3943–3948. [CrossRef] [PubMed]
177. Tisserand, R.; Balacs, T. *Essential Oil Safety—A Guide for Health Care Professionals*; Harcourt: Glasgow, UK, 1999.

178. Cavanagh, H.M.A.; Wilkinson, J.M. Biological activities of lavender essential oil. *Phyther. Res.* **2002**, *16*, 301–308. [CrossRef] [PubMed]
179. Williamson, E.M.; Priestley, C.M.; Burgess, I.F. An investigation and comparison of the bioactivity of selected essential oils on human lice and house dust mites. *Fitoterapia* **2007**, *78*, 521–525. [CrossRef] [PubMed]
180. Da Silva, J.K.R.; Maia, J.G.S.; Dosoky, N.S.; Setzer, W.N. Antioxidant, antimicrobial, and cytotoxic properties of *Aniba parviflora* essential oils from the Amazon. *Nat. Prod. Commun.* **2016**, *11*, 1025–1028.
181. Matura, M.; Skold, M.; Borje, A.; Andersen, K.E.; Bruze, M.; Frosch, P.; Goossens, A.; Johansen, J.D.; Svedman, C.; White, I.R.; et al. Selected oxidized fragrance terpenes are common contact allergens. *Contact Dermat.* **2005**, *52*, 320–328. [CrossRef] [PubMed]
182. Bickers, D.; Calow, P.; Greim, H.; Hanifin, J.M.; Rogers, A.E.; Saurat, J.H.; Sipes, I.G.; Smith, R.L.; Tagami, H. A toxicologic and dermatologic assessment of linalool and related esters when used as fragrance ingredients. *Food Chem. Toxicol.* **2003**, *41*, 919–942. [CrossRef]
183. Jenner, P.M.; Hagan, E.C.; Taylor, J.M.; Cook, E.L.; Fitzhugh, O.G. Food flavorings and compounds of related structure. I. acute oral toxicity. *Food Cosmet. Toxicol.* **1964**, *2*, 327–343. [CrossRef]
184. Letizia, C.S.; Cocchiara, J.; Lalko, J.; Api, A.M. Fragrance material review on linalool. *Food Chem. Toxicol.* **2003**, *41*, 943–964. [CrossRef]
185. Powers, K.A.; Beasley, V.R. Toxicolgical aspects of linalool: A review. *Vet. Hum. Toxicol.* **1985**, *27*, 484–486. [PubMed]
186. Fujii, T.; Furukawa, S.; Suzuki, S. Studies on compounded perfumes for toilet goods. On the non-irritative compounded perfumes for soaps. *Yukagaku* **1972**, *21*, 904–908.
187. Bicas, J.L.; Neri-Numa, I.A.; Ruiz, A.L.; De Carvalho, J.E.; Pastore, G.M. Evaluation of the antioxidant and antiproliferative potential of bioflavors. *Food Chem. Toxicol.* **2011**, *49*, 1610–1615. [CrossRef] [PubMed]
188. Placzek, M.; Frömel, W.; Eberlein, B.; Gilbertz, K.P.; Przybilla, B. Evaluation of phototoxic properties of fragrances. *Acta Derm. Venereol.* **2007**, *87*, 312–316. [CrossRef] [PubMed]
189. Gonçalves, M.J.; Cruz, M.T.; Tavares, A.C.; Cavaleiro, C.; Lopes, M.C.; Canhoto, J.; Salgueiro, L. Composition and biological activity of the essential oil from *Thapsia minor*, a new source of geranyl acetate. *Ind. Crop. Prod.* **2012**, *35*, 166–171. [CrossRef]
190. Kakarla, S.; Ganjewala, D. Antimicrobial activity of essential oils of four lemongrass (*Cymbopogon flexuosus* Steud) varieties. *Med. Aromat. Plant Sci. Biotechnol.* **2009**, *3*, 107–109.
191. Mortelmans, K.; Haworth, S.; Lawlor, T.; Speck, W.; Tainer, B.; Zeiger, E. *Salmonella* mutagenicity tests: II. Results from the testing of 270 chemicals. *Environ. Mutagen.* **1986**, *8*, 1–119. [CrossRef] [PubMed]
192. Shelby, M.D.; Erexson, G.L.; Hook, G.J.; Tice, R.R. Evaluation of a three-exposure mouse bone marrow micronucleus protocol: Results with 49 chemicals. *Environ. Mol. Mutagen.* **1993**, *21*, 160–179. [CrossRef] [PubMed]
193. Kim, H.J.; Chen, F.; Wu, C.; Wang, X.; Chung, H.Y.; Jin, Z. Evaluation of antioxidant activity of Australian tea tree (*Melaleuca alternifolia*) oil and its components. *J. Agric. Food Chem.* **2004**, *52*, 2849–2854. [CrossRef] [PubMed]
194. Li, Y.L.; Yeung, C.M.; Chiu, L.C.; Cen, Y.Z.; Ooi, V.E. Chemical composition and antiproliferative activity of essential oil from the leaves of a medicinal herb, *Schefflera heptaphylla*. *Phytother. Res.* **2009**, *23*, 140–142. [CrossRef] [PubMed]
195. Pirila, V.; Siltanen, E.; Pirila, L. On the chemical nature of the eczematogenic agent in oil of turpentine. IV. the primary irritant effect of terpenes. *Dermatologica* **1964**, *128*, 16–21. [CrossRef]
196. Schlede, E.; Aberer, W.; Fuchs, T.; Gerner, I.; Lessmann, H.; Maurer, T.; Rossbacher, R.; Stropp, G.; Wagner, E.; Kayser, D. Chemical substances and contact allergy—244 substances ranked according to allergenic potency. *Toxicology* **2003**, *193*, 219–259. [CrossRef]

International Journal of
Molecular Sciences

MDPI

Review

Natural Products for Drug Discovery in the 21st Century: Innovations for Novel Drug Discovery

Nicholas Ekow Thomford [1,2,†], Dimakatso Alice Senthebane [3,4], Arielle Rowe [3], Daniella Munro [1], Palesa Seele [5], Alfred Maroyi [6] and Kevin Dzobo [3,4,*,†]

1. Pharmacogenomics and Drug Metabolism Group, Division of Human Genetics, Department of Pathology and Institute of Infectious Disease and Molecular Medicine, Faculty of Health Sciences, University of Cape Town, Anzio Road, Observatory, Cape Town 7925, South Africa; nicholas.thomford@uct.ac.za (N.E.T.); MNRDAN002@myuct.ac.za (D.M.)
2. School of Medical Sciences, University of Cape Coast, PMB, Cape Coast, Ghana
3. International Centre for Genetic Engineering and Biotechnology (ICGEB), Cape Town Component, Wernher and Beit Building (South), University of Cape Town Medical Campus, Anzio Road, Observatory, Cape Town 7925, South Africa; SNTDIM001@myuct.ac.za (D.A.S.); arielle.rowe@icgeb.org (A.R.)
4. Division of Medical Biochemistry and Institute of Infectious Disease and Molecular Medicine, Faculty of Health Sciences, University of Cape Town, Anzio Road, Observatory, Cape Town 7925, South Africa
5. Division of Chemical and Systems Biology, Department of Integrative Biomedical Sciences, Faculty of Health Sciences, University of Cape Town, Anzio Road, Observatory, Cape Town 7925, South Africa; SLXPAL001@myuct.ac.za
6. Department of Botany, University of Fort Hare, Private Bag, Alice X1314, South Africa; amaroyi@ufh.ac.za

* Correspondence: kd.dzobo@uct.ac.za; Tel.: +27-21-404-7689; Fax: +27-21-406-6060

† These authors contributed equally to this work.

Received: 27 April 2018; Accepted: 18 May 2018; Published: 25 May 2018

Abstract: The therapeutic properties of plants have been recognised since time immemorial. Many pathological conditions have been treated using plant-derived medicines. These medicines are used as concoctions or concentrated plant extracts without isolation of active compounds. Modern medicine however, requires the isolation and purification of one or two active compounds. There are however a lot of global health challenges with diseases such as cancer, degenerative diseases, HIV/AIDS and diabetes, of which modern medicine is struggling to provide cures. Many times the isolation of "active compound" has made the compound ineffective. Drug discovery is a multidimensional problem requiring several parameters of both natural and synthetic compounds such as safety, pharmacokinetics and efficacy to be evaluated during drug candidate selection. The advent of latest technologies that enhance drug design hypotheses such as Artificial Intelligence, the use of 'organ-on chip' and microfluidics technologies, means that automation has become part of drug discovery. This has resulted in increased speed in drug discovery and evaluation of the safety, pharmacokinetics and efficacy of candidate compounds whilst allowing novel ways of drug design and synthesis based on natural compounds. Recent advances in analytical and computational techniques have opened new avenues to process complex natural products and to use their structures to derive new and innovative drugs. Indeed, we are in the era of computational molecular design, as applied to natural products. Predictive computational softwares have contributed to the discovery of molecular targets of natural products and their derivatives. In future the use of quantum computing, computational softwares and databases in modelling molecular interactions and predicting features and parameters needed for drug development, such as pharmacokinetic and pharmacodynamics, will result in few false positive leads in drug development. This review discusses plant-based natural product drug discovery and how innovative technologies play a role in next-generation drug discovery.

Keywords: natural products; drug design and development; innovation; automation; computational softwares; bioinformatics; precision medicine; omics; global health

1. Introduction

The scourge of communicable and non-communicable diseases and the challenges of finding drug candidates that can treat these diseases with little or no side effects is a huge challenge. Despite the development of drugs for treating and managing diseases such as HIV/AIDS, malaria, hypertension, diabetes and cancer, these diseases continue to plague diverse populations worldwide with significant associated-mortalities. There is need for innovative drug discovery strategies that skew from the current "blockbuster" Pharma R&D strategies. Currently, a viable approach will be to revert to "nature" for answers since it has worked for drug discovery in the past. Anticancer drugs such as Taxol (*Taxus brevifolia*), Vinblastine (*Catharanthus roseus*) and antimalarial drugs such as quinine (*Cinchona* spp.) and Artemisinin (*Artemisia annua*) were all discovered from natural products and are effective in treating these diseases. In the face of global public health challenges, natural products research and development (R&D) potentially plays a pivotal role in innovative drug discovery.

Plants are found in every habitable environment with most found on land. Faced with many stresses and challenges, coupled with being sedentary, plants have developed many molecules to ward off attacks from animals and environmental insults [1]. These same molecules give plants their ability to give off fragrances, colours and indeed toxicity. Many historical findings report on early use of plants for medicinal purposes [2]. The discovery of medicinal plants by early humans must have been a trial and error exercise necessitated by the need to ease disease manifestations. Before the advent of writing and recording of history, such knowledge was passed through generations through word of mouth. Many plants were recorded in the early years of having medicinal properties and were used to treat many pathological conditions [3–8]. Natural products from plants and animals have been the go-to source of drugs especially for anticancer and antimicrobial agents [9–13]. Traditional medicine has been overshadowed by modern medicine as the means of treatment for human diseases [14–16]. However, the past few decades have seen an increase in the use of medicinal plants for health promotion and treatment of diseases in many countries including developed countries [17–22]. Indeed, many medicinal plant extracts are now used as prescription drugs in numerous developed countries such as the UK, Germany, China and France [23,24].

About a quarter of all Food and Drug Administration (FDA) and/or the European Medical Agency (EMA) approved drugs are plant based, with well-known drugs such as Paclitaxel and Morphine having been isolated from plants (Figure 1) [25,26]. About a third of FDA-approved drugs over the past 20 years are based on natural products or their derivatives [27,28]. The discovery of penicillin from fungus led to the screening of many microorganisms for potential antibiotics [29]. Indeed, drug discovery from natural products revolutionised medicine. These include tetracycline from *Streptomyces aureofaciens*, artemisinin from *Artemisia afra*, doxorubicin from *Streptomyces peucetius* and cyclosporine from *Tolypocladium inflatum* [27,29,30]. Traditionally, plant extracts are used as concoctions made of combinations of different ingredients. Individually some of the ingredients do not have therapeutic activities, but require their synergistic activities [31].

Current challenges to the use of natural products and difficulty in accepting their therapeutic efficacy include: (1) lack of standardization procedures (2) lack of isolation of pure chemical products or compounds (3) lack of elucidation of biological mechanisms and rarely undergoing so-called controlled and (4) documented clinical trials according to "standards". Historically, there is scientific evidence on the therapeutic efficacy of natural products and as previously mentioned this led to development of some blockbuster conventional medicines. Searching for new drug candidates from natural products is often made difficult by the complexity of the molecular mixtures. The therapeutic activity of plant extracts is usually because of the synergistic and simultaneous action of several chemicals [30,32]. Given the complex nature of many diseases including cancer and degenerative diseases, it is not surprising that the reliance on single compound-based drug discovery has failed to provide effective cures. Plant-based drug discovery therefore must start with a combinatorial approach when evaluating candidate compounds. The advent of novel technologies including quantum computing, profiling techniques, computational biology techniques, big data, microfluidics and artificial intelligence will enable scientists to use a combinatorial approach to harness the therapeutic properties of plant-based natural products and simultaneously study their molecular effects in physiological conditions [33,34].

It is however possible that not all components of plant extracts have measurable effects. It has been suggested that one way to improve screening and simplify extracts is through the removal of possible interfering components such as polyphenolic tannins [35]. There are several reported innovative strategies which can be used to achieve this and these include pre-fractionation and extraction methods [36,37]. Indeed, these extraction strategies have resulted in higher hit leads during drug discovery [12,38–40]. Innovative extraction technologies including semi-bionic extraction [41], supercritical fluid extraction [42–44], microwave-assisted, ultrasonic-assisted and enzyme-assisted extraction [45], molecular distillation methods [46,47] and membrane separation technology [48,49] can be used to extract natural compounds efficiently from plants. These extractions strategies have been shown to have similar simulation to traditional methods allowing the extraction process to get most compounds from the natural product.

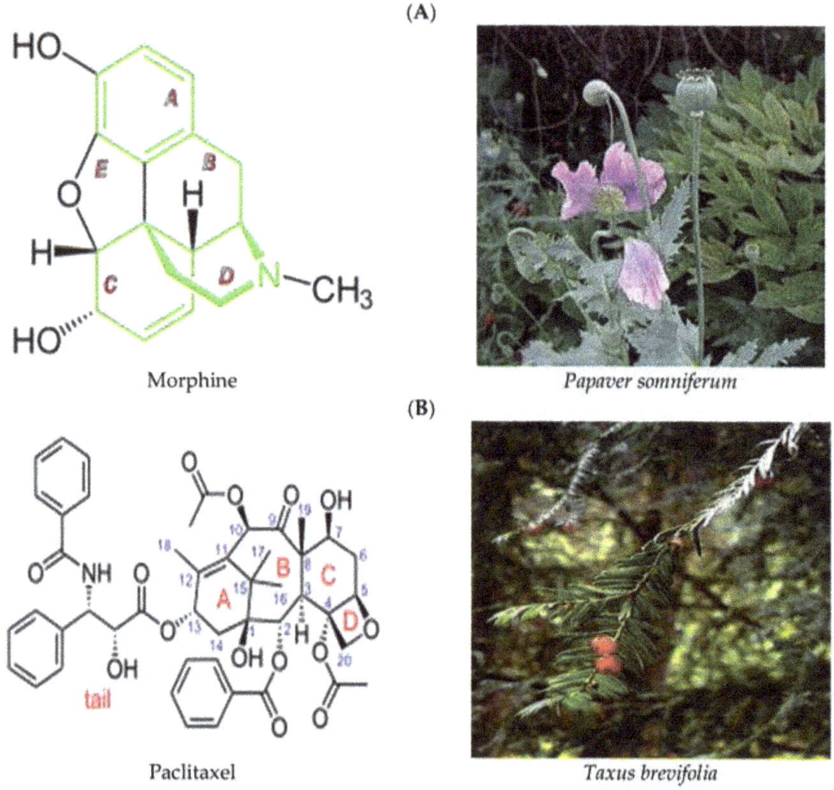

Figure 1. Two examples of successful stories of plant natural products that are being used in hospitals and clinics for disease treatment. (**A**) Morphine is isolated from *Papaver somniferum* also called opium poppy (**B**) Paclitaxel is isolated from *Taxus brevifolia* also called pacific yew. (Images credit: https://en.wikipedia.org/wiki).

Technologies such as high-performance liquid chromatography, nuclear magnetic resonance spectroscopy, mass spectrometry, microfluidics and computational algorithms have seen major advances in the field of medicinal chemistry especially in the 20th century [50,51]. This has allowed the determination of chemical components of plants and their utilisation in drug discovery. High throughput assays using bioreactors and microfluidics systems has led to many drug discoveries using plant natural products. Some of these natural products include opium and morphine [52,53]. Several structural analogues of these compounds are used in clinics and hospitals today. Several new plant-based compounds are emerging as promising anti-cancer remedies. In one of our studies we investigated the anticancer activities of extracts from African lettuce (*Launaea taraxacifolia*), a plant cultivated extensively in Africa, especially West Africa. *L. taraxacifolia* extract caused WHCO1 cell cycle arrest at the G0/G1 phase by affecting differential expression of genes involved in cell cycle regulation, presenting its potential beneficial effects [22]. The medicinal plant *Brucea javanica* (L.) Merr. (Simaroubaceae) has been shown to have many properties and activities. Through both phytochemical and biological investigations, it was shown that *Brucea javanica* (L.) Merr. contains many compounds with medicinal properties. For example the seeds of *Brucea javanica* contain several compounds such as quassinoids that show many biological properties, such as antitumour and antimalarial effects [54]. A well-known malarial drug Artemisinin is a natural product from *Artemisia annua* also known as Sweet Wormwood [55,56]. Artemisinin and its structural derivatives are also used for diseases such as type I diabetes and cancer [57–59]. High throughput screening assays face many challenges. For example, the Rio Convention on Biodiversity is aimed at limiting the use of natural products and deals with intellectual property rights. This has the effect of limiting access to natural products as there are fears of extinction of natural species [29,60–65].

Current drug discovery strategies and modern medicine discard the use of whole plant extracts and are driven by single compound-based medicine. Taking the whole plant or extracts with no isolation of components as practised in traditional medicine, produces a better therapeutic effect than individual compounds. This is important as most of the plant metabolites likely work in a synergistic fashion or concurrently to give the plant extract its therapeutic effect. Research into the use of whole plant extracts must be done as this will allow scientists to determine the molecular basis of the therapeutic effect of the plant extracts. For example, anti-asthma herbal medicine made from extracts from *Ganoderma lucidum*, *Glycyrrhiza uralensis* and *Sophora flavescens* alleviates bronchoconstriction in an animal model whilst restoring cytokines balance, contributing to longer lasting anti-asthma benefit after treatment [66]. The therapeutic effect only emanates from the synergistic effect of chemical components of the three herbal ingredients [67,68]. The adoption of Good Manufacturing Practises has allowed the increased use of plant-based medicines and many are now undergoing clinical trial for FDA approval [69]. Skroza and colleagues showed that catechin and resveratrol have synergistic effects as confirmed by different antioxidant assays [70]. The same study also showed the synergistic effects of caffeic acid and resveratrol by the ferric reducing ability of plasma (FRAP) antioxidant assay [70]. Another study showed the synergistic effects of ethnomedicinal plants of the *Apocynaceae* family and antibiotics against clinical isolates of *Acinetobacter baumannii* [71]. Several other studies showed the synergistic effect of different plant extracts and conventional drugs including doxorubicin [72].

Innovative drug design from natural products is needed to combat global health challenges with the assistance of technological innovation. Most importantly is the need for new and innovative computational and analytical methods to identify chemical components of crude plant extracts in order to identify compounds causing the desired therapeutic effect and optimize extraction to exclude interfering components. Ultimately, more research should be focussing on combinatorial effects of chemicals from plant extracts and not just single compounds. How these combinations affect genes and proteins involved in many cellular processes must be investigated through available "-omics" platforms. Developments in the field of microfluidics and computational analysis have allowed for the designing and testing of plant extract chemicals in drug discovery. Technological advances, such as the development of new analytical and bio-informatic techniques, will aid the design of new structures, the synthesis of these new compounds and the biological testing of such compounds [73,74]. Natural products, offer an endless source of compounds to help in the design of pharmacologically important molecular products [75–77]. Below we discuss some of the major innovations currently taking place in these areas. We focus on the need for the use of "-omics" technologies, automation and big data during drug design and testing to allow for the rapid production of drugs and computer aided drug design from plant-based natural products.

2. Multidisciplinary Approach to Natural Products Drug Discovery Using Innovative Technologies

Innovative drug discovery from natural products requires a multidisciplinary approach utilising available and innovative technologies to package such natural product compounds for medical practice and drug development (Figure 2). The successful use of such an approach will allow the development of next-generation drugs to combat the ever-increasing health challenges of today and the future.

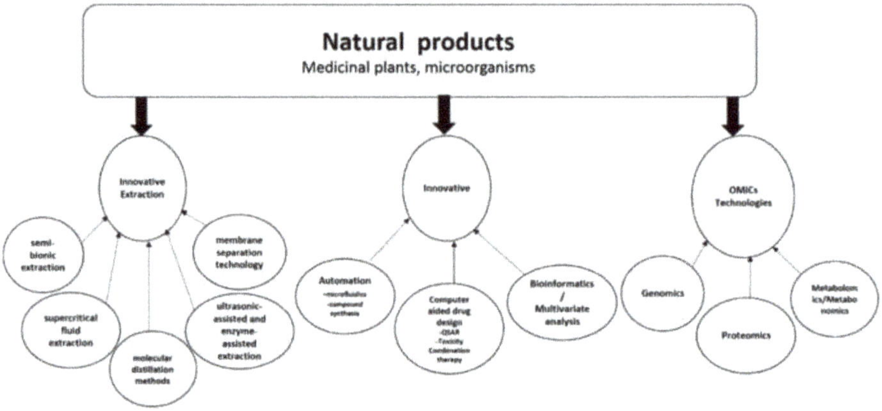

Figure 2. Innovative technologies for natural product drug discovery. Application of these technologies can potentially lead to novel drug candidates from natural products.

Most medicinal extract components often work in a synergistic manner to elicit their therapeutic effects so isolating individual components may be counter-productive. Innovative approaches are needed to study and to harness such compounds that can effectively lead to innovative drugs. In addition, a systems biology guided approach provides a different angle in natural products pharma-sciences [78]. This transcends looking for a specific molecule with a specific target and espousing the complete equilibrium of a physiological system undergoing synchronized mechanisms on multiple molecular targets. A systems biology approach coupled with application of available technologies such as genomics, transcriptomics, proteomics, metabolomics/metabonomics, automation and computational strategies will potentially pave the way for innovative drug design leading to better drug candidates. Molecular libraries of lead compounds from natural products R&D will serve as sources of lead compounds/herbal tinctures for innovative drugs. In the application of innovative technologies combined with systems biology, the focus should not be a reductionist approach of trying to source a single active compound but to consider the synergistic effects of compounds. It is important to emphasise that innovative drug discovery from natural products will require a non-reductionist strategy to understand their complex mechanisms of action at the molecular level.

3. Natural Products Drug Discovery Research and Development and Omics (Genomics Proteomics and Metabolomics/Metabonomics)

3.1. *Genomics in Plant-Based Natural Products Identification and Biomarker Identification*

The quality, precise identification and reliability in the plant species from which the natural product is obtained and to which the therapeutic properties are ascribed is very critical for successful innovative drug discovery. The use of a different or wrong plant species will likely affect the therapeutic properties due to different compounds and quantities that will be found in the species. Genomic methods are important in establishing an accurate identification method for plants and natural product species [78]. Genomic techniques such as DNA barcoding are established techniques that rely on sequence diversity in short, standard DNA regions (400–800 bp) for species-level identification [79]. DNA barcoding utilising genomics will provide a more robust and precise identification compared to traditional methods of morphological identification and local traditional (vernacular) names [80]. DNA barcoding of natural products has been applied in biodiversity inventories [81] and authentication of herbal products [82–84]. DNA barcoding was used in an integrative approach for identification of plant species such as *Amaranthus hybridus* L. and crude drugs recorded in the Japanese pharmacopoeia using *ITS2* or *psbA-trnH* sequence amplification [80,85]. Genomic-based techniques represent an effective platform for natural product identification but different parts of the same plant with similar sequences may have different qualities, clinical utilities and indications due to the diverse conditions under which they grow.

To show consistency in the species and pharmacological molecules from natural products, bio-farming can be used to ensure consistency after the traditional species have been authenticated through DNA barcoding [86]. Markers developed from species through genomic techniques can be incorporated into DNA chips to provide an effective, high-throughput tool for genotyping and also plant species authentication [78,87]. Gene expression using microarray analysis is an innovative transcriptomic technology that allows a fast and effective analysis of many transcripts [78,88,89]. This transcriptomic analysis makes it possible to concurrently evaluate variations in multiple gene expressions [90]. This represents a robust tool for elucidating the molecular mechanisms of therapeutic natural products and biological networks underlying their pharmacological actions.

Besides its use in natural products identification, genomics can also be used in natural product or compound targeting. Whole genome sequencing combined with transcriptomic analyses has allowed the exploration of drug or compound targeting as never before. Transcription factor binding sites, protein modifications, alterations of the DNA structure as well as methylation patterns can now be analysed and measured at the genome level [91–96]. Several studies including our own have identified deletions, insertions, copy number variations, splicing variants and translocations associated with certain cancers, and in so doing identified new drug targets [97–102]. The development of novel and unrivalled technologies, allowing genome-wide analysis, has enabled the unbiased discovery of drug targets. These technologies together with the availability of huge databases of chemicals or compounds have enabled the shortening of the time required for the whole process of drug discovery from drug design all the way to clinical trials [103–109].

3.2. Proteomics in Natural Product Validation and Biomarker Identification

Complimentary to genomic and transcriptomic approaches to quality control and sample variation is the use of proteomic platforms in describing the mechanism of action of many natural products. Proteomic approaches to innovative drug discovery from natural products have the potential to elucidate the protein expression, protein function, metabolic and biosynthetic pathways based on therapeutic effects translating to consistency in quality and profile of the product [110,111]. Approaches such as mass-spectrometry utilising isotope tags and two-dimensional electrophoresis will give insight into quantitative protein profiling which generates quantitative data on a scale and sensitivity comparable to what is generated at the genomic level. Proteomics application has been successfully used in identifying species of Chinese herbal medicine, *Panax ginseng* versus *Panax quinquefolium* [112,113]. The therapeutic effects of natural products can be elucidated using proteomics and imaging techniques to successfully study the metabolism of natural products and their compounds [114,115]. Proteomics is an effective way to elucidate multi-target effects of complex natural product preparations as well as the discovery of multiple compounds and fractions, characterisation of natural products and ultimately a molecular diagnostic platform [78,116].

For natural products to be used as drugs it is crucial that their target proteins be identified. Several methods including affinity chromatography have been in use to identify target proteins with relative success. The advent of technologies allowing for target protein identification without the modification of the natural product has resulted in natural products with increased activity. Such methods include cellular thermal shift assay which is based on the stabilisation of target protein when it binds to its ligand, thermal proteome profiling a method based on the stability of target proteins at high temperatures, bioinformatic-based analysis of connectivity and drug affinity responsive target stability. Due to their many structures and complexity, natural products do show a wide range of biological activities. This is probably due to their abilities to bind to several ligands. Every potential drug will have to be tested for side effects and this is due to its off-target effects. Complex natural compounds with potential target proteins will have to be evaluated properly to identify all its potential target proteins. One of the most utilised methods to identify target proteins and their biological activities is affinity chromatography [117–123]. This method is a pull-down method in which the natural product is immobilized on a physical solid support [124]. The identification of bound proteins is done using mass spectrometry. Modification of natural products however, can lead to reduced or loss of activity. The development of novel and innovative approaches, devoid of any modification, is paramount for the success of target identification [125,126]. Of late, several methods have been able to identify target proteins using label-free natural products. These new and improved methods measure the responses of natural product-target protein complex to proteomic and thermal treatment [127–129]. Using this new approach, it is possible to identify several target proteins for an individual natural product using proteomic analysis [13,130].

Methods for Target Identification of Label-Free Natural Products

Drug affinity responsive target stability (DARTS) is one of the direct methods used to identify target proteins using label free natural products [124]. This methods takes advantage of the changes in stability of a natural product-bound protein versus an unbound protein when subjected to proteolytic treatment [130]. This method has been used to validate several target proteins for compounds such as resveratrol and rapamycin [129,131]. It is however difficult to use DARTS to identify low abundance protein targets in cell lysates [132]. Another method that takes advantage of ligand-induced changes to target proteins is stability of proteins from rates of oxidation (SPROX) [124,133,134]. This method measures the irreversible oxidation of methionine residues on target proteins [124]. A mixture of candidate drug compound and proteins is incubated with an oxidising agent and guanidinium hydrochloride in order to oxidise methionine. Generated peptides are then analysed through mass spectrometry to evaluate selective methionine oxidation. Analyses of oxidised and non-oxidised methionine-containing peptides versus the guanidinium hydrochloride concentration reveal that proteins bound to ligands show a larger transition midpoint shift than control samples [13,135–137]. Indeed, several target proteins of compounds such as resveratrol and cyclophilin A were verified using SPROX [133,137,138]. This method however requires highly concentrated proteins for analysis. Modifications of the SPROX method, named stable isotope labelling with amino acids in cell culture (SILAC)-based SPROX is an improvement of the original method and has the advantage of covering more target proteins [130,139–144]. This method is limited to only identifying of methionine containing proteins.

Cellular Thermal Shift Assay (CETSA) is a recently introduced method based on stabilisation of a target protein by binding to its ligand [145–147]. Cell lysates and intact cells are treated with the candidate drug compound and heated to several temperatures and target protein is separated from destabilised protein and analysed by Western blot analysis. Shifts or changes in melting curves are detected when ligand–target interactions are plotted against temperature. This method has been useful in identifying target proteins of many anti-cancer therapeutic agents such as raltitrexed and methotrexate [145]. The advantage of this method is the obvious use of intact cells with no need for treatments or preparations. Due to the use of Western blot step it can be very selective. Some target proteins with unfolded binding sites, however, may not be detected. In addition, due to non-specificity of some antibodies used in Western blot step, off-target proteins may also be identified as false positives. Thermal Proteome Profiling (TPP) is an advanced modification of the CETSA method. This method identifies target proteins displaying thermal stability at high temperatures induced by ligand binding and the use of mass spectrometry to measure ligand–target protein interaction at cellular level [148–150]. This method uses isobaric mass tagging in for high resolution mass spectrometry. Most expressed soluble proteins will show melting curves resulting in the identification of both target and off-target proteins [13,127,148,151,152]. By identifying off-targets TPP can be used to study possible side effects of candidate drug compounds [150]. This method is very costly and is labour intensive.

Small interfering RNA and short hairpin RNA are obvious choices for target gene manipulation to functionally validate target protein and natural product interactions [153,154]. By knocking down target protein using interfering RNA it is possible to study off-target effects of candidate compounds. Recently clustered regularly interspaced short palindromic repeats-Cas9 (CRISPR-Cas9) genome editing approaches have been used to overcome off-target effects of candidate compounds and to delineate how many natural compounds work [155,156]. CRISPR-Cas9 based genome editing combined with high throughput sequencing and computer-based mutation analysis, referred to as DrugTargetSeqR, has been used to study drug resistance and for validation of several anti-cancer therapeutic agents [157–159].

3.3. Metabolomics and Metabonomics Approach to Natural Products Drug Discovery

Untargeted metabolomics and metabonomics approaches of discovering compounds of therapeutic interest from natural products have the potential to lead to innovative drugs for global health. Metabolomic profiling of natural products seeks to identify and quantify the complete set of its characteristic metabolites [160,161] while metabonomics broadly aims to evaluate the global and dynamic metabolic response of living systems to biological stimuli or genetic manipulation [162–165]. Drug discovery has traditionally focussed on metabolomics to identify metabolites but recently, the term metabonomics (although used interchangeably) has been reviewed to incorporate a systems biology guided approach to study the functions and perturbations of a biological system following a pharmacological effect. This elucidates a complete biological mechanism of both the natural product and its effect on a living system (Figure 3).

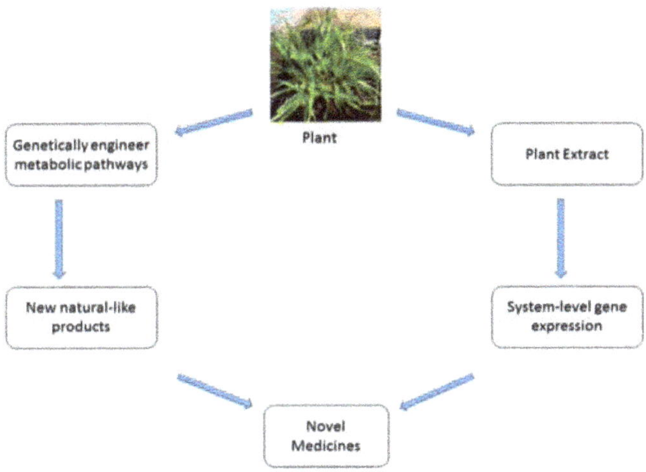

Figure 3. Exploiting the properties of plant extracts in the development of novel medicines inspired by compounds found in medicinal plant extracts.

Metabolomic profiling of natural products using technologies such as ultra-performance high performance liquid chromatography–quadruple TOF MS (UPLC–MS) has enabled identification of compounds that confer therapeutic properties on herbs such as *Newbouldia laevis*, *Cassia abbreviata*, *Hyptis suaveolens* and *Panax* herbs [166–168]. As a quality control measure and to show consistency in species usage, metabolomics has been used in identification of processed *Panax* species (*Panax ginseng* and *Panax quinquefolius*) using Nuclear Magnetic Resonance (NMR) based metabolomics, UPLC–QTOF MS and multivariate statistical analysis [169]. Metabonomics approach to profiling natural products for drug discovery has been hailed as a critical phenotyping tool. The systems biology approach of this technique positions the profiling of natural products in an all-inclusive manner in terms of metabolite and biology systems effect (Figure 3). Metabolomic and metabonomics profiling using NMR, MS and UPLC can potentially elucidate the pharmacodynamic, pharmacokinetic and toxicological value of natural products.

3.4. Big Data in Drug Development for Natural Product Drug Development and Precision Medicine

Omics analysis, like genomics, transcriptomics, proteomics, metabolomics and metabolomics, results in a generation of a complex multivariate dataset that requires computational and chemometric tools for interpretation. The use of computational platforms such as bioinformatics and multivariate statistical tools, will allow the application of omics multidata to elucidate pathophysiological effects, target specificity and molecular effects, as well as elucidate the pharmacodynamic, pharmacokinetic and toxicological characterisation of natural products and their compounds. Applications used during the drug discovery process such as docking and virtual screening can make use of novel machine learning algorithms such as deep learning. Machine learning methods can be used for virtual screening of thousands of compounds allowing the utilisation of data from high throughput screening [170,171].

Computer-based screening of candidate compounds for drug discovery makes use of big databases especially to identify compounds of similar activity. Similarity in structure is equated to similarity in biological activity, with results not always supporting this idea. Knowledge of the chemical structure of candidate compounds together with knowledge about the target protein is utilised to study possible interactions between the two. Transcriptomic data, used as gene signature, can be used to compare differences and similarities in response to candidate compounds [172–176]. For example, the connectivity map allows scientists to associate disease-associated gene signatures with drug signatures resulting in the identification of drugs that can potentially reverse the disease gene signature [177–181]. Generating a lot of data can have the consequence of losing the ability to understand its meaning. Big data must be useful and put into action. For big data to be useful during drug discovery it must be summarised into a little actionable information [182–184]. There are several data sources used for drug identification. These include ChemBank, PubChem, ChEMBL, DrugBank, UniProt, STITCH and the NIH Small Molecule Repository [185–188].

Connectivity Map (CMap) is a bioinformatic application that allows the study of diseases at the molecular level with the help of computers [189–191]. Established by the Broad Institute, the CMap is a collection of transcriptional data of many compounds-treated human cells [172–175,192]. The CMap associates gene expression signatures with compounds, genes and disease response allowing for its utilisation to show connections between compounds with the same modes of action and same physiological processes [172–174,192]. The CMap also allows associations to be made between diseases and drugs. The same pattern-matching analysis can be used for natural products, gene expression and diseases [173–176].

Using electronic databases of chemicals and protein targets and clinical data such as patient to patient variations in response to treatment, several strategies are being employed to reduce the cost of drug development and to increase the speed at which drugs are developed [193]. There are obvious challenges to the efficient development of drugs and these include the lack of models that can recapitulate the human body properly in terms of response to candidate compounds, the heterogeneity of individuals in terms of their response to candidate compounds and the inability to analyse biological processes properly during testing of candidate compounds [194–196]. Despite a heavy investment in research and development, most candidate compounds show weakened efficacy as the stages of drug development move towards clinical trials [197–201]. This strategy whereby information is collected without applying a hypothesis or any bias, analysed and then used to come up with new and innovative ideas is called Big Data [202–206]. Big data is now integrated with compound chemical structures, protein structures, compound toxicity and clinical trials and this has led to the development of complex algorithms needed for such analysis [207,208].

One major challenge with the use of big data-driven drug discovery is the relative low presence of similar somatic alterations in cancer patients enrolled in a study. This is caused by tumour heterogeneity, a chief cause of chemoresistance and drug treatment failure. A challenge to scientists using big data to inform drug development and testing is how to integrate a lot of information into a meaningful and manageable unit. For "omics" data to be meaningful and to revolutionise clinical medicine, clinical phenotype data has to be integrated with genomic, transcriptomic, proteomic and epigenomic data [33,193,209].

4. Automating Natural Product Drug Discovery

Automation is usually associated with negative feelings, with many people associating automation with loss of jobs and unfounded consequences such as robots taking over the world. In terms of drugs discovery automation, however, it has been used successfully to speed-up the process. Indeed many pharmaceutical companies already have high-throughput assays robustly used in the drug discovery process [210]. The design of most synthetic compounds is aided by computers using various softwares, as well as the synthesis of the compounds. Examples of softwares used during drug design include ADAM and EVE, used in target and hit finding [211,212]. New softwares and devices are being made to reduce problematic false positives an also to reduce material consumption during compound design, synthesis and biological testing [213]. For example, integrated microfluidics systems, with the ability to handle liquids and heat necessary for during-synthesis analyses and purification, are being designed by laboratories and pharmaceutical companies, for compound screening and synthesis of compounds [214,215]. This has allowed testing of several hypotheses within days. Even more advanced technologies through the use of artificial intelligence (AI) and 'organ-on-chip' technologies are now fully integrated in the drug discovery process, aiding scientists during drug design and optimisation of the drug discovery process [213,216–219]. All these technologies have allowed the reduction of human mistakes and bias commonly made during drug design and optimisation, reduction in the amount of candidate compound needed for the testing, have reduced the time needed for testing of candidate compounds to days and allowed the recapitulation of disease biology more effectively than in vitro assays [220,221]. Many times, innovation and technological advances have raised false hopes and never lived up to expectations. Automation and innovation in drug discovery must be fast, but also sustainable in the long run [33,222].

Several factors are taken into consideration during compound or molecule design. These include absorption, distribution, metabolism, excretion and toxicity (ADMET) properties and the final biological activity of the products. Thus, the optimisation of the drug discovery process is multidimensional. In the end, a balance has to be achieved in order to get the best in terms of compound activity and properties [213]. Automation will allow scientists to make the best decision regarding the best compound design with relevant biological activity whilst at the same time having desirable ADMET properties. Several concepts such as the diversity-oriented synthesis (DOS) and biology-oriented synthesis (BIOS) have been developed over the past few years to aid compound design and increasing compound collections with new chemical structures and constituents [223–228]. An even advanced concept is the function-oriented synthesis which seeks to mimic the function of a promising compound in order to get simple scaffolds and make their synthesis easier and simple [213,229,230]. Several automated compound generators that use deep learning techniques have been made and have allowed automated analysis of generated compounds to obtain even better designs of compounds with desired properties and biological activity [216,217,231,232]. Although deep learning models are used mainly to predict drug-target interactions and in the generation of new molecules, these models are also useful to predict ADMET properties of novel candidate drugs [233,234]. Several deep learning models have also been used to predict the binding affinity for candidate compounds during drug discovery [234]. Several compounds based on the imidazopyridine scaffold have been synthesised using automated computer-assisted de novo design resulting in the discovery of many ligands for G protein-coupled receptors antagonists [213,235,236]. It is also possible to use a virtual library enumeration parallel to target panel prediction to design a compound library and building block selection. Using integration of computational activity prediction and microfluidics-assisted synthesis enabled scientists to identify ligands with different binding profiles [236–239]. Thus, microfluidics synthesis and computer-aided target prediction can be used to generate bioactivity-focussed compound libraries rapidly and efficiently [235].

An important part of automation of compound synthesis is the availability and use of building blocks and chemical reactions that can result in diverse by-products. The use of small volumes of the starting compounds and compact synthesis coupled with in-line purification and analyses ultimately led to the development of novel machines to synthesise complex structures recapitulating the biosynthesis of most natural compounds [240–242]. Importantly, 3D printing can allow for the building of different microfluidic devices with several sophisticated and specialised algorithms to monitor product synthesis. 3D printing is very important for microfluidics platforms as most microfluidics systems are custom made for a specific function. Some of the latest approaches using automated robotic synthesis are remotely controlled making it even more efficient [243,244]. Some automated compound synthesis approaches are very versatile with only a small set of building blocks being needed to generate a diverse group of by-products [245]. Microfluidics based synthesis of compounds allows the continuous synthesis of compounds and not batch-wise. Cytochrome P450-catalysed drug oxidation can now be simulated meaning that in future on-chip chemotransformations of compounds can replace in vitro metabolite identification [246,247]. Microfluidics synthesis of compounds, coupled with in-process analysis and purification, is revolutionising drug discovery automation [248]. Besides the obvious avoidance of human exposure to chemicals and dangerous solutions, microfluidics also allows the use of minimum amounts of compounds and reagents [249–251]. Given that most animal models are very poor predictors of human response to drugs and biological testing, microfluidic systems can aid in recapitulating human- and species-specific functions by incorporating organoid-based approaches. This allows for the generation of physiological relevant environments within the microfluidic devices and these can be stable over some time [252,253]. Several systems incorporating cancer cells or 3D cancer models have been developed and allow for the recapitulation of human tumours and their microenvironments [254–256]. Several constraints do exist for continuous flow systems such as microfluidics synthesis of compounds. The synthesis and eventual deposition of reactive reagents and by-products brings about the danger of fluidic surfaces instability as some of the reagents and solutions used in compound synthesis are incompatible with the microfluidic systems. In addition, clogging of channels of the microfluidic system is a major problem.

Several integrated microfluidics-assisted synthesise and test platforms are now available combining the reagent and compound selection and can adapt based on materials available for the subsequent steps during synthesis and testing of compounds. Several computational tools and networks (containing millions of reactions and pathways for compound synthesis) used for automated compound synthesis have been developed and aid in finding the optimal and innovative route to compound synthesis [257–260]. Drug design with the help of artificial intelligence is a requirement to have a sustainable drug discovery process [261–264]. Hypothesis generation if done by machines can result in the designing of compounds using several criteria at the same time. Such criteria can be biological activity, side-effects and synthesizability. Machine-guided hypothesis or generation of compound structures is also much faster and can generate different designs at the same time. Artificial intelligence is therefore an enabling technology, aiding the scientist in pattern recognition and can be optimised to do pattern recognition [265–267].

5. Computer-Aided Drug Design from Natural Products

Synthetic compounds with structures inspired by natural products can help solve many global health challenges while in many instances some of the new synthetic compounds would have been discarded as not suitable for drug designs. The so called "rule of three" and "rule of five" criteria often used for decision making with regard to drug leads is too strict and some of the new designs would have been failed [268–272]. In fact, many of the guidelines used during drug designing show human bias and therefore are limited in their scope and effectiveness, especially when applied to natural products [269–272]. Many therapeutic synthetic compounds have been developed using computer-aided designs and these include several anticancer agents [273–276]. The Scaffold Hunter software for example was used to simplify complex natural products to generate virtual fragments of small chemically attractive molecules [277]. The simple molecules visualised by such computational software must retain the same biological activity as the mother compound. Indeed, this method was already used to identify inhibitors and activators of pyruvate kinase [278]. However, it is also possible that natural-product derived simple molecules will exhibit weaker activities than the parent compound [275,276]. The PASS software has been used to predict the biological activities of simple structures or chemical structures obtained from the mother compound with considerable success [279,280]. The PASS software has predicted the anti-tumour activities of several marine alkaloids [278–280].

Indeed several individual compounds from St John's wort were also predicted rightly to have cytochrome P450 modulating effects [278]. Several computational softwares, databases and web servers have been developed that can predict compound-target associations. Most if not all of these softwares use the similarity of new compound to known drugs to infer target and normal ligand–receptor docking. In the absence of any similarity between new compound and any known drug, the SPIDER software can compare computed features between natural products and new compound to predict the target of the new compound [281,282]. The identification of G-protein coupled receptor ligands was one of the success stories of the SPIDER software [282]. The use of computational drug design and target prediction is now tangible and will continue to influence drug development in the near future. However only previously studied targets or proteins can be predicted. Computer based quantitative structure activity approaches can be employed in natural product drug discovery to explain the molecular basis of their therapeutic values and to predict possible derivatives that would improve activity [283]. The positive aspect of computer-based drug designs is that it guides optimization of lead compounds as to whether to increase their affinity or pharmacodynamic and pharmacokinetic properties.

New systems are being developed in order to detect candidate or lead compound toxicity at early stages of drug discovery [284–287]. Strategies employing in silico methods can be used to detect drug toxicity early on along the drug discovery process. Such approaches if combined with in vitro and in vivo biological testing can drastically decrease the time and cost of drug discovery and improve safety evaluation. Quantitative structure–activity relationship models aim to understand the relationship between the structure of a compound and its toxicity [288–291]. To understand the possible accumulation of the drug and its metabolism properties such as adsorption, distribution, metabolism and excretion must be evaluated [292–295]. To compound the issue of candidate compound toxicity, one has to consider environmental toxicity. So, during drug discovery the potential risk of having a drug in the environment must be addressed. These candidate compounds or lead compounds may have toxic effects on other animals.

The advent of advanced technologies has allowed scientists to discover the magnitude of tumour heterogeneity and the different patients' responses to treatment [296–299]. Drug discovery however is based on the "one drug-one target" strategy. It is a fact that combination therapy is the gold standard nowadays. Thus, drug design must take a combinatorial approach, where two or more drugs either target the same pathway or act synergistically to achieve a cure. Conventional chemotherapeutic agents may be combined with targeted therapies such as kinase inhibitors [300–304]. Now, a few approaches for computer-based screening for combinatorial drug design and treatment are under development.

6. Natural Products and Precision Medicine

The past few years have seen genomics informing drug discovery but overall the clinical efficacy of the resultant drugs has been poor. This is largely due to the complex nature of diseases. Advances in technological and analytical tools used in genomics now allow for the rapid identification and interpretation of genetic differences driving patient specific features of disease (Figure 4) [33,222]. Precision medicine would then target these specific features to obtain a cure. At the heart of the Human Genome project lies the need to understand how genetics impacts disease and vice versa. For oncologists and cancer scientists, how genetics can transform drug discovery has generated a lot of excitement. The rapid development of many new techniques now allows the analysis of patients' and healthy individuals genomes (Figure 4). Importantly it is possible to link a patient's genome and clinical presentation [305]. Investigations of whether specific proteins are drug targets culminated in many drugs in use today. Over time however, productivity in terms of drugs produced declined as there were no more definite new drug targets. The "gene to screen" approach was based on the realisation that genes expressed within a cell are the main contributor to the overall cellular phenotype [306,307]. Genome-wide association studies (GWAS) is a cost-effective and unbiased way of genotyping and comparison of genomic variations between patients with disease and healthy individuals. GWAS has led to the identification of genetic determinants of diseases and underlying mechanisms driving disease development.

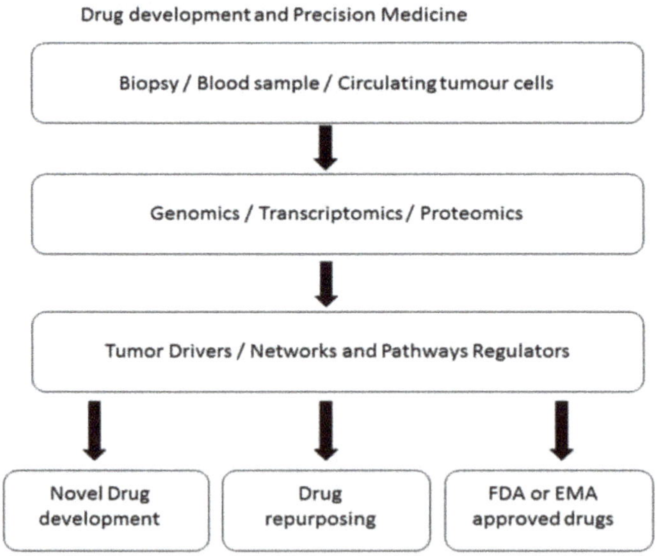

Figure 4. Precision therapies in oncology can be designed to only affect cancer cells. Biomarkers can be identified through next generation sequencing, gene expression profiling and proteomics. Drivers and regulators of important pathways involved in cancer cell proliferation, survival and chemoresistance can be identified. Only with this knowledge can the development of novel drugs be achieved.

7. Conclusions

The low success rate of drug discovery requires a paradigm shift for innovative drug development strategies. Innovative drug discovery starts by deriving inspiration from natural products for effective treatment of disease conditions. The relevance of natural products in providing innovative drugs to find solutions to communicable and non-communicable diseases cannot be over-emphasized. Technological advances have made it possible to understand the profiles of these complex natural products with the potential to discover new drugs for use. An impressive number of blockbuster drugs have been isolated or synthesized from natural product lead compounds. This positions natural product drug discovery as a very successful strategy for the development of novel therapeutic drugs. In this era of advancing scientific technology, innovative drug discovery from natural products will potentially increase the success rate of new therapeutic moieties. Natural product drug discovery stands as a major contributor to solving global health challenges and achieving sustainable development goals on health.

Author Contributions: N.E.T. and K.D. wrote the main body of the Review manuscript. All authors reviewed and commented the manuscript.

Acknowledgments: The funding for this research was provided by the National Research Foundation (NRF) of South Africa (Grant Number: 91457: RCA13101656402), International Centre for Genetic Engineering and Biotechnology (ICGEB) (Grant Number: 2015/0001), Faculty of Health Sciences, UCT and the University of Cape Town.

Conflicts of Interest: The authors declare no conflict of interest.

References

1. Weng, J.K.; Philippe, R.N.; Noel, J.P. The rise of chemodiversity in plants. *Science* **2012**, *336*, 1667–1670. [CrossRef] [PubMed]
2. Lietava, J. Medicinal plants in a Middle Paleolithic grave Shanidar IV? *J. Ethnopharmacol.* **1992**, *35*, 263–266. [CrossRef]
3. Ernst, M.; Grace, O.M.; Saslis-Lagoudakis, C.H.; Nilsson, N.; Simonsen, H.T.; Ronsted, N. Global medicinal uses of *Euphorbia* L. (*Euphorbiaceae*). *J. Ethnopharmacol.* **2015**, *176*, 90–101. [CrossRef] [PubMed]
4. Gozubuyuk, G.S.; Aktas, E.; Yigit, N. An ancient plant *Lawsonia inermis* (henna): Determination of in vitro antifungal activity against dermatophytes species. *J. Mycol. Med.* **2014**, *24*, 313–318. [CrossRef] [PubMed]
5. Hotwani, K.; Baliga, S.; Sharma, K. Phytodentistry: Use of medicinal plants. *J. Complement. Integr. Med.* **2014**, *11*, 233–251. [CrossRef] [PubMed]
6. Liu, Q.; Lawrence, A.J.; Liang, J.H. Traditional Chinese medicine for treatment of alcoholism: From ancient to modern. *Am. J. Chin. Med.* **2011**, *39*, 1–13. [CrossRef] [PubMed]
7. Mannangatti, P.; Naidu, K.N. Indian herbs for the treatment of neurodegenerative disease. *Adv. Neurobiol.* **2016**, *12*, 323–336. [PubMed]
8. McGovern, P.E.; Mirzoian, A.; Hall, G.R. Ancient Egyptian herbal wines. *Proc. Natl. Acad. Sci. USA* **2009**, *106*, 7361–7366. [CrossRef] [PubMed]
9. Blunt, J.W.; Carroll, A.R.; Copp, B.R.; Davis, R.A.; Keyzers, R.A.; Prinsep, M.R. Marine natural products. *Nat. Prod. Rep.* **2018**, *35*, 8–53. [CrossRef] [PubMed]
10. Harvey, A.L. Natural products in drug discovery. *Drug Discov. Today* **2008**, *13*, 894–901. [CrossRef] [PubMed]
11. Harvey, A.L.; Clark, R.L.; Mackay, S.P.; Johnston, B.F. Current strategies for drug discovery through natural products. *Expert Opin. Drug Discov.* **2010**, *5*, 559–568. [CrossRef] [PubMed]
12. Harvey, A.L.; Edrada-Ebel, R.; Quinn, R.J. The re-emergence of natural products for drug discovery in the genomics era. *Nat. Rev. Drug Discov.* **2015**, *14*, 111–129. [CrossRef] [PubMed]
13. Chang, J.; Kim, Y.; Kwon, H.J. Advances in identification and validation of protein targets of natural products without chemical modification. *Nat. Prod. Rep.* **2016**, *33*, 719–730. [CrossRef] [PubMed]
14. Tansaz, M.; Tajadini, H. Comparison of leiomyoma of modern medicine and traditional Persian medicine. *J. Evid.-Based Complement. Altern. Med.* **2016**, *21*, 160–163. [CrossRef] [PubMed]
15. Xu, Q.; Bauer, R.; Hendry, B.M.; Fan, T.P.; Zhao, Z.; Duez, P.; Simmonds, M.S.; Witt, C.M.; Lu, A.; Robinson, N.; et al. The quest for modernisation of traditional Chinese medicine. *BMC Complement. Altern. Med.* **2013**, *13*, 132. [CrossRef] [PubMed]
16. Yuan, H.; Ma, Q.; Ye, L.; Piao, G. The traditional medicine and modern medicine from natural products. *Molecules* **2016**, *21*, 559. [CrossRef] [PubMed]
17. Banjari, I.; Misir, A.; Savikin, K.; Jokic, S.; Molnar, M.; De Zoysa, H.K.S.; Waisundara, V.Y. Antidiabetic effects of *Aronia melanocarpa* and its other therapeutic properties. *Front. Nutr.* **2017**, *4*, 53. [CrossRef] [PubMed]

18. Yatoo, M.I.; Dimri, U.; Gopalakrishnan, A.; Karthik, K.; Gopi, M.; Khandia, R.; Saminathan, M.; Saxena, A.; Alagawany, M.; Farag, M.R.; et al. Beneficial health applications and medicinal values of pedicularis plants: A review. *Biomed. Pharmacother.* **2017**, *95*, 1301–1313. [CrossRef] [PubMed]
19. Thomford, N.E.; Awortwe, C.; Dzobo, K.; Adu, F.; Chopera, D.; Wonkam, A.; Skelton, M.; Blackhurst, D.; Dandara, C. Inhibition of cyp2b6 by medicinal plant extracts: Implication for use of efavirenz and nevirapine-based highly active anti-retroviral therapy (HAART) in resource-limited settings. *Molecules* **2016**, *21*, 211. [CrossRef] [PubMed]
20. Thomford, N.E.; Dzobo, K.; Chopera, D.; Wonkam, A.; Maroyi, A.; Blackhurst, D.; Dandara, C. In vitro reversible and time-dependent cyp450 inhibition profiles of medicinal herbal plant extracts *Newbouldia laevis* and *Cassia abbreviata*: Implications for herb-drug interactions. *Molecules* **2016**, *21*, 891. [CrossRef] [PubMed]
21. Thomford, N.E.; Dzobo, K.; Chopera, D.; Wonkam, A.; Skelton, M.; Blackhurst, D.; Chirikure, S.; Dandara, C. Pharmacogenomics implications of using herbal medicinal plants on African populations in health transition. *Pharmaceuticals* **2015**, *8*, 637–663. [CrossRef] [PubMed]
22. Thomford, N.E.; Mkhize, B.; Dzobo, K.; Mpye, K.; Rowe, A.; Parker, M.I.; Wonkam, A.; Skelton, M.; September, A.V.; Dandara, C. African lettuce (*Launaea taraxacifolia*) displays possible anticancer effects and herb-drug interaction potential by CYP1A2, CYP2C9, and CYP2C19 inhibition. *Omics* **2016**, *20*, 528–537. [CrossRef] [PubMed]
23. Ji, S.; Fattahi, A.; Raffel, N.; Hoffmann, I.; Beckmann, M.W.; Dittrich, R.; Schrauder, M. Antioxidant effect of aqueous extract of four plants with therapeutic potential on gynecological diseases; semen persicae, *Leonurus cardiaca*, *Hedyotis diffusa*, and *Curcuma zedoaria*. *Eur. J. Med. Res.* **2017**, *22*, 50. [CrossRef] [PubMed]
24. Ruhsam, M.; Hollingsworth, P.M. Authentication of eleutherococcus and rhodiola herbal supplement products in the United Kingdom. *J. Pharm. Biomed. Anal.* **2017**, *149*, 403–409. [CrossRef] [PubMed]
25. Patridge, E.; Gareiss, P.; Kinch, M.S.; Hoyer, D. An analysis of FDA-approved drugs: Natural products and their derivatives. *Drug Discov. Today* **2016**, *21*, 204–207. [CrossRef] [PubMed]
26. Wani, M.C.; Taylor, H.L.; Wall, M.E.; Coggon, P.; McPhail, A.T. Plant antitumor agents. VI. The isolation and structure of taxol, a novel antileukemic and antitumor agent from *Taxus brevifolia*. *J. Am. Chem. Soc.* **1971**, *93*, 2325–2327. [CrossRef] [PubMed]
27. Newman, D.J.; Cragg, G.M. Natural products as sources of new drugs over the 30 years from 1981 to 2010. *J. Nat. Prod.* **2012**, *75*, 311–335. [CrossRef] [PubMed]
28. Carter, G.T. Natural products and Pharma 2011: Strategic changes spur new opportunities. *Nat. Prod. Rep.* **2011**, *28*, 1783–1789. [CrossRef] [PubMed]
29. Li, J.W.; Vederas, J.C. Drug discovery and natural products: End of an era or an endless frontier? *Science* **2009**, *325*, 161–165. [CrossRef] [PubMed]
30. Li, F.S.; Weng, J.K. Demystifying traditional herbal medicine with modern approach. *Nat. Plants* **2017**, *3*, 17109. [CrossRef] [PubMed]
31. Kiyohara, H.; Matsumoto, T.; Yamada, H. Combination effects of herbs in a multi-herbal formula: Expression of juzen-taiho-to's immuno-modulatory activity on the intestinal immune system. *Evid.-Based Complement. Altern. Med.* **2004**, *1*, 83–91. [CrossRef] [PubMed]
32. Leonti, M.; Verpoorte, R. Traditional Mediterranean and European herbal medicines. *J. Ethnopharmacol.* **2017**, *199*, 161–167. [CrossRef] [PubMed]
33. Ozdemir, V.; Hekim, N. Birth of industry 5.0: Making sense of big data with artificial intelligence, "the internet of things" and next-generation technology policy. *Omics* **2018**, *22*, 65–76. [CrossRef] [PubMed]
34. Özdemir, V. Omics 2.0: An accelerator for global science, systems medicine and responsible innovation. *Omics* **2015**, *19*, 579–580. [CrossRef] [PubMed]
35. Wall, M.E.; Wani, M.C.; Brown, D.M.; Fullas, F.; Olwald, J.B.; Josephson, F.F.; Thornton, N.M.; Pezzuto, J.M.; Beecher, C.W.; Farnsworth, N.R.; et al. Effect of tannins on screening of plant extracts for enzyme inhibitory activity and techniques for their removal. *Phytomedicine* **1996**, *3*, 281–285. [CrossRef]
36. Eldridge, G.R.; Vervoort, H.C.; Lee, C.M.; Cremin, P.A.; Williams, C.T.; Hart, S.M.; Goering, M.G.; O'Neil-Johnson, M.; Zeng, L. High-throughput method for the production and analysis of large natural product libraries for drug discovery. *Anal. Chem.* **2002**, *74*, 3963–3971. [CrossRef] [PubMed]
37. Wu, S.; Liang, J. Counter-current chromatography for high throughput analysis of natural products. *Comb. Chem. High Throughput Screen.* **2010**, *13*, 932–942. [CrossRef] [PubMed]

38. Bugni, T.S.; Richards, B.; Bhoite, L.; Cimbora, D.; Harper, M.K.; Ireland, C.M. Marine natural product libraries for high-throughput screening and rapid drug discovery. *J. Nat. Prod.* **2008**, *71*, 1095–1098. [CrossRef] [PubMed]
39. Koehn, F.E. High impact technologies for natural products screening. In *Natural Compounds as Drugs Volume I*; Birkhäuser: Basel, Switzerland, 2008; Volume 65, pp. 175–210.
40. Wong, W.R.; Oliver, A.G.; Linington, R.G. Development of antibiotic activity profile screening for the classification and discovery of natural product antibiotics. *Chem. Biol.* **2012**, *19*, 1483–1495. [CrossRef] [PubMed]
41. He, G.; Yin, Y.; Yan, X.; Wang, Y. Semi-bionic extraction of effective ingredient from fishbone by high intensity pulsed electric fields. *J. Food Process Eng.* **2017**, *40*, e12392. [CrossRef]
42. Yoshioka, T.; Nagatomi, Y.; Harayama, K.; Bamba, T. Development of an analytical method for polycyclic aromatic hydrocarbons in coffee beverages and dark beer using novel high-sensitivity technique of supercritical fluid chromatography/mass spectrometry. *J. Biosci. Bioeng.* **2018**. [CrossRef] [PubMed]
43. Hofstetter, R.; Fassauer, G.M.; Link, A. Supercritical fluid extraction (SFE) of ketamine metabolites from dried urine and on-line quantification by supercritical fluid chromatography and single mass detection (on-line SFE–SFC–MS). *J. Chromatogr. B* **2018**, *1076*, 77–83. [CrossRef] [PubMed]
44. Morales, D.; Piris, A.J.; Ruiz-Rodriguez, A.; Prodanov, M.; Soler-Rivas, C. Extraction of bioactive compounds against cardiovascular diseases from *Lentinula edodes* using a sequential extraction method. *Biotechnol. Prog.* **2018**. [CrossRef] [PubMed]
45. Joana Gil-Chávez, G.; Villa, J.A.; Fernando Ayala-Zavala, J.; Basilio Heredia, J.; Sepulveda, D.; Yahia, E.M.; González-Aguilar, G.A. Technologies for extraction and production of bioactive compounds to be used as nutraceuticals and food ingredients: An overview. *Compr. Rev. Food Sci. Food Saf.* **2013**, *12*, 5–23. [CrossRef]
46. De Morais, S.R.; Oliveira, T.L.; de Oliveira, L.P.; Tresvenzol, L.M.; da Conceicao, E.C.; Rezende, M.H.; Fiuza, T.S.; Costa, E.A.; Ferri, P.H.; de Paula, J.R. Essential oil composition, antimicrobial and pharmacological activities of *Lippia sidoides* cham. (verbenaceae) from Sao Goncalo do Abaete, Minas Gerais, Brazil. *Pharmacogn. Mag.* **2016**, *12*, 262–270. [PubMed]
47. Gan, Z.; Liang, Z.; Chen, X.; Wen, X.; Wang, Y.; Li, M.; Ni, Y. Separation and preparation of 6-gingerol from molecular distillation residue of Yunnan ginger rhizomes by high-speed counter-current chromatography and the antioxidant activity of ginger oils in vitro. *J. Chromatogr. B Anal. Technol. Biomed. Life Sci.* **2016**, *1011*, 99–107. [CrossRef] [PubMed]
48. Zhang, L.; Mei, J.; Xie, Y.; Li, M.; Liu, D.; He, C. Application of membrane separation technology in extraction process of Chuanxiong Chatiao granules. *Zhongguo Zhong yao za zhi = Zhongguo zhongyao zazhi = China J. Chin. Mater. Med.* **2012**, *37*, 934–936.
49. Williams, S.; Oatley, D.; Abdrahman, A.; Butt, T.; Nash, R. Membrane technology for the improved separation of bioactive compounds. *Procedia Eng.* **2012**, *44*, 2112–2114. [CrossRef]
50. Wang, H.; Jiang, Y.; Ding, M.; Li, J.; Hao, J.; He, J.; Wang, H.; Gao, X.M.; Chang, Y.X. Simultaneous determination and qualitative analysis of six types of components in Naoxintong capsule by miniaturized matrix solid-phase dispersion extraction coupled with ultra high-performance liquid chromatography with photodiode array detection and quadrupole time-of-flight mass spectrometry. *J. Sep. Sci.* **2018**. [CrossRef]
51. Zhang, L.; Ge, Y.; Li, J.; Hao, J.; Wang, H.; He, J.; Gao, X.M.; Chang, Y.X. Simultaneous determination of columbianetin-beta-d-glucopyranoside and columbianetin in a biological sample by high-performance liquid chromatography with fluorescence detection and identification of other columbianetin-beta-d-glucopyranoside metabolites by ultra high-performance liquid chromatography coupled with quadrupole-time of flight mass spectrometry. *J. Pharm. Biomed. Anal.* **2018**, *153*, 221–231. [PubMed]
52. Manglik, A.; Kruse, A.C.; Kobilka, T.S.; Thian, F.S.; Mathiesen, J.M.; Sunahara, R.K.; Pardo, L.; Weis, W.I.; Kobilka, B.K.; Granier, S. Crystal structure of the micro-opioid receptor bound to a morphinan antagonist. *Nature* **2012**, *485*, 321–326. [CrossRef] [PubMed]
53. Edwards, G. Forces of habit: Drugs and the making of the modern world. *Addiction* **2002**, *97*, 608–609. [CrossRef]
54. Zhao, L.; Li, C.; Zhang, Y.; Wen, Q.; Ren, D. Phytochemical and biological activities of an anticancer plant medicine: *Brucea javanica*. *Anti-Cancer Agents Med. Chem.* **2014**, *14*, 440–458. [CrossRef]

55. Tu, Y. The discovery of artemisinin (qinghaosu) and gifts from Chinese medicine. *Nat. Med.* **2011**, *17*, 1217–1220. [CrossRef] [PubMed]
56. Tu, Y. Artemisinin—A gift from traditional Chinese medicine to the world (Nobel lecture). *Angew. Chem. Int. Ed. Engl.* **2016**, *55*, 10210–10226. [CrossRef] [PubMed]
57. Li, J.; Casteels, T.; Frogne, T.; Ingvorsen, C.; Honoré, C.; Courtney, M.; Huber, K.V.M.; Schmitner, N.; Kimmel, R.A.; Romanov, R.A.; et al. Artemisinins target $GABA_A$ receptor signaling and impair α cell identity. *Cell* **2017**, *168*, 86–100. [CrossRef] [PubMed]
58. Lai, H.; Singh, N.P. Oral artemisinin prevents and delays the development of 7,12-dimethylbenz[a]anthracene (dmba)-induced breast cancer in the rat. *Cancer Lett.* **2006**, *231*, 43–48. [CrossRef] [PubMed]
59. Lai, H.C.; Singh, N.P.; Sasaki, T. Development of artemisinin compounds for cancer treatment. *Investig. New Drugs* **2013**, *31*, 230–246. [CrossRef] [PubMed]
60. Return to Rio: Second chance for the planet. *Nature* **2012**, *486*, 19.
61. Barbault, R. 2010: A new beginning for biodiversity? *C.R. Biol.* **2011**, *334*, 483–488. [CrossRef] [PubMed]
62. Salazar, R.; Cabrera, J.A. Intellectual property rights in Costa Rica in the light of the biodiversity convention. *J. Ethnopharmacol.* **1996**, *51*, 177–193. [CrossRef]
63. Samper, C. Taxonomy and environmental policy. *Philos. Trans. R. Soc. Lond. B Biol. Sci.* **2004**, *359*, 721–728. [CrossRef] [PubMed]
64. Seidl, P.R. Pharmaceuticals from natural products: Current trends. *Anais da Academia Brasileira de Ciencias* **2002**, *74*, 145–150. [CrossRef] [PubMed]
65. Tollefson, J.; Gilbert, N. Earth summit: Rio report card. *Nature* **2012**, *486*, 20–23. [CrossRef] [PubMed]
66. Wen, M.C.; Wei, C.H.; Hu, Z.Q.; Srivastava, K.; Ko, J.; Xi, S.T.; Mu, D.Z.; Du, J.B.; Li, G.H.; Wallenstein, S.; et al. Efficacy and tolerability of anti-asthma herbal medicine intervention in adult patients with moderate-severe allergic asthma. *J. Allergy Clin. Immunol.* **2005**, *116*, 517–524. [CrossRef] [PubMed]
67. Srivastava, K.; Sampson, H.A.; Charles, W.; Emala, S.; Li, X.-M. The anti-asthma herbal medicine ashmi acutely inhibits airway smooth muscle contraction via prostaglandin e2 activation of ep2/ep4 receptors. *Am. J. Physiol.-Lung Cell. Mol. Physiol.* **2013**, *305*, L1002–L1010. [CrossRef] [PubMed]
68. Yang, N.; Liang, B.; Srivastava, K.; Zeng, J.; Zhan, J.; Brown, L.; Sampson, H.; Goldfarb, J.; Emala, C.; Li, X.M. The *Sophora flavescens* flavonoid compound trifolirhizin inhibits acetylcholine induced airway smooth muscle contraction. *Phytochemistry* **2013**, *95*, 259–267. [CrossRef] [PubMed]
69. Chan, K.; Shaw, D.; Simmonds, M.S.; Leon, C.J.; Xu, Q.; Lu, A.; Sutherland, I.; Ignatova, S.; Zhu, Y.P.; Verpoorte, R.; et al. Good practice in reviewing and publishing studies on herbal medicine, with special emphasis on traditional Chinese medicine and Chinese materia medica. *J. Ethnopharmacol.* **2012**, *140*, 469–475. [CrossRef] [PubMed]
70. Skroza, D.; Generalić Mekinić, I.; Svilović, S.; Šimat, V.; Katalinić, V. Investigation of the potential synergistic effect of resveratrol with other phenolic compounds: A case of binary phenolic mixtures. *J. Food Compos. Anal.* **2015**, *38*, 13–18. [CrossRef]
71. Chusri, S.; Siriyong, T.; Na-Phatthalung, P.; Voravuthikunchai, S.P. Synergistic effects of ethnomedicinal plants of *Apocynaceae* family and antibiotics against clinical isolates of *Acinetobacter baumannii*. *Asian Pac. J. Trop. Med.* **2014**, *7*, 456–461. [CrossRef]
72. Sharma, G.; Tyagi, A.K.; Singh, R.P.; Chan, D.C.; Agarwal, R. Synergistic anti-cancer effects of grape seed extract and conventional cytotoxic agent doxorubicin against human breast carcinoma cells. *Breast Cancer Res. Treat.* **2004**, *85*, 1–12. [CrossRef] [PubMed]
73. Medema, M.H.; Fischbach, M.A. Computational approaches to natural product discovery. *Nat. Chem. Biol.* **2015**, *11*, 639–648. [CrossRef] [PubMed]
74. Kim, E.; Moore, B.S.; Yoon, Y.J. Reinvigorating natural product combinatorial biosynthesis with synthetic biology. *Nat. Chem. Biol.* **2015**, *11*, 649–659. [CrossRef] [PubMed]
75. Akbulut, Y.; Gaunt, H.J.; Muraki, K.; Ludlow, M.J.; Amer, M.S.; Bruns, A.; Vasudev, N.S.; Radtke, L.; Willot, M.; Hahn, S.; et al. (-)-Englerin A is a potent and selective activator of TRPC4 and TRPC5 calcium channels. *Angew. Chem. Int. Ed. Engl.* **2015**, *54*, 3787–3791. [CrossRef] [PubMed]
76. Ludlow, M.J.; Gaunt, H.J.; Rubaiy, H.N.; Musialowski, K.E.; Blythe, N.M.; Vasudev, N.S.; Muraki, K.; Beech, D.J. (-)-Englerin A-evoked cytotoxicity is mediated by Na^+ influx and counteracted by Na^+/K^+-atpase. *J. Biol. Chem.* **2017**, *292*, 723–731. [CrossRef] [PubMed]

77. Muraki, K.; Ohnishi, K.; Takezawa, A.; Suzuki, H.; Hatano, N.; Muraki, Y.; Hamzah, N.; Foster, R.; Waldmann, H.; Nussbaumer, P.; et al. Na(+) entry through heteromeric TRPC4/C1 channels mediates (-)Englerin A-induced cytotoxicity in synovial sarcoma cells. *Sci. Rep.* **2017**, *7*, 16988. [CrossRef] [PubMed]
78. Buriani, A.; Garcia-Bermejo, M.L.; Bosisio, E.; Xu, Q.; Li, H.; Dong, X.; Simmonds, M.S.; Carrara, M.; Tejedor, N.; Lucio-Cazana, J.; et al. Omic techniques in systems biology approaches to traditional Chinese medicine research: Present and future. *J. Ethnopharmacol.* **2012**, *140*, 535–544. [CrossRef] [PubMed]
79. Ganie, S.H.; Upadhyay, P.; Das, S.; Prasad Sharma, M. Authentication of medicinal plants by DNA markers. *Plant Gene* **2015**, *4*, 83–99. [CrossRef]
80. Ghorbani, A.; Saeedi, Y.; de Boer, H.J. Unidentifiable by morphology: DNA barcoding of plant material in local markets in Iran. *PLoS ONE* **2017**, *12*, e0175722. [CrossRef] [PubMed]
81. Thompson, K.A.; Newmaster, S.G. Molecular taxonomic tools provide more accurate estimates of species richness at less cost than traditional morphology-based taxonomic practices in a vegetation survey. *Biodivers. Conserv.* **2014**, *23*, 1411–1424. [CrossRef]
82. Cao, M.; Wang, J.; Yao, L.; Xie, S.; Du, J.; Zhao, X. Authentication of animal signatures in traditional Chinese medicine of Lingyang Qingfei Wan using routine molecular diagnostic assays. *Mol. Biol. Rep.* **2014**, *41*, 2485–2491. [CrossRef] [PubMed]
83. Newmaster, S.G.; Grguric, M.; Shanmughanandhan, D.; Ramalingam, S.; Ragupathy, S. DNA barcoding detects contamination and substitution in North American herbal products. *BMC Med.* **2013**, *11*, 222. [CrossRef] [PubMed]
84. Mishra, P.; Kumar, A.; Nagireddy, A.; Mani, D.N.; Shukla, A.K.; Tiwari, R.; Sundaresan, V. DNA barcoding: An efficient tool to overcome authentication challenges in the herbal market. *Plant Biotechnol. J.* **2016**, *14*, 8–21. [CrossRef] [PubMed]
85. Chen, X.; Xiang, L.; Shi, L.; Li, G.; Yao, H.; Han, J.; Lin, Y.; Song, J.; Chen, S. Identification of crude drugs in the Japanese pharmacopoeia using a DNA barcoding system. *Sci. Rep.* **2017**, *7*, 42325. [CrossRef] [PubMed]
86. Pulice, G.; Pelaz, S.; Matías-Hernández, L. Molecular farming in *Artemisia annua*, a promising approach to improve anti-malarial drug production. *Front. Plant Sci.* **2016**, *7*, 329. [CrossRef] [PubMed]
87. Gantait, S.; Debnath, S.; Nasim Ali, M. Genomic profile of the plants with pharmaceutical value. *3 Biotech* **2014**, *4*, 563–578. [CrossRef] [PubMed]
88. Lv, C.; Wu, X.; Wang, X.; Su, J.; Zeng, H.; Zhao, J.; Lin, S.; Liu, R.; Li, H.; Li, X.; et al. The gene expression profiles in response to 102 traditional Chinese medicine (TCM) components: A general template for research on TCMs. *Sci. Rep.* **2017**, *7*, 352. [CrossRef] [PubMed]
89. Lee, K.-H.; Lo, H.-L.; Tang, W.-C.; Hsiao, H.H.-Y.; Yang, P.-M. A gene expression signature-based approach reveals the mechanisms of action of the Chinese herbal medicine Berberine. *Sci. Rep.* **2014**, *4*, 6394. [CrossRef] [PubMed]
90. Kiyama, R. DNA microarray-based screening and characterization of traditional Chinese medicine. *Microarrays* **2017**, *6*, 4. [CrossRef] [PubMed]
91. Jones, M.J.; Goodman, S.J.; Kobor, M.S. DNA methylation and healthy human aging. *Aging Cell* **2015**, *14*, 924–932. [CrossRef] [PubMed]
92. Kelly, T.K.; Liu, Y.; Lay, F.D.; Liang, G.; Berman, B.P.; Jones, P.A. Genome-wide mapping of nucleosome positioning and DNA methylation within individual DNA molecules. *Genome Res.* **2012**, *22*, 2497–2506. [CrossRef] [PubMed]
93. Nordlund, J.; Backlin, C.L.; Wahlberg, P.; Busche, S.; Berglund, E.C.; Eloranta, M.L.; Flaegstad, T.; Forestier, E.; Frost, B.M.; Harila-Saari, A.; et al. Genome-wide signatures of differential DNA methylation in pediatric acute lymphoblastic leukemia. *Genome Biol.* **2013**, *14*, r105. [CrossRef] [PubMed]
94. Su, J.; Wang, Y.; Xing, X.; Liu, J.; Zhang, Y. Genome-wide analysis of DNA methylation in bovine placentas. *BMC Genom.* **2014**, *15*, 12. [CrossRef] [PubMed]
95. Zykovich, A.; Hubbard, A.; Flynn, J.M.; Tarnopolsky, M.; Fraga, M.F.; Kerksick, C.; Ogborn, D.; MacNeil, L.; Mooney, S.D.; Melov, S. Genome-wide DNA methylation changes with age in disease-free human skeletal muscle. *Aging Cell* **2014**, *13*, 360–366. [CrossRef] [PubMed]
96. Barbosa, S.; Carreira, S.; Bailey, D.; Abaitua, F.; O'Hare, P. Phosphorylation and SCF-mediated degradation regulate CREB-H transcription of metabolic targets. *Mol. Biol. Cell* **2015**, *26*, 2939–2954. [CrossRef] [PubMed]
97. Bose, P.; Vachhani, P.; Cortes, J.E. Treatment of relapsed/refractory acute myeloid leukemia. *Curr. Treat. Options Oncol.* **2017**, *18*, 17. [CrossRef] [PubMed]

98. Ley, T.J.; Miller, C.; Ding, L.; Raphael, B.J.; Mungall, A.J.; Robertson, A.; Hoadley, K.; Triche, T.J., Jr.; Laird, P.W.; Baty, J.D.; et al. Genomic and epigenomic landscapes of adult de novo acute myeloid leukemia. *N. Engl. J. Med.* **2013**, *368*, 2059–2074. [PubMed]
99. Brat, D.J.; Verhaak, R.G.; Aldape, K.D.; Yung, W.K.; Salama, S.R.; Cooper, L.A.; Rheinbay, E.; Miller, C.R.; Vitucci, M.; Morozova, O.; et al. Comprehensive, integrative genomic analysis of diffuse lower-grade gliomas. *N. Engl. J. Med.* **2015**, *372*, 2481–2498. [PubMed]
100. Eckel-Passow, J.E.; Lachance, D.H.; Molinaro, A.M.; Walsh, K.M.; Decker, P.A.; Sicotte, H.; Pekmezci, M.; Rice, T.; Kosel, M.L.; Smirnov, I.V.; et al. Glioma groups based on 1p/19q, *IDH*, and *TERT* promoter mutations in tumors. *N. Engl. J. Med.* **2015**, *372*, 2499–2508. [CrossRef] [PubMed]
101. Mwapagha, L.M.; Tiffin, N.; Parker, M.I. Delineation of the HPV11e6 and HPV18e6 pathways in initiating cellular transformation. *Front. Oncol.* **2017**, *7*, 258. [CrossRef] [PubMed]
102. Vogelsang, M.; Wang, Y.; Veber, N.; Mwapagha, L.M.; Parker, M.I. The cumulative effects of polymorphisms in the DNA mismatch repair genes and tobacco smoking in oesophageal cancer risk. *PLoS ONE* **2012**, *7*, e36962. [CrossRef] [PubMed]
103. Fishilevich, S.; Nudel, R.; Rappaport, N.; Hadar, R.; Plaschkes, I.; Iny Stein, T.; Rosen, N.; Kohn, A.; Twik, M.; Safran, M.; et al. Genehancer: Genome-wide integration of enhancers and target genes in genecards. *Database* **2017**, *2017*. [CrossRef] [PubMed]
104. Guo, X.; Long, J.; Zeng, C.; Michailidou, K.; Ghoussaini, M.; Bolla, M.K.; Wang, Q.; Milne, R.L.; Shu, X.O.; Cai, Q.; et al. Fine-scale mapping of the 4q24 locus identifies two independent loci associated with breast cancer risk. *Cancer Epidemiol. Biomark. Prev.* **2015**, *24*, 1680–1691. [CrossRef] [PubMed]
105. Ombrello, M.J.; Sikora, K.A.; Kastner, D.L. Genetics, genomics, and their relevance to pathology and therapy. *Best Pract. Res. Clin. Rheumatol.* **2014**, *28*, 175–189. [CrossRef] [PubMed]
106. Simmonds, P.; Loomis, E.; Curry, E. DNA methylation-based chromatin compartments and CHIP-seq profiles reveal transcriptional drivers of prostate carcinogenesis. *Genome Med.* **2017**, *9*, 54. [CrossRef] [PubMed]
107. Yang, T.Y.; Hsu, L.I.; Chiu, A.W.; Pu, Y.S.; Wang, S.H.; Liao, Y.T.; Wu, M.M.; Wang, Y.H.; Chang, C.H.; Lee, T.C.; et al. Comparison of genome-wide DNA methylation in urothelial carcinomas of patients with and without arsenic exposure. *Environ. Res.* **2014**, *128*, 57–63. [CrossRef] [PubMed]
108. Mehta, G.; Jalan, R.; Mookerjee, R.P. Cracking the encode: From transcription to therapeutics. *Hepatology* **2013**, *57*, 2532–2535. [CrossRef] [PubMed]
109. Tragante, V.; Moore, J.H.; Asselbergs, F.W. The encode project and perspectives on pathways. *Genet. Epidemiol.* **2014**, *38*, 275–280. [CrossRef] [PubMed]
110. Bumpus, S.B.; Evans, B.S.; Thomas, P.M.; Ntai, I.; Kelleher, N.L. A proteomics approach to discovery of natural products and their biosynthetic pathways. *Nat. Biotechnol.* **2009**, *27*, 951–956. [CrossRef] [PubMed]
111. Martínez-Esteso, M.J.; Martínez-Márquez, A.; Sellés-Marchart, S.; Morante-Carriel, J.A.; Bru-Martínez, R. The role of proteomics in progressing insights into plant secondary metabolism. *Front. Plant Sci.* **2015**, *6*, 504. [CrossRef] [PubMed]
112. Lum, J.H.; Fung, K.L.; Cheung, P.Y.; Wong, M.S.; Lee, C.H.; Kwok, F.S.; Leung, M.C.; Hui, P.K.; Lo, S.C. Proteome of oriental ginseng *Panax ginseng C.A. Meyer* and the potential to use it as an identification tool. *Proteomics* **2002**, *2*, 1123–1130. [CrossRef]
113. Kim, S.W.; Lee, S.H.; Min, C.W.; Jo, I.H.; Bang, K.H.; Hyun, D.-Y.; Agrawal, G.K.; Rakwal, R.; Zargar, S.M.; Gupta, R.; et al. Ginseng (*Panax* sp.) proteomics: An update. *Appl. Biol. Chem.* **2017**, *60*, 311–320. [CrossRef]
114. Li, Z.H.; Alex, D.; Siu, S.O.; Chu, I.K.; Renn, J.; Winkler, C.; Lou, S.; Tsui, S.K.; Zhao, H.Y.; Yan, W.R.; et al. Combined in vivo imaging and omics approaches reveal metabolism of icaritin and its glycosides in zebrafish larvae. *Mol. BioSyst.* **2011**, *7*, 2128–2138. [CrossRef] [PubMed]
115. Hung, M.W.; Zhang, Z.J.; Li, S.; Lei, B.; Yuan, S.; Cui, G.Z.; Man Hoi, P.; Chan, K.; Lee, S.M.Y. From omics to drug metabolism and high content screen of natural product in zebrafish: A new model for discovery of neuroactive compound. *Evid.-Based Complement. Altern. Med.* **2012**, *2012*, 605303. [CrossRef] [PubMed]
116. Lao, Y.; Wang, X.; Xu, N.; Zhang, H.; Xu, H. Application of proteomics to determine the mechanism of action of traditional Chinese medicine remedies. *J. Ethnopharmacol.* **2014**, *155*, 1–8. [CrossRef] [PubMed]
117. Guan, D.; Chen, Z. Challenges and recent advances in affinity purification of tag-free proteins. *Biotechnol. Lett.* **2014**, *36*, 1391–1406. [CrossRef] [PubMed]
118. Novick, D.; Rubinstein, M. Ligand affinity chromatography, an indispensable method for the purification of soluble cytokine receptors and binding proteins. *Methods Mol. Biol.* **2012**, *820*, 195–214. [PubMed]

119. Pfaunmiller, E.L.; Paulemond, M.L.; Dupper, C.M.; Hage, D.S. Affinity monolith chromatography: A review of principles and recent analytical applications. *Anal. Bioanal. Chem.* **2013**, *405*, 2133–2145. [CrossRef] [PubMed]
120. Rix, U.; Gridling, M.; Superti-Furga, G. Compound immobilization and drug-affinity chromatography. *Methods Mol. Biol.* **2012**, *803*, 25–38. [PubMed]
121. Wang, H.Z.; Chu, Z.Z.; Chen, C.C.; Cao, A.C.; Tong, X.; Ouyang, C.B.; Yuan, Q.H.; Wang, M.N.; Wu, Z.K.; Wang, H.H.; et al. Recombinant passenger proteins can be conveniently purified by one-step affinity chromatography. *PLoS ONE* **2015**, *10*, e0143598. [CrossRef] [PubMed]
122. Zhang, X.; Wang, T.; Zhang, H.; Han, B.; Wang, L.; Kang, J. Profiling of drug binding proteins by monolithic affinity chromatography in combination with liquid chromatography-tandem mass spectrometry. *J. Chromatogr. A* **2014**, *1359*, 84–90. [CrossRef] [PubMed]
123. Schenone, M.; Dancik, V.; Wagner, B.K.; Clemons, P.A. Target identification and mechanism of action in chemical biology and drug discovery. *Nat. Chem. Biol.* **2013**, *9*, 232–240. [CrossRef] [PubMed]
124. McFedries, A.; Schwaid, A.; Saghatelian, A. Methods for the elucidation of protein-small molecule interactions. *Chem. Biol.* **2013**, *20*, 667–673. [CrossRef] [PubMed]
125. Rix, U.; Superti-Furga, G. Target profiling of small molecules by chemical proteomics. *Nat. Chem. Biol.* **2009**, *5*, 616–624. [CrossRef] [PubMed]
126. Lee, H.; Lee, J.W. Target identification for biologically active small molecules using chemical biology approaches. *Arch. Pharm. Res.* **2016**, *39*, 1193–1201. [CrossRef] [PubMed]
127. Franken, H.; Mathieson, T.; Childs, D.; Sweetman, G.M.; Werner, T.; Togel, I.; Doce, C.; Gade, S.; Bantscheff, M.; Drewes, G.; et al. Thermal proteome profiling for unbiased identification of direct and indirect drug targets using multiplexed quantitative mass spectrometry. *Nat. Protoc.* **2015**, *10*, 1567–1593. [CrossRef] [PubMed]
128. Jafari, R.; Almqvist, H.; Axelsson, H.; Ignatushchenko, M.; Lundback, T.; Nordlund, P.; Martinez Molina, D. The cellular thermal shift assay for evaluating drug target interactions in cells. *Nat. Protoc.* **2014**, *9*, 2100–2122. [CrossRef] [PubMed]
129. Lomenick, B.; Hao, R.; Jonai, N.; Chin, R.M.; Aghajan, M.; Warburton, S.; Wang, J.; Wu, R.P.; Gomez, F.; Loo, J.A.; et al. Target identification using drug affinity responsive target stability (darts). *Proc. Natl. Acad. Sci. USA* **2009**, *106*, 21984–21989. [CrossRef] [PubMed]
130. Schirle, M.; Bantscheff, M.; Kuster, B. Mass spectrometry-based proteomics in preclinical drug discovery. *Chem. Biol.* **2012**, *19*, 72–84. [CrossRef] [PubMed]
131. Lomenick, B.; Olsen, R.W.; Huang, J. Identification of direct protein targets of small molecules. *ACS Chem. Biol.* **2011**, *6*, 34–46. [CrossRef] [PubMed]
132. Dejonghe, W.; Russinova, E. Target identification strategies in plant chemical biology. *Front. Plant Sci.* **2014**, *5*, 352. [CrossRef] [PubMed]
133. West, G.M.; Tucker, C.L.; Xu, T.; Park, S.K.; Han, X.; Yates, J.R., 3rd; Fitzgerald, M.C. Quantitative proteomics approach for identifying protein-drug interactions in complex mixtures using protein stability measurements. *Proc. Natl. Acad. Sci. USA* **2010**, *107*, 9078–9082. [CrossRef] [PubMed]
134. West, G.M.; Tang, L.; Fitzgerald, M.C. Thermodynamic analysis of protein stability and ligand binding using a chemical modification- and mass spectrometry-based strategy. *Anal. Chem.* **2008**, *80*, 4175–4185. [CrossRef] [PubMed]
135. Jin, L.; Wang, D.; Gooden, D.M.; Ball, C.H.; Fitzgerald, M.C. Targeted mass spectrometry-based approach for protein-ligand binding analyses in complex biological mixtures using a phenacyl bromide modification strategy. *Anal. Chem.* **2016**, *88*, 10987–10993. [CrossRef] [PubMed]
136. Saxena, C. Identification of protein binding partners of small molecules using label-free methods. *Expert Opin. Drug Discov.* **2016**, *11*, 1017–1025. [CrossRef] [PubMed]
137. Strickland, E.C.; Geer, M.A.; Hong, J.; Fitzgerald, M.C. False-positive rate determination of protein target discovery using a covalent modification- and mass spectrometry-based proteomics platform. *J. Am. Soc. Mass Spectrom.* **2014**, *25*, 132–140. [CrossRef] [PubMed]
138. Dearmond, P.D.; Xu, Y.; Strickland, E.C.; Daniels, K.G.; Fitzgerald, M.C. Thermodynamic analysis of protein-ligand interactions in complex biological mixtures using a shotgun proteomics approach. *J. Proteome Res.* **2011**, *10*, 4948–4958. [CrossRef] [PubMed]

139. Tran, D.T.; Adhikari, J.; Fitzgerald, M.C. Stableisotope labeling with amino acids in cell culture (SILAC)-based strategy for proteome-wide thermodynamic analysis of protein-ligand binding interactions. *Mol. Cell. Proteom.* **2014**, *13*, 1800–1813. [CrossRef] [PubMed]
140. Geiger, T.; Wisniewski, J.R.; Cox, J.; Zanivan, S.; Kruger, M.; Ishihama, Y.; Mann, M. Use of stable isotope labeling by amino acids in cell culture as a spike-in standard in quantitative proteomics. *Nat. Protoc.* **2011**, *6*, 147–157. [CrossRef] [PubMed]
141. Hoedt, E.; Zhang, G.; Neubert, T.A. Stable isotope labeling by amino acids in cell culture (SILAC) for quantitative proteomics. *Adv. Exp. Med. Biol.* **2014**, *806*, 93–106. [PubMed]
142. Larance, M.; Bailly, A.P.; Pourkarimi, E.; Hay, R.T.; Buchanan, G.; Coulthurst, S.; Xirodimas, D.P.; Gartner, A.; Lamond, A.I. Stable-isotope labeling with amino acids in nematodes. *Nat. Methods* **2011**, *8*, 849–851. [CrossRef] [PubMed]
143. Ong, S.E.; Mann, M. A practical recipe for stable isotope labeling by amino acids in cell culture (SILAC). *Nat. Protoc.* **2006**, *1*, 2650–2660. [CrossRef] [PubMed]
144. Zhang, L.; Jin, J.; Zhang, L.; Hu, R.; Gao, L.; Huo, X.; Liu, D.; Ma, X.; Wang, C.; Han, J.; et al. Quantitative analysis of differential protein expression in cervical carcinoma cells after zeylenone treatment by stable isotope labeling with amino acids in cell culture. *J. Proteom.* **2015**, *126*, 279–287. [CrossRef] [PubMed]
145. Martinez Molina, D.; Jafari, R.; Ignatushchenko, M.; Seki, T.; Larsson, E.A.; Dan, C.; Sreekumar, L.; Cao, Y.; Nordlund, P. Monitoring drug target engagement in cells and tissues using the cellular thermal shift assay. *Science* **2013**, *341*, 84–87. [CrossRef] [PubMed]
146. Schirle, M.; Jenkins, J.L. Identifying compound efficacy targets in phenotypic drug discovery. *Drug Discov. Today* **2016**, *21*, 82–89. [CrossRef] [PubMed]
147. Tang, H.; Duggan, S.; Richardson, P.L.; Marin, V.; Warder, S.E.; McLoughlin, S.M. Target identification of compounds from a cell viability phenotypic screen using a bead/lysate-based affinity capture platform. *J. Biomol. Screen.* **2016**, *21*, 201–211. [CrossRef] [PubMed]
148. Huber, K.V.; Olek, K.M.; Muller, A.C.; Tan, C.S.; Bennett, K.L.; Colinge, J.; Superti-Furga, G. Proteome-wide drug and metabolite interaction mapping by thermal-stability profiling. *Nat. Methods* **2015**, *12*, 1055–1057. [CrossRef] [PubMed]
149. Reinhard, F.B.; Eberhard, D.; Werner, T.; Franken, H.; Childs, D.; Doce, C.; Savitski, M.F.; Huber, W.; Bantscheff, M.; Savitski, M.M.; et al. Thermal proteome profiling monitors ligand interactions with cellular membrane proteins. *Nat. Methods* **2015**, *12*, 1129–1131. [CrossRef] [PubMed]
150. Savitski, M.M.; Reinhard, F.B.; Franken, H.; Werner, T.; Savitski, M.F.; Eberhard, D.; Martinez Molina, D.; Jafari, R.; Dovega, R.B.; Klaeger, S.; et al. Tracking cancer drugs in living cells by thermal profiling of the proteome. *Science* **2014**, *346*, 1255784. [CrossRef] [PubMed]
151. Becher, I.; Werner, T.; Doce, C.; Zaal, E.A.; Togel, I.; Khan, C.A.; Rueger, A.; Muelbaier, M.; Salzer, E.; Berkers, C.R.; et al. Thermal profiling reveals phenylalanine hydroxylase as an off-target of panobinostat. *Nat. Chem. Biol.* **2016**, *12*, 908–910. [CrossRef] [PubMed]
152. Mateus, A.; Maatta, T.A.; Savitski, M.M. Thermal proteome profiling: Unbiased assessment of protein state through heat-induced stability changes. *Proteome Sci.* **2016**, *15*, 13. [CrossRef] [PubMed]
153. Ho, C.H.; Magtanong, L.; Barker, S.L.; Gresham, D.; Nishimura, S.; Natarajan, P.; Koh, J.L.Y.; Porter, J.; Gray, C.A.; Andersen, R.J.; et al. A molecular barcoded yeast ORF library enables mode-of-action analysis of bioactive compounds. *Nat. Biotechnol.* **2009**, *27*, 369–377. [CrossRef] [PubMed]
154. Jung, H.J.; Kwon, H.J. Target deconvolution of bioactive small molecules: The heart of chemical biology and drug discovery. *Arch. Pharm. Res.* **2015**, *38*, 1627–1641. [CrossRef] [PubMed]
155. Bassik, M.C.; Kampmann, M.; Lebbink, R.J.; Wang, S.; Hein, M.Y.; Poser, I.; Weibezahn, J.; Horlbeck, M.A.; Chen, S.; Mann, M.; et al. A systematic mammalian genetic interaction map reveals pathways underlying ricin susceptibility. *Cell* **2013**, *152*, 909–922. [CrossRef] [PubMed]
156. Shalem, O.; Sanjana, N.E.; Hartenian, E.; Shi, X.; Scott, D.A.; Mikkelson, T.; Heckl, D.; Ebert, B.L.; Root, D.E.; Doench, J.G.; et al. Genome-scale crispr-cas9 knockout screening in human cells. *Science* **2014**, *343*, 84–87. [CrossRef] [PubMed]
157. Kasap, C.; Elemento, O.; Kapoor, T.M. Drugtargetseqr: A genomics- and CRISPR-Cas9-based method to analyze drug targets. *Nat. Chem. Biol.* **2014**, *10*, 626–628. [CrossRef] [PubMed]

158. Ipsaro, J.J.; Shen, C.; Arai, E.; Xu, Y.; Kinney, J.B.; Joshua-Tor, L.; Vakoc, C.R.; Shi, J. Rapid generation of drug-resistance alleles at endogenous loci using CRISPR-Cas9 indel mutagenesis. *PLoS ONE* **2017**, *12*, e0172177. [CrossRef] [PubMed]
159. Neggers, J.E.; Vercruysse, T.; Jacquemyn, M.; Vanstreels, E.; Baloglu, E.; Shacham, S.; Crochiere, M.; Landesman, Y.; Daelemans, D. Identifying drug-target selectivity of small-molecule CRM1/XPO1 inhibitors by CRISPR/Cas9 genome editing. *Chem. Biol.* **2015**, *22*, 107–116. [CrossRef] [PubMed]
160. Liu, X.; Locasale, J.W. Metabolomics: A primer. *Trends Biochem. Sci.* **2017**, *42*, 274–284. [CrossRef] [PubMed]
161. Clish, C.B. Metabolomics: An emerging but powerful tool for precision medicine. *Cold Spring Harb. Mol. Case Stud.* **2015**, *1*, a000588. [CrossRef] [PubMed]
162. Nicholson, J.K.; Lindon, J.C. Systems biology: Metabonomics. *Nature* **2008**, *455*, 7216. [CrossRef] [PubMed]
163. Perez-Pinera, P.; Ousterout, D.G.; Gersbach, C.A. Advances in targeted genome editing. *Curr. Opin. Chem. Biol.* **2012**, *16*, 268–277. [CrossRef] [PubMed]
164. Siminovitch, L. Genetic manipulation: Now is the time to consider controls. *Sci. Forum* **1973**, *6*, 7–11. [PubMed]
165. Yarmush, M.L.; Banta, S. Metabolic engineering: Advances in modeling and intervention in health and disease. *Ann. Rev. Biomed. Eng.* **2003**, *5*, 349–381. [CrossRef] [PubMed]
166. Yan, T.; Fu, Q.; Wang, J.; Ma, S. UPLC-MS/MS determination of ephedrine, methylephedrine, amygdalin and glycyrrhizic acid in beagle plasma and its application to a pharmacokinetic study after oral administration of Ma Huang Tang. *Drug. Test. Anal.* **2015**, *7*, 158–163. [CrossRef] [PubMed]
167. Ekow Thomford, N.; Dzobo, K.; Adu, F.; Chirikure, S.; Wonkam, A.; Dandara, C. Bush mint (*Hyptis suaveolens*) and spreading hogweed (*Boerhavia diffusa*) medicinal plant extracts differentially affect activities of CYP1A2, CYP2D6 and CYP3A4 enzymes. *J. Ethnopharmacol.* **2018**, *211*, 58–69. [CrossRef] [PubMed]
168. Xie, G.; Plumb, R.; Su, M.; Xu, Z.; Zhao, A.; Qiu, M.; Long, X.; Liu, Z.; Jia, W. Ultra-performance LC/TOF MS analysis of medicinal *Panax* herbs for metabolomic research. *J. Sep. Sci.* **2008**, *31*, 1015–1026. [CrossRef] [PubMed]
169. Park, H.-W.; In, G.; Kim, J.-H.; Cho, B.-G.; Han, G.-H.; Chang, I.-M. Metabolomic approach for discrimination of processed ginseng genus (*Panax ginseng* and *Panax quinquefolius*) using UPLC-QTOF MS. *J. Ginseng Res.* **2014**, *38*, 59–65. [CrossRef] [PubMed]
170. Korotcov, A.; Tkachenko, V.; Russo, D.P.; Ekins, S. Comparison of deep learning with multiple machine learning methods and metrics using diverse drug discovery data sets. *Mol. Pharm.* **2017**, *14*, 4462–4475. [CrossRef] [PubMed]
171. Oprea, T.I.; Matter, H. Integrating virtual screening in lead discovery. *Curr. Opin. Chem. Biol.* **2004**, *8*, 349–358. [CrossRef] [PubMed]
172. Beck, A.; Eberherr, C.; Hagemann, M.; Cairo, S.; Haberle, B.; Vokuhl, C.; von Schweinitz, D.; Kappler, R. Connectivity map identifies HDAC inhibition as a treatment option of high-risk hepatoblastoma. *Cancer Biol. Ther.* **2016**, *17*, 1168–1176. [CrossRef] [PubMed]
173. Brum, A.M.; van de Peppel, J.; van der Leije, C.S.; Schreuders-Koedam, M.; Eijken, M.; van der Eerden, B.C.; van Leeuwen, J.P. Connectivity map-based discovery of parbendazole reveals targetable human osteogenic pathway. *Proc. Natl. Acad. Sci. USA* **2015**, *112*, 12711–12716. [CrossRef] [PubMed]
174. Cheng, J.; Yang, L.; Kumar, V.; Agarwal, P. Systematic evaluation of connectivity map for disease indications. *Genome Med.* **2014**, *6*, 95. [CrossRef] [PubMed]
175. Lamb, J. The connectivity map: A new tool for biomedical research. *Nat. Rev. Cancer* **2007**, *7*, 54–60. [CrossRef] [PubMed]
176. Lamb, J.; Crawford, E.D.; Peck, D.; Modell, J.W.; Blat, I.C.; Wrobel, M.J.; Lerner, J.; Brunet, J.P.; Subramanian, A.; Ross, K.N.; et al. The connectivity map: Using gene-expression signatures to connect small molecules, genes, and disease. *Science* **2006**, *313*, 1929–1935. [CrossRef] [PubMed]
177. Hahn, C.K.; Berchuck, J.E.; Ross, K.N.; Kakoza, R.M.; Clauser, K.; Schinzel, A.C.; Ross, L.; Galinsky, I.; Davis, T.N.; Silver, S.J.; et al. Proteomic and genetic approaches identify Syk as an AML target. *Cancer Cell* **2009**, *16*, 281–294. [CrossRef] [PubMed]
178. Nair, M.; Sandhu, S.S.; Sharma, A.K. Prognostic and predictive biomarkers in cancer. *Curr. Cancer Drug Targets* **2014**, *14*, 477–504. [CrossRef] [PubMed]
179. Narayanan, R. Druggable cancer secretome: Neoplasm-associated traits. *Cancer Genom. Proteom.* **2015**, *12*, 119–131.

180. Roti, G.; Stegmaier, K. Genetic and proteomic approaches to identify cancer drug targets. *Br. J. Cancer* **2012**, *106*, 254–261. [CrossRef] [PubMed]
181. Verma, M.; Wright, G.L., Jr.; Hanash, S.M.; Gopal-Srivastava, R.; Srivastava, S. Proteomic approaches within the NCI early detection research network for the discovery and identification of cancer biomarkers. *Ann. N. Y. Acad. Sci.* **2001**, *945*, 103–115. [CrossRef] [PubMed]
182. Awale, M.; Visini, R.; Probst, D.; Arus-Pous, J.; Reymond, J.L. Chemical space: Big data challenge for molecular diversity. *Chimia* **2017**, *71*, 661–666. [CrossRef] [PubMed]
183. Denny, J.C.; Van Driest, S.L.; Wei, W.Q.; Roden, D.M. The influence of big (clinical) data and genomics on precision medicine and drug development. *Clin. Pharmacol. Ther.* **2018**, *103*, 409–418. [CrossRef] [PubMed]
184. Singh, G.; Schulthess, D.; Hughes, N.; Vannieuwenhuyse, B.; Kalra, D. Real world big data for clinical research and drug development. *Drug Discov. Today* **2018**, *23*, 650–660. [CrossRef] [PubMed]
185. Bento, A.P.; Gaulton, A.; Hersey, A.; Bellis, L.J.; Chambers, J.; Davies, M.; Kruger, F.A.; Light, Y.; Mak, L.; McGlinchey, S.; et al. The ChEMBL bioactivity database: An update. *Nucleic Acids Res.* **2014**, *42*, D1083–D1090. [CrossRef] [PubMed]
186. Gaulton, A.; Bellis, L.J.; Bento, A.P.; Chambers, J.; Davies, M.; Hersey, A.; Light, Y.; McGlinchey, S.; Michalovich, D.; Al-Lazikani, B.; et al. Chembl: A large-scale bioactivity database for drug discovery. *Nucleic Acids Res.* **2012**, *40*, D1100–D1107. [CrossRef] [PubMed]
187. Gaulton, A.; Hersey, A.; Nowotka, M.; Bento, A.P.; Chambers, J.; Mendez, D.; Mutowo, P.; Atkinson, F.; Bellis, L.J.; Cibrian-Uhalte, E.; et al. The ChEMBL database in 2017. *Nucleic Acids Res.* **2017**, *45*, D945–D954. [CrossRef] [PubMed]
188. Kruger, F.A.; Rostom, R.; Overington, J.P. Mapping small molecule binding data to structural domains. *BMC Bioinform.* **2012**, *13*, S11.
189. Roos, D.S. Computational biology. Bioinformatics—Trying to swim in a sea of data. *Science* **2001**, *291*, 1260–1261. [CrossRef] [PubMed]
190. Jennings, A.; Tennant, M. Discovery strategies in a pharmaceutical setting: The application of computational techniques. *Expert Opin. Drug Discov.* **2006**, *1*, 709–721. [CrossRef] [PubMed]
191. Chen, Y.P.; Chen, F. Identifying targets for drug discovery using bioinformatics. *Expert Opin. Ther. Targets* **2008**, *12*, 383–389. [CrossRef] [PubMed]
192. Segal, M.R.; Xiong, H.; Bengtsson, H.; Bourgon, R.; Gentleman, R. Querying genomic databases: Refining the connectivity map. *Stat. Appl. Genet. Mol. Biol.* **2012**, *11*. [CrossRef] [PubMed]
193. Kim, R.S.; Goossens, N.; Hoshida, Y. Use of big data in drug development for precision medicine. *Expert Rev. Precis. Med. Drug Dev.* **2016**, *1*, 245–253. [CrossRef] [PubMed]
194. Cappon, G.D. Nonclinical support of pediatric drug development in a global context: An industry perspective. *Birth Defects Res. Part B Dev. Reprod. Toxicol.* **2011**, *92*, 269–272. [CrossRef] [PubMed]
195. Kaneko, T.; Cooper, C.; Mdluli, K. Challenges and opportunities in developing novel drugs for TB. *Future Med. Chem.* **2011**, *3*, 1373–1400. [CrossRef] [PubMed]
196. Morford, L.L.; Bowman, C.J.; Blanset, D.L.; Bogh, I.B.; Chellman, G.J.; Halpern, W.G.; Weinbauer, G.F.; Coogan, T.P. Preclinical safety evaluations supporting pediatric drug development with biopharmaceuticals: Strategy, challenges, current practices. *Birth Defects Res. Part B Dev. Reprod. Toxicol.* **2011**, *92*, 359–380. [CrossRef] [PubMed]
197. Beggs, N.F.; Dobrovolny, H.M. Determining drug efficacy parameters for mathematical models of influenza. *J. Biol. Dyn.* **2015**, *9*, 332–346. [CrossRef] [PubMed]
198. Hwang, W.; Choi, J.; Kwon, M.; Lee, D. Context-specific functional module based drug efficacy prediction. *BMC Bioinform.* **2016**, *17* (Suppl. 6). [CrossRef] [PubMed]
199. Jimenez-Diaz, M.B.; Viera, S.; Fernandez-Alvaro, E.; Angulo-Barturen, I. Animal models of efficacy to accelerate drug discovery in malaria. *Parasitology* **2014**, *141*, 93–103. [CrossRef] [PubMed]
200. Nelson, M.R.; Johnson, T.; Warren, L.; Hughes, A.R.; Chissoe, S.L.; Xu, C.F.; Waterworth, D.M. The genetics of drug efficacy: Opportunities and challenges. *Nat. Rev. Genet.* **2016**, *17*, 197–206. [CrossRef] [PubMed]
201. Tsugawa, J.; Onozawa, R.; Fukae, J.; Mishima, T.; Fujioka, S.; Tsuboi, Y. Impact of insufficient drug efficacy of antiparkinson agents on patient's quality of life: A cross-sectional study. *BMC Neurol.* **2015**, *15*, 105. [CrossRef] [PubMed]
202. Gange, S.J.; Golub, E.T. From smallpox to big data: The next 100 years of epidemiologic methods. *Am. J. Epidemiol.* **2016**, *183*, 423–426. [CrossRef] [PubMed]

203. Docherty, A.B.; Lone, N.I. Exploiting big data for critical care research. *Curr. Opin. Crit. Care* **2015**, *21*, 467–472. [CrossRef] [PubMed]
204. Greene, C.S.; Tan, J.; Ung, M.; Moore, J.H.; Cheng, C. Big data bioinformatics. *J. Cell. Physiol.* **2014**, *229*, 1896–1900. [CrossRef] [PubMed]
205. Tan, S.S.; Gao, G.; Koch, S. Big data and analytics in healthcare. *Methods Inf. Med.* **2015**, *54*, 546–547. [CrossRef] [PubMed]
206. Wasser, T.; Haynes, K.; Barron, J.; Cziraky, M. Using 'big data' to validate claims made in the pharmaceutical approval process. *J. Med. Econ.* **2015**, *18*, 1013–1019. [CrossRef] [PubMed]
207. Reshef, D.N.; Reshef, Y.A.; Finucane, H.K.; Grossman, S.R.; McVean, G.; Turnbaugh, P.J.; Lander, E.S.; Mitzenmacher, M.; Sabeti, P.C. Detecting novel associations in large data sets. *Science* **2011**, *334*, 1518–1524. [CrossRef] [PubMed]
208. Omberg, L.; Ellrott, K.; Yuan, Y.; Kandoth, C.; Wong, C.; Kellen, M.R.; Friend, S.H.; Stuart, J.; Liang, H.; Margolin, A.A. Enabling transparent and collaborative computational analysis of 12 tumor types within the cancer genome atlas. *Nat. Genet.* **2013**, *45*, 1121–1126. [CrossRef] [PubMed]
209. Chen, R.; Mias, G.I.; Li-Pook-Than, J.; Jiang, L.; Lam, H.Y.; Chen, R.; Miriami, E.; Karczewski, K.J.; Hariharan, M.; Dewey, F.E.; et al. Personal omics profiling reveals dynamic molecular and medical phenotypes. *Cell* **2012**, *148*, 1293–1307. [CrossRef] [PubMed]
210. Chapman, T. Lab automation and robotics: Automation on the move. *Nature* **2003**, *421*, 661–666. [CrossRef] [PubMed]
211. King, R.D.; Rowland, J.; Oliver, S.G.; Young, M.; Aubrey, W.; Byrne, E.; Liakata, M.; Markham, M.; Pir, P.; Soldatova, L.N.; et al. The automation of science. *Science* **2009**, *324*, 85–89. [CrossRef] [PubMed]
212. Sparkes, A.; Aubrey, W.; Byrne, E.; Clare, A.; Khan, M.N.; Liakata, M.; Markham, M.; Rowland, J.; Soldatova, L.N.; Whelan, K.E.; et al. Towards robot scientists for autonomous scientific discovery. *Autom. Exp.* **2010**, *2*, 1. [CrossRef] [PubMed]
213. Meanwell, N.A. Improving drug design: An update on recent applications of efficiency metrics, strategies for replacing problematic elements, and compounds in non-traditional drug space. *Chem. Res. Toxicol.* **2016**, *29*, 564–616. [CrossRef] [PubMed]
214. MacConnell, A.B.; Price, A.K.; Paegel, B.M. An integrated microfluidic processor for DNA-encoded combinatorial library functional screening. *ACS Comb. Sci.* **2017**, *19*, 181–192. [CrossRef] [PubMed]
215. Baranczak, A.; Tu, N.P.; Marjanovic, J.; Searle, P.A.; Vasudevan, A.; Djuric, S.W. Integrated platform for expedited synthesis-purification-testing of small molecule libraries. *ACS Med. Chem. Lett.* **2017**, *8*, 461–465. [CrossRef] [PubMed]
216. Gupta, A.; Muller, A.T.; Huisman, B.J.H.; Fuchs, J.A.; Schneider, P.; Schneider, G. Generative recurrent networks for de novo drug design. *Mol. Inform.* **2017**. [CrossRef] [PubMed]
217. Merk, D.; Friedrich, L.; Grisoni, F.; Schneider, G. De novo design of bioactive small molecules by artificial intelligence. *Mol. Inform.* **2018**. [CrossRef] [PubMed]
218. Zhang, L.; Tan, J.; Han, D.; Zhu, H. From machine learning to deep learning: Progress in machine intelligence for rational drug discovery. *Drug Discov. Today* **2017**, *22*, 1680–1685. [CrossRef] [PubMed]
219. Duch, W.; Swaminathan, K.; Meller, J. Artificial intelligence approaches for rational drug design and discovery. *Curr. Pharm. Des.* **2007**, *13*, 1497–1508. [CrossRef] [PubMed]
220. Esch, E.W.; Bahinski, A.; Huh, D. Organs-on-chips at the frontiers of drug discovery. *Nat. Rev. Drug Discov.* **2015**, *14*, 248–260. [CrossRef] [PubMed]
221. Eglen, R.M.; Randle, D.H. Drug discovery goes three-dimensional: Goodbye to flat high-throughput screening? *Assay Drug Dev. Technol.* **2015**, *13*, 262–265. [CrossRef] [PubMed]
222. Ozdemir, V.; Patrinos, G.P. David bowie and the art of slow innovation: A fast-second winner strategy for biotechnology and precision medicine global development. *Omics* **2017**, *21*, 633–637. [CrossRef] [PubMed]
223. Burke, M.D.; Lalic, G. Teaching target-oriented and diversity-oriented organic synthesis at Harvard University. *Chem. Biol.* **2002**, *9*, 535–541. [CrossRef]
224. Schreiber, S.L. Target-oriented and diversity-oriented organic synthesis in drug discovery. *Science* **2000**, *287*, 1964–1969. [CrossRef] [PubMed]
225. Maier, M.E. Design and synthesis of analogues of natural products. *Org. Biomol. Chem.* **2015**, *13*, 5302–5343. [CrossRef] [PubMed]

226. Basu, S.; Ellinger, B.; Rizzo, S.; Deraeve, C.; Schurmann, M.; Preut, H.; Arndt, H.D.; Waldmann, H. Biology-oriented synthesis of a natural-product inspired oxepane collection yields a small-molecule activator of the Wnt-pathway. *Proc. Natl. Acad. Sci. USA* **2011**, *108*, 6805–6810. [CrossRef] [PubMed]
227. Kaiser, M.; Wetzel, S.; Kumar, K.; Waldmann, H. Biology-inspired synthesis of compound libraries. *Cell. Mol. Life Sci.* **2008**, *65*, 1186–1201. [CrossRef] [PubMed]
228. Wetzel, S.; Bon, R.S.; Kumar, K.; Waldmann, H. Biology-oriented synthesis. *Angew. Chem. Int. Ed. Engl.* **2011**, *50*, 10800–10826. [CrossRef] [PubMed]
229. Wender, P.A.; Quiroz, R.V.; Stevens, M.C. Function through synthesis-informed design. *Acc. Chem. Res.* **2015**, *48*, 752–760. [CrossRef] [PubMed]
230. Wender, P.A.; Verma, V.A.; Paxton, T.J.; Pillow, T.H. Function-oriented synthesis, step economy, and drug design. *Acc. Chem. Res.* **2008**, *41*, 40–49. [CrossRef] [PubMed]
231. Zhu, Q.; Sun, Y.; Challa, S.; Ding, Y.; Lajiness, M.S.; Wild, D.J. Semantic inference using chemogenomics data for drug discovery. *BMC Bioinform.* **2011**, *12*, 256. [CrossRef] [PubMed]
232. White, D.; Wilson, R.C. Generative models for chemical structures. *J. Chem. Inf. Model.* **2010**, *50*, 1257–1274. [CrossRef] [PubMed]
233. Rubio, D.M.; Schoenbaum, E.E.; Lee, L.S.; Schteingart, D.E.; Marantz, P.R.; Anderson, K.E.; Platt, L.D.; Baez, A.; Esposito, K. Defining translational research: Implications for training. *Acad. Med.* **2010**, *85*, 470–475. [CrossRef] [PubMed]
234. Jing, Y.; Bian, Y.; Hu, Z.; Wang, L.; Xie, X.S. Deep learning for drug design: An artificial intelligence paradigm for drug discovery in the big data era. *AAPS J.* **2018**, *20*, 58. [CrossRef] [PubMed]
235. Reutlinger, M.; Rodrigues, T.; Schneider, P.; Schneider, G. Combining on-chip synthesis of a focused combinatorial library with computational target prediction reveals imidazopyridine GPCR ligands. *Angew. Chem. Int. Ed. Engl.* **2014**, *53*, 582–585. [CrossRef] [PubMed]
236. Schneider, G. Automating drug discovery. *Nat. Rev. Drug Discov.* **2018**, *17*, 97–113. [CrossRef] [PubMed]
237. Reutlinger, M.; Rodrigues, T.; Schneider, P.; Schneider, G. Multi-objective molecular de novo design by adaptive fragment prioritization. *Angew. Chem. Int. Ed. Engl.* **2014**, *53*, 4244–4248. [CrossRef] [PubMed]
238. Schneider, P.; Rothlisberger, M.; Reker, D.; Schneider, G. Spotting and designing promiscuous ligands for drug discovery. *Chem. Commun.* **2016**, *52*, 1135–1138. [CrossRef] [PubMed]
239. Wang, L.; Wu, Y.; Deng, Y.; Kim, B.; Pierce, L.; Krilov, G.; Lupyan, D.; Robinson, S.; Dahlgren, M.K.; Greenwood, J.; et al. Accurate and reliable prediction of relative ligand binding potency in prospective drug discovery by way of a modern free-energy calculation protocol and force field. *J. Am. Chem. Soc.* **2015**, *137*, 2695–2703. [CrossRef] [PubMed]
240. Besnard, J.; Ruda, G.F.; Setola, V.; Abecassis, K.; Rodriguiz, R.M.; Huang, X.P.; Norval, S.; Sassano, M.F.; Shin, A.I.; Webster, L.A.; et al. Automated design of ligands to polypharmacological profiles. *Nature* **2012**, *492*, 215–220. [CrossRef] [PubMed]
241. Koppitz, M.; Eis, K. Automated medicinal chemistry. *Drug Discov. Today* **2006**, *11*, 561–568. [CrossRef] [PubMed]
242. Sutherland, J.D.; Tu, N.P.; Nemcek, T.A.; Searle, P.A.; Hochlowski, J.E.; Djuric, S.W.; Pan, J.Y. An automated synthesis-purification-sample-management platform for the accelerated generation of pharmaceutical candidates. *J. Lab. Autom.* **2014**, *19*, 176–182. [CrossRef] [PubMed]
243. Godfrey, A.G.; Masquelin, T.; Hemmerle, H. A remote-controlled adaptive medchem lab: An innovative approach to enable drug discovery in the 21st century. *Drug Discov. Today* **2013**, *18*, 795–802. [CrossRef] [PubMed]
244. Nicolaou, C.A.; Watson, I.A.; Hu, H.; Wang, J. The proximal lilly collection: Mapping, exploring and exploiting feasible chemical space. *J. Chem. Inf. Model.* **2016**, *56*, 1253–1266. [CrossRef] [PubMed]
245. Li, J.; Ballmer, S.G.; Gillis, E.P.; Fujii, S.; Schmidt, M.J.; Palazzolo, A.M.; Lehmann, J.W.; Morehouse, G.F.; Burke, M.D. Synthesis of many different types of organic small molecules using one automated process. *Science* **2015**, *347*, 1221–1226. [CrossRef] [PubMed]
246. Stalder, R.; Roth, G.P. Preparative microfluidic electrosynthesis of drug metabolites. *ACS Med. Chem. Lett.* **2013**, *4*, 1119–1123. [CrossRef] [PubMed]
247. Genovino, J.; Sames, D.; Hamann, L.G.; Toure, B.B. Accessing drug metabolites via transition-metal catalyzed c-h oxidation: The liver as synthetic inspiration. *Angew. Chem. Int. Ed. Engl.* **2016**, *55*, 14218–14238. [CrossRef] [PubMed]

248. LaPorte, T.L.; Wang, C. Continuous processes for the production of pharmaceutical intermediates and active pharmaceutical ingredients. *Curr. Opin. Drug Discov. Dev.* **2007**, *10*, 738–745.
249. Chin, P.; Barney, W.S.; Pindzola, B.A. Microstructured reactors as tools for the intensification of pharmaceutical reactions and processes. *Curr. Opin. Drug Discov. Dev.* **2009**, *12*, 848–861.
250. Saaby, S.; Knudsen, K.R.; Ladlow, M.; Ley, S.V. The use of a continuous flow-reactor employing a mixed hydrogen-liquid flow stream for the efficient reduction of imines to amines. *Chem. Commun.* **2005**, 2909–2911. [CrossRef] [PubMed]
251. Brzozowski, M.; O'Brien, M.; Ley, S.V.; Polyzos, A. Flow chemistry: Intelligent processing of gas-liquid transformations using a tube-in-tube reactor. *Acc. Chem. Res.* **2015**, *48*, 349–362. [CrossRef] [PubMed]
252. Loskill, P.; Sezhian, T.; Tharp, K.M.; Lee-Montiel, F.T.; Jeeawoody, S.; Reese, W.M.; Zushin, P.H.; Stahl, A.; Healy, K.E. Wat-on-a-chip: A physiologically relevant microfluidic system incorporating white adipose tissue. *Lab Chip* **2017**, *17*, 1645–1654. [CrossRef] [PubMed]
253. Eyer, K.; Stratz, S.; Kuhn, P.; Kuster, S.K.; Dittrich, P.S. Implementing enzyme-linked immunosorbent assays on a microfluidic chip to quantify intracellular molecules in single cells. *Anal. Chem.* **2013**, *85*, 3280–3287. [CrossRef] [PubMed]
254. Ferrari, M. Frontiers in cancer nanomedicine: Directing mass transport through biological barriers. *Trends Biotechnol.* **2010**, *28*, 181–188. [CrossRef] [PubMed]
255. Zhang, Y.S.; Zhang, Y.N.; Zhang, W. Cancer-on-a-chip systems at the frontier of nanomedicine. *Drug Discov. Today* **2017**, *22*, 1392–1399. [CrossRef] [PubMed]
256. Galler, K.; Brautigam, K.; Grosse, C.; Popp, J.; Neugebauer, U. Making a big thing of a small cell–recent advances in single cell analysis. *Analyst* **2014**, *139*, 1237–1273. [CrossRef] [PubMed]
257. Kayala, M.A.; Azencott, C.A.; Chen, J.H.; Baldi, P. Learning to predict chemical reactions. *J. Chem. Inf. Model.* **2011**, *51*, 2209–2222. [CrossRef] [PubMed]
258. Reynolds, C.R.; Muggleton, S.H.; Sternberg, M.J. Incorporating virtual reactions into a logic-based ligand-based virtual screening method to discover new leads. *Mol. Inform.* **2015**, *34*, 615–625. [CrossRef] [PubMed]
259. Kowalik, M.; Gothard, C.M.; Drews, A.M.; Gothard, N.A.; Weckiewicz, A.; Fuller, P.E.; Grzybowski, B.A.; Bishop, K.J. Parallel optimization of synthetic pathways within the network of organic chemistry. *Angew. Chem. Int. Ed. Engl.* **2012**, *51*, 7928–7932. [CrossRef] [PubMed]
260. Szymkuc, S.; Gajewska, E.P.; Klucznik, T.; Molga, K.; Dittwald, P.; Startek, M.; Bajczyk, M.; Grzybowski, B.A. Computer-assisted synthetic planning: The end of the beginning. *Angew. Chem. Int. Ed. Engl.* **2016**, *55*, 5904–5937. [CrossRef] [PubMed]
261. Baker, M. Europe bets on drug discovery. *Nature* **2013**, *494*, 20. [CrossRef] [PubMed]
262. Lopez-Rubio, E.; Elizondo, D.A.; Grootveld, M.; Jerez, J.M.; Luque-Baena, R.M. Computational intelligence techniques in medicine. *Comput. Math. Methods Med.* **2015**, *2015*, 196976. [CrossRef] [PubMed]
263. Montanez-Godinez, N.; Martinez-Olguin, A.C.; Deeb, O.; Garduno-Juarez, R.; Ramirez-Galicia, G. QSAR/QSPR as an application of artificial neural networks. *Methods Mol. Biol.* **2015**, *1260*, 319–333. [PubMed]
264. Wesolowski, M.; Suchacz, B. Artificial neural networks: Theoretical background and pharmaceutical applications: A review. *J. AOAC Int.* **2012**, *95*, 652–668. [CrossRef] [PubMed]
265. Baskin, I.I.; Winkler, D.; Tetko, I.V. A renaissance of neural networks in drug discovery. *Expert Opin. Drug Discov.* **2016**, *11*, 785–795. [CrossRef] [PubMed]
266. Nikolsky, Y.; Nikolskaya, T.; Bugrim, A. Biological networks and analysis of experimental data in drug discovery. *Drug Discov. Today* **2005**, *10*, 653–662. [CrossRef]
267. LeCun, Y.; Bengio, Y.; Hinton, G. Deep learning. *Nature* **2015**, *521*, 436–444. [CrossRef] [PubMed]
268. Lipinski, C.A. Drug-like properties and the causes of poor solubility and poor permeability. *J. Pharmacol. Toxicol. Methods* **2000**, *44*, 235–249. [CrossRef]
269. Congreve, M.; Carr, R.; Murray, C.; Jhoti, H. A 'rule of three' for fragment-based lead discovery? *Drug Discov. Today* **2003**, *8*, 876–877. [CrossRef]
270. Van Molle, I.; Thomann, A.; Buckley, D.L.; So, E.C.; Lang, S.; Crews, C.M.; Ciulli, A. Dissecting fragment-based lead discovery at the von Hippel-Lindau protein: Hypoxia inducible factor 1alpha protein-protein interface. *Chem. Biol.* **2012**, *19*, 1300–1312. [CrossRef] [PubMed]

271. Zuegg, J.; Cooper, M.A. Drug-likeness and increased hydrophobicity of commercially available compound libraries for drug screening. *Curr. Top. Med. Chem.* **2012**, *12*, 1500–1513. [CrossRef] [PubMed]
272. Ntie-Kang, F.; Lifongo, L.L.; Judson, P.N.; Sippl, W.; Efange, S.M. How "drug-like" are naturally occurring anti-cancer compounds? *J. Mol. Model.* **2014**, *20*, 2069. [CrossRef] [PubMed]
273. Grabowski, K.; Baringhaus, K.H.; Schneider, G. Scaffold diversity of natural products: Inspiration for combinatorial library design. *Nat. Prod. Rep.* **2008**, *25*, 892–904. [CrossRef] [PubMed]
274. Elumalai, N.; Berg, A.; Natarajan, K.; Scharow, A.; Berg, T. Nanomolar inhibitors of the transcription factor STAT5b with high selectivity over STAT5a. *Angew. Chem. Int. Ed. Engl.* **2015**, *54*, 4758–4763. [CrossRef] [PubMed]
275. Bon, R.S.; Waldmann, H. Bioactivity-guided navigation of chemical space. *Acc. Chem. Res.* **2010**, *43*, 1103–1114. [CrossRef] [PubMed]
276. Renner, S.; van Otterlo, W.A.; Dominguez Seoane, M.; Mocklinghoff, S.; Hofmann, B.; Wetzel, S.; Schuffenhauer, A.; Ertl, P.; Oprea, T.I.; Steinhilber, D.; et al. Bioactivity-guided mapping and navigation of chemical space. *Nat. Chem. Biol.* **2009**, *5*, 585–592. [CrossRef] [PubMed]
277. Wetzel, S.; Klein, K.; Renner, S.; Rauh, D.; Oprea, T.I.; Mutzel, P.; Waldmann, H. Interactive exploration of chemical space with scaffold hunter. *Nat. Chem. Biol.* **2009**, *5*, 581–583. [CrossRef] [PubMed]
278. Rodrigues, T.; Reker, D.; Schneider, P.; Schneider, G. Counting on natural products for drug design. *Nat. Chem.* **2016**, *8*, 531–541. [CrossRef] [PubMed]
279. Lagunin, A.; Stepanchikova, A.; Filimonov, D.; Poroikov, V. Pass: Prediction of activity spectra for biologically active substances. *Bioinformatics* **2000**, *16*, 747–748. [CrossRef] [PubMed]
280. Stepanchikova, A.V.; Lagunin, A.A.; Filimonov, D.A.; Poroikov, V.V. Prediction of biological activity spectra for substances: Evaluation on the diverse sets of drug-like structures. *Curr. Med. Chem.* **2003**, *10*, 225–233. [CrossRef] [PubMed]
281. Reker, D.; Rodrigues, T.; Schneider, P.; Schneider, G. Identifying the macromolecular targets of de novo-designed chemical entities through self-organizing map consensus. *Proc. Natl. Acad. Sci. USA* **2014**, *111*, 4067–4072. [CrossRef] [PubMed]
282. Schneider, G.; Reker, D.; Rodrigues, T.; Schneider, P. Coping with polypharmacology by computational medicinal chemistry. *Chimia* **2014**, *68*, 648–653. [CrossRef] [PubMed]
283. Sliwoski, G.; Kothiwale, S.; Meiler, J.; Lowe, E.W. Computational methods in drug discovery. *Pharmacol. Rev.* **2014**, *66*, 334–395. [CrossRef] [PubMed]
284. DiMasi, J.A.; Feldman, L.; Seckler, A.; Wilson, A. Trends in risks associated with new drug development: Success rates for investigational drugs. *Clin. Pharmacol. Ther.* **2010**, *87*, 272–277. [CrossRef] [PubMed]
285. DiMasi, J.A.; Reichert, J.M.; Feldman, L.; Malins, A. Clinical approval success rates for investigational cancer drugs. *Clin. Pharmacol. Ther.* **2013**, *94*, 329–335. [CrossRef] [PubMed]
286. Hay, M.; Thomas, D.W.; Craighead, J.L.; Economides, C.; Rosenthal, J. Clinical development success rates for investigational drugs. *Nat. Biotechnol.* **2014**, *32*, 40–51. [CrossRef] [PubMed]
287. Loong, H.H.; Siu, L.L. Selecting the best drugs for phase I clinical development and beyond. In *American Society of Clinical Oncology Educational Book. American Society of Clinical Oncology. Meeting*; American Society of Clinical Oncology: Alexandria, VA, USA, 2013; pp. 469–473.
288. Chavan, S.; Nicholls, I.A.; Karlsson, B.C.; Rosengren, A.M.; Ballabio, D.; Consonni, V.; Todeschini, R. Towards global qsar model building for acute toxicity: Munro database case study. *Int. J. Mol. Sci.* **2014**, *15*, 18162–18174. [CrossRef] [PubMed]
289. Cherkasov, A.; Muratov, E.N.; Fourches, D.; Varnek, A.; Baskin, I.I.; Cronin, M.; Dearden, J.; Gramatica, P.; Martin, Y.C.; Todeschini, R.; et al. Qsar modeling: Where have you been? Where are you going to? *J. Med. Chem.* **2014**, *57*, 4977–5010. [CrossRef] [PubMed]
290. Devillers, J. Methods for building QSARs. *Methods Mol. Biol.* **2013**, *930*, 3–27. [PubMed]
291. Sullivan, K.M.; Manuppello, J.R.; Willett, C.E. Building on a solid foundation: SAR and QSAR as a fundamental strategy to reduce animal testing. *SAR QSAR Environ. Res.* **2014**, *25*, 357–365. [CrossRef] [PubMed]
292. Kirchmair, J.; Goller, A.H.; Lang, D.; Kunze, J.; Testa, B.; Wilson, I.D.; Glen, R.C.; Schneider, G. Predicting drug metabolism: Experiment and/or computation? *Nat. Rev. Drug Discov.* **2015**, *14*, 387–404. [CrossRef] [PubMed]

293. Mukherjee, G.; Lal Gupta, P.; Jayaram, B. Predicting the binding modes and sites of metabolism of xenobiotics. *Mol. BioSyst.* **2015**, *11*, 1914–1924. [CrossRef] [PubMed]
294. Xiao, X.; Min, J.L.; Lin, W.Z.; Liu, Z.; Cheng, X.; Chou, K.C. Idrug-target: Predicting the interactions between drug compounds and target proteins in cellular networking via benchmark dataset optimization approach. *J. Biomol. Struct. Dyn.* **2015**, *33*, 2221–2233. [CrossRef] [PubMed]
295. Zhang, W.; Liu, F.; Luo, L.; Zhang, J. Predicting drug side effects by multi-label learning and ensemble learning. *BMC Bioinform.* **2015**, *16*, 365. [CrossRef] [PubMed]
296. Bastian, L.; Hof, J.; Pfau, M.; Fichtner, I.; Eckert, C.; Henze, G.; Prada, J.; von Stackelberg, A.; Seeger, K.; Shalapour, S. Synergistic activity of bortezomib and hdaci in preclinical models of b-cell precursor acute lymphoblastic leukemia via modulation of p53, pi3k/akt, and nf-kappab. *Clin. Cancer Res.* **2013**, *19*, 1445–1457. [CrossRef] [PubMed]
297. Stanciu-Herrera, C.; Morgan, C.; Herrera, L. Anti-cd19 and anti-cd22 monoclonal antibodies increase the effectiveness of chemotherapy in pre-b acute lymphoblastic leukemia cell lines. *Leukemia Res.* **2008**, *32*, 625–632. [CrossRef] [PubMed]
298. Dzobo, K.; Senthebane, D.A.; Rowe, A.; Thomford, N.E.; Mwapagha, L.M.; Al-Awwad, N.; Dandara, C.; Parker, M.I. Cancer stem cell hypothesis for therapeutic innovation in clinical oncology? Taking the root out, not chopping the leaf. *Omics* **2016**, *20*, 681–691. [CrossRef] [PubMed]
299. Dzobo, K.; Senthebane, D.A.; Thomford, N.E.; Rowe, A.; Dandara, C.; Parker, M.I. Not everyone fits the mold: Intratumor and intertumor heterogeneity and innovative cancer drug design and development. *Omics* **2018**, *22*, 17–34. [CrossRef] [PubMed]
300. Baselga, J.; Cortes, J.; Kim, S.B.; Im, S.A.; Hegg, R.; Im, Y.H.; Roman, L.; Pedrini, J.L.; Pienkowski, T.; Knott, A.; et al. Pertuzumab plus trastuzumab plus docetaxel for metastatic breast cancer. *N. Engl. J. Med.* **2012**, *366*, 109–119. [CrossRef] [PubMed]
301. Kawajiri, H.; Takashima, T.; Kashiwagi, S.; Noda, S.; Onoda, N.; Hirakawa, K. Pertuzumab in combination with trastuzumab and docetaxel for HER2-positive metastatic breast cancer. *Expert Rev. Anticancer Ther.* **2015**, *15*, 17–26. [CrossRef] [PubMed]
302. Swain, S.M.; Baselga, J.; Kim, S.B.; Ro, J.; Semiglazov, V.; Campone, M.; Ciruelos, E.; Ferrero, J.M.; Schneeweiss, A.; Heeson, S.; et al. Pertuzumab, trastuzumab, and docetaxel in HER2-positive metastatic breast cancer. *N. Engl. J. Med.* **2015**, *372*, 724–734. [CrossRef] [PubMed]
303. Swain, S.M.; Baselga, J.; Miles, D.; Im, Y.H.; Quah, C.; Lee, L.F.; Cortes, J. Incidence of central nervous system metastases in patients with HER2-positive metastatic breast cancer treated with pertuzumab, trastuzumab, and docetaxel: Results from the randomized phase iii study cleopatra. *Ann. Oncol.* **2014**, *25*, 1116–1121. [CrossRef] [PubMed]
304. Swain, S.M.; Kim, S.B.; Cortes, J.; Ro, J.; Semiglazov, V.; Campone, M.; Ciruelos, E.; Ferrero, J.M.; Schneeweiss, A.; Knott, A.; et al. Pertuzumab, trastuzumab, and docetaxel for HER2-positive metastatic breast cancer (cleopatra study): Overall survival results from a randomised, double-blind, placebo-controlled, phase 3 study. *Lancet Oncol.* **2013**, *14*, 461–471. [CrossRef]
305. National Academy of Sciences (US). The national academies collection: Reports funded by national institutes of health. In *Toward Precision Medicine: Building a Knowledge Network for Biomedical Research and a New Taxonomy of Disease*; National Academies Press (US), National Academy of Sciences: Washington, DC, USA, 2011.
306. Debouck, C. Integrating genomics across drug discovery and development. *Toxicol. Lett.* **2009**, *186*, 9–12. [CrossRef] [PubMed]
307. Debouck, C.; Metcalf, B. The impact of genomics on drug discovery. *Ann. Rev. Pharmacol. Toxicol.* **2000**, *40*, 193–207. [CrossRef] [PubMed]

International Journal of
Molecular Sciences

Review

Copaifera of the Neotropics: A Review of the Phytochemistry and Pharmacology

Rafaela da Trindade [1], Joyce Kelly da Silva [1,2] and William N. Setzer [3,4,*]

1 Programa de Pós-Graduação em Biotecnologia, Universidade Federal do Pará, 66075-900 Belém, Brazil; rcabral@ufpa.br (R.d.T.); joycekellys@ufpa.br (J.K.d.S.)
2 Programa de Pós-Graduação em Química, Universidade Federal do Pará, 66075-900 Belém, Brazil
3 Department of Chemistry, University of Alabama in Huntsville, Huntsville, AL 35899, USA
4 Aromatic Plant Research Center, 615 St. George Square Court, Suite 300, Winston-Salem, NC 27103, USA
* Correspondence: wsetzer@chemistry.uah.edu or wsetzer@aromaticplant.org; Tel.: +1-256-824-6519

Received: 25 April 2018; Accepted: 15 May 2018; Published: 18 May 2018

Abstract: The oleoresin of *Copaifera* trees has been widely used as a traditional medicine in Neotropical regions for thousands of years and remains a popular treatment for a variety of ailments. The copaiba resins are generally composed of a volatile oil made up largely of sesquiterpene hydrocarbons, such as β-caryophyllene, α-copaene, β-elemene, α-humulene, and germacrene D. In addition, the oleoresin is also made up of several biologically active diterpene acids, including copalic acid, kaurenoic acid, alepterolic acid, and polyalthic acid. This review presents a summary of the ecology and distribution of *Copaifera* species, the traditional uses, the biological activities, and the phytochemistry of copaiba oleoresins. In addition, several biomolecular targets relevant to the bioactivities have been implicated by molecular docking methods.

Keywords: copaiba; oleoresin; essential oil; sesquiterpenoids; diterpenoids; biological activity; molecular targets

1. Introduction to the Genus *Copaifera*

The copaiba trees belong to the genus *Copaifera*, family Fabaceae, and subfamily Caesalpinoideae. The genus was described the first time by Marcgraf and Piso in 1638, who employed the name "Copaiba" without designating the species [1]. In 1760, Nicolaus Joseph Von Jacquin described the species *Copaiva officinalis* in the work *Enumeratio Systematica Plantarum* [2]. Afterwards, in the year 1764, Carl von Linnaeus did a more detailed study of the genus in the work *Species Plantarum*, in which he described the type species *Copaifera officinalis* (Jacq.) L. [3]. There are more than 70 *Copaifera* species distributed throughout the world, with widespread occurrence in Central and South America; there are also four species found in Africa and one species found on the island of Borneo, situated in the Pacific Ocean [4]. Brazil is the country with the greatest biodiversity of *Copaifera* with 26 species and 8 varieties [5].

The vernacular name copaîba probably originated from the Tupi-Guarani and alludes to the names used by indigenous peoples, copaíva and copahu (kupa'iwa and kupa'u, respectively), which refers to the tree exudate, in reference to the oil stored in its interior [6]. Sixteenth-century records produced by chroniclers during the Brazilian colonization report the widespread use of copaiba oil among the natives as anti-inflammatory and healing agents, and also for esoteric purposes, such as aphrodisiac and contraceptive [4,6,7]. This natural product is known and valued to the present day, mainly in the Amazon region, where the rural population has little access to industrialized pharmaceutical products and public health care [6,8].

The copaiba trees have shrub or arboreal habits, can reach up to 40 m height and 4 m diameter at breast height (dbh), have slow growth, and can live up to 400 years [6]. Their cylindrical trunks contain intercellular secretory channels arranged in bands of marginal axial parenchyma, the lumen from secretory cells is formed schizogenously, and the oleoresin is synthesized in parenchyma cells of the canal. The species have alternate leaves, which are pinnate with 2–12 pairs of leaflets (opposite, alternate, or subopposite), usually glabrous, and may have translucent points and glands at the base of the marginal vein; they have small and interpetiolar stipules and are generally deciduous. The inflorescences are alternate panicles and the flower buds are protected by small bracts; they have small flowers, numerous and sessile, which are monoclamids with a tetramer chalice that forms short tubes and contains internally hirsute sepals. The androecium holds 10 free stamens, glabrous fillets, and oblong and rimose anther; and the gynoecium presents a sessile ovary with two elongate ovules, filiform style, and globular and papillary stigma. The fruits are bivalved, dehiscent, laterally compressed, and monospermic. The seed is a pendulum, oblong-globose, covered by abundant white or yellow aril, and lacking endosperm [1,9–11].

Although the *Copaifera* genus has been extensively studied taxonomically, there are still difficulties in identifying some species, mainly due to their intricate floral morphology and absence of reproductive structures in the samples studied. With regard to the Amazonian species, the scarcity of field information and illustrations of specimens comprise the main limitations for botanical descriptions of the group. These taxonomic problems have restricted the advance of chemical and pharmacological research, limited the industrial and rational uses of resin oils and wood, and have also hampered the development of projects, plans for sustainable management, and conservation of commercially targeted species [9,12].

The main economic contributions of *Copaifera* species have been wood and oleoresins. Among *Copaifera* species that are used in the production of oleoresins, *C. reticulata* is the most frequent, representing 70% of the production [6]. Copaiba oleoresin is one of the most important renewable natural remedies for the indigenous people from the Amazon region and its use is widely diffused due its various pharmacological properties [13]. The oleoresin is a transparent, colored liquid with variable viscosity, and is constituted by a nonvolatile fraction composed of diterpenes and a volatile fraction composed of sesquiterpenes [14,15]. Its chemical profile may vary according to species, seasonal and climatic characteristics of the environment, soil type and composition, and rainfall index. Biotic pressures, such as insect predation and pathogen infection, also cause differences in oleoresin composition [16,17]. The extraction of copaiba oil is done through the perforation of the trunk with a punch, and the resin is collected with the help of a polyvinyl chloride (PVC) pipe, through which the oil flows and is then stored. This practice is mainly done by plant extraction; therefore, the product of several trees is often mixed, resulting in an additional obstacle to the botanical identity of the copaiba trees. In addition, the lack of parameters to characterize the oil and to perform quality control of the botanical drug also constitutes an obstacle for the registration and exportation of herbal products containing copaiba [18,19].

2. Ecology and Distribution of *Copaifera*

The genus *Copaifera* is native to tropical regions of Latin America, an area of great species diversity [1]. Distributed widely in the Americas, stretching from Mexico to northern Argentina, the genus also occurs in West Africa and Asia [20]. The greatest richness of species occurs in Brazil, where they are distributed from the north to the south of the country. The most common species are *C. multijuga* Hayne, which is found in the Amazonas, Pará and Rondônia states; *C. reticulata* Ducke that occurs in Amapá, Pará and Roraima;, and *C. langsdorffii* Desf., which can occur from the northern to southern regions of Brazil [5]. Other species have more restricted distribution, such as *C. guyanensis* Desf. (Amazonas), *C. majorina* Dwyer (Bahia), *C. cearensis* Huber ex Ducke (Ceará, Bahia, Piauí and Rio de Janeiro), *C. elliptica* Mart. (Goias and Mato Grosso), *C. paupera* (Herzog) Dwyer (Acre), and *C. lucens* Dwyer (Bahia, Espírito Santo, Minas Gerais, Rio de Janeiro, São Paulo) [5]. Although many species of *Copaifera* have wide occurrence within the Brazilian territory, and may occur in different phytogeographic domains (e.g., *C. langsdorffii*), some feature endemism, such as *C. trapezifolia* Hayne, which occurs in an extremely disturbed region of the Atlantic rainforest, of which only 11.6% of the natural vegetation cover remains [21]. Thus, morphological, physiological, and ecological studies are highly relevant for the preservation of species and their natural environment [11]. A study conducted in the Minas Gerais state on the geographical distribution and environmental characteristics of arboreal species showed that *C. langsdorffii* has wide occurrence throughout the whole state, where latosol type soil predominates, but additionally has a preference for ustic soils (62%) [22].

In relation to the ecological group, copaíba are classified as long-living, late secondary, and climax tree species, demanding of light but tolerant to shade [23]. They are considered generalists because they are adapted to a wide variety of environments. They can occur in floodplains, riparian forest, and streams of the Amazon basin and the forests of the Cerrado in the center of Brazil [24]. *C. langsdorffii*, for example, has great ecological plasticity, occurring in several biomes, such as Cerrado, Atlantic Forest, Caatinga, and Amazon rainforest [23]. *Copaifera* species have great plasticity in relation to edaphic conditions; they occur in areas with fertile soil and well-drained soil and in areas with very poor acidic soils, such as Cerrado fields. They grow well on sandy and clayey soils and generally occupy the forest canopy [25,26].

Phenological studies on *Copaifera* are important for the rational use of the species and for the preparation of management plans [27]. The reproduction of copaibas occurs from the fifth year of growth after planting in a climax forest ecosystem [6]. *C. multijuga*, commonly found in the Amazon, blooms in the rainy season—between the months of December–April—and fructifies between April and July [27]. Blooming of *C. reticulata* occurs from January to March, with fruiting from March to August, lasting into October [26,28]. *C. langsdorffii*, observed in the Tijuca Forest, Rio de Janeiro, blooms between March and April and fructifies between August and September. Another survey carried out near Campinas, São Paulo state, showed that flowering of *C. langsdorffii* occurs in the middle of the rainy season (December–February), with development of fruit during the dry season (April–September) [29,30]. The phenophases of *C. officinalis* were monitored in the municipality of Boa Vista (Roraima state, Brazil), and showed that the flowering of the species occurs between the months of September and November and the fruiting from November to March. Depending on the stage of fruit ripening, the dehiscence can begin in January, in which the seeds enveloped by the aril are exposed, allowing for their dispersal [28].

Copaifera is a hermaphrodite plant of mixed reproduction with a predominance of allogamy. The trees are generally bee pollinated (melittophily), and *Apis mellifera* and *Trigona* spp. are its main pollinating agents [25]. *C. langsdorffii* has high fecundity, producing large quantity of fruits in a short period of time. Its seeds have low nutritional value, mainly composed of carbohydrates, but can attract a wide variety of animals with a general diet [30]. The dispersion of the copaiba seeds occurs mainly in zoocoric and barocoric forms [27,28]. Some vertebrates, such as birds and mammals, have been observed visiting the fruits of *Copaifera* [31]. Its seeds have morphological characteristics that fit the ornithocoria syndrome, mainly because they are black with colored, fleshy arils, which, after being swallowed, can be regurgitated intact and remain viable for germination [32]. A study revealed that 10 species of Passeriformes, such as *Ramphastos toco*, *Cyanocorax cristatellus*, and *Turdus rufiventris*, visited the fruits of *C. langsdorffii*. Likewise, monkeys of the species *Eriodes arachnoides* and *Cebus paella* also eat the fruits of *C. langsdorffii* [31]. Copaiba seeds may also present hydrocoric dispersion due to their frequent occurrence near waterways [25]. Copaiba seeds are of conventional behavior and may be conserved in the long term ex situ, with dormancy due to the deposition of coumarin in the tegument, and its germination is of the epigene type [25]. A tree can produce from 2 to 3 kg of seeds [33].

The population density of copaiba trees in an area is usually very low. It is possible to find only one tree every 5 ha, but they may occur in densities of one to two trees per hectare. The production of oleoresin by species is fairly variable and can be influenced by genetic differences among species, habitat, soil, and intensity of exploitation [34]. The production of oleoresin per tree ranges from 100 mL to 60 L per year. In addition, not all trees produce oil [24]. Therefore, detailed investigations regarding extraction methods and equipment that do not harm the plant, correlation of genetic data to botanical identification of species, floristic inventory of copaiba populations, and ecological studies on its ecosystems are indispensable for the sustainable and rational use of this resource [35,36].

3. Traditional Uses of *Copaifera*

3.1. Medicinal Uses

In Pará state (Amazon region, Brazil), people of all ages and social classes consider copaiba one of the most important natural remedies from the Amazon region. Several parts and preparations of the plant are used in folk medicine [24]. The oleoresin or bark decoction is used as an anti-inflammatory and contraceptive by native people from the Brazilian Amazon. The topical application of oil on the skin serves to heal wounds. It is used in massages on the head to cure paralysis, pains, and convulsions. In Amapá state, it is recommended to soak a cotton ball in oil and place on tumors, ulcers, or hives. The daily intake of two drops of oil mixed with one tablespoon of honey is indicated for inflammation, syphilis, bronchitis, and cough [6,37,38]. In Venezuela, the oil is used to prepare a patch that is applied to heal ulcers and wounds, and the decoction of the bark in the form of a bath is used to combat rheumatism, to wash infected wounds such as dog bites, and to use as an anti-tetanus [37,38]. A tea from the seeds is also used as a purgative and for treatment of asthma. In northern Brazil, the practice of "embrocation" (applying oil directly to the throat) is common to treat throat infections [39]. In Belém, the "garrafada"—an infusion of the bark sold in bottles—is currently used as a substitute for the oleoresin due to the difficulty in obtaining the oil in the city [38].

Copaiba has a wide range of ethnopharmacological indications, including for the treatment of: cystitis, urinary incontinence, gonorrhea, and syphilis; respiratory ailments, including bronchitis, strep throat, hemoptysis, pneumonia, and sinusitis; infections in the skin and mucosa, such as dermatitis, eczema, psoriasis, and wounds; ulcers and lesions of the uterus; leishmaniasis and leucorrhea; anemia; headaches; and snake bites. It is also used for its aphrodisiac, stimulant, anti-inflammatory, antiseptic, anti-tetanus, antirheumatic, antiherpetic, anthelminthic, anticancer, antitumor (prostate tumors), and antiparalytic properties [4,6,26,38,40]. *Copaifera* species are used by people of Igarapé Miri (Pará state) for healing wounds [41].

Studies have shown that the ingestion of high doses of copaiba oil can cause adverse side effects, such as gastrointestinal irritation, sialorrhea, and central nervous system depression. A dose of 10 g may cause symptoms of intolerance, nausea, vomiting, colic and diarrhea, and exanthema. Prolonged use may cause kidney damage and topical reactions in susceptible individuals [39,42]. Thus, the advance in pharmacological and quality control studies of copaiba formulations sold at herbal markets is indispensable for the safe use of this plant drug.

3.2. Human Nutrition

Copaiba oil was approved in the United States as a food additive and is used in small amounts as a flavoring agent in foods and beverages [43].

3.3. Cosmetic Uses

The species of *Copaifera* are intensively pursued for inclusion in the cosmetics market due to their therapeutic properties and fragrant value of their oils [44]. Copaiba oil is currently used in the cosmetic industry as a fixative for perfumes and perfuming soaps [38]. As an emollient, bactericidal, and anti-inflammatory agent, copaiba oil is used in the production of soaps, lotions, creams and moisturizers, bath foams, shampoos, and hair conditioners [6,24]. In addition, it aids in the treatment of dandruff and acne [38,45]. Despite its fragrant value, little information regarding its odorant potential is available in the literature [44].

3.4. Fuel

As a renewable source of hydrocarbons, the use of copaiba oil as an ecologically clean fuel has been evaluated. Experimental plantations were started in the early 1980s near Manaus, Brazil to test its viability as an alternative energy source to fossil fuels [7]. For potential use as fuel, a combination with diesel oil in a ratio of 9:1 (diesel oil to copaiba) has been recommended [6]. Various reports indicate that the liquid can be poured directly into the fuel tank of a diesel-powered car and the vehicle will run normally, with a bluish exhaust smoke being the only noticeable difference [46]. Traditionally, the oil is used in lamps as fuel for lighting [24].

3.5. Wood

The copaiba trees are considered hardwoods with high demand due to their properties of strength, as well as insect and xylophagous fungi repellency. The wood is saturated with oil and resin and has been used in both shipbuilding and civil construction, especially in the manufacture of steam caves, pool cues, and decorative and furniture coverings. It is also used in the preparation of lumbers, rafters, door and window frames, and boards in general, including for agricultural implements, general carpentry, flooring furniture, coatings, lamination, plywood sheets. The wood has a high content of lignin and is very good for the production of alcohol and charcoal. *C. langsdorffii* has traditionally been exploited extensively for charcoal in the Cariri Region, south of Ceará [24,47].

3.6. Veterinary Uses

In southern Pará state, farmers have used copaiba oil to prevent foot-and-mouth infection in cattle. The oil is poured on the floor next to the salt lick so that when cattle approach to eat salt, they step in oil soaking their feet [24]. When wounded, some animals lick and rub their bodies in the oil that flows from the trees [24].

3.7. Other Uses

Hunters often hunt under the copaiba tree during fruiting because the seeds and oil attract animals [24]. The oleoresin is used in the photographic industry to improve image clarity in areas of low contrast and resolution. The resin has also been used in paper making, as an additive for butadiene in the production of synthetic rubber, as a source of a chiral substrate in the synthesis of biomarkers of sediment and oil residues, and as fixative in the manufacture of varnish, perfume, and paints used in the painting of porcelain, fabrics, and for dying cotton yarn [6,24,38].

4. Essential Oil Chemistry of *Copaifera*

The major components of the essential oils from *Copaifera* species are summarized in Table 1. In general, copaiba oils derived from *Copaifera* oleoresins are rich in sesquiterpene hydrocarbons and often dominated by β-caryophyllene [15]. Some copaiba oils, however, also show significant concentrations of diterpene acids, which are generally analyzed as their methyl esters [15]. A perusal of internet sources of copaiba oil suggests that the most important commercial sources of copaiba oil are *C. langsdorffii*, *C. officinalis*, and *C. reticulata*, and the most prized copaiba oils are rich in β-caryophyllene. The oleoresin essential oils from these three *Copaifera* species can have as much as 33% (*C. langsdorffii*), 87% (*C. officinalis*), and 68% (*C. reticulata*) β-caryophyllene (see Table 1).

Table 1. Major components of the essential oils of *Copaifera* species.

Copaifera spp.	EO Source	Major Components (>5%)	Ref.
C. cearensis Huber ex Ducke	oleoresin	α-copaene (8.2%), β-caryophyllene (19.7%), δ-cadinene (7.2%), β-bisabolol (8.2%), hardwickiic acid (6.2%), clorechinic acid (11.3%)	[13]
C. cearensis Huber ex Ducke	oleoresin	α-copaene (8.2%), β-caryophyllene (19.7%), hardwickiic acid (6.2%)	[48]
C. duckei Dwyer	oleoresin	β-caryophyllene (0.7–6.2%), *trans*-α-bergamotene (3.4–7.9%), β-selinene (5.5–7.3%), β-bisabolene (8.9–12.1%), kaur-16-en-19-oic acid (19.8–24.5%), polyalthic acid (17.1–27.7%), hardwickiic acid (0–24.3%)	[8]
C. duckei Dwyer	oleoresin	β-elemene (8.3–9.4%), β-caryophyllene (13.0–15.5%), *trans*-α-bergamotene (8.3–10.6%), β-selinene (13.8–15.4%), α-selinene (8.8–9.9%), β-bisabolene (15.7–17.6%)	[49]
C. duckei Dwyer	oleoresin	β-caryophyllene (25.1–50.2%), *trans*-α-bergamotene (6.4–12.0%), (*E*)-β-farnesene (2.9–5.8%), β-selinene (1.8–6.7%), β-bisabolene (5.2–33.6%)	[49]
C. guianensis Desf.	oleoresin	*trans*-α-bergamotene (7.2%), caryophyllene oxide (19.1%), kaur-16-en-19-oic acid (17.5%), polyalthic acid (10.6%), hardwickiic acid (11.0%)	[8]
C. langsdorffii Desf.	oleoresin	β-caryophyllene (32.8%), kaurenoic acid (44.3%), copalic acid (5.6%), hardwickiic acid (8.2%)	[48]
C. langsdorffii Desf.	oleoresin	cyclosativene (5.0%), β-elemene (5.1%), β-caryophyllene (5.5%), *trans*-α-bergamotene (48.4%), β-selinene (5.0%), α-himachalene (11.2%)	[50]
C. langsdorffii Desf.	oleoresin	α-copaene (5.8%), γ-muurolene (22.7%), eremophilone (6.8%), kaurene (6.8%), methyl oleate (26.5%)	[51]
C. langsdorffii Desf.	oleoresin	β-elemene (8.0%), β-caryophyllene (31.4%), *trans*-α-bergamotene (10.2%), γ-muurolene (16.1%)	[52]
C. langsdorffii Desf.	oleoresin	β-caryophyllene (1.1–9.0%), germacrene D (4.0–18.0%), bicyclogermacrene (1.5–5.7%), spathulenol (12.6–35.7%), caryophyllene oxide (7.4–16.6%), α-cadinol (3.2–7.9%)	[53]
C. langsdorffii Desf.	pericarp	α-copaene (3.2–14.4%), β-elemene (0–11.1%), β-caryophyllene (2.7–10.5%), germacrene D (1.9–10.7%), bicyclogermacrene (0–6.3%), spathulenol (2.2–16.2%), caryophyllene oxide (4.0–5.1%), *iso*-spathulenol (5.6–21.6%)	[54]

Table 1. *Cont.*

Copaifera spp.	EO Source	Major Components (>5%)	Ref.
C. langsdorffii Desf.	leaf	α-copaene (1.8–6.9%), β-elemene (0–8.4%), β-caryophyllene (5.7–17.5%), germacrene D (0–17.3%), bicyclogermacrene (0–11.5%), δ-cadinene (1.6–6.1%), spathulenol (3.8–12.4%), caryophyllene oxide (0–15.6%), α-muurolol (4.8–6.2%), α-cadinol (4.9–6.8%)	[54]
C. langsdorffii Desf.	leaf	β-caryophyllene (10.1–16.8%), germacrene D (9.1–45.2%), bicyclogermacrene (4.8–21.1%), spathulenol (4.9–29.4%), caryophyllene oxide (3.8–18.8%)	[55]
C. langsdorffii Desf.	seed	coumarin (0–12.6%), spathulenol (19.4–38.9%), caryophyllene oxide (0–21.8%), humulene epoxide II (0–5.1%), *iso*-spathulenol (6.9–25.8%), τ-muurolol (1.3–5.0%), α-cadinol (2.0–10.4%)	[54]
C. langsdorffii Desf.	stem	β-caryophyllene (2.4–13.9%), germacrene D (0–19.1%), bicyclogermacrene (0–8.0%), δ-cadinene (0–5.7%), spathulenol (3.6–13.7%), caryophyllene oxide (4.9–13.3%), *iso*-spathulenol (0–7.9%), τ-muurolol (3.4–7.9%), α-cadinol (4.9–11.5%)	[54]
C. lucens Dwyer	oleoresin	polyalthic acid (69.8%), copalic acid (11.1%)	[48]
C. martii Hayne	oleoresin	α-copaene (36.4–51.2%), β-elemene (4.1–6.2%), *allo*-aromadendrene (4.2–5.0%), δ-cadinene (13.7–17.2%)	[56]
C. martii Hayne	oleoresin	β-bisabolene (10.7%), zingiberene (7.2%), kaurenoic acid (7.9%), kovalenic acid (29.0%)	[48]
C. multijuga Hayne	oleoresin	α-copaene (2.1–5.2%), β-caryophyllene (42.9–60.3%), *trans*-β-bergamotene (2.0–7.0%), caryophyllene oxide (tr–8.8%), copalic acid (1.9–11.0%), 3-acetoxycopalic acid (0.8–6.2%)	[8]
C. multijuga Hayne	oleoresin	β-caryophyllene (57.5%), α-humulene (8.3%), copalic acid (6.2%)	[57]
C. multijuga Hayne	oleoresin	β-caryophyllene (57.5%), α-humulene (8.3%), copalic acid (6.2%)	[13]
C. multijuga Hayne	oleoresin	β-caryophyllene (60.2%), *trans*-α-bergamotene (6.4%), α-humulene (8.6%), copalic acid (9.5%)	[44]
C. multijuga Hayne	oleoresin	β-caryophyllene (57.5%), copalic acid (6.2%)	[48]
C. multijuga Hayne	oleoresin	α-copaene (18.8%), β-caryophyllene (36.0%), *trans*-α-bergamotene (7.0%), β-bisabolene (8.5%), δ-cadinene (6.1%)	[58]
C. multijuga Hayne	oleoresin	α-copaene (2.0–15.0%), β-caryophyllene (5.1–64.0%), α-humulene (0–8.9%), germacrene D (0–16.7%), δ-cadinene (0–5.4%), caryophyllene oxide (0.2–31.5%), copalic acid (1.7–7.1%)	[17]

Table 1. *Cont.*

Copaifera spp.	EO Source	Major Components (>5%)	Ref.
C. multijuga Hayne	oleoresin	β-caryophyllene (57.1%), α-humulene (10.2%), β-sesquiphellandrene (9.9%)	[59]
C. multijuga Hayne	oleoresin	α-copaene (2.5–14.9%), β-caryophyllene (10.6–62.7%), α-humulene (2.4–8.7%), germacrene D (0–18.9%), caryophyllene oxide (0.2–32.5%), copalic acid (1.1–5.2%)	[60]
C. multijuga Hayne	oleoresin	α-copaene (5.0%), β-gurjunene (5.3%), β-caryophyllene (29.6%), α-humulene (5.7%), caryophyllene alcohol (5.8%), caryophyllene oxide (13.0%)	[61]
C. multijuga Hayne	oleoresin	β-caryophyllene (58.4%), α-humulene (8.4%), copalic acid (6.3%)	[61]
C. officinalis (Jacq.) L.	oleoresin	β-caryophyllene (8.5%), copalic acid (13.9%), hardwickiic acid (30.7%)	[48]
C. officinalis (Jacq.) L.	oleoresin	β-caryophyllene (24.9%), *allo*-aromadendrene (7.5%), germacrene B (5.1%), β-bisabolene (6.3%), δ-cadinene (15.3%), α-cadinene (5.6%)	[62]
C. officinalis (Jacq.) L.	oleoresin	β-caryophyllene (62.7%), *trans*-α-bergamotene (7.6%), α-humulene (8.1%)	Setzer [a]
C. officinalis (Jacq.) L.	oleoresin	β-caryophyllene (87.3%)	Setzer [b]
C. paupera (Herzog) Dwyer	oleoresin	β-bisabolene (20.2%), zingiberene (19.4%), kaurenoic acid (13.3%), copalic acid (6.1%)	[48]
C. paupera (Herzog) Dwyer	oleoresin	α-cubebene (5.5%), α-copaene (42.5%), β-caryophyllene (14.1%), δ-cadinene (10.4%)	[63]
C. piresii Ducke	oleoresin	α-copaene (45.5%), β-caryophyllene (10.3%), δ-cadinene (13.7%)	[63]
C. publflora Benth.	oleoresin	β-caryophyllene (65.9%), α-humulene (7.3%), β-selinene (10.2%), α-selinene (5.5%)	[63]
C. reticulata Ducke	oleoresin	β-caryophyllene (40.9%), α-humulene (6.0%), germacrene D (5.0%)	[13]
C. reticulata Ducke	oleoresin (Pará)	β-caryophyllene (40.9%)	[48]
C. reticulata Ducke	oleoresin (Acre)	α-copaene (25.1%), β-caryophyllene (13.1%), copalic acid (7.7%), kaurenoic acid (7.5%), hardwickiic acid (6.9%)	[48]
C. reticulata Ducke	oleoresin	β-elemene (0.5–5.6%), β-caryophyllene (1.4–68.0%), *trans*-α-bergamotene (2.4–29.6%), α-humulene (1.1–9.7%), β-selinene (0–20.6%), α-selinene (0–13.2%), β-bisabolene (3.7–42.4%), caryophyllene oxide (0.1–15.2%)	[64]

Table 1. *Cont.*

Copaifera spp.	EO Source	Major Components (>5%)	Ref.
C. reticulata Ducke	oleoresin	β-elemene (0–6.0%), β-caryophyllene (0–43.4%), *trans*-α-bergamotene (12.0–32.8%), α-guaiene (0–9.5%), α-humulene (0–7.0%), β-selinene (0–17.1%), α-selinene (0–10.4%), *trans*-β-guaiene (0–5.8%), β-bisabolene (24.2–50.3%)	[65]
C. reticulata Ducke	oleoresin	β-caryophyllene (25.1–50.2%), *trans*-α-bergamotene (6.4–12.0%), α-humulene (4.1–5.8%), β-selinene (1.8–6.7%), β-bisabolene (5.2–17.4%)	[66]
C. reticulata Ducke	oleoresin	β-caryophyllene (37.3%), *trans*-α-bergamotene (9.0%), α-humulene (5.4%), β-bisabolene (14.5%)	[67]
C. reticulata Ducke	oleoresin	β-caryophyllene (7.7%), *trans*-α-bergamotene (22.0%), β-selinene (12.2%), α-selinene (11.4%), β-bisabolene (24.9%)	[68]
C. trapezifolia Hayne	leaf	β-caryophyllene (33.5%), α-humulene (6.2%), germacrene D (11.0%), spathulenol (7.6%)	[69]

[a] Unpublished analysis of a commercial essential oil from New Directions Aromatics (Sydney, Australia).
[b] Unpublished analysis of a commercial essential oil from Améo Essential Oils/Zija International (Lehi, Utah).

5. Nonvolatile Chemistry of *Copaifera*

The oleoresins of several *Copaifera* species have been shown to be rich sources of clerodane, kaurane, and labdane triterpenoids (Figures 1–3, Table 2). In particular, *C. langsdorffii* resin is composed of biologically active copalic acid [70,71] and kaurenoic acid [72–74]. *C. multijuga* [74] and *C. paupera* [75] resins are also good sources of copalic acid.

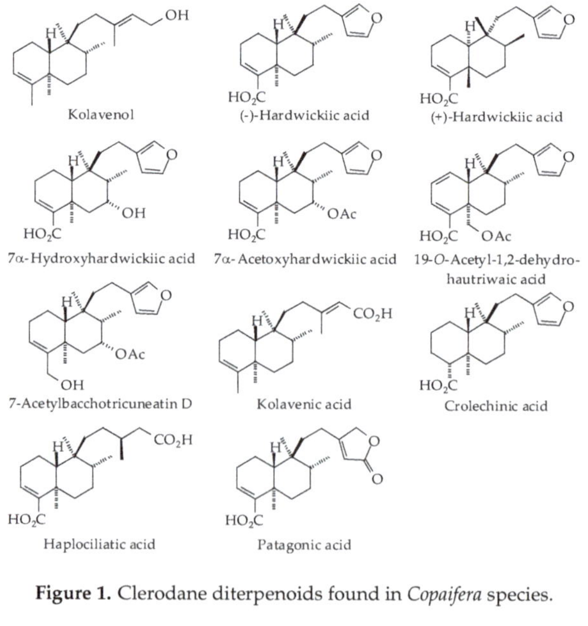

Figure 1. Clerodane diterpenoids found in *Copaifera* species.

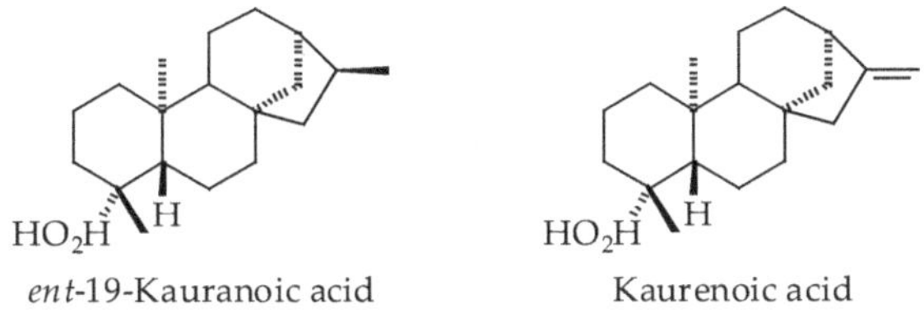

Figure 2. Kaurane diterpenoids found in *Copaifera* species.

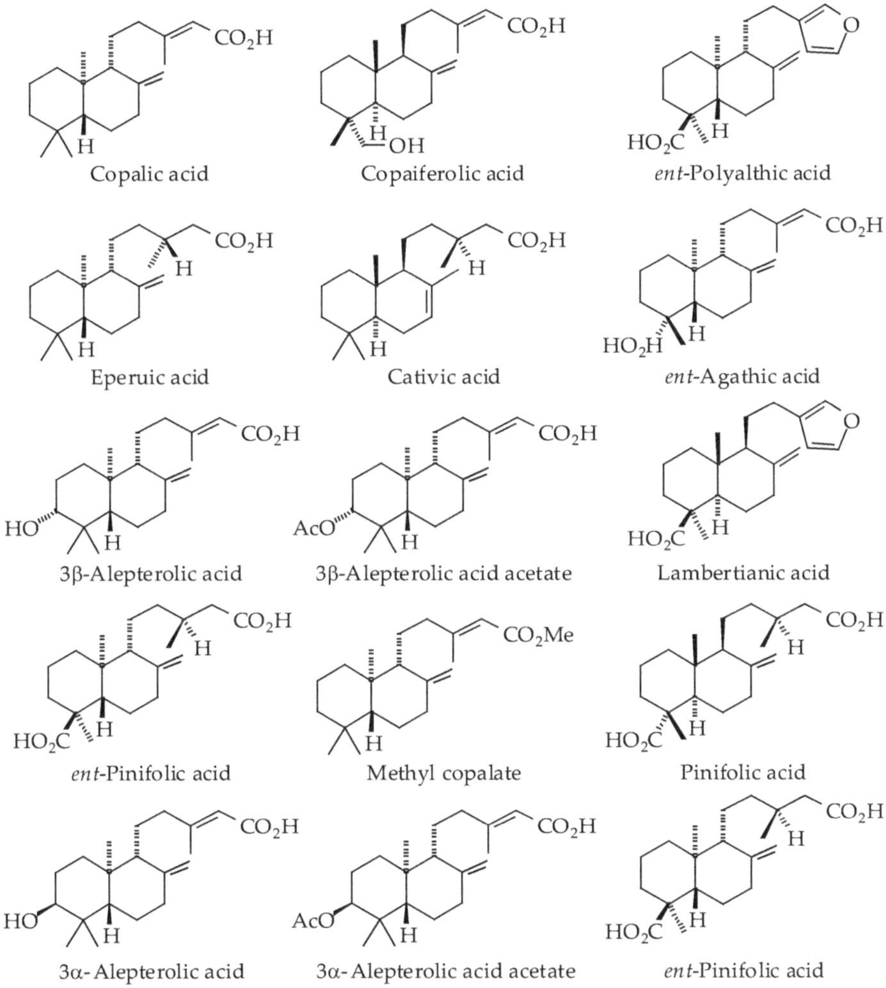

Figure 3. Labdane diterpenoids found in *Copaifera* species.

Table 2. Nonvolatile components isolated and/or identified from *Copaifera* species.

Copaifera spp.	Plant Part	Compounds Isolated and/or Identified	Ref.
C. cearensis Huber ex Ducke	oleoresin	epuric acid, cativic acid, copalic acid, kolavenic acid, crolechinic acid, hardwickiic acid, haplociliatic acid, labdanolic acid, patagonic acid.	[76]
C. guianensis Desf.	oleoresin	methyl copalate	[74]
C. langsdorffii Desf.	oleoresin	copalic acid, kaurenoic acid, acetoxycopalic acid (=3α-alepterolic acid acetate), *ent*-agathic acid, hydroxycopalic acid (=3α-alepterolic acid)	[71]
C. langsdorffii Desf.	oleoresin	copalic acid, acetoxycopalic acid (=3α-alepterolic acid acetate), 3-hydroxy-14,15-dinorlabd-8(17)-en-13-one, *ent*-agathic acid, hydroxycopalic acid (=3α-alepterolic acid)	[70]
C. langsdorffii Desf.	oleoresin	kaurenoic acid	[72]
C. langsdorffii Desf.	oleoresin	kaurenoic acid	[73]
C. langsdorffii Desf.	oleoresin	kaurenoic acid	[74]
C. langsdorffii Desf.	oleoresin	sclareol, manool, copalic acid, acetoxycopalic acid (=3α-alepterolic acid acetate), hydroxycopalic acid (=3α-alepterolic acid), *ent*-agathic acid	[77]
C. langsdorffii Desf.	leaves	kaurenoic acid, quercitrin, afzelin	[78]
C. langsdorffii Desf.	leaves	rutin, quercetin-3-*O*-α-L-rhamnopyranoside, kaempferol-3-*O*-α-L-rhamnopyranoside, quercetin, kaempferol	[79]
C. langsdorffii Desf.	fruit	gallic acid, epicatechin gallate, catechin, epicatechin, isoquercitrin	[80]
C. langsdorffii Desf.	leaves	kaurenoic acid, quercitrin, afzelin, eupatorin, galloyl quinic acid, gallic acid 4-*O*-glucoside	[81]
C. multijuga Hayne	oleoresin	copalic acid, 3-hydroxycopalic acid (=3α-alepterolic acid), 3-acetoxycopalic acid (=3α-alepterolic acid acetate)	[74]
C. paupera (Herzog) Dwyer	oleoresin	copalic acid, methyl copalate, agathic acid 15-methyl ester, agathic acid 15,19-dimethyl ester, *ent*-polyalthic acid, methyl *ent*-polyalthate, *ent*-pinifolic acid, methyl 3β-hydroxy-labda-8(17),13-dien-15-ate, methyl 18-hydroxy-copaiferolate, 14,15-bisnorlabd-8(17)-en-13-one, *ent*-kaurenic acid, 16β-kauran-19-oic acid, 3-methyl-5-(2,2,6-trimethyl-6-hydroxycyclohexyl)- pentanoic acid, pauperol	[75]
C. reticulata Ducke	oleoresin	3β-alepterolic acid, 3β-alepterolic acid acetate, 3β-hydroxylabdan-8(17)-en-15-oic acid, *ent*-agathic acid	[82]

6. Biological Activities of *Copaifera*

Copaifera oleoresins have shown remarkable biological activities, many of which have been attributed to diterpenoid acids (see Table 3). Generally, *Copaifera* oleoresins and their diterpenoid constituents have shown antibacterial, anti-inflammatory, antileishmanial, antiproliferative, antitrypanosomal, and wound-healing activities.

Table 3. Biological activities of *Copaifera* oleoresins, essential oils, and isolated components.

Copaifera spp.	Material	Biological Activity	Ref.
C. cearensis Huber ex Ducke	oleoresin	Anti-inflammatory: At a concentration of 50 μg/mL, in vitro NO production in mouse peritoneal macrophages was significantly reduced by *C. cearensis* oil.	[13]
C. cearensis Huber ex Ducke	oleoresin	Antileishmanial: *L. amazonensis* promastigotes (IC_{50} = 18.0 μg/mL).	[48]
C. cearensis Huber ex Ducke	oleoresin	Antibacterial: Methicillin-resistant *Staphylococcus aureus* (MRSA, MIC = 125 μg/mL), *B. subtilis* (MIC = 62.5 μg/mL), *Enterococcus faecalis* (MIC = 62.5 μg/mL)	[83]
C. duckei Dwyer	oleoresin	Anti-inflammatory: Carrageenin-induced paw edema test (rats, 18% edema inhibition with dose of 1802 mg/kg; granuloma test, 42% inhibition with dose of 1802 mg/kg); croton oil-induced dermatitis test (mice, IC_{50} = 663 mg/kg)	[84]
C. duckei Dwyer	oleoresin	Antinociceptive: Mouse model (acetic acid-induced writhing test, IC_{50} = 704 mg/kg)	[84]
C. duckei Dwyer	oleoresin	Antiproliferative: In vivo hepatocellular proliferation, partial hepatectomy, rats. Hepatocellular proliferation and liver mitochondrial respiration were significantly lower in *C. duckei* treated rats compared to control (saline solution).	[85]
C. duckei Dwyer	oleoresin	Antitrypanosomal: *T. evansi*, in vivo mouse model, doses of 0.63 mL/kg/day over 5 days showed no curative effects. *T. evansi*, in vitro trypomastigotes, 0.5% solution of *C. duckei* oil showed 100% killing after 6 h.	[86]
C. langsdorffii Desf.	oleoresin	Anti-inflammatory: Preincubation of LPS-stimulated human THP-1 monocytes with diterpenoid-rich oleoresin reduced the release of proinflammatory cytokines (IL-1β, IL-6, TNFα).	[50]
C. langsdorffii Desf.	oleoresin	Antifungal: *Tricophyton mentagrophytes* (MIC = 170 μg/mL). Scanning electron microscopic (SEM) analysis revealed physical damage and morphological alterations of the fungi upon exposure to copaiba oleoresin.	[52]
C. langsdorffii Desf.	oleoresin	Antipsoriatic: Human clinical trial, topical application of copaiba resin exhibited a significant improvement of the typical signs of psoriasis.	[50]
C. langsdorffii Desf.	oleoresin	Gastroprotective: Ethanol or indomethacin-induced ulcer in rats, oral administration of copaiba resin at doses of 400 mg/kg provided dose-dependent significant protection against gastric damage caused by ethanol or indomethacin.	[87]
C. langsdorffii Desf.	oleoresin	Gastroprotective: Mesenteric ischemia/reperfusion (I/R) in rats: Copaiba resin treatment caused significant attenuations in I/R-associated increases of myeloperoxidase, malondialdehyde, and catalase, and effectively prevented the I/R-associated depletion of glutathione.	[88]

Table 3. *Cont.*

Copaifera spp.	Material	Biological Activity	Ref.
C. langsdorffii Desf.	oleoresin	Wound-healing: Rat incision wounds, 4% oleoresin topically applied showed significant wound contraction and tensile strength compared to controls.	[89]
C. langsdorffii Desf.	oleoresin	Wound healing: Rat dorsal skin flaps, oral administration of copaiba oleoresin (400 mg/kg), copaiba-treatment presented discrete anti-lipoperoxidation action, intense antioxidant action, and anti-inflammatory activity during the ischemia and reperfusion of randomized cutaneous flaps.	[90]
C. langsdorffii Desf.	oleoresin	Anti-inflammatory: Rat model of experimental endometriosis. Copaiba oil caused a marked reduction in endometrial growth.	[91]
C. langsdorffii Desf.	oleoresin	Antileishmanial: *L. amazonensis* promastigotes (IC_{50} = 20.0 μg/mL).	[48]
C. langsdorffii Desf.	oleoresin	Antibacterial: *B. subtilis* (MIC = 62.5 μg/mL)	[83]
C. langsdorffii Desf.	10% copaiba oil ointment	Wound-healing: Rat dorsal skin flaps, topical copaiba oil ointment favors angiogenesis and accelerates the viability of random skin flaps in rats.	[51]
C. langsdorffii Desf.	10% oleoresin cream	Antibacterial: Open wounds on rats inoculated with *Streptococcus pyogenes* or *Staphylococcus aureus*. Treatment with 10% copaiba cream reduced bacterial populations to 0.02% (*S. pyogenes*) and 0.3% (*S. aureus*) after 14 days.	[92]
C. langsdorffii Desf.	10% oleoresin cream	Wound-healing: Rabbit ears, 10% oleoresin cream-treated wounds presented better clinical outcomes, confirmed by histology with evidence of fibroblastic activity by day 7 and organized collagen fibers observed from day 14.	[93]
C. langsdorffii Desf.	10% oleoresin cream	Wound-healing: Rat skin biopsy punch on dorsal surface, 10% oleoresin cream-treated wounds showed a faster wound-healing rate compared to saline or cream only controls, by regulating matrix metalloproteinase, (MMP)-2 and MMP-9 activities, stimulating collagen synthesis, and promoting tissue remodeling and re-epithelialization.	[94]
C. langsdorffii Desf.	3α-alepterolic acid acetate	Antibacterial: Cariogenic *Streptococcus* spp.; MIC range 12.0–60.0 μg/mL	[70]
C. langsdorffii Desf.	aqueous leaf extract	Insecticidal: 5% Extract inhibited *Bemisia tabaci* infestation of tomato plants in the field.	[95]
C. langsdorffii Desf.	copalic acid	Antibacterial: Gram-positive bacteria (MIC range 0.5 μg/mL to 15.0 μg/mL)	[71]
C. langsdorffii Desf.	copalic acid	Antibacterial: Cariogenic *Streptococcus* spp.; MIC range 2.0–6.0 μg/mL	[70]
C. langsdorffii Desf.	copalic acid	Antibacterial: Periodontal anaerobic bacteria: *Actinomyces naeslundii* (MIC 6.2 μg/mL), *Bacteroides fragilis* (MIC 25.0 μg/mL), *Peptostreptococcus anaerobius* (MIC 3.1 μg/mL), *Porphyromonas gingivalis* (MIC 3.1 μg/mL).	[77]
C. langsdorffii Desf.	copalic acid	Antiproliferative: In vitro cytotoxicity on MO59J (human glioblastoma cells, IC_{50} = 68.3 μg/mL) and HeLa (human cervical adenocarcinoma cells, IC_{50} = 44.0 μg/mL).	[71]

Table 3. *Cont.*

Copaifera spp.	Material	Biological Activity	Ref.
C. langsdorffii Desf.	EtOH/H_2O leaf extract	Gastroprotective: Ethanol/HCl-induced ulcer in mice, the extract (500 mg/kg) showed a significant decrease in the total gastric juice acidity and an increase in mucus production; isolated compounds (30 mg/kg) α-humulene, β-caryophyllene and caryophyllene oxide showed greater gastroprotective activity in the ethanol/HCl induced ulcer model.	[78]
C. langsdorffii Desf.	kaurenoic acid	Anti-inflammatory: Rat model of acetic acid-induced colitis. A marked reduction in gross damage score (52% and 42%) and wet weight of damaged colon tissue (39% and 32%) were observed in rats that received 100 mg/kg kaurenoic acid, respectively, by rectal and oral routes.	[72]
C. langsdorffii Desf.	kaurenoic acid	Antibacterial: Gram-positive bacteria (MIC range 5.0 μg/mL to 100.0 μg/mL)	[71]
C. langsdorffii Desf.	kaurenoic acid	Antiproliferative: In vitro cytotoxicity, 78 μM concentration, on CEM (human leukemia, 95% growth inhibition), MCF-7 (human breast tumor, 45% growth inhibition), and HCT-8 (human colon tumor, 45% growth inhibition) cells.	[73]
C. langsdorffii Desf.	kaurenoic acid	Antiproliferative: In vitro cytotoxicity, 20 μM concentration, on AGP01 (human gastric cancer, 28% growth inhibition) and SF-295 (human glioblastoma, 28% growth inhibition) cells.	[74]
C. langsdorffii Desf.	kaurenoic acid	Smooth muscle relaxant: Rat uterine muscle ex vivo: kaurenoic acid, exerts a uterine relaxant effect acting principally through calcium blockade and in part, by the opening of ATP-sensitive potassium channels.	[96]
C. lucens Dwyer	oleoresin	Antileishmanial: *L. amazonensis* promastigotes (IC_{50} = 20.0 μg/mL).	[48]
C. lucens Dwyer	oleoresin	Antibacterial: *S. aureus* (MIC = 125 μg/mL), *B. subtilis* (MIC = 125 μg/mL)	[83]
C. martii Hayne	oleoresin	Antileishmanial: *L. amazonensis* promastigotes (IC_{50} = 14.0 μg/mL).	[48]
C. martii Hayne	oleoresin	Antileishmanial: In vivo mouse model, copaiba oil oral treatment (100 mg/kg/day) caused a significant reduction in the average lesion size (1.1 ± 0.4 mm) against *Leishmania amazonensis* lesions compared with untreated mice (4.4 ± 1.3 mm).	[97]
C. martii Hayne	oleoresin	Antibacterial: *S. aureus* (MIC = 62.5 μg/mL), MRSA (MIC = 62.5 μg/mL), *B. subtilis* (MIC = 15.6 μg/mL), *S. epidermidis* (MIC = 62.5 μg/mL), *Enterococcus faecalis* (MIC = 62.5 μg/mL)	[83]
C. multijuga Hayne	oleoresin	Antiproliferative: In vitro cytotoxicity, B16F10 (murine melanoma cells, IC_{50} = 457 μg/mL).	[57]
C. multijuga Hayne	oleoresin	Antiproliferative: In vivo lung metastasis and tumor growth, mouse model: Oral administration of *C. multijuga* oleoresin (at 2 g/Kg in the days 3, 5, 7, 10, 12, and 14 after inoculation of tumoral cells) reduced tumor growth by 58% and tumor weight by 76% and reduced the number of lung nodules by 47.1%.	[57]

Table 3. *Cont.*

Copaifera spp.	Material	Biological Activity	Ref.
C. multijuga Hayne	oleoresin	Antiproliferative: In vivo Ehrlich ascitic and solid tumor, mouse model: *C. multijuga* oleoresin (doses varying between 100 and 200 mg/kg) showed antineoplastic properties against Ehrlich ascitic tumor (EAT) and solid tumor during 10 consecutive days of treatment.	[98]
C. multijuga Hayne	oleoresin	Insecticidal: Mosquito larvicidal activity (*Anopheles darlingi*, LC_{50} = 31 μg/mL; *Aedes aegypti*, LC_{50} = 93 μg/mL)	[59]
C. multijuga Hayne	oleoresin	Anti-inflammatory: The β-caryophyllene-rich oleoresin oil of *C. multijuga*, at a dose of 100 mg/kg, inhibited zymosan-induced pleurisy in a mouse model, reducing total leukocytes by 45% and neutrophil accumulation by 73%. *C. multijuga* oil also showed in vitro reduction of NO production in mouse peritoneal macrophages at a concentration of 5 μg/mL.	[13]
C. multijuga Hayne	oleoresin	Anti-inflammatory: Rat pleurisy model, doses of 100 mg/kg and 200 mg/kg presented in vivo anti-inflammatory effects.	[58]
C. multijuga Hayne	oleoresin	Antileishmanial: *L. amazonensis* promastigotes (IC_{50} = 10.0 μg/mL).	[48]
C. multijuga Hayne	oleoresin	Antibacterial: MRSA (MIC = 125 μg/mL), *B. subtilis* (MIC = 125 μg/mL)	[83]
C. multijuga Hayne	oleoresin	Antinociceptive: Mouse model (acetic acid-induced writhing, tail flick, hot plate), oral administration of *C. multijuga* oil with doses of 30–150 mg/kg significantly showed antinociception, which was reversed with naloxone.	[99]
C. multijuga Hayne	oleoresin	Insecticidal: Mosquito larvicidal activity (*Anopheles darlingi*, LC_{50} = 128 μg/mL; *Aedes aegypti*, LC_{50} = 18 μg/mL)	[59]
C. multijuga Hayne	oleoresin extracts	Anti-inflammatory: The CH_2Cl_2 and MeOH fractions obtained from *C. multijuga* oleoresin, given by the intraperitoneal route, caused a significant inhibition of carrageenan-induced rat paw edema with inhibition of 49 ± 13% and 64 ± 9%, respectively.	[61]
C. multijuga Hayne	oleoresin extracts	Anti-inflammatory: The hexane, chloroform and methanol fractions obtained from *C. multijuga* oleoresin, given by the oral gavage, caused a significant inhibition of carrageenan-induced rat paw edema.	[100]
C. multijuga Hayne	oleoresin extracts	Antinociceptive: The hexane, chloroform and methanol fractions obtained from *C. multijuga* oleoresin, given by the oral gavage, caused a significant inhibition (in a concentration-dependent way) the number of contortions induced by acetic acid and the second phase of formalin-induced licking response. Similar results were observed in the tail flick model; administration of naloxone inhibited the antinociceptive effect of the fractions indicating that copaiba resin maybe acting on opioid receptors.	[100]
C. multijuga Hayne	3β-alepterolic acid	Antiproliferative: In vitro cytotoxicity, 20 μM concentration, on AGP01 (human gastric cancer, 8.5% growth inhibition) and SF-295 (human glioblastoma, 21% growth inhibition) cells.	[74]

Table 3. *Cont.*

Copaifera spp.	Material	Biological Activity	Ref.
C. multijuga Hayne	3β-alepterolic acid acetate	Antiproliferative: In vitro cytotoxicity, 20 μM concentration, on AGP01 (human gastric cancer, 13% growth inhibition) and SF-295 (human glioblastoma, 18% growth inhibition) cells.	[74]
C. officinalis (Jacq.) L.	oleoresin	Antiproliferative: In vivo Walker 256 carcinoma inoculated into the vagina and uterine cervix of female rats, *C. officinalis* oleoresin stimulated tumor growth by 70%.	[101]
C. officinalis (Jacq.) L.	oleoresin EO	Anti-inflammatory: Dias and coworkers investigated the immunomodulatory effects of *C. officinalis* oleoresin essential oil on inflammatory cytokines (NO, H_2O_2, TNF-α, IFN-γ, and IL-17) in a murine model of experimental autoimmune encephalomyelitis. At a concentration of 100 μg/mL, *C. officinalis* oil inhibited the in vitro production of the inflammatory cytokines, modulating the immune response.	[62]
C. officinalis (Jacq.) L.	oleoresin	Antileishmanial: *L. amazonensis* promastigotes (IC_{50} = 20.0 μg/mL).	[48]
C. officinalis (Jacq.) L.	oleoresin	Antibacterial: *S. aureus* (MIC = 62.5 μg/mL), MRSA (MIC = 125 μg/mL), *B. subtilis* (MIC = 31.3 μg/mL), *S. epidermidis* (MIC = 31.3 μg/mL), *Enterococcus faecalis* (MIC = 31.3 μg/mL)	[83]
C. officinalis (Jacq.) L.	oleoresin	Antibacterial: *Streptococcus mutans* (MIC = 780 μg/mL)	[102]
C. officinalis (Jacq.) L.	oleoresin	Antibacterial: *Staphylococcus aureus* (MIC = 312.5 μg/mL)	[103]
C. officinalis (Jacq.) L.	agathic acid	Antileishmanial: *L. amazonensis* promastigotes (IC_{50} = 28.0 μg/mL), amastigotes (IC_{50} = 17.0 μg/mL)	[104]
C. officinalis (Jacq.) L.	alepterolic acid (=hydroxycopalic acid)	Antileishmanial: *L. amazonensis* promastigotes (IC_{50} = 2.5 μg/mL), amastigotes (IC_{50} = 18.0 μg/mL)	[104]
C. officinalis (Jacq.) L.	kaurenoic acid	Antileishmanial: *L. amazonensis* promastigotes (IC_{50} = 28.0 μg/mL), amastigotes (IC_{50} = 3.5 μg/mL)	[104]
C. officinalis (Jacq.) L.	methyl copalate	Antileishmanial: *L. amazonensis* promastigotes (IC_{50} = 6.0 μg/mL), amastigotes (IC_{50} = 14.0 μg/mL)	[104]
C. officinalis (Jacq.) L.	pinifolic acid	Antileishmanial: *L. amazonensis* promastigotes (IC_{50} = 70.0 μg/mL), amastigotes (IC_{50} = 4.0 μg/mL)	[104]
C. officinalis (Jacq.) L.	*ent*-polyalthic acid	Antileishmanial: *L. amazonensis* promastigotes (IC_{50} = 35.0 μg/mL), amastigotes (IC_{50} = 15.0 μg/mL)	[104]
C. paupera (Herzog) Dwyer	oleoresin	Antileishmanial: *L. amazonensis* promastigotes (IC_{50} = 11.0 μg/mL).	[48]
C. paupera (Herzog) Dwyer	oleoresin	Antibacterial: *B. subtilis* (MIC = 62.5 μg/mL), *Enterococcus faecalis* (MIC = 62.5 μg/mL)	[83]

Table 3. *Cont.*

Copaifera spp.	Material	Biological Activity	Ref.
C. paupera (Herzog) Dwyer	copalic acid	Antibacterial: *Bacillus subtilis* (MIC = 3.1–6.3 μg/mL), *Staphylococcus aureus* (MIC = 8–10 μg/mL), *Staphylococcus epidermidis* (MIC = 4–5 μg/mL).	[75]
C. paupera (Herzog) Dwyer	*ent*-polyalthic acid	Antibacterial: *Bacillus subtilis* (MIC = 20–30 μg/mL), *Staphylococcus aureus* (MIC = 40–50 μg/mL), *Staphylococcus epidermidis* (MIC = 40 μg/mL).	[75]
C. paupera (Herzog) Dwyer	kaurenoic acid	Antibacterial: *Bacillus subtilis* (MIC = 2.5–5 μg/mL), *Staphylococcus aureus* (MIC = 6–8 μg/mL), *Staphylococcus epidermidis* (MIC = 4–6 μg/mL).	[75]
C. paupera (Herzog) Dwyer	methyl copalate	Antiproliferative: In vitro cytotoxicity, P-388 (murine lymphoma, IC_{50} = 2.5 μg/mL), A-549 (human lung carcinoma, IC_{50} = 5 μg/mL), HT-29 (human colon carcinoma, IC_{50} = 5 μg/mL), MEL-28 (human melanoma, IC_{50} = 10 μg/mL).	[75]
C. reticulata Ducke	oleoresin	Antibacterial: *Porphyromonas gingivalis* (MIC = 6.25 μg/mL), *Streptococcus* spp. (MIC 25–50 μg/mL)	[68]
C. reticulata Ducke	oleoresin	Antiproliferative: In vitro cytotoxicity, GM07492-A (human lung fibroblast cells, IC_{50} = 51.85 μg/mL)	[68]
C. reticulata Ducke	oleoresin	Anxiolytic: elevated plus-maze test with rats: Oral doses of 100, 400, and 800 mg/kg produced a dose-dependent anxiolytic-like effect over the dose range tested.	[105]
C. reticulata Ducke	oleoresin	Insecticidal: Mosquito larvicidal activity (*Culex quinquefasciatus*, LC_{50} = 0.4, 0.9, 39, and 90 μg/mL against the 1st, 2nd, 3rd, and 4th larval instars, respectively)	[106]
C. reticulata Ducke	oleoresin	Insecticidal: Mosquito larvicidal activity (*Aedes aegypti*, LC_{50} = 8.9 μg/mL against the 3rd larval instar)	[107]
C. reticulata Ducke	oleoresin	Neuroprotective: Rat model of motor cortex excitotoxic injury, *C. reticulata* resin treatment induces neuroprotection by modulating inflammatory response following an acute damage to the central nervous system.	[67]
C. reticulata Ducke	oleoresin	Acaricidal: *Rhipicephalus* (*Boophilus*) *microplus* (LC_{50} = 1579 μg/mL)	[108]
C. reticulata Ducke	oleoresin	Anti-inflammatory: At a concentration of 500 μg/mL, *C. reticulata* oleoresin oil showed 85% inhibition of NO production in mouse peritoneal macrophages in vitro.	[13]
C. reticulata Ducke	oleoresin	Antileishmanial: A β-caryophyllene-rich *C. reticulata* (from Pará state) oleoresin oil showed remarkable activity against *L. amazonensis* promastigotes with IC_{50} of 5.0 μg/mL. Another sample of *C. reticulata* oil (from Acre) with lower concentration of β-caryophyllene was less active (IC_{50} = 22.0 μg/mL).	[48]
C. reticulata Ducke	oleoresin EO	Antileishmanial: *C. reticulata* oleoresin essential oil showed significant antileishmanial activity against axenic amastigotes (IC_{50} = 15.0 μg/mL) and intracellular amastigotes (IC_{50} = 20 μg/mL) of *L. amazonensis*. Note that the major component of the oil, β-caryophyllene, was inactive against the amastigotes. Interference with the mitochondrial membrane was suggested as the mechanism for antileishmanial activity.	[109]

Table 3. *Cont.*

Copaifera spp.	Material	Biological Activity	Ref.
C. reticulata Ducke	oleoresin	Antinociceptive: Mouse model (acetic acid-induced writhing, tail flick, hot plate), oral administration of *C. reticulata* oil with doses of 30–150 mg/kg significantly showed antinociception, which was reversed with naloxone.	[99]
C. reticulata Ducke	oleoresin	Antitrypanosomal: *T. evansi*, in vivo mouse model, doses of 0.63 mL/kg/day over 5 days showed no curative effects. *T. evansi*, in vitro trypomastigotes, 0.5% solution of *C. reticulata* oil showed 100% killing after 6 h.	[86]
C. reticulata Ducke	oleoresin EO (Acre)	Antibacterial: *S. aureus* (MIC = 62.5 µg/mL), MRSA (MIC = 125 µg/mL), *B. subtilis* (MIC = 31.3 µg/mL), *S. epidermidis* (MIC = 62.5 µg/mL), *Enterococcus faecalis* (MIC = 62.5 µg/mL)	[83]
C. reticulata Ducke	3β-alepterolic acid	Insecticidal: Mosquito larvicidal activity (*Aedes aegypti*, LC_{50} = 87.3 µg/mL against the 3rd larval instar)	[82]
C. reticulata Ducke	3β-alepterolic acid acetate	Insecticidal: Mosquito larvicidal activity (*Aedes aegypti*, LC_{50} = 0.8 µg/mL against the 3rd larval instar)	[82]
Copaifera spp.	oleoresin	Antibacterial: Oleoresin oils from unidentified species of *Copaifera* showed remarkable antibacterial activity against the Gram-positive *Bacillus subtilis* and *Staphylococcus aureus* (MIC = 5 µg/mL). The oils were inactive against Gram-negative organisms.	[110]
Copaifera spp.	agathic acid	Antitrypanosomal: *T. cruzi* epimastigotes (IC_{50} = 86.8 µM), trypomastigotes (IC_{50} = 823 µM), amastigotes (IC_{50} = 14.9 µM)	[111]
Copaifera spp.	copalic acid	Antitrypanosomal: *T. cruzi* epimastigotes (IC_{50} = 47.2 µM), trypomastigotes (IC_{50} = 444 µM), amastigotes (IC_{50} = 1.3 µM). Note: β-caryophyllene + copalic acid showed a significant synergistic effect against *T. cruzi* trypomastigotes.	[111]
Copaifera spp.	alepterolic acid (=hydroxycopalic acid)	Antitrypanosomal: *T. cruzi* epimastigotes (IC_{50} = 41.2 µM), trypomastigotes (IC_{50} = 453 µM), amastigotes (IC_{50} = 1.8 µM)	[111]
Copaifera spp.	kaurenoic acid	Antitrypanosomal: *T. cruzi* epimastigotes (IC_{50} = 167 µM), trypomastigotes (IC_{50} = 596 µM), amastigotes (IC_{50} = 16.5 µM)	[111]
Copaifera spp.	methyl copalate	Antitrypanosomal: *T. cruzi* epimastigotes (IC_{50} = 83.3 µM), trypomastigotes (IC_{50} = 377 µM), amastigotes (IC_{50} = 2.5 µM)	[111]
Copaifera spp.	pinifolic acid	Antitrypanosomal: *T. cruzi* epimastigotes (IC_{50} = 854 µM), trypomastigotes (IC_{50} = 1630 µM), amastigotes (IC_{50} = 18.6 µM)	[111]
Copaifera spp.	*ent*-polyalthic acid	Antitrypanosomal: *T. cruzi* epimastigotes (IC_{50} = 168 µM), trypomastigotes (IC_{50} = 965 µM), amastigotes (IC_{50} = 28.4 µM)	[111]
Copaifera spp.	β-caryophyllene	Antileishmanial: *L. amazonensis* amastigotes (IC_{50} = 1.3 µg/mL)	[112]
Copaifera spp.	β-caryophyllene	Antitrypanosomal: *T. cruzi* epimastigotes (IC_{50} = 78.4 µM), trypomastigotes (IC_{50} = 1593 µM), amastigotes (IC_{50} = 63.7 µM)	[111]

6.1. Antiparasitic Activity of Copaiba

Several *Copaifera* oleoresin oils have shown in vitro antiparasitic activity against *Leishmania amazonensis* promastigotes, including *C. cearensis*, *C. langsdorffii*, *C. lucens*, *C. martii*, *C. multijuga*, *C. officinalis*, *C. paupera*, and *C. reticulata* [48]. The resin oil of *C. martii* showed in vivo antileishmanial activity in a mouse model [97] and *C. reticulata* resin oil showed activity against *L. amazonensis* axenic amastigotes (IC_{50} = 15.0 μg/mL) and intracellular amastigotes (IC_{50} = 20 μg/mL) [109]. Diterpenoids isolated from *C. officinalis*—agathic acid, alepterolic acid, kaurenoic acid, methyl copalate, pinifolic acid, and *ent*-polyalthic acid—showed antileishmanial activity against *L. amazonensis* promastigotes [104].

Copaifera oleoresins and diterpene acids have also shown antitrypanosomal activities. *C. duckei* and *C. reticulata* resins showed in vitro activity against *T. evansi* trypomastigotes [86]. The diterpene acids—agathic acid, copalic acid, alepterolic acid, kaurenoic acid, methyl copalate, pinifolic acid, and *ent*-polyalthic acid—all showed antitrypanosomal activity against *T. cruzi*, including in the epimastigote, trypomastigote, and amastigote forms of the protozoan [111].

A number of parasitic protozoal proteins have been identified as potential targets for antiparasitic chemotherapy [113]. In conjunction with this review, we have examined the potential parasitic targets of *Copaifera* diterpenoids using molecular docking. It is currently not known what biomolecular targets from *Leishmania* or *Trypanosoma* may be responsible for the antiprotozoal activities of copaiba. The *Copaifera* diterpenoids (Figures 1–3) were screened, in silico, against *Leishmania* drug targets [114–116] and *Trypanosoma cruzi* protein targets [117] using Molegro Virtual Docker v. 6.0.1 as previously described [114–117]. The docking energies are summarized in Tables 4 and 5.

The *Leishmania* protein target with the best overall docking properties with *Copaifera* diterpenoids was *L. major* dihydroorotate dehydrogenase (average E_{dock} = −109.2 kJ/mol). These docking energies were better than the docking energy for the normal substrate, dihydroorotate (E_{dock} = −72.1 kJ/mol) and comparable to the co-crystallized ligand for this protein, nitroorotate (E_{dock} = −104.2 kJ/mol). Docking energies for *Copaifera* diterpenoids with TcDHODH (average −92.5 kJ/mol) were also better than the normal substrate (dihydroorotate, E_{dock} = −64.2 kJ/mol), but worse than the synthetic TcDHODH inhibitor, 5-[2-(5-carboxynaphthalen-2-yl)ethyl]-2,6-dioxo-1,2,3,6-tetrahydro-pyrimidine-4-carboxylic acid (TT2-2-199, E_{dock} = −140.7 kJ/mol). Similarly, *Copaifera* diterpenoids docked with *L. donovani* DHODH (average E_{dock} = −89.9 kJ/mol) better than dihydroorotate (E_{dock} = −60.9 kJ/mol). Based on these docking energies, protozoal dihydroorotate dehydrogenases are likely targets for *Copaifera* diterpenoids.

Leishmania major methionyl-tRNA synthetase was another *Leishmania* protein target with good docking energies. Although the docking energies with this protein were excellent (average E_{dock} = −106.9 kJ/mol), they are much poorer than the docking energy of the normal substrate, methionyl adenylate (E_{dock} = −168.1 kJ/mol). Similarly, the *T. cruzi* target protein with the best docking was UDP-galactose mutase (average E_{dock} = −104.5 kJ/mol), but the normal substrate and co-crystallized ligand, uridine diphosphate (UDP), had a much superior docking energy (E_{dock} = −232.8 kJ/mol). Likewise, *L. major* UDP-glucose pyrophosphorylase showed an average docking energy of −99.9 kJ/mol, which was much worse than UDP itself (E_{dock} = −145.9 kJ/mol). The diterpenoids showed good docking to *T. cruzi* spermidine synthase, with an average docking energy of −96.8 kJ/mol; however, these are much worse than the docking energy of the co-crystallized ligand, *S*-adenosyl methionine, with a docking energy of −133.0 kJ/mol. Thus, although they exhibited good docking properties, it is unlikely that *Copaifera* diterpenoids can compete with the normal substrate ligands for these proteins.

Table 4. MolDock docking energies (kJ/mol) of *Copaifera* diterpenoids with *Leishmania* protein targets.

Leishmania Targets	PDB[a]	E_{dock} (ave)	E_{dock} (min)	Best-Docking Diterpenoid Ligand
Cathepsin B (LdonCatB)	homology	−84.6	−100.6	3α-Alepterolic acid acetate
Cathepsin B (LmajCatB)	homology	−80.8	−93.7	7α-Acetoxyhardwickiic acid
Cyclophilin A (LdonCypA)	3EOV	−83.3	−102.6	*ent*-Pinifolic acid
Deoxyuridine triphosphate nucleotidohydrolase (LmajdUTPase)	2YAY	−85.3	−103.8	19-*O*-Acetyl-1,2-dehydrokautriwaic acid
Dihydroorotate dehydrogenase (LdonDHODH)	3GYE	−89.9	−102.7	7α-Acetoxyhardwickiic acid
Dihydroorotate dehydrogenase (LmajDHODH)	3MHU	−109.2	−126.7	7α-Acetoxyhardwickiic acid
Glucose-6-phosphate isomerase (LmexGPI)	1Q50	−73.0	−85.3	19-*O*-Acetyl-1,2-dehydrokautriwaic acid
Glyceraldehyde-3-phosphate dehydrogenase (LmexGAPDH)	1A7K	−74.2	−83.0	19-*O*-Acetyl-1,2-dehydrokautriwaic acid
Glycerol-3-phosphate dehydrogenase (LmexGPDH)	1N1E	−100.4	−114.3	3α-Alepterolic acid acetate
Methionyl-tRNA synthetase (LmajMetRS)	3KFL	−106.9	−123.0	3α-Alepterolic acid acetate
Nicotinamidase (LinfPnC1)	3R2J	−61.3	−75.9	3β-Alepterolic acid
N-Myristoyl transferase (LmajNMT)	4A30	−92.3	−104.0	19-*O*-Acetyl-1,2-dehydrokautriwaic acid
Nucleoside diphosphate kinase b (LmajNDKb)	3NGS	−83.9	−105.8	7α-Acetoxyhardwickiic acid
Nucleoside hydrolase (LmajNH)	1EZR	−80.5	−90.5	7-Acetylbacchotricuneatin D
Oligopeptidase B (LmajOPB)	2XE4	−97.8	−106.1	7α-Acetoxyhardwickiic acid
Phosphodiesterase B1 (LmajPDEB1)	2R8Q	−89.5	−105.8	3β-Alepterolic acid acetate
Phosphomannumutase (LmexPMM)	2I55	−94.2	−117.5	19-*O*-Acetyl-1,2-dehydrokautriwaic acid
Pteridine reductase 1 (LmajPTR1)	1E7W	−93.8	−110.7	Copaiferolic acid
Pyruvate kinase (LmexPYK)	1PKL	−103.4	−113.5	7α-Acetoxyhardwickiic acid
Sterol 14α-demethylase (LinfCYP51)	3L4D	−90.2	−111.3	19-*O*-Acetyl-1,2-dehydrokautriwaic acid
Thiol-dependent reductase I (LinfTDR1)	4AGS	−78.7	−88.8	19-*O*-Acetyl-1,2-dehydrokautriwaic acid
Triosephosphate isomerase (LmexTIM)	2VXN	−90.7	−101.5	3α-Alepterolic acid acetate
Trypanothione reductase (LinfTR)	4APN	−92.5	−109.0	19-*O*-Acetyl-1,2-dehydrokautriwaic acid
Tyrosyl-tRNA synthetase (LmajTyrRS)	3P0J	−92.4	−102.9	Patagonic acid
Uridine diphosphate-glucose pyrophosphorylase (LmajUGPase)	2OEG	−99.9	−113.9	Patagonic acid

[a] PDB = Protein Data Bank.

Table 5. MolDock docking energies (kJ/mol) of *Copaifera* diterpenoids with *Trypanosoma cruzi* protein targets.

***Trypanosoma cruzi* Targets**	**PDB**	E_{dock} **(ave)**	E_{dock} **(min)**	**Best-Docking Diterpenoid Ligand**
Cruzain	3IUT	−80.2	−92.6	Patagonic acid
Cyclophilin (TcCyp19)	1XQ7	−78.9	−92.0	3β-Alepterolic acid acetate
Deoxyuridine triphosphatase (TcUTPase)	1OGK	−83.4	−101.0	3β-Alepterolic acid acetate
Dihydrofolate reductase—thymidylate synthase (TcDHFR-TS)	3IRN	−93.2	−110.7	7α-Acetoxyhardwickiic acid
Dihydroorotate dehydrogenase (TcDHODH)	3W6Y	−92.5	−109.7	7α-Acetoxyhardwickiic acid
Farnesyl diphosphate synthase (TcFPPS)	3ICZ	−96.2	−109.8	7α-Acetoxyhardwickiic acid
Glyceraldehyde-3-phosphate dehydrogenase (TcGAPDH)	1QXS	−70.3	−85.3	Copaiferolic acid
Hypoxanthine phosphoribosyltransferase (TcHPRT)	1P19	−82.1	−94.4	7α-Hydroxyhardwickiic acid
Nucleoside diphosphate kinase B (TcNDKb)	3PRV	−71.6	−88.4	Crolechinic acid
Old yellow enzyme (=Prostaglandin F2α synthase) (TcPGFS)	3ATY	−85.6	−97.3	Patagonic acid
Pteridine reductase 2 (TcPTR2)	1MXH	−96.8	−118.4	(+)-Hardwickiic acid
Pyruvate kinase (TcPYK)	3QV9	−80.3	−87.4	(−)-Hardwickiic acid
Spermidine synthase (TcSpdSyn)	3BWC	−96.8	−106.8	19-*O*-Acetyl-1,2-dehydrokautriwaic acid
Sterol 14α-demethylase (TcCYP51)	3KLO	−89.5	−101.8	19-*O*-Acetyl-1,2-dehydrokautriwaic acid
Triosephosphate isomerase (TcTIM)	1SUX	−88.2	−100.7	*ent*-Polyalthic acid
Trypanothione reductase (TcTR)	1BZL	−81.9	−95.8	Copaiferolic acid
UDP-galactose mutase (TcUGM)	4DSH	−104.5	−115.7	Copaiferolic acid

Copaifera diterpenoids showed excellent docking to *L. mexicana* pyruvate kinase (average $E_{dock} = -103.4$ kJ/mol), much better than the normal substrate, phosphoenolpyruvate ($E_{dock} = -59.8$ kJ/mol). Docking energies with *T. cruzi* pyruvate kinase were not as impressive (average −80.3 kJ/mol), but still better than phosphoenolpyruvate ($E_{dock} = -48.6$ kJ/mol) and comparable to the TcPYK inhibitor, ponceau S ($E_{dock} = -83.6$ kJ/mol). Parasite pyruvate kinases can be expected to be target proteins for *Copaifera* diterpenoids.

Protozoal triosephosphate isomerases (LmexTIM and TcTIM) are expected to be targeted by *Copaifera* diterpenoids. The average docking energy with LmexTIM (−90.7 kJ/mol) was much better than either the normal substrate (dihydroxyacetone phosphate, $E_{dock} = -52.4$ kJ/mol) or the co-crystallized ligand, phosphoglycolohydroxamic acid ($E_{dock} = -61.1$ kJ/mol). Likewise, docking energies with TcTIM (average −88.2 kJ/mol) were better than the dihydroxyacetone phosphate ($E_{dock} = -59.7$ kJ/mol) and comparable to the TcTIM inhibitor, 3-(2-benzothiazolylthio)-1-propanesulfonic acid ($E_{dock} = -85.5$ kJ/mol).

Both *L. major* pteridine reductase and *T. cruzi* pteridine reductase had docking properties with *Copaifera* diterpenoids with comparable energies (average $E_{dock} = -93.8$ and −96.8 kJ/mol, respectively) with the normal substrate dihydrobiopterin ($E_{dock} = -96.9$ and −100.1 kJ/mol, respectively). Thus, *Copaifera* diterpenoids may compete with dihydrobiopterin for pteridine reductase.

Sterols are the normal substrates for sterol 14α-demethylase (CYP51), and triterpenoids are expected to also target this protein as inhibitors [118]. Nevertheless, *Copaifera* diterpenoids showed docking energies that may compete with normal sterols for these protein targets. *L. infantum* CYP51 had an average docking energy with the diterpenoids of −90.2 kJ/mol, which was generally not as good as a normal sterol substrate (obtusifoliol, $E_{dock} = -104.4$ kJ/mol), but comparable to the known LinfCYP51 inhibitor fluconazole ($E_{dock} = -87.5$ kJ/mol). Likewise, *T. cruzi* CYP51 had an average diterpenoid docking energy of −89.5 kJ/mol, but substrate (obtusifoliol) docking of −105.6 kJ/mol, and fluconazole docking energy of −90.9 kJ/mol.

Copaifera diterpenoids generally showed weak docking energies against the parasite cysteine proteases, *L. donovani* cathepsin B, *L. major* cathepsin B, or cruzain. This docking behavior of diterpenoids with *Leishmania* cathepsin B [114] and cruzain [117] was previously observed. *Leishmania donovani* and *T. cruzi* cyclophilins also showed weak docking energies.

Although *Copaifera* diterpenoids showed only weak docking to parasite glyceraldehyde-3-phosphate dehydrogenases, they may still target these proteins. LmexGAPDH had an average E_{dock} of −73.0 kJ/mol and TcGAPDH had an average E_{dock} of −70.3 kJ/mol, but these docking energies are better than the docking energies of the normal substrate, glyceraldehyde-3-phosphate ($E_{dock} = -58.9$ and −52.6 kJ/mol, respectively).

Additional *Leishmania* proteins expected to be targeted by *Copaifera* diterpenoids include glycerol-3-phosphate dehydrogenase, which showed excellent docking energies (average −100.4 kJ/mol) to LmexGPDH, better than the normal substrate, glycerol-3-phosphate ($E_{dock} = -62.5$ kJ/mol). Also targeted with a weak docking energy are: glucose-6-phosphate isomerase (Lmex GPI E_{dock} average = −73.0 kJ/mol), though better than the docking energy of the normal substrate (glucose-6-phosphate, $E_{dock} = -62.0$ kJ/mol); and phosphomannomutase (LmexPMM E_{dock} average = −94.2 kJ/mol), which is better compared to the normal substrate (mannose-6-phosphate, $E_{dock} = -72.5$ kJ/mol).

Additional *T. cruzi* protein targets may be dihydrofolate reductase—thymidylate synthase (TcDHFR–TS), which showed an average docking energy with *Copaifera* diterpenoids of −93.2 kJ/mol, comparable to the docking energy of the normal substrate (dihydrofolate, −99.3 kJ/mol), as well as the TcDHFR–TS inhibitor cycloguanil ($E_{dock} = -83.1$ kJ/mol); farnesyl diphosphate synthase (TcFPPS), with docking energies that averaged −96.2 kJ/mol, which is comparable to the docking energy of the normal substrate, isopentenyl diphosphate ($E_{dock} = -98.9$ kJ/mol); and hypoxanthine phosphoribosyltransferase (TcHPRT), having an average $E_{dock} = -82.1$ kJ/mol, compared to the normal substrate, hypoxanthine, with E_{dock} of −65.9 kJ/mol.

6.2. Antibacterial Activity of Copaiba

Copaiba oleoresin has shown antibacterial activity against several strains, in particular, Gram-positive *Bacillus subtilis* and *Staphylococcus aureus* with minimum inhibitory concentration (MIC) values of 5 μg/mL for both organisms [110]. Copalic acid, isolated from *C. langsdorffii*, showed excellent antibacterial activity against *Bacillus cereus* (MIC 8.0 μg/mL), *B. subtilis* (MIC 5.0 μg/mL), *Kocuria rhizophila* (MIC 5.0 μg/mL), *Streptococcus pyogenes* (MIC 3.0 μg/mL), *S. pneumoniae* (MIC 3.0 μg/mL), *S. agalactiae* (MIC 2.0 μg/mL), *S. dysgalactiae* (MIC 1.0 μg/mL), *S. epidermidis* (MIC 0.5 μg/mL) [71], *S. salivarius* (MIC 2.0 μg/mL), *S. mutans* (MIC 3.0 μg/mL), *S. mitis* (MIC 5.0 μg/mL), *S. sobrinus* (MIC 3.0 μg/mL), and *S. sanguinis* (MIC 6.0 μg/mL) [70]. Likewise, kaurenoic acid showed remarkable activity against *S. pyogenes* (MIC 5.0 μg/mL), *S. pneumoniae* (MIC 5.0 μg/mL), *S. dysgalactiae* (MIC 8.0 μg/mL) [71], *S. epidermidis* (MIC 4–5 μg/mL), *B. subtilis* (MIC 3.1–6.3 μg/mL), and *S. aureus* (MIC 8–10 μg/mL) [75]. 3α-Alepterolic acid acetate (acetoxycopalic acid) showed moderate antibacterial activity against cariogenic *Streptococcus* bacteria, with MIC values ranging from 12.0 to 60.0 μg/mL [70]. *ent*-Polyalthic acid also showed moderate antibacterial activity against *B. subtilis* (MIC 20–30 μg/mL), *S. aureus* (MIC 40–50 μg/mL), and *S. epidermidis* (MIC 40 μg/mL) [75].

In order to provide some insight into the mechanisms of activity, a virtual screening of copaiba diterpenoids has been carried out against several bacterial protein targets, including peptide deformylase, DNA gyrase, topoisomerase IV, UDP-galactopyranose mutase, protein tyrosine phosphatase, cytochrome P450 CYP 121, and nicotinamide adenine dinucleotide (NAD^+)-dependent DNA ligase [119] (see Table 6). The best bacterial target for copalic acid was *Mycobacterium tuberculosis* DNA gyrase B (PDB 3ZKD) with a docking energy (E_{dock}) of −105.7 kJ/mol. The protein with the best docking energy with kaurenoic acid was *S. pneumoniae* peptide deformylase (PDB 2AIE, E_{dock} = −89.7 kJ/mol). 3α-Alepterolic acid acetate was the best docking ligand to *Escherichia coli* topoisomerase IV (PDB 1S16) and *M. tuberculosis* DNAGyrB (PDB 3ZKD) with docking energies of −118.8 and −118.3 kJ/mol, respectively. 3β-Alepterolic acid acetate also showed excellent docking to these two proteins with docking energies of −117.1 and −117.3 kJ/mol, respectively. The best bacterial target for *ent*-polyalthic acid was *M. tuberculosis* protein tyrosine phosphatase (PDB 2OZ5, E_{dock} = −107.2 kJ/mol). The copaiba diterpenoid ligand with the best docking properties was 7α-acetoxyhardwickiic acid with *S. aureus* peptide deformylase (PDB 3U7M, E_{dock} = −120.6 kJ/mol).

6.3. Antiproliferative Activity of Copaiba

Copaiba oleoresins have exhibited both in vitro and in vivo antiproliferative activities (Table 3). *Copaifera reticulata* oleoresin, for example, has shown in vitro cytotoxic activity against GM07492-A human lung fibroblast cells with an IC_{50} of 51.85 μg/mL [68]. The oleoresin of *C. multijuga* has shown in vitro cytotoxic activity against B16F10 murine melanoma cells with an IC_{50} of 457 μg/mL [57]. Furthermore, in a mouse model of lung metastasis and tumor growth, oral administration of *C. multijuga* oleoresin reduced tumor growth, tumor mass, and number of lung nodules after inoculation of B16F10 tumor cells [57]. Likewise, *C. multijuga* oleoresin, in doses varying between 100 and 200 mg/kg, showed antineoplastic properties against Ehrlich ascetic tumors and solid tumors in an in vivo mouse model [98]. On the other hand, *C. officinalis* oleoresin actually stimulated growth of Walker 256 carcinoma by 70% in an in vivo rat model [101].

Diterpenoids isolated from *Copaifera* species have shown cytotoxic activities (Table 3). Copalic acid, isolated from *C. langsdorffii*, showed in vitro cytotoxicity on MO59J human glioblastoma cells and HeLa human cervical adenocarcinoma cells with IC_{50} of 68.3 and 44.0 μg/mL, respectively [71]. Kaurenoic acid has demonstrated cytotoxicity against several human tumor cell lines, including CEM leukemia, MCF-7 breast tumor, HCT-8 colon tumor [73], AGP01 gastric tumor, and SF-295 glioblastoma [74]. Growth inhibition of AGP01 and SF-295 cells was also demonstrated by 3β-alepterolic acid and 3β-alepterolic acid acetate [73]. Methyl copalate showed remarkable cytotoxic activity on P-388 murine lymphoma (IC_{50} = 2.5 μg/mL), A-549 human lung carcinoma (IC_{50} = 5 μg/mL), HT-29 human colon carcinoma (IC_{50} = 5 μg/mL), and MEL-28 human melanoma (IC_{50} = 10 μg/mL) cells [75].

Molecular docking (Molegro Virtual Docker, Aarhus, Denmark) has been carried out with *Copaifera* diterpenoids on cancer molecular targets, including androgen receptor, aromatase, caseine kinase II, cyclin-dependent kinases 2, 4, and 6, cyclooxygenase 2, DNA (cytosine-5)-methyltransferase-1 and -3A, epidermal growth factor receptor, estrogen receptor α, estrogen receptor β, heat shock protein 90, insulin-like growth factor 1 receptor, 5-lipoxygenase, mitogen-activated protein kinase 1, NF-κB, p90 ribosomal protein S6 kinase, P-glycoprotein, phosphatidylinositol-4,5-bisphosphate 3-kinase, topoisomerase I, topoisomerase IIα, topoisomerase IIβ, tubulin, and vascular endothelial growth factor receptor (Table 7). The best overall cancer targets for the copaiba diterpenoids were human DNA (cytosine-5)-methyltransferase-1 (HsDNMT1), human estrogen receptor β (HsERβ), and human mitogen-activated protein kinase 1 (HsMEK1), with average MolDock docking energies of −102.7, −99.2, and −101.5 kJ/mol, respectively. DNA (cytosine-5)-methyltransferase-1 (DNMT1) is the enzyme responsible for DNA methylation of carbon-5 of cytosine within CpG dinucleotides [120]. The enzyme is required for embryonic development [121], but is overexpressed in lung, liver, colorectal, gastric, breast, and lung tumors [122]. Thus, DNMT1 has emerged as an attractive target for cancer chemotherapy [123,124]. The mitogen-activated protein kinase (MAPK) signaling cascade is one of the most important pathways involved in cellular proliferation and differentiation [125] and, therefore, inhibition of components of this pathway, such as MEK1, can potentially target tumors that depend on MAPK signaling [126]. Agonism of estrogen receptor α (ERα) stimulates proliferation of breast, uterus, and prostate tissues, whereas ERβ agonism inhibits proliferation of these tissues [127]. Thus, compounds that can selectively bind and activate ERβ, but not ERα, could represent effective antitumor agents for treatment of prostate and breast cancer [128]. Copalic acid and methyl copalate both targeted HsMEK1, with docking energies of −108.2 and −111.0 kJ/mol, respectively, while 3β-alepterolic acid and 3β-alepterolic acid acetate showed excellent docking with HsDNMT1 (E_{dock} = −107.2 and −121.7 kJ/mol, respectively). Kaurenoic acid was a relatively weakly docking ligand but did show selective docking to aromatase (E_{dock} = −93.7 kJ/mol). The best-docking ligand was patagonic acid, which had a docking energy of −121.8 kJ/mol with HsDNMT1.

6.4. Anti-Inflammatory Activity of Copaiba

Inflammation is the biological response of body tissues to detrimental stimuli, such as pathogenic microorganisms, chemical or physical irritants, or injury. Inflammation is manifested by redness, swelling, heat, and sometimes pain. While acute inflammation is a normal part of the healing process, chronic inflammation often plays a role in chronic diseases such as osteoarthritis, lupus, and inflammatory bowel disease, and can be problematic. Several copaiba oleoresins have shown anti-inflammatory activity, including *C. cearensis* [13], *C. duckei* [84], *C. langsdorffii* [50,91], *C. multijuga* [13,58,61,100], *C. officinalis* [62], and *C. reticulata* [13] (Table 3).

The immune response is a complex cascade of interacting cytokines and reactions, and there are several biomolecular targets important in treating chronic inflammation. We have carried out virtual screening of copaiba diterpenoids against soluble epoxide hydrolase (EPHX2), fibroblast collagenase, phospholipase A2 (PLA2), 5-lipoxygenase, inducible nitric oxide synthase, phosphoinositide 3-kinase, interleukin-1 receptor-associated kinase 4, glutathione *S*-transferase ω-1, cyclooxygenase-1, cyclooxygenase-2, c-Jun *N*-terminal kinase, nuclear factor κ-light-chain-enhancer of activated B cells (NF-κB), inhibitor of κB kinase β, NF-κB essential modulator, lipid binding protein MD-2, myeloperoxidase, p38 mitogen-activated protein kinase, peroxisome proliferator-activated receptor γ, and cAMP-specific 3′,5′-cyclic phosphodiesterase 4D (Table 8). The overall best target proteins were murine soluble epoxide hydrolase and murine phospholipase A2, with average docking energies of −108.3 and −100.0 kJ/mol. Secretory phospholipase A2 and cytosolic phospholipase A2 are both targets for anti-inflammatory drug development [129]. Soluble epoxide hydrolase has been identified as a molecular target not only for inflammatory diseases, but also as a target for neurodegenerative diseases and for treatment of pain [130]. Thus, targeting EPHX2 and/or PLA2 by copaiba diterpenoids may explain the anti-inflammatory activities of copaiba oleoresins.

Table 6. MolDock docking energies (kJ/mol) of *Copaifera* diterpenoids with bacterial protein targets.

Bacterial Protein Targets	PDB	E_{dock} (ave)	E_{dock} (min)	Best Docking Diterpenoid Ligand
Pseudomonas aeruginosa peptide deformylase (PaPDF)	1LRY	−96.3	−113.5	(+)-Hardwickiic acid
Streptococcus pneumoniae peptide deformylase (SpPDF)	2AIE	−100.2	−115.4	7α-Acetoxyhardwickiic acid
Mycobacterium tuberculosis peptide deformylase (MtPDF)	3E3U	−95.7	−107.3	(+)-Hardwickiic acid
Escherichia coli topoisomerase IV (EcTopoIV)	1S16	−100.5	−118.8	7α-Acetoxyhardwickiic acid
Mycobacterium tuberculosis DNA gyrase B (MtDNAGyrB)	3ZKD	−101.3	−118.3	3α-Alepterolic acid acetate
Mycobacterium tuberculosis protein tyrosine phosphatase (MtPTPB)	2OZ5	−89.2	−107.2	*ent*-Polyalthic acid
Mycobacterium tuberculosis UDP-galactopyranose mutase (MtUGM)	4RPL	−92.2	−104.4	19-*O*-Acetyl-1,2-dehydrokautriwaic acid
Mycobacterium tuberculosis mycocyclosin synthase (MtCYP121)	5IBE	−87.0	−108.2	19-*O*-Acetyl-1,2-dehydrokautriwaic acid
Escherichia coli DNA ligase (EcLigA)	2OWO	−97.8	−108.5	19-*O*-Acetyl-1,2-dehydrokautriwaic acid
Mycobacterium tuberculosis DNA ligase (MtLigA)	1ZAU	−89.0	−107.2	19-*O*-Acetyl-1,2-dehydrokautriwaic acid
Staphylococcus aureus DNA ligase (SaLigA)	4CC6	−85.2	−97.8	Methyl copalate
Streptococcus pneumoniae DNA ligase (SpLigA)	4GLW	−88.1	−109.5	Cativic acid

Table 7. MolDock docking energies (kJ/mol) of *Copaifera* diterpenoids with cancer-relevant protein targets.

Cancer-Relevant Protein Targets	PDB	E_{dock} (ave)	E_{dock} (min)	Best Docking Ligand
Human androgen receptor (HsAR)	5VO4	−67.6	−103.2	Cativic acid
Human aromatase (HsCYP19A1)	5JKW	−97.1	−112.7	*ent*-Pinifolic acid
Human casein kinase II (HsCK2)	5N9K	−83.3	−101.0	3α-Alepterolic acid acetate
Human cyclin-dependent kinase 2 (HsCDK2)	5JQ8	−91.1	−104.1	7α-Acetoxyhardwickiic acid
Human cyclin-dependent kinase 4 (HsCDK4)	2W96	−95.2	−117.6	3α-Alepterolic acid acetate
Human cyclin-dependent kinase 6 (HsCDK6)	5L2S	−87.3	−99.0	(+)-Hardwickiic acid
Murine cyclooxygenase 2 (MmCOX-2)	6COX	−93.7	−106.9	Kolavenic acid
Human DNA (cytosine-5)-methyltransferase 1 (HsDNMT1)	3SWR	−102.7	−121.8	Patagonic acid
Human DNA (cytosine-5)-methyltransferase 3A (HsDNMT3A)	2QRV	−94.3	−113.4	7α-Hydroxyhardwickiic acid
Human epidermal growth factor receptor (HsEGFR)	1XKK	−81.2	−98.8	19-*O*-Acetyl-1,2-dehydrokautriwaic acid
Human estrogen receptor α (HsERα)	1X7E	−96.5	−107.5	19-*O*-Acetyl-1,2-dehydrokautriwaic acid
Human estrogen receptor β (HsERβ)	1U3S	−99.6	−120.1	19-*O*-Acetyl-1,2-dehydrokautriwaic acid
Human heat shock protein HSP 90-α	5J2X	−83.8	−92.6	Cativic acid
Human insulin-like growth factor 1 receptor (HsIGF1R)	3LW0	−86.1	−94.2	Copaiferolic acid
Human 5-lipoxygenase (Hs5-LOX)	3V99	−89.9	−106.2	3α-Alepterolic acid acetate
Human mitogen-activated protein kinase kinase 1 (HsMEK1)	3OS3	−101.5	−113.5	3β-Alepterolic acid acetate
Murine nuclear factor κ-light-chain-enhancer of activated B cells (MmNF-κB)	1VKX	−74.2	−87.7	3α-Alepterolic acid acetate
Human p90 ribosomal protein S6 kinase (HsRSK2) *C*-terminal domain	4D9U	−75.3	−90.7	3β-Alepterolic acid acetate
Human p90 ribosomal protein S6 kinase (HsRSK2) *N*-terminal domain	4NW6	−86.4	−99.7	7α-Acetoxyhardwickiic acid
Murine P-glycoprotein	3G60	−97.6	−116.1	Patagonic acid

Table 7. *Cont.*

Cancer-Relevant Protein Targets	PDB	E_{dock} (ave)	E_{dock} (min)	Best Docking Ligand
Human phosphatidylinositol-4,5-bisphosphate 3-kinase (HsPI3K)	2A5U	−84.5	−97.6	7α-Acetoxyhardwickiic acid
Human topoisomerase I (HsTOPO-I)	1NH3	−83.7	−99.6	Copaiferolic acid
Human topoisomerase IIα (HsTOPO-IIα)	4FM9	−94.2	−105.2	19-*O*-Acetyl-1,2-dehydrokautriwaic acid
Human topoisomerase IIβ (HsTOPO-IIβ)	4J3N	−85.6	−98.9	3α-Alepterolic acid acetate
Bovine tubulin (colchicine binding site)	1SA1	−94.2	−103.8	3α-Alepterolic acid acetate
Bovine tubulin (paclitaxel binding site)	1JFF	−79.1	−88.6	7α-Acetoxyhardwickiic acid
Bovine tubulin (vinblastine binding site)	1Z2B	−89.1	−101.0	(+)-Hardwickiic acid
Human vascular endothelial growth factor receptor (HsVEGFR)	4ASE	−92.9	−105.5	7-acetylbacchotricuneatin D

Table 8. MolDock docking energies (kJ/mol) of *Copaifera* diterpenoids with cancer-relevant protein targets.

Inflammation-Relevant Protein Targets	PDB	E_{dock} (ave)	E_{dock} (min)	Best Docking Ligand
Murine soluble epoxide hydrolase (MmEPHX2)	1CR6	−108.3	−125.6	19-*O*-Acetyl-1,2-dehydrokautriwaic acid
Human soluble epoxide hydrolase (HsEPHX2)	4HAI	−95.1	−104.5	*ent*-Agathic_acid
Human fibroblast collagenase (HsMMP-1)	1CGL	−96.5	−109.0	19-*O*-Acetyl-1,2-dehydrokautriwaic acid
Porcine phospholipase A2 (SsPLA2)	2B03	−100.0	−112.4	(+)-Hardwickiic acid
Human phospholipase A2 (HsPLA2)	1J1A	−95.4	−109.5	7α-Acetoxyhardwickiic acid
Human 5-lipoxygenase (Hs5-LOX)	3V99	−89.9	−106.2	3α-Alepterolic acid acetate
Murine inducible nitric oxide synthase (MmiNOS)	1M8D	−87.5	−110.4	Copaiferolic acid
Human phosphatidylinositol-4,5-bisphosphate 3-kinase γ (HsPI3Kγ)	2A5U	−84.5	−97.6	7α-Acetoxyhardwickiic acid
Human interleukin-1 receptor-associated kinase 4 (HsIRAK4)	5T1S	−90.7	−100.6	7α-Acetoxyhardwickiic acid
Human glutathione *S*-transferase ω-1 (HsGSTO1)	5V3Q	−82.7	−94.2	19-*O*-Acetyl-1,2-dehydrokautriwaic acid
Ovine cyclooxygenase-1 (OaCOX-1)	3N8Z	−62.1	−92.0	Crolechinic acid
Murine cyclooxygenase-2 (MmCOX-2)	6COX	−93.7	−106.9	Kolavenic acid
Human c-Jun *N*-terminal kinase (HsJNK)	4Y46	−83.7	−97.7	19-*O*-Acetyl-1,2-dehydrokautriwaic acid
Xenopus laevis inhibitor of κB kinase β (XlIKKB)	3RZF	−88.1	−100.9	Patagonic acid
Human NF-κB essential modulator (HsNEMO)	3BRT	−85.9	−105.3	3α-Alepterolic acid acetate
Human lipid binding protein MD-2 (HsMD-2)	2E59	−71.2	−84.3	19-*O*-Acetyl-1,2-dehydrokautriwaic acid
Human myeloperoxidase (HsMPO)	4C1M	−84.3	−98.8	(+)-Hardwickiic acid
Murine nuclear factor κ-light-chain-enhancer of activated B cells (MmNF-κB)	3DO7	−72.7	−85.9	(+)-Hardwickiic acid
Human p38 mitogen-activated protein kinase (Hsp38MAPK)	1OZ1	−91.3	−116.4	19-*O*-Acetyl-1,2-dehydrokautriwaic acid
Human peroxisome proliferator-activated receptor γ (HsPPARγ)	3ADV	−91.9	−107.6	Copaiferolic acid
Human cAMP-specific 3′,5′-cyclic phosphodiesterase 4D (HsPDE4D)	5K32	−90.2	−107.3	7α-Acetoxyhardwickiic acid

7. Computational Methods—Molecular Docking

Molecular docking analyses were carried out using Molegro Virtual Docker (v. 6.0.1, Molegro ApS, Aarhus, Denmark) against known bacterial [119], *Leishmania* [114–116], *Trypanosoma cruzi* [117], and cancer-relevant and inflammation-relevant protein targets [131], as previously described [114–117,119,132].

8. Conclusions

The oleoresins from *Copaifera* species (copaiba) have been used by native peoples of the Amazon region for thousands of years. These materials have shown remarkable biological activities, including antibacterial, antiparasitic, antineoplastic, and anti-inflammatory activities. Copaiba resins have been distilled to give essential oils that are largely composed of sesquiterpenoids, particularly β-caryophyllene. The resins are also composed of diterpene acids, which are responsible for many of the observed biological activities. Molecular docking of copaiba diterpene acids with documented protein targets has revealed potential mechanisms of activity for these bioactive constituents. Future research to validate the molecular mechanisms of copaiba diterpenoids is encouraged.

Author Contributions: R.d.T., J.K.d.S. and W.N.S. authors contributed equally to literature searching and manuscript writing, review and editing; W.N.S. carried out the molecular docking.

Funding: W.N.S. is grateful to dōTERRA International (Available online: https://www.doterra.com/US/en) for financial support of the Aromatic Plant Research Centers (APRC, Available online: https://aromaticplant.org/).

Conflicts of Interest: The authors declare no conflict of interest.

References

1. Dwyer, J.D. The Central American, West Indian, and South American species of *Copaifera* (Caesalpiniaceae). *Brittonia* **1951**, *7*, 143–172. [CrossRef]
2. Jacquin, N.J. *Enumeratio Systematica Plantarum*; Apud Theodorum Haak: Leiden, The Netherlands, 1760.
3. Linné, C. *Species Plantarum*; Joannis Thomae de Trattner: Vienna, Austria, 1764.
4. Joyce, B.L.; Al-Ahmad, H.; Chen, F.; Stewart, C.N. Diesel Trees. In *Handbook of Bioenergy Crop Plants*; Kole, C., Joshi, C.P., Shonnard, D.R., Eds.; CRC Press: Boca Raton, FL, USA, 2012; pp. 619–629.
5. Costa, J.A.S.; Copaifera. In Flora do Brasil 2020, em Construção. Available online: http://floradobrasil.jbrj.gov.br/reflora/floradobrasil/FB22895 (accessed on 6 March 2018).
6. Veiga Junior, V.F.; Pinto, A.C. O gênero *Copaifera* L. *Quim. Nova* **2002**, *25*, 273–286. [CrossRef]
7. Plowden, C. The ethnobotany of copaiba (*Copaifera*) oleoresin in the Amazon. *Econ. Bot.* **2004**, *58*, 729–733. [CrossRef]
8. Cascon, V.; Gilbert, B. Characterization of the chemical composition of oleoresins of *Copaifera guianensis* Desf., *Copaifera duckei* Dwyer and *Copaifera multijuga* Hayne. *Phytochemistry* **2000**, *55*, 773–778. [CrossRef]
9. Martins-da-Silva, R.C.V.; Pereira, J.F.; de Lima, H.C. O gênero *Copaifera* (Leguminosae—Caesalpinioideae) na Amazônia Brasileira. *Rodriguésia* **2008**, *59*, 455–476.
10. Souza, V.C.; Lorenzi, H. *Botânica Sistemática: Guia Ilustrado para Identificação das Famílias de Angiospermas da Flora Brasileira, Baseado na APG III*, 3rd ed.; Instituto Plantarum: Nova Odessa, Brazil, 2012.
11. Milani, J.F.; Rocha, J.F.; de Pádua Teixeira, S. Oleoresin glands in copaíba (*Copaifera trapezifolia* Hayne: Leguminosae), a Brazilian rainforest tree. *Trees* **2012**, *26*, 769–775. [CrossRef]
12. Soares, N.S.; Goncalves, C.A.; Araujo, G.M.; Lomonaco, C. Floristic composition and abundance in forest fragments: A case study from southern Goias, Brazil. *Biosci. J.* **2015**, *31*, 1238–1252. [CrossRef]
13. Veiga Junior, V.F.; Rosas, E.C.; Carvalho, M.V.; Henriques, M.G.M.O.; Pinto, A.C. Chemical composition and anti-inflammatory activity of copaiba oils from *Copaifera cearensis* Huber ex Ducke, *Copaifera reticulata* Ducke and *Copaifera multijuga* Hayne—A comparative study. *J. Ethnopharmacol.* **2007**, *112*, 248–254. [CrossRef] [PubMed]
14. Langenheim, J.H. *Plant Resins: Chemistry, Evolution, Ecology, and Ethnobotany*; Timber Press, Inc.: Portland, OR, USA, 2003.

15. Leandro, L.M.; de Sousa Vargas, F.; Barbosa, P.C.S.; Neves, J.K.O.; da Silva, J.A.; da Veiga-Junior, V.F. Chemistry and biological activities of terpenoids from copaiba (*Copaifera* spp.) oleoresins. *Molecules* **2012**, *17*, 3866–3889. [CrossRef] [PubMed]
16. Langenheim, J.H. Higher plant terpenoids: A phytcentric overview of their ecological roles. *J. Chem. Ecol.* **1994**, *20*, 1223–1280. [CrossRef] [PubMed]
17. Barbosa, P.C.S.; Medeiros, R.S.; Sampaio, P.T.B.; Vieira, G.; Wiedemann, L.S.M.; Veiga-Junior, V.F. Influence of abiotic factors on the chemical composition of copaiba oil (*Copaifera multijuga* Hayne): Soil composition, seasonality and diameter at breast height. *J. Braz. Chem. Soc.* **2012**, *23*, 1823–1833. [CrossRef]
18. Biavatti, M.W.; Dossin, D.; Deschamps, F.C.; Lima, M.D.P. Análise de óleos-resinas de copaíba: Contribuição para o seu controle de qualidade. *Rev. Bras. Farmacogn.* **2006**, *16*, 230–235. [CrossRef]
19. Pieri, F.A.; Mussi, M.C.; Moreira, M.A.S. Óleo de copaíba (*Copaifera* sp.): Histórico, extração, aplicações industriais e propriedades medicinais. *Rev. Bras. Plantas Med.* **2009**, *11*, 465–472. [CrossRef]
20. Rosa, J.C.; da Silva Gomes, A.M. Os aspectos etnobotânicos da copaíba. *Rev. Geogr.* **2009**, *4*, 59–77. [CrossRef]
21. Ribeiro, R.D.; de Lima, H.C. Riqueza e distribuição geográfica de espécies arbóreas da família Leguminosae e implicações para conservação no Centro de Diversidade Vegetal de Cabo Frio, Rio de Janeiro, Brasil. *Rodriguésia* **2009**, *60*, 111–127. [CrossRef]
22. Carvalho, M.C.; Gomide, L.R.; Santos, R.M.D.; Scolforo, J.R.S.; Carvalho, L.M.T.D.; Mello, J.M.D. Modeling ecological niche of tree species in Brazilian tropical area. *Cerne* **2017**, *23*, 229–240. [CrossRef]
23. Carvalho, P.E.R. *Espécies Arbóreas Brasileiras, Vol. 1*; EMBRAPA Informação Tecnológica: Brasilia, Brazil, 2003.
24. Shanley, P.; Leite, A.; Alechandre, A.; Azevedo, C. Copaíba: *Copaifera* spp. In *Frutíferas e Plantas Úteis na Vida Amazônica*; Shanley, P., Medina, G., Eds.; CIFOR and IMAZON: Belém, Brazil, 2005; pp. 85–94.
25. Carvalho, P.E.R. *Espécies Florestais Brasileiras: Recomendações Silviculturais, Potencialidades e Uso da Madeira*; EMBRAPA-CNPF: Colombo, Brazil, 1994.
26. Rigamonte-Azevedo, O.C.; Wadt, P.G.S.; Wadt, L.D.O. *Copaíba: Ecologia e Produção de Óleo-Resina*; Embrapa Acre: Rio Branco, Brazil, 2004.
27. Alencar, J.D.C. Estudos silviculturais de uma população natural de *Copaifera multijuga* Hayne—Leguminosae, na Amazônia central. IV. Interpretação de dados fenológicos em relação a elementos climáticos. *Acta Amaz.* **1988**, *18*, 199–209. [CrossRef]
28. Muniz, F.H. Padrões de floração e frutificação de árvores da Amazônia Maranhense. *Acta Amaz.* **2008**, *38*, 617–626. [CrossRef]
29. Dos Santos, N. Fenologia. *Rodriguésia* **1979**, *31*, 223–226.
30. Pedroni, F.; Sanchez, M.; Santos, F.A.M. Fenologia da copaíba (*Copaifera langsdorffii* Desf.—Leguminosae, Caesalpinioideae) em uma floresta semidecídua no sudeste do Brasil. *Rev. Bras. Botânica* **2002**, *25*, 183–194. [CrossRef]
31. Pedroni, F. *Ecologia da Copaíba (Copaifera langsdorffii Desf. Caelsapiniaceae) na Reserva Municipal de Santa Genebra, Campinas, SP*; Universidade Estadual de Campinas: Barão Geraldo, Brazil, 1993.
32. Motta Junior, C.J.; Lombardi, J.A. Aves como agentes dispersores da copaiba (*Copaifera langsdorffii*, Caesalpiniaceae) em São Carlos, estado de São Paulo. *Rev. Bras. Ornitol.* **1990**, *1*, 105–106.
33. Brum, H.D.; Camargo, J.L.C.; Ferraz, I.D.K. Copaíba-roxa, *Copaifera mutlijuga* Hayne. In *Manual de Sementes da Amazônia*; Ferraz, I.D.K., Camargo, J.L.C., Eds.; INPA: Manaus, Brazil, 2009; p. 12.
34. Pinto, A.; Amaral, P.; Gaia, C.; de Oliveira, W. *Boas Práticas para Manejo Florestal e Agroindustrial de Produtos Florestais Não Madeireiros: Açaí, Andiroba, Babaçu, Castanha-do-Brasil, Copaíba e Unha-de-Gato*; Sebrae-AM: Belém, Brazil, 2010.
35. Dos Santos, J.C.; Leite, A.C.P.; Wadt, L.H.O.; Borges, K.H.; Andrade, F.G.; Menezes, R.S.; Muniz, P.S.B. *Demandas Tecnologicas para o Sistema Produtivo de Óleo de Copaíba (Copaifera spp.) no Estado do Acre*; Embrapa Acre: Rio Branco, Brazil, 2001.
36. Newton, P.; Watkinson, A.R.; Peres, C.A. Determinants of yield in a non-timber forest product: *Copaifera* oleoresin in Amazonian extractive reserves. *For. Ecol. Manag.* **2011**, *261*, 255–264. [CrossRef]
37. Estrella, E. *Plantas Medicinales Amazónicas: Realidad y Perspectivas*; Tratado de Cooperación Amazónica: Lima, Peru, 1995.
38. Rios, M.N.D.S.; Pastore Junior, F. *Plantas da Amazônia: 450 Espécies de Uso Geral*; Universidade de Brasília: Brasilia, Brazil, 2011.

39. Maciel, M.A.M.; Pinto, A.C.; Veiga Junior, V.F. Plantas medicinais: A necessidade de estudos multidisciplinares. *Quim. Nova* **2002**, *25*, 429–438. [CrossRef]
40. Luz, F.J.F. Plantas medicinais de uso popular em Boa Vista, Roraima, Brasil. *Hortic. Bras.* **2001**, *19*, 88–96. [CrossRef]
41. De Albuquerque, K.C.O.; da Veiga, A.D.S.S.; da Silva e Silva, J.V.; Brigido, H.P.C.; Ferreira, E.P.D.R.; Costa, E.V.S.; Marinho, A.M.D.R.; Percário, S.; Dolabela, M.F. Brazilian Amazon traditional medicine and the treatment of difficult to heal leishmaniasis wounds with *Copaifera*. *Evid.-Based Complement. Altern. Med.* **2017**, *2017*. [CrossRef] [PubMed]
42. Basile, A.C.; Sertié, J.A.; Freitas, P.C.; Zanini, A.C. Anti-inflammatory activity of oleoresin from Brazilian *Copaifera*. *J. Ethnopharmacol.* **1988**, *22*, 101–109. [CrossRef]
43. Taylor, L. *The Healing Power of Rainforest Herbs: A Guide to Understanding and Using Herbal Medicinals*; Square One Publishers: Garden City Park, NY, USA, 2005.
44. Sant'Anna, B.M.P.; Fontes, S.P.; Pinto, A.C.; Rezende, C.M. Characterization of woody odorant contributors in copaiba oil (*Copaifera multijuga* Hayne). *J. Braz. Chem. Soc.* **2007**, *18*, 984–989. [CrossRef]
45. Revilla, J. *Apontamentos para a Cosmética Amazônica*; SEBRAE-INPA: Manaus, Brazil, 2002.
46. Shanley, P.; Pierce, A.R.; Laird, S.A.; Guillén, A. *Tapping the Green Market: Certification & Management of Non-Timber Forest Products*; Earthscan: London, UK, 2002.
47. Gonzaga, A.L. *Madeira: Uso e Conservação*; IPHAN/MONUMENTA: Brasilia, Brazil, 2006.
48. Santos, A.O.; Ueda-Nakamura, T.; Dias Filho, B.P.; Veiga Junior, V.F.; Pinto, A.C.; Nakamura, C.V. Effect of Brazilian copaiba oils on *Leishmania amazonensis*. *J. Ethnopharmacol.* **2008**, *120*, 204–208. [CrossRef] [PubMed]
49. Lameira, O.A.; Martins-da-Silva, R.C.V.; Zoghbi, M.D.G.B.; Oliveira, E.C.P. Seasonal variation in the volatiles of *Copaifera duckei* Dwyer growing wild in the state of Pará—Brazil. *J. Essent. Oil Res.* **2009**, *21*, 105–108. [CrossRef]
50. Gelmini, F.; Beretta, G.; Anselmi, C.; Centini, M.; Magni, P.; Ruscica, M.; Cavalchini, A.; Maffei Facino, R. GC-MS profiling of the phytochemical constituents of the oleoresin from *Copaifera langsdorffii* Desf. and a preliminary in vivo evaluation of its antipsoriatic effect. *Int. J. Pharm.* **2013**, *440*, 170–178. [CrossRef] [PubMed]
51. Estevão, L.R.M.; de Medeiros, J.P.; Baratella-Evêncio, L.; Simões, R.S.; Mendonça, F.D.S.; Evêncio-Neto, J. Effects of the topical administration of copaiba oil ointment (*Copaifera langsdorffii*) in skin flaps viability of rats. *Acta Cirúrgica Bras.* **2013**, *28*, 863–869. [CrossRef]
52. Zimmermam-Franco, D.C.; Bolutari, E.B.; Polonini, H.C.; do Carmo, A.M.R.; Chaves, M.D.G.A.M.; Raposo, N.R.B. Antifungal activity of *Copaifera langsdorffii* Desf oleoresin against dermatophytes. *Molecules* **2013**, *18*, 12561–12570. [CrossRef] [PubMed]
53. De Almeida, L.F.R.; Portella, R.D.O.; Bufalo, J.; Marques, M.O.M.; Facanali, R.; Frei, F. Non-oxygenated sesquiterpenes in the essential oil of *Copaifera langsdorffii* Desf. increase during the day in the dry season. *PLoS ONE* **2016**, *11*, e0149332. [CrossRef] [PubMed]
54. Do Nascimento, M.E.; Zoghbi, M.D.G.B.; Pinto, J.E.B.P.; Bertolucci, S.K.V. Chemical variability of the volatiles of *Copaifera langsdorffii* growing wild in the southeastern part of Brazil. *Biochem. Syst. Ecol.* **2012**, *43*, 1–6. [CrossRef]
55. De Almeida, L.F.R.; Portella, R.D.O.; Facanali, R.; Marques, M.O.M.; Frei, F. Dry and wet seasons set the phytochemical profile of the *Copaifera langsdorffii* Desf. essential oils. *J. Essent. Oil Res.* **2014**, *26*, 292–300. [CrossRef]
56. Zoghbi, M.D.G.B.; Lameira, O.A.; Oliveira, E.C.P. Seasonal variation of oleoresin and volatiles from *Copaifera martii* Hayne growing wild in the State of Pará, Brazil. *J. Essent. Oil Res.* **2007**, *19*, 504–506. [CrossRef]
57. Lima, S.R.M.; Veiga Junior, V.F.; Christo, H.B.; Pinto, A.C.; Fernandes, P.D. In vivo and in vitro studies on the anticancer activity of *Copaifera multijuga* Hayne and its fractions. *Phyther. Res.* **2003**, *17*, 1048–1053. [CrossRef] [PubMed]
58. Kobayashi, C.; Fontanive, T.O.; Enzweiler, B.G.; de Bona, L.R.; Massoni, T.; Apel, M.A.; Henriques, A.T.; Richter, M.F.; Ardenghi, P.; Suyenaga, E.S. Pharmacological evaluation of *Copaifera multijuga* oil in rats. *Pharm. Biol.* **2011**, *49*, 306–313. [CrossRef] [PubMed]
59. Trindade, F.T.T.; Stabeli, R.G.; Pereira, A.A.; Facundo, V.A.; Silva, A.D.A. *Copaifera multijuga* ethanolic extracts, oil-resin, and its derivatives display larvicidal activity against *Anopheles darlingi* and *Aedes aegypti* (Diptera: Culicidae). *Braz. J. Pharmacogn.* **2013**, *23*, 464–470. [CrossRef]

60. Souza Barbosa, P.C.; Moreira Wiedemann, L.S.; da Silva Medeiros, R.; Barbosa Sampaio, P.D.T.; Vieira, G.; da Veiga-Junior, V.F. Phytochemical fingerprints of copaiba oils (*Copaifera multijuga* Hayne) determined by multivariate analysis. *Chem. Biodivers.* **2013**, *10*, 1350–1360. [CrossRef] [PubMed]
61. Veiga Junior, V.F.; Luciano, Z.; Patitucci, M.L.; Pinto, A.C.; Calixto, J.B. The inhibition of paw oedema formation caused by the oil of *Copaifera multijuga* Hayne and its fractions. *J. Pharm. Pharmacol.* **2006**, *58*, 1405–1410. [CrossRef] [PubMed]
62. Dias, D.S.; Fontes, L.B.A.; Crotti, A.E.M.; Aarestrup, B.J.V.; Aarestrup, F.M.; da Silva Filho, A.A.; Corrêa, J.O.A. Copaiba oil suppresses inflammatory cytokines in splenocytes of C57Bl/6 mice induced with experimental autoimmune encephalomyelitis (EAE). *Molecules* **2014**, *19*, 12814–12826. [CrossRef] [PubMed]
63. Zoghbi, M.D.G.B.; Martins-da-Silva, R.C.V.; Trigo, J.R. Volatiles of oleoresins of *Copaifera paupera* (Herzog) Dwyer, *C. piresii* Dwyer and *C. pubiflora* Benth. (Leguminosae). *J. Essent. Oil Res.* **2009**, *21*, 403–405. [CrossRef]
64. Zoghbi, M.D.G.B.; Andrade, E.H.A.; Martins-Da-Silva, R.C.V.; Trigo, J.R. Chemical variation in the volatiles of *Copaifera reticulata* Ducke (Leguminosae) growing wild in the states of Pará and Amapá, Brazil. *J. Essent. Oil Res.* **2009**, *21*, 501–503. [CrossRef]
65. Herrero-Jáuregui, C.; Casado, M.A.; Zoghbi, M.D.G.B.; Martins-Da-Silva, R.C. Chemical variability of *Copaifera reticulata* Ducke oleoresin. *Chem. Biodivers.* **2011**, *8*, 674–685. [CrossRef] [PubMed]
66. Sachetti, C.G.; de Carvalho, R.R.; Paumgartten, F.J.R.; Lameira, O.A.; Caldas, E.D. Developmental toxicity of copaiba tree (*Copaifera reticulata* Ducke, Fabaceae) oleoresin in rat. *Food Chem. Toxicol.* **2011**, *49*, 1080–1085. [CrossRef] [PubMed]
67. Guimarães-Santos, A.; Santos, D.S.; Santos, I.R.; Lima, R.R.; Pereira, A.; de Moura, L.S.; Carvalho, R.N.; Lameira, O.; Gomes-Leal, W. Copaiba oil-resin treatment is neuroprotective and reduces neutrophil recruitment and microglia activation after motor cortex excitotoxic injury. *Evid.-Based Complement. Altern. Med.* **2012**, *2012*. [CrossRef] [PubMed]
68. Bardají, D.K.R.; da Silva, J.J.M.; Bianchi, T.C.; de Souza Eugênio, D.; de Oliveira, P.F.; Leandro, L.F.; Rogez, H.L.G.; Venezianni, R.C.S.; Ambrosio, S.R.; Tavares, D.C.; et al. *Copaifera reticulata* oleoresin: Chemical characterization and antibacterial properties against oral pathogens. *Anaerobe* **2016**, *40*, 18–27. [CrossRef] [PubMed]
69. Veiga, V.F.; Pinto, A.C.; de Lima, H.C. The essential oil composition of *Copaifera trapezifolia* Hayne leaves. *J. Essent. Oil Res.* **2006**, *18*, 430–431. [CrossRef]
70. Souza, A.B.; Martins, C.H.G.; Souza, M.G.M.; Furtado, N.A.J.C.; Heleno, V.C.G.; de Sousa, J.P.B.; Rocha, E.M.P.; Bastos, J.K.; Cunha, W.R.; Veneziani, R.C.S.; et al. Antimicrobial activity of terpenoids from *Copaifera langsdorffii* Desf. against cariogenic bacteria. *Phyther. Res.* **2011**, *25*, 215–220. [CrossRef] [PubMed]
71. Abrão, F.; de Araújo Costa, L.D.; Alves, J.M.; Senedese, J.M.; de Castro, P.T.; Ambrósio, S.R.; Veneziani, R.C.S.; Bastos, J.K.; Tavares, D.C.; Martins, C.H.G. *Copaifera langsdorffii* oleoresin and its isolated compounds: Antibacterial effect and antiproliferative activity in cancer cell lines. *BMC Complement. Altern. Med.* **2015**, *15*, 1–10. [CrossRef] [PubMed]
72. Paiva, L.A.F.; Gurgel, L.A.; Silva, R.M.; Tomé, A.R.; Gramosa, N.V.; Silveira, E.R.; Santos, F.A.; Rao, V.S.N. Anti-inflammatory effect of kaurenoic acid, a diterpene from *Copaifera langsdorffii* on acetic acid-induced colitis in rats. *Vascul. Pharmacol.* **2003**, *39*, 303–307. [CrossRef]
73. Costa-Lotufo, L.V.; Cunha, G.M.A.; Farias, P.A.M.; Viana, G.S.B.; Cunha, K.M.A.; Pessoa, C.; Moraes, M.O.; Silveira, E.R.; Gramosa, N.V.; Rao, V.S.N. The cytotoxic and embryotoxic effects of kaurenoic acid, a diterpene isolated from *Copaifera langsdorffii* oleo-resin. *Toxicon* **2002**, *40*, 1231–1234. [CrossRef]
74. Vargas, F.D.S.; de Almeida, P.D.O.; Aranha, E.S.P.; Boleti, A.P.D.A.; Newton, P.; de Vasconcellos, M.C.; Veiga Junior, V.F.; Lima, E.S. Biological activities and cytotoxicity of diterpenes from *Copaifera* spp. oleoresins. *Molecules* **2015**, *20*, 6194–6210. [CrossRef] [PubMed]
75. Tincusi, B.M.; Jiménez, I.A.; Bazzocchi, I.L.; Moujir, L.M.; Mamani, Z.A.; Barroso, J.P.; Ravelo, A.G.; Hernández, B.V. Antimicrobial terpenoids from the oleoresin of the Peruvian medicinal plant *Copaifera paupera*. *Planta Med.* **2002**, *68*, 808–812. [CrossRef] [PubMed]
76. Pinto, A.C.; Braga, W.F.; Rezende, C.M.; Garrido, F.M.S.; Veiga, V.F.; Bergter, L.; Patitucci, M.L.; Antunes, O.A.C. Separation of acid diterpenes of *Copaifera cearensis* Huber ex Ducke by flash chromatography using potassium hydroxide impregnated silica gel. *J. Braz. Chem. Soc.* **2000**, *11*, 355–360. [CrossRef]

77. Souza, A.B.; de Souza, M.G.M.; Moreira, M.A.; Moreira, M.R.; Furtado, N.A.J.C.; Martins, C.H.G.; Bastos, J.K.; dos Santos, R.A.; Heleno, V.C.G.; Ambrosio, S.R.; et al. Antimicrobial evaluation of diterpenes from *Copaifera langsdorffii* oleoresin against periodontal anaerobic bacteria. *Molecules* **2011**, *16*, 9611–9619. [CrossRef] [PubMed]
78. Lemos, M.; Santin, J.R.; Mizuno, C.S.; Boeing, T.; de Sousa, J.P.B.; Nanayakkara, D.; Bastos, J.K.; de Andrade, S.F. *Copaifera langsdorffii*: Evaluation of potential gastroprotective of extract and isolated compounds obtained from leaves. *Braz. J. Pharmacogn.* **2015**, *25*, 238–245. [CrossRef]
79. De Sousa, J.P.B.; Brancalion, A.P.S.; Junior, M.G.; Bastos, J.K. A validated chromatographic method for the determination of flavonoids in *Copaifera langsdorffii* by HPLC. *Nat. Prod. Commun.* **2012**, *7*, 25–28. [PubMed]
80. Batista, Â.G.; Ferrari, A.S.; da Cunha, D.C.; da Silva, J.K.; Cazarin, C.B.B.; Correa, L.C.; Prado, M.A.; de Carvalho-Silva, L.B.; Esteves, E.A.; Maróstica Júnior, M.R. Polyphenols, antioxidants, and antimutagenic effects of *Copaifera langsdorffii* fruit. *Food Chem.* **2016**, *197*, 1153–1159. [CrossRef] [PubMed]
81. Costa, A.R.M.; Freitas, L.A.P.; Mendiola, J.; Ibáñez, E. *Copaifera langsdorffii* supercritical fluid extraction: Chemical and functional characterization by LC/MS and in vitro assays. *J. Supercrit. Fluids* **2015**, *100*, 86–96. [CrossRef]
82. Geris, R.; da Silva, I.G.; da Silva, H.H.G.; Barison, A.; Rodrigues-Filho, E.; Ferreira, A.G. Diterpenoids from *Copaifera reticulata* Ducke with larvicidal activity against *Aedes aegypti* (L.) (Diptera, Culicidae). *Rev. Inst. Med. Trop. Sao Paulo* **2008**, *50*, 25–28. [PubMed]
83. Dos Santos, A.O.; Ueda-Nakamura, T.; Prado Dias Filho, B.; da Veiga Junior, V.F.; Pinto, A.C.; Nakamura, C.V. Antimicrobial activity of Brazilian copaiba oils obtained from different species of *Copaifera*. *Mem. Inst. Oswaldo Cruz* **2008**, *103*, 277–281. [CrossRef]
84. Carvalho, J.C.T.; Cascon, V.; Possebon, L.S.; Morimoto, M.S.S.; Cardoso, L.G.V.; Kaplan, M.A.C.; Gilbert, B. Topical antiinflammatory and analgesic activities of *Copaifera duckei* Dwyer. *Phyther. Res.* **2005**, *19*, 946–950. [CrossRef] [PubMed]
85. Castro-e-Silva, O., Jr.; Zucoloto, S.; Ramalho, F.S.; Ramalho, L.N.Z.; Reis, J.M.C.; Bastos, A.A.C.; Brito, M.V.H. Anti-proliferative activity of oleoresin from Brazilian *Copaifera duckei* oleoresin on liver regeneration in rats. *Phyther. Res.* **2004**, *18*, 92–94. [CrossRef] [PubMed]
86. Dorneles, F.D.S.; Da Silva, A.S.; Oliveira, C.B.; Zimmermann, C.E.P.; Rosa, L.D.; Tonin, A.A.; de Oliveira, E.C.P.; Santurio, J.M.; Monteiro, S.G. Susceptibility of *Trypanosoma evansi* in the Copaiba oil: In vitro test and in mice experimentally infected with the parasite. *Acta Sci. Vet.* **2013**, *41*, 1136.
87. Paiva, L.A.F.; Rao, V.S.N.; Gramosa, N.V.; Silveira, E.R. Gastroprotective effect of *Copaifera langsdorffii* oleo-resin on experimental gastric ulcer models in rats. *J. Ethnopharmacol.* **1998**, *62*, 73–78. [CrossRef]
88. Paiva, L.A.F.; Gurgel, L.A.; Campos, A.R.; Silveira, E.R.; Rao, V.S.N. Attenuation of ischemia/reperfusion-induced intestinal injury by oleo-resin from *Copaifera langsdorffii* in rats. *Life Sci.* **2004**, *75*, 1979–1987. [CrossRef] [PubMed]
89. Paiva, L.A.F.; de Alencar Cunha, K.M.; Santos, F.A.; Gramosa, N.V.; Silveira, E.R.; Rao, V.S.N. Investigation on the wound healing activity of oleo-resin from *Copaifera langsdorffii* in rats. *Phyther. Res.* **2002**, *16*, 737–739. [CrossRef] [PubMed]
90. De Lima Silva, J.J.; Guimarães, S.B.; da Silveira, E.R.; de Vasconcelos, P.R.L.; Lima, G.G.; Torres, S.M.; de Vasconcelos, R.C. Effects of *Copaifera langsdorffii* Desf. on ischemia-reperfusion of randomized skin flaps in rats. *Aesthet. Plast. Surg.* **2009**, *33*, 104–109. [CrossRef] [PubMed]
91. Neto, J.N.; Lindoso, M.J.D.S.; Coelho, L.F.; Antonio, R.; Carvalho, R.A.F.; Rodrigues, T.G.P.D.M.; de Araújo, A.G.P.; Girão, M.J.B.C.; Schor, E. Changes in the volume and histology of endometriosis foci in rats treated with copaiba oil (*Copaifera langsdorffii*). *Acta Cirúrgica Bras.* **2011**, *26*, 20–24. [CrossRef]
92. Masson-Meyers, D.S.; Enwemeka, C.S.; Bumah, V.; Andrade, T.A.M.; Cashin, S.E.; Frade, M.A.C. Antimicrobial effects of *Copaifera langsdorffii* oleoresin in infected rat wounds. *Int. J. Appl. Microbiol. Sci.* **2013**, *2*, 9–20.
93. Masson-Meyers, D.S.; Andrade, T.A.M.; Leite, S.N.; Frade, M.A.C. Cytotoxicity and wound healing properties of *Copaifera langsdorffii* oleoresin in rabbits. *Int. J. Nat. Prod. Sci.* **2013**, *3*, 10–20.
94. Masson-Meyers, D.; Enweme, C.S.; Bumah, V.; Andrade, T.; Frade, M.A. Topical treatment with *Copaifera langsdorffii* oleoresin improves wound healing in rats. *Int. J. Phytomed.* **2013**, *5*, 378–386.

95. Barbosa, F.S.; Leite, G.L.D.; Alves, S.M.; Nascimento, A.F.; D'Ávila, V.D.A.; da Costa, C.A. Insecticide effects of *Ruta graveolens*, *Copaifera langsdorffii* and *Chenopodium ambrosioides* against pests and natural enemies in commercial tomato plantation. *Acta Sci. Agron.* **2011**, *33*, 37–43.
96. De Alencar Cunha, K.M.; Paiva, L.A.; Santos, F.A.; Gramosa, N.V.; Silveira, E.R.; Rao, V.S. Smooth muscle relaxant effect of kaurenoic acid, a diterpene from *Copaifera langsdorffii* on rat uterus in vitro. *Phyther. Res.* **2003**, *17*, 320–324. [CrossRef] [PubMed]
97. Dos Santos, A.O.; Costa, M.A.; Ueda-Nakamura, T.; Dias-Filho, B.P.; da Veiga-Júnior, V.F.; de Souza Lima, M.M.; Nakamura, C.V. *Leishmania amazonensis*: Effects of oral treatment with copaiba oil in mice. *Exp. Parasitol.* **2011**, *129*, 145–151. [CrossRef] [PubMed]
98. Gomes, N.D.M.; Rezende, C.D.M.; Fontes, S.P.; Hovell, A.M.C.; Landgraf, R.G.; Matheus, M.E.; Pinto, A.D.C.; Fernandes, P.D. Antineoplasic activity of *Copaifera multijuga* oil and fractions against ascitic and solid Ehrlich tumor. *J. Ethnopharmacol.* **2008**, *119*, 179–184. [CrossRef] [PubMed]
99. Gomes, N.M.; Rezende, C.M.; Fontes, S.P.; Matheus, M.E.; Fernandes, P.D. Antinociceptive activity of Amazonian copaiba oils. *J. Ethnopharmacol.* **2007**, *109*, 486–492. [CrossRef] [PubMed]
100. Gomes, N.D.M.; de Rezende, C.M.; Fontes, S.P.; Matheus, M.E.; Pinto, A.D.C.; Fernandes, P.D. Characterization of the antinociceptive and anti-inflammatory activities of fractions obtained from *Copaifera multijuga* Hayne. *J. Ethnopharmacol.* **2010**, *128*, 177–183. [CrossRef] [PubMed]
101. Brito, N.M.B.; Brito, M.V.H.; Carvalho, R.D.K.V.; Matos, L.T.D.M.B.; Lobato, R.C.; Correa, S.C.; Brito, R.B. The effect of copaiba balsam on Walker 256 carcinoma inoculated into the vagina and uterine cervix of female rats. *Acta Cir. Bras.* **2010**, *25*, 176–180. [CrossRef] [PubMed]
102. Pieri, F.A.; Mussi, M.C.M.; Fiorini, J.E.; Moreira, M.A.S.; Schneedorf, J.M. Bacteriostatic effect of copaiba oil (*Copaifera officinalis*) against *Streptococcus mutans*. *Braz. Dent. J.* **2012**, *23*, 36–38. [CrossRef] [PubMed]
103. Guimarães, A.L.; Cunha, E.A.; Matias, F.O.; Garcia, P.G.; Danopoulos, P.; Swikidisa, R.; Pinheiro, V.A.; Nogueira, R.J. Antimicrobial activity of copaiba (*Copaifera officinalis*) and pracaxi (*Pentaclethra macroloba*) oils against *Staphylococcus aureus*: Importance in compounding for wound care. *Int. J. Pharm. Compd.* **2016**, *20*, 58–62. [PubMed]
104. Dos Santos, A.O.; Izumi, E.; Ueda-Nakamura, T.; Dias-Filho, B.P.; da Veiga-Júnior, V.F.; Vataru Nakamura, C. Antileishmanial activity of diterpene acids in copaiba oil. *Mem. Inst. Oswaldo Cruz* **2013**, *108*, 59–64. [CrossRef]
105. Curio, M.; Jacone, H.; Perrut, J.; Pinto, Â.C.; Veiga Filho, V.F.; Silva, R.C.B. Acute effect of *Copaifera reticulata* Ducke copaiba oil in rats tested in the elevated plus-maze: An ethological analysis. *J. Pharm. Pharmacol.* **2009**, *61*, 1105–1110. [CrossRef] [PubMed]
106. Silva, I.G.; Zanon, V.O.M.; Silva, H.H.G. Larvicidal activity of *Copaifera reticulata* Ducke oil-resin against *Culex quinquefasciatus* Say (Diptera: Culicidae). *Neotrop. Entomol.* **2003**, *32*, 729–732. [CrossRef]
107. Da Silva, H.H.G.; Geris, R.; Rodrigues Filho, E.; Rocha, C.; da Silva, I.G. Larvicidal activity of oil-resin fractions from the Brazilian medicinal plant *Copaifera reticulata* Ducke (Leguminosae-Caesalpinoideae) against *Aedes aegypti* (Diptera, Culicidae). *Rev. Soc. Bras. Med. Trop.* **2007**, *40*, 264–267. [CrossRef] [PubMed]
108. Fernandes, F.D.F.; Freitas, E.D.P.S. Acaricidal activity of an oleoresinous extract from *Copaifera reticulata* (Leguminosae: Caesalpinioideae) against larvae of the southern cattle tick, *Rhipicephalus* (*Boophilus*) *microplus* (Acari: Ixodidae). *Vet. Parasitol.* **2007**, *147*, 150–154. [CrossRef] [PubMed]
109. Dos Santos, A.O.; Ueda-Nakamura, T.; Dias Filho, B.P.; da Veiga Junior, V.F.; Nakamura, C.V. Copaiba oil: An alternative to development of new drugs against leishmaniasis. *Evid.-Based Complement. Altern. Med.* **2012**, *2012*. [CrossRef] [PubMed]
110. Pacheco, T.A.R.C.; Barata, L.E.S.; Duarte, M.C.T. A ntimicrobial activity of copaiba (*Copaifera* spp.) balsams. *Rev. Bras. Plantas Med.* **2006**, *8*, 123–124.
111. Izumi, E.; Ueda-Nakamura, T.; Veiga, V.F.; Pinto, A.C.; Nakamura, C.V. Terpenes from *Copaifera* demonstrated in vitro antiparasitic and synergic activity. *J. Med. Chem.* **2012**, *55*, 2994–3001. [CrossRef] [PubMed]
112. Soares, D.C.; Portella, N.A.; Ramos, M.F.D.S.; Siani, A.C.; Saraiva, E.M. *trans*-β-Caryophyllene: An effective antileishmanial compound found in commercial copaiba oil (*Copaifera* spp.). *Evid.-Based Complement. Altern. Med.* **2013**, *2013*. [CrossRef] [PubMed]
113. Ogungbe, I.V.; Setzer, W.N. The potential of secondary metabolites from plants as drugs or leads against protozoan neglected diseases-Part III: In-silico molecular docking investigations. *Molecules* **2016**, *21*, 1389. [CrossRef] [PubMed]

114. Ogungbe, I.V.; Setzer, W.N. In-silico *Leishmania* target selectivity of antiparasitic terpenoids. *Molecules* **2013**, *18*, 7761–7847. [CrossRef] [PubMed]
115. Ogungbe, I.V.; Ng, J.D.; Setzer, W.N. Interactions of antiparasitic alkaloids with *Leishmania* protein targets: A molecular docking analysis. *Future Med. Chem.* **2013**, *5*, 1777–1799. [CrossRef] [PubMed]
116. Ogungbe, I.V.; Erwin, W.R.; Setzer, W.N. Antileishmanial phytochemical phenolics: Molecular docking to potential protein targets. *J. Mol. Graph. Model.* **2014**, *48*, 105–117. [CrossRef] [PubMed]
117. Mcculley, S.F.; Setzer, W.N. An in-silico investigation of anti-Chagas phytochemicals. *Curr. Clin. Pharmacol.* **2014**, *9*, 205–257. [CrossRef] [PubMed]
118. Warfield, J.; Setzer, W.N.; Ogungbe, I.V. Interactions of antiparasitic sterols with sterol 14α-demethylase (CYP51) of human pathogens. *SpringerPlus* **2014**, *3*, 679. [CrossRef] [PubMed]
119. Setzer, M.S.; Sharifi-Rad, J.; Setzer, W.N. The search for herbal antibiotics: An in-silico investigation of antibacterial phytochemicals. *Antibiotics* **2016**, *5*, 30. [CrossRef] [PubMed]
120. Veeck, J.; Esteller, M. Breast cancer epigenetics: From DNA methylation to microRNAs. *J. Mammary Gland Biol. Neoplasia* **2010**, *15*, 5–17. [CrossRef] [PubMed]
121. Chen, T.; Hevi, S.; Gay, F.; Tsujimoto, N.; He, T.; Zhang, B.; Ueda, Y.; Li, E. Complete inactivation of DNMT1 leads to mitotic catastrophe in human cancer cells. *Nat. Genet.* **2007**, *39*, 391–396. [CrossRef] [PubMed]
122. Lin, R.K.; Wu, C.Y.; Chang, J.W.; Juan, L.J.; Hsu, H.S.; Chen, C.Y.; Lu, Y.Y.; Tang, Y.A.; Yang, Y.C.; Yang, P.C.; et al. Dysregulation of p53/Sp1 control leads to DNA methyltransferase-1 overexpression in lung cancer. *Cancer Res.* **2010**, *70*, 5807–5817. [CrossRef] [PubMed]
123. Medina-Franco, J.L.; Caulfield, T. Advances in the computational development of DNA methyltransferase inhibitors. *Drug Discov. Today* **2011**, *16*, 418–425. [CrossRef] [PubMed]
124. Maldonado-Rojas, W.; Olivero-Verbel, J.; Marrero-Ponce, Y. Computational fishing of new DNA methyltransferase inhibitors from natural products. *J. Mol. Graph. Model.* **2015**, *60*, 43–54. [CrossRef] [PubMed]
125. Isshiki, Y.; Kohchi, Y.; Iikura, H.; Matsubara, Y.; Asoh, K.; Murata, T.; Kohchi, M.; Mizuguchi, E.; Tsujii, S.; Hattori, K.; et al. Design and synthesis of novel allosteric MEK inhibitor CH4987655 as an orally available anticancer agent. *Bioorg. Med. Chem. Lett.* **2011**, *21*, 1795–1801. [CrossRef] [PubMed]
126. Weekes, C.D.; Von Hoff, D.D.; Adjei, A.A.; Leffingwell, D.P.; Eckhardt, S.G.; Gore, L.; Lewis, K.D.; Weiss, G.J.; Ramanathan, R.K.; Dy, G.K.; et al. Multicenter phase I trial of the mitogen-activated protein kinase 1/2 inhibitor BAY 86-9766 in patients with advanced cancer. *Clin. Cancer Res.* **2013**, *19*, 1232–1243. [CrossRef] [PubMed]
127. Warner, M.; Gustafsson, J.Å. The role of estrogen receptor β (ERβ) in malignant diseases—A new potential target for antiproliferative drugs in prevention and treatment of cancer. *Biochem. Biophys. Res. Commun.* **2010**, *396*, 63–66. [CrossRef] [PubMed]
128. Warner, M.; Huang, B.; Gustafsson, J.A. Estrogen receptor β as a pharmaceutical target. *Trends Pharmacol. Sci.* **2017**, *38*, 92–99. [CrossRef] [PubMed]
129. Tibes, U. Phospholipase A2 inhibitors in development. *Expert Opin. Investig. Drugs* **1997**, *6*, 279–298. [CrossRef] [PubMed]
130. Wagner, K.M.; McReynolds, C.B.; Schmidt, W.K.; Hammock, B.D. Soluble epoxide hydrolase as a therapeutic target for pain, inflammatory and neurodegenerative diseases. *Pharmacol. Ther.* **2017**, *180*, 62–76. [CrossRef] [PubMed]
131. Setzer, W.N.; Byler, K.G. In-silico approaches to natural products drug discovery: A review of the recent literature. In *Natural Products and Drug Discovery: From Pharmacochemistry to Pharmacological Approaches*; Diniz, M.F.F.M., Scotti, M.T., Scotti, L., Alves, M.F.E., Eds.; Editora UFPB: João Pessoa, Brazil, 2018.
132. Setzer, M.S.; Byler, K.G.; Ogungbe, I.V.; Setzer, W.N. Natural products as new treatment options for trichomoniasis: A molecular docking investigation. *Sci. Pharm.* **2017**, *85*, 5. [CrossRef] [PubMed]

International Journal of
Molecular Sciences

MDPI

Review

Antimalarial Activity of Plant Metabolites

Wen-Hui Pan [1], Xin-Ya Xu [1,2], Ni Shi [1], Siu Wai Tsang [1] and Hong-Jie Zhang [1,*]

1 School of Chinese Medicine, Hong Kong Baptist University, 7 Baptist University Road, Kowloon Tong, Kowloon, Hong Kong SAR, China; 13480448@life.hkbu.edu.hk (W.-H.P.); xuxinya@scsio.ac.cn (X.-Y.X.); 14252252@life.hkbu.edu.hk (N.S.); tsang@hkbu.edu.hk (S.W.T.);

2 CAS Key Laboratory of Tropical Marine Bio-resources and Ecology, Guangdong Provincial Key Laboratory of Applied Marine Biology, South China Sea Institute of Oceanology, Chinese Academy of Science, Guangzhou 510070, China

* Correspondence: zhanghj@hkbu.edu.hk; Tel.: +852-3411-2956; Fax: +852-3411-2461

Received: 13 April 2018; Accepted: 2 May 2018; Published: 6 May 2018

Abstract: Malaria, as a major global health problem, continues to affect a large number of people each year, especially those in developing countries. Effective drug discovery is still one of the main efforts to control malaria. As natural products are still considered as a key source for discovery and development of therapeutic agents, we have evaluated more than 2000 plant extracts against *Plasmodium falciparum*. As a result, we discovered dozens of plant leads that displayed antimalarial activity. Our phytochemical study of some of these plant extracts led to the identification of several potent antimalarial compounds. The prior comprehensive review article entitled "Antimalarial activity of plant metabolites" by Schwikkard and Van Heerden (2002) reported structures of plant-derived compounds with antiplasmodial activity and covered literature up to the year 2000. As a continuation of this effort, the present review covers the antimalarial compounds isolated from plants, including marine plants, reported in the literature from 2001 to the end of 2017. During the span of the last 17 years, 175 antiplasmodial compounds were discovered from plants. These active compounds are organized in our review article according to their plant families. In addition, we also include ethnobotanical information of the antimalarial plants discussed.

Keywords: anti-malaria activity; plants; natural products; ethnopharmacology; *Plasmodium* parasites

1. Introduction

Malaria is still considered as a major global health problem, affecting a large population of the world. According to World Health Organization (WHO), there were about 216 million malaria cases globally and 445,000 deaths in 2016. Most of the cases and the deaths occurred in the WHO African region and affected primarily children and pregnant women [1].

P. falciparum, *P. vivax*, *P. ovale*, *P. malariae* and *P. knowlesi* are the five *Plasmodium* species that cause malaia disease in humans. *P. falciparum* is the deadliest strain that causes malaria and this form of parasite predominates in Africa [2,3]. Humans get infected with malaria parasites through the bites of female anopheline mosquitoes [4]. The *Plasmodium* parasites travel through blood and become mature and reproduce in the liver, leading to malaria disease. The common symptoms of malaria are fever and headache, and in severe cases, malaria causes death [5].

Currently, there is no commercially available malaria vaccine, though efforts to develop vaccines are still ongoing. The most promising vaccine candidate is RTS, S/AS01, which is in clinical trials for treatment of malaria caused by *P. falciparum* [1]. Several medications are available to prevent malaria for travellers in malaria-endemic countries, and a number of drugs are available for treatment of those who have the disease [6].

In 1820, French scientists Pelletier and Caventou discovered quinine (**I**) as the first antimalarial drug, which was originally isolated from the barks of *Cinchona* species (Rubiaceae) (Figure 1). *Cinchona* plants are used as folk medicines in South America by Peruvian Indians, and they were introduced to Europe in the 1700s [7]. Quinine is commercially obtained by solvent extraction from wild-growing *Cinchona* species in South America, or the plants cultivated in Indonesia [8].

Chloroquine (**II**) and its derivative 4-aminoquinoline were developed in the 1940s. They are widely used as antimalarial drugs, even today. The effectiveness of the drugs, however, has declined rapidly since the 1960s, which was due to the development of drug resistance by *P. falciparum* strains, leading to a significant malaria-associated death rate [9]. Mefloquine (**III**), is a 4-quinolinemethanol derivative obtained via total synthesis. It was introduced as a new antimalarial drug in 1985. The drug can be used to treat mild or moderate malaria but should not be used to treat severe malaria [10].

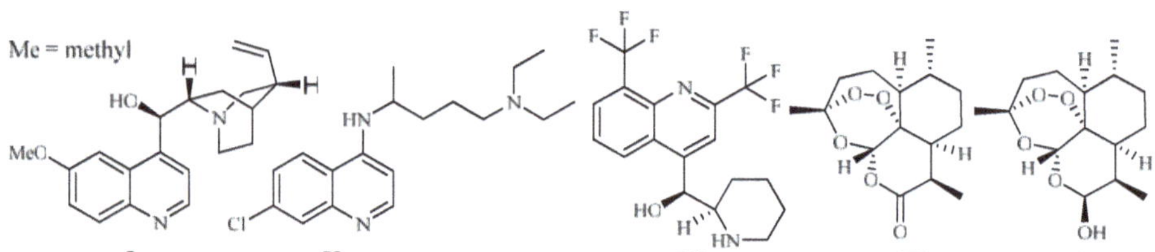

Figure 1. Antimalarial drugs developed from plants.

The current antimalarial drug of choice is artemisinin (Qinghaosu, **IV**), which was originally obtained from the leaves of Qinghao [*Artemisia annua* L. (Asteraceae)] in the 1970s. The compound is clinically effective against chloroquine-resistant malaria strains [11]. The plant Qinghao has been used as a traditional medicine in China for the treatment of fever of malaria origin for about 2000 years [12]. A large number of artemisinin analogs have also been synthesized. The best known among these derivatives are artemether, arteether (artemotil), artesunate and artenimol (β-dihydroartemisinin, DHA) [13]. Artemisinin and its semi-synthetic derivatives have shown better efficacy than quinine for both children and adults patients [14].

Although the anti-parasitic mechanism of action of artemisinin is still in question [15], the endoperoxide bridge is regarded as the key functional group responsible for eliciting free radical-mediated parasite killing mechanisms. According to one school of thought, *Plasmodium* parasites live and reproduce in the host by ingesting red blood cell hemoglobin. This results in an accumulation of heme Fe^{2+} in the parasite. Fe^{2+} firstly interacts and cleaves the peroxide bridge of artemisinin to form highly reactive free radicals, which in turn cause a series of parasite molecular events and eventually kill the parasites [16]. The most used artemisinin derivative today is the prodrug, dihydroartemisinin (**V**), which is metabolized into the pharmacologically active artimisinin (**IV**) in the body [17]. Artesunate was investigated as a potential inhibitor of the essential *P. falciparum* exported protein 1 (EXP1), a membrane glutathione *S*-transferase [18].

Clinically, it is unwise to use artemisinin as the lone therapy due to the potential risk of the parasites to develop resistance to this drug. Indeed, artemisinin drug resistance has been already detected in some Southern Asian countries: Lao People's Democratic Republic, Cambodia, Thailand, Myanmar and Viet Nam [1]. This risk has led to the withdrawal of artemisinin monotherapy from clinical applications.

At present, the use of artemisinins in combination with other drugs, known as artemisinin-based combination therapy (ACT), is the most effective to treat malarial disease caused by *P. falciparum* infection. Five currently available ACTs are artemether in combination with lumefantrine, and four other forms based on artesunate in combination with amodiaquine (two formulations), mefloquine and sulfadoxine+pyrimethamine [1]. Unfortunately, resistance has already been detected to both artemisinin and artesunate components of the multiple ACTs, as well as the non-artemisinin-based combination comprising atovaquone and proguanil. The current availbale antimalarial drugs are listed in Table 1 [1,19,20].

Table 1. Available antimalarial drugs.

Chemical Class	Generic Names	Chemical Class	Generic Names
4-Aminoquinolines	chloroquine amodiaquine piperaquine	Antibiotics	azythromycin clindamycin doxycycline
8-Aminoquinoline	primaquine bulaquine		artemether-lumefantrine artesunate
Arylamino-alcohols	quinine quinidine mefloquine halofantrine lumefantrine	Artemisinin-based combination therapy (ACT)	artesunate/sulfadoxine/pyrimethamine artesunate/sulfadoxine-pyrimethamine/primaquine artesunate/amodiaquine artesunate/mefloquine artesunate/pyronaridine
Biguanides	proguanil chlorproguanil		chloroquine/primaquine dihydroartemisinin/piperaquine
Glycosylamines	pyrimethamine proguanil cycloguanil chlorproguanil chlorcycloguanil	Antibiotics-antimalarial drug combination	doxycyclin/quinine doxycycline/artesunate doxycyclin/mefloquine clindamycin/quinine clindamycin/artesunate
Naphthoquinone	atovaquone		clindamycin/mefloquine
Sesquiterpene lactones	artemisinin arteether artemether artesunate dihydroartemisinin	Other combination therapy	sulfadoxine/pyrimethamine bulaquine/chloroquine dapsone/chlorproguanil atovaquone/proguanil
Sulfonamides/Sulfones	sulfadoxine sulfalene dapsone		

In the search for drug candidates, the initial step is the employment of appropriate bioassays to evaluate the antiplasmodial activity of a candidate. Several strains of *P. falciparum* have been used for this purpose in the past. The strains of *P. falciparum* that are sensitive and resistant to chloroquine are frequently used for antimalarial drug discovery programs. D6, D10, 3D7, TM4 and PoW are chloroquine-sensitive strains, whereas, W2, FCR-3, FcB1 and Dd2 represent chloroquine-resistant strains, and K1 is a multidrug resistant strain.

The need to discover effective and non-drug resistant antimalarial drugs is urgent as *Plasmodium* strains have already developed resistance to all of today's available drugs including artemisinin. In that regard, it should be noted that natural products have proven to be a valuable source for the discovery of novel antimalarial therapeutic agents since the discovery of the first antimalarial drug in 1800s [20]. We, thus, pursued this approach in the search for new antimalarial potential drug leads.

In our antimalarial drug discovery program, we have evaluated more than 2000 plant extracts against D6 and W2 strains of *P. falciparum*. Dozens of these plants displayed antimalarial activity. Several of these plant leads were investigated further to uncover their antimalarial constituents. Phytochemical separation of these plant leads guided by bioassays led to the identification of ten new and 13 known active compounds [21]. Some of these compounds demonstrated potent antimalarial activity [22–29]. For example, polysyphorin (**1**) and rhaphidecurperoxin (**2**), isolated from *Rhaphidophora decursiva* (Araceae), showed antimalarial activities of 1.5 and 1.4 μM against the W2 clones of *P. falciparum*, respectively (Figure 2) [22]. Two trichothecenes, roridin E (**3**) from *R. decursiva* (Araceae) and verrucarin L acetate (**4**) from *Ficus fistulosa* (Moraceae), were found to potently inhibit the parasite growth with IC_{50} values in the sub-nano molar range [24].

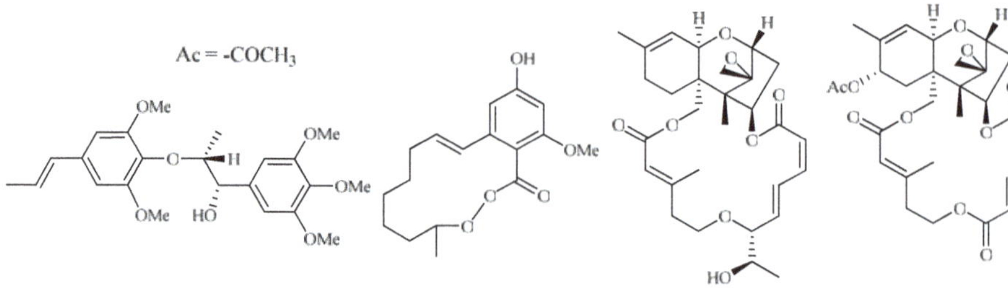

Figure 2. Compounds from *R. decursiva* and *F. fitulosa*.

De-replication to avoid duplication of previous efforts is an essential step in drug discovery protocols. To that end, we conducted a thorough review of the published literature on natural products possessing antimalarial activity. Previously, a literature review by Schwikkard and Van Heerden [30], covered plant-derived antiplasmodial active natural compounds up to the year 2000. The compounds were organized according to the origins of their corresponding plant families. The current review seeks to supplement the review of Schwikkard and Van Heerden. Compounds with antimalarial activity will also be organized according to their plant family of origin (Table 2). Literature published between 2001 and 2017 have been covered. In addition, we also included the ethnobotanic information of plants that have been used as folk medicines for the treatment of malarial disease (Table 3).

Table 2. Antiplasmodial activities and toxicities of compounds isolated from terrestrial plants.

Family	Species	Extract Solvent	Compound	Antiplasmodial IC_{50} (μM) [a] (*P. falciparum*)	Cytotoxicity, ED_{50} (μM) [b] (Cell Line)	References
Annonaceae	*Friesodielsia discolor*	EtOAc	30-formyl-20,40-dihydroxy-60-methoxychalcone (**5**)	9.2 (K1)	21.8 (KB); 13.9 (MCF-7)	[31]
			8-formyl-7-hydroxy-5-methoxyflavanone (**6**)	9.3 (K1)	41.9 (KB); 34.5 (MCF-7)	
			tectochrysin (**7**)	7.8 (K1)	59.1 (KB); 16.8 (MCF-7)	
	Mitrephora diversifolia	CH_2Cl_2/MeOH	5-hydroxy-6-methoxyonychine (**8**)	9.9 (3D7); 11.4 (Dd2)	120.0 (HEK293)	[32]
	Miliusa cuneata	Acetone	miliusacunines A (**9**)	19.3 (TM4)	–	[33]
			miliusacunines B (**10**)	10.8 (K1)	–	
Araceae	*Rhaphidophora decursiva*	MeOH	polysyphorin (**1**)	1.7 (D6); 1.5 (W2)	8.3 (KB)	[22,23]
			rhaphidecurperoxin (**2**)	1.8 (D6); 1.4 (W2)	13.1 (KB)	
			rhaphidecursinol A (**11**)	7.2 (D6); 4.2 (W2)	28.7 (KB)	
			rhaphidecursinol B (**12**)	12.9 (D6); 11.2 (W2)	23.9 (KB)	
			grandisin (**13**)	3.5 (D6); 3.4 (W2)	32.4 (KB)	
			epigrandisin (**14**)	>23 (D6); 7.7 (W2)	37.0 (KB)	
			decursivine (**15**)	11.2 (D6); 12.6 (W2)	–	[22,23]
			Roridin E (**3**)	0.0004 (D6); 0.001 (W2)	0.0004 (KB)	[24]
Asclepiadaceae	*Gongronema napalense*	EtOH	gongroneside A (**16**)	1.6 (D6); 1.4 (W2)	>13.7 (KB)	[25]
Asteraceae	*Achillea millefolium*	MeOH	apigenin 7-*O*-glucoside (**17**)	25.3 (D10); 15.3 (W2)	–	[34]
			luteolin 7-*O*-glucoside (**18**)	61.1 (D10); 62.5 (W2)	–	
	Carpesium divaricatum	MeOH	2-isopropenyl-6-acetyl-8-methoxy-1,3-benzodioxin-4-one (**19**)	2.3 (D10)	63.2 (SK-OV-3)	[35]
	Microglossa pyrifolia	Petroleum ether-EtOAc (1:1, *v*/*v*)	*E*-phytol (**20**)	8.5 (PoW); 11.5 (Dd2)	–	[36]
			6*E*-geranylgeraniol-19-oic acid (**21**)	12.9 (PoW); 15.6 (Dd2)	–	
	Echinops hoehnelii	CH_2Cl_2	5-(penta-1,3-diynyl)-2-(3,4-dihydroxybut-1-ynyl)-thiophene (**22**)	50.2% (100 mg/kg)	–	[37]
			5-(penta-1,3-diynyl)-2-(3-chloro-4-acetoxy-but-1-yn)-thiophene (**23**)	32.7% (100 mg/kg)	–	
Buxaceae	*Buxus semperviren*	MeOH	compound (**24**)	0.5–3.0 (HB3)	7.0 (Hela)	[38]
			compound (**25**)	0.5–3.0 (HB3)	>20 (Hela)	
			23-*O*-(*trans*)-feruloyl-23-hydroxybetulin (**26**)	0.5–3.0 (HB3)	>20 (Hela)	
			compound (**27–31**)	0.5–3.0 (HB3)	>20 (Hela)	
Cecropiaceae	*Cecropia pachystachya*	EtOH	β-sitosterol (**32**)	>120 (W2)	–	[39]
			tormentic acid (**33**)	19.0–25.2 (W2)	–	

Table 2. *Cont.*

Family	Species	Extract Solvent	Compound	Antiplasmodial IC_{50} (μM) [a] (*P. falciparum*)	Cytotoxicity, ED_{50} (μM) [b] (Cell Line)	References
Chloranthaceae	*Chloranthus. fortunei*	EtOH	fortunilide A (**34**)	0.005 (Dd2)	8.8 (WI-38)	[40]
			fortunilide B (**35**)	0.02 (Dd2)	3.1 (WI-38)	
			fortunilide C (**36**)	0.2 (Dd2)	-	
			fortunilide D (**37**)	0.03 (Dd2)	0.5 (WI-38)	
			fortunilide E (**38**)	0.04 (Dd2)	>100 (WI-38)	
			fortunilide F (**39**)	5.3 (Dd2)	-	
			fortunilide G (**40**)	0.05 (Dd2)	1.2 (WI-38)	
			fortunilide H (**41**)	0.2 (Dd2)	-	
			fortunilide I (**42**)	0.09 (Dd2)	-	
			fortunilide J (**43**)	9.9 (Dd2)	-	
			fortunilide K (**44**)	4.7 (Dd2)	-	
			fortunilide L (**45**)	0.1 (Dd2)	15.5 (WI-38)	
			sarglabolide I (**46**)	4.6 (Dd2)	-	
			sarglabolide J (**47**)	0.007 (Dd2)	4.0 (WI-38)	
			shizukaol K (**48**)	0.9 (Dd2)	-	
			shizukaol I (**49**)	0.1 (Dd2)	-	
			shizukaol C (**50**)	0.02 (Dd2)	0.8 (WI-38)	
			schizukaol M (**51**)	0.10 (Dd2)	4.5 (WI-38)	
			chlorahololide D (**53**)	0.01 (Dd2)	0.2 (WI-38)	
	C. multisachys	-	chloramultilide B (**65**)	7.1 (Dd2)	-	
	C. serratus and *C. spicatus*	-	chlorajaponilide C (**52**)	0.001 (Dd2)	5.4 (WI-38)	
			shizukaol N (**54**)	0.1 (Dd2)	10.0 (WI-38)	
			shizukaol E (**58**)	1.8 (Dd2)	-	
			shizukaol D (**59**)	0.6 (Dd2)	-	
			shizukaol F (**60**)	0.01 (Dd2)	0.2 (WI-38)	
			shizukaol G (**61**)	0.01 (Dd2)	1.7 (WI-38)	
			shizukaol B (**62**)	0.03 (Dd2)	16.7 (WI-38)	
			spicachlorantin D (**63**)	0.5 (Dd2)	-	
			shizukaol A (**64**)	1.5 (Dd2)	-	
	Sarcandra glabra	-	sarcandrolide B (**55**)	0.27 (Dd2)	-	
			sarcandrolide A (**56**)	0.3 (Dd2)	-	
			sarcandrolide J (**57**)	11.4 (Dd2)	-	

Table 2. *Cont.*

Family	Species	Extract Solvent	Compound	Antiplasmodial IC_{50} (μM) [a] (*P. falciparum*)	Cytotoxicity, ED_{50} (μM) [b] (Cell Line)	References
Chrysobalanceae	*Parinari capensis*	Petroleum ether and CH_2Cl_2	10,13-dihydroxy-9-methyl-15-oxo-20-norkaur-16-en-18-oic acid γ-lactone (**66**)	1.7 (FCR-3)	5.5 (Graham)	[41]
			10-hydroxy-13-methoxy-9-methyl-15-oxo-20-norkaur-16-en-18-oic acid γ-lactone (**37**)	1.9 (FCR-3)	3.2 (Graham)	
			10-hydroxy-9-methyl-15-oxo-20-norkaur-16-en-18-oic acid γ-lactone (**68**)	5.0 (FCR-3)	9.6 (Graham)	
Clusiaceae	*Garcinia mckeaniana*	Acetone	mckeanianones A (**69**)	6.2 (TM4)	–	[42]
			mckeanianones B (**70**)	6.7 (TM4)	12.9 (Vero)	
			mckeanianones C (**71**)	6.0 (TM4)	29.5 (Vero)	
			bannaxanthones I (**72**)	8.5 (TM4)	–	
			bannaxanthones E (**73**)	8.3 (TM4)	–	
Connaraceae	*Rourea minor* (Gaertn.) Aubl.	$CHCl_3$	rourinoside (**74**)	3.7 (D6); 2.1 (W2)	KB: ED_{50}: >35.1	[26]
			rouremin (**75**)	5.1 (D6); 4.5 (W2)	KB: ED_{50}: >25.5	
			1-(26-hydroxyhexacosanoyl)-glycerol (**76**)	9.5 (D6); 12.7 (W2)	KB: ED_{50}: >41.2	
Cornaceae	*Cornus florida* L.	EtOH	ergosta-4,6,8,22-tetraene-3-one (**77**)	61.0 (D10)	27.0 (L6)	[43]
			3-epideoxyflindissol (**78**)	128.0 (D10)	14.7 (L6)	
			3β-*O*-*cis*-coumaroyl betulinic acid (**79**)	10.4 (D10)	5.6 (L6)	
			3β-*O*-*trans*-coumaroyl betulinic acid (**80**)	15.3 (D10)	9.3 (L6)	
Cucurbitaceae	*Cogniauxia podolaena* Baill.	CH_2Cl_2	cucurbitacin B (**81**)	2.9 (FcM29 strain)	94% inhibition of KB at 1.8 μM	[44]
			cucurbitacin D (**82**)	7.8 (FcM29 strain)	95% inhibition of KB at 1.9 μM	
			20-epibryonolic acid (**83**)	4.4 (FcM29 strain)	20% inhibition of KB at 2.2 μM	
Ebenaceae	*Diospyros quaesita* Thw.	$CHCl_3$	betulinic acid 3-caffeate (**84**)	1.4 (D6); 1.0 (W2)	4.0 (KB)	[27]
Euphorbiaceae	*Jatropha isabelli*	-	compound **85**	–	–	[45]
			compound **86**	–	–	
	Strophioblachia fimbricalyx	MeOH	9-*O*-demethyltrigonostemone (**87**)	8.7 (K1)	2.6 (KB)	[46]
			3,6,9-trimethoxyphenanthropolone (**88**)	9.9 (K1)	12.3 (KB)	
Fabaceae	*Cajanus cajan* L.	-	cajachalcone (**89**)	7.4 (K1)	–	[47]
	Piptadenia pervillei	EtOAc	(+)-catechin 5-gallate (**70**)	1.2 (FcB1)	>75 (MRC-5)	[48]
			(+)-catechin 3-gallate (**91**)	1.0 (FcB1)	>75 (MRC-5)	
	Prosopis glandulosa var. *glandulosa*	EtOH	prosopilosidine (**92**)	0.1 (D6); 0.3 (W2)	20.2 (KB)	[49]
			isoprosopilosidine (**93**)	0.1 (D6); 0.3 (W2)	18.8 (KB)	
Fagaceae	*Quercus laceyi*	MeOH	kaempferol 3-*O*-glucosides (**94**–**97**)	0.6–2.1 (HB3)	<3.0 (Hela)	[38]
Hypericaceae	*Vismia orientalis*	-	vismione D (**98**)	2.4 (K1)	10.0 (L6 cell)	[50]
	Psorospermum glaberrimum	Hexane	3-geranyloxyemodin anthrone (**99**)	1.7 (W2)	–	[51]
			acetylvismione D (**100**)	0.1 (W2)	–	

Table 2. *Cont.*

Family	Species	Extract Solvent	Compound	Antiplasmodial IC_{50} (μM) [a] (*P. falciparum*)	Cytotoxicity, ED_{50} (μM) [b] (Cell Line)	References
Lamiaceae	*Ocimum sanctum*	EtOAc	compound **101**	0.1 (3D7)	-	[52]
	Phlomis brunneogaleata	MeOH	luteolin 7-*O*-β-D-glucopyranoside (**102**)	5.4 (K1)	>200	[53]
			chrysoeriol 7-*O*-β-D-glucopyranoside (**103**)	12.7 (K1)	>194	
	Salvia radula	MeOH:$CHCl_3$ = 1:1	betulafolientriol oxide (**104**)	10.4 (FCR-3)	-	[54]
			salvigenin (**105**)	75.0 (FCR-3)	207 (MCF-7)	
Loganiaceae	*Strychnos icaja*	EtOAc-EtOH-NH_4OH (96:3:1)	15-hydroxyvomicine (**106**)	101.0 (W2)	-	[55]
			N-methyl-sec-iso-pseudostrychnine (**107**)	110.6 (W2)	-	
Lythraceae	*Ammannia multiflora, A. baccifera*	MeOH	4-hydroxy-α-tetralone (**108**)	194.0 (NF-54)	-	[56]
			tetralone-4-*O*-β-D-glucopyranoside (**109**)	124.0 (NF-54)	-	
			ammaniol (**110**)	88.3 (NF-54)	-	
Malvaceae	*Thespesia danis.*	Acetone–water (7:3)	(*R*)-(−)-gossypol (**111**)	4.5 (3D7)	-	[57]
Monimiaceae	*Doryphora sassafras*	CH_2Cl_2/MeOH	1-(4-hydroxybenzyl)-6,7-methylenedioxy-2-methylisoquinolinium trifluoroacetate (**112**)	3.0 (3D7); 4.4 (Dd2)	120.0 (HEK293)	[58]
	Glossocalyx brevipes Benth.	$CHCl_3$/MeOH (1/1)	methyl 2-(1′β-geranyl-5′β-hydroxy-2′-oxocyclohex-3′-enyl) acetate (**113**)	2.2 (D6); 6.6 (W2)	-	[59]
			2-(1′β-geranyl-5′β-hydroxy-2′-oxocyclohex-3′-enyl) acetic acid (**114**)	4.8 (D6); 8.3 (W2)	-	
Moraceae	*Ficus fistulosa*	-	verrucarin L acetate (**4**)	0.001 (D6); 0.001 (W2)	0.2 (KB)	[24]
	F. septica	MeOH	dehydrotylophorine (**115**)	0.4 (3D7)	8.2 (L929)	[60]
			dehydroantofine (**116**)	0.03 (3D7)	>55 (L929)	
			tylophoridicine D (**117**)	0.06 (3D7)	>56 (L929)	
Myristicaceae	*Knema glauca*	EtOAc	malabaricone A (**118**)	8.5 (K1)	>61 (KB); 55.4 (NCI-H187)	[61]
Piperaceae	*Piper sarmentosum*	Hexane-MeOH	sarmentine (**119**)	85.5 (K1)	-	[62]
			1-piperettyl pyrrolidine (**120**)	21.9 (K1)	-	
	P. tricuspe	Petroleum ether	dictyochromenol (**121**)	9.6 (FcB1)	7.7 (L-6)	[63]
			3-farnesyl-*p*-hydroxy benzoic acid (**122**)	29.8 (FcB1)	40.9 (L-6)	
			2′*E*,6′*E* 2-farnesyl hydroquinone (**123**)	1.4 (FcB1)	1.1 (L-6)	
Platanaceae	*Platanus occidentalis*	MeOH	kaempferol 3-*O*-rhamnosides (**124**–**127**)	0.5–1.8 (HB3)	9.3–20.0 (Hela)	[38]
Rubiaceae	*Nauclea orientalis*	MeOH	naucleaorine (**128**)	6.9 (D6); 8.0 (W2)	38.0 (KB)	[28]
			epimethoxynaucleaorine (**129**)	12.4 (D6); 13.2 (W2)	>37.9 (KB)	
			3α,23-dihydroxyurs-12-en-28-oic acid (**130**)	9.7 (D6); 12.7 (W2)	>42.2 (KB)	
			oleanolic acid (**131**)	4.6 (D6); 5.1 (W2)	46.0 (KB)	

Table 2. *Cont.*

Family	Species	Extract Solvent	Compound	Antiplasmodial IC_{50} (μM) [a] (*P. falciparum*)	Cytotoxicity, ED_{50} (μM) [b] (Cell Line)	References
Rutaceae	*Citropsis articulata*	MeOH	5-hydroxynoracronycine (**132**)	2.8 (FcB1)	28.8 (Vero)	[64]
			1,5-dihydroxy-2,3-dimethoxy-10-methyl-9-acridone (**133**)	10.0 (FcB1)	101 (Vero)	
	Zanthoxylum chiloperone var. *angustifolium* Engl.	CH_2Cl_2	*trans*-avicennol (**134**)	7.8 (K1); 1.5 (F32); 3.5 (PFB); 6.4 (FcB1)	12.8 (MCR5)	
			canthin-6-one (**135**)	24.1 (K1); 9.1 (F32); 14.6 (PFB); 18.2 (FcB1)	42.7 (MCR5)	[65]
			5-methoxycanthin-6-one (**136**)	20.4 (K1); 41.6 (F32)	–	
Simaroubaceae	*Eurycoma longifolia*	CH_2Cl_2	eurycomanone (**137**)	0.06 (D6); 0.04 (W2)	0.02 (A-549); <0.006 (MCF-7)	[66,67]
			pasakbumin B (**138**)	0.08 (D6); 0.05 (W2)	0.02 (A-549); <0.006 (MCF-7)	
	Picrolemma sprucei	Hexane/H_2O	neosergeolide (**139**)	0.002 (K1)	–	[68]
Apocynaceae	*Aspidosperma vargasii*	EtOH	ellipticine (**140**)	0.07 (K1)	–	
	A. desmanthum	EtOH	aspidocarpine (**141**)	0.02 (K1)	–	
Piperaceae	*Pothomorphe peltata*	$CHCl_3$/EtOH	4-nerolidylcatechol (**142**)	0.7 (K1)	–	
Theaceae	*Camellia sinensis*		mefloquine (**143**)	–	–	[69]
			gallocatecin (**144**)	–	–	
Tiliaceae	*Grewia bilamellata*	MeOH	3α,20-lupandiol (**145**)	19.8 (D6); 19.1 (W2)	>90 (KB)	[29]
			grewin (**146**)	11.2 (D6); 5.5 (W2)	>107.5 (KB)	
			nitidanin (**147**)	21.2 (D6); 18.4 (W2)	>90 (KB)	
			2α,3β-dihydroxyolean-12-en-28-oic acid (**148**)	21.1 (D6); 8.6 (W2)	51.5 (KB)	
			2,6-dimethoxy-1-acetonylquinol (**149**)	42.2 (D6); 23.0 (W2)	169 (KB)	
Verbenaceae	*Lippia javanica*	EtOAc (aerial parts)	lippialactone (**150**)	23.8 (D10)	–	[70]

[a] IC_{50}: Concentration that resulted in 50% death of *Plasmodium falciparum*. [b] ED_{50}: Concentration that resulted in 50% cell death.

Table 3. The ethnology of plants.

Family	Ethnologic Plant	Country	Plant Part	Antiplasmodial Activity (IC_{50}) (μg/mL, Unless Indicated) [a] (*P. falciparum*)	Cytotoxicity (CC_{50} for Cells, LD_{50} for Brine Shrimp) (μg/mL, Unless Indicated) [b,c] (Cell Line)	References
Acanthaceae	*Justilia schimperand* (Hochst ex Nees) T. Alnder		Roots	–	–	[71]
Anacardiaceae	*Mangifera indica* L.	Africa	Leaves	% parasitaemia reduced from 8.9 at 60 mg/kg to 7.2 at 240 mg/kg (mice)	208.3 mg/kg (mice)	[72]
		Nigeria	Leaves	–	3079.1 (brine shrimp)	[73]
		Nigeria	Stem barks	–	2456.0 (brine shrimp)	[73,74]
	Pseudoprotorhus longifolius H. Perr.	Madagascar	Leaves	–	–	[75]
	Rhus taratana (Bak.) H. Perr.	Madagascar	Leaves	–	–	[75]
	Sclerocarya birrea (A. Rich) Hochst.	South Africa	Stem-bark (MeOH)	5.91 (D6)	–	[76]
	S. caffra Sond.	Madagascar	Leaves	–	–	[75]
Annonaceae	*Annona senegalensis* Rolyns &Gh	Nigeria	Leaves	–	6811.0 (brine shrimp)	[73]
	Enantia chlorantha Oliv.	Nigeria	Stem barks	–	214.3 (brine shrimp)	[73,74]
Apocynaceae	*Alstonia boonei* DeWild	Nigeria	Leaves; stem barks	% parasitaemia reduced from 19.4% (negative control) to 5.5% at 240 mg/kg (mice)	78.77 mg/kg (mice)	[72,74]
	Aspidosperma cylindrocarpon Müll. Arg.	Brazil	Trunk woods (EtOH)	44.0 (W2); 39.0 (3D7)	>500 (Vero)	[7]
	A. parvifolium A. DC.	Brazil	Trunk barks (EtOH)	32.8 (W2); 20.5 (3D7)	>500 (Vero)	[7]
	A. olivaceum Müll. Arg.	Brazil	Leaves (CH_2Cl_2)	7.0 (W2); 25.5 (3D7)	>500 (Vero)	[7]
			Leaves (EtOH)	7.0 (W2); 5.0 (3D7)	–	
			Trunk wood (CH_2Cl_2)	<6 (W2); <6 (3D7)	>500 (Vero)	
			Trunk bark (CH_2Cl_2)	<6 (W2); <6 (3D7)	–	
			Trunk bark (EtOH)	5.0 (W2); 7.0 (3D7)	>500 (Vero)	
	A. ramiflorum Müll. Arg.	Brazil	Leaves (EtOH)	32.8 (W2); 20.5 (3D7)	–	[7]
			Leaves (CH_2Cl_2)	<6 (W2); <6 (3D7)	–	
			Trunk woods (EtOH)	36.5 (W2); 48.0 (3D7)	–	
			Trunk woods (CH_2Cl_2)	9.5 (3D7)	>500 (Vero)	
			Trunk woods (EtOH)	19.8 (W2); 1.0 (3D7)	–	
			Trunk barks (CH_2Cl_2)	<6 (W2); <6 (3D7)	>500 (Vero))	

Table 3. *Cont.*

Family	Ethnologic Plant	Country	Plant Part	Antiplasmodial Activity (IC_{50}) (μg/mL, Unless Indicated) [a] (*P. falciparum*)	Cytotoxicity (CC_{50} for Cells, LD_{50} for Brine Shrimp) (μg/mL, Unless Indicated) [b,c] (Cell Line)	References
	A. spruceanum Benth. ex Müll. Arg.	Brazil	Leaves (EtOH)	65.0 (W2); >100 (3D7)	–	[7]
			Leaves (CH_2Cl_2)	23.25 (W2); 47.0 (3D7)	–	
			Trunk woods (EtOH)	29.5 (W2); 41.5 (3D7)	–	
			Trunk woods (CH_2Cl_2)	<6 (W2); <6 (3D7)	109.6 (Vero))	
			Trunk woods ($CHCl_3$)	37.0 (W2); >100 (3D7)	–	
			Trunk barks (EtOH)	26.3 (W2); 14.0 (3D7)	–	
			Trunk barks (CH_2Cl_2)	<6 (W2); <6 (3D7)	–	
			Trunk barks (EtOH)	28.0 (W2); 19.0 (3D7)	–	
	A. tomentosum Mart.	Brazil	Trunk woods (EtOH)	26.5 (W2); 25.0 (3D7)	–	[7]
			Leaves (EtOH)	23.8 (W2); 27.0 (3D7)	–	
			Fruits (EtOH)	20.5 (W2); 38.6 (3D7)	–	
			Seeds (EtOH)	24.5 (W2); 3.0 (3D7)	>500 (Vero))	
Aristolochiaceae	*Aristolochia acuminata* Lamk.	Madagascar	Roots, stems, leaves	–	–	[75]
Asteraceae	*Artemisia annua* L.	China	Whole plants	–	–	[77]
	Tithonia diversifolia A. Gray	Nigeria	Leaves	–	2304 (brine shrimp)	[73]
	Vernonia amygdalina Del.		Leaves	–	–	[71]
Avicenniaceae	*Avicennia marina* (Forsk) Vierh.	Madagascar	Aerial parts	–	–	[78]
	A. basilicum L.	Madagascar	Aerial parts	–	–	[75]
Bignoniaceae	*Fernandoa* sp.	Madagascar	Aerial parts	–	–	[75]
	Kigelianthe madagascariensis Sprague var. hidebrandtii	Madagascar	Leaves	–	–	[75]
Brassicaceae	*Brassica nigra* (L.) Koch.		Seeds	–	–	[71]
Caricaceae	*Carica papaya* L.		Leaves, fruits, roots		–	[71,79]
Celastraceae	*Maytenus acuminata* (L.f.) Loes	Kenya	leaves, root barks	36.6–41.5%	–	[80]
Combretaceae	*Combretu raimbaulti* Heckel	Madagascar	Leaves		–	[75]
	Terminalia catappa	Nigeria	Leaves (EtOAc)	3.1 (K1)	159.9 μg/L (L6)	[81]
	T. latifolia Engl.	Nigeria	leaves	–	272.9 (brine shrimp)	[73]
Commelinaceae	*Commelina benghalensis* L.	Madagascar	Aerial parts	–	–	[75]

Table 3. *Cont.*

Family	Ethnologic Plant	Country	Plant Part	Antiplasmodial Activity (IC_{50}) (µg/mL, Unless Indicated) [a] (*P. falciparum*)	Cytotoxicity (CC_{50} for Cells, LD_{50} for Brine Shrimp) (µg/mL, Unless Indicated) [b,c] (Cell Line)	References
Compositae	*Brachylaena ramiflora* (DC.) H. Humb	Madagascar	Aerial parts	–	–	[75]
	Conyza aegytiaca Ait. Var *lineariloba*	Madagascar	Aerial parts	–	–	[75]
	Inula perrieri H. Humb.	Madagascar	Leaves	–	–	[75]
	Parthenium hysterophorus L.	Madagascar	Aerial parts	–	–	[75]
	Senecio ompricaefolius (ex DC.) H. Humb.	Madagascar	Aerial parts	–	–	[75]
	Stenocline inuloides DC.	Madagascar	Leaves	–	–	[75]
	Tagetes erecta L.	Madagascar	Leaves	–	–	[75]
	T. patula L.	Madagascar	Leaves	–	–	[75]
	Vernonia lasiopus O. Hoffm.	Kenya	Root barks	–	–	[75]
	V. pectoralis Bak.	Madagascar	Aerial parts	–	–	[75]
	V. trichodesma Bak.	Madagascar	Leaves	–	–	[75]
	V. chapelieri Drak.	Madagascar	Aerial parts	–	–	[75]
	V. sp. (Dr. Hely)	Madagascar	Aerial parts	–	–	[75]
	V. ampandrandavensis Bak.	Madagascar	Aerial parts	–	–	[75]
Cucurbitaceae	*Momordica charantia* L.	Madagascar	Aerial parts	–	–	[75]
	Zehneria scabra (Lf.) Sond.		Roots	–	–	[71]
Euphorbiaceae	*Bridelia micrantha* Benth.	Nigeria	Leaves	–	>90,000 (brine shrimp)	[73]
	Croton goudoti H. Bn.	Madagascar	Leaves	–	–	[75]
	C. macrostachyus Hochst. Ex Del.		Leaves/barks/roots	–	–	[71]
	Euphorbia hirta	Nigeria	Whole plants (Hexane)	4.3 (K1)	14.2 (L6)	[81,82]
	Flueggea microcarpa Blume	Madagascar	Aerial parts		–	[75]
	Jatropha curcas L.	Nigeria	Leaves (EtOAc)	2.4 (K1)	126.5 (L6)	[75,81,82]
		Madagascar	leaves, roots			
	Manihot utilisma Pohl.	Madagascar	Leaves	–	–	[75]
	Phyllanthus amarus Schum. & Thonn.	Brazil, Cuba, Haiti, Nigeria, Elsewhere	Whole plants (MeOH)	5.0 (3D7)	–	[83,84]
			Whole plants (CH_2Cl_2)	14.5 (3D7)	–	
		India	Whole plants	–	–	[85]
		Nigeria	Leaves (EtOAc)	5.6 (K1)	77.7 (L6)	[81,82]
		Ghana	Whole plants	–	–	[85]
		West Africa	Aerial parts	–	–	
	Phyllanthus sp.	Madagascar	Aerial parts	–	–	[75]

Table 3. *Cont.*

Family	Ethnologic Plant	Country	Plant Part	Antiplasmodial Activity (IC_{50}) (μg/mL, Unless Indicated) [a] (*P. falciparum*)	Cytotoxicity (CC_{50} for Cells, LD_{50} for Brine Shrimp) (μg/mL, Unless Indicated) [b,c] (Cell Line)	References
Fabaceae	*Acacia nilotica* L.	Pakistan	Leaves (EtOH)	1.3 (3D7)	–	[86]
	Caesalpinia benthamiana	Guinea	Leaves (MeOH)	4.0 (Ghana)	32.0 (MRC-5)	[79]
	Cajanus cajan Mill sp.	Nigeria	Leaves	–	988.5 (brine shrimp)	[73,74]
	Calliandra haematocephala Hassk	Nigeria	Roots	–	–	
	Calpurna ourea (Ait.) Benth		Leaves	–	–	[71]
	Cassia siamea	Nigeria	Stem barks (EtOAc)	2.70 (K1)	988.5 (stem bark), 8232.2 (brine shrimp)	[73]
			leaves	–		
	Piliostigma thonnigii Schum	Nigeria	Leaves	–	7958.0 (brine shrimp)	[73]
Flacourtiaceae	*Homalium* sp.	Madagascar	Aerial parts	–	–	[75]
Gramineae	*Phragmites mauritianus* Kunth	Madagascar	Aerial parts	–	–	[75]
Hydrengeaceae	*Dichroa febrifuga*	China	Roots	–	–	[87]
Icacinaceae	*Cassinopsis madagascariensis* (Baill.) H. Bn.	Madagascar	Leaves, stem barks	–	–	[75]
Lamiaceae	*Hyptispectinata* Poit.	Madagascar	Leaves	–	–	[75]
	Ocimum canum Sims.	Nigeria	Leaves (EtOAc)	1.8 (K1)	60.1 (L6)	[75,81]
		Madagascar	Stems, seeds	–		
	O. lamiifolium Hochst. ex Benth.		Leaves	–	–	[71]
	Cassytha filiformis L.	Nigeria	Vines	–	–	[74]
	Cinnamomum camphora (L.) Sieb	Madagascar	Leaves	–	–	[75]
Leguminosae	*Abrus precatorius* L.	Madagascar	Leaves	–	–	[75]
	Albizzia lebbek Benth.	Madagascar	Aerial parts	–	–	[75]
	Caesalpinia bonducella Fleming	Madagascar	Seeds, roots	–	–	[75]
	Cassia occidentalis L.	Madagascar	Aerial parts	–	–	[75]
	Crotalaria spinosa Hochst.	Madagascar	Leaves	–	–	[75]
	Erythryna indica Lamk.	Madagascar	Aerial parts	–	–	[75]
	Piliostigma thonningii	Nigeria	Leaves (EtOAc)	3.6 (K1)	56.1 (L6)	[81]
	Pongamia pinnata L.	India	Barks (MeOH)	11.7 (CQ-sensitive)	>200 (THP-1)	[88]
Lilliaceae	*Allium sativum* L.		Bulbs	–	–	[71]
Loganiaceae	*Anthocleista amplexicaulus* Bak.	Madagascar	Aerial parts	–	–	[75]
	A. rhizophoroides Bak.	Madagascar	Roots, leaves	–	–	[75]
	Strychnos mostuoides Leeuwenberg	Madagascar	Aerial parts	–	–	[75]

Table 3. *Cont.*

Family	Ethnologic Plant	Country	Plant Part	Antiplasmodial Activity (IC_{50}) (μg/mL, Unless Indicated) [a] (*P. falciparum*)	Cytotoxicity (CC_{50} for Cells, LD_{50} for Brine Shrimp) (μg/mL, Unless Indicated) [b,c] (Cell Line)	References
Malvaceae	*Gossypium arboreum* L.	Nigeria	Leaves	–	94.1 (brine shrimp)	[73]
	G. barbadense L.	Nigeria	Leaves	–	3585.0 (brine shrimp)	[73]
	G. hirsitum L.	Nigeria	Leaves	–	257.2 (brine shrimp)	[73]
Meliaceae	*Azadirachta indica* A. Juss	Africa	leaves	The percentage parasitaemia reduced from 15.7 % to 4.8 % at 240 mg/kg (in vivo)	140.0 mg/kg (mice)	[72]
	Swietenia macrophylla King	Indonesia	Seeds	–	–	[89]
			Barks	78% inhibition at 100 (Indo)	–	[90]
Melianthaceae	*Bersama abyssinica* Fresen.		Leaves, root barks and stems	–	–	[71]
Menispermaceae	*Burasaia australis* Sc. Elliot	Madagascar	Root barks	–	–	[75]
	B. congesta Decne	Madagascar	Root barks	–	–	[75]
	B. gracilis Decne	Madagascar	Root barks	–	–	[75]
	Burasaia madagascariensis Thou.	Madagascar	Root barks	–	–	[75]
	B. nigrescens R. Cap.	Madagascar	Root barks	–	–	[75]
	Chasmanthera uviformis Baill.	Madagascar	Stem barks	–	–	[75]
	Cissampelos pareira L.	Madagascar	Roots	–	–	[75]
	C. madagascariensis (Baill.) Diels.	Madagascar	Roots	–	–	[75]
	Spirospermum penduliflorum Thou.	Madagascar	Roots, stem barks	–	–	[75]
	Strychnopsis thouarsii Baill.	Madagascar	Leaves, root barks	–	–	[75]
	Triclisia macrocarpa (Baill.) Diels	Madagascar	Root barks, stem barks	–	–	[71]
Mimosaceae	*Acacia catechu* (L.f.) Willd.		Leaves	–	–	[71]
Moraceae	*Ficus elastica* Roxb. ex Hornem.	Cameroon	Roots (MeOH)	9.5	–	[91]
	F. sur Forssk.	Kenya	Leaves, stem barks, root barks	34.1–48.4% Inhibition	–	[80]
	F. thonningii Blume	Nigeria	Leaves (Hexane)	2.7 (NF54); 10.4 (K1)	>20 (KB)	[90]
Myrtaceae	*Psidium guajava* L.	Nigeria	Stem barks	–	707.2 (brine shrimp)	[72]
Ochnaceae	*Lophira alata* Banks	Nigeria	Leaves (Hexane)	2.5 (NF54); 2.5 (K1)	>20 (KB)	[90]
Papilionaceae	*Pericopsis elata* Harms	Nigeria	leaves	–	601.8 (brine shrimp)	[73]
	Pterocarpus osun Craib	Nigeria	Stem barks	–	–	[74]
Periplocaceae	*Cryptolepts sanguinolenta*	West Africa	Roots	–	13.9 (MCF7)	[92]
	Parquetina nigrescens (Afz.) Bullock	Nigeria	Root barks	–	–	[74]

Table 3. *Cont.*

Family	Ethnologic Plant	Country	Plant Part	Antiplasmodial Activity (IC_{50}) (μg/mL, Unless Indicated) [a] (*P. falciparum*)	Cytotoxicity (CC_{50} for Cells, LD_{50} for Brine Shrimp) (μg/mL, Unless Indicated) [b,c] (Cell Line)	References
Phytolaccacaa	*Phytolacca dodecandra* L'Hér.		Leaves	–	–	[71]
Polygonaceae	*Rumex abyssinicus* Jacq.		Leaves and stems	–	–	[71]
Potamogetonaceae	*Potamogeton javanicus* Hass Karl	Madagascar	Aerial parts	–	–	[75]
Ranunculaceae	*Clematis mauritiana* Lamk. Var. *normalis*	Madagascar	Aerial parts	–	–	[75]
Rhamnaceae	*Rhamnus prinoides* L' H'erit	Kenya	Leaves, root barks	34.1–43.9% Inhibition	–	[80]
	R. staddo A. Rich.	Kenya	Root barks	11.1% Inhibition	–	[80]
Rubiaceae	*Anthospermum emirnense* Bak.	Madagascar	Aerial parts	–	–	[75]
	Cinchona ledgeriana Muens	Madagascar	Stem barks	–	–	[75]
	C. officinalis L.	Madagascar	Stem barks	–	–	[75]
	C. succirubra Pavon et Kiutzsch	Madagascar	Stem barks	–	–	[75]
	Cephalanthus spathelliferus Bak.	Madagascar	Leaves	–	–	[75]
	Danais fragrans Gaertn.	Madagascar	Roots	–	–	[75]
	D. gerrardii Bak.	Madagascar	Roots	–	–	[75]
	D. verticillata Bak.	Madagascar	Roots	–	–	[75]
	D. breviflora Bak.	Madagascar	Roots	–	–	[75]
	D. cernua Bak.	Madagascar	Roots	–	–	[75]
	Hymenodyction lohavato baill.	Madagascar	Root barks, stem barks	–	–	[75]
	Morinda lucida Benth	Africa	Leaves	The percentage parasitaemia reduced from 14.0 % to 5.8 % at 240 mg/kg (in vivo)	134.5 mg/kg (mice)	[72]
		Nigeria	Stem barks	*P. berghei*	2.6 (brine shrimp)	[73]
		Nigeria	Leaves	–	383.9 (brine shrimp)	[73]
	Nauclea latifolia S.M.	Nigeria	Stem barks	–	9368.0 (brine shrimp)	[73]
	Saldinia sp. (andriambavifoy)	Madagascar	Aerial part	–	–	[75]
	Sarcocephalus latifolius (J. E. Smith) E. A. Bruce	Nigeria	Root barks	–	–	[74]
	Schismatoclada concinna Bak.	Madagascar	Root barks	–	–	[75]
	S. farahimpensis Bak.	Madagascar	Root barks	–	–	[75]
	S. viburnoides Bak.	Madagascar	Root barks	–	–	[75]
	Citropsis articulata (Willd. ex Spreng.) Swingle & Kellerman	Uganda	Roots	77% inhibition at 10 (FcB1)	12% inhibition at 10 (Vero)	[64]
			Demethylsuberosin	16.7	>50% inhibition at 16.7 (Vero)	
			5-hydroxynoracronycine	0.9	9.3% inhibition at 0.9 (Vero)	
			1,5-dihydroxy-2,3-dimethoxy-10-methyl-9-acridone	3.0	30.5% inhibition at 3.0 (Vero)	
			7α-obacunyl acetate	9.3	>50% inhibition at 9.3 (Vero)	

Table 3. *Cont.*

Family	Ethnologic Plant	Country	Plant Part	Antiplasmodial Activity (IC_{50}) (µg/mL, Unless Indicated) [a] (*P. falciparum*)	Cytotoxicity (CC_{50} for Cells, LD_{50} for Brine Shrimp) (µg/mL, Unless Indicated) [b,c] (Cell Line)	References
Rutaceae	*Evodia fatraina* H. Perr	Madagascar	Root barks, stem barks	–	–	[75]
	Toddalia asiatica (L.) Lam.	Kenya; Madagascar	Root barks; root barks, stem barks	–	–	[75,80]
	Zanthoxylum tsihanimpotsa H. Perr.	Madagascar	Stem barks	–	–	[75]
Santalaceae	*Okoubaka aubrevillei* Phelleg & Nomand	Nigeria	Stem barks	–	–	[74]
Sapindaceae	*Dodonaea viscosa* Jacq.	Madagascar	Leaves	–	–	[75]
	D. madagascariensis Rdlk.	Madagascar	Leaves	–	–	[75]
Selaginellaceae	*Salaginella vogelli*	Cameroon	Leaves (MeOH)	32.2	–	[91]
Schizaeaceae	*Mohria caffrorum* (L.) Desv.	Madagascar	Aerial parts	–	–	[75]
Simaroubaceae	*Brucea antidysenterica* J.F. Mill.		Stems, barks seeds	–	–	[71]
Ulmaceae	*Trema commersonii* Boj.	Madagascar	Aerial part	–	–	[75]
	T. orientalis Blume	Madagascar	Root barks	2.0 (K1)	32.5 (L6)	[75]
Verbanaceae	*Lippia multiflora* Moldenke	Nigeria	Aerial part	–	1.1 (brine shrimp)	[73]
	Clerodendrum myricoides (Hochst.) Vatke	Kenya	Root barks	9.8% (*Plasmodium berghei* NK65)	–	[71,80]
	Vitex doniana	Nigeria	Leaves (Hexane)	3.6 (K1)	431.4	[81,82]
			Stem barks (Hexane)	6.8 (K1)	ND	[81]
Zingiberaceae	*Curcuma longa* L.	Madagascar	Leaves	–	–	[75]
	Zingiber officinale Roscoe		Rhizome	–	–	[71]

[a] IC_{50}: Concentration that resulted in 50% death of *Plasmodium falciparum*. [b] LD_{50}: Concentration that was lethal to 50% of test animals. [c] CC_{50}: Concentration that resulted in 50% cell death.

2. Plant-derived Antimalarial Compounds

2.1. Annonaceae–Asteraceae Families

2.1.1. Annonaceae Family

Annonaceae is a family of flowering plants consisting of about 2400 species. Two plants in this family have been phytochemically investigated for their antiplasmodial and cytotoxic activities. From the leaves of *Friesodielsia discolor*, Prawat et al. isolated two new flavonoids, 3′-formyl-2′,4′-dihydroxy-6′-methoxychalcone (**5**), 8-formyl-7-hydroxy-5-methoxyflava-none (**6**), and the known tectochrysin (**7**) (Figure 3) [31]. They displayed antiplasmodial activity against the K1 multidrug resistant strain of *P. falciparum* with IC_{50} values of 9.2, 9.3 and 7.8 μM, respectively. However, these compounds also exhibited cytotoxicity against the cancer cell lines KB and MCF-7, with the IC_{50} values ranging from 13.9–34.5 μM.

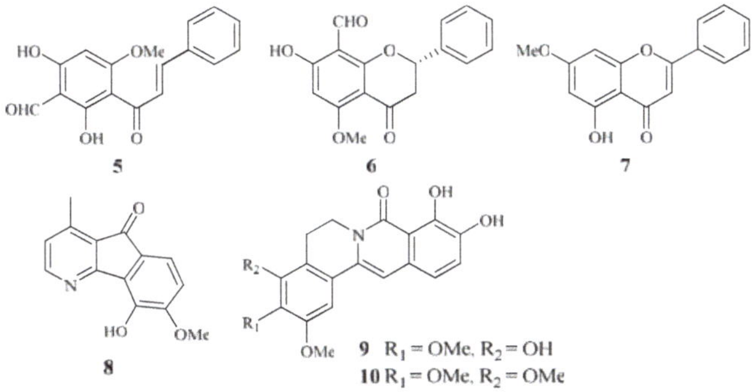

Figure 3. Compounds from Annonaceae plants.

According to Mueller et al. [32], 5-hydroxy-6-methoxyonychine (**8**), an alkaloid obtained from the roots of the Australian tree plant *Mitrephora diversifolia*, showed IC_{50} values of 9.9 and 11.4 μM against the 3D7 and Dd2 clones of *P. falciparum*, respectively.

Miliusacunines A (**9**) and B (**10**) were identified from an acetone extract of the leaves and twigs of *Miliusa cuneatas* [33]. Compound **9** demonstrated inhibitory activity against the TM4 malarial strain (IC_{50} 19.3 μM), and compound **10** displayed activity against the K1 malarial strain (IC_{50} 10.8 μM). Both isolates showed no toxicity to the Vero cells at the elevated concentrations.

2.1.2. Araceae Family

Zhang et al. [22,23] performed extensive research on *Rhaphidophora decursiva*, a vine growing in Vietnam. The MeOH extract of the plant leaves and stems showed antimalarial activity against both D6 and W2 clones with no apparent cytotoxicity at a concentration of 20 μg/mL. Seven compounds were identified from the stems and leaves of the plant through a bioassay-guided separation (Figure 4). Polysyphorin (**1**) and rhaphidecurperoxin (**2**) were among the most active compounds, which demonstrated antimalarial activity with IC_{50} values of 1.4–1.8 μM against the D6 and W2 strains and cytotoxicity with ED_{50} values of 8.3–13.1 μM against KB cells (Figure 2). Rhaphidecursinols A (**11**) and B (**12**), grandisin (**13**), epigrandisin (**14**) and decursivine (**15**) also showed activities against *P. falciparum* (D6 and W2) with IC_{50} values of 3.4–12.9 μM and cytotoxicity of ED_{50} values of 23.9–37.0 μM against KB cells with an exception of compound **14**, which showed no antimalarial activity against D6 strain at 23 μM.

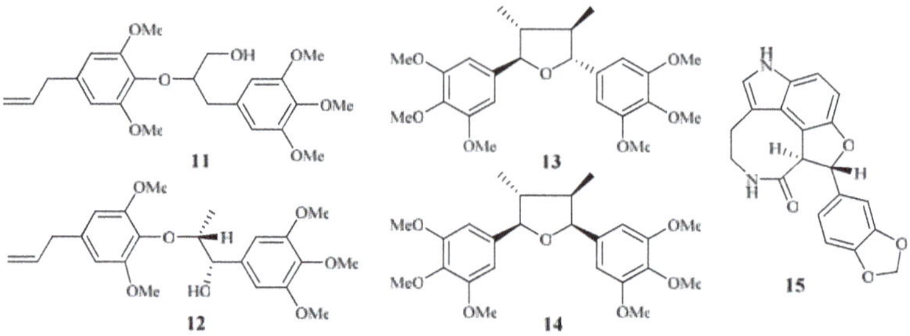

Figure 4. Compounds from an Araceae plant.

According to the further investigation of Zhang et al. [24], a potent but toxic trichothecene compound, roridin E (**3**), was identified from the same plant extract (Figure 2). The investigators determined that the compound was able to inhibit parasite growth with IC_{50} values in the sub-nano molar range. However, roridin E was also very cytotoxic against KB cells. Interestingly, these researchers reported another trichothecene compound (**4**) from a plant in a different family, and the compound showed equally potent antimalarial activities as that of roridin E, but with much less cytotoxicity (see Section 2.8.3).

2.1.3. Asclepiadaceae Family

Libman et al. reported the antimalarial bioassay-directed separation of *Gongronema napalense*, leading to the identification of a new steroidal glycoside, gongroneside A (**16**) (Figure 5) [25]. The compound showed inhibitory activity against the D6 and W2 clones with IC_{50} values of 1.6 and 1.4 μM, respectively. Gongroneside A showed no cytotoxicity against KB cells at a concentration of 13.7 μM.

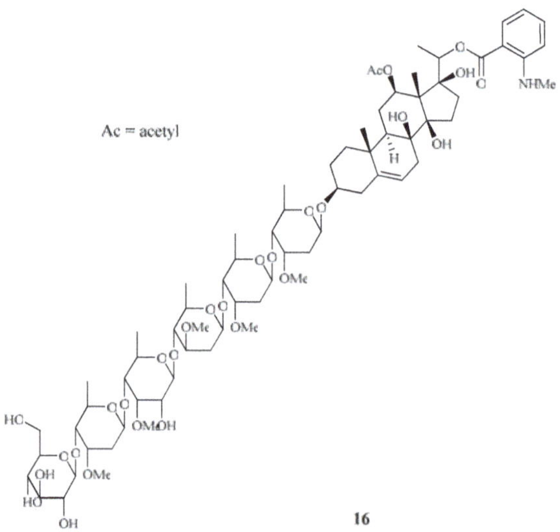

Figure 5. Compound from an Asclepiadaceae plant.

2.1.4. Asteraceae Family

Apigenin 7-*O*-glucoside (**17**) and luteolin 7-*O*-glucoside (**18**), two flavonoid glycosides obtained from the aerial parts of *Achillea millefolium*, showed antiplasmodial activities against D10 and W2 strains with IC_{50} values in the range of 15.3–62.5 μM [34] (Figure 6).

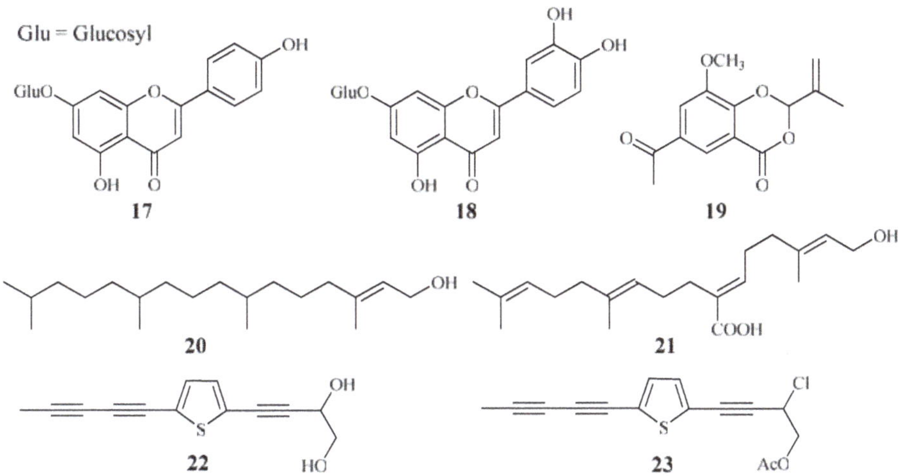

Figure 6. Compounds from Asteraceae plants.

2-Isopropenyl-6-acetyl-8-methoxy-1,3-benzodioxin-4-one (**19**), isolated from the whole plants of the Korean folk medicine *Carpesium divaricatum*, was reported to show antimalarial activity [35,93] (Figure 6). The compound exhibited activity against D10 with an IC_{50} value of 2.3 μM.

Microglossa pyrifolia, a medicinal plant used against malaria in Ghana, was tested against both PoW and Dd2 strains of *P. falciparum* by Köhler et al. [36]. Two diterpenes, *E*-phytol (**20**) (IC_{50}: 8.5 μM (PoW); 11.5 μM (Dd2)), and 6*E*-geranylgeraniol-19-oic acid (**21**) (IC_{50}: 12.9 μM (PoW); 15.6 μM (Dd2)) were shown to be the most active compounds in their test system (Figure 6).

A *Plasmodium berghei*-infected mouse model was used to evaluate the antimalarial activity of the 80% methanol extract of the roots of the traditionally used antimalarial plant *Echinops hoehnelii*. The methanol extract could suppress the parasite growth by 68.5% at a dose of 200mg/kg. No acute oral toxicity was observed in the animal study, indicating the safety use of the plant extract. Further phytochemical separation of the plant led to the isolation of two acetylenicthiophenes, 5-(penta-1,3-diynyl)-2-(3,4-dihydroxybut-1-ynyl)-thiophene (**22**) and 5-(penta-1,3-diynyl)-2-(3-chloro-4-acetoxy-but-1-yn)-thiophene (**23**), which displayed significant growth suppression of the *Plasmodium* parasite by 50.2% and 32.7% at 100 mg/kg, respectively [37] (Figure 6).

2.2. *Buxaceae Family*

Cai et al. identified several new antimalarial compounds from *Buxus sempervirens* [38], the native and introduced plant species in the United States. The traditionally used plants have received scant attention as potential source materials for drug discovery research as compared to the botanical materials from tropical and semitropical areas of the world. The eight lupane triterpenes (**24–31**), isolated from the *Buxus* plant (Figure 7), were evaluated for their activity against multi-drug-resistant malaria parasites (HB3, IC_{50} 0.5–3.0 μM) and counterscreened against HeLa cells (IC_{50} 7 μM for **24**; >20 μM for **25–31**). Strikingly, 23-*O*-(*trans*)-feruloyl-23-hydroxybetulin (**26**) displayed antimalarial activity at a concentration that was 75-fold more selective to the drug-resistant parasite strain than to HeLa cells.

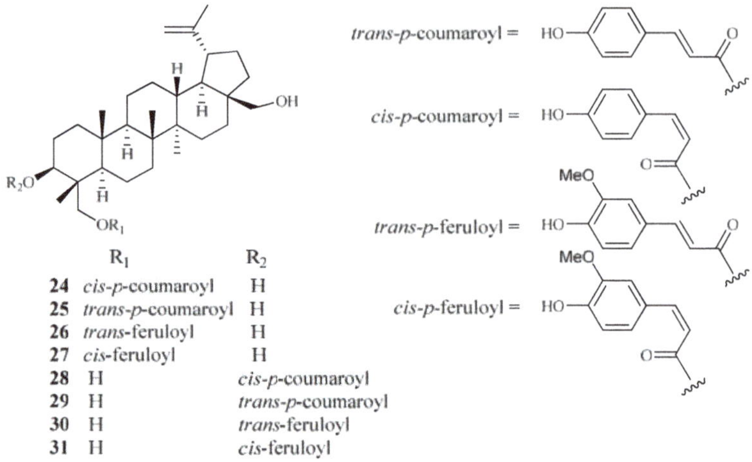

Figure 7. Compounds from a Buxaceae plant.

2.3. Cecropiaceae–Cucurbitaceae Families

2.3.1. Cecropiaceae Family

Cecropia pachystachya is a medicinal plant, which has been used in Brazil. The ethanol extracts of the different parts of the plants were evaluated for their activity against *P. falciparum* in vitro and *P. berghei* in vivo [39]. The parasitemia of malaria-infected mice was reduced by 35–66% with treatment of the ethanol extracts of the wood, root, and leaf materials in comparison with the non-treated control group. The plant root extracts were further analyzed and fractionated to provide subfractions, which were also active in an in vivo study. Two compounds, β-sitosterol (**32**) and tormentic acid (**33**), were identified from the subfractions (Figure 8). Both compounds showed plasmodial inhibitory activity. However, only tormentic acid (**33**) demonstrated inhibitory activity against *P. falciparum* chloroquine-resistant parasites (W2) (IC_{50} 19.0–25.2 μM).

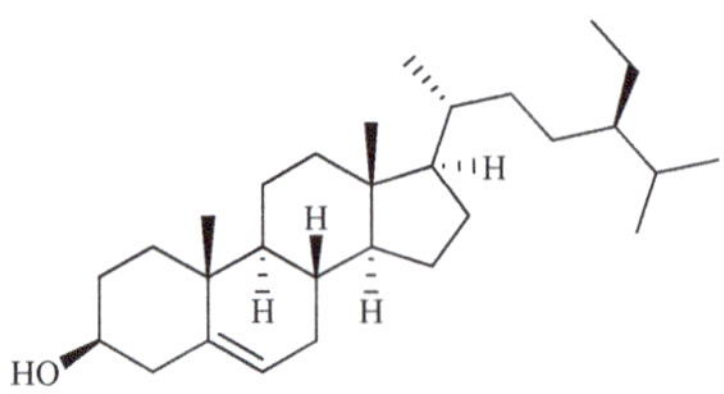

32

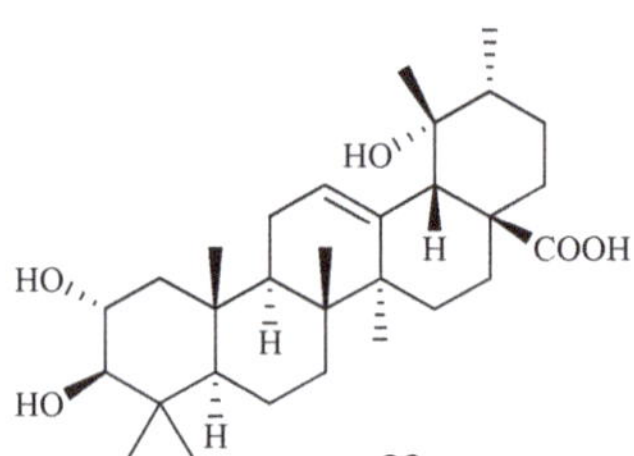

33

Figure 8. Compounds from a Cecropiaceae plant.

2.3.2. Chloranthaceae Family

Yue et al. [40] recently reported the isolation of 32 antimalarial lindenane-type sesquiterpenoids (**34–65**) from several plants in Chloranthaceae family with IC_{50} values lower than 11.4 μM against *P. falciparum* strain Dd2. The 12 new sesquiterpenoid dimers fortunilides A−L (**34–45**), along with 7 known isolates (**46–51** and **53**) were isolated from *C. fortune*. Compounds **52**, **54**, **58**, **59** and **60–64** were obtained from *C. serratus* and *C. spicatus*, and compounds **55–57** were separated from *Sarcandra glabra*. Compound **65** was originated from *C. multisachys*. Among these isolates, fortunilide A (**34**), sarglabolide J (**47**) and chlorajaponilide C (**52**) exhibited low nanomolar activities with IC_{50} values of 5.2, 7.2 and 1.1 nM, respectively, and their selectivity index values toward mammalian cells were greater than 500 (Figure 9).

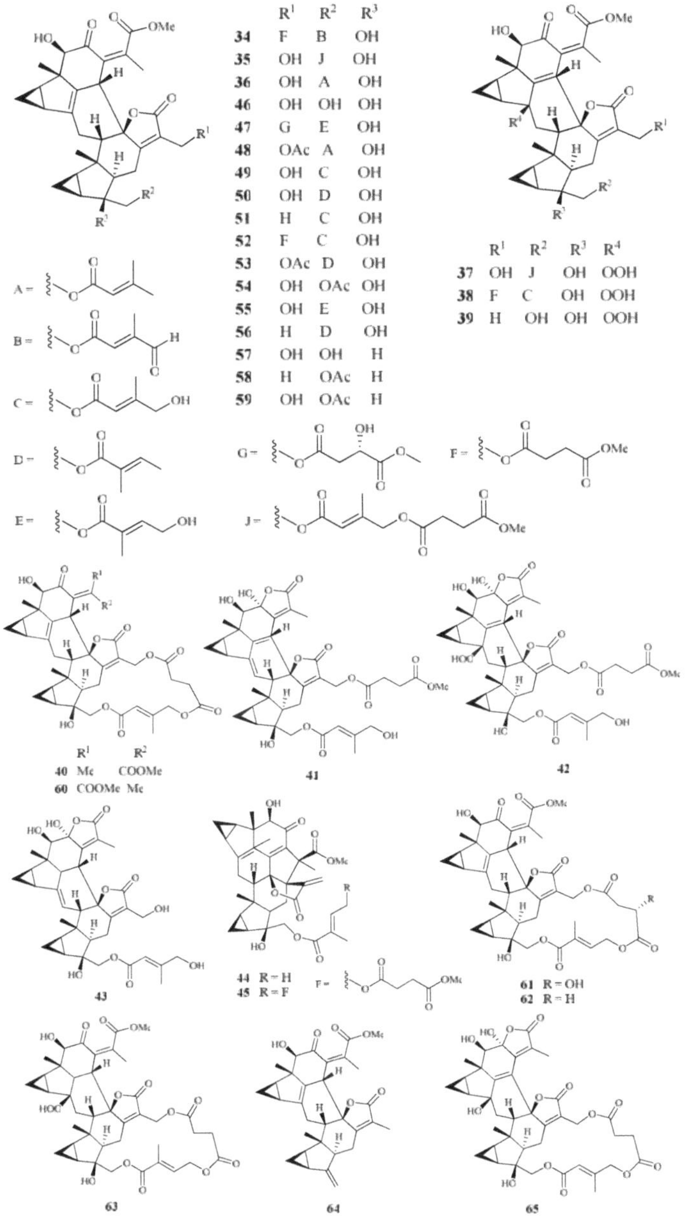

Figure 9. Compounds from Chloranthaceae plants.

2.3.3. Chrysobalanaceae Family

From the Petroleum ether/CH_2Cl_2 extracts of the stems of *Parinari capensis*, three kaurene diterpene lactones, 10, 13-dihydroxy-9-methyl-15-oxo-20-norkaur-16-en-18-oic acid γ-lactone (**66**), 10-hydroxy-13-methoxy-9-methyl-15-oxo-20-norkaur-16-en-18-oic acid γ-lactone (**67**) and 10-hydroxy-9-methyl-15-oxo-20-norkaur-16-en-18-oic acid γ-lactone (**68**) were isolated (Figure 10) [41]. They possess antimalarial activity against FCR-3 with IC_{50} values of 1.7, 1.9 and 5.0 μM, respectively.

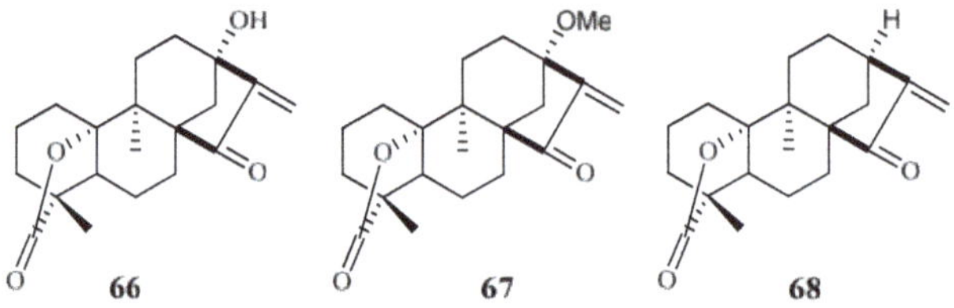

Figure 10. Compounds from a Chrysobalanaceae plant.

The three compounds (**66–68**) also displayed cytotoxicity against Graham cells with ED_{50} values in the range of 3.2–9.2 μM, which preclude them from further biological investigation. They could, however, be used effectively as lead compounds for drug optimization through synthesis.

2.3.4. Clusiaceae Family

Phytochemical separation of the concentrated acetone extract of the dried leaves and branches of *Garcinia mckeaniana* has led to the identification of three new xanthones, mckeanianones A-C (**69–71**), and two known ones, bannaxanthones I (**73**) and E (**73**) (Figure 11). These compounds all contain two isoprene units. They were evaluated for their activity against the TM4 and K1 strains of *P. falciparum* with IC_{50} values in the range of of 6.0–8.5 and 3.6–7.3 μM, respectively, and compounds **70**, **71** and **73** showed cytotoxicity against Vero cells with the IC_{50} values in the range of 12.6–29.5 μM [42].

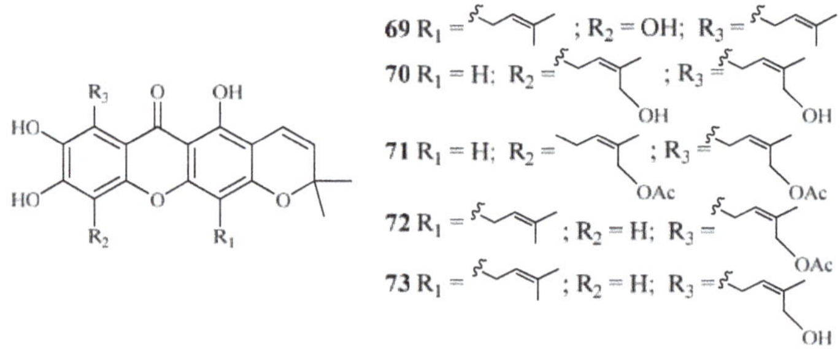

Figure 11. Compounds from a Clusiaceae plant.

2.3.5. Connaraceae Family

From the work of He et al. [26], bioassay-guided separation of the chloroform extract of the stems of *Rourea minor* (Gaertn.) Aubl. led to the identification of three active compounds including two new neolignan glycosides, rourinoside (**74**) and rouremin (**75**), and the known 1-(26-hydroxyhexacosanoyl)-glycerol (**76**) (Figure 12). The three compounds showed weak to moderate in vitro activities against the D6 and W2 clones of *P. falciparum*. Compound **74** demonstrated IC_{50} values at 3.7 (D6) and 2.1 (W2) μM; **75** at IC_{50} values of 5.1 (D6) and 4.5 (W2) μM, and **76** at IC_{50} values of 9.5 (D6) and 12.7 (W2) μM. These compounds exhibited no cytotoxicity against KB cells at 20 μg/mL.

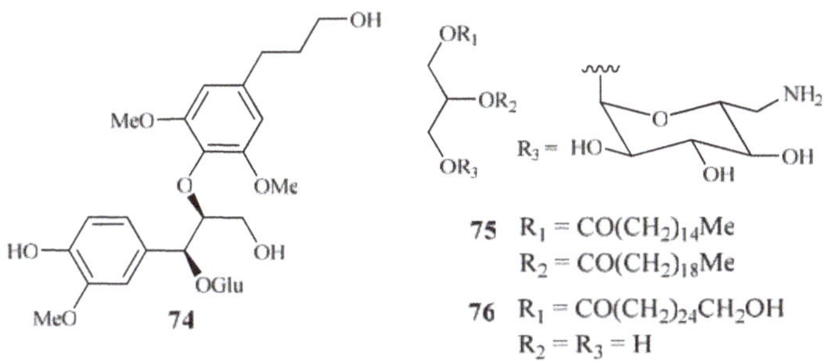

Figure 12. Compounds from a Connaraceae plant.

2.3.6. Cornaceae Family

In vitro IC_{50} values against the *P. falciparum* D10 strain were determined for ergosta-4,6,8,22-tetraene-3-one (**77**) (61.0 μM), 3-epideoxyflindissol (**78**) (128.0 μM), 3β-*O*-*cis*-coumaroyl betulinic acid (**79**) (10.4 μM) and 3β-*O*-*trans*-coumaroyl betulinic acid (**80**) (15.3 μM) (Figure 13), which were separated from the leaves of *Cornus florida* L. by Graziose et al. for the first time [43].

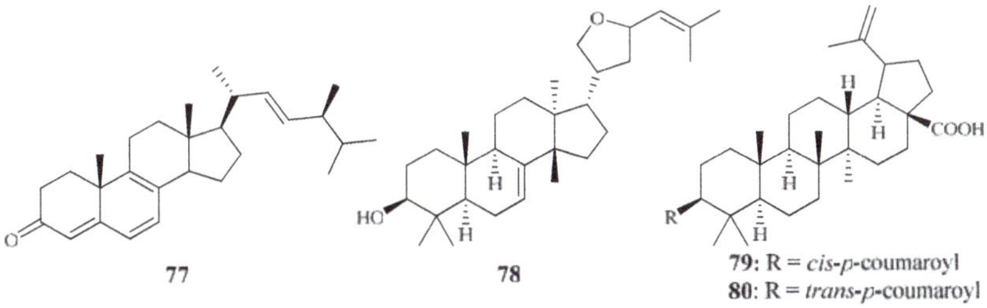

Figure 13. Compounds from a Cornaceae plant.

2.3.7. Cucurbitaceae Family

Cogniauxia podolaena Baill. is a folk medicine that has been traditionally used to treat malaria in Congo Brazzaville. Banzouzi et al. [44] identified cucurbitacins B (**81**) and D (**82**), and 20-epibryonolic acid (**83**), the three triterpenes from the stems of this plant (Figure 14). These compounds exhibited inhibitory activity against FcM29 strain with IC_{50} values of 2.9, 7.8 and 4.4 μM, respectively. Both cucurbitacins B and D showed a high cytotoxicity with approximately 95% inhibition against KB cells at 1 μg/mL, while 20-epibryonolic acid displayed a better selectivity index (20% inhibition of KB cells at 1 μg/mL).

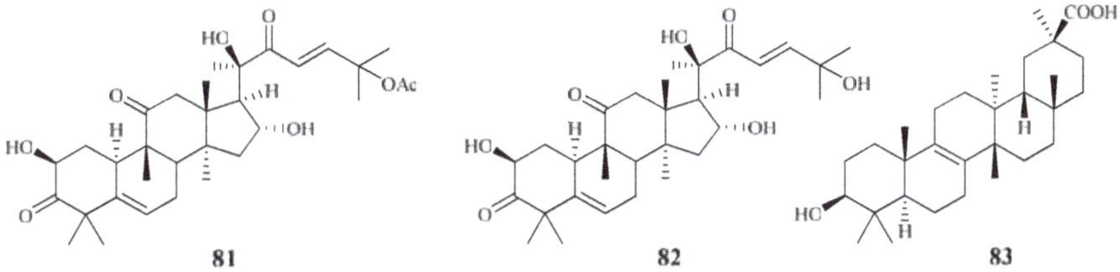

Figure 14. Compounds from a Cucurbitaceae plant.

2.4. Ebenaceae–Euphorbiaceae Families

2.4.1. Ebenaceae Family

Ma et al. [27] investigated the plant *Diospyros quaesita* Thw., known as "Muang Kout" in Laos. Of the isolates from the up parts of this plant, betulinic acid 3-caffeate (**84**) demonstrated antiplasmodial activity against the D6 and W2 clones with IC_{50} values of 1.40 and 0.98 μM, respectively (Figure 15). The compound was cytotoxic to KB cells with an ED_{50} value of 4.0 μM.

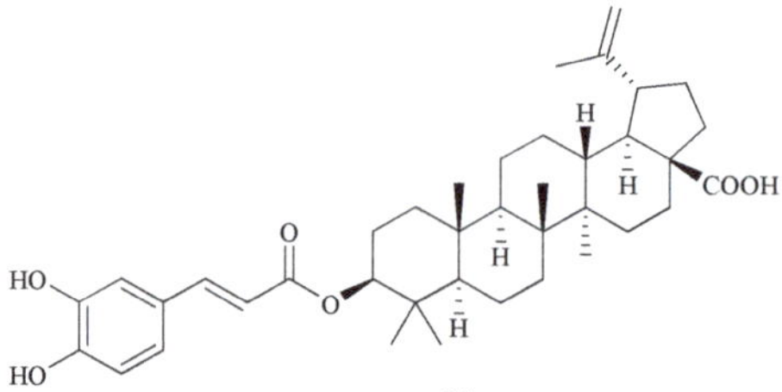

84

Figure 15. Compounds from an Ebenaceae plant.

2.4.2. Euphorbiaceae Family

Through the screening of a natural product-based synthetic compound library, Hadi et al. [45] discovered that jatrophones (the natural products from *Jatropha isabelli*) possess significant antiplasmodial activity. The jatrophone diterpene derivatives **85** and **86** displayed antiplasmodial activities against strains 3D7 and K1 of *P. falciparum* with IC_{50} values of 5.7/5.9 and 6.1/5.9 μM, respectively (Figure 16). The two compounds showed low cytotoxicities against the human HepG2, RAJI, BJ and HEK293 cells with EC_{50} values at around 26 μM.

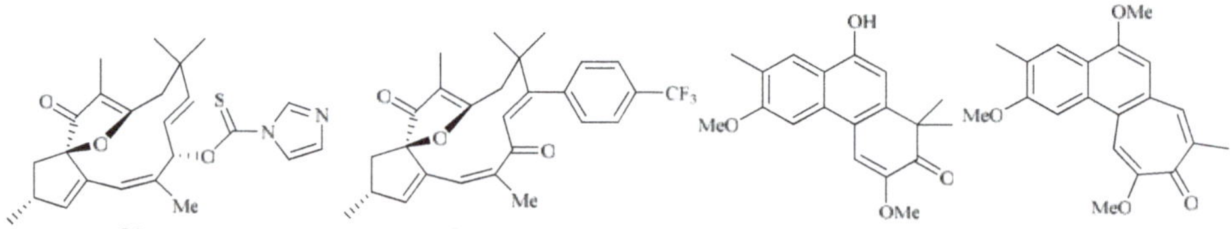

85 **86** **87** **88**

Figure 16. Compounds from Euphorbiaceae plants.

Seephonkai et al. [46] studied the Thai traditional medicinal plant *Strophioblachia fimbricalyx*, and isolated 9-*O*-demethyltrigonostemone (**87**) and a new phenanthropolone, 3,6,9-trimethoxyphenanthropolone (**88**), which exhibited antimalarial activity against the multiresistant K1 strain of *P. falciparum* with IC_{50} values of 8.7 and 9.9 μM, respectively (Figure 16).

2.5. Fabaceae–Fagaceae Families

2.5.1. Fabaceae Family

According to Nigerian ethnobotany, the plant *Cajanus cajan* L. (Fabaceae) can be used for treatment of malaria. From the methanol extract of the leaves of this plant, 2′,6′-dihydroxy-4-methoxy chalcone (**89**), a cajachalcone, was isolated through bioassay-guided fractionation, which used the parasite lactate dehydrogenase assay by targeting the K1 strain of *P. falciparum* (Figure 17). The cajachalcone showed an IC_{50} value of 7.4 μM [47].

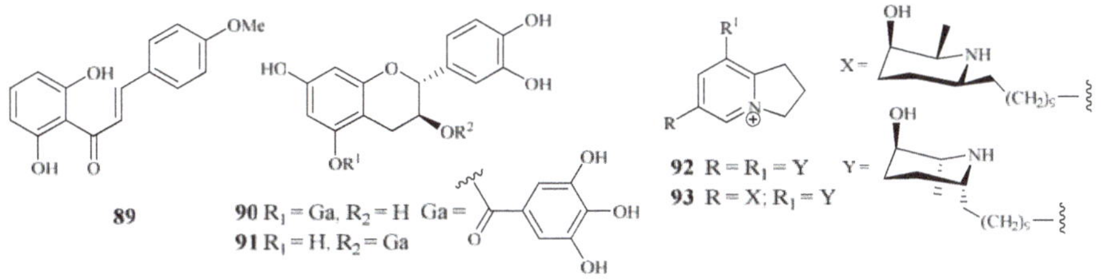

Figure 17. Compounds from Fabaceae plants.

From the work of Ramanandraibe et al. [48], *Piptadenia pervillei* Vatke was prioritized as an active plant lead identified through a screening program, which was dedicated to discovering antimalarial compounds from the plants in Madagascar. Separation of the EtOAc extract of the leaves of this plant led to the identification of the bioactive compounds (+)-catechin 5-gallate (**90**) and (+)-catechin 3-gallate (**91**). The two compounds showed antimalarial activity against FcB1 strain with IC_{50} values of 1.2 and 1.0 μM, respectively (Figure 17), and no significant cytotoxicity was observed at 75 μM for the two compounds against the human embryonic lung cells MRC-5.

According to the work of Samoylenko et al. [49], prosopilosidine (**92**) and isoprosopilosidine (**93**), isolated from the leaves of *Prosopis glandulosa* var. *glandulosa*, showed potent antimalarial activity against the D6 and W2 strains of *P. falciparum* with high selectivity index (SI) values (Figure 17). Compound **92** exhibited IC_{50} values of 0.1 (D6) and 0.3 (W2) μM, while **93** demonstrated IC_{50} values of 0.1 (D6) and 0.3 (W2) μM. Compounds **92** and **93** showed much lower cytotoxicity to KB cells with ED_{50} values of 20.2 and 18.8 μM, respectively.

2.5.2. Fagaceae Family

Subsequent bioassay-guided fractionation work by Cai et al. [38] yielded four kaempferol 3-*O*-glucosides (**94–97**) from *Quercus laceyi* (Figure 18). The IC_{50} values for these compounds against multi-drug-resistant malaria parasites HB3 are 0.6–2.1 μM, and the IC_{50} value against HeLa cells was <3 μM.

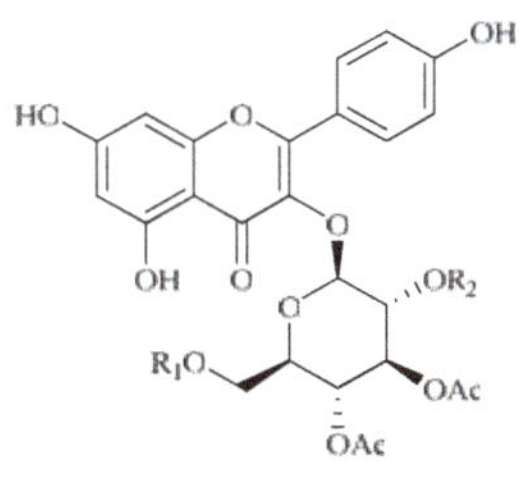

94 $R_1 = R_2 =$ *trans-p*-coumaroyl
95 $R_1 =$ *trans-p*-coumaroyl, $R_2 =$ *cis-p*-coumaroyl
96 $R_1 =$ *cis-p*-coumaroy, $R_2 =$ *trans-p*-coumaroyl
97 $R_1 = R_2 =$ *cis-p*-coumaroyl

Figure 18. Compounds from a Fagaceae plant.

2.6. Hypericaceae Family

Vismia orientalis, a traditional medicine used in Tanzania, was studied by Mbwambo et al. [50]. Vismione D (**98**), isolated from the stem barks of this plant, exhibited activity against the K1 strain with an IC_{50} value of 2.4 μM (Figure 18). However, the compound also showed cytotoxicity against human L6 cells with an IC_{50} value of 10.0 μM.

Pure isolates from the hexane extract of the stem barks of the African plant *Psorospermum glaberrimum* were evaluated for their antimalarial activity against the W2 clone of *P. falciparum* by Ndjakou Lenta et al. [51]. The isolates 3-geranyloxyemodin anthrone (**99**) and acetylvismione

D (**100**) displayed inhibition activity against the W2 strain with IC_{50} values of 1.7 and 0.1 μM, respectively (Figure 19).

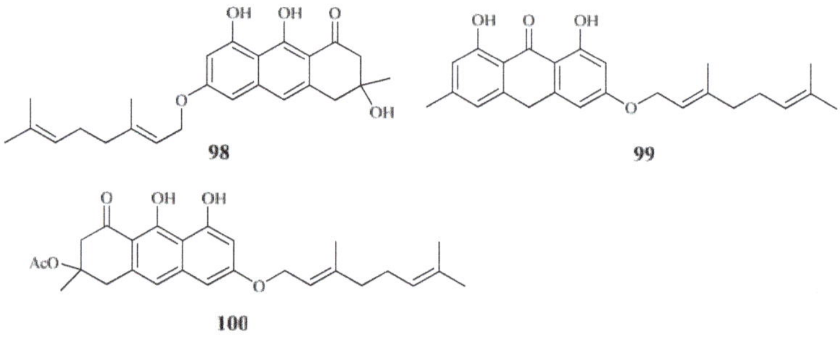

Figure 19. Compounds from Hypericaceae plants.

2.7. *Lamiaceae–Lythraceae Families*

2.7.1. Lamiaceae Family

An EtOH extract of the dried root barks of *Ocimum sanctum* exhibited considerable in vitro antimalarial activity. Bioactivity-directed separation of the EtOH extract resulted in the isolation of a new antimalarial natural compound (**101**) (Figure 20). The compound showed comparable activity to the positive controls, chloroquine and amodiaquine, against the *P. falciparum* 3D7 strains with an IC_{50} value of 0.1 μM [52].

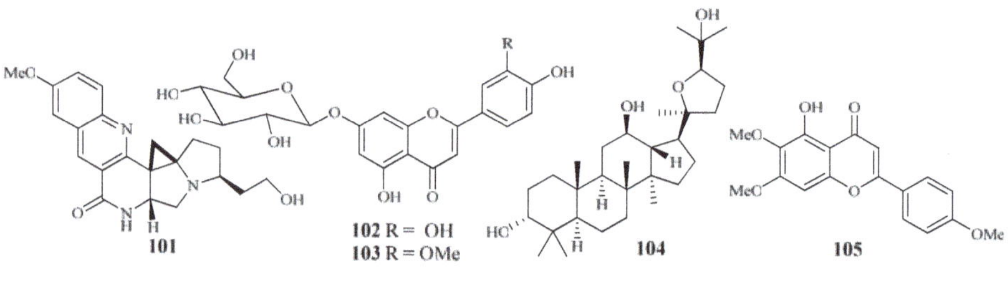

Figure 20. Compounds from Lamiaceae plants.

From the study of Kirmizibekmez et al. [53], luteolin 7-*O*-β-D-glucopyranoside (**102**) and chrysoeriol 7-*O*-β-D-glucopyranoside (**103**), two flavonoid glycosides isolated as the major antimalarial constituents from *Phlomis brunneogaleata* through an activity-directed separation (Figure 20), showed activity with IC_{50} values of 5.4 and 12.7 μM against the K1 clones, respectively.

The extracts of 17 *Salvia* species, which are used as folk medicines in South Africa, were subjected to biological testing by Kamatou et al. [54]. The potential activity of the *Salvia* plant extracts against the FCR strain of *P. falciparum* and their cytotoxic effects against MCF-7 cells were investigated. These extracts showed antiplasmodial activity with IC_{50} values in the range of 3.9–26.0 μg/mL. The extracts from *S. radula* demonstrated the most potent activities. Two compounds, betulafolientriol oxide (**104**) and salvigenin (**105**), were subsequently isolated (Figure 20), and they showed antimalarial activity with IC_{50} values of 10.4 and 75.0 μM, respectively.

2.7.2. Loganiaceae Family

A phytochemical study was carried out for the stem barks of *Strychnos icaja* for the first time by Tchinda et al. [55], which led to the isolation of the monomers 15-hydroxyvomicine (**106**) and

N-methyl-sec-iso-pseudostrychnine (**107**). The isolates were evaluated against the *P. falciparum* 3D7 strain with IC_{50} values of 101.0 and 110.6 μM, respectively (Figure 21).

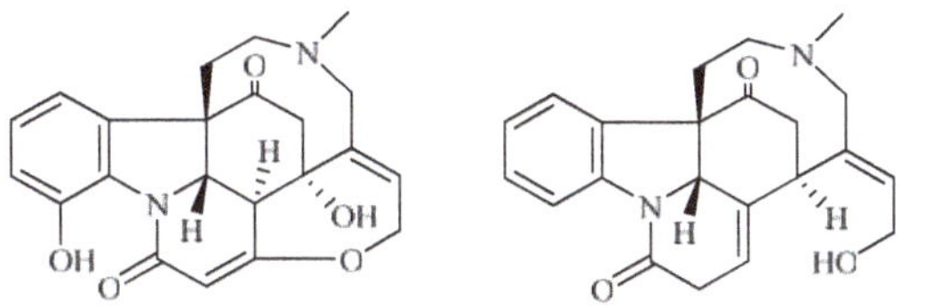

106 **107**

Figure 21. Compounds from a Loganiaceae plant.

2.7.3. Lythraceae Family

The plants in the genus of *Ammannia* are frequently used in China and India as folk medicines for treatment of various diseases. Upadhyay et al. [56] investigated the compounds in four species of this genus (*Ammannia*: *A. multiflora*, *A. verticillata*, *A. Baccifera* and *A. coccinea*) for their antimalarial activities. Among the isolated compounds, 4-hydroxy-α-tetralone (**108**) and tetralone-4-O-β-D-glucopyranoside (**109**) from *A. multiflora*, and ammaniol (**110**) from *A. baccifera* displayed antimalarial activities against the *P. falciparum* NF-54 strain with IC_{50} values of 194.0, 124.0 and 88.3 μM, respectively (Figure 22).

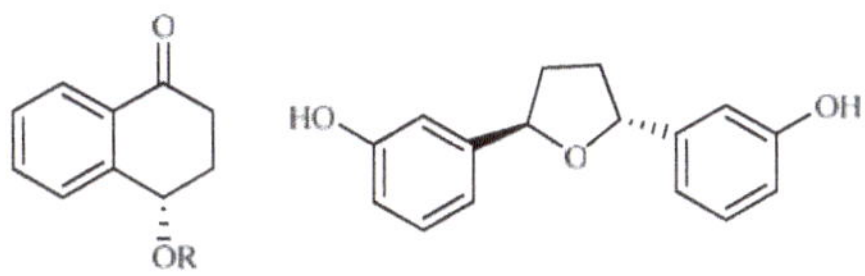

108 R = H
109 R = Glu

110

Figure 22. Compounds from Lythraceae plants.

2.8. Malvaceae–Myristicaceae Families

2.8.1. Malvaceae Family

LC-PDA-MS-SPE-NMR technique was used by Sprogøe et al. in combination with CD to detect (*R*)-(−)-gossypol [(*R*)-1] (**111**) in the twigs of *Thespesia danis* (Figure 23) [57]. (*R*)-1 demonstrated antimalarial activity with an IC_{50} value of 4.5 μM. However, its enantiomer was inactive up to a concentration of 20 μM.

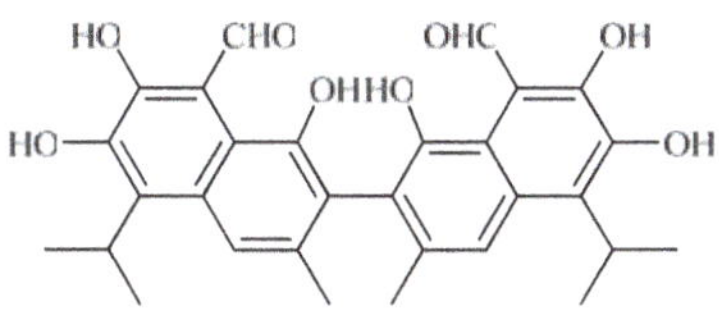

111

Figure 23. Compounds from a Malvaceae plant.

2.8.2. Monimiaceae Family

The compound 1-(4-hydroxybenzyl)-6,7-methylenedioxy-2-methylisoquinolinium trifluoroacetate (**112**), a new benzylisoquinoline alkaloid isolated by mass-guided separation of the CH_2Cl_2/MeOH extract of *Doryphora sassafras* (Figure 24) [58]. Compound **112** showed antiplasmodial activity against two different strains (3D7 and Dd2) of *P. falciparum* with IC_{50} values of 3.0 and 4.4 μM, respectively. The compound did not exhibit inhibitory activity against the human embryonic kidney cell line (HEK293) at a concentration of 120 μM.

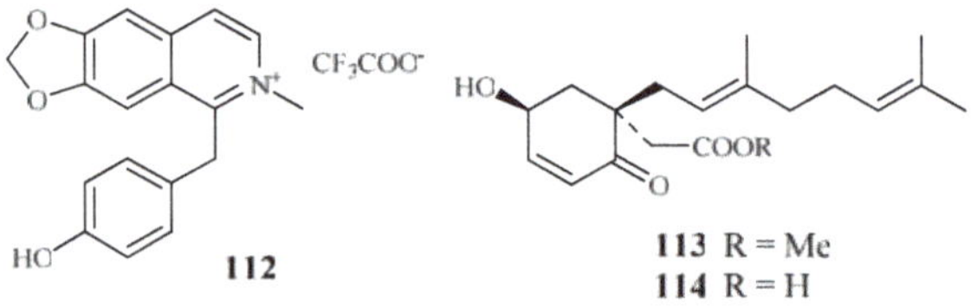

Figure 24. Compounds from Monimiaceae plants.

A phytochemical study of the leaves of *Glossocalyx brevipes* Benth. led to isolation of two new homogentisic acid derivatives of methyl 2-(1′β-geranyl-5′β-hydroxy-2′-oxocyclohex-3′-enyl) acetate (**113**) and 2-(1′β-geranyl-5′β-hydroxy-2′-oxocyclohex-3′-enyl) acetic acid (**114**), which displayed antiplasmodial activity against D6/W2 clones with IC_{50} values of 2.2/6.6 and 4.8/8.3 μM, respectively (Figure 24) [59].

2.8.3. Moraceae Family

According to the investigation of Zhang et al. [24], an antimalarial trichothecene compound, verrucarin L acetate (**4**), was identified from *Ficus fistulosa* (Figure 2). The antimalarial potency of **4** was equivalent to that of roridin E (**3**) isolated from *Rhaphidophora decursiva*, a plant from a different family. However, **4** was observed to be much less cytotoxic to KB cells (ED_{50} 0.2 μM) than **3**.

Bioassay-directed separation of the MeOH extract of the twigs of *Ficus septica* afforded three known phenanthroindolizine alkaloids, dehydrotylophorine (**115**), dehydroantofine (**116**) and tylophoridicine D (**117**) by Kubo et al. (Figure 25) [60]. They showed antiplasmodial activity against the *P. falciparum* 3D7 strain with IC_{50} values in the range of 0.03–0.4 μM. Compound **115** also displayed cytotoxicity against the mouse fibroblast cells L929 with an IC_{50} value of 8.2 μM, while the other two compounds showed no toxicity at a concentration of 50 μM.

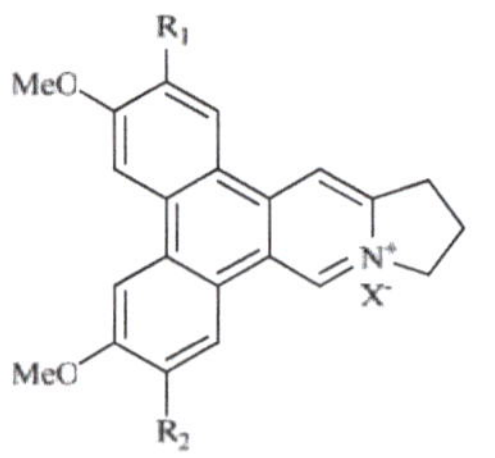

Figure 25. Compounds from a Moraceae plant.

2.8.4. Myristicaceae Family

Phytochemical investigation of the fruits of *Knema glauca* by Rangkaew et al. [61] led to the isolation of malabaricone A (**118**) as an active compound against the *P. falciparum* K1 strain with an IC_{50} value of 8.5 μM (Figure 26). The compound was cytotoxic towards KB cell with an ED_{50} value of >61 μM.

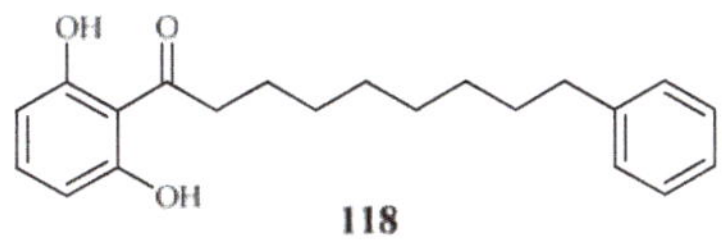

118

Figure 26. Compound from a Myristicaceae plant.

2.9. Piperaceae–Platanaceae Families

2.9.1. Piperaceae Family

The *Piperaceae* family consists of many plants that are used by the native populations in Thailand as traditional medicines for the treatment of various diseases. Sarmentine (**119**) and 1-piperettyl pyrrolidine (**120**) were isolated from the fruits of *Piper sarmentosum* by Rukachaisirikul et al. [62], and they exhibited antiplasmodial activity against the K1 strain with IC_{50} values of 85.5 and 21.9 μM, respectively (Figure 27).

From the whole plant of *Piper tricuspe*, dictyochromenol (**121**), 3-farnesyl-*p*-hydroxy benzoic acid (**122**) and 2′*E*,6′*E*-2-farnesyl hydroquinone (**123**) were isolated by Saez Vega et al. [63] (Figure 27). The compounds are active against several strains of *P. falciparum* with IC_{50} values ranging from 1.4 to 29.8 μM. Cytotoxic effects were also observed for the compounds with EC_{50} values in the range of 1.1–41.0 μM. The results suggest that the antimalarial activity of the compounds was most probably the direct result of their cytotoxicity.

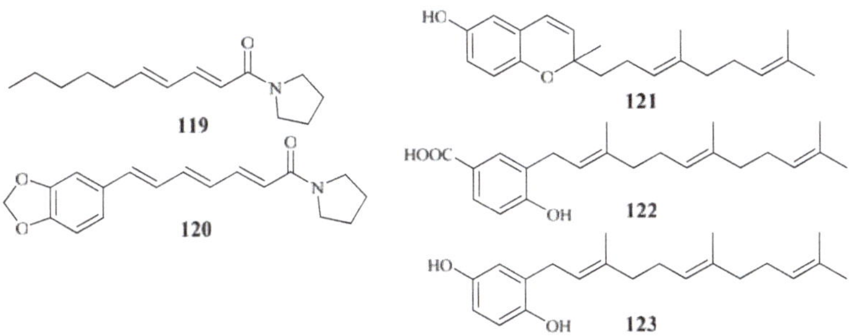

Figure 27. Compounds from Piperaceae plants.

2.9.2. Platanaceae Family

Bioactivity-guided fractionation of *Platanus occidentalis* by Cai et al. [38] yielded four kaempferol 3-*O*-rhamnosides (**124**–**127**) (Figure 28). The IC_{50} values for these compounds against multi-drug-resistant malaria parasites HB3 ranged from 0.5 to 1.8 μM. The IC_{50} values against HeLa cells were in the range of 9.3–20.0 μM.

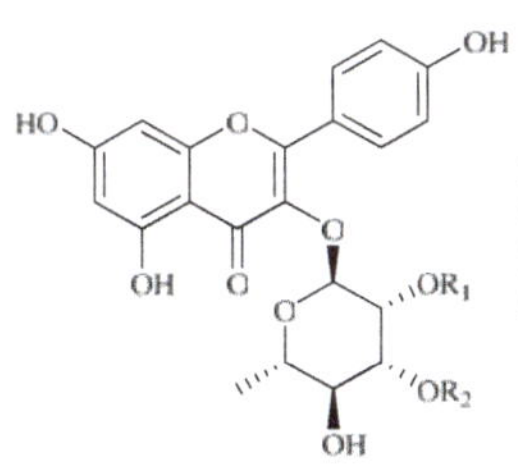

124 $R_1 = R_2$ = *trans-p*-coumaroyl
125 R_1 = *trans-p*-coumaroyl, R_2 = *cis-p*-coumaroyl
126 R_1 = *cis-p*-coumaroyl, R_2 = *trans-p*-coumaroyl
127 $R_1 = R_2$ = *cis-p*-coumaroyl

Figure 28. Compounds from a Platanaceae plant.

2.10. Rubiaceae-Rutaceae Families

2.10.1. Rubiaceae Family

Naucleaorine (**128**), epimethoxynaucleaorine (**129**), 3α,23-dihydroxyurs-12-en-28-oic acid (**130**) and oleanolic acid (**131**) were identified from the stems of *Nauclea orientalis* by He et al. [28] (Figure 29). The compounds showed antiplasmodial activities against the *P. falciparum* D6(*)/W2(**) strains with the IC_{50} values shown as below: compound **128** (IC_{50} 6.9*/6.0** μM); **129** (IC_{50} 12.4*/13.2** μM); **130** (IC_{50} 9.7*/12.7** μM) and **131** (IC_{50} 4.6*/5.1** μM). Compounds **128–131** displayed cytotoxicity against KB cells with ED_{50} values of 38.0, >37.9, >42.2 and 46.0 μM, respectively.

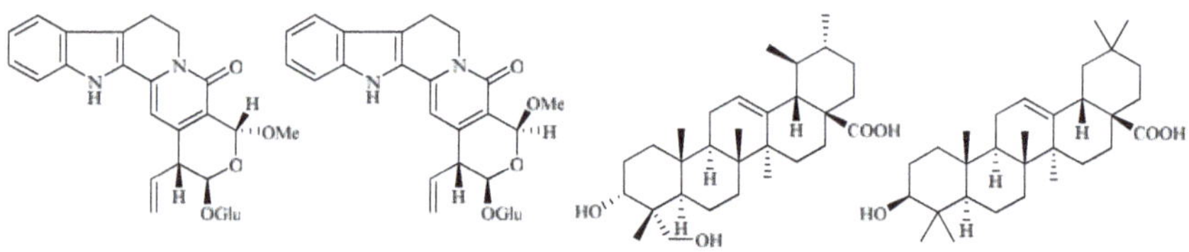

128 139 130 131

Figure 29. Compounds from a Rubiaceae plant.

2.10.2. Rutaceae Family

Based on an ethnomedicinal survey of the plants in Uganda, *Citropsis articulata* was selected for phytochemical study to investigate its antimalarial constituents [64]. From the ethyl acetate extract of the root barks of this plant, two known alkaloids, 5-hydroxynoracronycine (**132**) and 1,5-dihydroxy-2,3-dimethoxy-10-methyl-9-acridone (**133**), were identified as the best growth inhibitors of *P. falciparum* with IC_{50} values of 2.8 and 10.0 μM, respectively. The compounds were cytotoxic towards Vero cells at EC_{50} values of 28.8 and 101.0, respectively.

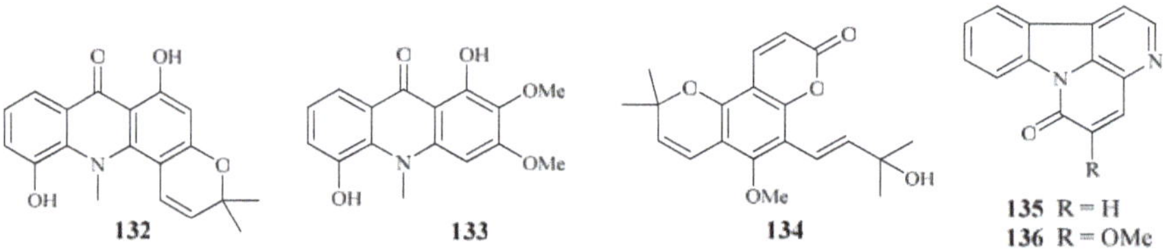

132 133 134 135 R = H 136 R = OMe

Figure 30. Compounds from Rutaceae plants.

The roots and stem barks of *Zanthoxylum chiloperone* have been used as a folk medicine for the treatment of malaria and for its emmenagogue and antirheumatic properties. The pyranocoumarin *trans*-avicennol (**134**) and two canthinone alkaloids, canthin-6-one (**135**) and 5-methoxycanthin-6-one (**136**), were identified from the stem barks of this plant by Cebrián-Torrejón et al. [65] (Figure 30). These compounds possessed antiplasmodial IC_{50} values against chloroquine/mefloquine resistant and sensitive strains of *P. falciparum* (F32, K1, PFB and FcB1 cells) in the range of 1.4–41.6 μM. Compounds **134** and **135** were cytotoxic towards MCR5 cells with EC_{50} values of 12.8 and 42.7 μM, respectively.

2.11. Simaroubaceae Family

Kuo et al. [66] found that among the isolates from the roots of *Eurycoma longifolia*, eurycomanone (**137**) and pasakbumin B (**138**) [67] displayed potent antimalarial activity against the *P. falciparum* W2/D6 strains with IC_{50} values of 0.04/0.06 and 0.05/0.08 μM, respectively (Figure 31). The compounds also exhibited strong cytotoxicity toward human breast cancer (MCF-7) and lung cancer (A549) cells at low concentrations.

De Andrade-Neto et al. [68] studied a number of Simaroubaceous plants, resulting in the isolation of the following compounds: the quassinoid neosergeolide (**139**) from the roots and stems of *Picrolemma spruce* (Figure 31); the indole alkaloids ellipticine (**140**) and aspidocarpine (**141**) from the barks of *Aspidosperma vargasii* and *A. desmanthum* (Apocynaceae), respectively; and 4-nerolidylcatechol (**142**) from the roots of *Pothomorphe peltata* (Piperaceae). Compounds **139–141** presented significant inhibitory activity against the multi-drug resistant K1 strain with IC_{50} values of 0.002, 0.07, 0.02 and 0.7 μM, respectively, and these compoundsdisplayed antimalarial potency greater than those of quinine and chloroquine.

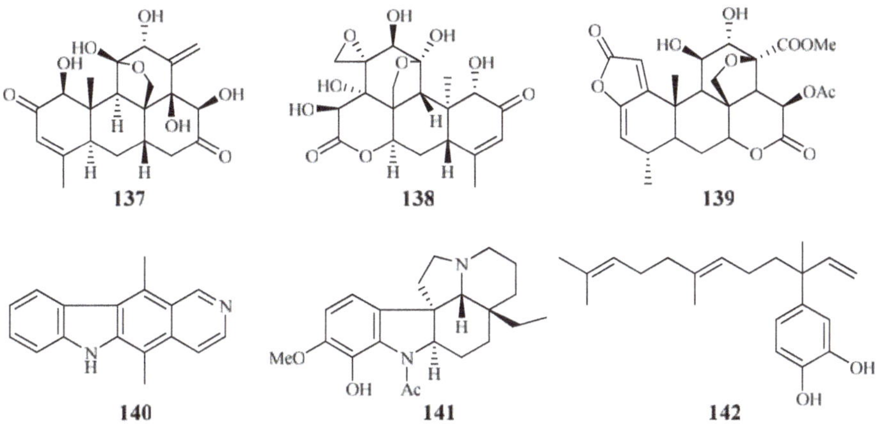
137 138 139 140 141 142

Figure 31. Compounds from Simaroubaceae plants.

2.12. Theaceae–Tiliaceae Families

2.12.1. Theaceae Family

Gallocatecin (**143**) is a flavonoid contained in the tea leaf extract of *Camellia sinensis* (Figure 32). Based on molecular docking studies, Tegar et al. [69] found that gallocatecin has stronger antimalarial potency than mefloquine (**144**), a synthetic drug with antimalarial activity.

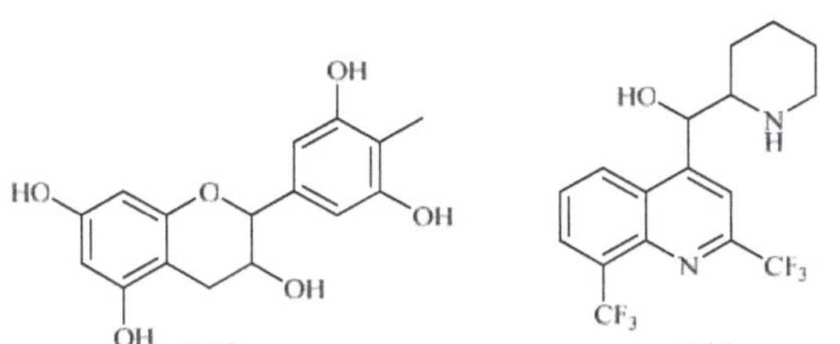
143 144

Figure 32. Compound from Theaceae plants.

2.12.2. Tiliaceae Family

According to the study of Ma et al. [29], five isolates from the leaves, stems and twigs of *Grewia bilamellata*, 3α,20-lupandiol (**145**), grewin (**146**), nitidanin (**147**), 2α,3β-dihydroxyolean-12-en-28-oic acid (**148**) and 2,6-dimethoxy-1-acetonylquinol (**149**), displayed antimalarial activity against the *P. falciparum* D6 and W2 clones with IC_{50} values in the range of 5.5–42.2 μM (Figure 33). These compounds showed no cytotoxicity towards KB carcinoma cell line at a concentration of 50 μM.

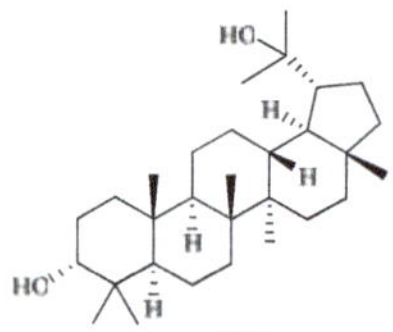
145

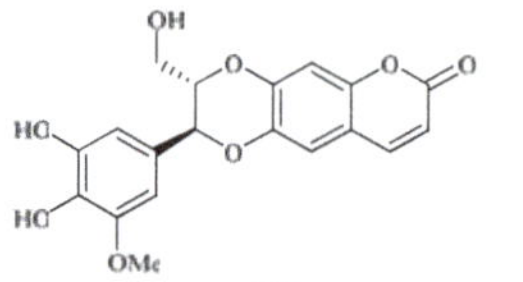
146

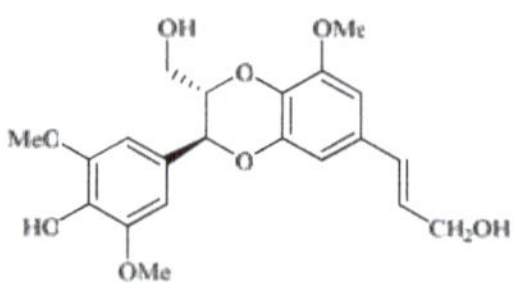
147

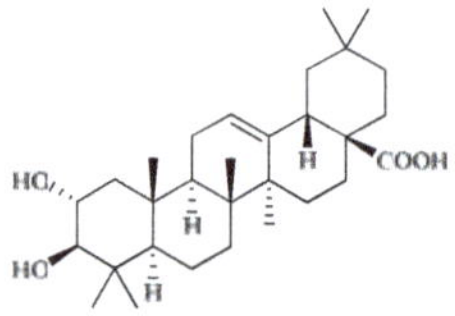
148

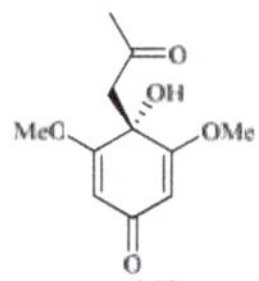
149

Figure 33. Compounds from a Tiliaceae plant.

2.13. *Verbenaceae Family*

Chromatographic separation of the ethyl acetate extract of the aerial parts of *Lippia javanica* yielded a new antimalarial α-pyrone, lippialactone (**150**) (Figure 34). This compound is active against the D10 strain with an IC_{50} value of 23.8 µM. Compound **119** is also mildly cytotoxic [70].

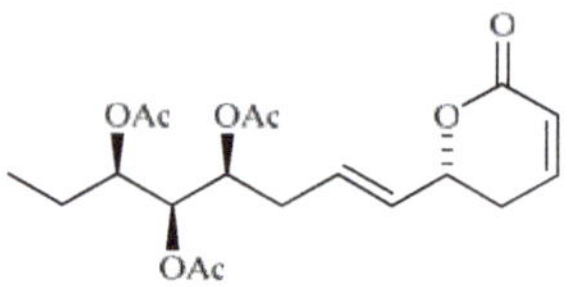
150

Figure 34. Compound from a Verbenaceae plant.

3. Marine Plant-Derived Antimalarial Compounds

Marine organisms offer unique opportunity to discover lead compounds for the treatments of malaria.

Separation of the extracts of Fijian red alga *Callophycus serratus* by Lane et al. led to the isolation of bromophycolides J-Q (**151–158**) [94] (Figure 35), the macrolide diterpene-benzoate derivatives represented as two novel carbon skeletons. These diterpenes, together with the previously reported ten bromophycolides, bromophycolides A-I (**159–167**) and debromophycolide A (**168**) from this alga (Figure 36) [95], were evaluated for their antimalarial activity against *P. falciparum*. The IC_{50} values of bromophycolides A, D, E, H and M (**159, 162, 163, 164** and **154**) were observed to be 0.9, 0.3, 0.8, 0.9 and 0.5 µM, respectively. Some of these compounds also exhibited strong cytotoxicity toward DU4475, a human breast cancer cell line. The ED_{50} values of bromophycolides N and Q (**155** and **158**) were 1.5 and 2.0 µM, respectively.

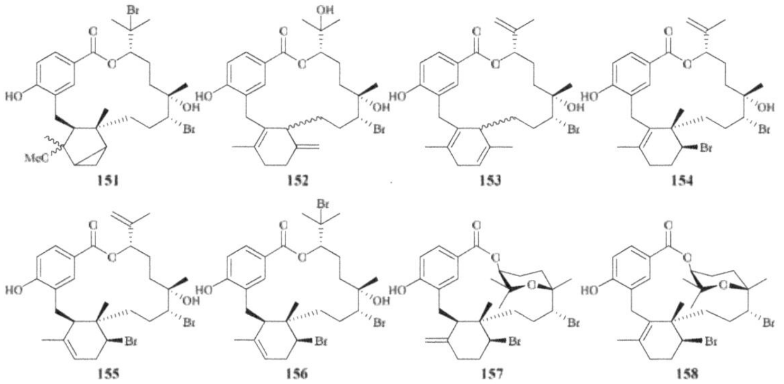

Figure 35. Compounds (**151–158**) from the red alga *Callophycus serratus*.

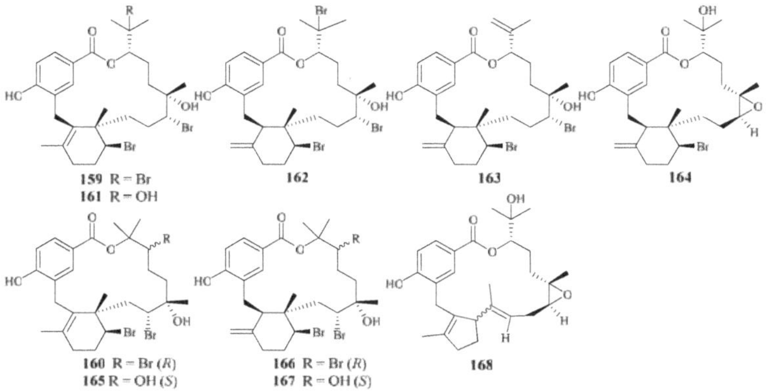

Figure 36. Compounds (**159–168**) from the red alga *Callophycus serratus*.

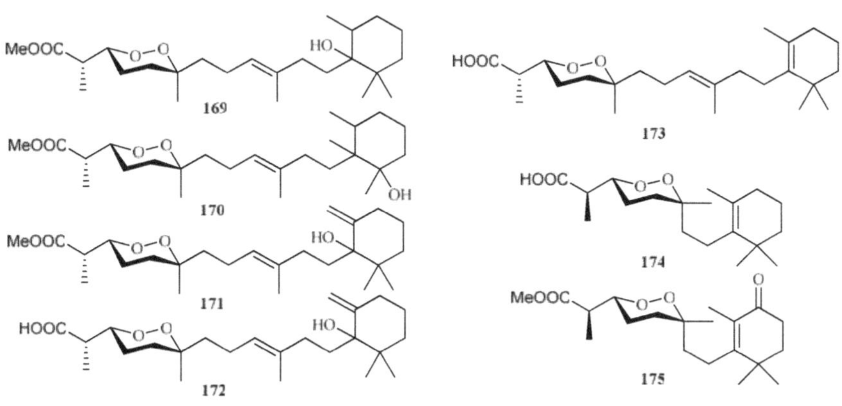

Figure 37. Compounds from the sponge *Diacarnus megaspinorhabdosa*.

From the sponge *Diacarnus megaspinorhabdosa* collected in Xisha Islands, four new norterpene cyclic peroxides, diacarnuperoxides M (**169**) and N (**170**), (+)-2, 3, 6-epihurghaperoxide (**171**) and (+)-2,3,6-epihurghaperoxide acid (**172**), together with the known norterpene cyclic peroxides,

(−)-muqubilin A (**173**), nuapapuin A (**174**) and diacarperoxide A (**175**) were isolated by Yang et al. [96] (Figure 37). They exhibited inhibitory activity against W2 clones of the malaria parasite *P. falciparum* with IC_{50} values of 4.2, 3.0, 1.6, 4.9, 5.6, 5.5 and 1.6 μM, respectively.

4. Ethnologic Antimalarial Compounds

At present, more than 80% of the world's population relies on ethnopharmacologic healing modalities and plants for their primary health care and wellness [97]. In Africa and many other developing countries, ethnomedicines are often regarded as their primary choice to treat diseases as they are obtained most affordable and accessible from locally available plants or other natural sources [78]. Plants are the major resource for the treatment of malaria infections in sub-Saharan Africa, where health care facilities are limited [98]. Ethnomedicinal plants have played a pivotal role in the treatment of malarial for centuries [71,99].

Early writing of over 6000 years ago in Egypt and China, and those of the Vedic civilisation dated 1600 B.C. in India, indicate that malaria has afflicted humans since antiquity, and there is ample evidence that antimalarial traditional medicaments have been used in virtually all cultures as the mainstay for the treatment of this disease. In the 5th century B.C., Hippocrates rejected superstition as a cause for the fevers that afflicted ancient Greeks. He instead recognized the seasonality of fevers and described the early clinical manifestations and complication of malaria [71].

The widely used antimalarial drug, artemisinin, was isolated from the traditional Chinese herb *Artemisia annua* L. (Qinghao) [11], which has been used in China as an ethnomedicine for close to 2000 years. The treatment of malaria with Qinghao was first recorded in "Zhouhou Bei Ji Fang", the handbook of prescriptions for emergencies in 243 A.D. [71,77].

The use of ethnomedicine such as herbs for the treatment of malaria varies by region, environment and population subgroups. It may be more preferred in some areas than in others. In order to explore the ethnologic basis of these antimalarial plants, several hundred species from 50 families are presently reviewed and listed in Table 3. These plants were collected from 13 countries and areas, exemplified by Madagascar, Nigeria, South Africa and India. The antimalarial activity and toxicity of these plants are also presented in the table [7,64,72–76,79–92,100].

5. Conclusions

It is imperative that the search for new antimalarial agents continues at an unabated pace in order to meet the challenges posed by the development of antimalarial drug resistance. During the last decade, numerous antimalarial compounds have been isolated from plants, and many of these compounds exhibit significant activity against *P. falciparum* in vitro. It is, therefore, evident that plant secondary metabolites continue to play an important role in pre-clinical antimalarial drug discovery.

We present in this comprehensive review, the structures of 175 plant-derived antiplasmodial compounds that have been published during the period of 2001–2017. The relevant plants are organized according to the geographical origins of their corresponding plant families.

Among the 175 plant-derived antiplasmodial compounds, several classes of compounds that showed nanomolar range of activity can be regarded as lead compounds to further explore their antimalarial potential. The trichothecene roridin E (**3**) from *Rhaphidophora decursiva* (Araceae family) showed potent inhibitory effects against the parasite growth with IC_{50} values in the sub-nano molar range (IC_{50}: 0.4 nM (D6), 1 nM (W2)) with high cytotoxicity against KB cells (ED_{50}: 0.4 nM). However, its closely related structural analog, verrucarin L acetate (**4**), identified from *Ficus fistulosa* (Moraceae family), displayed much lower cytotoxicity to KB cells (ED_{50} 200 nM) while retaining the same level of the antiplasmodial activity as **3**. Identified from the plant (*Ficus septica*) in the same genus as that of **4**, the phenanthroindolizine alkaloids dehydroantofine (**116**) and tylophoridicine D (**117**) demonstrated potent antiplasmodial activity against the *P. falciparum* 3D7 strain with IC_{50} values of 30 and 60 nM, respectively, and the compounds showed no toxicity at a concentration of 50 μM. A recent study found that the lindenane-type sesquiterpenoids fortunilide A (**34**), sarglabolide J (**47**) and chlorajaponilide C

(**52**) from the plant in Chloranthaceae family displayed potent antiplasmodial activity against Dd2 strain of with IC_{50} values of 5.2, 7.2 and 1.1 nM, respectively, and these compounds also showed low cytotoxicity to the mammalian cells WI-38 with IC_{50} values of 8.8, 4.0 and 5.4 μM, respectivley. More prominently, fortunilide E (**38**) containing a peroxide group showed antiplasmodial activity of 43 nM with no cytotoxicity at 100 μM.

This review also describes 25 antimalarial compounds that were reported from marine plants during the time period covered. In addition, we included ethnologic information on antimalarial plants from 50 families that are used as folk medicines for the treatment of malaria. Taken together, all the information presented attests to the fact that the phytochemical investigation of terrestrial plants coupled with the biological validation of ethnomedicines constitute proven strategies for the discovery of potential lead compounds for antimalarial drug development.

Author Contributions: All authors contributed to surveying the literature, preparation and editing of the manuscript.

Acknowledgments: This work was supported by the Research Grants Council of the Hong Kong Special Administrative Region, China (Project No. HKBU 12103014) and the Hong Kong Baptist University (HKBU) Interdisciplinary Research Matching Scheme (RC-IRMS/15-16/02).

Conflicts of Interest: The authors declare no conflict of interest.

References

1. World Health Organization. *World Malaria Report 2017*; WHO Press: Geneva, Switzerland, 2017.
2. Mueller, I.; Zimmerman, P.A.; Reeder, J.C. *Plasmodium malariae* and *Plasmodium ovale*—The "bashful" malaria parasites. *Trends Parasitol.* **2007**, *23*, 278–283. [CrossRef] [PubMed]
3. Collins, W.E. *Plasmodium knowlesi*: A malaria parasite of monkeys and humans. *Annu. Rev. Entomol.* **2012**, *57*, 107–121. [CrossRef] [PubMed]
4. Kajfasz, P. Malaria prevention. *Int. Marit. Health* **2009**, *60*, 67–70. [PubMed]
5. Beare, N.A.; Taylor, T.E.; Harding, S.P.; Lewallen, S.; Molyneux, M.E. Malarial retinopathy: A newly established diagnostic sign in severe malaria. *Am. J. Trop. Med. Hyg.* **2006**, *75*, 790–797. [PubMed]
6. Mehlhorn, H. *Encyclopedia of Parasitology*, 3rd ed.; Springer: New York, NY, USA, 2008.
7. Dolabela, M.F.; Oliveira, S.G.; Peres, J.M.; Nascimento, J.M.; Póvoa, M.M.; Oliveira, A.B. In vitro antimalarial activity of six Aspidosperma species from the state of Minas Gerais (Brazil). *An. Acad. Bras. Ciênc.* **2012**, *84*, 899–910. [CrossRef] [PubMed]
8. Boulos, M.; Dutra, A.P.; DiSanti, S.M.; Shiroma, M.; Amato, N.V. The clinical evaluation of quinine for the treatment of *Plasmodium falciparum* malaria. *Rev. Soc. Bras. Med. Trop.* **1997**, *30*, 211–213. [CrossRef] [PubMed]
9. Guerin, P.J.; Olliaro, P.; Nosten, F.; Druilhe, P.; Laxminarayan, R.; Binka, F.; Kilama, W.L.; Ford, N.; White, N.J. Malaria: Current status of control, diagnosis, treatment, and a proposed agenda for research and development. *Lancet Infect. Dis.* **2002**, *2*, 564–573. [CrossRef]
10. Fidock, D.A.; Rosenthal, P.J.; Croft, L.; Brun, R.; Nwaka, S. Antimalarial drug discovery: Efficacy models for compound screening. *Nat. Rev. Drug. Discov.* **2004**, *3*, 509–520. [CrossRef] [PubMed]
11. Tu, Y. The discovery of artemisinin (qinghaosu) and gifts from Chinese medicine. *Nat. Med.* **2011**, *17*, 1217–1220. [CrossRef] [PubMed]
12. Klayman, D. Qinghaosu (artemisinin): An antimalarial drug from China. *Science* **1985**, *228*, 1049. [CrossRef] [PubMed]
13. Sriram, D.; Rao, V.S.; Chandrasekhara, K.V.; Yogeeswari, P. Progress in the research of artemisinin and its analogues as antimalarials: An update. *Nat. Prod. Res.* **2004**, *18*, 503–527. [CrossRef] [PubMed]
14. Zhang, Y.K.; Ge, M.; Plattner, J.J. Recent Progress in the synthesis of antimalarial agents. *Org. Prep. Proced. Int.* **2012**, *44*, 340–374. [CrossRef]
15. Kappe, S.H.; Vaughan, A.M.; Boddey, J.A.; Cowman, A.F. That was then but this is now: Malaria research in the time of an eradication agenda. *Science* **2010**, *328*, 862–866. [CrossRef] [PubMed]
16. Ginsburg, H.; Atamna, H. The redox status of malaria-infected erythrocytes: An overview with an emphasis on unresolved problems. *Parasite* **1994**, *1*, 5–13. [CrossRef] [PubMed]

17. Zani, B.; Gathu, M.; Donegan, S.; Olliaro, P.L.; Sinclair, D. Dihydroartemisinin-piperaquine for treating uncomplicated *Plasmodium falciparum* malaria. *Cochrane Database Syst. Rev.* **2014**, *1*, 1–160. [CrossRef] [PubMed]
18. Lisewski, A.M.; Quiros, J.P.; Ng, C.L.; Adikesavan, A.K.; Miura, K.; Putluri, N.; Eastman, R.T.; Scanfeld, D.; Regenbogen, S.J.; Altenhofen, L.; et al. Supergenomic network compression and the discovery of EXP1 as a glutathione transferase inhibited by artesunate. *Cell* **2014**, *158*, 916–928. [CrossRef] [PubMed]
19. Schlitzer, M. Antimalarial drugs—What is in use and what is in the pipeline. *Arch. Pharm. Chem. Life Sci.* **2008**, *341*, 149–163. [CrossRef] [PubMed]
20. Newman, D.J.; Cragg, G.M. Natural products as sources of new drugs from 1981 to 2014. *J. Nat. Prod.* **2016**, *79*, 629–661. [CrossRef] [PubMed]
21. Zhang, H.J.; Li, W.F.; Fong, H.H.S.; Soejarto, D.D. Discovery of bioactive compounds by UIC-ICBG drug discovery program in the 18 years since 1998. *Molecules* **2016**, *21*, 1448. [CrossRef] [PubMed]
22. Zhang, H.J.; Tamez, P.A.; Vu, D.H.; Ghee, T.T.; Nguyen, V.H.; Le, T.X.; Le, M.H.; Nguyen, M.C.; Do, T.T.; Soejarto, D.D.; et al. Antimalarial compounds from *Rhaphidophora decursiva*. *J. Nat. Prod.* **2001**, *64*, 772–777. [CrossRef] [PubMed]
23. Zhang, H.J.; Qiu, S.; Tamez, P.; Tan, G.T.; Aydogmus, Z.; Nguyen, V.H.; Nguyen, M.C.; Angerhofer, C.; Soejarto, D.D.; Pezzuto, J.M.; et al. Antimalarial agents from plants II. Decursivine, a new antimalarial indole alkaloid from *Rhaphidophora decursiva*. *Pharm. Biol.* **2002**, *40*, 221–224. [CrossRef]
24. Zhang, H.J.; Tamez, P.A.; Aydoqmus, Z.; Tan, G.T.; Saikawa, Y.; Hashimoto, K.; Nakata, M.; Hung, N.V.; Xuan, L.T.; Cuong, N.M.; et al. Antimalarial agents from plants. III. Trichothecenes from *Ficus fistulosa* and *Rhaphidophora decursiva*. *Planta Med.* **2002**, *68*, 1088–1091. [CrossRef] [PubMed]
25. Libman, A.; Zhang, H.; Ma, C.; Southavong, B.; Sydara, K.; Bouamanivong, S.; Tan, G.T.; Fong, H.H.; Soejarto, D.D. A first new antimalarial pregnane glycoside from *Gongronema napalense*. *Asian J. Tradit. Med.* **2008**, *3*, 203–210. [PubMed]
26. He, Z.D.; Ma, C.Y.; Tan, G.T.; Sydara, K.; Tamez, P.; Southavong, B.; Bouamanivong, S.; Soejarto, D.D.; Pezzuto, J.M.; Fong, H.H.; et al. Rourinoside and rouremin, antimalarial constituents from *Rourea minor*. *Phytochemistry* **2006**, *67*, 1378–1384. [CrossRef] [PubMed]
27. Ma, C.Y.; Musoke, S.F.; Tan, G.T.; Sydara, K.; Bouamanivong, S.; Southavong, B.; Soejarto, D.D.; Fong, H.H.; Zhang, H.J. Study of antimalarial activity of chemical constituents from *Diospyros quaesita*. *Chem. Biodivers.* **2008**, *5*, 2442–2448. [CrossRef] [PubMed]
28. He, Z.D.; Ma, C.Y.; Zhang, H.J.; Tan, G.T.; Tamez, P.; Sydara, K.; Bouamanivong, S.; Southavong, B.; Soejarto, D.D.; Pezzuto, J.M.; et al. Antimalarial constituents from *Nauclea orientalis* (L.) L. *Chem. Biodivers.* **2005**, *2*, 1378–1386. [CrossRef] [PubMed]
29. Ma, C.; Zhang, H.J.; Tan, G.T.; Hung, N.V.; Cuong, N.M.; Soejarto, D.D.; Fong, H.H. Antimalarial compounds from *Grewia bilamellata*. *J. Nat. Prod.* **2006**, *69*, 346–350. [CrossRef] [PubMed]
30. Schwikkard, S.; van Heerden, F.R. Antimalarial activity of plant metabolites. *Nat. Prod. Rep.* **2002**, *19*, 675–692. [CrossRef] [PubMed]
31. Prawat, U.; Phupornprasert, D.; Butsuri, A.; Salae, A.W.; Boonsri, S.; Tuntiwachwuttikul, P. Flavonoids from *Friesodielsia discolor*. *Phytochem. Lett.* **2012**, *5*, 809–813. [CrossRef]
32. Mueller, D.; Davis, R.A.; Duffy, S.; Avery, V.M.; Camp, D.; Quinn, R.J. Antimalarial activity of azafluorenone alkaloids from the Australian tree *Mitrephora diversifolia*. *J. Nat. Prod.* **2009**, *72*, 1538–1540. [CrossRef] [PubMed]
33. Promchai, T.; Jaidee, A.; Cheenpracha, S.; Trisuwan, K.; Rattanajak, R.; Kamchonwongpaisan, S.; Laphookhieo, S.; Pyne, S.G.; Ritthiwigrom, T. Antimalarial Oxoprotoberberine Alkaloids from the Leaves of *Miliusa cuneata*. *J. Nat. Prod.* **2016**, *79*, 978–983. [CrossRef] [PubMed]
34. Vitalini, S.; Beretta, G.; Iriti, M.; Orsenigo, S.; Basilico, N.; Dall'Acqua, S.; Iorizzi, M.; Fico, G. Phenolic compounds from *Achillea millefolium* L. and their bioactivity. *Acta Biochim. Pol.* **2011**, *58*, 203–209. [PubMed]
35. Chung, I.M.; Seo, S.H.; Kang, E.Y.; Park, W.H.; Park, S.D.; Moon, H.I. Antiplasmodial activity of isolated compounds from *Carpesium divaricatum*. *Phytother. Res.* **2010**, *24*, 451–453. [CrossRef] [PubMed]
36. Köhlera, I.; Jenett-Siems, K.; Kraft, C.; Siems, K.; Abbiw, D.; Bienzle, U.; Eich, E. Herbal remedies traditionally used against malaria in Ghana: Bioassay-guided fractionation of *Microglossa pyrifolia* (Asteraceae). *Z. Naturforsch. C* **2002**, *57*, 1022–1027. [CrossRef]

37. Bitew, H.; Mammo, W.; Hymete, A.; Yeshak, M.Y. Antimalatial activity of acetylenic thiophenes from *Echinops hoehnelii* Schweinf. *Molecules* **2017**, *22*, 1965. [CrossRef] [PubMed]
38. Cai, S.; Risinger, A.L.; Nair, S.; Peng, J.; Anderson, T.J.; Du, L.; Powell, D.R.; Mooberry, S.L.; Chichewicz, R.H. Identification of compounds with efficacy against malaria parasites from common North American plants. *J. Nat. Prod.* **2015**, *79*, 490–498. [CrossRef] [PubMed]
39. Uchôa, V.T.; de Paula, R.C.; Krettli, L.G.; Santan, A.E.G.; Krettli, A.U. Antimalarial activity of compounds and mixed fractions of *Cecropia pachystachya*. *Drug Dev. Res.* **2010**, *71*, 82–91. [CrossRef]
40. Zhou, B.; Wu, Y.; Dalal, S.; Merino, E.F.; Liu, Q.F.; Xu, C.H.; Tao, Y.; Ding, J.; Kingston, D.G.I.; Cassera, M.B.; et al. Nanomolar antimalarial agents against chloroquine-resistant *Plasmodium falciparum* from medicinal plants and their structure-activity relationships. *J. Nat. Prod.* **2017**, *80*, 96–107. [CrossRef] [PubMed]
41. Uys, A.C.; Malan, S.F.; van Dyk, S.; van Zyl, R.L. Antimalarial compounds from *Parinari capensis*. *Bioorg. Med. Chem. Lett.* **2002**, *12*, 2167–2169. [CrossRef]
42. Auranwiwat, C.; Laphookhieo, S.; Rattanajak, R.; Kamchonwongpaisan, S.; Pyne, S.G.; Ritthiwigrom, T. Antimalarial polyoxygenated and prenylated xanthones from the leaves and branches of *Garcinia mckeaniana*. *Tetrahedron* **2016**, *72*, 6837–6842. [CrossRef]
43. Graziose, R.; Rojas-Silva, P.; Rathinasabapathy, T.; Dekoc, C.; Grace, M.H.; Poulev, A.; Ann, L.M.; Smith, P.; Raskin, I. Antiparasitic compounds from *Cornus florida* L. with activities against *Plasmodium falciparum* and *Leishmania tarentolae*. *J. Ethnopharmacol.* **2012**, *142*, 456–461. [CrossRef] [PubMed]
44. Banzouzi, J.T.; Soh, P.N.; Mbatchi, B.; Cavé, A.; Ramos, S.; Retailleau, P.; Rakotonandrasana, O.; Berry, A.; Benoit-Vical, F. *Cogniauxia podolaena*: Bioassay-guided fractionation of defoliated stems, isolation of active compounds, antiplasmodial activity and cytotoxicity. *Planta Med.* **2008**, *74*, 1453–1456. [CrossRef] [PubMed]
45. Hadi, V.; Hotard, M.; Ling, T.; Salinas, Y.G.; Palacios, G.; Connelly, M.; Rivas, F. Evaluation of *Jatropha isabelli* natural products and their synthetic analogs as potential antimalarial therapeutic agents. *Eur. J. Med. Chem.* **2013**, *65*, 376–380. [CrossRef] [PubMed]
46. Seephonkai, P.; Sangdee, A.; Bunchalee, P.; Pyne, S.G. Cytotoxic and antiplasmodial compounds from the roots of *Strophioblachia fimbricalyx*. *J. Nat. Prod.* **2009**, *72*, 1892–1894. [CrossRef] [PubMed]
47. Ajaiyeoba, E.O.; Ogbole, O.O.; Abiodun, O.O.; Ashidi, J.S.; Houghton, P.J.; Wright, C.W. Cajachalcone: An Antimalarial Compound from *Cajanus cajan* Leaf Extract. *J. Parasitol. Res.* **2013**, *2013*, 703781. [CrossRef] [PubMed]
48. Ramanandraibe, V.; Grellier, P.; Martin, M.T.; Deville, A.; Joyeau, R.; Ramanitrahasimbola, D.; Mouray, E.; Rasoanaivo, P.; Mambu, L. Antiplasmodial phenolic compounds from *Piptadenia pervillei*. *Planta Med.* **2008**, *74*, 417–421. [CrossRef] [PubMed]
49. Samoylenko, V.; Ashfaq, M.K.; Jacob, M.R.; Tekwani, B.L.; Khan, S.I.; Manly, S.P.; Joshi, V.C.; Walker, L.A.; Muhammad, I. Indolizidine, antiinfective and antiparasitic compounds from *Prosopis glandulosa* var. Glandulosa. *J. Nat. Prod.* **2009**, *72*, 92–98. [CrossRef] [PubMed]
50. Mbwambo, Z.H.; Apera, S.; Moshi, M.J.; Kapingu, M.C.; Van Miert, S.; Claeys, M.; Brun, R.; Cos, P.; Pieters, L.; Vlietinck, A. Anthranoid compounds with antiprotozoal activity from *Vismia orientalis*. *Planta Med.* **2004**, *70*, 706–710. [CrossRef] [PubMed]
51. Ndjakou Lenta, B.; Devkota, K.P.; Ngouela, S.; Fekam Boyom, F.; Naz, Q.; Choudhary, M.I.; Tsamo, E.; Rosenthal, P.J.; Sewald, N. Anti-plasmodial and cholinesterase inhibiting activities of some constituents of *Psorospermum glaberrimum*. *Chem. Pharm. Bull.* **2008**, *56*, 222–226. [CrossRef] [PubMed]
52. Zhu, S. Small Molecules with Antimalarial Activity. U.S. Patent 2013/0023552 A1, 24 January 2013.
53. Kirmizibekmez, H.; Calis, I.; Perozzo, R.; Brun, R.; Dönmez, A.A.; Linden, A.; Rüedi, P.; Tasdemir, D. Inhibiting activities of the secondary metabolites of *Phlomis brunneogaleata* against *parasitic protozoa* and plasmodial enoyl-ACP Reductase, a crucial enzyme in fatty acid biosynthesis. *Planta Med.* **2004**, *70*, 711–717. [CrossRef] [PubMed]
54. Kamatou, G.P.P.; Van Zyl, R.L.; Davids, H.; Van Heerden, F.R.; Lourens, A.C.U.; Viljoen, A.M. Antimalarial and anticancer activities of selected South African Salviaspecies and isolated compounds from *S. radula*. *S. Afr. J. Bot.* **2008**, *74*, 238–243. [CrossRef]
55. Tchinda, A.T.; Tamze, V.; Ngono, A.R.N.; Ayimele, G.A.; Cao, M.; Angenot, L.; Frédérich, M. Alkaloids from the stem bark of *Strychnos icaja*. *Phytochem. Lett.* **2012**, *5*, 108–113. [CrossRef]

56. Upadhyaya, H.C.; Sisodia, B.S.; Agrawal, J.; Pal, A.; Darokar, M.P.; Srivastava, S.K. Antimalarial potential of extracts and isolated compounds from four species of genus Ammannia. *Med. Chem. Res.* **2014**, *23*, 870–876. [CrossRef]
57. Sprogøe, K.; Staek, D.; Ziegler, H.L.; Jensen, T.H.; Holm-Møller, S.B.; Jaroszewski, J.W. Combining HPLC-PDA-MS-SPE-NMR with circular dichroism for complete natural product characterization in crude extracts: Levorotatory gossypol in *Thespesia danis*. *J. Nat. Prod.* **2008**, *71*, 516–519. [CrossRef] [PubMed]
58. Buchanan, M.S.; Davis, R.A.; Duffy, S.; Avery, V.M.; Quinn, R.J. Antimalarial benzylisoquinoline alkaloid from the rainforest tree *Doryphora sassafras*. *J. Nat. Prod.* **2009**, *72*, 1541–1543. [CrossRef] [PubMed]
59. Mbah, J.A.; Tane, P.; Ngadjui, B.T.; Connolly, J.D.; Okunji, C.C.; Iwu, M.M.; Schuster, B.M. Antiplasmodial agents from the leaves of *Glossocalyx brevipes*. *Planta Med.* **2004**, *70*, 437–440. [PubMed]
60. Kubo, M.; Yatsuzuka, W.; Matsushima, S.; Harada, K.; Inoue, Y.; Miyamoto, H.; Matsumoto, M.; Fukuyama, Y. Antimalarial phenanthroindolizine alkaloids from *Ficus septica*. *Chem. Pharm. Bull.* **2016**, *64*, 957–960. [CrossRef] [PubMed]
61. Rangkaew, N.; Suttisri, R.; Moriyasu, M.; Kawanishi, K. A new acyclic diterpene acid and bioactive compounds from *Knema glauca*. *Arch. Pharm. Res.* **2009**, *32*, 685–692. [CrossRef] [PubMed]
62. Rukachaisirikul, T.; Siriwattanakit, P.; Sukcharoenphol, K.; Wongvein, C.; Ruttanaweang, P.; Wongwattanavuch, P.; Suksamrarn, A. Chemical constituents and bioactivity of *Piper sarmentosum*. *J. Ethnopharmacol.* **2004**, *93*, 173–176. [CrossRef] [PubMed]
63. Sáez Vega, A.; Rojanoa, B.; Blair, S.; Segura, C.; Figadere, B.; Seone, B.; Grellierf, P.; Sáeza, J. Antimalarials and antioxidants compounds from *Piper tricuspe* (Piperaceae). *Pharmacologyonline* **2008**, *1*, 1–8.
64. Lacroix, D.; Prado, S.; Kamoga, D.; Kasenene, J.; Bodo, B. Structure and in vitro antiparasitic activity of constituents of *Citropsis articulata* root bark. *J. Nat. Prod.* **2011**, *74*, 2286–2289. [CrossRef] [PubMed]
65. Cebrián-Torrejón, G.; Spelman, K.; Leblanc, K.; Muñoz-Durango, K.; Gutiérrez, S.T.; Ferreira, M.E.; de Arias, A.R.; Figadere, B.; Fournet, A.; Maciuk, A.; et al. The antiplasmodium effects of a traditional South American remedy: *Zanthoxylum chiloperone* var. angustifolium against chloroquine resistant and chloroquine sensitive strains of *Plasmodium falciparum*. *Rev. Bras. Farmacogn. Braz. J. Pharmacogn.* **2011**, *21*, 652–661. [CrossRef]
66. Kuo, P.C.; Damu, A.G.; Lee, K.H.; Wu, T.S. Cytotoxic and antimalarial constituents from the roots of *Eurycoma longifolia*. *Bioorg. Med. Chem.* **2004**, *12*, 537–544. [CrossRef] [PubMed]
67. Tada, H.; Yasuda, F.; Otani, K.; Doteuchi, M.; Ishihara, Y.; Shiro, M. New antiulcer quassinoids from *Eurycoma longifolia*. *Eur. J. Med. Chem.* **1991**, *26*, 345–349. [CrossRef]
68. De Andrade-Neto, V.F.; Pohlit, A.M.; Pinto, A.C.; Silva, E.C.; Nogueir, K.L.; Melo, M.R.; Henrique, M.C.; Amorim, R.C.; Silva, L.F.; Costa, M.R.; et al. In vitro inhibition of *Plasmodium falciparum* by substances isolated from Amazonian antimalarial plants. *Mem. Inst. Oswaldo Cruz* **2007**, *102*, 359–365. [CrossRef] [PubMed]
69. Tegar, M.; Purnomo, H. Tea leaves extracted as anti-malaria based on molecular docking plants. *Procedia Environ. Sci.* **2013**, *17*, 188–194. [CrossRef]
70. Ludere, M.T.; van Ree, T.; Vleggaa, R. Isolation and relative stereochemistry of lippialactone, a new antimalarial compound from *Lippia javanica*. *Fitoterapia* **2013**, *86*, 188–192. [CrossRef] [PubMed]
71. Karunamoorthi, K.; Tsehaye, E. Ethnomedicinal knowledge, belief and self-reported practice of local inhabitants on traditional antimalarial plants and phytotherapy. *J. Ethnopharmacol.* **2012**, *141*, 143–150. [CrossRef] [PubMed]
72. Adepiti, A.O.; Elujoba, A.A.; Bolaji, O.O. In vivo antimalarial evaluation of *MAMA* decoction on *Plasmodium berghei* in mice. *Parasitol. Res.* **2014**, *113*, 505–511. [CrossRef] [PubMed]
73. Ajaiyeoba, E.O.; Abiodun, O.O.; Falade, M.O.; Ogbole, N.O.; Ashidi, J.S.; Happi, C.T.; Akinboye, D.O. In vitro cytotoxicity studies of 20 plants used in Nigerian antimalarial ethnomedicine. *Phytomedicine* **2006**, *13*, 295–298. [CrossRef] [PubMed]
74. Ogunkunle, A.T.; Oyelakin, T.M.; Enitan, A.O.; Oyewole, F.E. A quantitative documentation of the composition of two powdered herbal formulations (antimalarial and haematinic) using ethnomedicinal information from ogbomoso, Nigeria. *Evid. Based Complement. Altern. Med.* **2014**, *2014*, 1–8. [CrossRef] [PubMed]
75. Rasoanaivo, P.; Petitjean, A.; Ratsimamanga-Urverg, S.; Rakoto-Ratsimamanga, A. Medicinal plants used to treat malaria in Madagascar. *J. Ethnopharmacol.* **1992**, *37*, 117–127. [CrossRef]

76. Ojewole, J.A.; Mawoza, T.; Chiwororo, W.D.; Owira, P.M. *Sclerocarya birrea* (A. Rich) Hochst. ['Marula'] (Anacardiaceae): A review of its phytochemistry, pharmacology and toxicology and its ethnomedicinal uses. *Phytother. Res.* **2010**, *24*, 633–639. [PubMed]
77. Qinghaosu Antimalaria Coordinating Research Group. Antimalaria studies on Qinghaosu. *Chin. Med. J.* **1979**, *92*, 811–816.
78. Kitua, A.Y.; Malebo, H.M. Malaria control in Africa and the role of traditional medicine. In *Traditional Medicinal Plants and Malaria*, 1st ed.; Willcox, M., Bodeker, G., Rasoanaivo, P., Addae-Kyereme, J., Eds.; CRC Press: Boca Raton, FL, USA, 2004; pp. 2–20.
79. Zeleke, G.; Kebebe, D.; Mulisa, E.; Gashe, F. In vivo antimalarial activity of the solvent fractions of fruit and root of *Carica papaya* Linn (Caricaceae) against *Plasmodium berghei* in Mice. *Evid. Based Complement. Altern. Med.* **2017**, *2017*, 3121050. [CrossRef] [PubMed]
80. Muregi, F.W.; Ishih, A.; Miyase, T.; Suzuki, T.; Kino, H.; Amano, T.; Mkoji, G.M.; Terada, M. Antimalarial activity of methanolic extracts from plants used in Kenyan ethnomedicine and their interactions with chloroquine (CQ) against a CQ-tolerant rodent parasite, in mice. *J. Ethnopharmacol.* **2007**, *111*, 190–195. [CrossRef] [PubMed]
81. Abiodun, O.O.; Gbotosho, G.O.; Ajaiyeoba, E.O.; Happi, C.T.; Falade, M.; Wittlin, S.; Sowunmi, A.; Brun, R.; Oduola, A. In vitro antiplasmodial activity and toxicity assessment of some plants from Nigerian ethnomedicine. *Pharm. Biol.* **2011**, *49*, 9–14. [CrossRef] [PubMed]
82. Abiodun, O.O.; Gbotosho, G.O.; Ajaiyeoba, E.O.; Happi, C.T.; Hofer, S.; Wittlin, S.; Sowunmi, A.; Brun, R.; Oduola, A.M. Comparison of SYBR Green I-, PicoGreen-, and [^3H]-hypoxanthine-based assays for in vitro antimalarial screening of plants from Nigerian ethnomedicine. *Parasitol. Res.* **2010**, *106*, 933–939. [CrossRef] [PubMed]
83. Patel, J.R.; Tripathi, P.; Sharma, V.; Chauhan, N.S.; Dixit, V.K. *Phyllanthus amarus*: Ethnomedicinal uses, phytochemistry and pharmacology: A review. *J. Ethnopharmacol.* **2011**, *138*, 286–313. [CrossRef] [PubMed]
84. Adjobimey, T.; Edaye, I.; Lagnika, L.; Gbenou, J.; Moudachirou, M.; Sanni, A. Activités antiplasmodiales in vitro de quelques plantes antipaludiques de la pharmacopée béninoise. *Comptes Rendus Chim.* **2004**, *7*, 1023–1027. [CrossRef]
85. Upadhyay, B.; Parveen Dhaker, A.K.; Kumar, A. Ethnomedicinal and ethnopharmaco-statistical studies of Eastern Rajasthan. *Indian J. Ethnopharmacol.* **2010**, *129*, 64–86. [CrossRef] [PubMed]
86. Sadiq, M.B.; Tharaphan, P.; Chotivanich, K.; Tarning, J.; Anal, A.K. In vitro antioxidant and antimalarial activities of leaves, pods and bark extracts of *Acacia nilotica* (L.) Del. *BMC Complement. Altern. Med.* **2017**, *17*, 372. [CrossRef] [PubMed]
87. Zhu, S.; Zhang, Q.; Gudise, C.; Wei, L.; Smith, E.; Zeng, Y. Synthesis and biological evaluation of febrifugine analogues as potential antimalarial agents. *Bioorg. Med. Chem.* **2009**, *17*, 4496–4502. [CrossRef] [PubMed]
88. Satish, P.V.V.; Sunita, K. Antimalarial efficacy of *Pongamia pinnata* (L) Pierre against *Plasmodium falciparum* (3D7 strain) and *Plasmodium berghei* (ANKA). *BMC Complement. Altern. Med.* **2017**, *17*, 458. [CrossRef] [PubMed]
89. Moghadamtousi, S.Z.; Goh, B.H.; Chan, C.K.; Shabab, T.; Kadir, H.A. Biological activities and phytochemicals of *Swietenia macrophylla* King. *Molecules* **2013**, *18*, 10465–10483. [CrossRef] [PubMed]
90. Falade, M.O.; Akinboye, D.O.; Gbotosho, G.O.; Ajaiyeob, E.O.; Happi, T.C.; Abiodun, O.O.; Oduola, A.M. In Vitro and In Vivo Antimalarial Activity of *Ficus thonningii* Blume (Moraceae) and *Lophira alata* Banks (Ochnaceae), Identified from the Ethnomedicine of the Nigerian Middle Belt. *J. Parasitol. Res.* **2014**, *2014*, 1–6. [CrossRef] [PubMed]
91. Teinkela, J.E.M.; Noundou, X.S.; Nguemfo, E.L.; Meyer, F.; Wintjens, R.; Isaacs, M.; Mpondo Mpondo, A.E.; Hoppe, H.C.; Krause, R.W.M.; Azebaze, A.G.B. Biological activities of plant extracts from *Ficus elastica* and *Selaginella vogelli:* An antimalarial, antitrypanosomal and cytotoxity evaluation. *Saudi J. Biol. Sci.* **2018**, *25*, 117–122. [CrossRef] [PubMed]
92. Ansah, C.; Gooderham, N.J. The popular herbal antimalarial, extract of *Cryptolepis sanguinolenta*, is potently cytotoxic. *Toxicol. Sci.* **2002**, *70*, 245–251. [CrossRef] [PubMed]
93. Kazuki, T.; Yasunori, Y.; Masao, K. Constituents of the leaves and roots of *Ligularia stenocephala* Matsum. *J. Nat. Med.* **2006**, *60*, 329–330.

94. Lane, A.L.; Stout, E.P.; Lin, A.S.; Prudhomme, J.; le Roch, K.; Fairchild, C.R.; Franzblau, S.G.; Hay, M.E.; Aalbersberg, W.; Kubanek, J. Antimalarial bromophycolides J-Q from the Fijian red alga *Callophycus serratus*. *J. Org. Chem.* **2009**, *74*, 2736–2742. [CrossRef] [PubMed]
95. Teasdale, M.E.; Prudhomme, J.; Torres, M.; Braley, M.; Cervantes, S.; Bhatia, S.C.; la Clair, J.J.; le Roch, K.; Kubanek, J. Pharmacokinetics, metabolism, and in vivo efficacy of the antimalarial natural product bromophycolide A. *ACS Med. Chem. Lett.* **2013**, *4*, 989–993. [CrossRef] [PubMed]
96. Yang, F.; Wang, R.P.; Xu, B.; Yu, H.B.; Ma, G.Y.; Wang, G.F.; Dai, S.W.; Zhang, W.; Jiao, W.H.; Song, S.J.; et al. New antimalarial norterpene cyclic peroxides from Xisha Islands sponge *Diacarnus megaspinorhabdosa*. *Bioorg. Med. Chem. Lett.* **2016**, *526*, 2084–2087. [CrossRef] [PubMed]
97. World Health Organization. *World Health Report 2002*; WHO Press: Geneva, Switzerland, 2002.
98. De Ridder, S.; van der Kooy, F.; Robert Verpoorte, R. *Artemisia annua* as a self-reliant treatment for malaria in developing countries. *J. Ethnopharmacol.* **2008**, *120*, 302–314. [CrossRef] [PubMed]
99. Dharani, N.; Rukunga, G.; Abiy Yenesew, A.; Mbora, A.; Mwaura, L.; Dawson, I.; Jamnadass, R. *Common Antimalarial Trees and Shrubs of East Africa*; World Agroforestry Centre and the Kenya Medical Research Institute: Nairobo, Kenya, 2010.
100. Loua, J.; Traore, M.S.; Camara, A.; Balde, M.A.; Maes, L.; Pieters, L.; Balde, A.M. Biological and phytochemical investigations on *Caesalpinia benthamiana*, a plant traditionally used as antimalarial in Guinea. *Evid. Based Complement. Altern. Med.* **2017**, *2017*, 9438607. [CrossRef] [PubMed]

MDPI
St. Alban-Anlage 66
4052 Basel
Switzerland
Tel. +41 61 683 77 34
Fax +41 61 302 89 18
www.mdpi.com

International Journal of Molecular Sciences Editorial Office
E-mail: ijms@mdpi.com
www.mdpi.com/journal/ijms

www.ingramcontent.com/pod-product-compliance
Lightning Source LLC
Chambersburg PA
CBHW041750220926
51847CB00014B/155
* 9 7 8 3 0 3 8 9 7 7 1 2 4 *